THE OSLER MEDICAL HANDBOOK

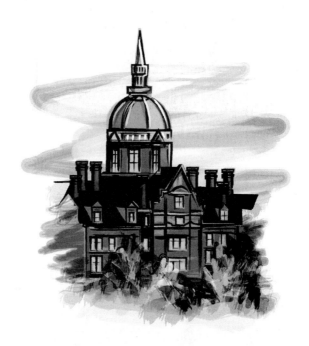

second
EDITION

THE OSLER MEDICAL HANDBOOK

The Osler Medical Service
The Johns Hopkins Hospital

EDITORS

Kent R. Nilsson, Jr., MD, MA
Jonathan P. Piccini, MD

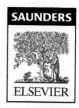

SAUNDERS

ELSEVIER

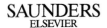

SAUNDERS
ELSEVIER

1600 John F. Kennedy Boulevard
Suite 1800
Philadelphia, Pennsylvania 19103-2899

THE OSLER MEDICAL HANDBOOK   ISBN-13: 978-0-323-03748-8
Second Edition   ISBN-10: 0-323-03748-8
Copyright © 2006 by The Johns Hopkins University.

Library of Congress Cataloging-in-Publication Data
The Osler medical handbook/Osler Medical Service, Johns Hopkins Hospital.—2nd ed./
    editors, Kent R. Nilsson, Jr., Jonathan Piccini.
        p. ; cm.
    Includes bibliographical references and index.
    ISBN 0-323-03748-8
    1. Clinical medicine—Handbooks, manuals, etc. 2. Primary care (Medicine)—Handbooks,
manuals, etc. 3. Medicine—Handbooks, manuals, etc. I. Nilsson, Kent R. II. Piccini,
Jonathan. III. Johns Hopkins Hospital. Osler Medical Service.
    [DNLM: 1. Clinical Medicine—Handbooks. WB 39 O825 2006]
RC55.O87 2006
616—dc22

                                                                        2005057670

Acquisitions Editor: Joanne Husovski
Developmental Editor: Patrick M. N. Stone
Senior Project Manager: Cecelia Bayruns
Design Direction: Karen O'Keefe Owens

Printed in the United States of America

Last digit is the print number: 9 8 7 6 5 4 3 2 1

Sir William Osler

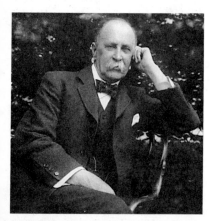

Sir William Osler (1849–1919)

Nearly a century after his death, Sir William Osler is still probably the most famous and oft-quoted physician in North America and in Europe. Over the course of his professional life at McGill University, the University of Pennsylvania, Johns Hopkins University, and Oxford University, he placed an indelible stamp on medical practice and teaching that persists to this day.

William Osler came to Johns Hopkins in 1889 as the first chief physician of the new Hospital and School of Medicine. He wanted to create a hospital and school that would be "a place of refuge for the sick and poor of the city—a place where the best that is known is taught to a group of the best students—a place where new thought is materialized in research—a school where men are encouraged to base the art upon the science of medicine—a fountain to which teachers in every subject would come for inspiration—a place with a hearty welcome to every practitioner who seeks help—a consulting center for the whole country in cases of obscurity." The spirit of dedication to patient care, teaching, and research that was instilled by Osler and his colleagues remains the mission of the Johns Hopkins Hospital and the School of Medicine.

It was during Osler's time at Johns Hopkins (1889–1905) that he wrote *Principles and Practice of Medicine*. Osler was a renowned author even before he took on the task of singlehandedly writing a state-of-the-art, comprehensive textbook of medicine. His book was "designed for the use of practitioners and students of medicine" and was the first modern textbook that took a scientific approach to the diagnosis and practice of medicine. *Principles and Practice of Medicine*, first published in 1892, was a worldwide success and greatly enhanced the professional stature of physicians because it rooted medicine in science and in rigorous observation.

The explosion of medical publishing over the past 100 years can be traced to the publication of this remarkable book.

Another of Osler's legacies is the Osler Medical Housestaff and the Osler Medical Service at the Johns Hopkins Hospital. Although in Osler's day medical training commonly included a period of residency, he was among the first to appoint residents to his own service based on their intellectual prowess as well as their personal characteristics. He valued collegial interactions and believed strongly that because the attending physician and resident would have frequent intense contact, they should have similar values and goals for improving health, understanding medicine, and communicating with patients. He led and taught by example, advising his students to "care more particularly for the individual patient, than for the special features of the disease" and frequently reminding them that "medicine is learned by the bedside and not in the classroom." These principles remain the foundation on which clinical education and housestaff training are based at Johns Hopkins. Osler did not minimize the value of scholarship and reading. His scholastic expectations for physicians and trainees were extremely high. He expected doctors to read about their cases and to have a current understanding of pathophysiology: "It is astonishing with how little reading a doctor can practice medicine, but it is not astonishing how badly he may do it."

It is the spirit of professionalism, scholarship, and collegiality that led to the creation of *The Osler Medical Handbook*. In 2002–2003, the year the first edition of this book was published, it was apparent that then-interns Kent Nilsson and Jon Piccini had all of the intellectual and personal characteristics to steward the second edition of our book. In addition to the monumental task of organizing a large group of housestaff and faculty colleagues, they identified and implemented a number of improvements to make the second edition of *The Osler Medical Handbook* even more usable for house officers and inpatient physicians. These improvements include a more usable and structured chapter design, a thinner book despite the inclusion of many new chapters and topics, and a continued dedication to providing evidence-based practical clinical recommendations. On behalf of the past, present, and future Osler Medical Housestaff, we offer this book to our colleagues in the spirit of a passion for patient care, scholarship, and education.

As the current Program Director of the Osler Medical Housestaff, I have immeasurable pride in our housestaff, who daily perpetuate the values that William Osler lived and taught at Johns Hopkins. We hope that this book, which is also "designed for the use of practitioners and students of medicine," is as useful and as successful as was his.

Charles M. Wiener, MD
Vice Chairman, Department of Medicine
Director, Osler Medical Training Program
Johns Hopkins School of Medicine

Foreword

Medical residencies as we now know them began at The Johns Hopkins Hospital in the 1890s. There were residency physicians in a literal sense—physicians who resided in hospitals—before The Johns Hopkins Hospital opened in 1889. The graduated residency program, however, was initiated at Hopkins by William Osler, the first physician-in-chief. The system included interns, junior and senior assistant residents, and a chief resident, called the resident physician, who had a long tenure. During his 16 years (1889–1905) at Hopkins, Osler had only five resident physicians.

From the beginning, major responsibility for the care of the patients was given to the resident staff. The graduated residency made this possible, with juniors learning from their seniors. It may not be facetious to suggest that the traditionally strong and independent character of the Osler Medical Service's residency program can be traced in part to the hot Baltimore summers. By the end of June most faculty had departed for cooler climates.

I was a member of the Osler Medical Housestaff as an intern for 15 months (April 1946 to June 1947) and a junior assistant resident from 1947 to 1948. After a 2-year interlude in cardiovascular research, I returned to the Osler Medical Service as senior assistant resident from 1950 to 1951 and then resident physician from 1951 to 1952.

When I was the resident physician, the Osler Medical Housestaff worked in the Osler Building. The patients were the responsibility of the resident staff, with the ultimate responsibility resting with the physician-in-chief. There were four general medical wards and no specialty wards; two additional wards were devoted to patients with infectious diseases requiring isolation and a metabolic research unit. Each of the four general medical units had accommodations for 29 patients and was staffed by two or three interns and a junior or senior assistant resident. Patients had long hospital stays, and most of the residency experience was with inpatients. Both interns and assistant residents "covered" the Emergency Department (then called the "Accident Room"), however. Admissions to the Osler Medical Service from the clinic or Emergency Department were determined by the senior residents, who rotated through the duty of admitting officer.

Each of the four major general medical units was the base for instruction for five or six fourth-year medical students. (Third-year medicine was taught in the outpatient clinics.) These medical students played a major role in patient care. In turn, the housestaff played a major role in the clinical education of the students. The only remuneration the assistant residents received for teaching was a paltry $200 a year, although room, board, and laundry were provided. Interns received no stipend. Each unit had a visiting physician whose role was advisory and pedagogical; he or she was not an attending physician in the sense of physician-of-record. Medical students spent 8 weeks in their senior year on one unit. Interns and junior assistant residents rotated monthly, whereas senior residents stayed with the student group for the entire 8 weeks.

The resident physician made rounds on each unit in the morning and more extensive rounds in the evening. After the morning tour through the Osler Building, the resident physician reported to the physician-in-chief. He or she had an opportunity to keep in touch with the patients passing through the clinic and was available for consultation on particular problems. In addition, the resident physician played a major role in consultations on the residency services in other departments, such as surgery, ophthalmology, gynecology, and psychiatry. Resident's rounds at 5 PM Monday through Friday were a major teaching event during which housestaff presented their most instructive or puzzling patients and thereby taught one another.

In the pyramidal system, each echelon learned from the more experienced. The unit's visiting physician made rounds with the students and resident staff for 2 hours three mornings a week. By hearing from the students (or sometimes the intern) about particular patients, the visiting physician maintained some familiarity with the patients on the unit. By rotation through the four teaching units the physician-in-chief made rounds for 2 hours three mornings a week, during which students usually presented two patients for detailed discussion. He was available at other times to consult on difficult problems.

I became director of the Department of Medicine in 1973, 21 years after I completed my residency. The Osler residency program had changed and was now overseen by two chief residents. The residency group was no longer a close-knit cadre whose members became well known to one another and to the chief resident, who could foster their development as physicians. The situation was less satisfactory, with fewer opportunities for juniors to learn from seniors and all to learn from one another.

Changes in medicine at that time included an increased awareness of the importance of outpatient experience in the training of physicians. Economic pressures were reducing the length of hospital stays. Public programs for support of medical care, such as Medicare, which was instituted in 1964, demanded clearer definition of the physician-of-record. By long tradition, on the Osler Medical Service the intern was the primary physician for the patients in his or her care. The intern was assisted by the medical student assigned to each patient, was supervised by the assistant resident(s) assigned to the ward, and received advice from the visiting physician. It was the intern who wrote medication and other orders for the patient. However, an intern or an assistant resident would not be acceptable as a physician-of-record. Designating the visiting physician as physician-of-record for patients on units that traditionally constitute the ward service was considered undesirable because this would erode the independence of the housestaff, which had been so important in their training.

These considerations led to the creation of the Osler Firm System in 1975. The system split the housestaff into four units, or firms (a term used for units in British teaching hospitals), each headed by an assistant chief of service (ACS). The ACS was physician-of-record for the patients in the firm. Each firm had one of the original Osler wards as a home base and also had responsibility for part of the Private Service.

It was originally planned that the ACS position would be a 2-year job, in imitation of the long-tenured chief residents of Osler's time. Two new ACSs would be appointed each year, giving useful overlap. However, the job was found to be too grueling and to require the ACS to be away too long from subspecialty training and research for a 2-year tenure to be acceptable.

Today the Osler Firm System is an established institution that has adapted well to socioeconomic change while preserving its advantages for clinical learning. It provides the camaraderie and collegiality that have been so important in the teaching of interns and junior residents by senior residents. The Firm System has been able to accommodate the shift toward greater involvement of physicians-in-training in ambulatory medicine.

This book has grown out of the Osler tradition of giving housestaff a pivotal role in educating colleagues and peers. Each chapter was written by a member of the Osler housestaff with direct supervision of a member of the Johns Hopkins faculty. Despite revolutionary changes in medicine and the U.S. health care system, we hold true to the core values Osler taught by precept and example, namely, that it is our mission to improve the health of our patients and as physicians to strive consistently to improve our knowledge and experience. The Osler housestaff offers *The Osler Medical Handbook* in that spirit.

Victor A. McKusick, MD
Former William Osler Professor
and Director
Department of Medicine
Johns Hopkins University
Physician-in-Chief,
The Johns Hopkins Hospital (1973–1985)

Preface

One hundred years after his tenure at the Johns Hopkins Hospital, Sir William Osler is most remembered for the method and vigor of his clinical practice. Today, his legacy of dedicated patient care, bedside education, and exhaustive investigation lives on in the traditions of the Osler Medical Housestaff. In the spirit of this tradition, Dr. Aimee Zaas and Dr. Alan Cheng recognized a need for a new bedside handbook that could provide both the essentials of diagnosis and treatment as well as the latest in evidence-based medicine. Under their leadership, the first edition of *The Osler Medical Handbook* was published in 2003 with resounding success.

In editing the second edition, we have striven to uphold the principles set forth in the first edition while at the same time including new material. To incorporate the suggestions of our readers, we have made several changes to the second edition. First, we added 39 new chapters on topics ranging from traditional acid-base disorders to more contemporary subjects such as solid organ transplantation. Second, we have included several chapters on common clinical problems whose subject matter is underrepresented in traditional bedside manuals. Such topics include evidence-based cardiac resuscitation, transfusion medicine, and inpatient radiology. Finally, in recognition of the proliferation of online and handheld pharmaceutical guides, the formulary was replaced with comparative drug tables, a feature we believe will provide useful point-of-care prescribing information not easily found elsewhere. We hope that you find these changes useful and that they eliminate the need for other pocket references.

Like the first edition, each chapter begins with a presentation of essential Fast Facts and concludes with Pearls and Pitfalls useful to the practicing internist. When possible, chapters are divided into sections: Epidemiology, Clinical Presentation, Diagnosis, and Management. To help the reader identify the type of information cited in the references, the references have been labeled with a "strength of evidence" grade. Category **A** describes studies that are randomized, placebo-controlled, and double-blinded. Category **B** describes articles that are prospective trials, retrospective trials, case reports, or basic science reports. Category **C** describes articles that are review papers, meta-analyses, or pooled analyses. Finally, category **D** describes articles that are guidelines or position papers from authoritative medical associations (e.g., Infectious Diseases Society of America, American College of Cardiology), editorials, or expert opinion.

At a time when popular culture and regulatory bodies have made it increasingly difficult to keep doctors at the bedside,[1,2] we would like to extend special thanks to Dr. Myron L. Weisfeldt, the current William Osler Professor

[1] Steinbrook R: The debate over residents' work hours, *N Engl J Med* 347:1296-1302, 2002.

[2] Charap M: Reducing resident work hours: unproven assumptions and unforeseen outcomes, *Ann Intern Med* 140:814-815, 2004.

of Medicine, and Dr. Charles M. Wiener, the director of the Osler Residency Training Program, for their extraordinary leadership and unfailing support in a time of change. Because of their tireless work, the Osler Medical Housestaff and tradition are stronger than ever.

We would like to thank everyone at Elsevier who assisted in the production of this manual, including Dolores Meloni, Elyse O'Grady, Theresa Dudas, Joanne Husovski, and Patrick Stone. We would also like to extend a special thank you to the section editors, Susan Arnold, Jeff Brewer, and the faculty advisors (denoted with an asterisk).

Finally, and most importantly, we would like to thank all of our contributors. This handbook truly is the product of the entire Osler Housestaff Training Program. Without the housestaff, program leadership, and faculty, this publication would not be possible. We would like to thank all of the authors for their inspiring dedication and scholarship.

We are honored and humbled to have worked with so many talented and dedicated physicians during this project. On behalf of the men and women of the Osler Medical Housestaff and faculty, we present the second edition of *The Osler Medical Handbook*. It is our hope that it enhances your clinical practice and fosters bedside patient care, as advocated by Sir William Osler, so many years ago.

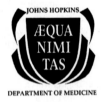

DEPARTMENT OF MEDICINE

Kent R. Nilsson, Jr., MD, MA
Jonathan P. Piccini, MD

Section Editors

Martin F. Britos, MD
Fellow, Pulmonary Diseases
Division of Pulmonary Medicine
Department of Medicine
Johns Hopkins University School of
   Medicine
Baltimore, Maryland
Nephrology and Electrolytes

Franco D'Alessio, MD
Fellow, Pulmonary Diseases
Division of Pulmonary Medicine
Department of Medicine
Johns Hopkins University School of
   Medicine
Baltimore, Maryland
Critical Care Medicine and
   Pulmonology

Christopher Hoffmann, MD, MPH
Fellow, Infectious Diseases
Division of Infectious Diseases
Department of Medicine
Johns Hopkins University School of
   Medicine
Baltimore, Maryland
Infectious Diseases and *HIV-
   Related Infectious Diseases*

Yuli Y. Kim, MD
Fellow, Cardiovascular Disease
Division of Cardiology
Department of Medicine
The Cleveland Clinic Foundation
Cleveland, Ohio
*Neurology, Psychiatry, and
   Substance Abuse*

James O. Mudd, MD
Fellow, Cardiovascular Disease
Division of Cardiology
Department of Medicine
Johns Hopkins University School of
   Medicine
Baltimore, Maryland
Cardiology

Kent R. Nilsson, Jr., MD, MA
Fellow, Cardiovascular Disease
Division of Cardiology
Department of Medicine
Duke University Medical Center
Durham, North Carolina
Transplantation

Jonathan P. Piccini, MD
Fellow, Cardiovascular Disease
Division of Cardiology
Department of Medicine
Duke University Medical Center
Durham, North Carolina
Gastroenterology

Jordan M. Prutkin, MD, MHS
Fellow, Cardiology
Division of Cardiology
Department of Medicine
University of Washington School of
   Medicine
Seattle, Washington
*Acute Management of the Adult
   Patient* and *Cardiology*

David Riedel, MD
Hospitalist
Greater Baltimore Medical Center
Baltimore, Maryland
Dermatology and *Rheumatology*

Amin Sabet, MD
Fellow, Endocrinology
Division of Endocrinology
Department of Medicine
Johns Hopkins University School of
  Medicine
Baltimore, Maryland
Endocrinology and Metabolism

Sara Tolaney, MD
Fellow, Hematology/Oncology
Department of Oncology
Dana Farber/Partners Cancer
  Institute
Harvard University
Boston, Massachusetts
Hematology and Oncology

Nicola Zetola, MD
Fellow, Infectious Diseases
Division of Infectious Diseases
Department of Medicine
University of California, San
  Francisco
San Francisco, California
Infectious Diseases

Contributors

Moeen Abedin, MD
Jacob Abraham, MD
N. Franklin Adkinson, Jr., MD*
Homaa Ahmad, MD
Neil Aggarwal, MD
Eric Aldrich, MD*
Carlos Alves, MD
Gregory B. Ang, MD
Hossein Ardehali, MD, PhD
Reza Ardehali, MD, PhD
Susan Arnold, PharmD*
Mohamed G. Atta, MD*
Paul Auwaerter, MD*
Lauren Averett, MD
Johan Bakken, MS
Matthew R. Baldwin, MD
Pennan Barry, MD, MPH
John Bartlett, MD*
Justin Bekelman, MD
Peter Belitsos, MD*
Sigrid Berg, MD, MPH
Ronald Berger, MD, PhD*
Gail V. Berkenblit, MD, PhD
Adam R. Berliner, MD
Rinky Bhatia, MD
Kenneth Bilchick, MD
Ari M. Blitz, MD
Gerald Bloomfield, MD, MPH
Bruce S. Bochner, MD*
P. Peter Borek, MD
Jeffrey Brewer, PharmD*
Martin F. Britos, MD
Robert Brodsky, MD*
Cynthia Brown, MD
Kelly Brungardt, MD
Tricia Brusco, MS, RD, LD*
Hugh Calkins, MD*
Paul Campbell, MD
Hetty Carraway, MD
Kerri L. Cavanaugh, MD

Hunter C. Champion, MD, PhD*
Nisha Chandra-Strobos, MD*
Katherine Chang, MD
Raquel Charles, MD
Tze-Ming (Benson) Chen, MD
Alan Cheng, MD
Susan Cheng, MD
Patti P. Chi, MD
Michael J. Choi, MD*
Sharon A. Chung, MD
Amanda M. Clark, RN, BSN, CWCN
Gregory O. Clark, MD
John Clarke, MD
David Cosgrove, MD
Sara Cosgrove, MD*
Deidra C. Crews, MD
Keliegh S. Culpepper, MD
Franco D'Alessio, MD
Rachel Damico, MD, PhD
Rachel Derr, MD
Sanjay Desai, MD
Ross C. Donehower, MD*
Mark Donowitz, MD*
John A. Dooley, MD
M. Bradley Drummond, MD
Kerry Dunbar, MD
Lynn B. Eckert, MD
Michelle Estrella, MD
Traci Thompson Ferguson, MD
Henry E. Fessler, MD*
Michael Field, MD
Derek M. Fine, MD*
John A. Flynn, MD, MBA*
Paul R. Forfia, MD
Paul F. Frey, MD, MPH
Linda Fried, MD*
John J. Friedewald, MD
Kelly Gebo, MD*
Allan C. Gelber, MD, MPH, PhD*

(* denotes faculty mentor)

Jonathan M. Gerber, MD
Gary Gerstenblith, MD*
Leslie S. Gewin, MD
Francis Giardiello, MD*
Reda Girgis, MD*
Jenna D. Goldberg, MD
Benjamin Greenberg, MD
Elizabeth Griffiths, MD
Patrick Ha, MD
David N. Hager, MD
Saptarsi Haldar, MD
Edward Haponik, MD
Rizwan Haq, MD, PhD
Mary L. Harris, MD*
Megan R. Haymart, MD
Anna Hemnes, MD
Laura B. Herpel, MD
Christopher Hoffmann, MD, MPH
Peter Holt, MD*
Andrew Holz, MD
Edward C. Hsiao, MD, PhD
Thomas V. Ingelsby, MD*
Nadine Jackson, MD, MPH
Suzanne Jan de Beur, MD*
Peter V. Johnston, MD
J. Dedrick Jordan, MD, PhD
Rosalyn Juergens, MD
Anthony N. Kalloo, MD*
Sergey Kantsevoy, MD*
David E. Kaplan, MD
Edward Kasper, MD*
Rebecca A. Kazin, MD
Esther S.H. Kim, MD
Matthew Kim, MD*
Scott Kim, MD
Yuli Y. Kim, MD
Landon S. King, MD*
Michael J. Klag, MD, MPH*
Ayman Koteish, MD*
Jerry A. Krishan, MD*
Amar Krishnaswamy, MD
David Kuperman, MD
Richard Lange, MD*
Sophie Lanzkron, MD*
Josh Lauring, MD, PhD
David Lim, MD, PhD

Susan Lee Limb, MD
Ronald Lesser, MD, PhD*
Thomas E. Lloyd, MD, PhD
Michael Londner, MD*
Vandana R. Long, MD
Julie-Aurore Losman, MD, PhD
Katarzyna J. Macura, MD, PhD*
Catherine S. Magid, MD
Andrew Mammen, MD, PhD
Ciro Martins, MD*
Nisa Maruthur, MD
Laura Y. McGirt, MD
Michal L. Melamed, MD
Alison Moliterno, MD*
David Moller, MD*
Daniel J. Mollura, MD
Majd Mouded, MD
James O. Mudd, MD
Ann Mullally, MD
Melissa A. Munsell, MD
Jonathan R. Murrow, MD
Jennifer S. Myers, MD
Avindra Nath, MD*
Geoffrey C. Nguyen, MD
John S. Nguyen, MD
Kent R. Nilsson, Jr., MD, MA
Sarah Noonberg, MD, PhD
Eric Nuermberger, MD*
Yngvild Olsen, MD, MPH*
Jonathan B. Orens, MD*
Anand K. Parekh, MD
Catherine Passaretti, MD
David Pearse, MD*
Trish M. Perl, MD, MS*
Jonathan P. Piccini, MD
Matthew Pipeling, MD
Albert J. Polito, MD*
Tatiana M. Prowell, MD
Jordan M. Prutkin, MD, MHS
Rudra Rai, MD*
Rita Rastogi, MD
Stuart Ray, MD*
Ann Reed, MD
David Riedel, MD
Anne Rompalo, MD, ScM*
Jason Rosenberg, MD*

Michol Rothman, MD
Amin Sabet, MD
Janet Sailor, MD
Assil Saleh, MD
Roberto Salvatori, MD*
Milagros Samaniego, MD*
Christopher D. Saudek, MD*
Paul Scheel, MD*
Joshua Schiffer, MD
Eric Schmidt, MD
Emily L. Schopick, MD
Steven P. Schulman, MD*
Julia Scialla, MD
Timothy Scialla, MD
Karen Scully, MD*
Cynthia L. Sears, MD*
Philip Seo, MD*
Anandi N. Sheth, MD
Vikesh K. Singh, MD
Stephen D. Sisson, MD*
Kevin Smith, MD
Philip L. Smith, MD*
Patrick Sosnay, MD*
Adam Spivak, MD
Jerry Spivak, MD*
Brady Stein, MD

R. Scott Stephens, MD
Nimalie Stone, MD
Michael Streiff, MD*
Aruna Subramanian, MD*
Adlah Sukkar, MD
Dechen Surkhang, RD, LD
Christopher Tehlirian, MD
Peter B. Terry, MD*
Chloe Thio, MD*
Erin Tiberio, RD, CNSD
Sabrina M. Tom, MD
Thomas Traill, MD*
Daniel Y. Wang, MD
Tracy J. Warner, MD
Myron L. Weisfeldt, MD*
Clifford R. Weiss, MD
Charles M. Wiener, MD*
Robert Wise, MD*
Lara Wittine, MD
Ilan Wittstein, MD*
Eric H. Yang, MD
Aimee Zaas, MD*
David Zaas, MD*
Nicola Zetola, MD
David A. Zidar, MD

Contents

S indicates supplemental PDA chapters, which are available through the handheld software download.

PART I   Acute Management of the Adult Patient
Section Editor: Jordan M. Prutkin, MD, MHS

1   Advanced Cardiopulmonary Life Support, 3
    *Jonathan P. Piccini, MD; Kent R. Nilsson, Jr., MD, MA; and
    Myron L. Weisfeldt, MD*

2   Procedures, 13
    *Jordan M. Prutkin, MD, MHS; Tze-Ming (Benson) Chen, MD; and
    Henry E. Fessler, MD*

3   Nutrition Support, 32
    *Erin Tiberio, RD, CNSD; Dechen Surkhang, RD, LD; and
    Tricia Brusco, MS, RD, LD*

4   Anaphylaxis and Drug Allergy, 37
    Franco D'Alessio, MD, and N. Franklin Adkinson, Jr., MD

5   Inpatient Radiology, 44
    *Clifford R. Weiss, MD; Janet Sailor, MD; Andrew Holz, MD;
    Daniel J. Mollura, MD; Nadine Jackson, MD, MPH; Ari M. Blitz, MD;
    Paul Campbell, MD; Kevin Smith, MD; and Katarzyna J. Macura, MD, PhD*

PART II   Diagnostic and Therapeutic Information

Cardiology
Section Editors: Jordan M. Prutkin, MD, MHS, and James O. Mudd, MD

6   Electrocardiogram Analysis, 57
    *Daniel Y. Wang, MD; Lauren Averett, MD; David Kuperman, MD; and
    Gary Gerstenblith, MD*

7   Chest Pain in the Emergency Department, 72
    *Yuli Y. Kim, MD; Paul R. Forfia, MD; Michael Londner, MD; and
    Steven P. Schulman, MD*

8   Acute Coronary Syndromes, 86
    Paul F. Frey, MD, MPH, and Richard Lange, MD

9   Hypertensive Urgency and Emergency, 107
    *Sharon A. Chung, MD; Edward C. Hsiao, MD, PhD; and
    Michael J. Klag, MD, MPH*

10   Syncope, 120
    Esther S.H. Kim, MD; Eric H. Yang, MD; and Hunter C. Champion, MD, PhD

11   Heart Failure, 131
    James O. Mudd, MD; Michael Field, MD; and Edward Kasper, MD

12 Valvular Heart Disease, 147
Reza Ardehali, MD, PhD; Hunter C. Champion, MD, PhD; and Thomas Traill, MD

13 Diseases of the Pericardium, 165
P. Peter Borek, MD; Sanjay Desai, MD; and Gary Gerstenblith, MD

14 Bradycardia and Pacemakers, 176
Jacob Abraham, MD; Kenneth Bilchick, MD; and Ronald Berger, MD, PhD

15 Tachyarrhythmias and Implantable Cardioverter-Defibrillators, 188
Jordan M. Prutkin, MD, MHS, and Ronald Berger, MD, PhD

16 Atrial Fibrillation, 197
Rinky Bhatia, MD; Moeen Abedin, MD; and Hugh Calkins, MD

S1 Pulmonary Artery Catheters, Intraaortic Balloon Pumps, and Transvenous Pacemakers (Supplemental PDA Chapter)
Gerald Bloomfield, MD, MPH; Sabrina M. Tom, MD; and Nisha Chandra-Strobos, MD

S2 Allograft Dysfunction in Heart Transplantation (Supplemental PDA Chapter)
Julia Scialla, MD, and Ilan Wittstein, MD

Critical Care Medicine
Section Editor: Franco D'Alessio, MD

17 Care of the Critically Ill, 211
Franco D'Alessio, MD, and Henry Fessler, MD

18 Acute Respiratory Failure, 218
Franco D'Alessio, MD; Kent R. Nilsson, Jr., MD, MA; Lara Wittine, MD; and Landon S. King, MD

19 Invasive and Noninvasive Ventilation, 228
Matthew Pipeling, MD; David N. Hager, MD; and Landon S. King, MD

20 Hypotension and Shock, 239
R. Scott Stephens, MD; Saptarsi Haldar, MD; and Charles M. Wiener, MD

21 Sepsis, 253
Nisa Maruthur, MD; Sarah Noonberg, MD, PhD; and Trish M. Perl, MD, MS

Dermatology
Section Editor: David Riedel, MD

22 Inpatient Dermatology, 263
Laura Y. McGirt, MD; Rebecca A. Kazin, MD; Keliegh S. Culpepper, MD; and Karen Scully, MD

23 Dermatologic Disorders in Human Immunodeficiency Virus, 275
Anandi N. Sheth, MD, and Ciro Martins, MD

24 Management of Chronic Wounds, 282
Amanda M. Clark, RN, BSN, CWCN

Endocrinology and Metabolism
Section Editor: Amin Sabet, MD

25 Inpatient Management of Endocrinologic Disorders, 292
Lauren Averett, MD, and Roberto Salvatori, MD

26 Adrenal Insufficiency, 302
Ann Reed, MD; Assil Saleh, MD; and Roberto Salvatori, MD

27 Diabetic Ketoacidosis and Hyperosmolar Hyperglycemic State, 312
Rita Rastogi, MD; Gregory O. Clark, MD; and Christopher D. Saudek, MD

28 Thyroid Disorders, 321
Amin Sabet, MD; Gail V. Berkenblit, MD, PhD; and Matthew Kim, MD

29 Disorders of Calcium Homeostasis, 335
Rachel Derr, MD, and Suzanne Jan de Beur, MD

Gastroenterology
Section Editor: Jonathan P. Piccini, MD

30 Approach to Abdominal Pain, 349
Jonathan M. Gerber, MD; Vandana R. Long, MD; and Francis Giardiello, MD

31 Acute Pancreatitis, 362
Melissa A. Munsell, MD; Geoffrey C. Nguyen, MD; and Mary L. Harris, MD

32 Biliary Tract Disease, 371
Vikesh K. Singh, MD; Jonathan P. Piccini, MD; and Anthony N. Kalloo, MD

33 Acute Liver Failure and Biochemical Liver Testing, 377
Christopher Hoffmann, MD, MPH; David E. Kaplan, MD; and Chloe Thio, MD

34 Viral Hepatitis, 389
Brady Stein, MD; Kelly Brungardt, MD; John Clarke, MD; and Rudra Rai, MD

35 End-Stage Liver Disease, 402
Carlos Alves, MD; Kelly Brungardt, MD; Brady Stein, MD; Jonathan P. Piccini, MD; and Rudra Rai, MD

S3 Allograft Dysfunction in Liver Transplantation (Supplemental PDA Chapter)
Timothy Scialla, MD, and Ayman Koteish, MD

36 Ascites, 418
Daniel J. Mollura, MD; Raquel Charles, MD; Michal L. Melamed, MD; and Rudra Rai, MD

37 Gastrointestinal Bleeding, 428
Elizabeth Griffiths, MD, and Sergey Kantsevoy, MD

38 Inflammatory Bowel Disease, 442
Lynn B. Eckert, MD; Geoffrey C. Nguyen, MD; and Mary L. Harris, MD

39 Diarrhea, 456
    Melissa A. Munsell, MD; Gregory B. Ang, MD; Mark Donowitz, MD; and Cynthia L. Sears, MD

Hematology and Oncology
Section Editor: Sara Tolaney, MD

40 Transfusion Medicine, 467
    Kent R. Nilsson, Jr., MD, MA; Johan Bakken, MS; and Jerry Spivak, MD

41 Anemia and Erythrocytosis, 475
    Sigrid Berg, MD, MPH; Julie-Aurore Losman, MD, PhD; Hetty Carraway, MD; and Michael Streiff, MD

42 Sickle Cell Anemia, 487
    Elizabeth Griffiths, MD; Rosalyn Juergens, MD; and Sophie Lanzkron, MD

43 Thrombocytopenia, 497
    Ann Mullally, MD; Susan Lee Limb, MD; and Alison Moliterno, MD

S4 Eosinophilia (Supplemental PDA Chapter)
    Rizwan Haq, MD, PhD, and Bruce S. Bochner, MD

44 Bone Marrow Failure, 510
    Catherine S. Magid, MD, and Robert Brodsky, MD

45 Bleeding Disorders, 516
    Susan Cheng, MD, and Michael Streiff, MD

46 Hypercoagulable States, 526
    Susan Cheng, MD, and Michael Streiff, MD

S5 Hematologic Malignancies (Supplemental PDA Chapter)
    Julie-Aurore Losman, MD, PhD, and Jerry Spivak, MD

47 Oncologic Emergencies, 537
    Justin Bekelman, MD; Nadine Jackson, MD, MPH; and Ross C. Donehower, MD

HIV-Related Infectious Diseases
Section Editor: Christopher Hoffmann, MD, MPH

48 Acute Retroviral Syndrome and General Management of the Human Immunodeficiency Virus, 561
    Christopher Hoffmann, MD, MPH, and John Bartlett, MD

49 Central Nervous System Involvement in Human Immunodeficiency Virus Infection, 569
    David Riedel, MD; Nimalie Stone, MD; and Avindra Nath, MD

50 Pulmonary Involvement in Human Immunodeficiency Virus, 577
    Catherine Passaretti, MD; Josh Lauring, MD, PhD; and Stuart Ray, MD

51 Gastrointestinal Disorders in Patients with the Human Immunodeficiency Virus, 587
Pennan Barry, MD, MPH, and Peter Belitsos, MD

52 Systemic Manifestations of the Human Immunodeficiency Virus, 600
David Riedel, MD, and Cynthia L. Sears, MD

Infectious Diseases
Section Editors: Christopher Hoffmann, MD, MPH, and Nicola Zetola, MD

53 Fever of Unknown Origin, 608
Scott Kim, MD; Rachel Damico, MD, PhD; and Paul Auwaerter, MD

54 Central Nervous System Infection, 619
Adam Spivak, MD; Alan Cheng, MD; Aimee Zaas, MD; and Paul Auwaerter, MD

S6 Inpatient Infections of the Ear, Nose, and Throat (Supplemental PDA Chapter)
Joshua Schiffer, MD; Patrick Ha, MD; and Kelly Gebo, MD

55 Pneumonia, 630
Nicola Zetola, MD; Aimee Zaas, MD; and John Bartlett, MD

56 Tuberculosis, 640
Joshua Schiffer, MD, and Eric Nuermberger, MD

57 Infective Endocarditis, 650
Nicola Zetola, MD; David A. Zidar, MD; and Stuart Ray, MD

58 Central Venous Catheter Infections, 658
Nicola Zetola, MD; Aimee Zaas, MD; and Stuart Ray, MD

59 Urinary Tract Infections, 663
Catherine Passaretti, MD; Hossein Ardehali, MD, PhD; and Eric Nuermberger, MD

S7 Sexually Transmitted Diseases (Supplemental PDA Chapter)
Pennan Barry, MD, MPH; Katherine Chang, MD; and Anne Rompalo, MD, ScM

60 Soft Tissue and Bone Infection, 672
Adam Spivak, MD; Patrick Sosnay, MD; and Sara Cosgrove, MD

61 Fungus, 681
Catherine Passaretti, MD, and Aruna Subramanian, MD

S8 Bioterrorism (Supplemental PDA Chapter)
Anand K. Parekh, MD, and Thomas V. Inglesby, MD

62 Infection in the Solid Organ Transplant Recipient, 692
David Lim, MD, PhD, and Aruna Subramanian, MD

Nephrology and Electrolytes
Section Editor: Martin F. Britos, MD

63 Urinalysis, 702
   Leslie S. Gewin, MD, and Derek M. Fine, MD

64 Approach to Acute Renal Failure, 709
   Julia Scialla, MD; John J. Friedewald, MD; and Michael J. Choi, MD

65 Glomerular Disease, 719
   Megan R. Haymart, MD, and Mohamed G. Atta, MD

66 Renal Tubulointerstitial Diseases, 731
   Adam R. Berliner, MD, and Michael J. Choi, MD

67 Renovascular Hypertension, 741
   Leslie S. Gewin, MD, and Paul Scheel, MD

68 Chronic Kidney Disease, 748
   Martin F. Britos, MD, and Mohamed G. Atta, MD

69 Dialysis, 756
   Michelle Estrella, MD; Jennifer S. Myers, MD; and Paul Scheel, MD

S9 Hematuria (Supplemental PDA Chapter)
   Deidra C. Crews, MD, and Michael J. Choi, MD

70 Acute Renal Colic, 762
   John A. Dooley, MD, and Michael J. Choi, MD

71 Acid-Base Disorders, 771
   John A. Dooley, MD, and Stephen D. Sisson, MD

72 Renal Tubular Acidosis, 784
   Adam R. Berliner, MD, and Michael J. Choi, MD

73 Disorders of Sodium Balance, 789
   Emily L. Schopick, MD; Kerri L. Cavanaugh, MD; and Derek M. Fine, MD

74 Disorders of Potassium Homeostasis, 800
   Deidra C. Crews, MD; Patty P. Chi, MD; and Michael J. Choi, MD

S10 Disorders of Magnesium and Phosphate Homeostasis (Supplemental
   PDA Chapter)
   Emily L. Schopick, MD; Peter V. Johnston, MD; and Milagros Samaniego, MD

75 Allograft Dysfunction in Renal Transplantation, 807
   Timothy Scialla, MD, and Milagros Samaniego, MD

Neurology, Psychiatry, and Substance Abuse
Section Editor: Yuli Y. Kim, MD

76 Delirium, 816
   *Susan Cheng, MD; Nadine Jackson, MD, MPH; Cynthia Brown, MD; and
   Linda Fried, MD*

77 Status Epilepticus, 826
Andrew Mammen, MD, PhD, and Ronald Lesser, MD, PhD

78 Stroke, 833
Thomas E. Lloyd, MD, PhD; Benjamin Greenberg, MD; and Eric Aldrich, MD

S11 Headache (Supplemental PDA Chapter)
J. Dedrick Jordan, MD, PhD, and Jason Rosenberg, MD

79 Substance Abuse, 847
*Jonathan R. Murrow, MD; Michol Rothman, MD; and
Yngvild Olsen, MD, MPH*

Pulmonology
Section Editor: Franco D'Alessio, MD

80 Pulmonary Function Tests, 858
Jenna D. Goldberg, MD; Anna Hemnes, MD; and Charles M. Wiener, MD

81 Asthma, 865
Anandi N. Sheth, MD; Tatiana M. Prowell, MD; and Jerry A. Krishnan, MD

82 Chronic Obstructive Pulmonary Disease, 877
David Cosgrove, MD; Majd Mouded, MD; and Robert Wise, MD

83 Pleural Effusions, 886
M. Bradley Drummond, MD, and Peter B. Terry, MD

84 Hemoptysis, 892
Adlah Sukkar, MD; Sarah Noonberg, MD, PhD; and Edward Haponik, MD

85 Pulmonary Hypertension, 900
Amar Krishnaswamy, MD; Reda Girgis, MD; and Hunter C. Champion, MD, PhD

86 Venous Thromboembolism, 911
Eric Schmidt, MD; David Zaas, MD; and David Pearse, MD

S12 Sleep-Disordered Breathing (Supplemental PDA Chapter)
Martin F. Britos, MD; Laura B. Herpel, MD; and Philip L. Smith, MD

87 Interstitial Lung Disease, 922
Neil Aggarwal, MD; Kerry Dunbar, MD; and Albert J. Polito, MD

88 Sarcoidosis, 933
Homaa Ahmad, MD, and David Moller, MD

S13 Allograft Dysfunction in Lung Transplantation (Supplemental PDA
Chapter)
Timothy Scialla, MD, and Jonathan B. Orens, MD

Rheumatology
Section Editor: David Riedel, MD

89 Approach to the Rheumatic Disorders, 939
Ann Reed, MD, and Philip Seo, MD

90 Vasculitis, 947
    John S. Nguyen, MD, and John A. Flynn, MD, MBA

91 Systemic Lupus Erythematosus, 960
    Ann Reed, MD; Traci Thompson Ferguson, MD; and Peter Holt, MD

92 Connective Tissue Diseases, 967
    Christopher Tehlirian, MD, and Allan C. Gelber, MD, MPH, PhD

PART III Comparative Pharmacology and Dosing Tables
    Susan Arnold, PharmD, and Jeffrey Brewer, PharmD

1   Equianalgesic Dosage Conversion for Selected Opiates, 979

2   Equivalent Dosing Steroid Table, 980

3   Proton Pump Inhibitors, 981

4   Weight-Based Unfractionated Heparin Dosing Algorithm, 982

5   Direct Thrombin Inhibitors, 983

6   Warfarin Initiation in the Hospital, 985

7   Warfarin Maintenance Dosing, 986

8   Management of Excessive Anticoagulation with Warfarin, 987

9   Comparison of Angiotensin-Converting Enzyme Inhibitors, 988

10 Comparison of Angiotensin II Receptor Antagonists, 990

11 Comparison of β-Blockers, 992

12 Combination Antihypertensives, 994

13 Comparison of Cholesterol Agents, 995

14 Comparison of Antidiabetic Medications, 1000

15 Comparison of Insulin Products, 1004

PART IV Rapid References, 1005
    Tracy J. Warner, MD, and Matthew R. Baldwin, MD

Index, 1017

Color plates follow p. 276

PART I

Acute Management of the Adult Patient

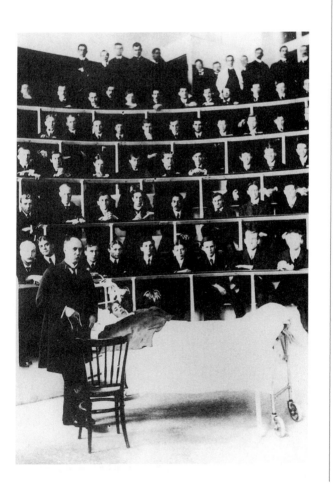

Reverse, Sir William Osler delivering a guest lecture at the Royal Victoria Hospital, McGill University, in 1906.

Advanced Cardiopulmonary Life Support

Jonathan P. Piccini, MD; Kent R. Nilsson, Jr., MD, MA;
and Myron L. Weisfeldt, MD

FAST FACTS

- The incidence of pulseless electrical activity (PEA) is increasing, whereas the incidence of ventricular tachycardia (VT) and ventricular fibrillation (VF) arrest is decreasing.[1]
- A hospitalized patient with an unwitnessed arrest who is found to be in PEA or asystole and who does not have return of spontaneous circulation (ROSC) within 10 minutes of the beginning of advanced cardiopulmonary life support has a 98.9% chance of not surviving to hospital discharge.[2]
- Time to defibrillation is the most important determinant of survival in VT and VF arrest.
- Therapeutic hypothermia improves neurologic recovery in patients who do not regain consciousness within 1 hour of out-of-hospital arrest.
- Cardiopulmonary arrest accounts for approximately 450,000 deaths per year in the United States. Recent research suggests a time-sensitive paradigm in which electrical rhythms are viewed on a continuum rather than as separate entities. Therefore interventions should be guided by time from the onset of cardiovascular compromise.[3]

I. VENTRICULAR TACHYCARDIA AND VENTRICULAR FIBRILLATION ARREST

A. EPIDEMIOLOGY

Despite an increasing incidence of PEA and asystolic arrest, VT and VF remain the most common dysrhythmia in adult cardiac arrests. The most important determinant of survival in VT and VF arrest is the time to defibrillation. According to the traditional paradigm of VT and VF, the chance of survival decreases by about 10% per minute, such that after 12 minutes less than 2% of patients survive. However, recent research has challenged this linear relationship.[4]

B. ETIOLOGY

Please see Table 1-1 for causes of ventricular arrhythmias.

C. PRESENTATION

The absence of pulses in an unresponsive patient confirms the diagnosis of cardiac arrest (Fig. 1-1). Basic life support should begin immediately, with the first priority of advanced cardiopulmonary life support being

TABLE 1-1		
CAUSES OF VT AND VF		
Monomorphic VT	**Polymorphic VT**	**VF**
Fixed reentry around scar	Medications	Degeneration of VT
Automaticity	Dilated cardiomyopathy	Ischemia
	Severe ischemia	
	Long QT syndrome	
	Channelopathies (e.g., Brugada syndrome)	

VF, ventricular fibrillation; *VT,* ventricular tachycardia.

identification of the underlying cardiac rhythm. See Chapter 6 for an approach to rhythm identification.

D. MANAGEMENT AND TREATMENT

Please see Fig. 1-2 for an algorithm for managing VT or VF arrest.

1. **Witnessed VT or VF should be treated with immediate defibrillation. However,** recent literature suggests that immediate defibrillation may be harmful if the time to first response is more than 4 to 5 minutes. In such situations, cardiopulmonary resuscitation should be performed for 1 to 3 minutes before the first defibrillation attempt. Delaying defibrillation increases the rate of ROSC and decreases the chance of post-countershock PEA or asystole.[2]

2. **Defibrillation** terminates ventricular arrhythmias through uniform depolarization of the myocardium, which prolongs the postshock refractory period. Biphasic defibrillation reverses current direction in the second half of the shock and is associated with greater efficacy and less myocardial injury. A meta-analysis of seven randomized control trials demonstrated that biphasic defibrillation decreased postshock asystole and persistent VF by 81% (RR 0.19; 95% CI, 0.06-0.60).[5]

3. **Vasopressors** should be administered as soon as possible during cardiac arrest because they increase aortic diastolic pressure and coronary perfusion. After 5 minutes of cardiac arrest without defibrillation, chest compression must be forceful and interrupted as little as possible to afford an aortic diastolic pressure of at least 15 mmHg and optimally 30 mmHg.

a. Vasopressin 40 U intravenous push and epinephrine 1 mg intravenous push are equally efficacious in VT or VF arrest.

b. In a recent randomized control trial comparing vasopressin and epinephrine, subgroup analysis suggests that the addition of vasopressin increased ROSC rates in patients without ROSC despite treatment with epinephrine (6.2% vs. 1.7% survival to discharge).[6]

4. **Therapeutic hypothermia** improves neurologic outcome in patients who have not regained consciousness after out-of-hospital VT or VF arrest.[7] Studies addressing whether these results are generalizable to inpatient arrests are under way.

a. Patients are sedated and cooled to 32° C to 34° C for 12 to 24 hours with a cooling blanket or ice packs.

b. Paralytic agents should be used if shivering limits hypothermia.

5. Conditions that warrant specific management include the following:

a. **Shock-refractory VT or VF** generally is treated with 300 mg intravenous amiodarone, although there is no evidence of long-term survival benefit.[8]

b. **Electrical storm** (more than two episodes of VT or VF in 24 hours) should be treated with aggressive beta-blockade (e.g., esmolol starting at 50 µg/kg/min) and intravenous amiodarone.[9]

c. **Torsade de pointes**, or twisting of the points, is defined by the presence of polymorphic VT in the setting of a prolonged QT interval. Immediate treatment includes defibrillation and empiric intravenous magnesium. Isoproterenol or overdrive pacing can be helpful during refractory torsade by increasing the heart rate and thereby shortening the QT interval. Serum potassium should be maintained at more than 4 mEq/dl.

II. PEA AND ASYSTOLE

A. EPIDEMIOLOGY

PEA and asystole are the final common pathway for a diverse group of physiologic insults. They account for 36% and 18% of in-hospital arrests, respectively, and mortality approaches 90%.[1] Therapy should be directed at both stabilizing the patient and correcting the underlying insult.

B. ETIOLOGY

Please see Table 1-2 for common causes.

C. PRESENTATION

History and physical examination should seek the cause of the arrest.

1. A **history** of renal failure (suggesting electrolyte derangements), venous thromboembolism (suggesting pulmonary embolism), medication ingestion, or surgery (suggesting exsanguination) should be determined quickly.

2. **Physical examination** should confirm a pulseless state (Fig. 1-1) before proceeding to a directed physical aimed at identifying the underlying pathophysiologic derangement (e.g., evidence of elevated jugular venous pressure (JVP), tracheal deviation, and asymmetric breath sounds suggesting a tension pneumothorax). In PEA arrest, it is important to note that the diagnosis of tamponade cannot be made on

Text continued on p. 11

TABLE 1-2	
CAUSES OF PULSELESS ELECTRICAL ACTIVITY AND ASYSTOLIC ARREST	
5 *Hs*	**5 *Ts***
Hypothermia	Tension pneumothorax
Hypoxia	Tamponade
Hypovolemia	Thrombosis (acute coronary syndrome)
Hyperkalemia and hypokalemia	Thromboembolism (pulmonary embolism)
Hydrogen ion excess	Tablet or toxin ingestion

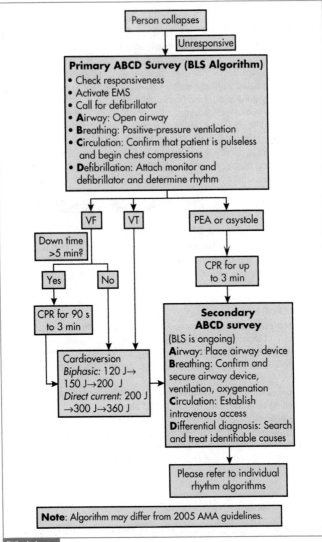

FIG. 1-1
Primary and secondary survey in advanced cardiopulmonary life support. *BLS*, basic life support; *CPR*, cardiopulmonary resuscitation; *EMS*, emergency medical services; *PEA*, pulseless electrical activity; *VF*, ventricular fibrillation; *VT*, ventricular tachycardia.

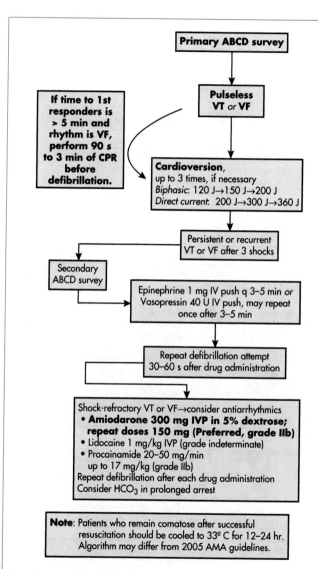

Primary ABCD survey

Pulseless VT *or* VF

If time to 1st responders is > 5 min and rhythm is VF, perform 90 s to 3 min of CPR before defibrillation.

Cardioversion, up to 3 times, if necessary
Biphasic: 120 J→150 J→200 J
Direct current: 200 J→300 J→360 J

Persistent or recurrent VT or VF after 3 shocks

Secondary ABCD survey

Epinephrine 1 mg IV push q 3–5 min or Vasopressin 40 U IV push, may repeat once after 3–5 min

Repeat defibrillation attempt 30–60 s after drug administration

Shock-refractory VT or VF→consider antiarrhythmics
• **Amiodarone 300 mg IVP in 5% dextrose; repeat doses 150 mg (Preferred, grade IIb)**
• Lidocaine 1 mg/kg IVP (grade indeterminate)
• Procainamide 20–50 mg/min up to 17 mg/kg (grade IIb)
Repeat defibrillation after each drug administration
Consider HCO_3 in prolonged arrest

Note: Patients who remain comatose after successful resuscitation should be cooled to 33° C for 12–24 hr. Algorithm may differ from 2005 AMA guidelines.

ADVANCED CARDIOPULMONARY LIFE SUPPORT

1

FIG. 1-2

Ventricular tachycardia and ventricular fibrillation. *CPR*, cardiopulmonary resuscitation; *IV*, intravenous; *primary ABCD*, airway, breathing, circulation, and defibrillation; *secondary ABCD*, airway, breathing, circulation, and differential diagnosis; *VF*, ventricular fibrillation; *VT*, ventricular tachycardia.

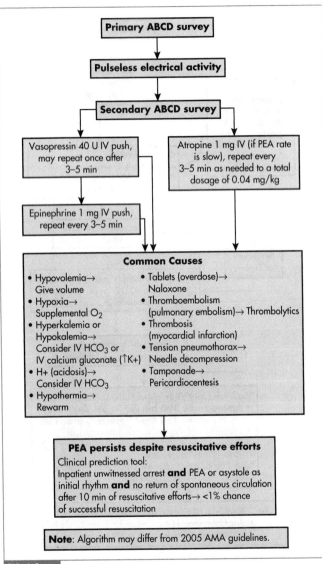

Primary ABCD survey

↓

Pulseless electrical activity

↓

Secondary ABCD survey

Vasopressin 40 U IV push, may repeat once after 3–5 min

Atropine 1 mg IV (if PEA rate is slow), repeat every 3–5 min as needed to a total dosage of 0.04 mg/kg

Epinephrine 1 mg IV push, repeat every 3–5 min

Common Causes

- Hypovolemia→ Give volume
- Hypoxia→ Supplemental O_2
- Hyperkalemia or Hypokalemia→ Consider IV HCO_3 or IV calcium gluconate (↑K+)
- H+ (acidosis)→ Consider IV HCO_3
- Hypothermia→ Rewarm
- Tablets (overdose)→ Naloxone
- Thromboembolism (pulmonary embolism)→ Thrombolytics
- Thrombosis (myocardial infarction)
- Tension pneumothorax→ Needle decompression
- Tamponade→ Pericardiocentesis

PEA persists despite resuscitative efforts

Clinical prediction tool:
Inpatient unwitnessed arrest **and** PEA or asystole as initial rhythm **and** no return of spontaneous circulation after 10 min of resuscitation efforts→ <1% chance of successful resuscitation

Note: Algorithm may differ from 2005 AMA guidelines.

FIG. 1-3

Pulseless electrical activity algorithm. *IV,* intravenous; *PEA,* pulseless electrical activity; *primary ABCD,* airway, breathing, circulation, and defibrillation; *secondary ABCD,* airway, breathing, circulation, and differential diagnosis.

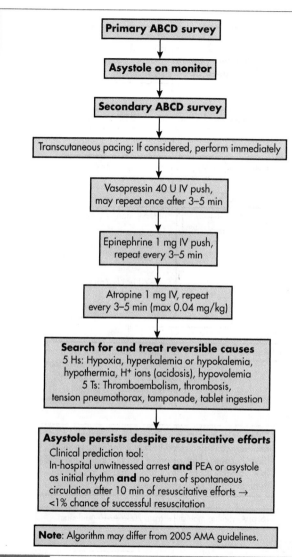

FIG. 1-4

Asystolic arrest. *IV,* intravenous; *PEA,* pulseless electrical activity; *primary ABCD,* airway, breathing, circulation, and defibrillation; *secondary ABCD,* airway, breathing, circulation, and differential diagnosis.

ADVANCED CARDIOPULMONARY LIFE SUPPORT

1

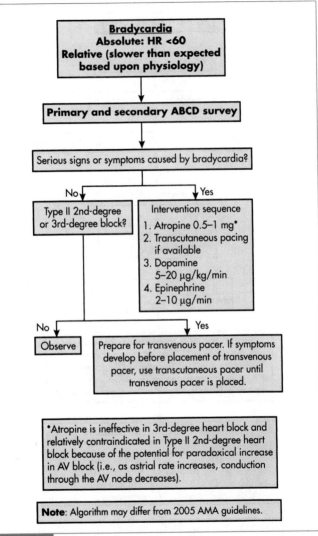

FIG. 1-5

Approach to bradycardia. *AV*, atrioventricular; *HR*, heart rate; *primary ABCD*, airway, breathing, circulation, and defibrillation; *secondary ABCD*, airway, breathing, circulation, and differential diagnosis. *(Adapted from Hazinski MF, Cummins RO, Field JM, eds:* 2000 Handbook of Emergency Cardiovascular Care for Healthcare Providers, *Dallas, 2000, American Heart Association.)*

physical examination. Rather, the diagnosis should be suspected based on history and excluded with emergent transthoracic echocardiography. If suspicion of pericardial tamponade is high and an echocardiogram is not immediately available, an emergent pericardiocentesis may be indicated.

3. **Continuous rhythm monitoring demonstrates either a nonperfusing organized rhythm or asystole.**

D. MANAGEMENT AND TREATMENT

Please see Figs. 1-3 and 1-4 for algorithms for managing PEA and asystole, respectively.

1. Vasopressin may be superior to epinephrine in asystole but equivalent to epinephrine in PEA.[5]
2. Given their synergistic properties, vasopressin should be given if ROSC has not been achieved after epinephrine administration.[7]

III. BRADYCARDIA

An approach to the acute management of bradycardia is detailed in Fig. 1-5.

PEARLS AND PITFALLS

- Minimize all interruptions of chest compression during cardiopulmonary resuscitation.[10]
- Recent clinical trials suggest that routine hyperventilation during cardiopulmonary arrest leads to auto–positive end-expiratory pressure, decreased coronary perfusion pressure, decreased rates of ROSC, and increased mortality.[11]
- Adequate chest compressions should produce a palpable carotid and femoral pulse. The absence of a pulse despite compressions implies ineffective forward flow and suggests tamponade, tension pneumothorax, or massive pulmonary embolism.
- Although the preferred route of administration is intravenous, epinephrine, atropine, naloxone, and lidocaine can be administered through an endotracheal tube at twice the normal dosage if there is a delay in establishing intravenous access.
- Treat all cardiac arrest in patients on hemodialysis as hyperkalemia until proven otherwise.
- Twenty percent to 40% of patients become bacteremic within 24 hours of successful resuscitation after arrest.
- Given its high volume of distribution, repeated loading doses of intravenous amiodarone can be given to the amiodarone-naive patient with recurrent ventricular arrhythmias.
- **Note:** Every attempt was made to incorporate the most up-to-date, evidence-based treatment in this chapter. At the time of publication, the 2005 American Medical Association resuscitation guidelines are forthcoming and should also be consulted.

REFERENCES

1. Parish DC, Dinesh Chandra KM, Dane FC: Success changes the problem: why ventricular fibrillation is declining, why pulseless electrical activity is emerging, and what to do about it, *Resuscitation* 58:31-35, 2003. D

2. van Walraven C, Forster AJ, Parish DC, et al: Validation of a clinical decision aid to discontinue in-hospital cardiac arrest resuscitations, *JAMA* 285(12):1602-1606, 2001. B

3. Weisfeldt ML, Becker LB: Resuscitation after cardiac arrest: a 3-phase time-sensitive model, *JAMA* 288(23):3035-3038, 2002. D

4. Wik L, Hansen TB, Fylling F, et al: Delaying defibrillation to give basic cardiopulmonary resuscitation to patients with out-of-hospital ventricular fibrillation: a randomized trial, *JAMA* 289(11):1389-1395, 2003. A

5. Faddy SC, Powell J, Craig JC: Biphasic and monophasic shocks for transthoracic defibrillation: a meta-analysis of randomised controlled trials, *Resuscitation* 58:9-16, 2003. C

6. Wenzel V, Krismer AC, Arntz HR, et al: A comparison of vasopressin and epinephrine for out-of-hospital cardiopulmonary resuscitation, *N Engl J Med* 350(2):105-113, 2004. A

7. Bernard SA, Gray TW, Buist MD, et al: Treatment of comatose survivors of out-of-hospital cardiac arrest with induced hypothermia, *N Engl J Med* 346(8):557-563, 2002. A

8. Dorian P, Cass D, Schwartz B, Cooper R, Gelaznikas R, Barr A: Amiodarone as compared with lidocaine for shock-resistant ventricular fibrillation, *N Engl J Med* 346:884-890, 2002. A

9. Nademanee K, Taylor R, Bailey WE, Rieders DE, Kosar EM: Treating electrical storm: sympathetic blockade versus advanced cardiac life support-guided therapy, *Circulation* 102:742-747, 2000. B

10. Yu T, Weil MH, Tang W, et al: Adverse outcomes of interrupted precordial compression during automated defibrillation, *Circulation* 106(3):368-372, 2002. B

11. Aufderheide TP, Sigurdsson G, Pirrallo RG, et al: Hyperventilation-induced hypotension during cardiopulmonary resuscitation, *Circulation* 109(16):1960-1965, 2004. B

Procedures

Jordan M. Prutkin, MD, MHS; Tze-Ming (Benson) Chen, MD; and Henry E. Fessler, MD

FAST FACTS

- Obtain informed consent before performing any elective procedure.
- Proper patient and physician positioning are key factors for successful and comfortable completion of all procedures.
- Sterile technique should be used for all procedures. Chlorhexidine is the preferred antiseptic solution because it has a lower rate of infection than povidone-iodine, although povidone-iodine may be used in lumbar punctures.[1]
- Always draw back on the syringe plunger when performing any procedure to determine whether the needle is in a blood vessel, especially if using lidocaine.
- A list of necessary equipment for each procedure is shown in Table 2-1.

Knee Arthrocentesis[2,3]

A. INDICATIONS
1. To evaluate a joint effusion.
2. To drain a joint effusion or hemarthrosis.
3. To inject medications.

B. CONTRAINDICATIONS
1. Infection of the overlying skin or soft tissue.
2. Bleeding diathesis, thrombocytopenia, or anticoagulant therapy.
3. Unstable joint from trauma.

C. COMPLICATIONS
Pain, infection, bleeding, hemarthrosis, and tendon rupture.

D. TECHNIQUE: ANTEROMEDIAL APPROACH
1. Place the patient in the supine position and flex the patient's knee approximately 160 degrees to open the joint space. Insert towels beneath the knee to support the leg.
2. Identify the medial edge of the patella and perform sterile preparation of the area with antiseptic solution. Drape accordingly.
3. Apply local anesthesia with 1% lidocaine using the 25-gauge needle. Start with a subcutaneous injection until a wheal forms, then insert the needle toward the inferior aspect of the patella, infiltrating the tissue with lidocaine (Fig. 2-1). Continue anesthetizing the soft tissue until the periosteum of the patella is reached. Anesthetize this area well because it is very sensitive. Withdraw the anesthesia needle.

TABLE 2-1	
EQUIPMENT NEEDED FOR BEDSIDE PROCEDURES	
Equipment Needed for All Procedures	
Skin Preparation and Draping	
Fenestrated sterile drape	
Towels	
Chlorhexidine solution	
Sterile gloves, sterile gown, sterile cap, surgical mask with eye shield	
Local Anesthesia	
1% lidocaine	
3-ml or 5-ml syringe	
Needles:	
$\quad$ 25 gauge × ⅝ inch	
$\quad$ 22 gauge × 1½ inch	
$\quad$ 20 gauge × 1½ inch	
Sterile 4 × 4 gauze and sterile dressing	

Procedure-Specific Equipment	
Knee arthrocentesis	18-gauge × 1½-inch needle
	10-ml or larger syringe
	Sterile specimen tubes
Lumbar puncture	3-way stopcock and manometer
	Spinal needle with stylet (20 gauge × 3½ inch)
	3-ml syringe
	≥4 sterile specimen tubes
Paracentesis	16- or 18-gauge Caldwell paracentesis needle
	Syringes (3 ml and 20 ml)
	Sterile specimen tubes
	High-pressure tubing line
	Vacutainer bottles
Thoracentesis	18-gauge × 2½-inch needle
	17-gauge × 6-inch thoracentesis needle with a 14-gauge Teflon catheter
	3-ml and two 20-ml syringes
	Scalpel
	3-way stopcock, 2-way valve
	Sterile specimen tubes
	1-L Vacutainer bottle
	High-pressure tubing line
Radial arterial line	20-gauge × 1-inch angiocatheter or radial artery catheterization kit (20-gauge × 1¾-inch cannula over a 22-gauge introducer needle with a spring wire guide)
	Arterial pressure transducer and pressure tubing
	3-0 skin suture, needle driver, and suture scissors
Central line	18-gauge × 2½-inch introducer needle
	Syringes (3 ml and 2 10 ml)
	Scalpel, skin dilator
	30 ml injectable saline
	Single-, double-, or triple-lumen catheter with associated guidewire
	Needleless or needle-adapted hub caps
	3-0 skin suture, needle driver, and suture scissors

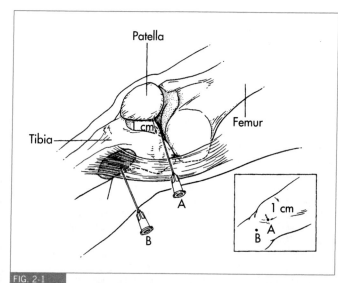

FIG. 2-1

Arthrocentesis: medial approach. The needle is inserted 1 cm below the patella, parallel to the plane of the table. *(From Salm TJV, Cutler BS, Wheeler HB, eds: Atlas of bedside procedures, Boston, 1979, Little, Brown.)*

4. Insert an 18- or 20-gauge needle attached to a 10- or 30-ml syringe and guide it to the inferior aspect of the patella.
5. After making contact with the patella, march the needle until it is just inferior to the patella.
6. Advance the needle into the joint space while gently aspirating back until joint fluid is obtained. A small pop may be felt when the needle enters the joint space.
7. Withdraw the needle after aspiration of the joint fluid and apply a sterile dressing over the insertion site.
8. Send aspirated fluid for cell count and differential, glucose, Gram stain and culture, and crystalline examination, as indicated.

PEARLS AND PITFALLS

- Consider orthopedic consultation for septic joints.
- Radiographic imaging of the joint before arthrocentesis is not routinely indicated unless trauma is suspected.
- See Chapter 89 for details on how to interpret synovial fluid.

Lumbar Puncture[3,4]

A. INDICATIONS

1. To assess for infectious meningitis, encephalitis, or neurosyphilis.
2. To assess for subarachnoid hemorrhage.

3. To assess for the meningeal carcinomatosis and staging of lymphoma.
4. To evaluate for multiple sclerosis.
5. To measure cerebrospinal fluid (CSF) pressure.
6. To administer intrathecal medication.

B. CONTRAINDICATIONS

1. Infection involving the path of the spinal needle (e.g., cellulitis, epidural abscess).
2. Elevated intracranial pressure.
3. Bleeding diathesis, thrombocytopenia, or anticoagulant therapy.

C. COMPLICATIONS

1. **Herniation syndrome.** High risk with supratentorial mass lesions.
2. **Infection.** Possible increased risk of meningitis if the patient is bacteremic.[5,6]
3. **Subdural or epidural hematoma.**
4. **Post–lumbar puncture headache.**[7]
   a. **Incidence.** Occurs in one in nine lumbar punctures performed with a 26-gauge spinal needle and one in three lumbar punctures performed with a 22-gauge spinal needle.[8]
   b. **Timing.** May start within minutes or up to 48 hours after completion of the lumbar puncture and may last a day to 2 weeks.
   c. **Risk factors.** Younger patients, female patients, prior lumbar puncture headache history.
5. **Minor backache.** Occurs in 90% of cases.
6. **Implantation of epidermoid tumors.** Occurs years after the procedure and is associated with the use of needles without stylets.[4]
7. **Aspiration of nerve roots.** Occurs with the use of needles without stylets.[4]
8. **Disk herniation.** Possible if the needle is advanced beyond the subarachnoid space into the anulus fibrosus.[2]

D. TECHNIQUE

1. Place the patient in the lateral decubitus position with knees drawn to the chest and a pillow to keep the head in line with the spinous processes, or seat the patient upright on the edge of the bed, leaning forward over a bedside table (Fig. 2-2).
2. Find the superior edge of the iliac crests and imagine a line across the back connecting these landmarks. The intersection of this line with the spinous processes localizes the L4 to L5 area. Palpate the space between the L4 and L5 spinous processes to identify the spinal needle insertion site.
3. Perform sterile preparation of the insertion site with chlorhexidine or Betadine and drape accordingly.
4. Apply local anesthesia with 1% lidocaine using the 25-gauge needle. After subcutaneous infiltration, direct the needle toward the umbilicus, along the sagittal plane, which includes the spinous process.
5. Continue anesthetizing the soft tissue until the periosteum of the vertebrae is reached. Anesthetize this area well because it is very sensitive. Withdraw the anesthesia needle.

2

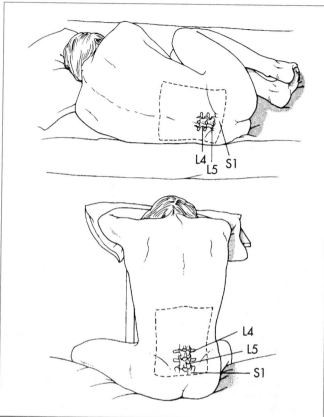

FIG. 2-2

Lumbar puncture: proper positioning. The patient is placed either in a lateral decubitus position *(above)* or sitting upright with the back slightly flexed forward *(below)*. An imaginary line drawn between the two superior iliac crests approximates the L4 to L5 intervertebral space. The patient should be prepped and draped to include the area in the dotted box. *(From Salm TJV, Cutler BS, Wheeler HB, eds: Atlas of bedside procedures, Boston, 1979, Little, Brown.)*

6. Insert the 20-gauge spinal needle (with the stylet inserted) along the previously described sagittal plane, angled toward the umbilicus (Fig. 2-3).
7. Advance the needle until a sudden slight yielding of the needle is noticed. If you encounter a bony process while advancing the needle, withdraw the needle until the tip is about 1 mm below the skin surface and then reinsert the needle after redirecting it a few degrees in the

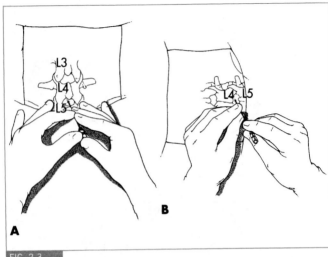

FIG. 2-3

Lumbar puncture: techniques in needle insertion. The needle should be advanced slowly with the bevel in the 12 o'clock position. **A,** Both hands are used to hold the needle. The ring fingers are positioned against the patient's back to help guide the needle into the intervertebral space. **B,** In another approach one hand is pressed against the patient's back while the other slowly advances the needle into the intervertebral space. *(From Salm TJV, Cutler BS, Wheeler HB, eds: Atlas of bedside procedures, Boston, 1979, Little, Brown.)*

   cephalad direction. If bone is encountered at a shallower level, redirect the needle caudally.
 8. Withdraw the stylet and attach the manometer with stopcock to measure opening pressure.
 9. After the opening pressure has been determined, switch the stopcock to direct CSF flow into the specimen tubes and remove the manometer.
10. When a sufficient amount of CSF has been collected, reinsert the stylet, and then withdraw the spinal needle. Closing pressure may also be measured with the manometer before the stylet is reinserted.
11. Send fluid for cell count and differential, glucose, protein, Gram stain and culture, mycobacterial culture and polymerase chain reaction (PCR), viral PCR, cryptococcal antigen, Venereal Disease Research Laboratory test, myelin basic protein, oligoclonal bands, and cytopathology, as indicated.

PEARLS AND PITFALLS

- Suggested treatment for post–lumbar puncture headaches includes prone positioning for 3 hours after the procedure, caffeine sodium benzoate

500 mg in 2 ml normal saline intravenous (IV) push,[9] aminophylline 5 to 6 mg IV over 20 minutes[10] (original study was performed in patients with hypertensive headaches), and blood patch for a prolonged low-pressure headache after conservative therapy has failed.

- Post–lumbar puncture headaches result from decreased CSF pressure caused by leakage of CSF from a persistent dural perforation. Infiltrating the tissue surrounding the perforation with 10 to 15 ml of autologous blood theoretically will tamponade the CSF leakage. However, spinal blood patches have a failure rate of 15% to 20% and are less effective if the headache has been present for more than 2 weeks.[11,12] This procedure is performed mainly by anesthesiologists.
- Computed tomography (CT) imaging of the head before a lumbar puncture has been advocated in the past because of concerns about post–lumbar puncture brainstem herniation. Clinical predictors for an abnormal CT scan of the head in adults with suspected meningitis include age older than 60 years, immunocompromised state, history of central nervous system disease, history of seizures within the week before presentation, abnormal level of consciousness, and abnormal neurologic examination.[13] If none of these features is present, the CT scan is unlikely to be abnormal (97% negative predictive value).
- Opening pressure is accurate only if obtained when the patient is in the lateral decubitus position.
- CSF abnormalities are detailed in Chapter 54.

Paracentesis[3,14,15]

A. INDICATIONS
1. To determine the cause of ascites.
2. To rule out spontaneous bacterial peritonitis.
3. To relieve cardiopulmonary and gastrointestinal complications of tense ascites.

B. CONTRAINDICATIONS
1. **Pregnancy, second or third trimester.** Recommend ultrasound guidance to avoid uterine laceration or perforation.
2. **Multiple previous abdominal surgeries.** Avoid inserting the needle into areas of the abdominal wall with prior surgical scars because of the high likelihood of adherent bowel in these areas.
3. **Infection of overlying skin or soft tissue.**
4. **Acute abdomen.**
5. **Bowel obstruction, unless bowel distension has been ruled out radiographically.**

Note: Coagulopathy is not a contraindication to paracentesis. *One study of paracentesis and thoracentesis demonstrated that among 608 patients, 71% of whom were coagulopathic, transfusion was provided in less than 0.2% (1 patient), but 3.1% had a decrease in hemoglobin level of 2 g/dl or more.*[16]

C. COMPLICATIONS

Pneumoperitoneum, peritonitis, perforated bladder, perforated bowel, intra-abdominal hemorrhage, abdominal wall hematoma, persistent fluid leak, infection, and renal insufficiency (controversial).

D. TECHNIQUE

1. Infraumbilical approach.
a. Place the patient in the lateral decubitus position.
b. Percuss the abdominal wall to determine where dullness is present. The insertion site for paracentesis is 3 to 4 cm below the umbilicus in the abdominal midline perpendicular to the skin (Fig. 2-4). The spot may also be marked using ultrasound.

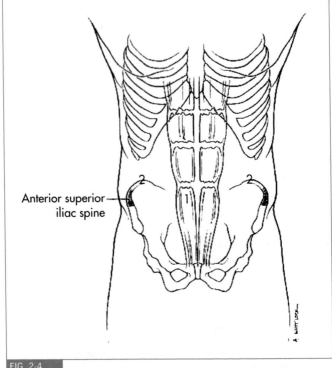

Anterior superior iliac spine

FIG. 2-4

Paracentesis: anterior abdominal anatomy. The anterior superior iliac crests *(2)* are noted as landmarks. The point of insertion for an infraumbilical approach is highlighted *(1)*. *(From Roberts JR, Hedges JR: Clinical procedures in emergency medicine, 4th ed, Philadelphia, 2004, WB Saunders.)*

c. Continue with step 3 for therapeutic paracentesis; continue with step 4 detailed as follows for diagnostic paracentesis.

2. Lower quadrant approach.

a. Place the patient in the supine position.

b. Examine the abdominal wall to assess for the presence of hepatosplenomegaly. If either organ is enlarged, the paracentesis insertion site should be on the opposite side of the organomegaly. If both hepatomegaly and splenomegaly are present, percuss the abdominal wall to determine the level of dullness. The insertion site is along the anterior axillary line lateral to the rectus sheath, halfway between the umbilicus and the anterior superior iliac spine or 1 to 2 cm lateral to the level of percussed dullness. The spot may also be marked using ultrasound.

3. Apply local anesthesia with 1% lidocaine using the 25-gauge needle and 22-gauge needle for deeper injection.

4. For the infraumbilical approach, pull the skin caudally 3 cm. For the lower quadrant approach, pull the skin medially 3 cm.

5. With the 20-ml syringe attached, insert an 18- or 20-gauge needle for a diagnostic paracentesis or a 16- or 18-gauge Caldwell needle for a therapeutic paracentesis, pulling back on the syringe plunger gently while advancing the needle slowly.

6. Release the skin after the needle has entered about 2 cm. This technique is called the Z-track approach.

7. Remove the Caldwell needle stylet and attach the high-pressure tubing line to a Vacutainer bottle for a therapeutic paracentesis.

8. If the ascitic fluid flow slows or ceases, stop the suction, readjust the needle by tilting the tip inferiorly, and reapply the suction. If this is unsuccessful, advance or withdraw the needle slowly 0.5 to 1 cm at a time.

9. Send ascitic fluid for protein, albumin, cell count with differential, culture, amylase, glucose, lactate dehydrogenase, and cytology, as indicated.

PEARLS AND PITFALLS

- Avoid inserting the needle into the rectus muscles because this is where the inferior epigastric arteries lie.
- There is some evidence that plasma expansion with intravenous albumin after large-volume paracentesis decreases the risk of acute renal insufficiency.[17-21] Use of 8 to 10 g IV albumin per liter of ascites removed is recommended.
- Persistent ascitic fluid leak is common and can be minimized by using the Z-track approach. If there is a fluid leak, cover the site with an ostomy bag because it usually closes spontaneously. If it does not, a stitch can be used to close it.
- See Chapter 36 for information on ascitic fluid abnormalities.

2

PROCEDURES

Thoracentesis[3,22]

A. INDICATIONS
1. To evaluate a pleural effusion of unknown origin.
2. For therapeutic drainage of a pleural effusion.

B. CONTRAINDICATIONS
1. Severe contralateral lung impairment.
2. Bleeding diathesis, thrombocytopenia, or anticoagulant therapy.
3. Infection of the overlying skin or soft tissue.
4. Positive-pressure ventilation.

C. COMPLICATIONS
Chest wall hematoma or hemothorax, pneumothorax, infection, lung, hepatic or splenic laceration or puncture, reexpansion pulmonary edema, and hypotension if volume depleted.

D. TECHNIQUE
1. Review chest radiograph of patient in the erect and lateral decubitus positions and confirm location of the pleural effusion.
2. Place the patient in a sitting position over the edge of the bed, leaning over a bedside table (Fig. 2-5). Percuss out the effusion by noting the superior edge of dullness on the posterior aspect of the chest wall. Confirm by auscultation, listening for diminished breath sounds. The effusion also may be marked using ultrasound.
3. Perform sterile preparation of the insertion site with antiseptic solution and drape accordingly.
4. Provide local anesthesia with 1% lidocaine.
5. Insert the needle, aiming for the middle of the rib just below the superior edge of percussed dullness in the posterior axillary line.
6. Once the needle has come in contact with the rib, march the needle *superiorly* over the edge of the rib, gently withdrawing on the syringe plunger and anesthetizing the area well (Fig. 2-6).
7. When the needle enters the pleural space, the syringe will fill with pleural fluid.
8. **Diagnostic thoracentesis.** Insert the 18-gauge needle attached to the 20-ml syringe into the pleural space, following the same path as the anesthesia needle, withdrawing gently on the syringe plunger as the needle is advanced. Once the needle enters the pleural space, fill the syringe with fluid and remove the needle.
9. **Therapeutic thoracentesis.**
a. Make a small nick in the skin using a scalpel at the site where the anesthesia needle entered the skin.
b. Insert the 17-gauge thoracentesis needle (with overlying Teflon catheter) attached to the 20-ml syringe into the pleural space, following the same path as the anesthesia needle, withdrawing gently on the syringe plunger as the needle is advanced.
c. Once the needle has entered the pleural space, have the patient perform a Valsalva maneuver to increase the intrapleural pressure. This

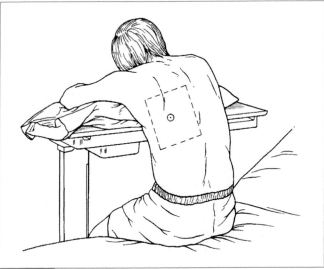

FIG. 2-5

Thoracentesis: proper positioning. The patient is positioned as shown, leaning forward against a pillow on a bedside table. The back should be examined to ensure that the anticipated entry site is dull to percussion before the patient is prepped and draped. After adequate local anesthesia the needle is inserted into the intercostal space over the superior aspect of the rib to avoid the vascular nerve bundle. *(From Salm TJV, Cutler BS, Wheeler HB, eds: Atlas of bedside procedures, Boston, 1979, Little, Brown.)*

   will decrease the likelihood of a pneumothorax developing while the
   syringe is being disconnected from the needle.
 d. Advance the Teflon catheter over the needle into the pleural space.
 e. Once the catheter is in place, remove the 17-gauge needle. Remove
   pleural fluid with the assistance of a three-way stopcock or two-way
   valve.
10. Send the pleural fluid for lactate dehydrogenase, albumin, protein,
   glucose, pH, cultures, hematocrit, adenosine deaminase, and gamma-
   interferon, as indicated.
11. Consider obtaining a chest radiograph to assess for the presence or
   absence of a pneumothorax. (There is debate as to whether this is
   necessary.)

PEARLS AND PITFALLS

- When performing a therapeutic thoracentesis, remove no more than 1 L
  fluid to minimize the risk of reexpansion pulmonary edema.
- Criteria for a transudative and exudative pleural effusion are described in
  Chapter 83.

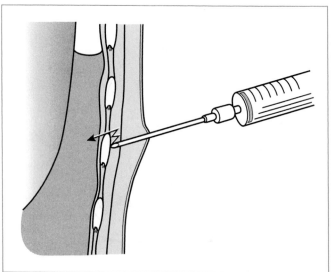

Thoracentesis: path of needle. The needle should be inserted aiming for the middle of the rib, then marched superiorly over the edge and into the pleural space. *(From Roberts JR, Hedges JR: Clinical procedures in emergency medicine, 4th ed, Philadelphia, 2004, WB Saunders.)*

Radial Arterial Line[3,23]

A. INDICATIONS
1. For continuous arterial blood pressure monitoring.
2. For frequent arterial blood sampling.

B. CONTRAINDICATIONS
1. Infection of the overlying skin or soft tissue.
2. Inadequate collateral arterial supply.
3. Bleeding diathesis, thrombocytopenia, or anticoagulant therapy.

C. COMPLICATIONS
Bleeding, infection, digital or hand ischemia, and retrograde air embolism.

D. TECHNIQUE
1. Allen test.
a. Occlude the radial and ulnar arteries by applying pressure with your thumbs.
b. Have the patient make a tight fist with that hand and then relax.
c. After observing the blanching of the hand, release the radial artery and watch for normalization of the hand color.

d. Repeat, but release the ulnar artery.
e. If both arteries provide adequate perfusion of the hand, release of each artery should result in normal hand color within 5 seconds.
f. If inadequate perfusion is demonstrated, do not cannulate either artery.
g. If evaluating for blanching is difficult, use a pulse oximetry tracing to provide evidence for distal perfusion during ulnar and radial artery compression.
2. Place the patient in the supine position, abduct the arm, supinate the forearm, and hyperextend the hand with a towel.
3. Place padding beneath the hand to help maintain this position.
4. Prepare the insertion site with chlorhexidine and anesthetize with 1% lidocaine.
5. Palpate the radial artery with two fingertips placed 2 cm apart.
6. Delineate a line between the fingertips and insert the angiocatheter along this line at a 45-degree angle from the skin into the radial artery.
7. Once a flash of red blood is seen in the needle hub, advance the guidewire into the artery. Advance the cannula over the wire into the artery.
8. Withdraw the needle and attached wire and confirm arterial placement with the presence of pulsatile blood flow out of the cannula hub.
9. Attach the pressure transducer and pressure tubing and suture the line in place.
10. Apply a sterile dressing over the insertion site and the cannula.

PEARLS AND PITFALLS
- Appropriate hyperextension of the hand minimizes inadvertent artery movement during the procedure.
- Confirm proper placement by observing the pressure wave on the cardiac monitor or by sending a sample of blood for an arterial blood gas analysis.

Central Line Placement[3,24-26]

A. INDICATIONS
1. To secure intravenous access for medications and blood products.
2. For phlebotomy.
3. To monitor central venous pressure.
4. To deliver parenteral nutrition.

B. CONTRAINDICATIONS
1. Infection of the area overlying the target vessel.
2. Thrombosis of the target vessel.
3. **Coagulopathy.** Avoid subclavian vein attempts, given the difficulty of compressing blood vessels in this area.
4. **Inferior vena cava filter.** Relative contraindication for femoral vein approaches. If necessary, use only single-lumen catheters because the guidewire for this device is the shortest available.

2

PROCEDURES

5. **Respiratory distress or impending respiratory failure.** Avoid the subclavian approach if a pneumothorax is likely to be fatal.

C. COMPLICATIONS

Pain, infection, bleeding, arterial or venous laceration, arterial cannulation, pneumothorax, hemothorax, cardiac arrhythmia, and air embolism.

D. SELDINGER TECHNIQUE

1. Place the patient in the supine position.
2. Examine the patient to determine the most appropriate location for the line.
3. **Internal jugular vein site** (Fig. 2-7):
   a. Turn the patient's head so the chin is directed away from the target vessel.
   b. Place the patient in a 15- to 20-degree Trendelenburg position.
   c. Identify the triangle formed by the anterior and posterior bellies of the sternocleidomastoid muscle and the clavicle. The insertion site is near the apex of this triangle, just lateral to the palpable pulsation of the carotid artery.
   d. Perform sterile preparation of the insertion site with antiseptic solution and apply local anesthesia with 1% lidocaine.
   e. Palpate the carotid artery in the triangle and retract it medially.
   f. Insert the 25-gauge needle at a 45-degree angle to the skin into the triangle apex just lateral to the carotid pulsation, with the bevel in the 12 o'clock position, advancing toward the ipsilateral nipple.
   g. Pull back on the syringe plunger gently while advancing the needle and infiltrate the tissue with lidocaine.
   h. Exchange the 25-gauge needle for a 22-gauge needle and continue to advance the needle.
   i. The internal jugular vein should be entered at a depth of approximately 3 cm (may be deeper with more obese patients). If it is not, withdraw the needle to just beneath the skin surface and redirect the needle laterally.
   j. Once the 22-gauge needle is in the internal jugular vein, maintain its position and take the 18-gauge needle attached to a 10-ml syringe and insert it following the path of the 22-gauge needle.
   k. Once the 18-gauge needle has entered the internal jugular vein, withdraw the 22-gauge needle.
   l. Continue with step 6.
4. **Subclavian vein site:**
   a. Turn the patient's head away from the target vessel (Fig. 2-8).
   b. Place the patient in a 10- to 15-degree Trendelenburg position.
   c. The insertion site is 2 to 3 cm caudal to the middle of the clavicle.
   d. Perform sterile preparation of the insertion site with antiseptic solution and apply local anesthesia with 1% lidocaine.
   e. Insert the 25-gauge needle almost parallel to the skin, with the bevel in the 12 o'clock position, aiming for the clavicle in the direction of the suprasternal notch.

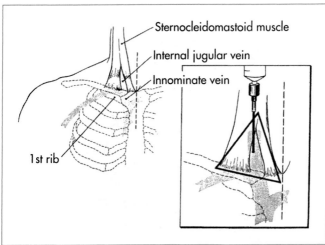

Sternocleidomastoid muscle

Internal jugular vein

Innominate vein

1st rib

FIG. 2-7

Central line placement into internal jugular vein: anatomy of the neck and upper chest and needle insertion point. *(From Roberts JR, Hedges JR: Clinical procedures in emergency medicine, 4th ed, Philadelphia, 2004, WB Saunders.)*

2

PROCEDURES

f. Pull back on the syringe plunger gently while advancing the needle and infiltrate the tissue with lidocaine.

g. Exchange the 25-gauge needle for a 22-gauge needle and continue to advance the needle until it hits the clavicle.

h. Anesthetize the periosteum well because it is very sensitive.

i. Pass the needle underneath the clavicle toward the suprasternal notch, parallel to the patient's back.

j. Remove the 22-gauge needle.

k. Using the 18-gauge needle attached to a 10-ml syringe, advance the needle toward the subclavian vein following the path of the 22-gauge needle. The desired insertion site into the vein is at the junction of the middle and medial thirds of the clavicle.

l. Draw back on the syringe as you are advancing.

m. Once the 18-gauge needle has entered the subclavian vein, continue with step 6.

5. **Femoral vein site:**

a. Identify the pulsation of the femoral artery.

b. The insertion site is just medial to the femoral artery pulsation and 1 cm inferior to the inguinal ligament.

c. Perform sterile preparation of the insertion site with antiseptic solution and apply local anesthesia with 1% lidocaine.

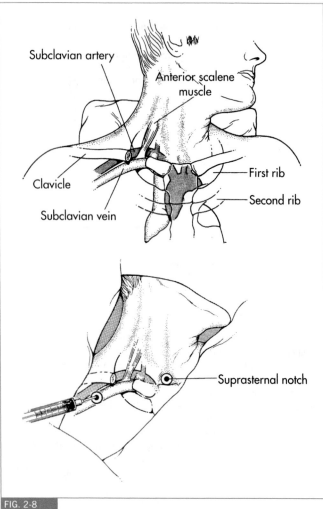

FIG. 2-8

Central line placement into the subclavian vein: anatomy of the upper chest. (*From Salm TJV, Cutler BS, Wheeler HB, eds: Atlas of bedside procedures, Boston, 1979, Little, Brown.*)

d. Insert the 25-gauge needle with the bevel in the 12 o'clock position at a 45- to 60-degree angle, aiming just medial to the femoral artery pulsation.

e. Pull back on the syringe plunger gently while advancing the needle and infiltrate the tissue with lidocaine.

f. Once the hub of the 25-gauge needle has been reached, change to the 22-gauge needle and continue to advance the needle.

g. If the femoral vein is not cannulated within a depth of 4 cm, withdraw the needle to just beneath the skin surface and redirect the needle medially. The depth may vary depending on the patient's body habitus.

h. Using the 18-gauge needle attached to a 10-ml syringe, advance the needle toward the femoral vein following the path of the 22-gauge needle.

i. Draw back on the syringe as you are advancing.

j. Once the 18-gauge needle has entered the femoral vein, continue with step 6.

6. When the needle enters a blood vessel, attempt to confirm that the needle is in the vein by detaching the syringe from the needle and observing the color of the blood and the absence of pulsatile flow.

7. If the vein has been cannulated, insert the curved end of the guidewire through the needle and advance it gently. To prevent embolization, do not insert more than half of the length of the guidewire.

8. If you feel resistance to the insertion of the guidewire, withdraw the wire, rotate the 18-gauge needle to change the bevel position, and reinsert the wire gently.

9. If the patient is on a cardiac monitor and an arrhythmia develops after the wire has been inserted, pull back on the wire and wait for resolution of the abnormal rhythm. If the abnormal rhythm persists, institute appropriate advanced cardiac life support.

10. Once the guidewire has been inserted, withdraw the needle.

11. Make a 2-mm nick in the skin at the wire entry site with the scalpel.

12. Place the dilator over the guidewire, insert the dilator while turning the instrument, and then withdraw it.

13. Insert the proximal end of the guidewire into the tip of the central venous catheter and pull back the wire until the wire tip protrudes from the proximal port of the catheter, making sure the cap has been removed from the proximal port. **Always maintain a hold on a section of the guidewire to prevent its embolization.**

14. While grasping the proximal end of the guidewire tip, insert the catheter into the insertion site over the guidewire using a twisting motion.

15. Insert the catheter to a depth of 15 cm for a right-sided internal vein jugular placement, to 17 cm for a left-sided internal jugular vein placement, to 15 cm for a right-sided subclavian vein placement, to

2

PROCEDURES

17 cm for a left-sided subclavian vein placement, and to the catheter hub for a femoral vein placement.

16. Withdraw the guidewire and check for blood return in all catheter ports.
17. Flush all ports with saline and suture the line in place.
18. Apply a sterile dressing.
19. For internal jugular and subclavian vein placements, obtain a chest radiograph to check for line position and assess for pneumothorax or hemothorax. Be sure the tip of the catheter is not in the right atrium.

PEARLS AND PITFALLS

- Ultrasound guidance reduces the number of mechanical complications, number of failed attempts, and duration of the procedure. It works best for internal jugular and femoral line attempts.[26]
- Introducer needles are cutting needles and should never be redirected unless they have been withdrawn to 1 to 2 mm below the skin. Doing so reduces the risk of a vascular laceration.
- The location of the line affects the risk of infection. Femoral lines have the highest incidence of infection, internal jugular the next highest, and subclavian the least.[26] As soon as the catheter is no longer needed it should be removed. See Chapter 58 for details on management of line infections.
- If in doubt as to whether the line is in the artery or the vein, consider sending a sample of blood for arterial blood gas analysis.
- If the femoral artery is cannulated, remove the catheter promptly and apply direct pressure for at least 15 minutes proximal to the point where the artery was cannulated. Confirm that the lower extremity appears well perfused during and after compression. Arterial puncture is more likely to occur with a femoral attempt than with an internal jugular or subclavian attempt.[26]
- If the carotid artery is cannulated, consider surgical consultation before removing the catheter. Otherwise, apply pressure for at least 10 minutes at the point in which the artery is cannulated.
- Antibiotic ointments should not be used at the insertion site because they might promote antibiotic resistance, they allow colonization by fungi, and they have not been shown to reduce bloodstream infections.[26]

REFERENCES

1. Centers for Disease Control and Prevention: Guidelines for the prevention of intravascular catheter-related infections, *MMWR* 51(RR-10):1-29, 2002. D
2. Haist SA, Robbins JB, Gomella LG: *Internal medicine on call,* 2nd ed, Stamford, Conn, 1997, Appleton & Lange. D
3. Roberts JR, Hedges JR: *Clinical procedures in emergency medicine,* 4th ed, Philadelphia, 2004, WB Saunders. D
4. Davidson RI: Lumbar puncture. In Salm TJV, Cutler BS, Wheeler HB, eds: *Atlas of bedside procedures,* Boston, 1979, Little, Brown. D

5. Petersdorf RG, Swarner DR, Garcia M: Studies on the pathogenesis of meningitis. II. Development of meningitis during pneumococcal bacteremia, *J Clin Invest* 41:320, 1962. B

6. Teele DW et al: Meningitis after lumbar puncture in children with bacteremia, *N Engl J Med* 305:1079, 1981. B

7. Brocker RJ: Technique to avoid spinal-tap headache, *JAMA* 168:261, 1958. B

8. Tourtellotte WW et al: A randomized double-blind clinical trial comparing the 22- versus 26-gauge needle in the production of the post–lumbar puncture syndrome in normal individuals, *Headache* 12:73, 1972. A

9. Sechzer PH, Abel L: Post–spinal anesthesia headache treated with caffeine: evaluation with demand method. I, *Curr Ther Res* 24:307, 1978. C

10. Moyer JH et al: The effect of theophylline with ethylenediamine (aminophylline) and caffeine on cerebral hemodynamics and cerebrospinal fluid pressure in patients with hypertensive headaches, *Am J Med Sci* 224:377, 1952. C

11. Bradsky JB: Epidural blood patch: a safe effective treatment for post–lumbar puncture headaches, *West J Med* 129:85, 1978. C

12. Olsen KS: Epidural blood patch in the treatment of post–lumbar headache, *Pain* 30:293, 1987. C

13. Hasbun R et al: Computed tomography of the head before lumbar puncture in adults with suspected meningitis, *N Engl J Med* 345:1727, 2001. B

14. Silva WE: Diagnostic paracentesis and lavage. In Salm TJV, Cutler BS, Wheeler HB, eds: *Atlas of bedside procedures*, Boston, 1979, Little, Brown. D

15. Runyon BA: Paracentesis of ascitic fluid: a safe procedure, *Arch Intern Med* 146:2259, 1986. B

16. McVay PA, Toy PTCY: Lack of increased bleeding after paracentesis and thoracentesis in patients with mild coagulation abnormalities, *Transfusion* 31:164, 1991. C

17. Planas R et al: Dextran-70 versus albumin as plasma expanders in cirrhotic patients with tense ascites treated with total paracentesis: results of a randomized study, *Gastroenterology* 99:1736, 1990. B

18. Altman C et al: Randomized comparative multicenter study of hydroxyethyl starch versus albumin as a plasma expander in cirrhotic patients with tense ascites treated with paracentesis, *Eur J Gastroenterol* 10:5, 1998. B

19. Wilkinson SP: Treatment options for cirrhotic ascites, *Eur J Gastroenterol* 10:1, 1998. D

20. Wong PY, Carroll RE, Lipinski TL, et al: Studies on the renin-angiotensin-aldosterone system in patients with cirrhosis and ascites: effect of saline and albumin infusion, *Gastroenterology* 77:1171, 1979. B

21. Vermeulen LC Jr et al: A paradigm for consensus: the University Hospital Consortium guidelines for the use of albumin, nonprotein colloid, and crystalloid solutions, *Arch Intern Med* 155:373, 1995. C

22. Salm TJV: Thoracentesis. In Salm TJV, Cutler BS, Wheeler HB, eds: *Atlas of bedside procedures,* Boston, 1979, Little, Brown. D

23. Salm TJV: Arterial cannula insertion, percutaneous. In Salm TJV, Cutler BS, Wheeler HB, eds: *Atlas of bedside procedures,* Boston, 1979, Little, Brown. D

24. Salm TJV: Subclavian vein cannulation. In Salm TJV, Cutler BS, Wheeler HB, eds: *Atlas of bedside procedures,* Boston, 1979, Little, Brown. D

25. Salm TJV: Internal jugular vein cannulation. In Salm TJV, Cutler BS, Wheeler HB, eds: *Atlas of bedside procedures,* Boston, 1979, Little, Brown. D

26. McGee DC, Gould MK: Preventing complications of central venous catheterization, *N Engl J Med* 348:1123-1133, 2003. C

2

PROCEDURES

Nutrition Support

Erin Tiberio, RD, CNSD; Dechen Surkhang, RD, LD;
and Tricia Brusco, MS, RD, LD

FAST FACTS

- The prevalence of malnutrition in hospitalized patients is 20% to 50%.[1,2]
- Malnutrition is associated with poor wound healing, longer length of stay, and increased morbidity and mortality.
- Nutrition support should be considered when volitional intake consistently fails to meet 50% of nutritional needs as determined by calorie counts.

I. NUTRITIONAL ASSESSMENT

1. **Evaluation of a patient's nutritional status** includes a review of the medical history, diet history, physical examination, anthropometric data, weight, and biochemical data.
2. The **Hamwii method** is used to determine ideal body weight for height and is calculated as follows: For men, 5 ft = 106 lb, and add 6 lb for each inch above 5 ft; for women, 5 ft = 100 lb, and add 5 lb for each inch above 5 ft.
3. **The patient's current body weight should be compared with his or her ideal body weight and usual body weight.** Determining the extent and duration of the patient's weight loss provides important insight into the severity of the malnourished state and helps determine the patient's nutritional needs.[3]
4. **Estimation of caloric needs.**
a. Basal energy expenditure (BEE) or basal metabolic rate (BMR) is the minimum energy needed for a person to maintain basic vital functions. BEE or BMR is determined by the Harris-Benedict equation:

$$\text{Women: BEE or BMR} = 655.1 + 9.56W + 1.85H - 4.68A$$
$$\text{Men: BEE or BMR} = 66.5 + 13.75W + 5.0H - 6.78A$$

where W is weight in kilograms, H is height in centimeters, and A is age. Adjustments are made to the Harris-Benedict equation for a patient's condition by multiplying the BMR by a stress factor ranging from 1.2 to as high as 2.0 for major stress (e.g., trauma, burns).
b. Caloric needs can also be estimated by body weight. Adults up to 69 years of age need 25 to 35 calories/kg. Adults 79 years and older need 25 to 28 calories/kg. Ideally, caloric needs should be estimated according to lean body mass.
5. **Estimation of protein needs.**

a. **The human body has no protein stores;** all body protein serves vital functions, so any depletion without replacement will impair protein's functional role. A healthy person needs 0.8 g/kg/day. A protein intake of 1 to 1.5 g/kg/day meets the needs of most hospitalized patients; those with severe stress may need as much as 2 g/kg/day.

b. A **24-hour urinary urea nitrogen** (UUN) is the most direct method of estimating protein need, which can be used to determine the nitrogen balance. Nitrogen balance is not reliable for patients on oral diets because of difficulty in obtaining precise protein intake data. Nitrogen balance = (24-hour protein intake/6.25) − (UUN [g/day] + 4).

II. FEEDING MODALITIES[4,5]

1. **Oral nutrition** includes specialized diets and supplements based on underlying pathological conditions, such as congestive heart failure or renal failure. When volitional intake consistently fails to meet 50% of nutritional needs, as determined by calorie counts, nutrition support should be considered.

2. **Enteral nutrition** is the provision of nutrients through the gastrointestinal (GI) tract. It is the preferred route of nutrition support because it is more "physiologic," less expensive, safer, and associated with fewer side effects than parenteral nutrition. Enteral nutrition is indicated when a patient consistently fails to consume at least half of his or her oral diet or when the patient is unable to tolerate an oral diet.

a. **Contraindications to enteral feeding** include diffuse peritonitis, intestinal obstruction, intractable vomiting, paralytic ileus, and severe diarrhea. Relative contraindications include severe pancreatitis, enterocutaneous fistulas, and early stages of short gut syndrome or malabsorption.

b. **Feeding tubes.** Short-term enteral nutrition (<30 days) can be administered through a nasoenteric (nasogastric, nasoduodenal, or nasojejunal) tube. Percutaneous tubes (e.g., percutaneous endoscopic gastrostomy and jejunostomy) and surgically placed feeding tubes (e.g., open gastrostomy) should be placed for long-term therapy.

c. **Enteral formulas** are polymeric (nutrients are intact, normal GI function is necessary) or monomeric or elemental (partially hydrolyzed nutrients, appropriate for compromised digestion and absorption). Specialty formulas are available and are designed for specific disease states, including renal failure, liver disease, and trauma (Table 3-1).

d. **Administration.** Continuous administration is preferred in patients unable to tolerate large-volume infusion, fed through the small intestine, or at high aspiration risk. Continuous feeds can be initiated at 30 ml/hr and increased as tolerated (based on gastric residuals and patient tolerance) every 8 to 12 hours to determined goal rate. Intermittent feeding is reserved for more stable patients. A typical regimen is 200 to 400 ml infused over 30 to 40 minutes every 3 to 4 hours. Bolus feedings are reserved for more stable patients. A syringe is used to infuse up to 500 ml within a few minutes.

TABLE 3-1

COMMONLY USED ENTERAL FEEDING FORMULAS

	Ensure	Osmolite	Jevity 1 Cal	Nutren 2.0	Nepro	Trauma Cal	Peptamen 1.5
Type	Oral supplement	Isotonic formula	Fiber-fortified formula	Concentrated formula	Specialty formula	Specialty formula	Semielemental formula
Serving size	8 fluid oz	1 L	1 L	1 L	1 L	1 L	1 L
Calories/ml	1.06	1.06	1.06	2	2	1.5	1.5
Carbohyd rate (% calories)	63.9	57	54.3	39	43	38	49
Protein (% calories)	14.1	14	16.7	16	14	22	18
Fat (% calories)	22	29	29	45	43	40	33
Na (mg/serving)	200	640	930	1300	845	1180	1020
K (mg/serving)	370	1020	1570	1920	1055	1390	1860
Water (ml/serving)	200	841	829	700	699	750	771
Osmolality (mOsm/kg H_2O)	590	300	300	745	665	560	550
Amount needed to meet 100% daily values for key vitamins and minerals (ml)	948	1887	1321	750	947	2000	1000
Features	Variety of flavors Ultratrace minerals	Low residue Moderate protein	Isotonic with fiber	For fluid-restricted patients	For dialyzed patients with acute or chronic renal failure Low in vitamins A and D	High in vitamin C, B-complex, E, Cu, Zn for wound healing	Peptide based

e. During enteral nutrition, the head of the bed should be raised by more than 30 degrees to decrease the risk of aspiration.

3. **Parenteral nutrition** is the provision of nutrients intravenously when the GI tract is not functional, accessible, or safe to use.

a. **Parenteral nutrition is indicated in the following clinical situations:** intestinal obstruction or ileus, severe necrotizing pancreatitis, failed enteral nutrition (high gastric residuals, inability to advance to goal), and short bowel syndrome.

b. Parenteral nutrition should not be used in the presence of a functioning GI tract, when the patient's prognosis does not warrant aggressive support, and when the risks outweigh the benefits.

c. **Peripheral parenteral nutrition** is a short-term (up to 7 days) supplemental therapy. Because peripheral veins are unable to tolerate hypertonic solutions with osmolarity greater than 900 mOsm/L, limited nutrients are provided in peripheral parenteral nutrition. Therefore a large volume of solution (up to 3 L) is necessary.

d. **Total parenteral nutrition** (TPN) is used to meet patients' full nutritional needs, including fluid restriction, and should be used for intermediate- and long-term intravenous nutrition. TPN osmolality may reach 1800 mOsm/L, and TPN is administered by central venous catheter. It can be administered with all nutrients (dextrose, amino acids, and lipids) mixed together (known as 3-in-1 or total nutrient admixture). Alternatively, the dextrose–amino acid solution can be infused separately from the lipid emulsion.

e. Parenteral nutrition components.

   (1) **Carbohydrate** is provided as dextrose monohydrate, which provides 3.4 kcal/g and is available in concentrations ranging from 2.5% to 70%, with concentrations greater than 10% reserved for TPN. Glucose administration should not exceed 5 mg/kg/min, and special attention should be paid to patient's serum glucose measurements during infusion.

   (2) **Lipid** emulsions are isotonic, concentrated sources of calories that provide 9 kcal/kg. Lipid infusions should not exceed 60% of total calories or more than 2 g/kg/day.

   (3) **Protein** is provided as essential, semiessential, and nonessential crystalline amino acids and provides 4 kcal/g.

f. **Additives.** Standard vitamin and mineral preparations are added daily to parenteral nutrition solutions. Requirements with parenteral nutrition are lower than the dietary reference intake levels because normal digestion and absorption are bypassed.

   (1) **Insulin** is commonly added to parenteral nutrition in patients with impaired glucose tolerance and diabetes. A minimum of 10 U should be added per day because of adherence to intravenous bags and tubing, and insulin should be increased in 5- to 10-U increments. The maximum insulin dosage in parenteral nutrition is 100 U/L.

(2) **H blockers** (ranitidine or famotidine) and **prokinetic agents** such as metoclopramide (maximum 40 mg/day) can also be added to parenteral nutrition.

g. **Weight and intake and output totals for patients on TPN should be recorded daily. Dexi-sticks should be taken every 6 hours initially.** The following laboratory tests should be reviewed every week or as needed: electrolytes, liver function tests, serum triglyceride levels, phosphorus, magnesium, and nitrogen balance. Serum prealbumin, transferrin, copper, zinc, and selenium should be assessed initially and periodically thereafter.

h. **Complications** of TPN include metabolic acidosis, hyperglycemia, electrolyte imbalances, hyperlipidemia, mineral deficiency, volume overload, cholestasis, respiratory failure, and sepsis.

PEARLS AND PITFALLS

- TPN must be administered through a dedicated TPN line. Nothing else should be infused through a TPN central venous line.
- If TPN must be stopped suddenly, 10% dextrose should be infused at the same rate.
- Patients on TPN are at elevated risk of developing fungemia.
- Refeeding syndrome consists of complications that occur when a chronically malnourished patient receives aggressive nutrition support, whether orally, enterally, or parenterally. It is characterized by severe fluid and electrolyte shifts that may lead to cardiac, pulmonary, and neuromuscular complications. After refeeding, a malnourished patient's energy source shifts from fat to carbohydrate. This shift results in increased insulin secretion with an increased cellular uptake of glucose, phosphorus, and magnesium and reduced excretion of sodium and water. The patient may present with hypokalemia, hypophosphatemia, hypomagnesemia, and edema.
- Provide nutrition slowly (begin at 20 kcal/kg of current weight) because excessive feeding increases morbidity and mortality.

REFERENCES

1. Bistrain BR et al: Prevalence of malnutrition in general medical patients, *JAMA* 253:1567, 1976. B
2. Butterworth CE: The skeleton in the hospital closet, *Nutr Today* 9:4, 1974. C
3. Shopbell JM, Hopkins B, Shronts EP: Nutrition screening and assessment. In Gottschlich MM et al, eds: *A case based core curriculum of the American Society for Parenteral and Enteral Nutrition,* Dubuque, Iowa, 2001, Kendall/Hunt. C
4. Bloch AS, Mueller C: Enteral and parenteral nutrition support. In Mahan LK, Escott-Stump S, eds: *Krause's food, nutrition and diet therapy,* 10th ed, Philadelphia, 2000, WB Saunders. C
5. Gorman RC, Morris JB: Minimally invasive access to the gastrointestinal tract. In Rombeau JC, Rolandelli RH, eds: *Clinical nutrition: enteral and tube feeding,* Philadelphia, 1997, WB Saunders. C

Anaphylaxis and Drug Allergy

Franco D'Alessio, MD; and N. Franklin Adkinson Jr., MD

FAST FACTS

- Anaphylaxis is a systemic, life-threatening immunoglobulin E (IgE)-dependent immediate hypersensitivity reaction that can lead to urticaria, bronchospasm, hypotension, and cardiovascular collapse.
- Secondary anaphylactoid (pseudoallergic) reactions to radiocontrast can be reduced by 80% using a premedication regimen of corticosteroids and antihistamines.
- Based on skin testing, 80% to 90% of those who report penicillin hypersensitivity are not truly allergic.[1]
- Angioedema without urticaria is a bradykinin-mediated pseudoallergic reaction that leads to deep tissue swelling of the eyes, lips, and oropharynx. Angioedema is commonly associated with the use of angiotensin-converting enzyme inhibitors.
- Stevens-Johnson syndrome is a severe drug-induced cutaneous reaction characterized by fever, erosive stomatitis, and disseminated dark red macules that can involve the ocular membranes. This highly morbid cutaneous reaction is most commonly associated with trimethoprim-sulfamethoxazole, sulfadoxine and pyrimethamine, and carbamazepine.[2]

4

I. EPIDEMIOLOGY

1. Anaphylaxis is a systemic, life-threatening acute hypersensitivity reaction caused by IgE-mediated release of histamine and other vasoactive mediators from mast cells and basophils. Anaphylactoid or pseudoallergic reactions are clinically similar but are not IgE mediated.
2. Adverse drug reactions can be classified as *predictable* (or type A; i.e., dose dependent, side effects, drug pharmacology, interactions) and *unpredictable* (or type B; i.e., intolerance, idiosyncrasy, immunologic) (Table 4-1).
3. Drugs, foods, and radiocontrast agents are among the most common causes of anaphylaxis.[3] Other causes include insect stings, natural rubber latex, exercise, and idiopathic reactions.
4. Beta-lactam antibiotics are the most common cause of anaphylaxis in the United States on the basis of retrospective reports.[4,5]
5. Angioedema occurs in about 0.1% to 1% of those treated with angiotensin-converting enzyme inhibitors, most after 2 to 6 months of treatment. The risk of angioedema persists with angiotensin II receptor blockers, but the risk is much lower.[6]
6. The cause of anaphylaxis remains unidentified in as many as two thirds of patients presenting to an allergist or immunologist for evaluation.[5]

TABLE 4-1[3]

CLASSIFICATION OF ADVERSE DRUG REACTIONS

Drug Reaction	Examples
REACTIONS OCCURRING IN MOST NORMAL PATIENTS, GIVEN SUFFICIENT DOSAGE AND DURATION OF THERAPY (TYPE A)	
Overdose	Hepatic failure (acetaminophen)
Side effects	Nausea, headache (with methylxanthines)
Secondary or indirect effects	Gastrointestinal bacterial overgrowth after antibiotics
Drug interactions	Erythromycin increasing theophylline and digoxin serum concentrations
DRUG HYPERSENSITIVITY REACTIONS LIMITED TO A SMALL SUBSET OF THE GENERAL POPULATION (TYPE B)	
Intolerance*	Tinnitus after a single aspirin tablet
Idiosyncrasy[†] (pharmacogenetics)	Glucose-6-phosphodehydrogenase deficiency: anemia after antioxidant drugs
Immunologic drug reactions (allergy)	Anaphylaxis from beta-lactam antibiotics

*Side effects at subtherapeutic dosages.
[†]Drug effect not attributable to known pharmacologic properties of drug and not immune mediated.

7. Drug allergies (immune-mediated drug hypersensitivity reactions) account for up to 230,000 hospital admissions in the United States and cost more than $600 million annually.[7]
8. Many risk factors influence the development of anaphylactic and other drug allergies, including age, atopy, exposure history, route of administration, prolonged or repeated courses of therapy, concomitant diseases, and previous drug allergies.

II. PRESENTATION

1. Patients with anaphylaxis usually develop symptoms within 30 minutes after exposure to an allergen, although symptoms may develop as late as 2 hours if the antigen is ingested. Recrudescence of symptoms up to 8 hours after the initial presentation is known as biphasic anaphylaxis and is caused by a late phase reaction. In addition, anaphylactic shock can persist for several days despite therapy.
2. The clinical manifestations of anaphylaxis are diverse (Fig. 4-1). The most common manifestations are dermatologic (90%), pulmonary (40% to 60%), and gastrointestinal (30%).
3. Hypotension or shock occurs in 30% of patients undergoing anaphylaxis and can occur without any cutaneous or respiratory symptoms.[8]
4. Drug allergy syndromes are manifested by the constellation of signs and symptoms identified with a particular mechanism of immunopathology (Table 4-2).

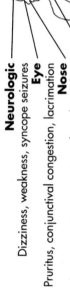

Neurologic
Dizziness, weakness, syncope seizures

Eye
Pruritus, conjunctival congestion, lacrimation

Nose
Pruritus, congestion, sneezing, clear rhinorrhea

Upper airway
Hoarseness, stridor, oropharyngeal or laryngeal edema, cough, complete obstruction

Cardiovascular
Tachycardia, hypotension, arrhythmias, cardiac arrest

Lower airways
Chest tightness, dyspnea, tachypnea, use of accessory muscles, cyanosis, bronchospasm, respiratory arrest

Skin
Sensation of warmth, flushing, erythema, general pruritus, urticaria, angioedema

Gastrointestinal
Nausea, vomiting, cramping, abdominal pain, diarrhea (often bloody)

FIG. 4-1

The manifestations of anaphylaxis. *(From Rakel RE, Bope ET: Conn's current therapy 2004, 56th ed, Philadelphia, 2004, Elsevier.)*

4

ANAPHYLAXIS AND DRUG ALLERGY

TABLE 4-2

GELL AND COOMBS CLASSIFICATION OF ALLERGIC REACTIONS

Reaction Type	Clinical Characteristics	Laboratory Testing	Future Use of Medication
I Immediate hypersensitivity	Urticaria, angioedema, wheezing hypersensitivity nausea, vomiting, abdominal pain, diarrhea	Skin testing, radioallergosorbent testing	Desensitization
II Antibody-dependent cytotoxicity	Hemolytic anemia, granulocytopenia, thrombocytopenia	Complete blood cell count, Coombs test	May be cautiously readministered
III Immune complex disease	Fever, urticaria, arthralgias, lymphadenopathy 2-21 days after therapy initiated	Complement levels, immune complex tests	May be cautiously readministered
IV Cell-mediated hypersensitivity	Skin erythema, skin blistering	Patch testing, delayed intradermal tests	Probably contraindicated
Morbilliform	Maculopapular rash becoming confluent	Possibly patch testing, intradermal skin testing (delayed reaction)	Use with caution
Erythema multiforme	Distinctive target lesions	None	Contraindicated
Stevens-Johnson or TEN	Target lesions, mucous membrane involvement, skin desquamation	None	Contraindicated (absolute)
Anaphylactoid (pseudoallergic)	Urticaria, wheezing, angioedema, hypotension	None	Pretreatment with prednisone and Benadryl for radiocontrast sensitivity
HSS/DRESS	Exfoliative dermatitis, fever, lymphadenopathy	Complete blood cell count, liver enzymes, creatinine, urinalysis	Contraindicated

Modified from Volcheck G: *Immunol Allergy Clin North Am* 24(3):357, 2004.
HSS/DRESS, hypersensitivity syndrome and drug rash with eosinophilia and systemic symptoms; *TEN,* toxic epidermal necrolysis.

III. DIAGNOSIS

1. Anaphylaxis is indicated by the presence of appropriate signs and symptoms after exposure to a suspected allergen. Exclusion of similar diagnoses should be considered (Table 4-3).
2. Laboratory diagnosis generally is of limited value. Serum tryptase, a mast cell protease, remains elevated for 2 to 6 hours after an anaphylactic reaction.
3. Skin tests, in vitro serum tests for IgE antibodies (radioallergosorbent testing), and alternatively graded rechallenge with the suspected agent may be useful in determining the diagnosis when insect stings, foods, and certain drugs are involved.
4. Skin testing for drug-mediated hypersensitivity has been validated only for beta-lactam antibiotics. A negative skin test does not rule out allergy to nonpenicillin medications.
5. The negative predictive value of penicillin skin testing is 97%, although testing has no predictive value for non–IgE-mediated reactions such as Stevens-Johnson syndrome, drug fever, hemolytic anemia, and maculopapular rashes.
6. The diagnosis of a drug allergy is made on the basis of a detailed history and physical examination. A list of all medications, including over-the-counter and herbal medications, with starting dates, dosage changes, temporal relationship between the drug reaction and administration of the drug, prior drug reactions, and associated comorbidities should be sought.

TABLE 4-3

DIFFERENTIAL DIAGNOSIS FOR ANAPHYLAXIS

Presentation	Differential Diagnosis
Hypotension	Septic shock
	Vasovagal reaction
	Cardiogenic shock
	Hypovolemic shock
Respiratory distress with wheezing or stridor	Airway foreign body
	Asthma and chronic obstructive pulmonary disease exacerbation
	Vocal cord dysfunction syndrome
Postprandial collapse	Airway foreign body
	Scombroid fish poisoning
Flush syndrome	Carcinoid
	Postmenopausal hot flushes
	Red man syndrome (vancomycin)
Miscellaneous	Panic attacks (upper airway closure; globus hystericus)
	Systemic mastocytosis
	Hereditary angioedema

Modified from Tang AW: *Am Fam Physician* 68:1325-1332, 1339-1340, 2003.

IV. MANAGEMENT

1. Initial management of anaphylaxis is outlined in Box 4-1.
2. For those with prior non–life threatening reactions to radiocontrast media, a regimen of diphenhydramine 50 mg 1 hour before and prednisone 50 mg 13 hours, 7 hours, and 1 hour before the procedure can substantially reduce allergic reactions.
3. The incidence and severity of anaphylactic reactions can be decreased by the following preventive measures:
   - Have patient wear warning identification tags (www.medicalert.org).
   - Instruct patients to read food labels and learn about cross-reacting medications.
   - Teach self-injection of epinephrine (EpiPen) and advise patients to keep an EpiPen close by at all times.
   - In high-risk patients, discontinue beta-adrenergic blocking agents and possibly angiotensin-converting enzyme inhibitors because they may impair treatment or affect the body's compensatory responses.
   - Use preventive techniques (e.g., gradual dosage escalation and desensitization) when patients encounter foods or drugs believed to entail risk.

PEARLS AND PITFALLS

- Skin tests for penicillin allergy may remain negative up to 6 weeks after a systemic allergic reaction to beta-lactam antibiotics. Skin testing should be repeated if clinically indicated.

BOX 4-1

THERAPY FOR ANAPHYLAXIS

1. Assess airway and vital signs. Intubation may be necessary in severe cases.
2. Administer oxygen.
3. **Immediate epinephrine 1:1000, 0.3-0.5 ml IM (adults), may be repeated after 5-10 min; EpiPen provides 0.3 ml.**
4. The patient should be supine, with legs elevated.
5. In the event of an insect sting, apply a tourniquet proximal to the sting site. Release the tourniquet for 3 min every 5 min (no more than 30 min total).
6. Administer intravenous fluids (rapid infusion of large volumes).
7. Administer H_1 and H_2 antagonists (putatively superior to either agent alone): diphenhydramine 50 mg IV and ranitidine 50 mg IV.
8. Administer corticosteroids (e.g., hydrocortisone 200 mg IV).
9. Administer vasopressors: epinephrine (the preferred agent) or dopamine.
10. Administer aminophylline for persistent airway resistance.
11. Administer glucagon 5-15 µg/min IV for patients on beta-blockers.

IM, intramuscularly; *IV,* intravenously.

- A history of penicillin-induced toxic epidermal necrolysis or Stevens-Johnson syndrome is an absolute contraindication to readministration, including penicillin skin testing.
- Intramuscular administration of epinephrine provides a more efficient absorption profile than subcutaneous injection. The lateral thigh is the preferred site of EpiPen injection to maximize absorption rates.[9]
- Unexplained hypotension in the perioperative period can be a presentation of anaphylaxis. Typically, there is cardiovascular collapse without observable dermatologic manifestations.
- Those allergic to natural rubber latex may also be sensitive to bananas, kiwis, avocados, and other fruits.
- Among those with documented penicillin hypersensitivity, only 4.4% have an allergic reaction to cephalosporin antibiotics. However, those with negative penicillin skin tests are not at elevated risk for IgE-dependent cephalosporin reactions.[10]
- The coexistence of urticaria and angioedema, which is common with allergic reactions, virtually eliminates the consideration of C1 inhibitor deficiency (hereditary angioedema), which *never* produces urticaria.

REFERENCES

1. Salkind AR, Cuddy PG, Foxworth JW: Is this patient allergic to penicillin? An evidence-based analysis of the likelihood of penicillin allergy, *JAMA* 285:2498-2505, 2001. C
2. Roujeau JC, Stern RS: Severe cutaneous reactions to drugs, *N Engl J Med* 331:1272-1285, 1994. C
3. Adkinson NF Jr: Drug allergy. In Adkinson NF, Yunginger JW, Busse WW, Bochner BS, Holgate ST, Simons FER, eds: *Middleton's allergy: principles and practice,* 6th ed, St. Louis, 2003, Mosby. C
4. Kemp SF, Lockey RF, Wolf BL, et al: Anaphylaxis: a review of 266 cases, *Arch Intern Med* 155:1749, 1995. B
5. Neugut AI, Ghatak AT, Miller RL: Anaphylaxis in the United States: an investigation into its epidemiology, *Arch Intern Med* 161(1):15-21, 2001. C
6. Cicardi M et al: Angioedema associated with angiotensin-converting enzyme inhibitor use: outcome after switching to a different treatment, *Arch Intern Med* 164:910-913, 2004. B
7. Coghlan-Johnston M, Lieberman P: Demographic and clinical characteristics of anaphylaxis, *J Allergy Clin Immunol* 107:557, 2001. C
8. Lieberman P: Unique clinical presentations of anaphylaxis, *Immunol Allergy Clin North Am* 21:813, 2001. C
9. Simons FE, Gu X, Simons KJ: Epinephrine absorption in adults: intramuscular versus subcutaneous injection, *J Allergy Clin Immunol* 108:871-873, 2001. A
10. Kelkar PS, Li JT-C: Cephalosporin allergy, *N Engl J Med* 345:804-809, 2001. C

4

ANAPHYLAXIS AND DRUG ALLERGY

Inpatient Radiology

Clifford R. Weiss, MD; Janet Sailor, MD; Andrew Holz, MD;
Daniel J. Mollura, MD; Nadine Jackson, MD, MPH; Ari M. Blitz, MD;
Paul Campbell, MD; Kevin Smith, MD; and
Katarzyna J. Macura, MD, PhD

FAST FACTS

- Radiographs done on stationary equipment in the radiology department generally are of higher quality than portable radiographs.
- Because radiographs are two-dimensional representations of three-dimensional structures, two orthogonal views should be obtained if possible.
- If one area of pathology is found on an image, continue thoroughly examining the whole film because there may be two or more important findings.
- For patients with prior non–life-threatening reactions to contrast media, a regimen of diphenhydramine 50 mg 1 hour before and prednisone 40 mg 24 hours, 12 hours, and 1 hour before the procedure can substantially reduce allergic reactions. (There are many variations of this regimen.)
- The risk of contrast-induced nephropathy can be significantly reduced by hydration with sodium bicarbonate and the administration of acetylcysteine.

Radiology is a powerful diagnostic and therapeutic tool. There are many diagnostic procedures for various conditions that may differ in sensitivity and specificity depending on the patient's underlying disease process. It is important to realize that many imaging findings are nonspecific and can be interpreted differently depending on the clinical setting. Clinical information should be provided to the radiologist because it may allow more focused radiologic evaluation and interpretation.

I. RADIOGRAPHS (PLAIN FILMS AND FLUOROSCOPY)

1. Plain film images use x-rays (ionizing radiation) to generate a shadowgram. Radiation absorption depends on tissue density: Denser tissues, such as bone, absorb more radiation and appear white; less dense tissues such as lung absorb less radiation and appear dark.
2. Chest radiography.
a. **Look thoroughly and systematically.** Examine all the structures, including intravenous catheters, tubes (endotracheal and nasogastric), lungs (together to judge symmetry and separately to screen for pathology), mediastinum, abdomen, and bones.
b. **Basic chest anatomy** (Fig. 5-1).

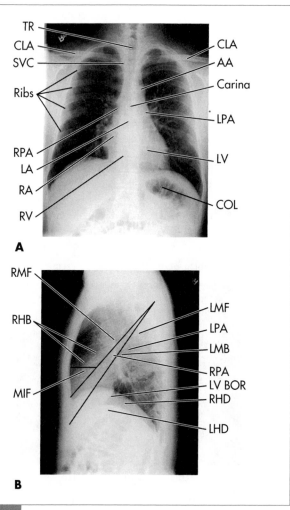

FIG. 5-1

Labeled posteroanterior and lateral chest radiographs with three-dimensional (3D) computed tomography (CT) correlation. **A,** Posteroanterior chest radiograph. *AA,* aortic arch; *CLA,* clavicle; *COL,* colon; *LA,* left atrium; *LPA,* left pulmonary artery; *LV,* left ventricle; *RA,* right atrium; *RPA,* right pulmonary artery; *RV,* right ventricle; *SVC,* superior vena cava; *TR,* trachea. **B,** Lateral chest radiograph. *LHD,* left hemidiaphragm; *LMB,* left mainstem bronchus; *LMF,* expected location of left major fissure; *LPA,* left pulmonary artery; *LV BOR,* left ventricular border; *MIF,* expected location of minor fissure; *RHB,* right heart border; *RHD,* right hemidiaphragm; *RMF,* expected location of right major fissure; *RPA,* right pulmonary artery.

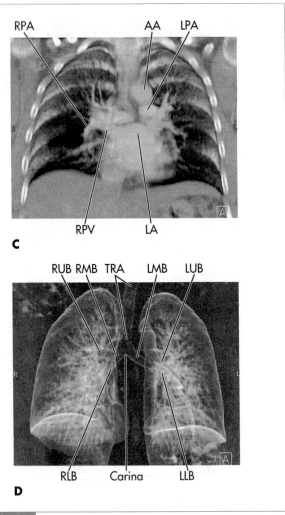

FIG. 5-1—cont'd
C, 3D volume-rendered CT scan of the chest (reconstructed for visualization of the vasculature). *AA,* aortic arch; *LA,* left atrium; *LPA,* left pulmonary artery; *RPA,* right pulmonary artery; *RPV,* right pulmonary vein. **D,** 3D volume-rendered CT scan of the chest (reconstructed for visualization of the lungs and bronchi). *LLB,* left lower lobe bronchus; *LMB,* left mainstem bronchus; *LUB,* left upper lobe bronchus; *RLB,* right lower lobe bronchus; *RMB,* right mainstem bronchus; *RUB,* right upper lobe bronchus; *TRA,* trachea.

- The right heart border is formed by the right atrium and is obscured (silhouetted) by right middle lobe processes unless only the lateral segment is involved.
- The left heart border is formed mainly by the left ventricle and is obscured by lingular processes (Fig. 5-1, *A*).
- The right middle lobe and lingular processes are projected over the heart on the lateral view.
- The right diaphragm is higher than left more than 95% of the time. On the lateral view, the left hemidiaphragm is anteriorly silhouetted by the inferior border of the heart (Fig. 5-1, *B*). In addition, it is possible to compare the distance of the gastric air bubble from the top of the left diaphragm, about 1 cm, to distinguish left and right hemidiaphragm on the lateral view.
- The right diaphragm is obscured by right lower lobe basal segment processes. The left diaphragm is obscured by left lower lobe basal segment processes.
- The major fissures are seen on the lateral view and have an oblique course (Fig. 5-1, *B*). The minor fissure is seen on the anterior view and has a horizontal course in the right lung.
- Hilar opacities are created predominantly by the pulmonary arteries and should be symmetric in size and density. The left hilum is higher than right more than 95% of the time (Fig. 5-1, *C*).
- The trachea is midline with slight rightward deviation from the aorta. There is a natural narrowing of the tracheal lumen in the laryngeal region (Fig. 5-1, *D*).
- The aortic knob is to the left of the trachea (unless a congenital right-sided arch is present), above the left hilum.
- The costophrenic angles should be very sharp on both frontal and lateral views.
- The heart size normally is less than or equal to 50% of the widest diameter of the thoracic cage.
- A healthy young person can take a breath deep enough to inflate the lungs to the level of the tenth rib posteriorly or the sixth rib anteriorly.
- Right and left lung opacification should be symmetric unless the patient is rotated (check position of the medial clavicles to judge rotation) or soft tissues are asymmetric (e.g., after mastectomy).
- Thoracic vertebral bodies appear more lucent (darker) inferiorly toward the diaphragm on the lateral view.

c. **Pleural effusion.** There is normally less than 10 ml of fluid in the pleural space. Depending on size, a pleural effusion may present as blunting of the posterior or lateral costophrenic angle, hemidiaphragm elevation, meniscus tracking up the lateral or posterior chest wall, opacity in an interlobar fissure, thickening of the pleural space, or total opacification of one hemithorax if very large. Anteroposterior portable films generally are not useful for detecting effusions. A lateral decubitus radiograph with the affected side down can demonstrate whether pleural fluid is free flowing. If the layering fluid is 1 cm thick, the effusion is amenable to thoracentesis. A posteroanterior (PA) film can detect 150 to 200 ml of pleural fluid, but a decubitus film can detect as little as 10 ml of pleural fluid. If an effusion is loculated, it can be confirmed on ultrasound, computed tomography (CT), or even magnetic resonance imaging (MRI).

d. **Pneumothorax.** A pneumothorax is seen as a thin white line with no lung markings peripheral to it. Subcutaneous air may be present. If it is a tension pneumothorax, the lung may be severely collapsed, with a mediastinal shift to the opposite side.

e. **Widened mediastinum.** In a patient with chest pain or history of trauma, a widened mediastinum (8 cm at the level of the aortic knob) may represent aortic aneurysm, dissection, or transection and warrants further evaluation. Widening of the superior mediastinum has a sensitivity of 64%, and an abnormal aortic contour has a sensitivity of 61% for the diagnosis of aortic dissection.[1]

f. **Congestive heart failure.**
   (1) **Minimal.** Cardiomegaly usually is present. There is cephalization, defined as redistribution of pulmonary blood flow to upper lungs, with upper lobe vessels equal to or larger than lower lobe vessels on an upright film. Congested pulmonary vessels often appear larger than their adjacent bronchi, another sign of vascular prominence.
   (2) **Moderate.** Interstitial edema causes peribronchial cuffing, indistinctness of blood vessel margins, pleural effusions (more often on the right), and Kerley B lines (fluid-thickened interlobular septa causing horizontal lines up to 1 cm long perpendicular to pleural surface, often seen in lateral costophrenic angles).
   (3) **Severe.** Alveolar edema leads to areas of increasing opacity (vessels no longer visible) in a basilar, perihilar, or diffuse distribution as blood-filled vessels are surrounded by fluid-filled alveoli rather than air-filled alveoli.

g. **Pneumonia** can have many different appearances but commonly presents as a focal area of increased opacity (whiteness) in a lobar, segmental, or subsegmental distribution. Other patterns of pneumonia include diffuse airspace or diffuse interstitial opacities.
   (1) Lines and tiny nodules represent the interstitial pattern of pneumonia.
   (2) Irregular ("fluffy") opacities and air bronchograms (black air-filled airways outlined by fluid-filled alveoli) represent the airspace pattern of pneumonia.
   (3) Spine sign. Inferior vertebral bodies should be darker than those in the upper thoracic spine on the lateral view; if they appear whiter, this may represent a superimposed alveolar opacity such as pneumonia.
   (4) **Aspiration pneumonia is distributed in the *dependent* portions of the lung.**

   (a) In an upright patient, aspirated material goes to medial basal segments and right middle lobe.

   (b) In a supine patient, aspirated material goes to superior segments of lower lobes and posterior segments of upper lobes.

   (c) Because of the anatomy of bronchus intermedius, it is common to have right middle lobe or right lower lobe opacity with left-sided sparing.

3. Abdominal radiography.

a. An upright PA chest and upright abdomen should be obtained after at least 5 minutes of upright positioning; the third view is the supine abdomen (Fig. 5-2).

b. **Look thoroughly and systematically.** Examine all the structures.

c. **Extraluminal gas** may represent pneumoperitoneum (sliver of air under diaphragm on upright radiograph or air adjacent to the liver on left lateral decubitus view, visualization of both sides of the bowel wall, or abnormally visible falciform ligament on supine or upright view), pneumatosis (gas in bowel wall, especially nondependent), portal venous gas (gas in the liver, usually distal or peripheral), pneumobilia (gas outlining the biliary tree and usually close to the porta hepatis), urinary tract gas (gas in the region of kidneys), retroperitoneal gas along the psoas muscles, abscess, or necrotic tumor.

d. **Dilated gas-filled bowel loops** are defined as those more than 3 cm in diameter for the small bowel and more than 6 cm in diameter for the large bowel. **The sensitivity of plain film for identifying small bowel obstruction is 46% to 80%.**

  (1) If the dilated loops are in the small bowel only, it is probably a small bowel obstruction.

  (2) If the dilated loops are in the large bowel only, it may be a large bowel obstruction or a cecal or sigmoid volvulus when the film shows a large bean-shaped loop of large bowel arising from the pelvis.

  (3) If the dilated loops are seen in the small and large bowel, it may be an adynamic ileus, a large bowel obstruction with an incompetent ileocecal valve, gastroenteritis, or excessive aerophagia.

e. **Calcified structures.** Renal calculi may appear as calcifications, but not all calculi are radiopaque. Bladder calculi often take on a lamellated appearance. Other calcified structures include arteriosclerotic calcifications; gallstones; fecaliths; splenic calcifications; pancreatic calcifications; nephrocalcinosis; and, in the pelvis, fibroids, phleboliths, and prostate calcifications.

f. **Small bowel series.** The patient swallows a contrast agent, such as barium. Multiple abdominal radiographs are taken after a contrast agent has reached the small bowel. Enteroclysis is similar examination, except that a tube is passed directly into the small intestine and a contrast agent mixed with methylcellulose is introduced for a see-through effect.

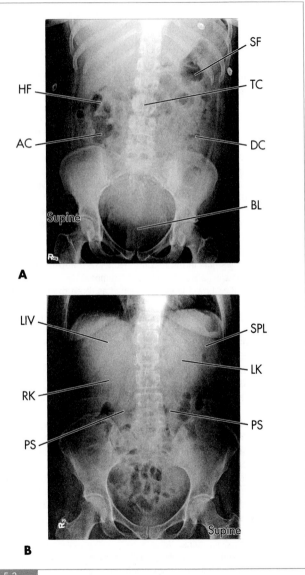

FIG. 5-2

Labeled abdominal radiographs. **A,** Supine abdominal radiograph. *AC,* ascending colon; *BL,* bladder; *DC,* descending colon; *HF,* hepatic flexure; *SF,* splenic flexure; *TC,* transverse colon. **B,** Supine abdominal radiograph. *LIV,* liver; *LK,* left kidney; *PS,* psoas muscle; *RK,* right kidney; *SPL,* spleen.

g. **Skeletal survey.** Radiographic evaluation of metastatic bone disease may include a lateral skull, lateral cervical spine, anteroposterior and lateral thoracic spine, anteroposterior bilateral shoulders, lateral lumbar spine, frontal pelvis, and bilateral hips films.

4. **Fluoroscopy** is a real-time, moving radiograph in which the patient is exposed to a continuous beam of x-ray radiation to generate a moving image, which is viewed on a TV monitor. Fluoroscopy can also be used to evaluate the motion of joints and mechanical heart valves and to guide biopsies and interventional procedures.

a. **Upper GI series** can be used to rule out esophageal perforation and motility disorders. Be aware that barium is dangerous to release into the mediastinum or peritoneum, and some water-soluble contrast agents can cause flash pulmonary edema when aspirated, so ensure that the proper contrast agent is used.

b. **Cine-esophagram** can assess pharyngeal motility in those who have had a stroke or have been extubated recently. It entails the use of barium of various thicknesses and a specialized cine-fluoroscopy unit.

II. COMPUTED TOMOGRAPHY (CT, CAT SCAN)

1. CT images are generated with rotational x-ray imaging. The scans from each 360-degree rotation are processed to produce cross-sectional images that can be processed to provide two- and three-dimensional reconstructions of body organs in different projections. This modality uses ionizing radiation (which is contraindicated in early pregnancy), which increases in dosage with patient weight.

2. Contrast.

a. **Oral.** Oral contrast agents include barium sulfate, iodinated contrast, and water. Oral contrast is safe, and unless there is increased mucosal permeability or leakiness, the contrast should pass through the bowel without being absorbed.

b. **Intravenous.** All intravenous contrast media are iodine based. Any contrast agent administered intravenously can cause an adverse reaction, from mild to severe. When patient has a history of a severe anaphylactoid reaction to intravenous contrast, iodine-based contrast is absolutely contraindicated. **For those with prior non–life threatening reactions to contrast media, a regimen of diphenhydramine 50 mg 1 hour before and prednisone 40 mg 24 hours, 12 hours, and 1 hour before the procedure can substantially reduce allergic reactions** (for similar regimens, see Chapter 4).

c. **Contrast-mediated nephrotoxicity.**

(1) Risk factors include congestive heart failure, diabetes, preexisting renal insufficiency, age older than 70, concurrent nephrotoxic medications, high-dose hyperosmolar intravenous contrast, diuretic medications, and dehydration.

(2) Intravenous 0.9% saline 1 ml/kg/hr 4 to 6 hours before contrast administration and 12 to 24 hours after exposure significantly

reduces the risk of contrast nephrotoxicity in patients with mild renal insufficiency.[2]

(3) **Recently, it has been shown that sodium bicarbonate is more effective than sodium chloride in preventing contrast-induced nephropathy. Sodium bicarbonate (154 mEq/L) should be infused at a rate of 3 ml/kg/hr for 1 hour before contrast exposure and 1 ml/kg/hr for 6 hours after contrast exposure.**[3]

(4) **Acetylcysteine, 600 mg orally twice daily for 24 hours before contrast administration and continued for 24 hours after contrast, along with hydration, is superior to hydration alone in preventing nephrotoxicity.**[4]

(5) When possible, it is beneficial to discontinue nephrotoxic medications and diuretics for at least 24 hours after contrast administration.

(6) Low-osmolarity contrast media are less nephrotoxic than high-osmolarity contrasts in patients with renal insufficiency.

(7) Alternative imaging modalities such as MRI, ultrasound, and nuclear scintigraphy should be considered in patients at high risk of developing contrast nephropathy.

III. ULTRASOUND (SONOGRAPHY)

Ultrasound uses the reflections (echoes) of high-frequency sound waves to construct an image of a body organ. It is an extremely powerful tool that can be tailored to many diagnostic and interventional uses. It does not use ionizing radiation to produce images, so it is safe even in early pregnancy, and it is completely portable. There are essentially no contraindications to ultrasound, although its usefulness may be limited in very obese people. The following are important considerations in ordering an ultrasound study.

1. **Right upper quadrant and abdominal ultrasounds** require that the patient have nothing by mouth (*nil per os,* NPO) 4 to 8 hours before the examination in order to allow the gallbladder to expand and to minimize abdominal gas.

2. **Pelvic ultrasounds** in female patients entail transabdominal and transvaginal scanning. For a transabdominal scan, a full bladder (filled by oral intake or via a Foley catheter) is required.

3. A quantitative serum beta human chorionic gonadotropin should be obtained to evaluate for ectopic pregnancy before pelvic ultrasounds.

IV. MAGNETIC RESONANCE IMAGING (MRI)

1. MRI uses magnetic fields and radiofrequency energy. MRI provides high contrast between different types of soft tissues. Because this modality uses a strong magnetic field, the presence of ferromagnetic foreign bodies and devices contraindicates MRI.

2. **Contraindications** vary from institution to institution. A representative list is shown in Table 5-1.

TABLE 5-1	
CONTRAINDICATIONS TO MAGNETIC RESONANCE IMAGING	
Absolute	Relative
Aneurysm clips placed in the last 6 mo	Claustrophobia
Surgical clips placed in the last 6 wk	Pregnancy
Neurostimulator device	Critical illness
Pacemaker or implantable defibrillator	Dependence on infusion pumps
Cochlear implant	
Metallic ocular foreign body (suspect this in patients with a welding history), metallic shrapnel	
Other metallic implanted devices such as insulin pumps	
Obesity (maximum table allowance usually is 350 lbs)	

3. **MRI contrast agents** are based on the inert metal gadolinium and are well tolerated without severe allergic reaction or nephrotoxic effects at diagnostic dosages. Gadolinium-based contrast agents can artifactually lower the serum calcium level by interfering with the laboratory assay.

V. NUCLEAR MEDICINE STUDIES

Nuclear medicine studies use small amounts of radioactive materials (radiopharmaceuticals), which are taken up by specific organs or tissues. Radiopharmaceuticals emit gamma rays, which are detected externally by gamma or positron emission tomography cameras. The following are important considerations in ordering a nuclear imaging study.

1. **Hepatobiliary** (HIDA) studies require the patient to be NPO for at least 4 hours and free from opioid medications 6 hours before the procedure.
2. **Positron emission tomography** requires the patient to be NPO for at least 4 hours before the procedure.
3. **Gastric emptying** studies require the patient to be NPO for at least 6 hours before the procedure.
4. **Meckel's diverticulum** studies require the patient to be NPO for at least 4 hours before the procedure.
5. **Thyroid imaging** studies require the patient to discontinue thyroxine (T_4) for 3 to 4 weeks and triiodothyronine (T_3) for 10 days before the procedure.
6. **Adrenal imaging with metaiodobenzylguanidine** cannot be completed while patients are taking beta-blockers, reserpine, tricyclic antidepressants, sympathomimetics, and many other agents.

PEARLS AND PITFALLS

- Always double-check the name and date on the film.
- Radiographs are excellent screening tools, are often diagnostic, and usually should be obtained before more expensive and time-consuming imaging modalities are used.

- When possible, always compare images with prior studies to assess for changes.
- The differential diagnosis of miliary infiltrates on chest radiography includes tuberculosis, histoplasmosis, varicella pneumonia, silicosis, sarcoidosis, eosinophilic granuloma, and pneumoconiosis.
- The differential diagnosis of cavitary lung lesions includes septic emboli, tuberculosis, bacterial pneumonia (especially *Staphylococcus aureus, Pseudomonas aeruginosa,* and *Nocardia*), and infected emphysematous bullae.
- On chest radiography, an enlarged right paratracheal stripe (> 4 mm) suggests mediastinal lymphadenopathy.
- **Unenhanced head CT often is normal or only subtly abnormal within the first 6 hours after ischemic infarction and therefore often is not useful during the therapeutic window to confirm or refute the clinical suspicion of acute infarction.** Nevertheless, a noncontrast head CT is ordered on many, if not all, patients with suspected ischemic stroke because it plays an important role in ruling out cerebral hemorrhage.
- MRI with gadolinium enhancement is the most sensitive imaging modality for detecting soft tissue characteristics of osteomyelitis and findings suggestive of early osteomyelitis, such as intraosseous marrow edema. Sensitivity ranges between 76% and 100% (average 91%). Specificity ranges between 65% and 96% (average 82%).[5]
- Plain film radiography should be obtained as the initial study in every patient with suspected avascular necrosis. Plain film radiography is most sensitive and specific for later stages of osteonecrosis, with findings that include bone sclerosis, bone cysts, subchondral fractures, and cortical deformity or loss of bone contour.[6]

REFERENCES

1. Klompas M: Does this patient have an acute thoracic aortic dissection? *JAMA* 287(17):2262-2272, 2002. C
2. Morcos SK, Thomsen HS, Webb JA, et al: Contrast-media induced nephrotoxicity: a consensus report, *Eur Radiol* 9:1602-1613, 1999. D
3. Merten GJ, Burgess WP, Gray LV, et al: Prevention of contrast-induced nephropathy with sodium bicarbonate: a randomized controlled trial, *JAMA* 291:2328-2334, 2004. A
4. Birck R et al: Acetylcysteine for prevention of contrast nephropathy: meta analysis, *Lancet* 303:598-603, 2003. C
5. Gilbert M: How to synthesize evidence for imaging guidelines, *Clin Radiol* 59(1):63-68, 2004. C
6. Assouline-Dayan Y, Chang C, Greenspan A, Shoenfeld Y, Gershwin E: Pathogenesis and natural history of osteonecrosis, *Semin Arthritis Rheum* 32(2):94-124, 2002. C

PART II

Diagnostic and Therapeutic Information

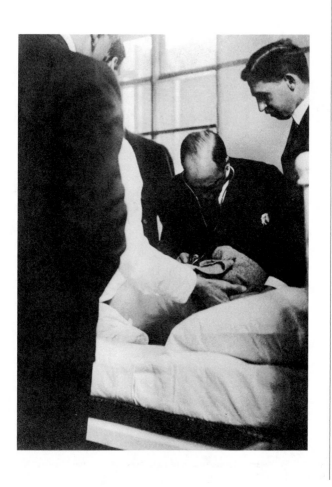

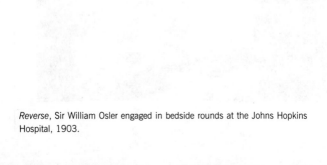

Reverse, Sir William Osler engaged in bedside rounds at the Johns Hopkins Hospital, 1903.

Electrocardiogram Analysis

Daniel Y. Wang, MD; Lauren Averett, MD; David Kuperman, MD;
and Gary Gerstenblith, MD

FAST FACTS

- Analysis of the electrocardiogram (ECG) should follow a systematic approach. This includes examination of the rate, rhythm, intervals, axis, and waveforms (P, Q, R, S, T, and U waves, QRS complexes, ST segments, R wave progression, and voltage).
- The sensitivity of the ECG for detecting chamber enlargement and hypertrophy is poor, but it is highly specific.
- When acute coronary syndrome is suspected, comparison with prior ECGs and examination of serial ECGs to detect dynamic changes are of great value.

6

The ECG is one of the most frequently ordered diagnostic tests in clinical medicine. It plays a crucial role in the diagnosis of arrhythmias, conduction defects, chamber enlargement and hypertrophy, ischemia and infarction, and numerous other clinical entities. As with all tests, its diagnostic accuracy is variable, depending on the disease and the population studied. ECGs must be reviewed in a systematic manner so that no findings are overlooked.

I. RATE

1. When the rhythm is regular, an easy way to calculate the rate is to divide into 300 the number of large, 5-mm boxes between consecutive R or P waves. For example, 1 large box corresponds to a rate of 300, 2 to 150, 3 to 100, 4 to 75, 5 to 60, etc. (This method assumes the standard paper speed of 25 mm/s.)
2. For irregular rhythms or very slow rates, the average rate can be estimated by counting the number of cycles in 6 seconds and multiplying by 10. The atrial and ventricular rates should be calculated separately when the number of P waves and QRS complexes differs, as in advanced atrioventricular (AV) block and other types of AV dissociation.

II. RHYTHM

1. The diagnosis of normal sinus rhythm requires a regular rate with a P wave preceding every QRS complex; a rate between 60 and 100; and an upright P wave in leads I, II, and aVF.
2. A common diagnostic dilemma is determining whether a wide complex tachycardia represents ventricular tachycardia (VT) or aberrant conduction of a supraventricular tachycardia. The presence of AV

dissociation, extreme axis deviation, or capture and fusion beats suggests a diagnosis of VT. In a patient with known coronary artery disease and no preexisting conduction delay, the finding of a wide complex tachycardia is 95% specific for the diagnosis of VT.

3. See Chapters 14 and 15 for more on the diagnosis of arrhythmias.

III. INTERVALS

1. The normal PR interval in adults is 0.12 to 0.2 seconds. Normal QRS duration ranges from 0.7 to 0.12 seconds.
2. The QT interval is inversely correlated to heart rate; the corrected QT or QTc (QT interval divided by the square root of the RR interval) adjusts for variations in rate. **Prolonged QTc is defined as more than 0.44 seconds in men and more than 0.46 seconds in women.**
3. Differential diagnoses of various interval abnormalities are presented in Table 6-1.

IV. AXIS

1. **The mean QRS electrical axis reflects the net direction of depolarization in the frontal plane.** It can be calculated by examining the predominant direction of the QRS complex in each limb lead: The QRS axis is oriented perpendicularly to leads in which the QRS is biphasic, toward leads in which the QRS is positive, and away from leads in which the QRS is negative.
2. A simple initial method to assess the QRS axis is to examine leads I and aVF. If the QRS complexes in leads I and aVF are predominantly positive, the axis is normal. In left axis deviation (−30 to −90 degrees) I is positive and aVF is negative, and in right axis deviation (100 to 180 degrees) I is negative and aVF is positive. Negative QRS complexes in both I and aVF correspond to an extreme axis.
3. Differential diagnoses of left and right axis deviation are presented in Table 6-1.
4. Mean P wave and T wave axes are calculated similarly to the QRS axis. In sinus rhythm the P wave axis is about 60 degrees (i.e., the P wave is positive in leads I, II, and aVF and negative in aVR). Ectopic atrial foci and retrograde P waves are typical causes of an abnormal P wave axis.

V. CHAMBER ENLARGEMENT AND HYPERTROPHY

1. **Atrial abnormalities.** Electrocardiographic criteria for atrial enlargement are highly specific but of variable sensitivity (Table 6-2). Biatrial enlargement is present when criteria for both left and right atrial enlargement are met.
2. **Left ventricular hypertrophy.** Numerous electrocardiographic criteria for left ventricular hypertrophy (LVH) exist (Table 6-3). Most are fairly

TABLE 6-1

DIFFERENTIAL DIAGNOSIS OF SELECTED ELECTROCARDIOGRAPHIC ABNORMALITIES

Abnormality	Differential Diagnosis
Q waves	Normal Q waves, MI, myocarditis, hyperkalemia, LBBB, LVH, RVH, hypertrophic cardiomyopathy, dilated cardiomyopathy, WPW pattern, infiltrative diseases of the myocardium (e.g., amyloidosis, sarcoidosis, tumors), chronic lung disease, left-sided pneumothorax, dextrocardia
Delayed precordial R wave progression[a]	Anterior or anteroseptal MI, LBBB, dilated cardiomyopathy, WPW pattern, LVH, right ventricular strain, chronic lung disease, left axis deviation
ST segment elevation	Normal or normal variant (early repolarization), transmural ischemia, ST elevation ACS, coronary vasospasm (Prinzmetal's angina), ventricular aneurysm, LBBB, LVH, acute pericarditis, acute myocarditis, hyperkalemia, Brugada's syndrome, arrhythmogenic right ventricular dysplasia, acute central nervous system injury, hypothermia (Osborn wave), pulmonary embolism, transthoracic cardioversion, tumor invasion of the left ventricle
ST segment depression	Normal variant (usually <1 mm), nontransmural ischemia, reciprocal ST depression in ST elevation ACS, left ventricular strain (e.g., in LVH), right ventricular strain (e.g., in pulmonary embolism or RVH), bundle branch block, cardiomyopathy, WPW pattern, digitalis effect, other drug effects, hypokalemia, hyperventilation
T wave inversion	Normal variant, myocardial ischemia, Wellens T waves, left ventricular strain, right ventricular strain, bundle branch block, WPW pattern, cerebrovascular accident, intracranial bleed, ventricular pacing, posttachycardia T wave inversion, stress cardiomyopathy
Peaked T waves[b]	Normal variant, hyperacute phase of transmural myocardial ischemia, hyperkalemia, LVH, LBBB, intracranial bleed
U waves	Hypokalemia, hypothermia, LVH, bradyarrhythmias, drug effects

ACS, acute coronary syndrome; *ASD,* atrial septal defect; *COPD,* chronic obstructive pulmonary disease; *LBBB,* left bundle branch block; *LVH,* left ventricular hypertrophy; *MI,* myocardial infarction; *RVH,* right ventricular hypertrophy; *WPW,* Wolff-Parkinson-White.
[a]Delayed R wave progression: failure of R/S to become >1 in progressive precordial leads by V_4.
[b]Peaked T wave: T wave >6 mV in limb leads or >10 mV in precordial leads.

cont'd

ELECTROCARDIOGRAM ANALYSIS

6

DIFFERENTIAL DIAGNOSIS OF SELECTED ELECTROCARDIOGRAPHIC ABNORMALITIES—cont'd

Abnormality	Differential Diagnosis
Tall R wave in V_1	Right bundle branch block, RVH, posterior MI, WPW pattern, Duchenne's muscular dystrophy, lead misplacement, dextrocardia, hypertrophic cardiomyopathy
Low-voltage QRS[c]	Normal variant, pericardial tamponade, pericardial effusion, pleural effusion, constrictive pericarditis, extensive MI, obesity, COPD, myxedema, dilated cardiomyopathy, cardiac infiltrative diseases (e.g., amyloidosis, sarcoidosis, hemochromatosis), adrenal insufficiency
Wide QRS (>0.12 s)	Ventricular beats, hyperkalemia or drug effect, bundle branch block or nonspecific intraventricular conduction delay, WPW pattern
Short PR interval (<0.12 s)	Normal variant, ventricular preexcitation (e.g., WPW pattern, Lown-Ganong-Levine syndrome), ectopic atrial beats, atrioventricular junctional rhythm with retrograde atrial activation
Long QT interval[d]	**Congenital long QT syndromes:** Romano-Ward syndrome (autosomal dominant), Jervell-Lange-Nielsen syndrome (autosomal recessive, associated with sensorineural deafness), Anderson's syndrome (hypokalemic periodic paralysis with cardiac arrhythmia) **Acquired long QT syndromes:** drugs (see www.torsades.org for a comprehensive list of drugs associated with QT prolongation), hypokalemia, hypocalcemia, hypomagnesemia, hypothermia, hypothyroidism, myocardial ischemia and MI, starvation, intracranial disease, bradyarrhythmias
Right axis deviation[e]	Normal variant, limb lead misplacement, right ventricular hypertrophy, COPD, right ventricular strain, left posterior fascicular block, lateral wall MI, ostium secundum ASD
Left axis deviation[f]	Normal variant, LVH, LBBB, left anterior fascicular block (≥45 degrees), inferior MI, ostium primum ASD

[c]Low-voltage QRS: QRS amplitude <0.5 mV in all limb leads, with or without <1 mV in all precordial leads.
[d]Long QT interval: QTc >0.44 s in men, >0.46 s in women.
[e]Right axis deviation: QRS axis 100 to 180 degrees.
[f]Left axis deviation: QRS axis −30 to −90 degrees.

TABLE 6-2

ELECTROCARDIOGRAPHIC CRITERIA FOR LEFT AND RIGHT
ATRIAL ABNORMALITY

Abnormality	Criteria
Left atrial abnormality	P wave duration ≥0.12 s in lead II (P mitrale)
	Terminal negative component of P wave in lead V_1 ≥1 mm deep and ≥0.04 s in duration
	P wave notching in leads I, II, or III with duration between peaks ≥0.04 s
Right atrial abnormality	Peaked P waves >2.5 mm in lead II (P pulmonale)
	P wave in lead V_2 >1.5 mm
	P wave axis >75 degrees

Modified from Mirvis D, Goldberger AL: Electrocardiography. In Braunwald E, Zipes DP, Libby P, eds: *Heart disease: a textbook of cardiovascular medicine*, 6th ed, Philadelphia, 2001, WB Saunders.

TABLE 6-3

ELECTROCARDIOGRAPHIC CRITERIA FOR LEFT VENTRICULAR HYPERTROPHY

Criterion	Definition	
Cornell voltage	$R_aVL + S_{V3}$ > 28 mm in men	
	$R_aVL + S_{V3}$ > 20 mm in women	
Cornell voltage duration product	Cornell voltage × QRS duration (ms) > 2436	
Sokolow-Lyon voltage	$S_{V1} + R_{V5}$ or R_{V6} > 35 mm	
Romhilt-Estes point score system*	Any limb lead R wave or S wave ≥20 mm or S_{V1} or S_{V2} ≥30 mm or R_{V5} or R_{V6} ≥30 mm	3 points
	Left ventricular strain (ST segment and T wave in opposite direction to QRS complex) without digitalis therapy	3 points
	Left ventricular strain with digitalis therapy	1 point
	Left atrial abnormality (terminal negativity of the P wave in lead V_1 ≥1 mm deep and ≥ 0.04 s in duration)	3 points
	Left axis deviation >−30 degrees	1 point
	QRS duration ≥0.09 s	1 point
	Intrinsicoid deflection in V_5 or V_6 ≥0.05 s	1 point
Other criteria	R_aVL ≥11 mm	
	R_{V5} or R_{V6} >26 mm	
	Maximum R wave + S wave in precordial leads > 45 mm	

*Left ventricular hypertrophy (LVH) is diagnosed if ≥5 points are present, and probable LVH is diagnosed if 4 points are present.

specific (generally >90%), but none is sensitive (all <50%).[1-3] Electrocardiographic evidence of LVH is an important finding because it is a predictor of heart failure and premature cardiovascular death.

3. **Right ventricular hypertrophy.** Various criteria for right ventricular hypertrophy (RVH) are presented in Table 6-4.

TABLE 6-4

ELECTROCARDIOGRAPHIC CRITERIA FOR RIGHT VENTRICULAR HYPERTROPHY

Criterion	Sensitivity (%)	Specificity (%)
R in V_1 ≥7 mm	<10	—
R/S in V_1 >1 (with R >5 mm)	25	89
S in V_5 or V_6 ≥7 mm	17	93
Right axis deviation (≥+90 degrees)	14	99
$S_1 Q_3$ pattern	11	93
P pulmonale	11	97

Modified from Mirvis D, Goldberger AL: Electrocardiography. In Braunwald E, Zipes DP, Libby P, eds: *Heart disease: a textbook of cardiovascular medicine,* 6th ed, Philadelphia, 2001, WB Saunders.

4. **Biventricular hypertrophy** is suggested by the presence of LVH criteria along with right axis deviation, by the presence of RVH criteria along with left atrial abnormality, or by tall R waves in both the right (V_1 to V_2) and left (V_5 to V_6) precordial leads.

VI. WAVEFORMS

A. MYOCARDIAL ISCHEMIA AND INFARCTION

1. The ECG provides critical information regarding the diagnosis, evolution, extent of injury, and prognosis in myocardial infarction (MI) and can assist in the identification of the infarct-related artery (IRA).

2. **Ischemia.** Acute ischemia decreases the myocyte action potential duration and resting membrane potential, thus creating a voltage gradient between ischemic and nonischemic myocardium. The resulting current (known as a current of injury) is reflected on the ECG as ST segment elevation.

a. **Transmural ischemia** (i.e., involving the full thickness of the myocardium) typically causes ST segment elevation (STE) or hyperacute T waves (upright T waves with T wave amplitude greater than R wave amplitude) (Fig. 6-1). Reciprocal ST depressions occur in the leads corresponding to the contralateral surface of the affected region. The degree of STE corresponds roughly with the severity of transmural ischemia.

b. **Nontransmural ischemia causes ST depression in multiple leads. ST depressions are not reliable in localizing ischemia.**

c. **T wave inversions** are common in ischemia; however, they are neither sensitive nor specific for ischemia. An exception is the finding of deep, symmetric, precordial T wave inversions called Wellens T waves (Fig. 6-2).

3. **Infarction** (see Chapter 8).

a. In acute ST segment elevation MI (STEMI), STE is present in two or more contiguous leads (STE at least 1 mm in the limb leads and at least 2 mm in the precordial leads). As the MI evolves, T wave

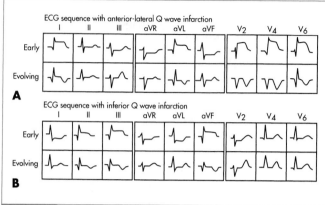

FIG. 6-1

Evolution of electrocardiographic changes in an anterolateral and inferior acute ST elevation myocardial infarction. *(From Braunwald E, Zipes DP, Libby P, eds:* Heart disease: a textbook of cardiovascular medicine, *6th ed, Philadelphia, 2001, WB Saunders.)*

inversions develop within hours to days, along with return of the ST segment toward baseline, with or without the development of Q waves (see Fig. 6-1). Early reperfusion, whether spontaneous, medical, or invasive, may alter the evolution of these changes.

b. Although Q waves classically indicate transmural infarctions, recent magnetic resonance studies indicate that their presence correlates better with increased total size of infarcted myocardium than with transmurality, as compared with non–Q wave MI.[4]

c. The exact definition of pathologic Q waves in MI is debated; however, they should be located in at least two contiguous leads. Isolated Q waves in III are not abnormal and are expected in aVR.

4. **Localization of injury and identification of the IRA.**

a. Table 6-5 summarizes the relationships between the standard electrocardiographic leads, anatomic territory, and epicardial coronary arteries.

b. Figures 6-3 and 6-4 show algorithms for predicting the IRA in **inferior and anterior acute MI.** Although V_1 through V_3 are called the anteroseptal leads, newer data show that Q waves in V_1 through V_3 correspond more reliably to the apex than to the septum.[5,6]

c. **Posterior wall injury.**

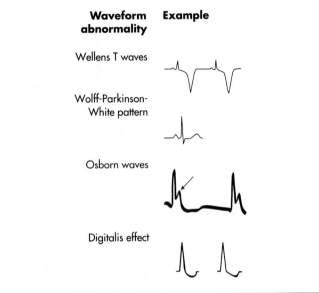

Waveform abnormality	Example
Wellens T waves	
Wolff-Parkinson-White pattern	
Osborn waves	
Digitalis effect	

FIG. 6-2

Miscellaneous waveform abnormalities. *(Osborn waves from Yoder E: Disorders due to heat and cold. In Goldman L, Ausiello D, eds: Cecil textbook of medicine, 22nd ed, Philadelphia, 2004, WB Saunders; Digitalis effect from Goldberger AL: Clinical electrocardiography: a simplified approach, 6th ed, St Louis, 1999, CV Mosby.)*

(1) Leads V_1 through V_3 also reflect reciprocal activity from the posterior left ventricular wall. In transmural inferoposterior ischemia, inferior STE may be accompanied by ST depression in V_1 through V_3.

(2) Prominent R waves in V_1 may represent reciprocal Q waves from the posterior wall and may extend up to V_3.

d. **RV injury.** Lead V_1 and the right-sided precordial leads (V_4R through V_6R) reflect right ventricular activity. All patients with evidence of inferior wall ischemia should undergo a right-sided ECG. STE of at least 1 mm in V_4R is 88% sensitive and 78% specific for concomitant RV infarction in patients with acute inferior MI.[7] The right coronary artery usually is the culprit vessel in these cases.

e. **Lead aVR.**

(1) Acute left main coronary artery occlusion was distinguished from left anterior descending artery (LAD) occlusion with 81% sensitivity

TABLE 6-5

ELECTROCARDIOGRAPHIC CHANGES OF ACUTE MYOCARDIAL INFARCTION*

Electrocardiographic Findings	Region of Cardiac Ischemia	Anatomy of Lesion
ST ↑ V_{1-6}, I, aVL, and fascicular or bundle branch block	Anterior-lateral plus septum	Proximal LAD (proximal to first septal perforator)
ST ↑ V_{1-6}, I, aVL	Anterior-lateral	Proximal LAD (proximal to any large diagonal supplying lateral wall)
ST ↑ V_{5-6}, I, aVL	Lateral	Distal LAD or large diagonal
ST ↑ II, III, aVF, and V_{5-6}	Inferior and possibly lateral	Proximal RCA or left circumflex (whichever is dominant)
ST ↑ II, III, aVF, and R > S in V_1 and V_2	Inferior-posterior	
ST ↑ II, III, aVF only	Inferior	Distal RCA or left circumflex (depending on coronary anatomy)

Modified from Topol EJ, Van de Werf FJ: Acute myocardial infarction: early diagnosis and management. In Topol EJ, ed: *Textbook of cardiovascular medicine*, New York, 1998, Lippincott-Raven.

LAD, left anterior descending artery; *RCA,* right circumflex artery.

*All patients received reperfusion therapy (mortality data from GUSTO I).

and 80% specificity when STE was present in aVR and exceeded the degree of elevation in V_1.[8]

   (2) In patients with their first non–ST segment elevation MI, STE in aVR predicted much higher in-hospital mortality (19.4%, 8.6%, and 1.3% for STE of at least 1 mm, 0.5 to 1 mm, or 0 mm, respectively) and greater likelihood of left main or three-vessel disease (66.4%, 42.6%, and 22%, respectively).[9]

f. **Wellens T waves** (see Fig. 6-2) are deeply inverted, symmetric T waves in V_2 and V_3 with or without involvement of contiguous precordial leads. **The presence of Wellens T waves in patients with unstable angina is highly predictive of high-grade proximal LAD disease and elevated risk of anterior MI.**[10] Similarly appearing T waves have also been described in acute pulmonary embolism (PE), acute intracranial injury, and stress cardiomyopathy. Biphasic T waves in V_2 and V_3 are a variant of Wellens T waves with similar implications.

5. **Ischemia and infarction in the setting of left bundle branch block (LBBB) or ventricular pacing.**

a. LBBB and electronic right ventricular pacing (which typically results in an LBBB pattern) cause STE and other depolarization and repolarization abnormalities, thereby limiting the accuracy of the ECG in the diagnosis of acute MI. The Sgarbossa criteria for diagnosis of evolving acute MI in patients with LBBB are three electrocardiographic criteria with independent value (Table 6-6).[11] Though highly specific (>90%), the

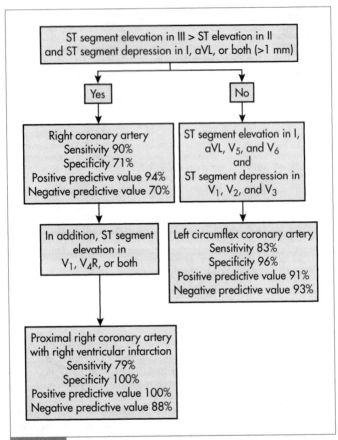

FIG. 6-3

Inferior myocardial infarction: algorithm for electrocardiographic identification of the infarct-related artery. *(From Zimetbaum PJ, Josephson ME:* N Engl J Med *348:933-940, 2003.)*

criteria have low sensitivity; therefore their absence cannot be used to rule out acute MI in the presence of LBBB.

B. WAVEFORM FEATURES OF OTHER CLINICAL DISORDERS

1. **Electrolyte abnormalities** result in alterations in depolarization and repolarization that produce characteristic waveform abnormalities. However, a normal ECG does not rule out a serious electrolyte disorder.

a. **Hyperkalemia** (Fig. 6-5). Acute hyperkalemia produces peaked T waves with a narrow base and may shorten the QT interval. Progressive

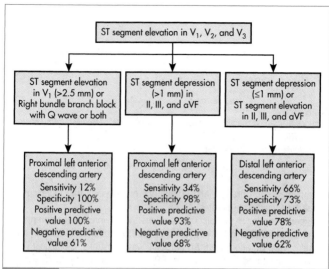

FIG. 6-4

Anterior myocardial infarction: algorithm for electrocardiographic identification of the infarct-related artery. *(From Zimetbaum PJ, Josephson ME: N Engl J Med 348:933-940, 2003.)*

TABLE 6-6

SGARBOSSA CRITERIA FOR DIAGNOSIS OF ACUTE MI IN THE PRESENCE OF LEFT BUNDLE BRANCH BLOCK

Criterion	Odds Ratio (95% CI)	Score*
ST ↑ ≥1 mm and concordant (in the same direction) with QRS complex	25.2 (11.6-54.7)	5
ST ↓ ≥1 mm in lead V_1, V_2, or V_3	6 (1.9-19.3)	3
ST ↑ ≥5 mm and discordant with QRS complex	4.3 (1.8-10.6)	2

Modified from Sgarbossa EB, Pinski SL, Barbagelata A, et al: *N Engl J Med* 334:481-487, 1996.
MI, myocardial infarction.
*A score of ≥3 is required to reach a specificity of ≥90% and sensitivity ≥36%. Therefore the third criterion should not be used alone to diagnose acute MI, and the absence of Sgarbossa criteria cannot be used to rule out an acute MI.

hyperkalemia causes P wave flattening, PR prolongation, and widening of the QRS complex. Severe hyperkalemia can lead to advanced AV block, diffuse intraventricular conduction delay, precordial STE (pseudoinfarction pattern), and asystole.

b. **Hypokalemia.** Common findings include T wave flattening or inversion, increased U wave prominence, ST depression, increased P wave

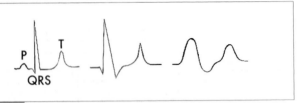

FIG. 6-5

Electrocardiographic changes in progressive hyperkalemia. (*Modified from Lobato E. In Kirby RR, ed.* Critical Care. Atlas of Clinical Anesthesiology series, *ed. Miller R. Philadelphia, 1997,* Current Medicine.)

   amplitude and duration, and QT interval prolongation that increases the
   risk for torsades de pointes.
c. **Hypercalcemia.** Hypercalcemia shortens the QT interval (beginning of
   the QRS complex to the beginning of the T wave) with little effect on
   the T wave duration itself. An abrupt T wave upstroke, biphasic T
   waves, increased QRS amplitude, PR prolongation, and Osborn waves
   have also been described in severe hypercalcemia.
d. **Hypocalcemia** prolongs the QT interval.
2. **Wolff-Parkinson-White syndrome (WPW)** is a preexcitation syndrome
   that is important to identify because patients are at risk for life-
   threatening paroxysmal tachycardia. The ECG in WPW is characterized
   by the classic triad of a short PR interval, widened QRS, and delta
   waves (see Fig. 6-2). See Chapter 15 for further discussion of WPW.
3. **Pericarditis** (See Chapter 13).
a. Diffuse STE is the earliest electrocardiographic manifestation of acute
   pericarditis. ST depression may be seen in aVR and V_1. The STE
   typically is concave, present in both limb and precordial leads, and
   without reciprocal ST depression. These features can help distinguish
   pericarditis from ST elevation acute coronary syndrome.
b. **PR depression (and PR elevation in aVR) is the most sensitive
   electrocardiographic feature for the diagnosis of pericarditis.**
4. **Pulmonary embolism.**
a. Electrocardiographic findings in acute PE are insensitive and
   nonspecific.
b. A prospective study of 28 electrocardiographic abnormalities in 212
   patients who were evaluated for PE found only tachycardia and
   incomplete right bundle branch block (RBBB) to occur significantly
   more often in patients with than without PE.[12] See Chapter 86.
5. **Hypothermia.** Pathologic J waves called Osborn waves, best seen in the
   precordial leads, may occur in severe hypothermia (see Fig. 6-2). Their
   amplitude corresponds with the degree of hypothermia, and they
   disappear with rewarming. QTc prolongation, sinus bradycardia, U

waves, atrial fibrillation, and other arrhythmias may also occur during hypothermia.

6. **Brugada's syndrome** is a familial syndrome of sudden cardiac death with characteristic electrocardiographic abnormalities during sinus rhythm in the right precordial leads, consisting of STE and a pseudo-RBBB pattern in V_1. The electrocardiographic changes may be transient and may be elicited by sodium channel blockade.

7. **Arrhythmogenic right ventricular dysplasia** is a hereditary cardiomyopathy characterized by fibrofatty replacement of the right ventricular myocardium that predisposes to VT and sudden cardiac death. Classic electrocardiographic abnormalities include complete or incomplete RBBB, T wave inversion in V_1 to V_3, epsilon waves (terminal notch in the QRS complex), and QRS prolongation in the right precordial leads.

8. **Digoxin.** The digitalis effect consists of coved ST depression (occurring more commonly in the lateral precordial leads), T wave flattening, and decreased QT interval (see Fig. 6-2). Digoxin toxicity can result in any of a large number of bradyarrhythmias, tachyarrhythmias, and conduction blocks.

C. DIFFERENTIAL DIAGNOSIS OF SELECTED ELECTROCARDIOGRAPHIC ABNORMALITIES

Numerous clinical disorders can result in similarly appearing waveform abnormalities. Taking into account the clinical context and the nuances of the specific waveform abnormality can help distinguish the cause. Table 6-1 lists differential diagnoses of some common electrocardiographic abnormalities.

PEARLS AND PITFALLS

- Always check the patient name, voltage standardization mark, and paper speed on each ECG. Conventional values are 1 mV for every 10-mm deflection for voltage standardization and 25 mm/s for paper speed (i.e., 0.04 seconds for each small, 1-mm box and 0.2 seconds for each large, 5-mm box).
- Suspect limb lead misplacement (or dextrocardia) when the P wave and QRS complex are negative in lead I. Precordial lead misplacement can cause abrupt changes in R wave progression.
- Whereas the electrocardiograph's rate, interval, and axis measurements generally are accurate, the diagnosis offered often is inaccurate or incomplete.
- Ischemia and infarction cause dynamic electrocardiographic changes. Therefore, obtaining serial ECGs is crucial in evaluating the patient with suspected acute coronary syndrome.
- The most common cause of left axis deviation is left anterior fascicular block.
- The specificity of LVH criteria that use voltage measurements in limb leads I or aVL is lower in younger patients or in the presence of LAD, as in left anterior fascicular block. In patients <40 years old, the diagnosis

of LVH should be made by both voltage and nonvoltage abnormalities, such as left ventricular strain pattern (ST depression with asymmetric T wave inversions V_4 to V_6), LAD, left atrial abnormality, delayed R wave progression, U waves, intraventricular conduction delay, and delayed onset of intrinsicoid (beginning of QRS to peak of R wave more than 0.05 seconds).

- Q waves, STE, and hyperacute T waves localize to specific myocardial regions, whereas ST depressions and T wave inversions are less reliable for localizing ischemia.
- Always obtain an ECG with right-sided leads when evidence of inferior ischemia is present.
- ST depression in V_1 to V_3 in the patient with chest discomfort may represent nontransmural ischemia, but it may also reflect posterior transmural ischemia.
- STE that does not resolve within 4 weeks after an STEMI suggests the development of ventricular aneurysm.
- Electrocardiographic findings in acute PE are insensitive and nonspecific.
- Atrial fibrillation with a wide QRS and a very rapid ventricular response (>200 beats per minute) should raise concern for the presence of an accessory pathway, as in WPW syndrome.
- Consider digitalis toxicity in the patient with a history of atrial fibrillation who develops a regular, junctional tachycardia.
- Digitalis toxicity does not necessarily correlate with the serum levels. Serious manifestations of digitalis toxicity include bradycardia, ventricular tachycardia, and ventricular fibrillation.
- Consider mitral stenosis in the patient with the triad of dyspnea, left atrial abnormality, and RVH.

REFERENCES

1. Casale PN, Devereux RB, Alonso DR, et al: Improved sex-specific criteria of left ventricular hypertrophy for clinical and computer interpretation of electrocardiograms: validation with autopsy findings, *Circulation* 75:565-572, 1987. B
2. Levy D, Labib SB, Anderson KM, et al: Determinants of sensitivity and specificity of electrocardiographic criteria for left ventricular hypertrophy, *Circulation* 81:815-820, 1990. B
3. Alfakih K, Walters K, Jones T, et al: New gender-specific partition values for ECG criteria of left ventricular hypertrophy: recalibration against cardiac MRI, *Hypertension* 44:175-179, 2004. B
4. Moon JC, De Arenaza DP, Elkington AG, et al: The pathologic basis of Q-wave and non–Q-wave myocardial infarction: a cardiovascular magnetic resonance study, *J Am Coll Cardiol* 44:554-560, 2004. B
5. Bogaty P, Boyer L, Rousseau L, et al: Is anteroseptal myocardial infarction an appropriate term? *Am J Med* 113:37-41, 2002. B
6. Shalev Y, Fogelman R, Oettinger M, et al: Does the electrocardiographic pattern of "anteroseptal" myocardial infarction correlate with the anatomic location of myocardial injury? *Am J Cardiol* 75:763-766, 1995. B

7. Zehender M, Kasper W, Kauder E, et al: Right ventricular infarction as an independent predictor of prognosis after acute inferior myocardial infarction, *N Engl J Med* 328:981-988, 1993. B

8. Yamaji H, Iwasaki K, Kusachi S, et al: Prediction of acute left main coronary artery obstruction by 12-lead electrocardiography. ST segment elevation in lead aVR with less ST segment elevation in lead V(1), *J Am Coll Cardiol* 38:1348-1354, 2001. B

9. Barrabés JA, Figueras J, Moure C, et al: Prognostic value of lead aVR in patients with a first non–ST-segment elevation acute myocardial infarction, *Circulation* 108:814-819, 2003. B

10. de Zwaan C, Bar FW, Wellens HJ: Characteristic electrocardiographic pattern indicating a critical stenosis high in left anterior descending coronary artery in patients admitted because of impending myocardial infarction, *Am Heart J* 103(4 Pt 2):730-736, 1982. B

11. Sgarbossa EB, Pinski SL, Barbagelata A, et al: Electrocardiographic diagnosis of evolving acute myocardial infarction in the presence of left bundle-branch block, *N Engl J Med* 334:481-487, 1996. B

12. Rodger M, Makropoulos D, Turek M, et al: Diagnostic value of the electrocardiogram in suspected pulmonary embolism, *Am J Cardiol* 86:807-809, 2000. B

6

ELECTROCARDIOGRAM ANALYSIS

Chest Pain in the Emergency Department

Yuli Y. Kim, MD; Paul R. Forfia, MD; Michael Londner, MD; and Steven P. Schulman, MD

FAST FACTS

- Chest pain is the most common complaint in the emergency department in patients older than 45 years.[1]
- Acute coronary syndromes (ACSs) account for an estimated 20% of all chest discomfort complaints presenting to the emergency department annually, representing by far the most common morbid cause of chest discomfort and the leading cause of death in the United States.[1]
- Aortic dissection should be considered in all patients with chest pain in the emergency department, both because of its inherent risks and because therapies such as thrombolytic agents and heparin may lead to catastrophic consequences if wrongfully implemented.
- Young, otherwise healthy people who have recently ingested cocaine have an estimated 24-fold higher risk of myocardial infarction (MI) within 24 hours of ingestion.[2]
- The purpose of immediate review of the 12-lead electrocardiogram (ECG) is to detect an ST elevation MI so that reperfusion strategies may begin immediately.
- Risk stratification of patients with non–ST elevation MI or unstable angina in the emergency department directs proper management and will identify those for whom early invasive therapy is appropriate.

Chest pain accounts for approximately 5.6 million visits to the emergency department in the United States annually, second only to abdominal pain.[3,4] The differential diagnoses are vast, as are the prognostic implications, varying from the benign to the life threatening (Box 7-1). This chapter focuses on the morbid causes of chest pain including ACS, pulmonary embolism (PE), aortic dissection, pneumothorax (PTX), and esophageal rupture. With the exception of ACS and PE, which are discussed in more detail in Chapters 8 and 86, each diagnostic possibility is discussed with regard to epidemiology, clinical presentation, diagnosis, and management.

Approach to the Patient

1. Initial evaluation of the patient with chest discomfort begins with a 12-lead ECG and a focused history and physical examination. Continuous

BOX 7-1	
DIFFERENTIAL DIAGNOSIS OF CHEST PAIN	
CARDIOVASCULAR	Mallory-Weiss tear
ST elevation myocardial infarction	Zenker's diverticulum
Non–ST elevation myocardial infarction or unstable angina	Plummer-Vinson syndrome
Aortic dissection	**CHEST WALL**
Sinus of Valsalva aneurysmal rupture	Costochondritis (Tietze's syndrome)
Aortic valve disease	Herpes zoster
Myocarditis	Breast cancer or infection
Pericarditis	Intercostal myositis or cramp
PULMONARY	**OTHER**
Pulmonary embolism	Nerve root and spinal pain
Spontaneous pneumothorax	Shoulder disorders
Pneumonia	Cervical disk disease
Pleuritis	Thoracic outlet syndrome
Primary pulmonary hypertension	Thyroiditis
GASTROINTESTINAL	Tabes dorsalis
Ruptured esophagus	Mediastinitis
Esophageal reflux and spasm	Subphrenic abscesses
Biliary diseases	Splenic infarct
Pancreatitis	Psychogenic or hyperventilatory
Peptic ulcer disease	syndrome

electrocardiographic monitoring should be initiated, intravenous access obtained, pulse oximetry measured, and blood pressures checked in both arms. The physician should first consider all morbid causes of chest pain, such as an acute MI, unstable angina, PE, aortic dissection, PTX, and esophageal rupture.

2. Signs of hemodynamic instability should be sought, including elevated jugular venous pressure, a left parasternal lift, gallop rhythms, rales, and cool extremities. A pulmonary examination should assess for equal breath sounds and adventitious breath sounds. The 12-lead ECG should be reviewed in conjunction with the primary survey, with particular emphasis on identifying ST segment elevations or a new left bundle branch block. The presence of ST segment elevation in this context identifies a well-defined, high-risk group of patients who benefit from immediate reperfusion therapy.

3. If this initial primary survey reveals neither a need for resuscitation nor evidence of an ST segment elevation MI, attention should then be directed to obtaining a more detailed history and physical examination. This secondary survey is essential to differentiate cardiac from noncardiac causes. It should focus on the description of the discomfort and an assessment of cardiac risk factors. Further diagnostic testing is conducted to further narrow the differential diagnosis.

4. If the initial evaluation does not yield a definitive diagnosis, focus on risk stratification and appropriate triage. A challenging aspect of chest pain management in the emergency department is determining who needs admission for further monitoring or stress testing and who can be safely discharged with follow-up as an outpatient.

Acute Coronary Syndromes

1. Clinical suspicion of acute coronary ischemia in a patient presenting with chest pain in the emergency department is shaped by elements of the patient's history (including cardiac risk factors), physical examination, ECG, and cardiac biomarkers (creatine kinase, creatine kinase myocardial band fraction, and troponin).
a. The ECG remains the cornerstone of diagnosis in ACS and may show ST segment elevations, ST segment depressions, and T wave inversions.
b. Box 7-2 reviews the differential diagnosis of ST segment elevation unrelated to acute MI.[5]
c. Elevations of serum troponin should be considered in the proper clinical context. Box 7-3 lists the conditions that result in elevated troponin.[6]
2. ACS versus demand ischemia.
a. ACS is caused by an unstable plaque, whereas demand ischemia often is caused by anemia or extremes of heart rate or blood pressure in the setting of fixed atherosclerotic plaques.

BOX 7-2[5]

CAUSES OF ST SEGMENT ELEVATION OTHER THAN ACUTE MYOCARDIAL INFARCTION

Normal (so-called male pattern)	Hyperkalemia
Early repolarization	Brugada's syndrome
ST elevation of normal variant	Pulmonary embolism
Left ventricular hypertrophy	Cardioversion
Left bundle branch block	Prinzmetal's angina
Acute pericarditis	

BOX 7-3[6]

CAUSES OF TROPONIN ELEVATION

Acute coronary syndrome	Cardioversion, radiofrequency ablation
Congestive heart failure	Chemotherapy (doxorubicin,
Pulmonary embolism	5-fluorouracil)
Myocarditis	Septic shock
Cardiac contusion	Extreme endurance athletics

b. Patients with demand ischemia may not benefit from (and may be harmed by) the therapeutic approaches aimed at treating ACS. Proper management of demand ischemia entails correction of the underlying cause, such as gastrointestinal hemorrhage or hypertensive emergency.

3. Patients with a normal or nondiagnostic ECG and normal initial cardiac biomarkers should undergo further evaluation depending on level of suspicion for ACS. Strategy options include continued monitoring, immediate provocative testing or imaging, or discharge from the emergency department with follow-up medical care.

4. Patients with possible ACS should be monitored for 6 to 24 hours in a chest pain observation unit, a stepdown or monitored bed, or the emergency department. Repeat ECG and cardiac biomarkers are obtained to complete a "rule-out MI" workup.

a. Observing patients in a chest pain unit can decrease the rate of missed MI to less than 1%.[7] They have been demonstrated to be a safe and cost-effective method of triaging patients appropriately.[8]

b. A 9- to 12-hour observation period for cocaine-associated chest pain in patients deemed to be at low to intermediate risk of cardiovascular events was recently demonstrated to be safe at 30-day follow-up.[9]

c. In a large randomized study, acute rest myocardial perfusion imaging was investigated in patients with suspected ischemia but nondiagnostic or normal ECG and no prior history of MI. Acute rest myocardial perfusion imaging significantly reduced unnecessary admissions without compromising care for those with an ACS[10] and has been given a class I recommendation for assessment of patients with possible ACS who have nondiagnostic initial serum markers and ECGs.[11]

d. If the pain has disappeared and tests remain normal, the physician may choose to pursue provocative testing. This can be performed in the emergency department or observation unit after acute MI has been excluded or immediately in low-risk patients. Otherwise, patients may be discharged with follow-up to pursue outpatient stress testing.

5. See Chapter 8 for evaluation and management of patients with ST elevation MI and non–ST elevation ACS.

Pulmonary Embolism

PE is the second most common cause of life-threatening chest pain in the emergency department. PE remains underdiagnosed, and its prevalence at autopsy has remained unchanged (12% to 15%) over the past 30 years.[12] It is critical to maintain a high clinical suspicion for PE in patients who present with chest discomfort because it is a common cause of preventable death. Anticoagulation should be initiated immediately after a patient is diagnosed with a PE because time to therapeutic level of anticoagulation is the most important determinant of survival. For a full discussion of the diagnosis and management of PE, see Chapter 86.

Aortic Dissection

I. BACKGROUND

1. Aortic dissection, defined as a separation of the intimal and medial layers of the aorta, is an uncommon but often fatal cause of chest pain in the emergency department. In a recent large prospective study, aortic dissection was present in 0.3% of patients with acute chest pain, outweighed by ACS by approximately 80:1.[13]

2. Acute aortic dissection is the most common aortic surgical emergency, surpassing ruptured abdominal aortic aneurysm. The majority of patients with this condition have an intimal flap identified on imaging, surgery, or autopsy. The remainder may have dissection caused by hemorrhage into the media from the vasa vasorum.

3. Risk factors for aortic dissection are outlined in Box 7-4. The typical patient is a 60- to 80-year-old man with a history of hypertension.[14]

4. The original system by DeBakey classified aortic dissections as type I (ascending and descending aortic involvement), type II (ascending aorta only), and type III (descending aorta only). Today the more commonly used Stanford classification divides aortic dissection into types A and B. Type A dissections involve the ascending aorta, and all others are type B (Fig. 7-1).

5. An aortic dissection is described as acute if symptoms are present for less than 2 weeks; otherwise, it is chronic.

II. CLINICAL PRESENTATION

A. SYMPTOMS

1. Tearing or ripping chest pain radiating to the back is the classic presentation; however, data from the International Registry of Acute Aortic Dissection show that the presentation is much more diverse.[14] Overall, pain in the chest, back, or abdomen was present in more than 95% of patients. Chest pain was present in only 73% of patients with dissection. Anterior pain was more likely in type A dissection, and back pain and abdominal pain were more common in type B dissection.

2. Ninety percent of patients described it as abrupt in onset, severe, or the worst pain they had ever experienced. Surprisingly, only 50% of patients reported ripping or tearing pain, with no difference between type A and B dissection.

BOX 7-4	
PREDISPOSING FACTORS FOR AORTIC DISSECTION	
Marfan's syndrome	Turner's syndrome
Ehlers-Danlos syndrome	Pregnancy
Cystic medial necrosis	Iatrogenic factors
Coarctation of the aorta	Weight lifting
Bicuspid aortic valve	Crack cocaine[22]

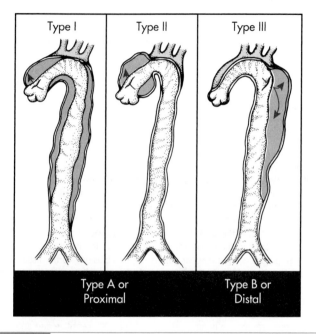

FIG. 7-1

Commonly used classification systems for aortic dissection. *(From Braunwald E et al: Heart disease, 6th ed, Philadelphia, 2001, WB Saunders.)*

3. Syncope was present in less than 10% of patients but was associated more often with type A dissection.

B. PHYSICAL EXAMINATION

1. The most common physical finding in acute dissection is hypertension, which is present in 50% of all patients and up to 70% of those with type B dissection.

2. The murmur of aortic insufficiency is present in up to 30% of patients with dissection and is more common with involvement of the ascending aorta. This murmur often is heard best not at the left lower sternal border (as noted when aortic insufficiency is caused by primary valvular disease) but at the right upper sternal border.

3. Proximal extension of a type A dissection may lead to coronary artery occlusion, and thus signs of myocardial ischemia, or rupture into the pericardium and lead to cardiac tamponade. Rupture into a hemithorax, most often the left, may produce signs of a pleural effusion.

4. Indications of aortic branch vessel occlusion, such as a focal neurologic deficit, a blood pressure differential in the upper extremities, signs of bowel ischemia, and lower limb pulse deficits, should be sought and can reveal the extent and location of the dissection along the length of the aorta. A blood pressure differential of more than 20 mmHg in the upper extremities was found to be an independent predictor of thoracic aortic dissections.[15]

III. DIAGNOSIS

1. The chest radiograph and ECG are abnormal in most patients with aortic dissection, but no single finding reliably establishes the diagnosis.
2. Chest radiography may reveal a widened mediastinum or abnormal aortic contour; however, in isolation these findings are nonspecific. In the setting of characteristic symptoms or blood pressure differential, mediastinal widening or abnormal aortic contour has a diagnostic sensitivity of 83% and 100%, respectively.[15]
3. The 12-lead ECG shows nonspecific ST and T wave abnormalities in up to 50% of patients. At presentation, 3% to 4% of patients with type A dissection have ST elevation, typically in the inferior leads as a consequence of right coronary artery ostial occlusion. **Aortic dissection should be considered whenever a patient is seen for acute chest pain because dissection is an absolute contraindication to almost all other therapies for acute chest pain in the emergency department.**
4. Transesophageal echocardiography, computed tomography (CT), and magnetic resonance imaging are more than 90% sensitive and specific in detecting an aortic dissection. However, each has its limitations and advantages (Table 7-1).

IV. MANAGEMENT

1. Management of acute aortic dissection includes initial medical stabilization and emergent cardiology and cardiothoracic surgery consultation.
2. **The goal of medical management is the rapid lowering of left ventricular contractility and arterial blood pressure.** This decreases the stress imposed on the aortic defect, which in turn reduces the likelihood of propagation or rupture of the dissection.
3. Initial treatment is intravenous beta-blockade, usually with labetalol or the short-acting agent esmolol. Once the heart rate is reduced to 50 to 60 beats per minute, if the systolic blood pressure remains above 100 mmHg, intravenous sodium nitroprusside should be added.
4. An arterial cannula should be inserted for continuous pressure monitoring, and urine output and mental status should be monitored to gauge the limits of blood pressure reduction.
5. In general, patients with acute type A dissection obtain the greatest reduction in mortality from emergency surgical intervention, whereas

TABLE 7-1		
TRANSESOPHAGEAL ECHOCARDIOGRAPHY, COMPUTED TOMOGRAPHY, AND MAGNETIC RESONANCE IMAGING IN THE DIAGNOSIS OF AORTIC DISSECTION		
	Pros	Cons
Transesophageal echocardiography	Rapid, portable Highly sensitive and specific Imaging modality of choice in patients with suspected dissection and hemodynamic instability	Potential need for intubation Operator dependent
Computed tomography	Widely available, rapid Can identify pericardial and pleural effusions Can visualize aorta and branches	Need for intravenous contrast May interrupt patient monitoring
Magnetic resonance imaging	Most accurate Imaging modality of choice for patients with stable type B dissection for documenting disease progression	Prolonged scanning time Interrupts patient monitoring

patients with type B dissection often are managed more successfully with blood pressure control and serial imaging of the aorta.

V. OUTCOME

Patient outcome varies depending on the type of dissection and the treatment used. For example, in-hospital mortality for patients with type A dissection who undergo surgery is approximately 25%, compared with 60% for patients who do not undergo surgery. In contrast, patients with type B dissection treated medically have a 10% in-hospital mortality, compared with 33% for those who undergo surgery.[14]

Spontaneous Pneumothorax

I. BACKGROUND

1. Primary spontaneous PTX occurs in patients with no clinically apparent lung disease. Secondary spontaneous PTX is a complication of preexisting lung disease. Primary and secondary spontaneous PTX have a similar incidence: approximately 6 cases per 100,000 men per year and 2 cases per 100,000 women per year.[16]

2. **Primary PTX** typically occurs in men between the ages of 10 and 30 years and is rare after the age of 40. The patient usually is tall and thin, although no clear relationship between body habitus and underlying pathophysiology has been shown. Primary PTX derives its name from the absence of clinical lung disease; however, thoracotomy or CT scanning shows that 80% to 100% of patients have subpleural bullae. An estimated 90% of patients are active cigarette smokers, and

those who smoke more than one pack per day increase their risk of PTX 70- to 100-fold.[17]

3. **Secondary PTX** usually occurs in patients older than the age of 60, in parallel with the peak rate of chronic lung disease in the general population. Predisposing conditions include chronic obstructive pulmonary disease, *Pneumocystis carinii* pneumonia, interstitial lung diseases such as pulmonary sarcoidosis, connective tissue disease, and underlying lung cancer.

II. CLINICAL PRESENTATION

A. SYMPTOMS

Most patients with spontaneous PTX have ipsilateral pleuritic chest pain or the abrupt onset of dyspnea. Pleuritic pain may be more prevalent in primary than in secondary PTX. Dyspnea, which varies from mild to severe in primary PTX, typically is severe in secondary PTX. Symptoms associated with primary PTX often resolve within 24 hours, even if untreated. This contrasts with the progressive nature of secondary PTX.

B. PHYSICAL EXAMINATION

1. In **primary PTX,** signs are variable and depend on the size of the PTX. Patients with a primary PTX occupying less than 15% of the hemithorax may have a normal physical examination. Tachycardia and tachypnea are the most common features. Hypoxemia, found on either pulse oximetry or an arterial blood gas analysis, is uncommon because most patients have enough alveolar reserve to preserve oxygenation. An abnormal A-a gradient is more common and is often caused largely by hypocapnia as a result of a rise in alveolar ventilation. As the size of the PTX increases, the expected signs emerge, such as diminished breath sounds, decreased fremitus, and hyperresonance to percussion on the involved side.

2. In **secondary PTX,** hypoxemia and hypercapnia are typical at presentation, reflecting both increased shunt and dead space physiology. Percussive and auscultatory findings are less reliable, especially in patients with severe chronic obstructive pulmonary disease.

3. In either case, hypotension with diminished breath sounds heralds tension PTX, which warrants emergency attention.

III. DIAGNOSIS

1. The diagnosis of PTX is confirmed by the identification of a thin visceral pleural line that is displaced from the chest wall on a standard chest radiograph. In patients with severe emphysema and bullous disease, the diseased areas of lung, or bullae, are hyperlucent and collapse to a lesser degree than normal areas of lung, making the pleural line more difficult to visualize. With a PTX, the pleural line runs parallel to and is convex toward the lateral chest wall, as opposed to the concave orientation of bullae.

2. Any uncertainty about the diagnosis can be resolved by a noncontrast CT scan of the chest.

IV. MANAGEMENT

1. Management of PTX should focus initially on evacuation of air from the pleural space, then on prevention of recurrence.
2. Current therapeutic options include observation, supplemental oxygen, simple aspiration, tube thoracostomy, pleurodesis, thoracoscopy, and thoracotomy. No hard evidence has been presented to support many of these therapies and their indications, although expert consensus dictates that the size and type of the PTX, severity of the clinical presentation, and persistence of an air leak determine which approaches are used.[18]
3. **In the event of tension PTX, emergency decompression is warranted, with insertion of an 18-gauge angiocatheter into the second intercostal space at the midclavicular line or into the fourth intercostal space at the anterior axillary line.**
4. Primary PTX
   a. A PTX less than 15% of the volume of the hemithorax can be treated with observation and supplemental oxygen. Supplemental oxygen creates a nitrogen diffusion gradient from the pleural space into pulmonary capillaries that accelerates the resorption of air from the pleural space fourfold to sixfold.
   b. If the PTX is more than 15% of hemithorax volume, simple aspiration or tube thoracostomy is indicated.
      (1) Simple aspiration. Absence of PTX on follow-up chest radiograph reflects successful management, and in most circumstances these patients can be discharged with close outpatient follow-up.
      (2) Most experts believe that tube thoracostomy should be reserved for patients in whom aspiration is unsuccessful or those who have recurrent primary PTX.
5. Patients with secondary PTX should be hospitalized. Because of the risk of respiratory decline in these patients, urgent chest tube insertion is recommended.
6. In both primary and secondary PTX, routine application of suction to the chest tube is not necessary or appropriate, although it is indicated if a PTX does not resolve when the chest tube is connected to water seal drainage or to a one-way Heimlich valve.
7. Recurrence can be prevented by chemical pleurodesis or surgery, with the particular approach tailored to the type of PTX and its likelihood of recurrence. Special emphasis is placed on secondary prevention in patients with secondary PTX because of the seriousness of primary and recurrent events.

V. OUTCOME

1. In general, patients with primary PTX have a benign clinical course, with an estimated case fatality rate of 0.1%. Those with larger PTXs or tension PTX have greater cardiopulmonary embarrassment and represent a high-risk subset of patients.

7

CHEST PAIN IN THE EMERGENCY DEPARTMENT

2. In comparison, patients with secondary PTX have a 20-fold higher risk of death, with an estimated 2% case fatality rate. These patients are much more likely to have hypotension and significant hypoxemia at presentation. At particularly high risk are patients with secondary PTX caused by underlying *Pneumocystis carinii* pneumonia, as shown by an in-hospital mortality rate of 25% and a median survival of 3 months.[19]

Esophageal Rupture

I. EPIDEMIOLOGY

1. Esophageal rupture is the least common cause of morbid chest pain, and more than half of these ruptures are iatrogenic. In a review of more than 500 patients from recent series, iatrogenic injury was the most common cause, accounting for 59% of all patients.[20]
2. Spontaneous esophageal rupture (Boerhaave's syndrome), or out-of-hospital perforation, classically occurs in the midst of retching or vomiting. These perforations are thought to be caused by muscular incoordination, which leads to failure of cricopharyngeus relaxation and critical elevations in intraesophageal pressure.
3. Spontaneous rupture typically occurs in men older than 50 years of age with a history of excessive dietary and alcohol intake. Occasionally, patients have an underlying esophageal defect such as Barrett's esophagitis or, in immunocompromised patients, infectious ulcers.

II. CLINICAL PRESENTATION

A. SYMPTOMS
Chest discomfort typically is retrosternal and severe. Many patients report epigastric pain, radiation to the back or left shoulder, and odynophagia. Because of potential communication between the esophagus and the pleural cavity, patients may report a cough or a cough precipitated by swallowing.

B. PHYSICAL EXAMINATION
Examination usually is not helpful, especially early in the course of the condition. Patients may present with frank dyspnea or shock, especially if the presentation has been delayed more than 24 hours.

1. Hypotension, tachycardia, and fever may reflect underlying sepsis and are more common in patients examined at least 24 hours after rupture.
2. Subcutaneous emphysema is present in only 30% of patients.
3. Signs of a pleural effusion may be present, usually on the left.
4. Patients may have abdominal rigidity or may have pneumoperitoneum caused by transdiaphragmatic rupture of the esophagus.

III. DIAGNOSIS

1. **Laboratory findings** are nonspecific, although presence of leukocytosis with a left shift is not uncommon. In addition, up to half of patients have a hematocrit value greater than 50%, reflecting

hemoconcentration caused by extracellular volume loss into pleural and tissue spaces. Pleural fluid analysis often reveals a pH less than 6 and elevated amylase content.

2. **Radiography.** A ruptured esophagus almost always produces abnormalities on routine chest radiography, including mediastinal air, pneumopericardium, pneumomediastinum, free peritoneal air, and unilateral left pleural effusion. Diagnosis of cervical esophageal perforation can be made with lateral radiograph of the neck, which may demonstrate air in the prevertebral fascial planes.

3. **Further imaging.** For practical reasons the next test often is thoracic CT, which shows mediastinal air in almost all cases; however, a Gastrografin esophagogram is necessary for diagnostic confirmation and for precise localization of the tear to determine a surgical approach. The use of barium is warranted only if the results of a water-soluble contrast study are negative and better definition is sought.

IV. MANAGEMENT

1. Timely surgical intervention is crucial in the management of ruptured esophagus. The goals of surgery are primary repair of the esophagus, mediastinal debridement, and pleural drainage.

2. Broad-spectrum intravenous antibiotics and fluid resuscitation should be started as soon as the diagnosis is suspected.

3. Nonoperative management may be an option for patients with well-contained perforations and minimal mediastinal or pleural contamination.

V. OUTCOME

In a retrospective review between 1990 and 2003, overall mortality was 18%. Mortality risk is influenced by the type of perforation, anatomic location, underlying disease, time to diagnosis, and choice of surgical or nonsurgical treatment.[20] Early diagnosis and treatment are essential to outcome and reduce mortality by at least 50%.

PEARLS AND PITFALLS

- Blood pressure should be measured in both arms during the evaluation of chest discomfort.
- Ischemic events related to occlusion of the left circumflex artery are electrocardiographically subtle.
- Relief of chest pain with nitroglycerin does not predict coronary artery disease in the acute setting and should not be used as a triage tool.[21]
- Troponin levels alone are unreliable in diagnosing recurrent MI. Always measure creatine kinase and creatine kinase myocardial band within the first 24 hours.
- Never forget to inquire about illicit drug use, especially in a young patient with chest pain.

7

CHEST PAIN IN THE EMERGENCY DEPARTMENT

- A history of chest discomfort suggesting an ACS and risk factors for atherosclerosis with persistently negative or normal electrocardiographic findings is highly suspicious for acute aortic dissection.
- Patients with intermediate or high clinical probability for PE should be given anticoagulation during the diagnostic workup.
- Secondary spontaneous PTX often is associated with a greater degree of cardiopulmonary embarrassment than occurs with primary spontaneous PTX.
- Mackler's triad consists of vomiting, lower thoracic pain, and subcutaneous emphysema and refers to signs and symptoms seen in barogenic esophageal rupture.

REFERENCES

1. Burt CW: Summary statistics for acute cardiac ischemia and chest pain visits to United States EDs, 1995-1996, *Am J Emerg Med* 17:552, 1999. C
2. Weber JE, Hollander JE: Cocaine-associated chest pain: how common is myocardial infarction? *Acad Emerg Med* 7:873, 2000. B
3. Goldman L, Kirtane AJ: Triage of patients with acute chest pain and possible cardiac ischemia: the elusive search for diagnostic perfection, *Ann Intern Med* 139:987, 2003. C
4. McCaig LF, Burt CW: National Hospital Ambulatory Medical Care Survey: 2002 emergency department summary, *Adv Data* (340):1, 2004. B
5. Wang K et al: ST-segment elevation in conditions other than acute myocardial infarction, *N Engl J Med* 349(22):2128, 2003. C
6. De Lemos JA, Morrow DA: Combining natriuretic peptides and necrosis markers in the assessment of acute coronary syndromes, *Rev Cardiovasc Med* 4(Suppl 4):S37, 2003. C
7. Graff LG et al: Impact on the care of the emergency department chest pain patient from the Chest Pain Evaluation Registry (CHEPER) Study, *Am J Cardiol* 80:563, 1997. B
8. Farkouh ME et al: A clinical trial of a chest-pain observation unit for patients with unstable angina. Chest Pain Evaluation in the Emergency Room (CHEER) Investigators, *N Engl J Med* 339:1882, 1998. B
9. Weber JE et al: Validation of a brief observation period for patients with cocaine-associated chest pain, *N Engl J Med* 348:510, 2003. B
10. Udelson JE et al: Myocardial perfusion imaging for evaluation and triage of patients with suspected acute cardiac ischemia: a randomized controlled trial, *JAMA* 288(21):2693, 2002. A
11. Klocke FJ et al: ACC/AHA/ASNC guidelines for the clinical use of cardiac radionuclide imaging: executive summary. A report of the American College of Cardiology/American Heart Association Task Force on Practice Guidelines (ACC/AHA/ASNC Committee to Revise the 1995 Guidelines for the Clinical Use of Cardiac Radionuclide Imaging), *Circulation* 108(11):1404, 2003. D
12. Goldhaber SZ: Pulmonary embolism, *N Engl J Med* 339:93, 1998. C
13. Dmowski AT et al: Aortic dissection, *Am J Emerg Med* 17:372, 1999. C
14. Hagan PG et al: The International Registry of Acute Aortic Dissection (IRAD), *JAMA* 283(7):897, 2000. B
15. von Kodolitsch et al: Clinical prediction of acute aortic dissection, *Arch Intern Med* 160:2977, 2000. B

16. Sahn SA, Heffner JE: Spontaneous pneumothorax, *N Engl J Med* 342(12):868, 2000. C
17. Bense L et al: Smoking and the increased risk of contracting spontaneous pneumothorax, *Chest* 92(6):1009, 1987. B
18. Baumann MH et al: Management of spontaneous pneumothorax: an American College of Chest Physicians Delphi Consensus Statement, *Chest* 119:590, 2001. C
19. Trachiotis GD et al: Management of AIDS-related pneumothorax, *Ann Thorac Surg* 62:1608, 1996. C
20. Brinster CJ et al: Evolving options in the management of esophageal perforation, *Ann Thorac Surg* 77:1475, 2004. C
21. Henrikson CA et al: Chest pain relief by nitroglycerin does not predict active coronary artery disease, *Ann Intern Med* 139(12):979-986, 2003. B
22. Hsue PY et al: Acute aortic dissection related to crack cocaine, *Circulation* 105:1592, 2002. B

Acute Coronary Syndromes

Paul F. Frey, MD, MPH; and Richard Lange, MD

1. Cardiovascular disease is the leading cause of death in the United States, accounting for more than 1 of every 5 deaths. Each year, approximately 1.7 million patients are hospitalized in the United States with ACS.[1]
2. ACS consists of the signs and symptoms of myocardial ischemia that occur at rest or with minimal exertion and usually is caused by rupture of a coronary atherosclerotic plaque, with subsequent platelet aggregation and coronary thrombosis.
3. The management of ACS depends on ECG findings. Patients with ST segment elevation probably have total occlusion of an epicardial coronary artery and should receive prompt reperfusion of the IRA, whereas patients with ACS and without ST segment elevation probably have subtotal occlusion of an epicardial coronary artery and should receive intense antiplatelet and anticoagulant therapy. Cardiac catheterization should be performed in those at high risk for myocardial infarction (MI) or death on the basis of risk stratification.

I. CLINICAL PRESENTATION

The history, physical examination, ECG findings, and cardiac biomarkers are used to determine whether the patient with chest pain has ACS (Table 8-1). Important historical features include the following:

TABLE 8-1

LIKELIHOOD THAT SIGNS AND SYMPTOMS REPRESENT ACUTE CORONARY SYNDROME SECONDARY TO CAD

	High Likelihood (any of the following)	Intermediate Likelihood (absence of high-likelihood features and presence of any of the following)	Low Likelihood (absence of high- or intermediate-likelihood features but may have the following)
History	Chest or left arm pain or discomfort as chief symptom reproducing prior documented angina Known history of CAD, including myocardial infarction	Chest or left arm pain or discomfort as chief symptom Age <70 yr Male sex Diabetes mellitus	Probable ischemic symptoms in absence of any of the intermediate-likelihood characteristics Recent cocaine use
Examination	Transient mitral regurgitation, hypotension, diaphoresis, pulmonary edema, or rales	Extracardiac vascular disease	Chest discomfort reproduced by palpation
Electrocardiogram	New, or presumably new, transient ST segment deviation (>0.05 mV) or T wave inversion (>0.2 mV) with symptoms	Fixed Q waves Abnormal ST segments or T waves not documented to be new	T wave flattening or inversion in leads with dominant R waves Normal electrocardiogram
Cardiac markers	Elevated cardiac troponin I, troponin T, or creatine kinase myocardial band	Normal	Normal

Modified from Braunwald E, Mark DB, Jones RH et al: *Unstable angina: diagnosis and management*, Rockville, Md, 1994, Agency for Health Care Policy and Research and the National Heart, Lung, and Blood Institute, U.S. Public Health Service, U.S. Department of Health and Human Services; AHCPR Publication No. 94-0602. *CAD*, coronary artery disease.

ACUTE CORONARY SYNDROMES

8

1. **Quality and frequency of chest discomfort.** Chest discomfort more severe than the patient's usual chest pain or occurring more frequently suggests ACS.
2. **Rest pain.** Chest discomfort occurring at rest or with minimal activity suggests ACS.
3. **Duration of chest pain.** Stable angina rarely causes chest discomfort longer than 10 minutes. Chest pain lasting longer is more likely to indicate ACS.
4. **Prior cardiac history.** Patients with chest pain within 2 months of an MI or coronary revascularization have ACS until proven otherwise.
5. **Associated symptoms.** Diaphoresis, shortness of breath, palpitations, and nausea often accompany chest pain caused by ACS.

II. DIAGNOSIS

All patients being evaluated for ACS should be placed on a cardiac monitor, and a 12-lead electrocardiogram should be obtained within 10 minutes of presentation and repeated if the chest discomfort changes. A careful physical examination (including assessment of blood pressure in both arms) should be performed and a chest film obtained. A blood sample should be sent for analysis of the comprehensive metabolic panel, troponin level, fractionated creatine kinase (CK) concentration, complete blood cell count, and prothrombin and activated partial thromboplastin times. Risk stratification of the patient should then be used.

A. ELECTROCARDIOGRAM

1. A 12-lead electrocardiogram should be obtained immediately for every patient with signs or symptoms suggestive of ACS and compared with a previous electrocardiogram if available.
2. The electrocardiogram differentiates ST segment elevation ACS from non–ST segment elevation ACS. This distinction is vital because treatment differs greatly between the two syndromes.
3. The current ECG criteria for the diagnosis of ST elevation ACS require more than 1 mm ST elevation in two or more anatomically contiguous limb leads, more than 2 mm ST elevation in two or more anatomically contiguous precordial leads, or a new or presumed new left bundle branch block.
4. Serial ECG analysis is essential because a suspected non–ST segment elevation ACS may evolve into an ST segment elevation ACS.
5. A right-sided electrocardiogram should be obtained in all patients with ST segment elevations in the inferior leads to determine whether right ventricular MI is present. ST segment elevation in V_4 of the right-sided leads suggests a right ventricular infarction.
6. When the electrocardiogram meets ST segment elevation ACS criteria, the patient becomes eligible for acute reperfusion therapy. The current recommendations are to administer thrombolytic therapy within 30 minutes or perform percutaneous coronary intervention (PCI) within 90 minutes of diagnosis.

7. Patients with non–ST segment elevation ACS may initially have a normal electrocardiogram or nonspecific ST-T wave changes. Thus a normal electrocardiogram does not exclude this diagnosis. ST segment depressions of more than 1 mm in two or more contiguous limb leads (or more than 2 mm in two or more contiguous precordial leads) may be present and predict adverse cardiac events.

B. CARDIAC BIOMARKERS

1. In patients with a non–ST segment elevation ACS, serum biomarkers (e.g., cardiac enzymes) indicative of myocardial necrosis are helpful in stratifying risk and differentiating ischemia from infarction. It takes several hours from the time myocardial injury occurs until biomarkers are detectable in the serum, so the patient with a non–ST segment elevation ACS may have normal values initially at presentation. Therefore blood samples should be obtained at the time of presentation and again 6 to 12 hours later.

2. Traditional biomarkers included CK, troponin I or T, and myoglobin. Based on current guidelines, the cardiac-specific troponins such as troponin T and troponin I are the preferred markers. Troponin T is detectable in the serum within 4 hours after myocardial injury, with elevated serum levels for 7 to 10 days. Troponin I is typically detectable within 6 hours of myocardial injury, and the serum levels remain elevated for 7 to 10 days. Troponin I is less likely to be associated with false elevations than troponin T in patients with renal insufficiency.

3. CK exists in three isoforms (MM, MB, BB), of which CK-MB is cardiac-specific. CK-MB serum levels typically increase 3 to 6 hours after myocardial injury, peak at 12 to 24 hours, and return to normal within 3 days. CK-MB is less cardiospecific than troponin, and serum levels may be elevated in the patient with trauma, surgery, rhabdomyolysis, sepsis, hypothyroidism, or renal dysfunction.

4. Myoglobin is a highly sensitive and early marker of myocardial damage. Serum myoglobin levels begin to increase within 2 hours of myocardial injury and peak at 24 hours. However, serum myoglobin has very low specificity because myoglobin increases with skeletal muscle injury, trauma, intramuscular injections, alcohol abuse, renal dysfunction, and hypothermia or hyperthermia. Therefore a negative myoglobin within 8 hours of the onset of chest pain may be useful to help rule out myocardial ischemia.

III. MANAGEMENT: NON–ST SEGMENT ELEVATION ACS

A. RISK STRATIFICATION

Risk stratification is integral in the management of a non–ST segment elevation ACS because not all patients with ACS are equally likely to have adverse cardiac events (i.e., death, MI, or urgent revascularization). Patients are classified as being at high, intermediate, or low risk of having an adverse cardiac event, and therapy is tailored to the patient's risk profile. The following clinical tools help risk stratify patients:

1. **Electrocardiogram and cardiac biomarkers.** ST segment depression and elevated cardiac biomarkers are associated with a higher risk of adverse outcomes. Patients with only one of the two are at intermediate risk, and those with neither are at low risk.

2. A list of **historical and physical findings** the American Heart Association has adopted in assisting with risk stratification is provided in Table 8-2.

3. **Thrombolysis in Myocardial Infarction (TIMI) risk score assessment.** The TIMI risk factor score predicts the probability of adverse cardiac outcomes in patients with non–ST segment elevation ACS based on data available at the bedside.[2] Seven variables are assessed (Box 8-1), with the likelihood of an adverse cardiac event predicted by the number of variables present. Patients with a score of less than 3 are at low risk, those with a score of 3 or 4 are at intermediate risk, and those with a score of 5 or higher are at high risk for having a cardiac event over the next 30 days.

B. **INTERVENTION: PHARMACOLOGIC AND NONPHARMACOLOGIC**

1. The management of non–ST segment elevation ACS is based on risk stratification. All patients initially are treated with aspirin, beta-blockers, nitrates, and anticoagulation unless contraindicated. Once these therapies are initiated, the first decision is whether the patient should undergo early invasive or noninvasive management. The next decision is whether the patient should receive clopidogrel or a glycoprotein (GP) IIb/IIIa inhibitor.

BOX 8-1

THROMBOLYSIS IN MYOCARDIAL INFARCTION RISK FACTOR SCORE

RISK FACTORS

Age >65 years

Three or more risk factors for coronary artery disease

Prior coronary stenosis ≥50%

Two or more anginal events in past 24 hr

Aspirin use in past 7 d

ST segment changes

Positive cardiac markers

30-DAY RISK OF ADVERSE CARDIAC EVENT*	
Number of Risk Factors	**Risk (%)**
0-1	4.7
2	8.3
3	13.2
4	19.9
5	26.2
6-7	41.0

Data from Antman E et al: *JAMA* 284:835, 2000.

*Defined as myocardial infarction, cardiac-related death, or persistent ischemia. Low risk, score 0-2; intermediate risk, score 3-4; high risk, score 5-7.

TABLE 8-2

SHORT-TERM RISK OF DEATH OR NONFATAL MYOCARDIAL INFARCTION IN PATIENTS WITH UNSTABLE ANGINA*

	High Risk (at least 1 of the following features must be present)	Intermediate Risk (no high-risk feature but must have 1 of the following)	Low Risk (no high- or intermediate-risk feature but may have any of the following features)
History	Accelerating tempo of ischemic symptoms in preceding 48 hr	Prior MI, peripheral or cerebrovascular disease, or coronary artery bypass graft; prior aspirin use	
Character of pain	Prolonged (>20 min) rest pain	Prolonged (>20 min) rest angina, now resolved, with moderate or high likelihood of CAD; rest angina (<20 min) or relieved with rest or sublingual nitroglycerin	New-onset Canadian Cardiovascular Society Class III or IV angina in the past 2 wk without prolonged (<20 min) rest pain but with moderate or high likelihood of CAD
Clinical findings	Pulmonary edema, probably due to ischemia; new or worsening mitral regurgitation murmur; S_3; or new or worsening rales Hypotension Bradycardia or tachycardia Age >75 years	Age >70 years	
Electrocardiogram	Angina at rest with transient ST segment changes >0.05 mV Bundle branch block, new or presumed new Sustained ventricular tachycardia	T wave inversions > 0.2 mV Pathological Q waves	Normal or unchanged electrocardiogram during an episode of chest discomfort
Cardiac markers	Markedly elevated (e.g., troponin T or troponin I > 0.1 ng/ml)	Slightly elevated (e.g., troponin T > 0.01 but < 0.1 ng/ml)	Normal

Modified from Braunwald E, Mark DB, Jones RH et al: *Unstable angina: diagnosis and management*, Rockville, Md, 1994, Agency for Health Care Policy and Research and the National Heart, Lung, and Blood Institute, U.S. Public Health Service, U.S. Department of Health and Human Services; AHCPR Publication No. 94-0602.
CAD, coronary artery disease; *MI*, myocardial infarction.
*Estimation of the short-term risks of death and nonfatal cardiac ischemic events in unstable angina is a complex multivariable problem that cannot be fully specified in a table such as this; therefore this table is meant to offer general guidance and illustration rather than rigid algorithms.

ACUTE CORONARY SYNDROMES 8

2. **Aspirin.** Platelet activation and aggregation play an important role in the pathophysiology of ACS. Aspirin inhibits the production of thromboxane, which is a potent mediator of platelet activation. As soon as ACS is suspected, 325 mg of non–enteric-coated aspirin should be administered. Patients with aspirin allergy can be given clopidogrel. Ticlopidine should not be used in lieu of clopidogrel because of its slow (3 to 5 days) onset of action.

3. **Beta-adrenergic blockers** reduce myocardial oxygen demand by exerting negative inotropic and chronotropic effects and protect against cardiac arrhythmias. Metoprolol is the preferred beta-adrenergic blocker because of its β_1-selective activity. It is initially given as a 5-mg intravenous (IV) bolus. If tolerated, the 5-mg dose is repeated twice at 10-minute intervals for a maximum dosage of 15 mg. The patient is then started on orally administered metoprolol. The dosage is titrated to achieve a mean systemic arterial pressure of 60 to 70 mmHg and a heart rate of 60 beats/min. If these hemodynamic goals are not tolerated, the lowest tolerated mean arterial pressure and pulse should be targeted.

4. **Nitrates** reduce myocardial oxygen demand (by reducing preload) and increase myocardial blood flow (by dilating coronary vessels). Sublingual nitroglycerin tablets or spray should be used initially if the patient is not hypotensive and has no other contraindications to these agents, such as sildenafil use in the previous 24 hours. If the patient's chest discomfort does not resolve after three 0.4-mg nitroglycerin tablets given 5 minutes apart, a continuous nitroglycerin IV infusion can be initiated at 10 μg/min and titrated upward by 10 μg every 3 to 5 minutes until the patient's discomfort resolves, the mean systemic arterial blood pressure drops below 25% of initial values in an initially hypertensive patient, or the systolic blood pressure drops below 110 mmHg in a normotensive patient. Common side effects include hypotension and headaches. Tachyphylaxis may occur with prolonged use. A reflex tachycardia can also occur in patients not receiving a beta-adrenergic blocker or other negative chronotropic therapy.

5. **Anticoagulation.** Plaque rupture exposes tissue factor, which initiates the clotting cascade and coronary thrombosis. Patients with a non–ST segment elevation ACS should receive anticoagulation unless a major contraindication exists. Two forms of heparin are approved for use in these patients: unfractionated heparin and low–molecular-weight heparin. For the patient with a history of heparin-induced thrombocytopenia who needs anticoagulation, lepirudin, a direct thrombin inhibitor, can be administered as a 0.4-mg/kg bolus followed by a 0.15-mg/kg/hr (maximum 16.5 mg/hr) infusion with a targeted activated partial thromboplastin time (aPTT) of 1.5 to 2.5 times the upper limit of normal.

   a. **Unfractionated heparin** is initiated as an IV bolus followed by a continuous infusion. The American Heart Association recommends a weight-based dosage regimen consisting of a 60- to 70-U/kg (maximum 5000-U) bolus followed by a maintenance infusion of 12 to 15 U/kg/hr. The aPTT should be measured 6 hours after every dosage adjustment and the infusion adjusted to reach an aPTT of 2 to 2.5 times the upper limit of normal. If the patient is receiving a GP IIb/IIIa inhibitor, the target aPTT is lower (1.8 to 2 times the upper end of normal) in order to minimize the risk of bleeding.

b. **Low–molecular-weight heparin** is also approved for use in the patient with a non–ST segment elevation ACS. Enoxaparin is administered initially as a 30-mg IV bolus, and then 1 mg/kg is administered subcutaneously twice daily. It has several advantages over heparin: It is easier to administer, does not necessitate aPTT monitoring, and is less likely to cause heparin-induced thrombocytopenia. Conversely, it is more expensive than heparin, it has a long half life, and its therapeutic effects cannot be reversed completely with protamine. Thus concerns have been raised regarding its use in patients referred for coronary revascularization. The dosage is reduced in the patient with renal failure or obesity (weight > 120 kg), and the patient with a history of heparin-induced thrombocytopenia should not receive low–molecular-weight heparin.

c. Two double-blind randomized trials—Efficacy and Safety of Subcutaneous Enoxaparin in Non–Q Wave Coronary Events (ESSENCE) and TIMI 11B—compared enoxaparin and unfractionated heparin therapy in 7081 patients with non–ST segment elevation ACS and demonstrated a significant reduction in the incidence of MI and urgent revascularization for recurrent angina with enoxaparin.[3,4] In these studies, patients were referred for catheterization if they had spontaneous or provocable ischemia (known as an ischemia-guided management strategy). The recent Superior Yield of the New Strategy of Enoxaparin, Revascularization, and Glycoprotein IIb/IIIa Inhibitors (SYNERGY) study compared low–molecular-weight heparin and unfractionated heparin therapy in 10,027 patients with non–ST segment elevation ACS who were treated with a GP IIb/IIIa inhibitor and an early invasive strategy.[5] The primary endpoint (incidence of death or MI at 30 days) was similar for the two treatments; however, patients receiving low–molecular-weight heparin had a higher rate of bleeding.

6. **Clopidogrel** is a thienopyridine antiplatelet agent that inhibits adenosine diphosphate–mediated activation of platelets. Clopidogrel has a quick onset of action when administered as a loading dose, and its benefits in non–ST segment elevation ACS have been demonstrated in several large-scale trials.

a. In the Clopidogrel in Unstable Angina to Prevent Recurrent Ischemic Events (CURE) trial, 12,562 patients with ACS were randomized to receive placebo or clopidogrel, 300 mg loading dose and then 75 mg daily.[6] All participants received daily aspirin and were followed for 3 to 12 months. The clopidogrel-treated patients were less likely to suffer a major adverse cardiovascular event (9.4% vs. 11.3%) but more likely to have major bleeding (3.7% vs. 2.7%, p = .001). Those who received clopidogrel within 5 days of coronary artery bypass surgery had a significantly higher risk of bleeding and need for transfusions perioperatively. For this reason, many surgeons delay cardiac surgery if the patient has received clopidogrel within 5 days of the planned procedure.

b. Two other studies address the use of clopidogrel in the setting of PCI and revascularization: the PCI CURE study[7] and the Clopidogrel for the Reduction of Events During Observation (CREDO) study.[8] The PCI CURE study, a subset of the CURE trial, evaluated the 2658 patients undergoing PCI who were pretreated with clopidogrel and received study drug or placebo for 4 weeks after the procedure. Compared with those in the placebo group, the clopidogrel-treated patients experienced a lower rate of the combined endpoint of cardiovascular death, MI, or urgent revascularization at 30 days (6.4% and 4.5%, respectively; p = .03). The CREDO trial randomly assigned 2116 patients to placebo or clopidogrel 3 to 24 hours before PCI and for up to 12 months afterward. The clopidogrel-treated patients were less likely to have an adverse ischemic event in the year after PCI. Thus prolonged therapy with clopidogrel after successful PCI reduces the risk of subsequent ischemic events.

c. Current American College of Cardiology and American Heart Association (ACC/AHA) recommendations for the use of clopidogrel include all patients not at high risk for bleeding in whom a noninterventional approach is planned. A 300-mg oral dose is administered initially, and then .75 mg is given daily for at least 1 month. Clopidogrel should also be used in patients in whom PCI is planned.[9] In these patients, a 300- to 600-mg oral loading dose should be given 4 to 6 hours before the procedure and 75 mg administered daily for up to 12 months afterward. Because clopidogrel therapy should be discontinued at least 5 to 7 days before elective coronary artery bypass grafting, many cardiologists avoid giving clopidogrel to the patient with ACS in whom cardiac catheterization and a determination regarding the need for coronary artery bypass grafting can be performed expeditiously (within 24 to 36 hours of presentation).

7. **Glycoprotein IIb/IIIa receptor inhibitors.** The final pathway in platelet aggregation is activation of the GP IIb/IIIa receptor, which allows platelets to bind to fibrinogen and von Willebrand factor. Three GP IIb/IIIa inhibitors are available: abciximab, a monoclonal antibody against the IIb/IIIa receptor; tirofiban, a peptidomimetic inhibitor; and eptifibatide, a cyclic peptide inhibitor. Several studies have shown the clinical efficacy of eptifibatide and tirofiban in the setting of ACS.[10-12] Subgroup analysis of the data in these studies shows that the greatest clinical benefit occurs in high- and intermediate-risk patients. Current data support the use of eptifibatide or tirofiban in high-risk patients, especially those with an elevated serum troponin in whom coronary

> **BOX 8-2**
>
> **CLASS I RECOMMENDATIONS FOR AN EARLY INVASIVE STRATEGY FOR UNSTABLE ANGINA AND NON–ST SEGMENT ELEVATION MYOCARDIAL INFARCTION**
>
> Recurrent angina or ischemia at rest or with low-level activities despite intensive antiischemic therapy
>
> Elevated troponin T or troponin I
>
> New or presumably new ST segment depression
>
> Recurrent angina or ischemia with congestive heart failure symptoms, S_3 gallop, pulmonary edema, worsening rales, or new mitral regurgitation
>
> High-risk findings on noninvasive stress testing
>
> Depressed left ventricular systolic function (e.g., ejection fraction < 0.4 on noninvasive testing)
>
> Hemodynamic instability
>
> Sustained ventricular tachycardia
>
> Percutaneous coronary intervention within 6 mo
>
> Prior coronary artery bypass graft

Modified from Braunwald E et al: *Circulation* 106:1893, 2002.

angiography is likely. An IV bolus of eptifibatide or tirofiban is followed by continuous IV infusion of the drug for 48 to 72 hours. If PCI is performed, the infusion is continued for 12 to 24 hours after the procedure. Abciximab is beneficial only in patients undergoing PCI,[13] in which case the IV infusion is initiated in the cardiac catheterization laboratory and continued for 12 hours after PCI.

8. **Early percutaneous coronary angiography compared with an ischemia-guided approach.** Three randomized, prospective studies have shown that an early invasive strategy in conjunction with aggressive medical management is superior to an ischemia-guided approach, in which angiography and PCI are reserved for patients with spontaneous or provocable ischemia.[14-16] Subgroup analysis has shown that high- and intermediate-risk patients benefit the most from an early invasive strategy. The current ACC/AHA recommendations include an early invasive strategy for any patient with high-risk features (Box 8-2). For intermediate- and low-risk patients without evidence of myocardial necrosis (elevation in cardiac biomarkers) a noninvasive stress test is a reasonable approach, with catheterization reserved for those with inducible ischemia. For patients with evidence of myocardial necrosis, most cardiologists would recommend early cardiac catheterization.

IV. MANAGEMENT: ST SEGMENT ELEVATION ACS

A. RISK STRATIFICATION

1. As with all forms of ACS, risk stratification is crucial to patient management. A classification scheme developed in the late 1960s by

Killip and Kimball correlates heart failure signs and outcome[17] (Table 8-3). Many studies have confirmed that the Killip classification predicts short- and long-term mortality after MI.

2. The TIMI study group developed a simple bedside stratification tool for patients with ST segment elevation ACS[18] (Table 8-4), assigning points for clinical risk indicators on the basis of patient history, physical examination, and features on presentation. When applied to the 84,029 patients in the National Registry of Myocardial Infarction 3 database, the scoring system reveals a graded risk in 30-day mortality ranging from 1.1% to 30% for scores ranging from 0 to more than 8, respectively.[19]

TABLE 8-3
RISK STRATIFICATION BASED ON KILLIP CLASS IN THE GISSI-1 TRIAL OF STREPTOKINASE AND PLACEBO IN ACUTE MYOCARDIAL INFARCTION

Killip Class	Definition	GISSI-1 (% of patients)		
		Incidence	Control Mortality	Lytic Mortality
I	No congestive heart failure	71	7.3	5.9
II	S_3 gallop or basilar rales	23	19.9	16.1
III	Pulmonary edema (rales more than halfway up)	4	39	33
IV	Cardiogenic shock (systolic blood pressure <90)	2	70.1	69.9

TABLE 8-4
THROMBOLYSIS IN MYOCARDIAL INFARCTION RISK SCORE FOR ST SEGMENT ELEVATION MYOCARDIAL INFARCTION

Clinical Risk Indicators	Points
HISTORY	
Age ≥75 yr	3
Age 65-74 yr	2
History of diabetes, hypertension, or angina	1
EXAMINATION	
Systolic blood pressure < 100 mmHg	3
Heart rate >100 beats/min	2
Killip class II-IV	2
Weight < 67 kg	1
PRESENTATION	
Anterior ST elevation or left bundle branch block	1
Time to reperfusion > 4 hr	1
Total possible points	14

Data from Morrow DA et al: *JAMA* 286:1356, 2001.

B. INTERVENTION: PHARMACOLOGIC AND NONPHARMACOLOGIC

1. Patients should be treated with an antiischemic drug regimen consisting of aspirin, beta-blockers, and nitroglycerin and considered for acute reperfusion therapy via administration of a thrombolytic agent or primary PCI. Early flow restoration in the infarct-related artery salvages myocardium and improves survival. The adequacy of coronary blood flow after reperfusion therapy can be assessed angiographically using the TIMI grading system (Table 8-5).

2. **Early recognition of ischemia and rapid reperfusion salvage myocardium and improve survival.** Initiation of thrombolytic therapy within 30 minutes of symptom onset can abort infarction. Although patients derive survival benefit if treated with a thrombolytic agent within 12 hours of symptom onset,[24] maximum benefit is obtained if a thrombolytic agent is administered within 2 hours of symptom onset.[20] With primary PCI, mortality rates increase significantly when door-to-balloon time exceeds 90 minutes.[21] Based on these data, current ACC/AHA recommendations are to administer thrombolytic therapy within 30 minutes or perform PCI within 90 minutes of arrival, with an overall goal of total ischemic time (from symptom onset to intervention) less than 120 minutes.[22]

3. **Thrombolytics** (fibrinolytic agents) act by converting plasminogen to plasmin, which digests fibrin and enhances thrombus dissolution. Large randomized controlled trials have demonstrated relative mortality benefits on the order of 20% to 30% when thrombolytic therapy is administered in a timely manner.

a. Multiple thrombolytic agents are available in the United States. When choosing an agent, one must consider factors such as efficacy, side effect profile, ease of administration, and cost. Several of the major thrombolysis trials are reviewed in Table 8-6.

b. Before a thrombolytic agent is administered, the patient must be screened for potential **contraindications** that increase the risk of intracranial hemorrhage and bleeding (Box 8-3).

8

ACUTE CORONARY SYNDROMES

TABLE 8-5

TIMI ANGIOGRAPHIC GRADING SYSTEM: ANGIOGRAPHIC ASSESSMENT OF RESTORATION OF FLOW TO THE IRA

TIMI Grade	Definition
0	Complete occlusion of the IRA
1	Some flow beyond the obstruction but none distally (e.g., penetration of blood without perfusion)
2	Reperfusion of the entire IRA but flow is delayed and slower than normal
3	Normal flow in the IRA

Modified from TIMI Study Group: *N Engl J Med* 312:932, 1985.
IRA, infarct-related artery; *TIMI*, Thrombolysis in Myocardial Infarction.

TABLE 8-6		
SELECT THROMBOLYTIC STUDIES		
Study	Year	Findings
ISIS-2	1988	This placebo-controlled, randomized trial of 17,187 patients demonstrated lower 30-day mortality with streptokinase (9.2%) or aspirin (9.4%) treatment than placebo (13.2%) ($p < .00001$) and lowest mortality when aspirin and streptokinase were combined (8%) ($p < .00001$).[23]
GUSTO-1	1993	In this 41,021 patient study, patients treated with t-PA and intravenous heparin had higher coronary patency rates and better 30-day survival (6.4%) than patients treated with streptokinase and subcutaneous or intravenous heparin (7.4%) or a combination of reduced-dose t-PA and streptokinase (7.2%).[24]
GUSTO-3	1997	This trial of 15,059 patients compared reteplase with alteplase. The 30-day mortality rates were similar for the two groups, as were the nonfatal stroke rates.[25]
ASSENT-2	1999	This trial of 16,949 patients compared tenecteplase and alteplase. Mortality at 30 days was equivalent (6.18% vs. 6.15%, respectively); however, the tenecteplase-treated group had fewer noncerebral bleeding events (26.4% vs. 28.9%, $p = .0003$) and transfusions (4.2% vs. 5.5%, $p = .0002$).[26]

t-PA, tissue plasminogen activator.

c. **Efficacy of thrombolytic therapy.** Patients with complete resolution of ST segment elevation at 90 minutes have a 93% likelihood of infarct-related artery patency and a nearly 80% probability of TIMI 3 flow.[27] Patients (approximately 20% to 30% of those receiving thrombolytic agents) who do not have improvement or resolution of chest discomfort or at least a 50% reduction in the degree of ST elevation within 60 minutes of thrombolytic administration should be considered for immediate coronary angiography.[28]

d. **Current recommendations** of the ACC and AHA regarding thrombolytic therapy are shown in Box 8-4.[29]

4. **PCI.** Primary PCI requires the immediate availability of a catheterization laboratory and skilled staff. High-volume (49 or more procedures per year) and intermediate-volume (17 to 48 procedures per year) centers have lower mortality rates than low-volume centers.[30] Despite these limitations, primary PCI is the preferred therapy for ST segment elevation MI when performed in a timely fashion and by skilled practitioners. Thrombolytic therapy restores normal blood flow to the infarct-related artery in 50% to 60% of patients,[31] and primary PCI does so in more than 90%.[32] A meta-analysis of 23 trials showed better outcomes for PCI than for thrombolytic therapy, with lower rates of short-term death (7% vs. 9%, $p = .0004$), nonfatal reinfarction (3% vs. 7%, $p < .0001$), stroke (1% vs. 2%, $p = .0004$), and the

BOX 8-3

ABSOLUTE AND RELATIVE CONTRAINDICATIONS TO THROMBOLYTIC THERAPY FOR MYOCARDIAL INFARCTION

ABSOLUTE CONTRAINDICATIONS

Any prior intracranial hemorrhage

Known structural cerebral vascular lesion (e.g., arteriovenous malformation)

Known malignant intracranial neoplasm (primary or metastatic)

Ischemic stroke within 3 mo except acute ischemic stroke within 3 hr

Suspected aortic dissection

Active bleeding or bleeding diathesis (excluding menses)

Significant closed head or facial trauma within 3 mo

RELATIVE CONTRAINDICATIONS

History of chronic, severe, poorly controlled hypertension

Severe uncontrolled hypertension on presentation (>180/110 mmHg)

History of prior ischemic stroke > 3 mo before, dementia, or known intracranial disorder not covered in contraindications

Traumatic or prolonged (> 10 min) cardiopulmonary resuscitation or major surgery (within 3 wk)

Noncompressible vascular punctures

Internal bleeding within 4 weeks

For streptokinase or anistreplase, prior exposure (especially within 2 yr) or prior allergic reaction

Pregnancy

Active peptic ulcer

Current use of anticoagulants (the higher the international normalized ratio, the higher the risk of bleeding)

Modified from Antman EM et al: *Circulation* 110:588-636, 2004. Available at www.acc.org.

BOX 8-4

RECOMMENDATIONS OF THE AMERICAN COLLEGE OF CARDIOLOGY AND AMERICAN HEART ASSOCIATION FOR THROMBOLYTIC THERAPY

CLASS I

ST elevation (>0.1 mm in 2 or more contiguous leads), time to therapy ≤12 hr

New or presumably new left bundle branch block within past 12 hr

CLASS IIA

12-lead electrocardiographic findings consistent with a true posterior MI within 12 hr of symptom onset

Patients with symptoms beginning within the past 12 to 24 hr with continued ST elevation (>0.1 mm in 2 or more contiguous leads) and ischemic symptoms

CLASS III

ST elevation with time to therapy >24 hr

ST segment depression unless true posterior MI suspected

Data from Antman EM et al: *Circulation* 110:588-636, 2004. Available at www.acc.org.
MI, myocardial infarction.

combined endpoint of death, nonfatal reinfarction, and stroke (8% vs. 14%, $p < .0001$).[33] Primary PCI is also associated with a significantly lower rate of long-term (5-year) mortality than streptokinase (13% vs. 24%, $p = .01$).[34]

a. **Transport to PCI sites.** Recognition of the advantages of PCI over thrombolytics has led investigators to explore whether the patient with acute MI who presents to a hospital without catheterization facilities should be transferred emergently to a site where PCI is available. If the triage and transport time is short ($\approx$90 minutes), then transfer of the patient to a center with catheterization facilities may be preferable. In the recent Danish Trial in Acute Myocardial Infarction (DANAMI-2) study, patients treated in this manner had a lower incidence of reinfarction than patients treated with thrombolysis.[35] A recent metaanalysis of 21 studies comparing PCI with thrombolytic therapy showed equivalence of the two reperfusion strategies with respect to 30-day mortality when the delay to PCI was 62 minutes or more and equivalence for the two strategies for composite endpoints of death, reinfarction, or stroke when the delay to PCI was 93 minutes or more.[36] Thus for institutions where timely administration of PCI is not practical, thrombolytics remain the treatment of choice for ST segment elevation ACS.

b. Current ACC/AHA recommendations for primary PCI are summarized in Box 8-5.

5. **GP IIb/IIIa receptor inhibitors.** The role of GP IIb/IIIa receptor inhibitors in ST segment elevation ACS is still being defined.

a. Many believe that administration of a GP IIb/IIIa receptor inhibitor **in conjunction with reduced-dose thrombolytic therapy** provides more complete macrovascular and microvascular reperfusion than thrombolytic monotherapy. Several small trials in which a thrombolytic agent and GP IIb/IIIa receptor inhibitor were given concomitantly showed improvements in early angiographic IRA patency and ST segment resolution.[37-39] Larger trials, such as ASSENT 3 (tenecteplase plus abciximab vs. tenecteplase)[40] and Global Use of Strategies to Open Occluded Arteries (GUSTO) V (reteplase plus abciximab vs. reteplase),[41] have shown that survival after therapy with a GP IIb/IIIa inhibitor and thrombolytic agent is no different than after a thrombolytic agent is given alone. However, the combination is associated with a higher incidence of bleeding complications and intracranial hemorrhage, particularly in older adults. Therefore combination therapy is not justified at this time.

b. **When coupled with primary PCI,** GP IIb/IIIa receptor inhibition reduces the composite endpoint of death, MI, and the need for urgent revascularization. The ADMIRAL trial ($n = 300$) demonstrated a significant reduction in the combined endpoint of death, reinfarction, and need for urgent repeat revascularization with abciximab in patients undergoing PCI for ST segment elevation ACS (6.0% vs.

BOX 8-5

RECOMMENDATIONS FOR PRIMARY PCI

CLASS I

As an alternative to thrombolytic therapy in patients with acute MI and ST segment elevation or new or presumed new LBBB who can undergo angioplasty of the infarct-related artery within 12 hr of onset of symptoms if performed in a timely fashion (balloon inflation within 90 min of presentation) by people skilled in the procedure and supported by experienced personnel in an appropriate laboratory environment.

Specific Considerations

PCI should be performed as quickly as possible, with a DTBT goal <90 min.

If symptom duration is <3 hr and the expected DTBT minus door-to-needle time is <1 hr, PCI is preferred; if DTBT minus door-to-needle time is >1 hr, fibrinolytic therapy is preferred.

If symptom duration is >3 hr, PCI is preferred, with goal DTBT <90 min.

PCI should be considered, if clinically suitable, for patients <75 yr old with STEMI or LBBB who develop shock within 36 hr of MI and can be revascularized within 18 hr of shock.

PCI should be performed in patients with severe CHF or pulmonary edema (Killip class III) and onset of symptoms within 12 hr, with DTBT as short as possible (i.e., goal <90 min).

CLASS IIA

PCI is reasonable for patients with good functional status who are 75 yr or older with STEMI or LBBB or who develop shock within 36 hr of MI and are suitable for revascularization that can be performed within 18 hr of shock.

It is reasonable to perform PCI with symptom onset in the past 12-24 hours when CHF or hemodynamic or electrical instability is present.

CLASS IIB

The benefit of primary PCI for patients with STEMI who are eligible for fibrinolysis is not well established when performed by operators with fewer than 75 PCI procedures per year.

CLASS III

PCI should not be performed in a noninfarcted artery at the time of primary PCI in patients without hemodynamic compromise.

Primary PCI should not be performed in asymptomatic patients more than 12 hr after onset of STEMI if they are hemodynamically and electrically stable.

Data from Antman EM et al: *Circulation* 110:588-636, 2004. Available at www.acc.org. *CHF,* congestive heart failure; *DTBT,* door-to-balloon time; *LBBB,* left bundle branch block; *MI,* myocardial infarction; *PCI,* percutaneous coronary intervention; *STEMI,* ST segment elevation myocardial infarction.

8

ACUTE CORONARY SYNDROMES

14.6%, p = .01).[42] The largest study of GP IIb/IIIa receptor inhibition during primary PCI for ST segment elevation ACS, the CADILLAC study, enrolled 2082 patients and demonstrated a significant benefit when abciximab was used with PCI (with or without stenting). Major adverse events occurred in 20% of patients in the primary PCI group, 16.5% with primary PCI plus abciximab, 11.5% with stenting alone, and 10.2% with stenting plus abciximab (p < .001). The majority of benefit seen with abciximab plus stenting was related to a lower risk of repeat revascularization procedures.[43] Nonetheless, as interventional techniques evolve, GP IIb/IIIa receptor inhibitors continue to demonstrate consistent benefits for patients treated with PCI reperfusion.

V. POST-ACS TREATMENT

A. COMPLICATIONS

Approximately 80% of in-hospital deaths after ST segment elevation ACS are caused by severe left ventricular pump failure. The remaining 20% of in-hospital deaths are caused by post-MI mechanical complications (Table 8-7), including mitral regurgitation from a ruptured papillary muscle, left ventricular free wall rupture, and acute ventricular septal defect.[44] Prompt clinical evaluation and bedside echocardiography of the patient with circulatory collapse are important in establishing the diagnosis and directing therapy.

Reperfusion arrhythmias are common after antegrade blood flow is successfully reestablished in the IRA. Premature ventricular contractions, nonsustained ventricular tachycardia, accelerated idioventricular rhythm, and heart block are common after successful reperfusion. In addition, the patient with an inferior infarct may have sinus bradycardia and transient hypotension (Bezold-Jarisch reflex).

B. SECONDARY PREVENTION

Once stabilized, patients with ACS should undergo risk factor assessment followed by the initiation of medications and lifestyle interventions for

TABLE 8-7

COMPLICATIONS OF MI

	Incidence (%)	Time to Onset After MI	Percentage of MI-Associated Mortality
Papillary rupture causing severe mitral regurgitation	<1	2-7 d	5
Left ventricular rupture	2	5-14 d	10
Acute ventricular septal defect	7	Any time	5
Severe left ventricular dysfunction and shock		Any time	80

Modified from Reeder GS: *Mayo Clin Proc* 70:880, 1995.
MI, myocardial infarction.

secondary prevention. Numerous studies document that medical therapies for secondary prevention of coronary artery disease remain underused and that practice patterns vary throughout the United States.[45,46] Initiation of secondary prevention techniques should occur *before* discharge to maximize patient compliance and to ensure that the patient is on an appropriate treatment regimen. Risk factor modification should include smoking cessation and dietary counseling. Patients should be encouraged to increase the amount of weekly exercise and to lose weight if necessary. Diabetic patients should maintain tight glucose control. Secondary prevention medications, including angiotensin-converting enzyme inhibitors, beta-blockers, aspirin, and lipid-lowering agents, should also be initiated.

PEARLS AND PITFALLS

- Non–ST segment elevation ACS encompasses the two prior terms *unstable angina* and *non–Q wave MI.*
- In the patient with ST segment elevation ACS, rapid reperfusion (via primary PCI or thrombolytic therapy) salvages myocardium and improves survival. This requires rapid assessment (including 12-lead electrocardiography), triage, and risk assessment.
- At presentation, the patient with ACS should be questioned about a history of cocaine or sildenafil use.
- Patients with heparin allergy or heparin-induced thrombocytopenia who need anticoagulation should be given lepirudin or another direct thrombin inhibitor.
- β_1-selective beta-adrenergic blockers can be used safely in the patient with a history of mild to moderate obstructive pulmonary disease.[47]

REFERENCES

1. American Heart Association: *Heart disease and stroke statistics: 2004 update.* Dallas, Tex, 2003, American Heart Association. D
2. Antman E et al: The TIMI risk score for unstable angina/non-ST elevation MI: a method for prognostication and therapeutic decision making, *JAMA* 284:835, 2000. B
3. Cohen M et al: A comparison of low-molecular weight heparin with unfractionated heparin for unstable coronary disease, *N Engl J Med* 337:447, 1997. A
4. Antman E et al: Enoxaparin prevents death and cardiac ischemic events in unstable angina/non-Q wave myocardial infarction, *Circulation* 100:1593, 1999. D
5. Ferguson JJ et al, SYNERGY Trial Investigators: Enoxaparin vs. heparin in high-risk patients with non–ST-segment elevation acute coronary syndromes managed with an intended early invasive strategy: primary results of the SYNERGY randomized trial, *JAMA* 292:45-54, 2004. A
6. Mehta SR, Yusuf S, Peters RJG et al for the Clopidogrel in Unstable Angina to Prevent Recurrent Events (CURE) Trial Investigators: The Clopidogrel in Unstable Angina to Prevent Recurrent Events (CURE) trial, *N Engl J Med* 345:494, 2001. A

7. Mehta SR, Yusuf S, Peters RJG et al, for the Clopidogrel in Unstable Angina to Prevent Recurrent Events (CURE) Trial Investigators: Effects of pretreatment with clopidogrel and aspirin followed by long-term therapy in patients undergoing percutaneous coronary intervention: the PCI-CURE study, *Lancet* 358:527, 2001. A

8. Steinhubl SR, Berger PB et al, for the CREDO Investigators: Early and sustained dual oral antiplatelet therapy following percutaneous coronary intervention: a randomized controlled trial, *JAMA* 288:2411, 2002. A

9. *ACC/AHA 2002 guideline update for the management of patients with unstable angina and non–ST-segment elevation myocardial infarction,* available at www.americanheart.org. D

10. Platelet Receptor Inhibition in Ischemic Syndrome Management (PRISM) Study Investigators: A comparison of aspirin plus tirofiban with aspirin plus heparin for unstable angina, *N Engl J Med* 338:1498, 1998. A

11. PRISM-PLUS Investigators: Inhibition of the platelet glycoprotein IIb/IIIa receptor with tirofiban in unstable angina and non–Q-wave myocardial infarction, *N Engl J Med* 338:1488, 1998. A

12. PURSUIT Investigators: Inhibition of platelet glycoprotein IIb/IIIa with eptifibatide in patients with acute coronary syndromes, *N Engl J Med* 339:436, 1998. A

13. Simoons M: Effect of glycoprotein IIb/IIIa receptor blocker abciximab on outcome in patients with acute coronary syndromes without early coronary revascularisation: the GUSTO IV–ACS randomised trial, *Lancet* 357:1915, 2001. A

14. Fragmin and Fast Revascularisation During Instability in Coronary Artery Disease (FRISC II) Investigators: Invasive compared with non-invasive treatment in unstable coronary-artery disease: FRISC II prospective randomised multicentre study, *Lancet* 354:708, 1999. A

15. Cannon C et al: Tactics: TIMI 18, *N Engl J Med* 344:1879, 2001. A

16. Fox KAA et al: Interventional versus conservative treatment for patients with unstable angina or non–ST-elevation myocardial infarction: the British Heart Foundation RITA 3 randomised trial, *Lancet* 360:743, 2002. A

17. Killip T, Kimball JT: Treatment of myocardial infarction in a coronary care unit, *Am J Cardiol* 20:457, 1967. B

18. Morrow DA et al: TIMI risk score for ST-elevation myocardial infarction: a convenient, bedside, clinical score for risk assessment at presentation: an InTIME II trial substudy, *Circulation* 102:2031, 2000. B

19. Morrow DA et al: Application of the TIMI risk score for ST-elevation MI in the National Registry of Myocardial Infarction 3, *JAMA* 286:1356, 2001. B

20. Boersma E et al: Early thrombolytic treatment in acute myocardial infarction: reappraisal of the golden hour, *Lancet* 348:771, 1996. D

21. Cannon CP et al: Relationship of symptom-onset-to-balloon time and door-to-balloon time with mortality in patients undergoing angioplasty for acute myocardial infarction, *JAMA* 283:2941, 2000. B

22. Antman EM et al: *ACC/AHA guidelines for management of patients with acute myocardial infarction.* A report of the American College of Cardiology/American Heart Association Task Force on Practice Guidelines (Writing Committee to Revise the 1999 Guidelines for Management of Patients with Acute Myocardial Infarction), 2004, available at www.acc.org. D

23. ISIS-2 (Second International Study of Infarct Survival) Collaborative Group: Randomised trial of intravenous streptokinase, oral aspirin, both, or neither

among 171,817 cases of suspected acute myocardial infarction: ISIS-2, *Lancet* 2:349, 1988. A

24. GUSTO Investigators: An international randomized trial comparing four thrombolytic strategies for acute myocardial infarction, *N Engl J Med* 329:673, 1993. A

25. A comparison of reteplase with alteplase for acute myocardial infarction. The Global Use of Strategies to Open Occluded Arteries (GUSTO III) Investigators, *N Engl J Med* 337:1118, 1997. A

26. Single-bolus tenecteplase compared with front-loaded alteplase in acute myocardial infarction: the ASSENT-2 double blind randomized trial, *Lancet* 354:716, 1999. A

27. de Lemos JA, Braunwald E: ST segment resolution as a tool for assessing the efficacy of reperfusion therapy, *J Am Coll Cardiol* 38:1283, 2001. C

28. Fernandez AR et al: ST segment tracking for rapid determination of patency of the infarct-related artery in acute myocardial infarction, *J Am Coll Cardiol* 26:675, 1995. B

29. Antman EM et al: ACC/AHA guidelines for management of patients with ST-elevation myocardial infarction: executive summary. A report of the American College of Cardiology/American Heart Association Task Force on Practice Guidelines (Committee to Revise the 1999 Guidelines for Management of Patients with Acute Myocardial Infarction), *Circulation* 110:588-636, 2004, available at www.acc.org. D

30. Magid DJ et al: Relation between hospital primary angioplasty volume and mortality for patients with acute MI treated with primary angioplasty vs thrombolytic therapy, *JAMA* 284:3131, 2000. B

31. The GUSTO Investigators: The effects of tissue plasminogen activator, streptokinase, or both on coronary-artery patency, ventricular function, and survival after acute myocardial infarction, *N Engl J Med* 329:1615, 1993. A

32. Henning RA et al: A comparison of coronary angioplasty with fibrinolytic therapy in acute myocardial infarction, *N Engl J Med* 349:733, 2003. A

33. Keeley EC et al: Primary angioplasty versus intravenous thrombolytic therapy for acute myocardial infarction: a quantitative review of 23 randomised trials, *Lancet* 361:13-20, 2003. C

34. Zijlstra F et al: Long-term benefit of primary angioplasty as compared to thrombolytic therapy for acute myocardial infarction, *N Engl J Med* 341:1431, 1999. B

35. Anderson HZ et al. DANAMI-2 Investigators. A comparison of acute coronary angioplasty with fibrinolytic therapy in acute myocardial infarction, *N Engl J Med* 349(18):733-747, 2003. A

36. Nallamothu BK, Bates ER: Percutaneous coronary intervention versus fibrinolytic therapy in acute myocardial infarction: is timing (almost) everything? *Am J Cardiol* 92:824, 2003. D

37. Kleiman NS et al: Profound inhibition of platelet aggregation with monoclonal antibody 7E3 Fab after thrombolytic therapy: results of the Thrombolysis and Angioplasty in Myocardial Infarction (TAMI)-8 pilot study, *J Am Coll Cardiol* 22:381, 1993. B

38. de Lemos J et al: Abciximab improves both epicardial flow and myocardial reperfusion in ST-elevation myocardial infarction: observations from the TIMI 14 trial, *Circulation* 101:239, 2000. B

39. Strategies for Patency Enhancement in the Emergency Department (SPEED) Group: Trial of abciximab with and without low dose reteplase for acute myocardial infarction, *Circulation* 100:2788, 2000. B

8

ACUTE CORONARY SYNDROMES

40. ASSENT-3 Investigators: Efficacy and safety of tenecteplase in combination with enoxaparin, abciximab, or unfractionated heparin: the ASSENT 3 randomised trial in acute myocardial infarction, *Lancet* 358:605, 2001. A

41. GUSTO-V Investigators: Reperfusion therapy for acute myocardial infarction with fibrinolytic therapy or combination reduced fibrinolytic therapy and platelet glycoprotein IIb/IIIa inhibition: the GUSTO-V randomised trial, *Lancet* 357:1905, 2001. A

42. Montalescot G et al: Abciximab before direct angioplasty and stenting in myocardial infarction regarding acute and long-term follow-up, *N Engl J Med* 344:1895, 2001. B

43. Stone GW et al: Comparison of angioplasty with stenting, with or without abciximab, in acute myocardial infarction, *N Engl J Med* 346:957, 2002. A

44. Reeder GS: Identification and treatment of complications of myocardial infarction, *Mayo Clin Proc* 70:880, 1995. B

45. O'Connor GT et al: Geographic variation in the treatment of acute myocardial infarction, *JAMA* 281:627, 1999. B

46. Stafford RS, DC Radley: The underutilization of cardiac medications of proven benefit, 1990 to 2002, *J Am Coll Cardiol* 41:56, 2003. B

47. Salpeter SR et al: Cardioselective β-blockers in patients with reactive airway disease: a meta-analysis, *Ann Intern Med* 137:715, 2002. C

Hypertensive Urgency and Emergency

Sharon A. Chung, MD; Edward C. Hsiao, MD, PhD;
and Michael J. Klag, MD, MPH

FAST FACTS

- When examining a hypertensive patient, the physician should always assess for end organ damage. The most commonly affected organs are the heart, brain, kidneys, and eyes.
- Hypertensive emergency may occur at any blood pressure but involves damage to at least one organ system. Mean arterial blood pressure should be reduced by no more than 25% in the first 2 hours and then to a blood pressure of 160/110 mmHg within the first 6 hours of treatment.
- Hypertensive urgency is usually defined as a diastolic pressure greater than 120 mmHg without evidence of end organ damage. Blood pressure can be reduced with oral medications, although close monitoring is necessary.
- The long-term blood pressure goal should be determined by the patient's concomitant conditions and risk factors for cardiovascular disease. Blood pressure should be controlled to 140/90 mmHg or lower for patients with uncomplicated hypertension and to 130/80 mmHg or lower for patients with diabetes and chronic kidney disease.[1]
- Patients who are hypertensive in the setting of acute stroke, mesenteric ischemia, or other vascular insufficiency may need a higher blood pressure to maintain adequate organ perfusion.

9

I. EPIDEMIOLOGY

1. See Table 9-1 for the Joint National Committee 7 classification of blood pressure in adults older than 18 years.[1]
2. According to the National Health and Nutrition Examination Survey (NHANES III) data, 28.7% of American adults, or approximately 58 million people, have hypertension. Approximately 30% of these people are unaware of their hypertension, and 47% of those who are treated continue to have uncontrolled hypertension.[2]
3. Hypertensive urgency and emergency can occur at any age and may be the patient's initial presentation with hypertension. However, many cases are the result of inadequately controlled and previously diagnosed hypertension.[3] Many of the risk factors for developing hypertension and hypertensive crises are the same as those for coronary artery disease. Major risk factors include dyslipidemia, diabetes mellitus, age older

TABLE 9-1		
CLASSIFICATION OF BLOOD PRESSURE IN ADULTS		
	Blood Pressure (mmHg)	
Blood Pressure Classification	Systolic	Diastolic
Normal	<120	<80
Prehypertension	120-139	80-89
Stage 1 hypertension	140-159	90-99
Stage 2 hypertension	≥160	≥100
Hypertensive urgency (no evidence of acute organ damage)	Usually >180	Usually >120
Hypertensive emergency (rapid increase in blood pressure or evidence of acute organ injury)	Usually >180	Usually >120

than 60 years, male sex, postmenopausal status, and family history (early hypertension in women before age 65 or in men before age 55). Other important risk factors include obesity, sedentary lifestyle, nutritional factors, and alcohol use.

4. Early diagnosis of hypertension and control of elevated blood pressure decrease morbidity and mortality from cardiovascular disease and other causes, even in young patients.[4] Previous trials, including the Hypertension Optimal Treatment (HOT) trial,[5] indicate that long-term aggressive control of hypertension using multiple medications decreases the incidence of cardiovascular events.

II. CLINICAL PRESENTATION

1. The initial evaluation of any patient with suspected hypertensive urgency or emergency should focus on determining whether end organ damage is present and whether rapid control of the blood pressure is necessary (i.e., whether an inpatient or intensive care unit admission is appropriate).

2. Patients should be asked about headache, visual changes (including blurry vision), chest discomfort, dyspnea, nausea, and vomiting. The presence of these symptoms suggests end organ injury.

3. Frequent vital signs, bilateral blood pressures, a funduscopic examination, and a thorough neurologic examination are essential. New neurologic deficits represent hypertensive emergency or stroke until proven otherwise. Box 9-1 reviews the laboratory assessment of the hypertensive patient. In addition, the evaluation should attempt to determine whether the elevated blood pressure is acute or chronic. Acute elevations in blood pressure may be associated with impaired autoregulation and pressure-dependent organ perfusion and should be managed with caution.

4. The four organs most commonly involved in hypertensive emergency are the heart, brain, kidneys, and eyes (Box 9-2). All hypertensive

---

BOX 9-1

LABORATORY AND RADIOLOGIC ASSESSMENT OF THE HYPERTENSIVE PATIENT

INITIAL EVALUATION

Electrocardiogram

Hematocrit, white blood cell count, and peripheral blood smear

Basic metabolic panel

Urinalysis with microscopic examination

Chest radiograph (if heart failure or aortic dissection is suspected)

Thyroid-stimulating hormone

Noncontrast computed tomography of the head (if neurologic findings are abnormal)

OTHER EVALUATION ONCE PATIENT IS STABLE

Echocardiogram (left ventricular dysfunction, valve abnormalities, wall motion abnormalities)

Lipid profile (preferably fasting)

Thyroid function studies

Renal artery imaging (if renal stenosis is suspected)

Other evaluations as guided by clinical presentation

BOX 9-2

COMMON TARGET ORGAN INVOLVEMENT IN SEVERE HYPERTENSION

CARDIOVASCULAR	Intracerebral or subarachnoid bleeding
Myocardial infarction	Stroke or transient ischemic attack
Angina	**RENAL**
Aortic dissection	Microhematuria
Aneurysmal dilation of large vessels	Proteinuria
Left ventricular failure	Acute renal failure
Congestive heart failure	**OPHTHALMOLOGIC**
Left ventricular hypertrophy	Retinal hemorrhages or exudates
Bleeding at vascular suture lines	Papilledema
Failure of vascular surgery or graft	Arteriovenous nicking
CENTRAL NERVOUS SYSTEM	**HEMATOLOGIC**
Cerebral edema	Microangiopathic hemolytic anemia
Altered mental status (hypertensive encephalopathy)	

9

HYPERTENSIVE URGENCY AND EMERGENCY

patients should undergo a thorough workup to identify signs and symptoms of secondary hypertension (Box 9-3).

5. The cause of hypertension may be difficult to separate from the sequelae of hypertension. In hypertensive patients with renal failure or acute stroke, the underlying process often must be treated to control the patient's blood pressure. As always, appropriate evaluation and treatment should be guided by the clinical picture.

BOX 9-3

POTENTIAL CAUSES OF HYPERTENSIVE URGENCY AND EMERGENCY

NEUROLOGIC

Intracranial hemorrhage

Stroke or transient ischemic attack

Head injury or brain tumor

Seizure, especially postictal state

Encephalitis

Cerebral vasculitis

Acute anxiety

ENDOCRINE

Hyperthyroidism

Hypercalcemia

Hyperparathyroidism

Mineralocorticoid or glucocorticoid
excess

Pheochromocytoma

Acute intermittent porphyria

OBSTETRIC

Eclampsia or preeclampsia

CARDIOVASCULAR

Essential hypertension

Myocardial infarction

Acute left ventricular failure

Vasculitis

Coarctation of the aorta

Aortic dissection

Volume overload (including
pulmonary edema)

RENAL

Renal artery stenosis

Renal parenchymal disease, including
vasculitis, acute glomerulonephritis,
hemolytic-uremic syndrome

Uremia, especially in setting of volume
overload

Erythropoietin use, particularly in setting
of hyperviscosity syndrome

Chronic lead intoxication

PHARMACOLOGIC

Drug ingestions, including cocaine,
amphetamines

Monoamine oxidase inhibitor
interactions

Cyclosporine

Clonidine withdrawal and rebound
hypertension

Noncompliance with outpatient
medications

Steroids, including synthetic
corticosteroids, mineralocorticoids,
exogenous steroids (e.g., licorice)

Anesthetics, including ketamine

Sympathomimetics, including
decongestants, antiemetics,
yohimbine, sildenafil

III. TREATMENT

Figure 9-1 presents an algorithm for triage of the hypertensive patient. In
all cases, treatment should be guided by the clinical presentation.
Important points to remember when treating hypertensive urgency or
emergency include:

1. Initial antihypertensive therapy should be based on the patient's clinical
   presentation, target organ involvement, and other comorbidities.
2. Avoid sudden and precipitous decreases in blood pressure. Short-acting
   calcium channel blockers should be used with caution. Oral or
   sublingual immediate-release nifedipine should not be used because it
   is associated with increased mortality and acute myocardial infarction.[6]
3. Optimal blood pressure control usually entails the use of several agents
   from different classes, including diuretics.
4. Hypertensive urgency and emergency warrant immediate pharmacologic
   therapy; however, patient education should also emphasize medication

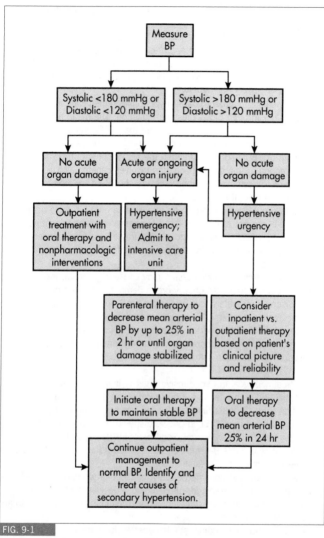

FIG. 9-1

Approach to the hypertensive patient. *BP,* blood pressure.

compliance and lifestyle modification, including abstinence from alcohol and salt restriction.

5. A secondary cause of hypertension is present in up to 5% of hypertensive patients. After blood pressure has been controlled in patients with hypertensive urgency or emergency, patients should be evaluated for causes of secondary hypertension (see Box 9-3).

A. HYPERTENSIVE EMERGENCY

1. The immediate treatment goal in hypertensive emergency is to limit end organ injury through blood pressure reduction. The mean arterial blood pressure should be reduced by no more than 25% within 2 hours using intravenous therapy (Tables 9-2 and 9-3) and then to a blood pressure of 160/110 mmHg within the first 6 hours of treatment.[1,3,7] An exception to this recommendation involves patients with aortic dissection, whose systolic blood pressure should be lowered to less than 100 mmHg if tolerated.

2. Patients should be admitted to an intensive care unit if acute organ damage is present or ongoing (e.g., hypertensive encephalopathy, myocardial infarction, acute stroke). An arterial line for continuous blood pressure monitoring usually is necessary for titration of parenteral medications.

3. Rapid decreases in blood pressure may cause vasospasm, leading to hypoperfusion and secondary organ damage, including new or worsening of acute stroke and acute renal failure. Disordered autoregulation may limit how quickly blood pressure can be reduced.

4. Once a patient with hypertensive emergency has been stabilized, the patient should be transitioned to oral antihypertensive medications based on the patient's risk factors and comorbidities.

B. HYPERTENSIVE URGENCY

1. The treatment goal in hypertensive urgency is to minimize the risk of potential end organ damage. Short-term blood pressure goals (e.g., in the first 6 to 12 hours) in this situation have not been well studied in large clinical trials.[8] Blood pressure should be reduced using oral therapy (Table 9-4) to normal blood pressure ranges as tolerated. Most medications in Table 9-4 may be titrated upward over 6 to 12 hours to achieve optimal blood pressure control.

2. Patients should be monitored closely for secondary organ damage from hypoperfusion or disordered autoregulation. Development of these complications may necessitate additional monitoring or admission to an intensive care unit.

3. Patients with long-standing, stable hypertension without evidence of end organ injury may be considered for outpatient management. Close follow-up of these patients is important, and patients who are discharged from acute care facilities with hypertensive urgency should have confirmed follow-up care within a few days.[1] Patients who may be noncompliant or are at risk for worsening sequelae from their hypertensive urgency should be treated in an inpatient setting.

TABLE 9-2
PARENTERAL VASODILATORS FOR USE IN HYPERTENSIVE CONTROL

Agent	Drug Type	Dosage	Onset/Duration of Action	Side Effects and Contraindications
Sodium nitroprusside	Direct peripheral vasodilator	0.25-10 µg/kg/min IV infusion	Immediate/2-3 min	Twitching, nausea, vomiting; monitor for thiocyanate toxicity, methemoglobinemia, increased intracerebral pressure.
Nitroglycerin	Venous and arterial dilator	5-100 µg/min IV infusion	2-5 min/5-10 min	Headache, tachycardia, vomiting, increased intracerebral pressure.
Hydralazine	Direct peripheral vasodilator	10-20 mg IV bolus or 10-40 mg intramuscularly q4-6hr	10-30 min/1-4 hr	Tachycardia, nausea, vomiting, headache, angina.
Nicardipine	Calcium channel blocker (arteriolar dilator)	5-15 mg/hr IV infusion	1-5 min/15-30 min; effects may linger for 12 hr at high dosages	Tachycardia, nausea, vomiting, headache.
Verapamil	Calcium channel blocker	5-10 mg IV bolus, then 3-25 mg/hr IV infusion	1-5 min/30-60 min	Bradycardia, heart block (especially when used with digitalis or β-blockers).
Enalaprilat	Angiotensin-converting enzyme inhibitor	0.625-5 mg IV bolus q6hr	15-60 min/12-24 hr	Renal failure in patients with renal artery stenosis.

IV, intravenous.

9

HYPERTENSIVE URGENCY AND EMERGENCY

TABLE 9-3

PARENTERAL ADRENERGIC INHIBITORS FOR USE IN HYPERTENSIVE CONTROL

Agent	Drug Type	Dosage	Onset/Duration of Action	Side Effects and Contraindications
Metoprolol	β-Blocker	5-15 mg IV bolus q30min	1 hr/3-6 hr	Bronchoconstriction, heart block, bradycardia.
Esmolol	β-Blocker	500 µg/kg IV bolus, then 25-100 µg/kg/min IV infusion	1-5 min/15-30 min	Bronchoconstriction, heart block, bradycardia.
Labetalol	α₁- and β-Blocker	20-80 mg IV bolus q10min, then 0.5-2 mg/min IV infusion	5-10 min/2-6 hr	Bronchoconstriction, heart block, bradycardia.
Phentolamine	α₁-Adrenergic antagonist	5-15 mg IV or intramuscular bolus	1-2 min/10-30 min	Tachycardia, hypotension.
Fenoldopam	Dopamine D1 and α₂ agonist	0.025-1.6 µg/kg/min IV infusion; do not give as bolus	5-15 min/1-4 hr	Headache, flushing, nausea, vomiting.

IV, intravenous.

TABLE 9-4

ORAL AGENTS COMMONLY USED FOR HYPERTENSIVE URGENCY

Agent	Drug Type	Starting Dosage/Maximum Dosage	Onset/Duration of Action	Side Effects and Contraindications
Labetalol	α- and β-Adrenergic blocker	100/1200 mg PO bid	30 min-2 hr/2-12 hr	Bronchoconstriction, heart block, bradycardia.
Metoprolol	β-Blocker	50/200 mg PO bid	1 hr/3-6 hr	Bronchoconstriction, heart block, bradycardia.
Captopril	Angiotensin-converting enzyme inhibitor	6.25/150 mg PO tid	15-30 min/2-6 hr	Hyperkalemia; may worsen renal function.
Clonidine	α_2 Agonist	0.1/1.2 mg PO bid	30-60 min/8-16 hr	Useful in cocaine-related hypertension; may cause rebound hypertension.
Methyldopa	α_2 Agonist	250/1500 mg PO bid	3-6 hr/24-48 hr	Hepatitis, cirrhosis; interacts with monamine oxidase inhibitors.
Nifedipine sustained release	Calcium channel blocker	30/120 mg PO qd	30 min/12-24 hr	May worsen liver function, congestive heart failure, aortic stenosis.
Hydralazine	Direct vasodilator	10/100 mg PO qid	1 hr/3-8 hr	Headache, tachycardia, palpitations, edema.
Minoxidil	Direct vasodilator	5/100 mg PO qd	30-60 min/10-12 hr	May worsen acute myocardial infarction, pericardial effusions.

PO, per os.

HYPERTENSIVE URGENCY AND EMERGENCY

9

4. After stabilization of the patient's hypertensive urgency, the long-term blood pressure goal should be determined by the patient's risk factors.

PEARLS AND PITFALLS

- Antihypertensive treatment should be individualized based on the patient's concomitant conditions.[1,7,9-11] Some common considerations are listed in Table 9-5.
- Use of a continuous nitroglycerin infusion and nitroprusside should be avoided in the acute management of hypertensive emergencies complicated by cerebral ischemia because these agents may worsen cerebral perfusion through an imbalance of cerebral arterial and venous dilation. Calcium channel blockers are the agents of choice in patients with elevated intracranial pressure.
- ACE inhibitors delay progression of renal disease in diabetic patients[12]

TABLE 9-5

SPECIAL CIRCUMSTANCES THAT MAY AFFECT THE CHOICE OF ANTIHYPERTENSIVE AGENTS

Condition	Useful Agents	Agents to Use with Caution
CARDIOPULMONARY DISEASE		
After myocardial infarction	β-Blockers, ACE inhibitors, angiotensin receptor blockers	Direct vasodilators (may worsen coronary insufficiency)
Congestive heart failure (systolic dysfunction)	ACE inhibitors, angiotensin receptor blockers, diuretics; β-Blockers (when euvolemic)	β-Blockers, calcium channel blockers
Tachyarrhythmias	β-Blockers (intrinsic antiarrhythmic effect), verapamil	
Angina	β-Blockers, calcium channel blockers (decrease cardiac O_2 requirement); nitrates (relax coronary vessels)	Direct vasodilators (decreased afterload may decrease coronary perfusion pressures)
Aortic dissection	Nitroprusside, β-Blockers	Drugs that increase cardiac output (increased shear stress)
Severe bronchospasm	Calcium channel blockers (may help relax airways)	β-Blockers (may induce flare of chronic obstructive pulmonary disease or asthma)
RENAL DISEASE		
Bilateral renal artery stenosis		ACE inhibitors, angiotensin receptor blockers (if serum creatinine > 2.5 mg/dl)

ACE, angiotensin-converting enzyme.

cont'd

TABLE 9-5

SPECIAL CIRCUMSTANCES THAT MAY AFFECT THE CHOICE
OF ANTIHYPERTENSIVE AGENTS—cont'd

Condition	Useful Agents	Agents to Use with Caution
Renal transplantation		ACE inhibitors and angiotensin receptor blockers (may worsen renal function)
CENTRAL NERVOUS SYSTEM		
Stroke or transient ischemic attack	ACE inhibitors (may allow reestablishment of central nervous system autoregulation)	Vasodilators (may increase intracranial pressure)
OTHER CONDITIONS		
Diabetes	ACE inhibitors (delay renal failure, decrease proteinuria)	
Pregnancy (preeclampsia, eclampsia)	Methyldopa, hydralazine; β-Blockers with caution (possible association with low birth weight)	ACE inhibitors, angiotensin receptor blockers (may cause renal agenesis), diuretics
Cocaine use	Verapamil, labetalol, clonidine	Pure β-Blockers (unopposed cocaine-induced α-agonism)
Pheochromocytoma	Combined α- and β-blockade	Selective β-Blockers (unopposed endogenous α-agonism)
Benign prostatic hypertrophy	α₁ antagonist	

ACE, angiotensin-converting enzyme.

and those with chronic renal insufficiency.[13] However, ACE inhibitors may worsen renal function in the setting of bilateral renal artery stenosis, dehydration, or acute renal failure.

- Renal artery stenosis should be considered when patients present with hypertension and flash pulmonary edema without evidence of systolic heart failure.
- In the setting of a myocardial infarction, β-blockers[14] and ACE inhibitors[15,16] have been shown to decrease morbidity and mortality.
- Although α₁ antagonists are beneficial in some patients, particularly those with benign prostatic hypertrophy, monotherapy with α₁ antagonists may be associated with increased morbidity and mortality from congestive heart failure with long-term use.[17] These drugs include doxazosin, prazosin, and terazosin.
- Endocrine disorders (Cushing's syndrome, hyperaldosteronism) should be considered when patients who are not being treated with diuretics or ACE inhibitors have elevated blood pressure and electrolyte abnormalities.
- Caution is necessary in restarting an outpatient antihypertensive regimen for patients with hypertensive urgency or emergency, particularly in

patients noncompliant with medication. These patients may not have been taking their medications as directed and are at risk for iatrogenic hypotension.
- Useful Web sites include those of the National Heart, Lung, and Blood Institute (www.nhlbi.nih.gov), American Heart Association (www.americanheart.org), and MICROMEDEX Healthcare Series (www.micromedex.com).

REFERENCES

1. Seventh report of the Joint National Committee on Prevention, Detection, Evaluation, and Treatment of High Blood Pressure, *Hypertension* 42(6):1206, 2003. D
2. Hajjar I et al: Trends in prevalence, awareness, treatment, and control of hypertension in the United States, 1988-2000, *JAMA* 290(2):199, 2003. B
3. Kaplan NM: Management of hypertensive emergencies, *Lancet* 344(8933):1335, 1994. C
4. Miura K et al: Relationship of blood pressure to 25-year mortality due to coronary heart disease, cardiovascular diseases, and all causes in young adult men: the Chicago Heart Association Detection Project in Industry, *Arch Intern Med* 161(12):1501, 2001. B
5. Hansson LA et al: Effects of intensive blood-pressure lowering and low-dose aspirin in patients with hypertension: principal results of the Hypertension Optimal Treatment (HOT) randomised trial. HOT Study Group, *Lancet* 351(9118):1755, 1998. A
6. Psaty BM et al: The risk of myocardial infarction associated with antihypertensive drug therapies, *JAMA* 274(8):620, 1995. B
7. Kaplan NM: Hypertensive crises, In *Clinical hypertension,* Baltimore, 1998, Williams & Wilkins. C
8. Cherney D et al: Management of patients with hypertensive urgencies and emergencies, *J Gen Intern Med* 17(12):937, 2002. C
9. Moser M: National recommendations for the pharmacological treatment of hypertension: should they be revised? *Arch Intern Med* 159(13):1403, 1999. D
10. Basile JN: Hypertension 2001: how will JNC VII be different from JNC VI? *South Med J* 94(9):889, 2001. D
11. Kaplan NM: Management of hypertension in patients with type 2 diabetes mellitus: guidelines based on current evidence, *Ann Intern Med* 135(12):1079, 2001. D
12. Lewis EJ et al: The effect of angiotensin-converting-enzyme inhibition on diabetic nephropathy. The Collaborative Study Group, *N Engl J Med* 329(20):1456, 1993. A
13. Randomised placebo-controlled trial of effect of ramipril on decline in glomerular filtration rate and risk of terminal renal failure in proteinuric, non-diabetic nephropathy. The GISEN Group (Gruppo Italiano di Studi Epidemiologici in Nefrologia), *Lancet* 349(9069):1857, 1997. A
14. Gottlieb SS et al: Effect of beta-blockade on mortality among high-risk and low-risk patients after myocardial infarction, *N Engl J Med* 339(8):489, 1998. B

15. Yusuf SP et al: Effects of an angiotensin-converting-enzyme inhibitor, ramipril, on cardiovascular events in high-risk patients. The Heart Outcomes Prevention Evaluation Study Investigators, *N Engl J Med* 342(3):145, 2000. A

16. Indications for ACE inhibitors in the early treatment of myocardial infarction: systematic overview of individual data from 100,000 patients in randomized trials. ACE Inhibitor Myocardial Infarction Collaborative Group, *Circulation* 97(22):2202, 1998. C

17. Furberg CD et al: Clinical implications of recent findings from the Antihypertensive and Lipid-Lowering Treatment to Prevent Heart Attack Trial (ALLHAT) and other studies of hypertension, *Ann Intern Med* 135(12): 1074, 2001. C

9

HYPERTENSIVE URGENCY AND EMERGENCY

Syncope

Esther S.H. Kim, MD; Eric H. Yang, MD; and Hunter C. Champion, MD, PhD

FAST FACTS

- Syncope is a sudden, brief loss of consciousness associated with a loss of postural tone from which recovery is spontaneous.
- In descending order of prevalence, the major causes of syncope are syncope of unknown origin, neurocardiogenic causes, cardiogenic causes, neurogenic causes, orthostatic hypotension, and psychiatric disorders.
- Prognosis is dictated by the cause of syncope; therefore it is important to distinguish between benign and life-threatening origins.
- The history and physical examination are the most important diagnostic tools in evaluating the patient with syncope.
- Neuroimaging and electroencephalography have a low diagnostic yield and should be used only when patients have a history suggestive of neurogenic syncope or focal neurologic signs on examination.
- All patients with suspected cardiogenic syncope should undergo electrocardiographic testing, Holter monitoring or inpatient telemetry, and echocardiography.
- Electrophysiologic studies should be reserved for patients with organic heart disease or conduction abnormalities.

A. EPIDEMIOLOGY

1. Syncope is a common problem resulting in 3% to 5% of all emergency department evaluations and 1% of all hospital admissions.[1]
2. Eleven percent of participants in the Framingham Heart Study followed for an average of 17 years experienced at least one episode of syncope.[2]
3. The common causes of syncope are shown in Table 10-1 and can be divided into five general categories: orthostatic hypotension, neurogenic, cardiogenic, neurocardiogenic, and syncope of unknown origin.
4. The incidence of syncope increases with age, and men are more likely than women to have cardiac causes of syncope.[2]
5. Cardiac syncope is associated with a mortality rate three times as high as that of those without syncope, whereas vasovagal syncope is not associated with a higher risk of death.[2]

B. CAUSES

1. Syncope of unknown origin is the most common type, accounting for 36% of syncopal episodes.

TABLE 10-1

CAUSES OF SYNCOPE

Cause of Syncope	Characteristics	Prevalence (%) Linzer et al.*	Prevalence (%) Schnipper et al.†
Unknown	Negative workup	34	39
Cardiogenic			
Organic heart disease (aortic stenosis, hypertrophic cardiomyopathy, pulmonary embolism, pulmonary hypertension, myxoma, myocardial infarction, coronary spasm, tamponade, aortic dissections)	Chest pain, exertional syncope, dyspnea	4	3
Arrhythmias (bradyarrhythmias, tachyarrhythmias)	Sudden syncope without prodrome, subsequent injury	14	14
Neurocardiogenic			
Vasovagal	Diaphoresis, nausea, lightheadedness, presence of clear precipitant, residual feelings of nausea and warmth present after syncope	18	14
Situational	Syncope during or immediately after micturition, cough, swallowing, or defecation	5	3
Carotid sinus sensitivity	Syncope occurring with pressure to carotid sinus: head turning, shaving, a tight collar, or neck mass	1	
Orthostatic hypotension	Occurs with standing	8	11
Neurogenic (migraines, transient ischemic attacks, seizures, subclavian steal)	Seizure activity, postictal state, hemiparesis, visual disturbances, headache	10	7
Medications	Symptoms associated with drug use	3	3
Psychiatric (anxiety disorder, panic disorder, major depression)	Frequent symptoms, lack of injury	2	1

Modified from Linzer M et al: *Ann Intern Med* 127:76, 1997; and Schnipper JL, Kapoor WN: *Med Clin North Am* 85:2, 2001.
*Based on five population-based studies in unselected patients with syncope.
†Based on six population-based studies in unselected patients with syncope.

10

SYNCOPE

2. Cardiogenic syncope is caused by a pathophysiologic cardiovascular condition: organic heart disease or dysrhythmia. The key feature of cardiogenic syncope is sudden loss of consciousness without a prodrome.

a. Organic heart disease causes 4% of syncopal episodes and includes coronary artery disease, valvular abnormalities, cardiomyopathy, and congenital heart disease.

b. Dysrhythmias account for 14% of syncopal episodes. Ventricular tachycardia is the most common arrhythmia associated with syncope.[3] Arrhythmias may also constitute a significant proportion of unexplained syncope but can be difficult to diagnose because of their paroxysmal or infrequent nature.

3. Neurocardiogenic syncope accounts for 24% of syncopal episodes and is caused by a neurally mediated reflex mechanism known as the Bezold-Jarish reflex. Inappropriate vasodilation results in an increase in venous pooling and a subsequent decrease in ventricular preload. To maintain cardiac output, the underfilled left ventricle contracts vigorously, resulting in an increase in left ventricular wall stress. To protect against excessive wall stress, there is an increase in cardiac vagal tone, which decreases heart rate and cardiac output, increasing the potential for syncope. A similar response occurs with the carotid sinus reflex, when an increase in blood pressure or extrinsic carotid sinus pressure causes an increase in cardiac vagal tone.

a. Neurocardiogenic syncope includes vasovagal syncope, situational syncope (e.g., cough syncope, micturition syncope), and carotid sinus hypersensitivity. Neurocardiogenic mechanisms are also implicated in syncope associated with ventricular outflow obstruction (e.g., aortic stenosis and pulmonary embolism) and supraventricular tachyarrhythmias.

4. Neurogenic syncope accounts for 10% of syncopal episodes. Common causes of neurogenic syncope include transient ischemic attacks, migraines, and seizures. Syncope may be accompanied by seizure activity, hemiparesis, visual disturbances, or headache.

5. Orthostatic hypotension accounts for 8% to 9% of syncopal episodes and can be caused by age-related physiologic changes, intravascular volume depletion, medications, and autonomic insufficiency. It occurs when a sudden rise from a seated or lying position results in pooling of blood in the legs, leading to decreased preload, cerebral hypoperfusion, and loss of consciousness.

C. CLINICAL PRESENTATION AND DIAGNOSIS

1. Diagnosing the cause of syncope can be costly and frustrating because there is no established gold standard test. Table 10-2 reviews the numerous diagnostic tools commonly used in a syncope workup and their diagnostic yields. A helpful algorithm for diagnosing syncope is shown in Figure 10-1.[4]

2. **History and physical examination.** The cause of a syncopal episode can be determined in 45% of cases on the basis of history and

TABLE 10-2

YIELD OF DIAGNOSTIC STUDIES IN SYNCOPE EVALUATION

Study	Cost ($)*	Yield (Range) (%)	Indications
History and physical examination	160	45 (32-74)	All patients
Electrocardiogram	90	5 (1-11)	Almost all patients
Echocardiography	580	(5-10)	Patients with known or suspected heart disease
Holter monitoring	468	19 (14-42) Positive yield 4[†] Negative yield 15[‡]	Patients with organic heart disease, abnormal ECG, or high suspicion for arrhythmia
External loop recorder[§]	284	34 (24-36) Positive yield 13 Negative yield 21	Patients with frequent syncope, suspected arrhythmia, and either no organic heart disease or heart disease or abnormal ECG with negative cardiac workup
Insertable loop recorder[§]		59 Positive yield 27 Negative yield 32	Negative cardiac workup, infrequent syncope, negative tilt table and psychiatric examinations
Electrophysiology studies[§]	4678	60 (18-75)	Organic heart disease and high suspicion for arrhythmia; clinically normal heart but high risk for bradyarrhythmia, especially if frail
Electroencephalography	493	1-2 (0-5)	Witnessed seizure, postevent confusion, history of seizure, focal neurologic symptoms or signs, seizure, or head trauma
Head computed tomography	888	4 (0-20)	Patients with focal neurologic symptoms or signs, seizure, or head trauma
Tilt table testing[§]	683	49 (26-90)	Recurrent unexplained syncope without evidence of organic heart disease or with negative cardiac workup

Modified from Linzer M et al: *Ann Intern Med* 127:76, 1997; and Schnipper JL, Kapoor WN: *Med Clin North Am* 85:2, 2001.

*Average of cost from University of Wisconsin, University of Pittsburgh Medical Center, New England Medical Center, and Duke University Medical Center.

[†]Positive yield indicates arrhythmia with symptoms.

[‡]Negative yield indicates symptoms without arrhythmia.

[§]Selected patients.

10

SYNCOPE

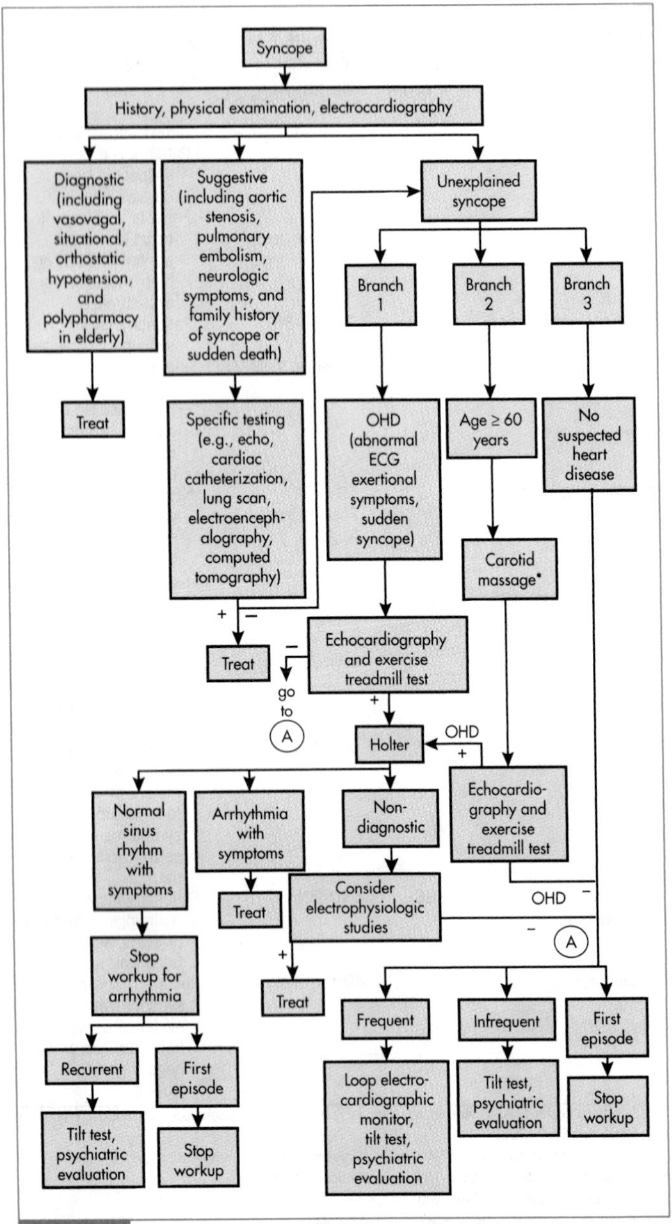

FIG. 10-1

See legend on the opposite page

physical examination alone. The history and physical examination can also help guide further diagnostic testing. Key historical features focus on what happened before, during, and after the syncopal event. Additional questions probe for potential triggers, whether any injury occurred during the event, frequency of syncopal episodes, underlying medical conditions predisposing to syncope, and a thorough review of prescription and nonprescription medications. A history taken from a family member or witness is helpful as well. Table 10-1 and Box 10-1 review key historical points and features for determining the cause of a syncopal episode. The physical examination should include an assessment of orthostatic vital signs (heart rate and blood pressure while the patient is supine, sitting, and standing at 5 minute intervals) and a thorough cardiovascular and neurologic examination.

3. **Basic laboratory testing.** Routine blood tests (complete blood cell count and chemistry) rarely identify the cause of syncope. They are not recommended, and in most cases they only confirm a clinical suspicion. Pregnancy testing is recommended for women of childbearing age, particularly if tilt table testing or electrophysiology testing is being considered.

4. **Electrocardiography.** Although the 12-lead electrocardiogram (ECG) provides a definitive diagnosis in only 5% of cases, it should be obtained in all cases of syncope. Structural or conduction abnormalities found on a resting ECG help guide more expensive and invasive evaluations for a cardiac cause.

5. **Neuroimaging and electroencephalography** are rarely diagnostic (≤ 2% cases) when used in unselected patients with syncope. These studies are recommended only for patients with histories suggestive of neurogenic syncope or focal neurologic signs on examination. Computed tomography of the head is recommended to rule out hemorrhage in patients with head trauma secondary to syncope.

6. **Echocardiography.** The efficacy of echocardiography in determining the cause of syncope is unknown. Echocardiography may not directly determine the cause of syncope, but it can identify patients with structural heart disease who are at increased risk for arrhythmias. Echocardiography reveals occult structural heart disease in 5% to 10% of unselected patients and should be part of the initial workup in all patients with suspected cardiogenic syncope.

7. **Exercise stress testing** has a diagnostic yield of less than 1% in the workup of syncope. Stress testing is recommended for evaluating exercise-associated syncope to assess for ischemia or exercise-induced

Diagnosis of syncope. *OHD,* organic heart disease. *(Modified from Linzer M et al: Ann Intern Med 126:989, 1997.)*

BOX 10-1

KEY HISTORICAL POINTS IN SYNCOPE EVALUATION

SITUATION
Sudden standing or sitting

Severe pain, fear, instrumentation

Micturition, defecation, severe coughing (especially in patients with chronic obstructive pulmonary disease)

During or immediately after exertion

PRODROME
Diaphoresis, nausea, warmth, lightheadedness

Diplopia, dysarthria, focal neurologic symptoms, headache

Chest pain, shortness of breath

Duration of prodrome

WITNESSED APPEARANCE
Tonic-clonic movements, cyanosis, urinary incontinence, tongue biting

POSTEVENT RESIDUA
Confusion

Fatigue, warmth, nausea

Neurologic symptoms

Injury from fall

Duration of recovery

PAST MEDICAL HISTORY
Previous syncopal episodes, number and frequency

Psychiatric disease

History of arrhythmias

Congestive heart failure, cardiomyopathy

Coronary disease risk factors

Cerebrovascular accident, transient ischemic attack

Pulmonary hypertension

Risk factors for pulmonary embolism

Recent dehydration, gastrointestinal bleeding

FAMILY HISTORY
Sudden death

MEDICATIONS
Antihypertensives

Antidepressants

Antianginals

Analgesics

Central nervous system depressants

QT-prolonging agents

Others (vincristine, digoxin, insulin, marijuana, alcohol, cocaine)

From Schnipper JL, Kapoor WN: *Med Clin North Am* 85:2, 2001.

arrhythmias. Echocardiography should be performed first to exclude hypertrophic cardiomyopathy or significant aortic valvular disease in all patients with exertional syncope.

8. **24-hour Holter monitoring and inpatient telemetry.**

a. The presence of an arrhythmia during monitoring is not diagnostic unless the disturbance reproduces the patient's symptoms or syncopal event. Holter monitoring or inpatient telemetry for 24 hours is recommended for all patients with suspected cardiogenic syncope, and when used for 24 hours, these tests can provide a diagnosis for syncope in 19% of patients. Monitoring for more than 24 hours may demonstrate more arrhythmias, but the yield of diagnostic, symptomatic arrhythmias does not increase.[5] In general, patients with nondiagnostic inpatient telemetry should not be sent home with further Holter monitoring.

b. The absence of arrhythmias or symptoms during monitoring does not necessarily exclude arrhythmic syncope given the episodic nature of arrhythmias. In patients with a high pretest likelihood of arrhythmias and negative Holter monitoring or inpatient telemetry, further evaluation for arrhythmias should be pursued through outpatient event monitoring, implantable loop recorders, or electrophysiologic studies.

9. **Electrophysiologic studies** are invasive studies that use electrical stimulation and monitoring to identify underlying conduction disorders and arrhythmias. These studies are safe but expensive, with diagnostic yields ranging from 32% to 60% in selected populations.[6,7] Patients with normal ECGs and no structural heart disease rarely need electrophysiologic studies. Invasive testing should be reserved for patients with known structural heart disease or conduction abnormalities. Electrophysiologic studies may be preferred over noninvasive testing in older adults with conduction disease who are at risk for morbid complications from syncope (e.g., hip fracture).

10. **Carotid sinus massage.** Carotid sinus hypersensitivity is a disease of older adults and is the cause of syncope in 1% of cases. Patients who are 60 years or older and have unexplained syncope should undergo carotid sinus massage as part of their workup unless contraindicated. A positive result is defined as symptomatic asystole for 3 or more seconds (cardioinhibitory response) or a decrease in systolic blood pressure of at least 50 mmHg (vasodepressor response) with a consistent history. Carotid sinus massage should be performed by trained staff with bedside cardiac monitoring and is contraindicated in patients with carotid bruits, history of arrhythmias, recent myocardial infarction, or stroke.

11. **Tilt table testing consists of two phases.** In the first, or passive, phase the patient is tilted from a supine position to a 60-degree angle. The patient is left in this position for several minutes in an effort to reproduce syncope or hypotension. If an endpoint (syncope or hypotension) is not reached, the patient is brought back to the supine

position and isoproterenol is infused at 1 µg/min. The patient is then retilted, and the isoproterenol infusion is continued. If an endpoint is not reached, the patient is returned to the supine position, the infusion rate is increased, and the patient is retilted. This protocol is repeated until an endpoint is obtained or the maximum infusion rate of 3 to 5 µg/min is reached.

a. Before tilt table testing, women of childbearing age should have a pregnancy test, and men older than 45 years and women older than 55 years should undergo stress testing.

b. The overall sensitivity of tilt table testing ranges from 67% to 83%, and specificity is approximately 75%. Tilt table testing should be used for patients with structurally normal hearts and infrequent syncope (less often than every 3 months). It should also be used for patients with nondiagnostic loop or Holter monitoring or symptoms suggesting vasovagal syncope but without an obvious precipitating event.

D. MANAGEMENT

1. The first decision in syncope management is whether to admit the patient. Box 10-2 provides some general indications for admission. Patients should be admitted to the hospital if rapid diagnostic evaluation is required due to suspicion for serious arrhythmias, sudden death, or newly diagnosed cardiac disease.

2. The next step is to treat the underlying cause of syncope. Fluid administration is the treatment of choice for orthostatic hypotension. Use of implantable pacemakers and defibrillators can be considered after appropriate evaluation in patients with cardiogenic syncope.

3. The effectiveness of drug therapy in preventing recurrent vasovagal syncope is open to debate. A large number of uncontrolled studies and one randomized trial[8] support use of beta-blockers, but several recent controlled trials did not show effectiveness.[9-11] No randomized studies have evaluated the effectiveness of fludrocortisone in preventing vasovagal syncope in adults, and only one small randomized, double-blind, placebo-controlled study showed midodrine to be beneficial.[12] A consensus algorithm[13] for treating vasovagal syncope suggests the use of beta-blockers for patients who have an increase in heart rate before syncope during tilt table testing. Those without significant increase in heart rate should be treated with fludrocortisone. If patients do not tolerate beta-blockers or fludrocortisone or if they are ineffective in preventing vasovagal syncope, empiric therapy with midodrine might be considered.

4. Most patients with vasovagal syncope do not need treatment beyond education and reassurance of the benign nature of their syncopal episodes. Some data suggest that orthostatic self-training and moderate exercise improve symptoms and may prevent recurrence of syncope.[14,15]

E. RISK STRATIFICATION, PROGNOSIS, AND MORTALITY

The Framingham study found that syncope (from any cause) was associated with a 31% increase in all-cause mortality. This mortality risk

---

BOX 10-2

CRITERIA FOR ADMISSION*

STRONG INDICATION

Cardiogenic syncope

Syncope in patients with heart disease (coronary artery disease, heart failure) and electrocardiographic findings (serious bradycardia or tachycardia, long QT interval, or bundle branch block)

Syncope with accompanying chest pain

Stroke or focal neurologic disorder

MODERATE INDICATION

Sudden loss of consciousness resulting in injury

Exertional syncope

Age >70 yr

Moderate to severe orthostatic hypotension

Frequent spells

From Linzer M et al: *Ann Intern Med* 127:76, 1997.
*Based on six population-based studies of patients with syncope seen in the emergency department.

---

appears to be driven mostly by a twofold increase in mortality caused by cardiogenic syncope. As mentioned previously, vasovagal syncope is not associated with an increase in the risk of death from any cause.[2]

PEARLS AND PITFALLS

- A history and physical examination can reveal the cause of syncope in approximately 45% of cases.
- Information should be obtained from witnesses of syncope whenever possible.
- Prognosis depends on the cause of syncope.
- Electrocardiography is recommended in all patients with syncope. Electrocardiographic abnormalities will guide further evaluation that may detect life-threatening disorders.

REFERENCES

1. Kapoor WN: Evaluation and outcome of patients with syncope, *Medicine* (Baltimore) 69:160-175, 1990. C
2. Soteriades E et al: Incidence and prognosis of syncope, *N Engl J Med* 347:878, 2002. B
3. Calkins H, Zipes DP: *Braunwald: heart disease—a textbook of cardiovascular medicine,* 6th ed, Philadelphia, 2001, WB Saunders. D
4. Linzer M et al: Diagnosing syncope. Part 1. Value of history, physical examination, and electrocardiography, *Ann Intern Med* 126:989, 1997. C
5. Bass EB et al: The duration of Holter monitoring in patients with syncope: is 24 hours enough? *Arch Intern Med* 150:1073-1078, 1990. B
6. Schnipper JL, Kapoor WN: Diagnostic evaluation and management of patients with syncope, *Med Clin North Am* 85:2, 2001. C
7. Linzer M et al: Diagnosing syncope. Part 2. Unexplained syncope, *Ann Intern Med* 127:76, 1997. C

8. Mahanonda N et al: Randomized double-blind, placebo-controlled trial of oral atenolol in patients with unexplained syncope and positive upright tilt table test results, *Am Heart J* 130:1250-1253, 1995. A

9. Sheldon R et al: Effects of beta blockers on the time to first syncope recurrence in patients after a positive isoproterenol tilt table test, *Am J Cardiol* 78:536-539, 1996. A

10. Madrid A et al: Lack of efficacy of atenolol for prevention of neurally-mediated syncope in highly symptomatic population: a prospective double-blind, randomized and placebo-controlled study, *J Am Coll Cardiol* 37:554-547, 2001. A

11. Sheldon R et al: *The Prevention of Syncope Trial*. Heart Rhythm Society 25th annual scientific sessions. Late breaking clinical trials 2004, San Francisco. A

12. Ward CR et al: Midodrine: a role in the management of neurocardiogenic syncope, *Heart* 79:45-49, 1998. A

13. Bloomfield DR et al: Putting it together: a new treatment algorithm for vasovagal syncope and related disorders, *Am J Cardiol* 84:33Q, 1999. C

14. Abe H et al: Usefulness of orthostatic self-training for the prevention of neurocardiogenic syncope, *Pacing Clin Electrophysiol* 25(10): 1454-1458, 2002. B

15. Mtinangi BL, Hainsworth R: Increased orthostatic tolerance following moderate exercise training in patients with unexplained syncope, *Heart* 80(6):596-600, 1998. B

Heart Failure

James O. Mudd, MD; Michael Field, MD; and Edward Kasper, MD

FAST FACTS

- The most common causes of heart failure (HF) in the United States are ischemic heart disease, hypertension, valvular heart disease, and idiopathic dilated cardiomyopathy.
- HF may result from impaired systolic function, impaired diastolic function, or a combination of the two.
- A patient's hemodynamic status can be classified based on the presence or absence of pulmonary congestion (wet or dry) and the presence or absence of poor perfusion (cold or warm).
- Diuretic therapy is the cornerstone of treatment in both acute and chronic HF.
- Angiotensin-converting enzyme (ACE) inhibitors are indicated in all cases of left ventricular dysfunction, improving both symptoms and survival.
- Beta-blocker therapy improves survival and symptoms in patients with New York Heart Association class II to IV HF.
- Digoxin therapy improves symptoms and rehospitalization rates but not mortality in patients with HF.
- Aldosterone blockade therapy improves survival and symptoms in selected patients with HF.
- Implantable cardioverter-defibrillators (ICDs) and cardiac resynchronization therapy provide survival benefit in patients with reduced left ventricular function.

11

I. EPIDEMIOLOGY

1. The prevalence of HF continues to grow, resulting in significant morbidity and mortality. Current estimates suggest that more than 5 million people have this syndrome, and another 400,000 to 700,000 develop HF each year.[1]
2. HF is a syndrome in which the heart cannot meet the metabolic demands of the body or fails to maintain adequate cardiac output in the face of rising filling pressures. Cardiomyopathy, on the other hand, is a disease of heart muscle that may or may not lead to HF. Box 11-1 lists the major forms of cardiomyopathy.
3. HF is further subclassified into systolic and nonsystolic (diastolic) HF. Approximately 30% to 50% of patients with HF have preserved left ventricular function.[2] Nonsystolic HF is defined as a clinical syndrome with signs and symptoms of HF in the setting of normal left ventricular ejection fraction (more than 50%) and the absence of valvular disease. Nonsystolic HF is heterogeneous and is caused by impaired left

---

BOX 11-1
CAUSES OF CARDIOMYOPATHY

Ischemic
Idiopathic and familial
Hypertensive disease
Valvular disease
Tachycardia-induced cardiomyopathy
Sleep apnea
Carcinoid tumor
Infiltrative disorders: amyloid, hemochromatosis, sarcoid
Connective tissue disorders: systemic lupus erythematosus, polyarteritis nodosa,
    rheumatoid arthritis, scleroderma, granulomatous disease, dermatomyositis
Endocrine and metabolic: thyrotoxicosis, hypothyroidism, pheochromocytoma,
    diabetes, myxedema, uremia, acromegaly, hypocalcemia, hypophosphatemia,
    porphyria, gout
Fabry's disease
Gaucher's disease
Glycogen storage diseases
Hematologic: polycythemia vera, sickle cell disease, leukemia, Loeffler's disease
Infectious and inflammatory: coxsackie B, human immunodeficiency virus,
    Chagas's disease, Lyme disease, adenovirus, cytomegalovirus
Medications and toxins: alcohol, cocaine, catecholamines, anthracyclines
    (doxorubicin), irradiation, cyclophosphamide, bleomycin, 5-fluorouracil, carbon
    monoxide, lithium, chloroquine, arsenic, cobalt, antimony, snake venom,
    methysergide, lead, antidepressants, disopyramide, phosphorus poisoning, sulfa
    drug hypersensitivity
Muscular dystrophies
Nutritional deficiencies: kwashiorkor, selenium, beriberi (thiamine), carnitine
    deficiency
Pericardial diseases (pseudocardiomyopathy)
Peripartum
Refsum's disease
Transplant rejection
Whipple's disease

---

ventricular relaxation, increased left ventricular stiffness, or impaired ventricular-arterial coupling. Often, both systolic and nonsystolic HF coexist. Furthermore, all patients with systolic HF have some degree of diastolic dysfunction.

II. CLINICAL PRESENTATION

1. The most common presenting symptom of HF is dyspnea.
2. Signs of HF include an accentuated S$_3$, pulmonary rales, pleural effusions, elevated jugular venous pressure, sustained abdominojugular reflux, lower extremity edema, Cheyne-Stokes respirations, a pulsatile

liver, and ascites. Subtle signs and symptoms of fluid overload from HF include low-grade fevers, slight increases in abdominal girth, nausea, and anorexia.

3. Elevated jugular venous pressure and an audible S_3 in patients with left ventricular dysfunction are associated with a higher risk of hospitalizations for HF and death.[3]

4. Quantification of symptoms is based on the New York Heart Association (NYHA) classification scheme (Box 11-2).

5. **Determining a patient's hemodynamic profile is the most important step in evaluating a patient with suspected HF;** the profile is based on evidence of congestion (wet vs. dry) or evidence of low perfusion (cold vs. warm). On the basis of this evaluation, patients can be placed into four hemodynamic profiles, as shown in Table 11-1.

a. Evidence of congestion.

   (1) Symptoms of left-sided congestion: dyspnea at rest or early in exertion, orthopnea, paroxysmal nocturnal dyspnea.

   (2) Symptoms of right-sided congestion: lower extremity edema, abdominal fullness and bloating, and anorexia.

   (3) Physical signs: elevated jugular venous pressure, pulmonary rales, loud P_2, new or worsening S_3, lower extremity edema, pulsatile liver. The most useful physical finding is elevation of the jugular venous pressure both in the acute setting and longitudinally when treating chronic HF.

b. Evidence of low perfusion.

   (1) Symptoms often are protean, including fatigue, somnolence, poor concentration, and anorexia.

   (2) Physical signs include pallor, cool extremities, low volume pulses, and a narrow pulse pressure.

   (3) A proportional pulse pressure ([systolic blood pressure (SBP) − diastolic blood pressure (DBP)]/SBP) less than 0.25 is 91%

BOX 11-2

NEW YORK HEART ASSOCIATION CLASSIFICATION

Class I: Symptoms of heart failure only at levels that would limit normal individuals

Class II: Symptoms of heart failure with ordinary exertion

Class III: Symptoms of heart failure on less than ordinary exertion

Class IV: Symptoms of heart failure at rest

TABLE 11-1

HEMODYNAMIC PROFILES IN HEART FAILURE

		Congestion at Rest?	
		No	Yes
Low Perfusion at Rest?	No	Dry-warm	Wet-warm
	Yes	Dry-cold	Wet-cold

Modified from Nohria A, Lewis E, Stevenson L: *JAMA* 287:628, 2002.

sensitive and 83% specific for a low output state (cardiac index of 2.2 L/min/m^2 or less).[4]

6. **Evidence of systolic or diastolic dysfunction.** Several features of the history and physical examination assist in determining whether HF is caused primarily by systolic or diastolic dysfunction. Clinical findings can be confirmed with the use of echocardiography.

a. **Systolic HF.** Evidence of cardiomegaly on chest radiograph, anterior Q waves on electrocardiogram, left bundle branch block, diffuse soft apical impulse, pulse greater than 100, and SBP less than 90.[5]

b. **Nonsystolic HF.** Hypertension during the HF episode with SBP greater than 160 mmHg or DBP greater than 100 mmHg. Other suggestive features include an S$_4$, female sex, history of hypertension, electrocardiographic evidence of left ventricular hypertrophy, tobacco use, advanced age, and no prior history of myocardial infarction (MI).

c. Although the aforementioned clinical findings are suggestive, in practice systolic and nonsystolic HF may be difficult to delineate because there is significant overlap in their clinical presentations.[6]

III. DIAGNOSIS

1. **Laboratory evaluation** should include a complete blood cell count, comprehensive metabolic panel, coagulation studies, thyroid-stimulating hormone, creatine kinase with isozymes, and troponin. Measurement of brain natriuretic peptide is useful in addressing new onset HF and potentially in following patients with chronic HF longitudinally, although such measurements should not be used in isolation but rather in combination with the history and physical examination.[7,8] In patients with newly diagnosed HF of unclear origin, assays for ferritin, total iron-binding capacity, antinuclear antibody, rheumatoid factor, urinary metanephrines, human immunodeficiency virus antibody testing, and serum and urine protein electrophoresis should be performed.

2. **Electrocardiogram.** An electrocardiogram should be obtained on all patients with new or chronic HF to assess for signs of myocardial ischemia, new conduction abnormalities, chamber enlargement, pericarditis, or right heart failure.

3. **Chest radiography.** Radiographic findings depend on the degree of HF and may include cardiomegaly, diffuse bilateral infiltrates extending from the hila, Kerley B lines, and pleural effusions. These findings may be absent in patients with chronic HF with isolated right heart failure or those who have adapted to elevated left ventricular filling pressures with enhanced pulmonary lymphatic clearance.

4. **Echocardiography.** All patients with a new-onset HF should undergo transthoracic echocardiography to assess systolic and diastolic function, valvular abnormalities, filling pressures, and pericardial disease.

5. **Right and left heart catheterization.** Coronary angiography is indicated for almost all patients with newly diagnosed HF to exclude ischemic

heart disease if a readily apparent explanation does not exist. Right heart catheterization (Swan-Ganz catheter) provides information about right- and left-sided filling pressures, pulmonary artery pressures, cardiac output, and systemic vascular resistance.

6. **Endomyocardial biopsy.** Some investigators have found right-sided endomyocardial biopsy helpful as it may help facilitate the diagnosis in 80% of patients with unexplained cardiomyopathy.[9]

7. **Exercise testing.** Exercise testing can be used to detect ischemic heart disease and provides an estimate of functional capacity for risk stratification and prognosis in patients with known HF. Measurement of maximal oxygen uptake is an objective index of functional severity and the best index of prognosis, and it can be used to determine the necessity and timing of cardiac transplantation in patients with chronic HF. The 6-minute walk test (distance the patient can walk in 6 minutes) is a simpler test used in clinical practice that correlates with maximal oxygen uptake.

IV. TREATMENT

A. ACUTE HF

A systematic search for precipitating causes must be performed in every patient with new-onset or worsening HF (Box 11-3). Therapy should be directed at the underlying cause (if identified and treatable) and standard HF therapy initiated on the basis of one of four clinical hemodynamic profiles (Table 11-1).

1. **Treatment goals by hemodynamic profile.**

a. **Wet and warm.** This is the most common hemodynamic profile in HF. These patients have congestion resulting from elevated filling pressures and volume overload. Congestion can be relieved with intravenous loop diuretics, and patients may benefit from intravenous or oral vasodilators such as nitroglycerin. Positive inotropic agents often are unnecessary and may be detrimental in patients who do not have evidence of low perfusion.

BOX 11-3

PRECIPITANTS OF ACUTE DECOMPENSATED HEART FAILURE

Myocardial ischemia

Hypertension

Infection (myocarditis)

Arrhythmia

Noncompliance with medication

Sodium and fluid indiscretion (dietary noncompliance)

Excessive alcohol intake

Pulmonary embolism

Thyrotoxicosis

High output (thyrotoxicosis, arteriovenous fistula, pregnancy, anemia)

b. **Wet and cold.** Patients with congestion and critically limited hypoperfusion often must be "warmed up" before they can be "dried out."[10] Perfusion may be improved through the use of vasodilators alone, although these patients may have therapy-limiting hypotension necessitating inotropic agents such as dopamine, milrinone, or dobutamine. In cases unresponsive to inotropic support, mechanical circulatory support with left ventricular assist devices or intraaortic balloon pump may be necessary as a lifesaving measure and a bridge to heart transplantation.

c. **Dry and warm.** This hemodynamic profile represents compensated HF, and many patients with this form do not need inpatient management. Efforts should be aimed at maintaining stable volume status and preventing disease progression, as outlined later in this chapter.

d. **Dry and cold.** This small subgroup of patients has a low cardiac output and evidence of poor perfusion but no clinical evidence of elevated filling pressures. Patients may respond transiently to inotropes, but long-term use has produced adverse effects. Careful management with ACE inhibitors, beta-blockers, and digoxin may lead to improvement in some patients, whereas others with unrecognized congestion may benefit from diuresis.

2. Pharmacologic agents in acute HF.

a. **Morphine** is a μ-opioid receptor agonist with both vascular and central effects providing symptomatic relief in acute pulmonary edema through venodilation and a decreased perception of dyspnea. Potential side effects include hypotension, somnolence, and respiratory depression.

b. **Diuretics.**

  (1) **Loop diuretics,** such as furosemide, are the cornerstone of therapy in acute decompensated HF. Furosemide produces acute venodilation and increases sodium excretion, thereby reducing preload and pulmonary vascular congestion.

    (a) In acute HF, patients who have been taking oral loop diuretics should be switched to intravenous therapy because intestinal absorption of oral agents may be limited by bowel wall edema. Patients with renal insufficiency may need higher dosages of loop diuretics, and some may respond better to a continuous infusion than intermittent doses.

    (b) The starting intravenous dosage typically is half of the home oral dosage. If there is not an adequate response (100 to 200 ml urine output) within 30 minutes, the dosage should be doubled until the patient responds. Once an effective dosage is identified, further diuresis can be accomplished by increasing the frequency of administration.

    (c) The diuretic effect of furosemide lasts 6 hours. Afterward, the kidneys are highly sodium avid, and diuretic efficacy will be lost if the patient is not maintained on a low-sodium diet as well.

    (d) Markers of adequate diuresis include resolution of dyspnea, decrease in jugular venous pressure, decrease in intensity of S_3, elevation of serum creatinine level, and attainment of dry weight. Side effects of loop diuretics include hypokalemia, hypomagnesemia, hyponatremia or hypernatremia, volume depletion, renal failure, and reversible ototoxicity.

(2) Adding a **thiazide diuretic** such as chlorothiazide can potentiate the effect of loop diuretics by preventing compensatory distal tubular reabsorption of sodium. Thiazide diuretics should be given approximately 30 minutes before a loop diuretic is administered.[11]

c. **Nesiritide,** or recombinant B-type natriuretic peptide, is a natriuretic peptide with potent vasodilator and natriuretic effects that reduce pulmonary capillary wedge pressure, right atrial pressure, and systemic vascular resistance and increase cardiac index.[12] Nesiritide is associated with a lower incidence of arrhythmias than that of other inotropes and may be particularly useful in patients with decompensated HF and tachyarrhythmias. The most common adverse effect of nesiritide is hypotension.

d. **Vasodilators.**

(1) **ACE inhibitors** are started at low dosages with short-acting agents such as captopril and titrated to the maximum tolerated dosage. Blood pressure response, symptoms, and serum potassium and creatinine levels should be monitored closely. Once short-acting agents are tolerated, patients should be transitioned to long-acting agents. About 10% to 30% of patients with advanced HF cannot tolerate ACE inhibitors because of hypotension or renal dysfunction.[8]

(2) **Organic nitrates** such as nitroglycerin are vasodilators (particularly of the systemic veins), resulting in decreased preload. Nitrates have a role in the management of acute pulmonary edema and HF in the setting of hypertension or angina. Contraindications include concurrent sildenafil use and severe aortic stenosis.

(3) **Hydralazine** is a potent short-acting arterial vasodilator that can be used alone or in combination with nitrates for rapid afterload reduction. It is often considered as an alternative to ACE inhibitors and angiotensin II receptor blockers (ARBs) in patients with acute renal failure and other conditions in which ACE inhibitors are contraindicated.

(4) **Nitroprusside** is a potent intravenous arterial vasodilator that may be warranted if further vasodilation and afterload reduction are necessary. Adverse effects include thiocyanate toxicity, particularly in patients with hepatic or renal dysfunction, and coronary steal phenomenon in patients with ischemic heart disease.

e. **Beta-blockers** should be used with caution in acute HF exacerbations. Patients naive to beta-blockade should be euvolemic and tolerating a stable dosage of ACE inhibitors before beginning beta-blocker therapy. Patients already on beta-blockers may have to have their dosage temporarily reduced, but beta-blockers should not be withdrawn unless hypotension or cardiogenic shock is present.

11

HEART FAILURE

f. **Inotropes** may be used for the temporary treatment of diuretic-refractory acute HF (i.e., cold and wet) and as a bridge to definitive treatment such as revascularization or cardiac transplantation. Inotropes may also be appropriate as a palliative measure in patients with end-stage HF. The routine use of inotropes is not indicated in either acute or chronic HF.[13]

   (1) **Dopamine** is an endogenous catecholamine that has distinct cardiovascular effects at escalating dosages: Low-dose dopamine (1 to 3 µg/kg/min) acts through dopaminergic receptors, leading to increased renal blood flow and natriuresis; intermediate dosages (2 to 10 µg/kg/min) result in predominant beta-adrenergic receptor stimulation, increasing cardiac output by augmenting contractility and heart rate; higher dosages (10 to 20 µg/kg/min) result in increased afterload through alpha-adrenergic stimulation, which may be detrimental in HF. Dopamine should be used primarily to stabilize hypotensive patients. Tachycardia may be an undesirable side effect, particularly in those with ischemic heart disease or diastolic dysfunction who depend on filling time. Low-dose dopamine in critically ill patients has not been shown to improve diuresis and does not provide renal protection in patients with renal dysfunction.[14]

   (2) **Dobutamine** is a beta-adrenergic agonist with a predominant hemodynamic effect of direct inotropic stimulation with reflex arterial vasodilation, resulting in afterload reduction and increased cardiac output. Side effects include hypotension, ventricular arrhythmias, and potentially worsening ischemic heart disease by increasing myocardial oxygen demand.

   (3) **Milrinone,** a phosphodiesterase inhibitor, increases contractility and produces vasodilation. As with dobutamine, hypotension and arrhythmias may occur.

3. **Response to therapy.** Once treatment has begun, careful attention should be paid to daily weights, urine output, jugular venous pressure, and pulse pressure. Use of Swan-Ganz catheters in patients with acute HF exacerbations who do not otherwise have an indication for a Swan-Ganz catheter is safe but does not alter length of stay, rehospitalization rates, or mortality.[15]

B. CHRONIC HF

1. Systolic HF.

Staging: HF is a continuum of stages progressing from asymptomatic to advanced disease (Fig. 11-1).

Stage A: Patients at high risk for left ventricular dysfunction.
The leading risk factor for HF is ischemic heart disease, accounting for approximately 60% of new cases.[16] Other risk factors include hypertension, diabetes mellitus, familial history, and presence of cardiotoxins such as excessive alcohol, radiation, and chemotherapy. Interventions include controlling hypertension[17] and hyperlipidemia;

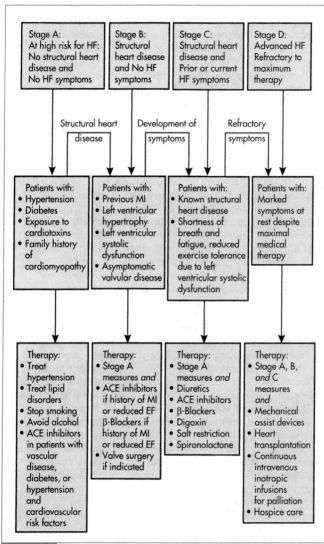

FIG. 11-1

Stages in the evolution of heart failure and recommended therapy by stage.[9] *ACE*, angiotensin-converting enzyme; *EF*, ejection fraction; *HF*, heart failure; *MI*, myocardial infarction.

discouraging smoking, excessive alcohol intake, and illicit drug use; and encouraging exercise and weight loss. ACE inhibitors are indicated for patients with atherosclerotic vascular disease (MI, cerebrovascular accident, peripheral vascular disease) or diabetes with associated risk factors.[18]

Stage B: Patients with structural heart disease in whom symptoms have not yet developed. Asymptomatic patients with a prior MI, evidence of left ventricular hypertrophy, left ventricular dysfunction, or valvular disease are at very high risk for HF. In addition to the recommendations for stage A, all patients with systolic dysfunction, regardless of symptoms, should receive ACE inhibitors. ACE inhibitors and beta-blockers are indicated for patients with a history of MI regardless of the ejection fraction. Beta-blockers may be used for patients with asymptomatic systolic dysfunction, although the evidence is not as strong as it is for symptomatic patients. Valvular repair or replacement should be performed according to published guidelines (see Chapter 12).[19]

Stage C: Patients with left ventricular dysfunction with current or prior symptoms. Readmission for HF occurs at a high rate (30% to 50%) in the 6 months after discharge. A number of criteria should be met before discharge, including transition to oral medications for 24 hours, achievement of dry weight, stable or improving renal function, and ambulation with decreased dyspnea and without symptomatic hypotension. During hospitalization patients should receive education about sodium and fluid restriction and recommendations for exercise. Patients should monitor their weight at home and may benefit from a sliding scale outpatient diuretic regimen based on their daily weight. Vaccination for pneumococcal infection and influenza is recommended. Use of nonsteroidal antiinflammatory drugs for patients with advanced HF should be avoided because it may lead to fluid retention and renal dysfunction. Recommendations listed under stage A and B apply as well.

Stage D: Patients with refractory end-stage HF. Recommendations include meticulous control of fluid retention with diuretics. ACE inhibitors and beta-blockers are beneficial, but these patients are at particular risk of developing hypotension and renal failure with ACE inhibitors and worsening HF with beta-blockers. Cardiac transplantation should be considered in eligible patients. Left ventricular assist devices provide hemodynamic support for patients awaiting heart transplantation and may be beneficial even for patients who are not candidates for heart transplantation.[20] Continuous intravenous inotropic infusions and hospice may be used as palliative measures in patients with end-stage HF.

2. Pharmacologic agents in chronic HF.

a. **ACE inhibitors** are indicated for all patients with systolic dysfunction as they improve survival, relieve symptoms, prevent hospitalization, and halt the progression of left ventricular remodeling.[21,22] They may have added benefit at higher dosages,[23] and attempts should be made to achieve target dosages reported in major clinical trials (lisinopril 20 to

40 mg/day, enalapril 10 mg twice a day, or captopril 50 mg three times a day). The benefit of ACE inhibitors in HF is independent of their blood pressure–lowering effect. Cough and angioedema are adverse effects most commonly associated with ACE inhibitors. Contraindications include symptomatic hypotension, acute renal failure, bilateral renal artery stenosis, hyperkalemia, and pregnancy.

b. **ARBs.** When patients are intolerant of ACE inhibitors, use of an ARB results in a significant reduction in mortality and HF hospitalizations.[24] As with ACE inhibitors, however, ARBs should not be used in the presence of acute renal failure or hyperkalemia and may produce symptomatic hypotension. Studies directly comparing ARBs and ACE inhibitors have shown no greater survival with use of ARBs.[25,26] Addition of an ARB to a regimen with an ACE inhibitor shows a trend toward improvement in mortality and reduced hospitalizations.[27] Given the greater experience with ACE inhibitors, they should be used as first-line agents, and ARBs should be reserved for patients who cannot tolerate ACE inhibitors.

c. **Nitrates and hydralazine.** Isosorbide dinitrate (40 mg four times a day) combined with hydralazine (75 mg four times a day) has been shown to improve survival in chronic HF.[28] Although inferior to ACE inhibitors, this combination should be considered for patients who cannot tolerate ACE inhibitors and ARBs.[29] A "nitrate-free" interval should be allowed to prevent the development of nitrate tolerance in patients on long-term therapy. This combination may be especially useful in African American patients with HF.[30]

d. **Beta-blockers.** Several beta-blockers have been shown to reduce mortality in patients with symptomatic HF and systolic dysfunction, including metoprolol, carvedilol, and bisoprolol.[31,32] All stable, euvolemic patients with NYHA class II to IV HF resulting from left ventricular dysfunction should receive a beta-blocker unless they cannot tolerate beta-blockers or have a contraindication. Usually an ACE inhibitor is titrated first, and the beta-blocker is added sequentially in the outpatient setting. Metoprolol extended release (metoprolol succinate) can be initiated at 25 mg per os (PO) daily (12.5 mg PO daily in NYHA class IV) and titrated slowly (monthly) to a maximum dosage of 200 PO daily. Carvedilol is begun at 3.125 mg PO twice daily and titrated (every 2 weeks) to a maximum dosage of 25 to 50 mg PO twice daily. Bisoprolol is begun at a dosage of 1.25 PO daily and titrated to 10 mg PO daily. Carvedilol has been shown to have a survival advantage over short-acting metoprolol[33] and better ejection fraction compared with extended-release metoprolol in a meta-analysis.[34] Contraindications to beta-blockade include acute decompensated HF, symptomatic bradycardia, advanced heart block, and severe bronchospastic disease. Although many patients take atenolol, no studies evaluating the use of atenolol in chronic HF have been presented.

11

HEART FAILURE

e. **Diuretics.**

    (1) **Loop diuretics.** In addition to their role in acute management of HF, loop diuretics have a central role in long-term management to attenuate progressive volume overload caused by compensatory sodium avidity. Diuretics are indicated for patients with symptomatic HF even after they have been rendered free of edema and generally are necessary indefinitely. Serum electrolytes should be monitored closely given the concern for increased risk of arrhythmic death in patients with HF taking non–potassium-sparing diuretics.[35]

    (2) **Aldosterone antagonism.** Aldosterone blockade provides a diuretic effect and modulates the harmful effects of aldosterone on the heart. Spironolactone, a potassium-sparing diuretic, has been shown to decrease both mortality and rehospitalization by one third in patients with primarily NYHA class III to IV HF.[36] Spironolactone is given as a once-daily dose of 25 mg to those without renal insufficiency or hyperkalemia. Patients should have stable serum creatinine levels less than 2.5 mg/dl and serum potassium less than 5 mmol/L, should undergo frequent electrolyte monitoring for hyperkalemia, and should not receive daily potassium supplementation.[37] Gynecomastia, breast pain, menstrual irregularities, and impotence are troubling side effects in about 10% of patients. Eplerenone is another alternative shown to reduce all-cause mortality in patients with reduced left ventricular ejection fraction after an MI.[38]

f. **Digoxin.** Digoxin is a glycoside shown to improve symptoms and prevent hospitalization in patients with systolic dysfunction.[39] It is indicated for patients with HF symptoms despite optimal therapy with ACE inhibitors and diuretics or for patients with coexisting atrial fibrillation. Toxic effects are more likely to occur in patients with renal insufficiency, electrolyte abnormalities, advanced age, and coadministration of other antiarrhythmic drugs (e.g., amiodarone, quinidine, verapamil, propafenone). Toxic manifestations include confusion, nonspecific gastrointestinal complaints, vision and color disturbances, and arrhythmia.

g. **Warfarin.** Anticoagulation with warfarin is warranted for patients with concomitant atrial fibrillation, visible thrombus on echocardiogram, or a previous cardioembolic event.[40] Although many consider anticoagulation for patients with a very low ejection fraction (< 20%), recent data from the Warfarin and Antiplatelet Therapy in Heart Failure (WATCH) trial suggest no short-term (23 months) benefit in reducing the incidence of nonfatal stroke, death, or nonfatal MI in patients with an ejection fraction of 35% or less randomized to aspirin, clopidogrel, or Coumadin.[41]

h. **Exercise.** A prescription for exercise may improve functional capacity and quality of life and prevent death from cardiovascular disease.[42]

i. **Maintenance of sinus rhythm.** Patients with HF benefit from normal sinus rhythm. Achieving this goal can be difficult with antiarrhythmic drugs in HF given potential drug interactions. Recent literature has shown an improvement in ejection fraction, symptoms, exercise capacity, and quality of life when patients are maintained in sinus rhythm by means of catheter ablation.[43]

3. Nonsystolic HF.

Acute exacerbations of nonsystolic HF generally are treated in a similar fashion as acute exacerbations of systolic HF. Few large trials have evaluated long-term treatment for nonsystolic HF. Based on the pathophysiology of diastolic dysfunction, four principles may be used to guide management.[9,44]

a. **Control of blood pressure.** Beta-blockers, ACE inhibitors, ARBs, and calcium channel blockers may be used to control SBP and DBP according to published guidelines. In the largest treatment trial for nonsystolic HF, the ARB candesartan, when added to traditional medical therapy, was associated with fewer hospitalizations for HF.[45]

b. **Control of tachycardia.** Patients with atrial fibrillation need rate control and may benefit from an attempt at cardioversion to optimize left ventricular filling.

c. **Control of pulmonary congestion and edema.** Patients may have rales and evidence of volume overload (elevated neck veins and peripheral edema). Loop diuretics such as furosemide decrease filling pressures and relieve pulmonary congestion. Care must be taken with diuresis because patients with diastolic HF are sensitive to preload reduction, and hypotension or prerenal azotemia may develop.

d. **Assessment and control of ischemia.** Revascularization should be considered for patients with evidence of ischemia.

4. **Device therapy for HF.** Patients with HF and reduced left ventricular function are at a higher risk for sudden cardiac death caused by ventricular arrhythmias. The Multicenter Automatic Defibrillator Implantation Trial II (MADIT II) showed a lower all-cause mortality for the use of ICDs as primary prevention in patients with a left ventricular ejection fraction less than 30% in cardiomyopathy of ischemic origin.[46] ICDs also provide a mortality benefit when used in patients with cardiomyopathy of nonischemic origin.[47] Combining ICD therapy with a biventricular pacemaker, known as cardiac resynchronization therapy, has also been shown to reduce all-cause mortality and hospitalizations in patients with ischemic or nonischemic cardiomyopathies.[48] Given these trials, ICDs with and without cardiac resynchronization therapy have become additional tools in the management of HF (see Chapter 15).

PEARLS AND PITFALLS

■ Patients already on beta-blocker therapy with HF exacerbations should remain on their current dosage (hemodynamics permitting) without escalation, whereas those who are naive to beta-blockers should not

11

HEART FAILURE

receive beta-blockade until clinically euvolemic and on a stable ACE inhibitor dosage.
- Accurate bedside determination of jugular venous pressure is crucial to successful management of HF.
- Frequent outpatient evaluation in chronic HF management helps to reduce hospitalizations.
- Care should be taken with the use of nonsteroidal antiinflammatory drugs, metformin, thiazolidinediones, sildenafil, and antiarrhythmic drugs because these medications may precipitate exacerbations of HF.
- Daily weight measurement at home allows patients to titrate diuretics to a goal weight.
- Atrial fibrillation can be deleterious to patients with systolic and nonsystolic HF.
- Patients who need positive inotropic support with dobutamine or dopamine may not receive the full benefit of these agents if on beta-blockers.

REFERENCES

1. American Heart Association: *Heart disease and stroke statistics: 2004 update,* Dallas, 2003, American Heart Association. C
2. Vasan RS, Benjamin EJ, Levy D: Prevalence, clinical features and prognosis of diastolic heart failure: an epidemiologic perspective, *J Am Coll Cardiol* 26:1565, 1995. B
3. Drazner MH et al: Prognostic importance of elevated jugular venous pressure and a third heart sound in patients with heart failure, *N Engl J Med* 345:574, 2001. B
4. Stevenson LW, Perloff JK: The limited reliability of physical signs for estimating hemodynamics in chronic heart failure, *JAMA* 261:884-888, 1989. C
5. Badgett RG, Lucey CR, Mulrow CD: Can the clinical examination diagnose left-sided heart failure in adults? *JAMA* 277(21):1712-1719, 1997. C
6. McDermott MM et al: Hospitalized congestive heart failure patients with preserved versus abnormal left ventricular systolic function: clinical characteristics and drug therapy, *Am J Med* 99:629, 1995. C
7. Maisel AS et al: Rapid measurement of B-type natriuretic peptide in the emergency diagnosis of heart failure, *N Engl J Med* 347:161, 2002. A
8. Packer ML: Should B-type natriuretic peptide be measured routinely to guide the diagnosis and management of chronic heart failure? *Circulation* 108:2950, 2003. C
9. Ardehali H et al: Endomyocardial biopsy plays a role in diagnosing patients with unexplained cardiomyopathy, *Am Heart J* 147(5):919-923, 2004. B
10. Nohria A, Lewis E, Stevenson L: Medical management of advanced heart failure, *JAMA* 287:628, 2002. C
11. Hunt S et al: ACC/AHA guidelines for the evaluation and management of chronic heart failure in the adult: executive summary. A report of the American College of Cardiology/American Heart Association Task Force on Practice Guidelines (Committee to Revise the 1995 Guidelines for the Evaluation and Management of Heart Failure), *J Am Coll Cardiol* 38(7):2101-2113, 2001. D
12. Colucci W et al: Intravenous nesiritide, a natriuretic peptide, in the treatment of decompensated congestive heart failure, *N Engl J Med* 343:246, 2000. A
13. Felker G et al: Inotropic therapy for heart failure: an evidence-based approach, *Am Heart J* 142:393, 2001. C

14. Australian and New Zealand Intensive Care Society Clinical Trials Group: Low-dose dopamine in patients with early renal dysfunction: a placebo-controlled randomized trial, *Lancet* 356:2139, 2000. A

15. Binanay C et al: Evaluation study of congestive heart failure and pulmonary artery catheterization effectiveness: the ESCAPE trial, *JAMA* 294:1625, 2005. A

16. He J et al: Risk factors for congestive heart failure in US men and women: NHANES I epidemiologic follow-up study, *Arch Intern Med* 161:996, 2001. B

17. Levy D et al: The progression from hypertension to congestive heart failure, *JAMA* 275:1557, 1996. C

18. Heart Outcomes Prevention Evaluation (HOPE) Investigators: Effects of an angiotensin-converting enzyme inhibitor, ramipril, on cardiovascular events in high risk patients, *N Engl J Med* 342:145, 2000. A

19. Bonow RO et al: ACC/AHA guidelines for the management of patients with valvular heart disease: a report of the American College of Cardiology/American Heart Association Task Force on Practice Guidelines (Committee on Management of Patients with Valvular Heart Disease), *J Am Coll Cardiol* 32:1486, 1998. D

20. Rose E et al: Long-term use of a left ventricular assist device for end-stage heart failure. Randomized Evaluation of Mechanical Assistance for the Treatment of Congestive Heart Failure (REMATCH) Study Group, *N Engl J Med* 345:1435, 2001. A

21. CONSENSUS Trial Study Group: Effects of enalapril on mortality in severe congestive heart failure: results of the Cooperative North Scandinavian Enalapril Survival Study, *N Engl J Med* 316:1429, 1987. A

22. SOLVD Investigators: Effect of enalapril on survival in patients with reduced left ventricular ejection fractions and congestive heart failure, *N Engl J Med* 325:293, 1991. A

23. Packer M et al: Comparative effects of low and high doses of the angiotensin-converting enzyme inhibitor, lisinopril, on morbidity and mortality in chronic heart failure. ATLAS Study Group, *Circulation* 100:2312, 1999. A

24. Coletta AP, Cleland JG, Freemantle N: Clinical trials update from the European Society of Cardiology: CHARM, BASEL, EUROPA and ESTEEM, *Eur J Heart Fail* 5:697, 2003. C

25. Pitt B et al: Randomized trial of losartan versus captopril in patients over 65 with heart failure. Evaluation of Losartan in the Elderly (ELITE) Study Investigators, *Lancet* 349:747, 1997. A

26. Pitt B et al: Effect of losartan compared with captopril on mortality in patients with symptomatic heart failure: randomised trial. The Losartan Heart Failure Survival Study ELITE II, *Lancet* 355:1582, 2000. A

27. McMurray JJV et al for the CHARM investigators and committees: Effects of candesartan in patients with chronic heart failure and reduced left-ventricular systolic function taking angiotensin converting enzyme inhibitors. The CHARM-Added trial, *Lancet* 362:767, 2003. A

28. Cohn JN et al: The effect of vasodilator therapy on mortality in chronic congestive heart failure: the results of the VA Cooperative Study. VA Cooperative Study Group, *N Engl J Med* 314:1547, 1986. A

29. Cohn JN et al: A comparison of enalapril with hydralazine-isosorbide dinitrate in the treatment of chronic congestive heart failure, *N Engl J Med* 325:303, 1991. A

30. Taylor AL, Ziesche S, Yancy C, et al: Combination of isosorbide dinitrate and hydralazine in blacks with heart failure, *N Engl J Med* 351:2049-2057, 2004. A

31. MERIT-HF Study Group: Effect of metoprolol CR/XL in chronic heart failure: metoprolol CR/XL randomized intervention trial in congestive heart failure, *Lancet* 353:2001, 1999. A

11

HEART FAILURE

32. CIBIS-II Investigators and Committees: The Cardiac Insufficiency Bisoprolol Study II: a randomised trial, *Lancet* 353:9, 1999. A
33. Poole-Wilson PA et al: Comparison of carvedilol and metoprolol on clinical outcomes in patients with chronic heart failure in the Carvedilol or Metoprolol European Trial (COMET): randomised controlled trial, *Lancet* 362:7, 2003. A
34. Packer M et al: Comparative effects of carvedilol and metoprolol on left ventricular ejection fraction in heart failure: results of a meta-analysis, *Am Heart J* 141:899, 2001. C
35. Cooper HA et al: Diuretics and risk of arrhythmic death in patients with left ventricular dysfunction, *Circulation* 100:1311-1315, 1999. B
36. RALES Investigators: Effectiveness of spironolactone added to an angiotensin-converting enzyme inhibitor and a loop diuretic for severe chronic congestive heart failure (the Randomized Aldactone Evaluation Study), *Am J Cardiol* 78:902, 1996. A
37. Juurlink DN et al: Rates of hyperkalemia after publication of the Randomized Aldactone Evaluation Study, *N Engl J Med* 351:543, 2004. B
38. Pitt B et al: Eplerenone, a selective aldosterone blocker, in patients with left ventricular dysfunction after myocardial infarction, *N Engl J Med* 348:1309-1321, 2003. A
39. Digitalis Investigators Group Study (DIG): The effect of digoxin on mortality and morbidity in patients with heart failure, *N Engl J Med* 336:525, 1997. A
40. Pulerwitz T et al: A rationale for the use of anticoagulation in heart failure management, *J Thromb Thrombolysis* 17(2):87, 2004. C
41. WATCH Trial, presented at the ACC 2004, New Orleans, La. A
42. Belardinelli R et al: Randomized controlled trial of long-term moderate exercise training in chronic heart failure: effects on functional capacity, quality of life, and clinical outcomes, *Circulation* 99:1173, 1999. A
43. Hsu Li-Fern et al: Catheter ablation for atrial fibrillation in congestive heart failure. *N Engl J Med* 352:2373, 2004. B
44. Aurigemma GP, Gaasch WH: Diastolic heart failure, *N Engl J Med* 351:1097, 2004. C
45. Yusuf S et al: Effects of candesartan in patients with chronic heart failure and preserved left-ventricular ejection fraction: the CHARM-Preserved Trial, *Lancet* 362:777, 2003. A
46. Moss AJ et al: Prophylactic implantation of a defibrillator in patients with myocardial infarction and reduced ejection fraction, *N Engl J Med* 346:877, 2002. A
47. Bardy GH et al: Amiodarone or an implantable cardioverter-defibrillator for congestive heart failure, *N Engl J Med* 352:225-237, 2005. A
48. Bristow MR et al: Cardiac-resynchronization therapy with or without an implantable defibrillator in advanced chronic heart failure, *N Engl J Med* 350:2140, 2004. A

Valvular Heart Disease

Reza Ardehali, MD, PhD; Hunter C. Champion, MD, PhD;
and Thomas Traill, MD

FAST FACTS

- In general, patients with valvular heart disease should undergo valve replacement or repair when they develop symptoms of left ventricular dysfunction.
- The symptoms of aortic stenosis are angina, exertional syncope, and congestive heart failure. Survival of patients with aortic stenosis is near normal until the onset of symptoms, at which time a precipitous increase in mortality occurs.
- Patients with chronic mitral regurgitation (MR) should undergo surgical intervention before left ventricular dysfunction develops (ejection fraction < 60% or end systolic dimension > 45 mm).
- Patients with mechanical valves should be examined carefully, especially for muffled opening and closing clicks and new murmurs, which herald valve dysfunction.
- Unexplained fever in a patient with a prosthetic valve should be presumed to be caused by endocarditis until proven otherwise.

12

Valvular heart disease has a substantial impact worldwide: The American Heart Association reported an estimated 82,000 valve replacement procedures in 2001, and approximately 275,000 procedures are performed globally each year.[1]

Valvular heart disease always leads to abnormal physical findings. Therefore clinicians can recognize valvular heart disease on the basis of the history and physical examination and then use appropriate diagnostic tools to further evaluate the extent of the disease.

When a patient has valvular heart disease, four major issues must be addressed: What is the nature of valvular disease, and what underlying cause contributed to its development? Is the structural failure leading to valvular disease severe enough to necessitate repair or replacement of the diseased valve? If so, then what are the best medical therapy and the best time for surgical intervention to minimize morbidity and mortality? If surgical intervention is warranted, then what type of prosthetic valve is most appropriate based on the patient's comorbidities? With this information, appropriate medical management and either serial follow-up examinations or surgical correction can be selected (Table 12-1).

TABLE 12-1

SUMMARY OF SEVERE VALVULAR HEART DISEASE

	Aortic Stenosis	Mitral Stenosis	Mitral Regurgitation	Aortic Regurgitation
Etiology	Idiopathic calcification of a bicuspid or tricuspid valve; congenital; rheumatic.	Rheumatic fever; annular calcification.	Mitral valve prolapse; ruptured chordae; endocarditis; ischemic papillary muscle dysfunction or rupture; collagen-vascular diseases and syndromes; result of LV myocardial diseases.	Annuloaortic ectasia; hypertension; endocarditis; Marfan's syndrome; ankylosing spondylitis; aortic dissection; syphilis; collagen-vascular disease.
Pathophysiology	Pressure overload on LV with compensation by LV hypertrophy; as disease advances, reduced coronary flow reserve causes angina; hypertrophy and afterload excess lead to both systolic and diastolic LV dysfunction.	Obstruction to LV inflow increases left atrial pressure and limits cardiac output, mimicking LV failure; mitral valve obstruction increases the pressure work of the right ventricle; right ventricular pressure overload is augmented further when pulmonary hypertension develops.	Places volume overload on the LV, which responds with eccentric hypertrophy and dilation, allowing increased stroke volume; eventually, LV dysfunction develops if volume overload is uncorrected.	*Chronic:* Total stroke volume causes hyperdynamic circulation, induces systolic hypertension, and thus causes both pressure and volume overload; compensation is by both concentric and eccentric hypertrophy. *Acute:* Because cardiac dilation had not developed, hyperdynamic findings are absent; high diastolic LV pressure causes mitral valve preclosure and potentiates LV ischemia and failure.

Symptoms	Angina, syncope, heart failure.	Dyspnea, orthopnea, PND, hemoptysis, hoarseness, edema, ascites.	Dyspnea, orthopnea, PND.	Dyspnea, orthopnea, PND, angina, syncope.
Signs	Systolic ejection murmur radiating to neck; delayed carotid upstroke; S_4, soft or paradoxical S_2.	Diastolic rumble following an opening snap; loud S_1; right ventricular lift; loud P_2.	Holosystolic apical murmur radiates to axilla, S_3; displaced PMI.	*Chronic:* Diastolic blowing murmur, hyperdynamic circulation; displaced PMI; Quincke pulse; Musset sign. *Acute:* Short diastolic blowing murmur; soft S_1.
Electrocardiogram Chest radiograph	LAA; LVH. Boot-shaped heart; aortic valve calcification on lateral view.	LAA; RVH. Straightening of left heart border; double density at right heart border; Kerley B lines; enlarged pulmonary arteries.	LAA; LVH. Cardiac enlargement.	LAA; LVH. *Chronic:* Cardiac enlargement; uncoiling of the aorta. *Acute:* Pulmonary congestion with normal heart size.
Echocardiographic changes	Concentric LVH; aortic valve cusp separation; Doppler shows mean gradient ≤ 50 mmHg in most severe cases.	Restricted mitral leaflet motion; valve area ≤ 1 cm² in most severe cases; tricuspid Doppler may reveal pulmonary hypertension.	LV and left atrial enlargement in chronic severe disease; Doppler; large regurgitant jet.	*Chronic:* LV enlargement; large Doppler jet; PHT <400 ms. *Acute:* Small LV; mitral valve preclosure.

Data from Goldman L, Bennett JC: *Cecil textbook of medicine,* 21st ed, Philadelphia, 2000, WB Saunders.
LAA, left atrial enlargement; *LV,* left ventricle; *LVH,* left ventricular hypertrophy; *PHT,* pressure half-time; *PMI,* point of maximal impulse; *PND,* paroxysmal nocturnal dyspnea; *RVH,* right ventricular hypertrophy.

12

VALVULAR HEART DISEASE

Aortic Stenosis

I. EPIDEMIOLOGY

1. **Aortic stenosis is the most common valvular disease in the developed world.** It is caused by progressive valvular calcification of a congenitally bicuspid valve or a normal valve. In the former group, presentation tends to occur in the fourth or fifth decade of life. In the latter group, the aortic valve becomes sclerotic and, with further calcification, stenotic during the sixth, seventh, or eighth decade of life.

2. Approximately 25% of people older than age 65 and 35% of those older than age 70 have echocardiographic evidence of sclerosis, and 2% to 3% exhibit hemodynamic evidence of stenosis.[2-4]

II. PATHOPHYSIOLOGY

1. The development of aortic stenosis is a complex biological process similar to atherosclerosis. Chronic inflammation with macrophage and T-lymphocyte involvement, accumulation of lipid particles, and the appearance of calcifying valve cells with osteoblast-like activities all contribute to aortic valve stenosis.[5]

2. **Progression of aortic stenosis narrows the valve orifice area, causes a pressure gradient between the left ventricle (LV) and aorta, and increases afterload.** Increased afterload causes concentric hypertrophy, impaired relaxation, and decreased compliance, leading to diastolic dysfunction. Systolic dysfunction (left ventricular dilation and decreased ejection fraction) develops in some patients with especially severe stenosis and is a particularly ominous sign.[6]

III. CLINICAL PRESENTATION

A. HISTORY AND NATURAL PROGRESSION

1. **The symptoms of aortic stenosis are angina, syncope, and congestive heart failure.** Angina develops because of both reduced coronary flow reserve and increased myocardial demand caused by high afterload. Syncope typically is related to exertion and may be caused by arrhythmias, hypotension, or decreased cerebral perfusion resulting from increased blood flow to exercising muscles without compensatory increase in cardiac output.

2. Approximately 75% of patients with symptomatic aortic stenosis will die 3 years after onset of symptoms unless the aortic valve is replaced. Heart failure carries the worst prognosis.[3]

B. PHYSICAL EXAMINATION

1. Mild or moderate aortic valve stenosis is characterized by a systolic ejection murmur at the aortic area, which is transmitted to the neck and apex, is preceded by an ejection sound, and peaks in early systole.

2. As the severity of stenosis increases, the ejection click disappears, the murmur peaks later in systole, and the murmur is softer because of

diminished cardiac output. A palpable left ventricular heave or thrill may be present, the second heart sound is reduced in intensity or is absent, and a soft early diastolic murmur of mild aortic regurgitation (AR) may be heard.

3. When the valve area is less than 1 cm^2 (normal 3 to 4 cm^2), ventricular systole becomes prolonged, and the typical carotid pulse pattern of delayed upstroke and low amplitude is present (parvus et tardus). The murmur may disappear over the sternum and then reappear in the apical area, mimicking MR (Gallavardin's phenomenon).[2,7]

IV. DIAGNOSIS

1. The severity of aortic stenosis usually can be evaluated by noninvasive techniques. Echocardiography provides accurate assessment of the transvalvular gradient and valve area and an estimate of left ventricular hypertrophy and ejection fraction.

2. **Typically, a valve area less than 0.8 cm^2 or a transvalvular gradient of more than 50 mmHg is considered critical stenosis and in the presence of symptoms would be sufficient to warrant valve replacement.**[2,3]

3. Cardiac catheterization is performed before surgery in older patients to exclude concomitant coronary artery disease.

V. MANAGEMENT

1. With the exception of prophylaxis against endocarditis, there is no proven medical therapy for aortic stenosis. Although recent studies suggest that lipid-lowering agents may provide a beneficial effect by slowing disease progression, the only effective relief of this mechanical obstruction to blood flow is aortic valve replacement. After onset of heart failure, angina, or syncope, the prognosis without surgery is very poor. Medical treatment may stabilize patients in heart failure, but **surgery is indicated for all symptomatic patients, including those with left ventricular dysfunction, which often improves postoperatively.**

2. Asymptomatic patients should be followed with serial echocardiograms every 2 to 5 years to detect declining left ventricular function, very severe left ventricular hypertrophy, and very high gradient (more than 80 mmHg) or severely reduced valve area (less than 0.7 cm^2).[2-4]

3. The surgical mortality rate for valve replacement is 2% to 5%, but it rises to 10% in people older than the age of 75. Bypass of severe coronary lesions usually is performed at the same time as valve replacement, although it is associated with higher postoperative mortality than valve surgery alone.

4. Except in adolescents, balloon valvuloplasty is considered largely as a palliative procedure or as a bridge to valve surgery in critically ill patients with advanced aortic stenosis. Recent development of

12

VALVULAR HEART DISEASE

percutaneous transcatheter aortic valve replacement may provide an alternative in the near future for patients with aortic stenosis.

5. Anticoagulation with warfarin is necessary for mechanical prosthesis but is not essential with bioprostheses. The majority of aortic valve operations in the United States involve the use of mechanical valves. The Ross procedure, which entails switching the patient's pulmonary valve to the aortic position and placing a bioprosthesis in the pulmonary position, is also an option in patients who are poor candidates for long-term anticoagulation.[8]

Aortic Regurgitation

I. EPIDEMIOLOGY

1. The most common congenital cause of AR is bicuspid aortic valve. Other causes include disorders that affect the valve itself (e.g., infective endocarditis, rheumatic heart disease, dietary medication) and those causing proximal ascending aorta dilation (e.g., Marfan's syndrome, Takayasu's arteritis, syphilis, ankylosing spondylitis, and Reiter's syndrome). Causes of acute AR include endocarditis and aortic root dissection.[4,9]

2. Approximately 10% of those with long-standing systemic hypertension may have evidence of AR caused by aortic valve ring dilation.

II. CLINICAL PRESENTATION AND PATHOPHYSIOLOGY

A. HISTORY AND NATURAL PROGRESSION

1. **The presentation of AR generally is determined by the rapidity with which regurgitation develops.**

a. In chronic AR, volume overload of the LV subsequently leads to increase in left ventricular radius and wall thickness. This allows the LV to eject an augmented stroke volume, which in turn causes low diastolic blood pressure in the setting of systolic hypertension, wide pulse pressure, and increased afterload. Left ventricular failure is a late event and may be sudden in onset. Exertional dyspnea and fatigue are the most common symptoms.

b. In acute AR the large regurgitant volume entering the normal-size LV results in a rapid increase in the left ventricular filling pressure, leading to premature mitral valve closure and acute pulmonary congestion. Severe regurgitation may impair cardiac output, leading to cardiogenic shock.[6]

2. Associated coronary artery disease and syncope are less common than in aortic stenosis.[4,10]

B. PHYSICAL EXAMINATION

1. **The pulse pressure usually is elevated because of a large stroke volume, a portion of which regurgitates back into the LV.** The pulse has a rapid rise and fall (Corrigan pulse), with an elevated systolic and a low diastolic pressure. The well-known peripheral signs include Quincke pulse (subungual capillary pulsation), Duroziez sign (diastolic

murmur over a partially compressed peripheral artery, commonly femoral), Musset sign (head bobbing), and Hill sign (systolic blood pressure at least 30 mmHg higher in the leg than in the arm). The apical impulse is prominent, laterally displaced, and usually hyperdynamic and may be sustained.

2. The hallmark of AR is a high-pitched decrescendo diastolic murmur, best heard along the left parasternal border. In advanced AR a mid-diastolic murmur or late diastolic low-pitched mitral murmur (Austin Flint murmur) may be heard.[10]

3. Patients with acute AR do not have the dilated LV of chronic AR. They also have a shorter diastolic murmur that may be minimal in intensity, and the pulse pressure may not be widened, making clinical diagnosis difficult. The rapid development of LV failure manifested primarily as pulmonary edema may warrant urgent surgical intervention.

III. DIAGNOSIS

1. Echocardiography can demonstrate whether the lesion involves the aortic root or whether valvular disease is present. Serial assessments of left ventricular size and function are critical in determining the timing for valve replacement. Doppler techniques can be used to estimate the severity of regurgitation, although mild regurgitation is not uncommon and should not be overinterpreted. Scintigraphic studies can be used to quantify left ventricular function and functional reserve during exercise.

2. Cardiac catheterization is seldom necessary to quantify severity but is used to evaluate the coronary and aortic root anatomy preoperatively.

IV. MANAGEMENT

1. **Patients with chronic AR may remain asymptomatic for many years; however, once symptoms develop, the prognosis is poor without surgery.**

2. Vasodilators such as hydralazine; angiotensin-converting enzyme inhibitors; and, in particular, nifedipine can lessen the severity of regurgitation by reducing afterload. Such prophylactic treatment may postpone or obviate surgery in asymptomatic patients.

3. Surgery usually is indicated once AR causes symptoms. Surgery is also indicated for patients who have few or no symptoms but have significant left ventricular dysfunction (ejection fraction < 45%) or who exhibit progressive deterioration of left ventricular function, irrespective of symptoms. Although the operative mortality rate is higher when left ventricular function is severely impaired, valve replacement or repair is still indicated because left ventricular function often improves somewhat and long-term prognosis is thereby enhanced.

4. The "55 rule" has been useful in gauging the timing of surgery for AR. Aortic valve surgery should be performed before the end-systolic dimension exceeds 55 mmHg.[4]

12

VALVULAR HEART DISEASE

Mitral Stenosis

I. EPIDEMIOLOGY
Mitral stenosis usually is associated with a history of rheumatic heart disease. The decline in the incidence of rheumatic heart disease has significantly reduced the incidence of mitral stenosis in the developed world.

II. PATHOPHYSIOLOGY
Rheumatic fever is a hypersensitivity reaction induced by group A streptococci in which antibodies directed against the M proteins of certain strains of streptococci cross-react with tissue glycoproteins in the valves. This chronic inflammatory reaction results in subsequent fibrous thickening and calcification of the valve leaflets, fusion of the commissures, and thickening of the chordae tendineae. As a result, the stenotic valve poses obstruction to left atrial emptying, leading to pulmonary hypertension and compromised right ventricular function.[11]

III. CLINICAL PRESENTATION
A. HISTORY AND NATURAL PROGRESSION
1. Symptoms typical of left-sided heart failure are observed in patients with mitral valve stenosis. These include dyspnea on exertion, orthopnea, and paroxysmal nocturnal dyspnea. Less common presenting symptoms include hemoptysis, hoarseness, and symptoms of right-sided heart failure.
2. Patients with mitral stenosis often are asymptomatic until the onset of atrial fibrillation or during pregnancy, when dyspnea and orthopnea are noted.[8,9]
3. The symptoms of mitral stenosis are caused by increased left atrial pressure and reduced cardiac output caused by mechanical obstruction of left ventricular filling. LV contractility usually is normal in mitral stenosis but may be impaired in patients with severe disease of the subvalvular apparatus. Right ventricular function is compromised first by the afterload imposed on it by high atrial pressure and then by the development of secondary pulmonary vasoconstriction.[8,9]

B. PHYSICAL EXAMINATION
1. On physical examination, mitral stenosis produces the classic diastolic rumble that follows an opening snap. In patients with a mobile but thickened valve, S_1 is characteristically loud, but in more advanced disease as the valve calcifies, the first sound becomes soft. S_2 is also loud because of an increased P_2 component thought to result from pulmonary hypertension. In severe mitral stenosis with low flow across the mitral valve, the murmur may be soft and difficult to hear, especially in patients with atrial fibrillation.
2. If the patient has both mitral stenosis and MR, the dominant features may be the systolic murmur of MR with or without a short diastolic murmur and

a delayed opening snap. With severe, long-standing disease the presence of a loud P_2 probably indicates that pulmonary hypertension is producing right ventricular overload. In such circumstances, a lift is present over the right ventricle and the pulmonary artery in the second, third, and fourth left intercostal space.[8,9]

IV. DIAGNOSIS

1. The electrocardiogram may demonstrate a prominent terminal portion of a biphasic P wave in lead V_1, indicating left atrial enlargement. In severe or long-standing mitral stenosis, right ventricular hypertrophy may be seen.
2. Echocardiography is used to assess the degree of mitral stenosis and determine the need for treatment with balloon mitral valvotomy or surgery. Planimetric calculation of valve area is performed, and the severity of stenosis can be estimated by measuring the decay of the transvalvular gradient. This "pressure half-time" is based on the principle that as the severity of stenosis worsens, the transmitral flow gradient takes longer to decay. In addition to valve area, left atrial size can be determined. Increased left atrial size denotes an increased likelihood of atrial fibrillation or systemic emboli.
3. Interestingly, atrial myxomas can have physical findings similar to those with mitral stenosis. Use of echocardiography is particularly helpful in this situation.[9]

V. MANAGEMENT

1. **Mitral stenosis is generally associated with a long asymptomatic phase, followed by subtle limitation of activity.** When mild symptoms appear, diuretics have been shown to be effective in lowering left atrial pressure and reducing symptoms.
2. The onset of atrial fibrillation often precipitates more severe symptoms. Conversion to sinus rhythm or ventricular rate control may be necessary for symptom relief (see Chapter 16). At the onset of atrial fibrillation the patient should receive warfarin anticoagulation even if sinus rhythm is restored because 20% to 30% of these patients have systemic embolization if untreated.
3. Indications for mechanical intervention include New York Heart Association class III or IV heart failure symptoms, evidence of pulmonary hypertension (pulmonary arterial systolic pressure > 50 mmHg at rest or > 60 mmHg with exercise), or limitation of activity despite ventricular rate control and medical therapy.
4. Balloon valvotomy is a treatment option for younger patients without accompanying MR. Initial success rates of balloon valvotomy are high, especially if valve calcification is not excessive. However, if valvular calcification, severe distortion of valvular components, or moderate MR exists, then open commissurotomy, valve reconstruction, or mitral valve replacement will be necessary.[6,8]

12

VALVULAR HEART DISEASE

Mitral Regurgitation

I. EPIDEMIOLOGY

The majority of MR in the United States results from mitral valve prolapse, which affects 3% to 5% of the population. Other causes include ischemic heart disease involving papillary muscle infarction with or without rupture (presenting as acute MR), annular dilation induced by left ventricular enlargement, endocarditis, dietary medications, collagen-vascular disorders, and rheumatic heart disease.[4,6]

II. PATHOPHYSIOLOGY

1. In mitral prolapse, the valve leaflets, particularly the posterior leaflet, are enlarged, and the normal dense collagen and elastin matrix of the valvular fibrosa is fragmented and replaced with loose, myxomatous connective tissue.
2. Papillary muscle dysfunction and rupture may occur 2 to 7 days after an acute myocardial infarction, which results in severe valvular incompetence. Total rupture generally leads to sudden death. Infective endocarditis also leads to acute valvular dysfunction (see Chapter 57).
3. Patients with coronary heart disease may also have stable **ischemic** papillary muscle dysfunction, leading to MR that is mild at rest but worse during exercise. **Functional** MR results from the malfunctioning of the mitral apparatus that is seen in patients with long-standing left ventricular failure. Anatomic changes that accompany chronic heart failure cause dilation of the mitral annulus, leading to mitral valve incompetency.

III. CLINICAL PRESENTATION

A. HISTORY AND NATURAL PROGRESSION

1. **The clinical presentation of MR depends on the rapidity with which the valvular incompetence develops.** Because blood is ejected both into the left atrium (LA) and through the aortic valve, MR leads to both low cardiac output and left ventricular diastolic volume overload.
2. In acute regurgitation, LA pressure rises abruptly; this is transmitted to the pulmonary circulation, resulting in pulmonary congestion. However, if the onset is more gradual, the LA enlarges progressively, but the pressure in the pulmonary veins and capillaries rises only transiently during exertion. As a result, exertional dyspnea and fatigue progress gradually over many years.
3. Like those with mitral stenosis, patients with MR are also predisposed to atrial fibrillation; however, this arrhythmia is less likely to provoke acute pulmonary congestion, and less than 5% of patients have peripheral arterial emboli. In addition, MR often predisposes to infective endocarditis.[9]

B. PHYSICAL EXAMINATION

On physical examination, MR is characterized by a pansystolic murmur, maximal at the apex, radiating to the axilla. A prominent third heart sound is an important clue to severity, although it does not necessarily indicate that the patient has congestive heart failure because the sound is produced when the large volume of blood from the enlarged LA rapidly fills the LV. Other signs of advanced disease include a hyperdynamic left ventricular impulse and a brisk carotid upstroke.[4,9]

IV. DIAGNOSIS

1. Echocardiography is useful in identifying the underlying pathologic process (rheumatic, infectious, prolapse, flail leaflet), and Doppler techniques provide qualitative and semiquantitative estimates of the degree of MR.
2. Cardiac catheterization allows accurate assessment of regurgitation, left ventricular function, and pulmonary artery pressure but is seldom advised unless the noninvasive methods provide contradictory results. Coronary angiography is indicated to determine the presence of coronary artery disease before valve surgery.

V. MANAGEMENT

1. Acute MR caused by endocarditis, myocardial infarction, and ruptured chordae tendineae often warrants emergency surgery. Some patients can be stabilized with vasodilators (nitroprusside) or the use of an intra-aortic balloon pump, both of which reduce regurgitant flow by lowering systemic vascular resistance.
2. In chronic MR, surgery usually is necessary if symptoms develop. Because progressive and irreversible deterioration of left ventricular function may occur before the onset of symptoms, **early operation is indicated in asymptomatic patients with a declining ejection fraction (< 60%) or marked left ventricular dilation (end-systolic left ventricular dimension > 45 mm) on echocardiography.**
3. Although vasodilators are used successfully to increase forward output and decrease left ventricular filling pressure in patients with acute MR, there are no data to suggest long-term benefit from their use, especially in asymptomatic patients.[9]

Tricuspid Regurgitation

I. EPIDEMIOLOGY

The most common cause of tricuspid valve regurgitation is right ventricular overload caused by left ventricular failure. Tricuspid regurgitation (TR) also occurs in association with right ventricular and inferior myocardial infarction. Tricuspid valve endocarditis and subsequent regurgitation are common in intravenous drug users. Other causes include pulmonary hypertension, carcinoid syndrome, lupus erythematosus, and myxomatous

12

VALVULAR HEART DISEASE

degeneration of the valve (associated with mitral valve prolapse). Ebstein's anomaly is a congenital defect of the tricuspid valve that often presents in adults as right-sided cardiomegaly caused by TR.

II. CLINICAL PRESENTATION

1. **The symptoms of TR are those of right ventricular failure.** TR can be suspected on the basis of an early onset of right-sided heart failure and the characteristic jugular pulsation.
2. Auscultation may reveal a systolic murmur along the lower left sternal border that increases in intensity during and just after inspiration (Carvallo's sign). Accentuation of the tricuspid murmur can be achieved at times by pressing down on the liver (Vitum sign).
3. Hemodynamic characteristics of TR include a prominent regurgitant systolic (v) wave in the right atrium and jugular venous pulse, with a rapid y descent and a small or absent x descent. The regurgitant wave, like the systolic murmur, increases with inspiration, and its size depends on the size of the right atrium. An S_3 may coincide with the trough of the y descent, and it may increase in intensity during inspiration.

III. DIAGNOSIS

As in other valvular disorders, echocardiography can be used to assess the presence and severity of TR. On the basis of this and a modified version of Bernoulli's equation, the right ventricular systolic pressure can be estimated as right atrial pressure $+ 4V_{TR}^2$, where V_{TR} = tricuspid jet velocity.

IV. MANAGEMENT

1. TR resulting from severe mitral valve disease or other left-sided lesions may regress when the underlying disease is corrected. Tricuspid valvular annuloplasty is indicated for patients who need mitral valve surgery and also have severe TR and pulmonary hypertension.
2. Surgical valve replacement is most commonly used for patients with severe TR and abnormal valve leaflets not amenable to valvuloplasty. Replacement of the tricuspid valve is infrequently performed today but may be lifesaving in patients with deteriorating right ventricular function after previous repair of congenital heart disease.[6]

Prosthetic Heart Valves

I. VALVE SELECTION

1. Fifty-five percent of implanted valves worldwide are mechanical, and the remaining 45% are bioprosthetic.
2. Mechanical valves normally have a lifespan of at least 20 years. The earliest successful devices were caged-ball models such as the Starr-Edwards, but these have given way to the single tilting disk valves

(Björk-Shiley) and the most frequently used bileaflet tilting disk models (St. Jude Medical or Carbomedics models) (Fig. 12-1).

3. Bioprosthetic heterograft valves are composed of porcine valves or bovine pericardium, mounted on a metal support structure, and include such models as Hancock, Carpentier-Edwards, Life Science–Edwards, and Ionescu-Shiley. Homograft valves are composed of preserved cadaveric human aortic valves.[12-14]

4. **The patient's clinical situation guides the selection of the valve.**

5. The advantage of mechanical valves is their extended durability, but the downfall is the need for long-term anticoagulation. Generally, mechanical valves are preferred for patients whose life expectancy is greater than 10 to 15 years and are best suited for those with another indication for long-term anticoagulation (e.g., atrial fibrillation).

6. The advantage of bioprosthetic valves is their low thromboembolic potential, which obviates long-term anticoagulation. The disadvantage is their reduced longevity: 10% to 20% of bioprosthetic valves fail within 15 years of implantation. Bioprosthetic valves are preferred for older adults whose life expectancy is less than 20 years, those for whom long-term anticoagulation therapy would be difficult, and women who plan pregnancy.[12-14]

II. EVALUATION OF THE PATIENT WITH A PROSTHETIC VALVE

1. Detailed history taking is paramount in determining patient's long-term compliance with anticoagulation in cases of mechanical valves.

2. Mechanical valves should produce crisp sounds of opening and closing and differ from bioprosthetic valves, whose sound should be similar to that of native valve. **On physical examination a change in the intensity or quality of the audible sound of the valve or the presence of a new valvular murmur may suggest a potential valve dysfunction.**

3. If prosthetic valve dysfunction is suspected, imaging of the valve should be performed to further assess its function. Transthoracic echocardiography is a reliable method for evaluating prosthetic valves

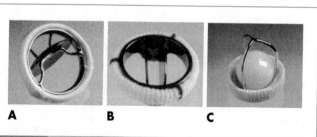

FIG. 12-1

Mechanical prosthetic valves. **A**, Bjork-Shiley. **B**, St. Jude's Medical.
C, Starr-Edwards. (*Courtesy Vincent Gott, MD.*)

12

VALVULAR HEART DISEASE

and permits the evaluation of sewing-ring stability, the absence or presence of valvular regurgitation and perivalvular leak, the prosthetic transvalvular gradient, and the motion of bioprosthetic leaflets. Transesophageal echocardiography provides better views of the mitral valve than does transthoracic echocardiography and is necessary if mitral prosthetic dysfunction is suspected.

4. Cinefluoroscopy can be used to assess mechanical valves by observation of the motion of the valve ring and leaflets.[12]
5. Structural failure of the mechanical prosthetic heart valve is rare but should be considered in the event of a rapid deterioration in hemodynamic stability.

III. RECOMMENDED ANTITHROMBOTIC THERAPY

1. Because of the risk of thromboembolism, patients with mechanical prosthetic valves need long-term anticoagulant therapy, which should be started within 12 hours after surgery. The degree of anticoagulation depends on the type of prosthetic valve and is summarized in Table 12-2.
2. To minimize thromboembolic complications, recent data indicate use of lower-dose aspirin (100 mg daily) in combination with warfarin (target international normalized ratio 3.0 to 4.5) for patients who have mechanical or bioprosthetic heart valves and also have atrial fibrillation or previous systemic embolization. The combination of aspirin and warfarin offers additional protection against thromboembolism, but a higher risk of complications from more frequent bleeding is the tradeoff. Therefore this combination should be reserved for patients with a history or high risk of systemic embolization or with other conditions in which it is indicated, such as coronary artery or peripheral vascular disease.[17,18]

IV. MANAGEMENT OF COMPLICATIONS IN THE PATIENT WITH A PROSTHETIC VALVE

A. VALVE THROMBOSIS

1. The reported annual incidence of prosthetic valve thrombosis ranges from 2% to 4%, with higher risk among those with subtherapeutic anticoagulation.[15]

TABLE 12-2

SUGGESTED THERAPEUTIC ANTICOAGULATION FOR PATIENTS WITH PROSTHETIC HEART VALVES

Type of Prosthetic Valve	Recommended International Normalized Ratio*
Bileaflet disk (St. Jude, Carbomedics)	2.5-3.5
Single tilting disk (Björk-Shiley)	2.5-3.5
Caged ball (Starr-Edwards)	3.0-4.5
Heterograft bioprosthetic	2.0-3.0 (for first 3 mo)
Homograft	Not required

*Target international normalized ratio is at the higher end of the recommended ranges for valves in the mitral position.

2. The risk of valve thrombosis is related to the type and location of the valve. Of the most commonly used mechanical prosthetic valves, the bileaflet tilting disk is the least thrombogenic, followed by the single tilting disk and the caged ball. **Mitral and tricuspid valve prostheses are associated with higher risk of valve thrombosis than aortic valves.**[15,16]

3. Thrombosis of a prosthetic valve can result in severe hemodynamic compromise. In some cases, however, the onset of symptoms is more gradual (days to weeks).

4. Presence of thrombus that interferes with valve function warrants surgical removal of the valve and thrombus.

B. EMBOLIC EVENTS

1. Without antithrombotic therapy, the incidence of death or a persistent neurologic deficit as a result of embolism in patients with mechanical valves is at least 4% per patient-year. With warfarin therapy, the risk falls to 1% per patient-year. Risk factors for thromboembolic complications are shown in Box 12-1.[12-15]

2. The majority of embolic events are manifested as embolic strokes, but emboli may also result in renal infarct, bowel infarct, splenic infarct, or lower extremity arterial occlusion. In patients who have prosthetic heart valves and signs of systemic embolism, the possibility of endocarditis or valve thrombosis should be considered.

3. Conflicting data are available regarding optimal timing for initiating or continuing anticoagulants when an embolus is the presumed cause of a stroke. Ideally, treatment should be started early to prevent recurrent emboli, but the early use of heparin (within 72 hours) is associated with a higher risk (15% to 25%) of converting an embolic stroke into a hemorrhagic stroke. Generally, if computed tomography of the brain provides no evidence of hemorrhagic conversion of stroke at 72 hours after the event, heparin is instituted with a goal-activated partial thromboplastin time of 40 to 50 seconds and maintained until the

12

VALVULAR HEART DISEASE

BOX 12-1

RISK FACTORS FOR THROMBOEMBOLIC COMPLICATIONS IN PATIENTS WITH PROSTHETIC VALVES

Age > 70 yr

Multiple prosthetic valves

Tricuspid or mitral position

Caged-ball valve

History of thromboembolic event

Atrial fibrillation

Left atrial enlargement

Left ventricular systolic dysfunction (ejection fraction < 45%)

Known left atrial thrombus

international normalized ratio is therapeutic for the valve position and model. If computed tomography demonstrates significant cerebral hemorrhage or if the systemic arterial pressure is significantly elevated, anticoagulation should be withheld until the bleeding is treated or has stabilized (7 to 14 days).[14,15]

C. HEMORRHAGE IN THE SETTING OF ANTICOAGULATION

1. Patients on anticoagulation are at a higher risk for hemorrhage. When significant bleeding occurs, regardless of the location, antithrombotic therapy should be stopped. If the patient is at high risk, drug effects should be reversed with fresh frozen plasma and vitamin K in the case of warfarin therapy and with protamine in the case of heparin therapy. If possible, the source of bleeding must be treated and antithrombotic therapy restarted as soon as possible.

2. No reliable data are available regarding the time to reinstitute anticoagulation, and decisions should be made on a case-by-case basis.[15]

D. ENDOCARDITIS

1. Endocarditis occurs at some point in 3% to 6% of patients with prosthetic valves. So-called early endocarditis (occurring < 60 days after valve replacement) usually results from perioperative bacteremia arising from skin or wound infections. Late prosthetic valve endocarditis (occurring > 60 days postoperatively) usually is secondary to organisms that cause traditional endocarditis. The risk of endocarditis is similar for mechanical and bioprosthetic valves.

2. In patients who have prosthetic valve endocarditis, fever is the most common symptom. **Unexplained fever in a patient with a prosthetic valve should be presumed to be caused by endocarditis until proven otherwise.** Both transthoracic and transesophageal echocardiography should be performed in patients with suspected prosthetic valve endocarditis.

3. Careful consideration must be given to replacing a prosthetic valve if blood cultures remain positive while the patient is receiving appropriate therapy.[15,17]

4. **Antibiotic prophylaxis against endocarditis** is advocated by the American Heart Association in all patients with prosthetic heart valves and certain valvular heart disease.

a. Box 12-2 lists the procedures in which endocarditis prophylaxis is indicated.[17]

b. Recommended regimens include oral amoxicillin 2 g 1 hour before the procedure or intravenous ampicillin 2 g 30 minutes before the procedure. High-risk patients undergoing nondental procedures should be treated with ampicillin and gentamicin. Patients allergic to penicillin can be treated with clindamycin 600 mg or azithromycin 500 mg 1 hour before the procedure.

c. Patients with mitral valve prolapse without valvular regurgitation or thickened leaflets do not need endocarditis prophylaxis.

BOX 12-2

PROCEDURES AND ENDOCARDITIS PROPHYLAXIS

ENDOCARDITIS PROPHYLAXIS RECOMMENDED

Dental procedures
  Periodontal surgery
  Endodontic instrumentation (root canal)
  Prophylactic cleaning
Airway and respiratory tract instrumentation
  Bronchoscopy with a rigid bronchoscope
  Tonsillectomy or adenoidectomy
  Thoracic surgery
Gastrointestinal procedures
  Sclerotherapy for esophageal varices
  Esophageal stricture dilation
  Endoscopic retrograde cholangiography
  Gastrointestinal or biliary surgery
Genitourinary procedures
  Cystoscopy
  Prostatic or urethral surgery

ENDOCARDITIS PROPHYLAXIS NOT RECOMMENDED

Restorative dentistry, including orthodontic appliance applications and adjustments
Genitourinary procedures
  Vaginal or cesarean delivery
  Urethral catheterization
Airway and respiratory tract instrumentation
  Endotracheal intubation
  Transesophageal echocardiography
  Flexible bronchoscopy with or without biopsy

PEARLS AND PITFALLS

- Patients with critical aortic stenosis have a fixed cardiac output and are exquisitely preload dependent; therefore diuretics and vasodilators should be used with caution because they may precipitate life-threatening hypotension.
- Bicuspid aortic valves are found in 1% to 2% of the population and are associated with valvular stenosis and regurgitation, aortic coarctation, dissection, and infective endocarditis.
- Whenever possible, valve replacement should be deferred until after a woman's childbearing years. Management of women who have mechanical valves and subsequently become pregnant remains challenging. Treatment with heparin has been tried but has proven to be logistically difficult. Use of warfarin during pregnancy increases the risk of fetal malformation. The current consensus is to continue warfarin during pregnancy because the risks of thromboembolic complications from inadequate anticoagulation outweigh the risks of impaired fetal development.

- Patients receiving long-term hemodialysis have a high incidence of early bioprosthetic valve failure.

REFERENCES

1. Heart disease and stroke statistics, 2004 update, www.americanheart.org. C
2. O'Rouke RA: Aortic valve stenosis: a common clinical entity, *Curr Probl Cardiol* 23:429, 1998. C
3. Carabello BA: Aortic stenosis, *N Engl J Med* 343:611, 2002. C
4. Sing JP et al: Prevalence and clinical determinants of mitral, tricuspid, and aortic regurgitation, *Am J Cardiol* 83:897, 1999. B
5. Chan KL: Is aortic stenosis a preventable disease? *J Am Coll Cardiol* 42:593, 2003. B
6. Reginelli JP, Griffin B: The challenge of valvular heart disease: when is it time to operate? *Cleve Clin J Med* 71:463, 2004. C
7. Rosenhek R et al: Predictors of outcome in severe, asymptomatic aortic stenosis, *N Engl J Med* 343:611, 2000. B
8. Goldsmith I et al: Valvular heart disease and prosthetic valve, *BMJ* 325:1228, 2002. C
9. Zoghbi WA: Valvular heart disease, *Cardiol Clin* 16:3, 1998. C
10. Segal BL: Valvular heart disease, part 1. Diagnosis and surgical management of aortic valve disease in older adults, *Geriatrics* 58:39, 2003. C
11. Yacoub MH et al: Novel approaches to cardiac valve repair: from structure to function, *Circulation* 109:942, 2004. B
12. McAnulty JH, Rahimtoola SH: Antithrombotic therapy and prosthetic valve disease. In Alexander RW et al, eds: *Hurst's the heart,* 11th ed, New York, 2004, McGraw-Hill. C
13. Bach DS: Choice of prosthetic heart valve for adult patients, *J Am Coll Cardiol* 42:1717, 2003. B
14. Garcia MJ: Prosthetic valve disease. In Topel EJ, ed: *Comprehensive cardiovascular medicine,* Philadelphia, 1998, Lippincott, Williams & Wilkins. C
15. Lengyel M: Management of prosthetic valve thrombosis, *J Heart Valve Dis* 13:329, 2004. D
16. Rahimtoola SH: Choice of prosthetic heart valve for adult patients, *J Am Coll Cardiol* 41:893, 2003. C
17. Sexton DJ, Spelman D: Current best practices and guidelines. Assessment and management of complications in infective endocarditis, *Infect Dis Clin North Am* 16:507, 2002. D
18. Fanikos J et al: Comparison of efficacy, safety, and cost of low-molecular-weight heparin with continuous-infusion unfractionated heparin for initiation of anticoagulation after mechanical prosthetic valve implantation, *Am J Cardiol* 58:39, 2004. A

Diseases of the Pericardium

P. Peter Borek, MD; Sanjay Desai, MD; and Gary Gerstenblith, MD

FAST FACTS

- Acute inflammation of the pericardium can occur in a vast array of systemic illnesses and is commonly associated with viral infection, autoimmune disorders, uremia, and myocardial infarction.
- Acute pericarditis is a clinical diagnosis that is supported largely by the patient's history, physical examination, and electrocardiography.
- Pericardial disease can compromise cardiac output through either cardiac tamponade or constrictive pericarditis.
- Cardiac tamponade should be suspected when hypotension, elevated jugular venous pressure, and muffled heart sounds develop in a patient with recent cardiac surgery, aortic dissection, myocardial infarction, or acute pericarditis. The diagnosis is supported by echocardiographic evidence of effusion, right ventricular diastolic collapse, and variation in transmitral and transtricuspid Doppler flow velocities.

The pericardium can be affected in a vast array of diseases, both primarily and secondarily. The most common clinical manifestation of pericardial involvement is inflammation, causing acute pericarditis. The other clinical manifestation of pericardial disease is hemodynamic compromise, resulting from either cardiac tamponade or constrictive pericarditis. This chapter reviews the diagnosis, evaluation, and treatment of these disorders.

Acute Pericarditis

I. EPIDEMIOLOGY

1. Accurate estimation of the incidence and prevalence of acute pericarditis is limited by underdiagnosis but may account for up to 5% of presentations for nonischemic chest pain.
2. Acute inflammation of the pericardium can be an isolated process but more commonly is the result of another systemic condition (Box 13-1).
3. Therapeutic radiation, percutaneous interventions, cardiothoracic instrumentation, and human immunodeficiency virus infection are becoming more prevalent causes of pericarditis in Western populations. Worldwide, however, mycobacterial disease remains the most common cause of pericarditis.[1]

II. CLINICAL PRESENTATION

Acute pericarditis classically presents with sharp pleuritic chest pain that is progressive. Often the pain is relieved by sitting up or leaning forward and exacerbated when lying supine. The chest discomfort may radiate to the

<table>
<tr><td colspan="2">BOX 13-1
COMMON CAUSES OF ACUTE PERICARDITIS</td></tr>
<tr><td>Idiopathic (often thought to be viral)</td><td>Metabolic</td></tr>
<tr><td>Infection</td><td> Renal failure</td></tr>
<tr><td> Common: cardiotropic viruses,</td><td> Hypothyroidism</td></tr>
<tr><td>   gram-positive bacteria,</td><td>Neoplastic</td></tr>
<tr><td>   *Mycobacterium tuberculosis*</td><td>Myocardial infarction</td></tr>
<tr><td> Less common: fungi, parasites,</td><td>Trauma</td></tr>
<tr><td>   spirochetes, rickettsiae</td><td>Aortic dissection</td></tr>
<tr><td></td><td>Esophageal fistula</td></tr>
<tr><td></td><td>Drugs and toxins</td></tr>
</table>

neck, arms, shoulder, and trapezius muscle ridge. The physician must hunt diligently for associated symptoms, which may be nonspecific signs of viral infection or systemic inflammation (including nonproductive cough, fever, and myalgias).

III. DIAGNOSIS

A. PHYSICAL EXAMINATION

1. The hallmark physical examination finding is a pericardial friction rub, heard in approximately 85% of patients with acute pericarditis.[2] The friction rub is "scratchy," superficial, and heard loudest in end-expiration with the patient leaning forward. The sound can be easier to detect and differentiated from pleural sounds if the patient suspends respirations. Classically, the rub has a triple cadence with atrial systolic, ventricular systolic, and early diastolic components. Often it is biphasic or monophasic, especially in patients with atrial or ventricular tachycardia, because of fusion of approximate sounds.

2. **Electrocardiography.** Although the pericardium itself has no detectable electrical activity, pericardial inflammation can lead to electrical changes in the epicardial tissue, which are detected by the surface electrocardiogram.

   a. The electrocardiographic changes associated with this epicardial inflammation typically evolve through four stages, which, when collectively present, are typical of pericarditis (Fig. 13-1).

      (1) **Phase I.**
         (a) Diffuse ST elevation (except for aVR).
         (b) PR depression in the inferolateral leads (II, III, aVF, V_5, V_6).
      (2) **Phase II.** ST and PR segment normalization.
      (3) **Phase III.** Diffuse T wave inversions (occasionally not present).
      (4) **Phase IV.** Resolution of electrocardiographic changes or persistence of T wave inversions, indicating "chronic" inflammation.

   b. **The electrocardiographic changes must be differentiated from acute myocardial infarction and other causes of ST elevation** (see Chapter 6).[3] Pericarditis typically does not involve Q waves, hyperacute T waves, and QT prolongation.

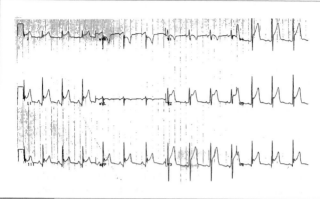

FIG. 13-1

Electrocardiographic changes with acute pericarditis.

c. **Low electrocardiographic voltage and electrical alternans are insensitive** indicators of small to moderate pericardial effusion, and when present they indicate a large effusion. When they are coupled with sinus tachycardia, pericardial tamponade should be suspected.
3. **Echocardiography** may be unremarkable (dry pericarditis) or show pericardial effusion.
4. The **chest radiograph** may show a newly enlarged cardiac silhouette and an associated pleural effusion, usually left sided.
5. **Laboratory evaluation** should include evaluation of renal function, erythrocyte sedimentation rate, C-reactive protein (CRP), antinuclear antibodies, lactate dehydrogenase, and complete blood cell count. Blood cultures should be drawn in febrile patients. Tuberculin skin test and evaluation of human immunodeficiency virus status are warranted. Routine viral studies are not indicated because they do not change management. Creatine kinase, creatine kinase myocardial band, and troponin should always be followed to rule out ischemia. In viral or idiopathic pericarditis, troponin elevation is common, but unlike acute coronary syndromes it is not a negative prognostic marker.[4]

IV. ETIOLOGY AND MANAGEMENT

The differential diagnosis of acute pericarditis is broad and diverse. The most common etiological categories are infectious, metabolic, rheumatic, neoplastic, and diseases of contiguous organs, most commonly myocardial infarction. Management is dictated by the cause of the effusion and the presence and extent of hemodynamic compromise.

A. INFECTIOUS PERICARDITIS

1. **Viral infections are the most common cause of infectious pericarditis,** including coxsackie virus, influenza virus, human immunodeficiency

virus, and the hepatitis A and B viruses. Clinical presentation is that of a viral syndrome with fever and leukocytosis. Nonsteroidal antiinflammatory drugs (NSAIDs) are the mainstay of therapy. Approximately 50% of patients have recurrence within 8 months, and, uncommonly, chronic inflammation develops.

2. **In recurrent idiopathic pericarditis, treatment is largely supportive.** NSAIDs are occasionally helpful; however, colchicine offers the best prophylaxis against recurrence.

3. **Bacterial infection of the pericardium is a more serious condition** with significant morbidity and mortality.

a. The offending organisms usually are gram-positive pathogens, including staphylococci, streptococci, and pneumococci. Less commonly, and usually in the setting of an immunocompromised state, other organisms such as *Escherichia coli, Salmonella, Clostridium*, and *Neisseria* have been implicated. Pericardial effusions make the pericardium particularly vulnerable to bacterial infection via hematogenous spread.[5] Similarly, surrounding bacterial infections, such as lobar pneumonia, mediastinitis, and bacterial endocarditis, predispose the pericardium to bacterial invasion.

b. Bacterial pericarditis has an acute presentation, usually with significant fever and pain. An inflammatory, exudative effusion almost always accompanies it.

c. Management involves intravenous antibiotics and drainage.[5] A combination of an antistaphylococcal antibiotic and an aminoglycoside should be initiated. Subxiphoid surgical pericardiotomy is preferred over percutaneous procedures. Pericardiectomy is necessary in patients with dense adhesions, loculated or thick effusion, recurrence of tamponade, or progression to constriction.[6,7]

4. *Mycobacterium tuberculosis* is particularly notable for its predilection for the pericardium. The illness usually arises in an indolent fashion, without evidence of extrapericardial tuberculous infection.

a. Diagnosis of tuberculous pericarditis can be difficult. Although identification of *M. tuberculosis* in pericardial fluid or tissue biopsy is specific, it is not sensitive. Extrapericardial tuberculosis and positive tuberculin skin tests can help support the diagnosis but are not confirmatory. The optimal test is *M. tuberculosis* DNA identification by polymerase chain reaction amplification in the pericardial fluid, which is 100% sensitive and more than 70% specific for tuberculous infection.[8,9]

b. Management involves prompt therapy with combination of three to four tuberculostatic drugs for 9 to 12 months and a prednisone taper starting at 1 mg/kg for the first week and tapered over 8 weeks.[10]

B. METABOLIC DERANGEMENTS

1. **Uremia** can cause pericarditis in patients with chronic renal failure, on hemodialysis with inadequate treatment, or less commonly with acute renal failure. No direct correlation exists between the level of uremia

and clinical manifestations. Treatment focuses on hemodialysis to correct the uremia. Pericardiocentesis should be performed early in patients with pretamponade physiology given increased risk of vascular collapse with acute fluid removal during dialysis.

2. Pericarditis has been observed in **other metabolic derangements,** notably diabetic ketoacidosis, hypothyroid myxedema, adrenal failure, gout, and hypercholesterolemia.[11,12] A clear pathogenesis, other than systemic inflammation, has yet to be described in these conditions.[5]

C. RHEUMATIC DISEASES

1. The majority of vasculitides and connective tissue disorders can have associated pericarditis. The same pathologic process that leads to blood vessel and tissue inflammation also leads to pericardial inflammation.
2. Rheumatoid arthritis is the most common rheumatologic disease associated with pericarditis, usually with fibrinous exudates. Systemic lupus erythematosus is also commonly associated with pericarditis as well. The pericardial inflammation tends to parallel systemic flares.

D. NEOPLASTIC DISEASE

1. Pericardial disease caused by primary pericardial neoplasms, mesotheliomas, and sarcomas is rare and typically develops in the third and fourth decades of life.[5]
2. Neoplastic involvement of the pericardium can occur through metastatic disease, usually via pericardial lymphatics, or from direct extension of malignant tissue from breast, lung, or chest wall. Because malignancies may initially manifest themselves as "idiopathic" pericarditis, a search for systemic neoplasms is warranted in certain situations.[13,14]
3. Management of neoplastic pericardial disease includes pericardial drainage, typically with pericardial windows or shunts. Surgical resection is necessary for recurrent pericardial constriction from malignancy. Conservative therapy with pericardial sclerosis may be appropriate as palliative treatment in poor surgical candidates.[5]

E. MYOCARDIAL INFARCTION

1. Myocardial infarction can be associated with pericarditis, either early (< 7 days) or late (weeks to months) after infarction. Almost half of transmural infarctions are associated with early pericarditis.
2. **Early postinfarction pericarditis** increases in incidence with infarct size and is a common cause of new chest pain during the first few days after infarction.[5,15,16] In-hospital outcomes do not seem to be affected by early postinfarction pericarditis.
a. Use of NSAIDs should be avoided in the first 7 to 10 days after infarction because, like corticosteroids, they have been linked to scar thinning, ventricular aneurysm, and free wall rupture, and they also increase aspirin resistance.
b. Early infarction pericarditis is not an absolute contraindication to anticoagulation, although caution should be used.
3. **Late postinfarction pericarditis,** also known as Dressler syndrome, is more common with larger infarcts but can also be associated with

nontransmural infarction.[5,17] The syndrome arises between 1 week and several months after infarction and is thought to be immune mediated. Presentation tends to be characteristic for acute pericarditis, and management is focused on antiinflammatory treatment with NSAIDs or corticosteroids, if necessary.

Cardiac Tamponade

I. CLINICAL PRESENTATION

1. Tamponade occurs when excess fluid accumulates in the pericardial sac, raising the intrapericardial pressure to levels that exceed intracardiac pressures. This impairs ventricular filling and cardiac output.

2. Tamponade can occur acutely, usually after traumatic rupture of cardiac structures or percutaneous misadventure, or it can evolve more slowly, as in inflammatory disorders. Although the former is a hemodynamic emergency, the latter may have a more subtle presentation with dyspnea, lightheadedness, and chest pain before severe hypotension develops.

II. DIAGNOSIS

A. PHYSICAL EXAMINATION

1. **Because tamponade is a clinical diagnosis, a thoughtful physical examination for pertinent findings is crucial.** Signs of low cardiac output, including hypotension and compensatory sinus tachycardia, are important. A careful examination of the jugular venous pulse shows an elevated jugular venous pressure, preserved x descent, and a dampened or absent y descent.

2. **Patients commonly have pulsus paradoxus, an abnormally large decrease (> 10 mmHg) in systolic blood pressure during inspiration.** As the patient breathes in a normal fashion, the blood pressure cuff should be inflated to a level 10 to 15 mmHg above the systolic pressure and then very slowly deflated into the systolic range. The examiner should first hear Korotkoff's sounds only during expiration because the inspiratory systolic pressure will be lower. Once the examiner obtains a precise measurement of this pressure, the cuff should be slowly depressurized until Korotkoff's sounds are heard throughout the respiratory cycle. The difference between the two measurements is the pulsus paradoxus.

B. ELECTROCARDIOGRAM

1. The changes most commonly associated with tamponade are nonspecific ST segment and T wave changes and the changes associated with acute pericarditis.

2. Less commonly, electrical alternans can be observed, reflected on the surface electrocardiogram as a beat-to-beat shift in electrical axis of the QRS complex, best seen in leads V_2 to V_4. Combined P wave and QRS complex alternation is specific for cardiac tamponade.[6]

C. ECHOCARDIOGRAPHY

1. Ultrasound examination of the heart is the test of choice for the rapid assessment of pericardial effusions.
2. **End-diastolic chamber collapse is the characteristic echocardiographic finding of tamponade.** End-diastolic right ventricular collapse is poorly sensitive but highly specific for tamponade; end-diastolic right atrial collapse is highly specific if inward movement lasts for more than 30% of cardiac cycle. Left atrial collapse occurs in up to 25% of patients and is a highly specific finding of cardiac tamponade.
3. Doppler studies may show respiratory variation in transvalvular velocities during passive diastolic filling. Transmitral respiratory variation of more than 25% and transtricuspid variation of more than 50% are characteristic of tamponade.
4. Dilation of the inferior vena cava and less than 50% reduction in diameter during inspiration represent elevated central venous pressures and may aid in the diagnosis of tamponade.[18]
5. It should be emphasized that these echocardiographic findings are not useful in terms of diagnosing tamponade in patients with pulmonary hypertension.

III. MANAGEMENT

1. Medical management of tamponade includes volume resuscitation only in patients who are hypovolemic because aggressive volume resuscitation in those who are normovolemic will increase cardiac size, thus increasing pericardial pressure and leading to further reduction in transmural pressures that support the circulation.[19]
2. Definitive intervention entails pericardial drainage, optimally performed in a cardiac catheterization laboratory under controlled conditions. An alternative to catheter drainage is open surgery.

Constrictive Pericarditis

I. CLINICAL PRESENTATION

1. Constrictive pericarditis occurs when the pericardial tissue becomes fibrotic and the pericardial space is totally or almost totally obliterated. This pericardial constriction markedly alters the ventricular pressure-volume relationship, impairing ventricular filling and increasing ventricular interdependence.
2. Well-demonstrated risk factors include a history of cardiac surgery, mediastinal radiation therapy (commonly for Hodgkin's lymphoma), neoplasm, infection, uremia, sarcoidosis, and connective tissue disease with pericardial involvement. A retrospective study of patients who needed pericardiectomy for constrictive pericarditis found that 42% of cases were idiopathic and 31% of the patients had received mediastinal radiation therapy a mean of 85 months before presentation.[20]
3. On initial examination patients often complain of chest pain, lower extremity swelling, and increased abdominal girth. Late presentation

13

DISEASES OF THE PERICARDIUM

can involve further symptoms of impaired cardiac output, including dyspnea on exertion, lightheadedness, and fatigue.

II. DIAGNOSIS

1. On **physical examination,** signs that mimic right-sided heart failure are helpful, including elevated jugular venous pressure with sharp x and y descents, ascites, and peripheral edema. Other associated signs on physical examination are muffled heart sounds, soft S_1 caused by premature closure of mitral and tricuspid valves, a third heart sound, and a pericardial friction rub. The "third heart sound" is not a typical S_3; it is louder, of a higher pitch, and sometimes called a pericardial knock. Pulsus paradoxus is less common in constrictive pericarditis than in tamponade, and when present it may indicate an effusive constrictive process. In addition, Kussmaul sign, described as a paradoxical increase in jugular venous pressure during inspiration caused by limited accommodation of volume by a pressure-constricted right ventricle in late diastole, may be present. Rales are a rare finding on pulmonary examination.

2. **Chest x-ray** examination can demonstrate pericardial calcification.

3. **Two-dimensional echocardiography** features include pericardial thickening, flattening of myocardial wall at end diastole, a septal bounce during atrial systole, and inferior vena cava plethora. Unfortunately, these findings carry a low sensitivity and specificity for constrictive pericarditis. Doppler interrogation of transvalvular velocities may reveal respiratory variation and preserved indexes of early ventricular relaxation.[21]

4. **Right heart catheterization** can be useful in the diagnosis of constrictive pericarditis. Common findings include an increase and equalization of all four cardiac chamber diastolic pressures, a dip and plateau pattern in ventricular pressure during diastole, and rapid x and y descents in atrial pressures. However, these findings are not specific for constrictive pericarditis and may be found in patients with restrictive disease. The most useful finding on cardiac catheterization is demonstration of ventricular interdependence and dynamic respiratory variation between intrathoracic and intracardiac pressure curves.

5. **Radiographic imaging** may aid in diagnosing constriction. Both computed tomography and magnetic resonance imaging can directly visualize pericardial thickness greater than 2 mm. Unfortunately, the presence of thickened pericardium does not necessarily imply constriction, and up to 20% of patients with surgically confirmed constriction may have a normal pericardium on imaging.[22]

6. **Differentiation from cardiac tamponade.**

a. It is important to recognize the hemodynamic differences between tamponade and constrictive pericarditis. **Tamponade involves decreased ventricular compliance throughout the cardiac cycle as the heart operates in a continuously high-pressure environment. However,** constrictive pericarditis creates a decreased ventricular compliance only when the cardiac diameter approaches that of the pericardium. This difference affects diastolic venous flow. Specifically, with tamponade, venous return confronts high pressure throughout diastole, producing a single venous return wave as opposed to the normal biphasic return. However, venous return in constrictive pericarditis is not impeded until right ventricular compliance is decreased, that is, in middle to late diastole. Therefore the venous return maintains bimodal flow, seen in jugular veins as the x and y descents and directly by hemodynamics. Echocardiography can aid in the differentiation of these entities by showing the presence or absence of an effusion and diastolic right ventricular collapse on two-dimensional images.

b. The mechanism of abnormal ventricular filling in tamponade differs from that in constriction. Ventricular interdependence caused by physiologic changes in the respiratory cycle is the primary pathophysiology in tamponade. In constriction, encasement of the heart by a rigid pericardium leads to dissociation of intracardiac and intrathoracic pressures during respiration. This leads to reduction of pulmonary vein to left atrium pressure gradient, decreasing flow into the left atrium and ventricle. This decrease in left ventricular filling allows the right ventricle to fill better, leading to further decrease in left-sided filling.

7. **Differentiation from restrictive cardiomyopathy.**

a. Differentiation between constrictive pericarditis and restrictive cardiomyopathy is also important because **treatment and outcomes for the two conditions are very different.** Restrictive cardiomyopathy is a condition in which the myocardium has intrinsically decreased compliance, often as the result of an infiltrative process such as amyloidosis and hemochromatosis.

b. The two pathologic entities have similar presentations, so differentiation on clinical grounds often is challenging. Both conditions lead to impairment of ventricular filling, thereby producing similar physical examination findings of elevated pressures in the right side of the heart and the typical square root sign seen on cardiac catheterization.

c. The overall history and diagnostic evaluation may lead to a collection of findings that together help identify the underlying disease. Clearly a previous history of acute pericarditis or conditions associated with pericarditis favors constriction, just as a history of an infiltrative disease suggests restriction. Physical examination has limited value because the jugular venous dynamics are identical. Electrocardiographic findings of conduction abnormalities, a pseudoinfarct pattern (poor R wave progression without evidence of prior infarct), and diffuse low voltage favor an infiltrative process.

d. Differentiating constrictive pericarditis from restrictive cardiomyopathy can be performed with a careful echocardiographic analysis. In both processes a restrictive Doppler mitral inflow velocity is present, often with an early to late diastolic filling ratio greater than 2. **With constriction, however, ventricular filling is exaggerated by respiratory variation, as demonstrated by a 25% reduction in Doppler mitral inflow velocity with inspiration. This is rarely present in restrictive disease.**[23,24] Simultaneous left and right heart catheterization may ultimately need to be performed to differentiate between constrictive and restrictive physiology.

III. MANAGEMENT

The majority of patients with constrictive pericarditis need surgical pericardiectomy. However, this treatment is associated with significant morbidity and mortality. Perioperative mortality ranges from 5.6% to 12% across different studies.[20,25] Although more than 80% of patients become symptom free, long-term survival is still a concern.

PEARLS AND PITFALLS

- Myocardial ischemia must be differentiated from acute pericarditis.
- Peri-infarct pericarditis with an effusion is a relative contraindication to anticoagulation because the fluid may represent hemopericardium.
- Moderate to large pericardial effusions raise the threshold for defibrillation and cardioversion.
- Positive airway pressure ventilation should be avoided in patients with tamponade.
- Cardiac tamponade should be managed with vigorous intravascular volume expansion (in patients who are hypovolemic) and pressure support until definitive pericardiocentesis is performed.
- The most useful diagnostic tool for identifying constriction is high clinical suspicion in a patient with clinical evidence of right heart failure that cannot be explained by degree of pulmonary hypertension or left-sided failure. Radiography, echocardiography, and cardiac catheterization may all be necessary for final diagnosis.

REFERENCES

1. Wragg A, Strang JI: Tuberculous pericarditis and HIV infection, *Heart* 84:127-128, 2000. C
2. Zayas R et al: Incidence of specific etiology and role of methods for specific etiologic diagnosis of primary acute pericarditis, *Am J Cardiol* 75:378, 1995. B
3. Chou TC: *Electrocardiography in clinical practice: adult and pediatric,* 4th ed, Philadelphia, 1996, WB Saunders. C
4. Imazio M et al: Cardiac troponin I in acute pericarditis, *J Am Coll Cardiol* 42:2114-2148, 2003. B
5. Spodick DH: *The pericardium: a comprehensive textbook,* New York, 1997, Marcel Dekker. C
6. Spodick DH: Pericardial diseases. In Braunwald E, Zipes DP, Libby P, eds: *Heart disease: a textbook of cardiovascular medicine,* 6th ed, Philadelphia, 2001, WB Saunders. C
7. Tirilomis T, Univerdorben S, von der Emde J: Pericardectomy for chronic constrictive pericarditis, *Ann Thorac Surg* 58:1171, 1994. B

8. Shah S et al: Rapid diagnosis of tuberculosis in various biopsy and body fluid specimens by the AMPLICOR *Mycobacterium tuberculosis* polymerase chain reaction test, *Chest* 113:1190, 1998. B

9. Rana BS, Jones RA, Simpson IA: Recurrent pericardial effusion: the value of polymerase chain reaction in the diagnosis of tuberculosis, *Heart* 82:246, 1999. B

10. Hakim JG et al: Double blind randomized placebo controlled trial of adjunctive prednisolone in the treatment of effusive tuberculous pericarditis in HIV seropositive patients, *Heart* 84:183-188, 2000. A

11. Spodick DH: Pericarditis in systemic disease, *Cardiol Clin* 8:709, 1990. C

12. Kabadi UM, Kumer SP: Pericardial effusion in primary hypothyroidism, *Am Heart J* 120:1393, 1990. C

13. Bardales RH et al: Secondary pericardial malignancies: a critical appraisal of the role of cytology, pericardial biopsy, and DNA ploidy analysis, *Am J Pathol* 106:29, 1996. C

14. Malamou-Mitsi VD, Zioga AP, Agnantis NJ: Diagnostic accuracy of pericardial fluid cytology: an analysis of 53 specimens from 44 consecutive patients, *Diagn Cytopathol* 15:197, 1996. B

15. Nagahama Y et al: The role of infarction-associated pericarditis on the occurrence of atrial fibrillation, *Eur Heart J* 19:287, 1998. B

16. Sugiura T et al: Frequency of pericardial friction rub ("pericarditis") after percutaneous transluminal coronary angioplasty in Q-wave myocardial infarction, *Am J Cardiol* 79:362, 1997. B

17. Spodick DH: Post-myocardial infarction syndrome (Dressler's syndrome), *ACC Curr J Rev* 4:35, 1995. C

18. Spodik DH: Acute cardiac tamponade, *N Engl J Med* 349:684-690, 2003. C

19. Cogswell TL et al: The shift in the relationship between intrapericardial fluid pressure and volume induced by acute left ventricular pressure overload during cardiac tamponade, *Circulation* 74:173-180, 1986. B

20. Cameron J et al: The etiologic spectrum of constrictive pericarditis, *Am Heart J* 113:354, 1987. C

21. Oh JK et al: Diagnostic role of Doppler echocardiography in constrictive pericarditis, *J Am Coll Cardiol* 23:154-162, 1994. B

22. Nishimura RA: Constrictive pericarditis in the modern era: a diagnostic dilemma, *Heart* 86:619-623, 2001. C

23. Gillam LD et al: Hydrodynamic compression of the right atrium: a new echocardiographic sign of cardiac tamponade, *Circulation* 68:294, 1983. B

24. Leimgruber P et al: The hemodynamic derangement associated with right ventricular diastolic collapse in cardiac tamponade: an experimental echocardiographic study, *Circulation* 68:612, 1983. B

25. DeValeria PA, Baumgartner WA, Casale AS: Current indications, risks, and outcome after pericardiectomy, *Ann Thorac Surg* 52:219, 1991. B

13

DISEASES OF THE PERICARDIUM

Bradycardia and Pacemakers

Jacob Abraham, MD; Kenneth Bilchick, MD; and Ronald Berger, MD, PhD

FAST FACTS

- Patients with symptomatic bradycardia need permanent pacemaker placement.
- Sinus node dysfunction and atrioventricular conduction disturbance are the most common indications for permanent pacing.
- Pacing modes are classified according to a three- to five-letter code that specifies (in the following order) the chamber paced (*A* for atrium, *V* for ventricle, *D* for dual or both chambers), the chamber sensed (*A, V, D* as before or *O* for none), the response of the pacemaker to a sensed signal (*I* for inhibited, *T* for triggered, or *D* for dual response), the presence of rate-responsive pacing (*R* if present), and a fifth letter if antitachycardia pacing features are present.
- The American College of Cardiology, American Heart Association, and North American Society of Pacing and Electrophysiology 2002 Guideline Update provide recommendations for the implantation of permanent pacemakers in the treatment of bradyarrhythmias and novel indications such as chronic heart failure with intraventricular conduction delay.

I. EPIDEMIOLOGY, PRESENTATION, AND DIAGNOSIS

1. Bradycardia, defined as a heart rate less than 60 beats per minute (bpm), is a common finding in healthy and ill patients. In some healthy patients, especially athletes, heart rates as low as 35 bpm and brief periods of asystole may be physiologic. Therefore bradycardia itself is not necessarily indicative of disease.

2. **The first step in evaluating the bradycardic patient is to determine whether the patient is symptomatic.**

a. Symptomatic bradycardia occurs when the inadequate heart rate causes a decrease in cardiac output (the product of heart rate and stroke volume) sufficient to produce symptoms of hypoperfusion.

b. Symptoms may occur at rest or with exertion, may be episodic and specific (e.g., syncope), or may be chronic and nonspecific (e.g., dizziness, fatigue, or exercise intolerance).

c. Less commonly, asymptomatic patients with advanced conduction disease (Mobitz type II and third-degree atrioventricular [AV] block) should be treated with a permanent pacemaker (class IIa indication).

3. The two most common indications for permanent pacemaker implantation are sinus node dysfunction and AV conduction block.

4. **Patients with symptomatic chronic inappropriate bradycardia are said to have sick sinus syndrome.** The electrocardiographic manifestations encompass sinus bradycardia, sinus pauses or sinus arrest, and sinoatrial exit block. Patients with sick sinus syndrome accompanied by paroxysmal tachycardia have tachy-brady syndrome.

5. **AV block is classified into three types.**

a. **First-degree block** is defined by prolongation of the PR interval over 0.2 seconds. Most patients are asymptomatic. There is no indication for pacing.

b. **Second-degree AV block** is characterized by a prolonged PR interval and intermittent failure of AV conduction. **Mobitz type I** second-degree AV block manifests as progressive prolongation of the PR interval with subsequent AV block and is caused by delay within the AV node. In **Mobitz type II** second-degree block, the PR interval is constant with intermittent AV block. Mobitz type II arises below the AV node and therefore is more likely to progress to complete heart block. When conduction is 2:1, the block cannot be definitively classified as either type, although the width of the QRS complex is suggestive (narrow QRS suggests Mobitz type I; wide QRS suggests Mobitz type II). Advanced second-degree block is diagnosed when P waves are conducted in a ratio of 3:1 or higher and the PR interval is constant.

c. **Third-degree heart block** (complete heart block) is characterized by the absence of AV nodal conduction and AV dissociation.

6. Both the sinus node and the AV conduction system are susceptible to injury from ischemia, infiltrative diseases, infection, and trauma (surgical or catheter related), but the most common cause of intrinsic conduction disease is age-related idiopathic degeneration (Lev's disease).

7. **Common reversible causes of bradycardia** (Box 14-1) including drug effects, sleep apnea, hypothyroidism, and electrolyte imbalances should be sought.

II. INDICATIONS FOR PERMANENT PACING

A joint task force of the American College of Cardiology, American Heart Association, and North American Society of Pacing and Electrophysiology published practice guidelines for the implantation of cardiac pacemakers in 1998 and an update in 2002.[1,2] The indications for pacing are summarized according to a standard American College of Cardiology and American Heart Association classification: class I indications, for which evidence or general agreement suggests benefit from treatment; class II indications, for which there is conflicting evidence or divergent opinion of benefit; and class III indications, for which evidence or opinion suggests inefficacy or harm. Class II indications are further subdivided into IIa

---

> **BOX 14-1**
>
> ## CAUSES OF ACQUIRED SINUS NODE DYSFUNCTION AND ATRIOVENTRICULAR BLOCK
>
> | **INTRINSIC CAUSES** | |
> | --- | --- |
> | Idiopathic degeneration (Lev's disease) | Infiltrative |
> | Coronary artery disease | Sarcoidosis |
> | Chest irradiation | Amyloidosis |
> | Infections | Hemochromatosis |
> | Syphilis | Malignancy |
> | Viral myocarditis | Neuromuscular |
> | Chagas's disease | Myotonic muscular dystrophy |
> | Tuberculosis | Limb-girdle dystrophy |
> | Toxoplasmosis | Charcot-Marie-Tooth disease |
> | Lyme disease | Surgery or trauma |
> | Infective endocarditis | AV node ablation |
> | Diphtheria | Valve surgery |
> | Collagen-vascular disease | **EXTRINSIC CAUSES** |
> | Rheumatoid arthritis | Drugs |
> | Scleroderma | Digoxin |
> | Dermatomyositis | β-Blockers |
> | Ankylosing spondylitis | Calcium channel blockers |
> | Polyarteritis nodosa | Antiarrhythmic drugs (amiodarone, |
> | Systemic lupus erythematosus | procainamide, class IC agents) |
> | Marfan's syndrome | Hypothermia |
> | | Hypothyroidism |
> | | Hypokalemia |
> | | Hyperkalemia |

Modified from Braunwald E et al, eds: *Braunwald's heart disease: a textbook of cardiovascular medicine*, 6th ed, Philadelphia, 2001, WB Saunders.

(weight of evidence or opinion suggests benefit of treatment) or IIb (benefit is less well established). The indications for permanent pacing in commonly encountered situations are summarized in Table 14-1.

1. Sinus node dysfunction.
a. Symptomatic **bradycardia** necessitates pacemaker placement. In patients with sick sinus syndrome, bradycardia or tachycardia may cause symptoms. Documenting a causal link between symptoms and arrhythmias often is difficult but is essential to avoid inappropriate therapy. Ambulatory electrocardiographic or event monitoring is useful for this purpose.
b. **Iatrogenic bradycardia resulting from essential drug therapy** (as may be necessary to treat tachycardia) is a class I indication for pacing.
c. **Chronotropic incompetence,** defined by an inadequate heart rate response to exercise or stress, is also a class I indication.
d. If the association between symptoms and bradycardia is not clear, the indication is class IIa.
2. **AV conduction disease.** Symptomatic third-degree heart block and Mobitz type II second-degree AV block are class I indications for pacing.

TABLE 14-1

INDICATIONS FOR PERMANENT PACING IN COMMONLY ENCOUNTERED CONDITIONS

Disorder	Indication for Pacing
Sinus node dysfunction	**Class I**
	Documented bradycardia, including frequent sinus pauses that cause symptoms.
	Symptomatic chronotropic incompetence.
	Class IIa
	Sinus node dysfunction occurring spontaneously or as a result of necessary drug therapy, with a heart rate ≤ 40 bpm, when a clear association between significant symptoms consistent with bradycardia and the actual presence of bradycardia has not been documented.
	Syncope of unexplained origin when major abnormalities of sinus node function are discovered or provoked in electrophysiologic studies.
	Class IIb
	In minimally symptomatic patients, chronic heart rate < 40 bpm while awake.
	Class III
	Sinus node dysfunction in asymptomatic patients including those in whom substantial sinus bradycardia (heart rate < 40 bpm) is a consequence of long-term drug treatment.
	Sinus node dysfunction in patients with symptoms suggestive of bradycardia that are clearly documented as not associated with a slow heart rate.
	Sinus node dysfunction with symptomatic bradycardia caused by nonessential drug therapy.
AV block in adults	**Class I**
	Third-degree and advanced second-degree AV block at any anatomic level, associated with symptomatic bradycardia caused by AV block, necessary drug therapy, documented periods of asystole ≥ 3 s or escape rate < 40 bpm in awake, symptom-free patients; AV node ablation or permanent postoperative AV block; or neuromuscular disease with AV block.
	Class IIa
	Asymptomatic third-degree AV block at any anatomic site with average awake ventricular rate of 40 bpm or higher, especially if cardiomegaly or LV dysfunction is present.
	Asymptomatic type II second-degree AV block with a narrow QRS. When type II second-degree AV block occurs with a wide QRS, pacing is a class I indication.

AV, atrioventricular; *bpm,* beats per minute; *LV,* left ventricular.

cont'd

14

BRADYCARDIA AND PACEMAKERS

TABLE 14-1

INDICATIONS FOR PERMANENT PACING IN COMMONLY
ENCOUNTERED CONDITIONS—cont'd

Disorder	Indication for Pacing
	Asymptomatic type I second-degree AV block at intra- or infra-His levels found at electrophysiologic study performed for other indications.
	First- or second-degree AV block with symptoms similar to those of pacemaker syndrome.
	Class IIb
	Marked first-degree AV block (> 0.30 s) in patients with LV dysfunction and symptoms of congestive heart failure in whom a shorter AV interval results in hemodynamic improvement.
	Neuromuscular disease such as myotonic muscular dystrophy, Kearns-Sayre syndrome, Erb's dystrophy (limb-girdle), and peroneal muscular dystrophy with any degree of AV block with or without symptoms.
	Class III
	Asymptomatic first-degree AV block.
	Asymptomatic type I second-degree AV block at the supra-His (AV node) level or not known to be intra- or infra-Hisian.
	AV block expected to resolve or unlikely to recur (e.g., drug toxicity, Lyme disease, or during hypoxia in sleep apnea syndrome in absence of symptoms).
Chronic bifascicular or trifascicular block	**Class I**
	Intermittent third-degree AV block.
	Type II second-degree AV block.
	Alternating bundle branch block.
	Class IIa
	Syncope not demonstrated to be caused by AV block when other likely causes have been excluded, specifically ventricular tachycardia.
	Class IIb
	Neuromuscular diseases such as myotonic muscular dystrophy, Kearns-Sayre syndrome, Erb's dystrophy, and peroneal muscular atrophy with any degree of fascicular block with or without symptoms, because there may be unpredictable progression of AV conduction disease.
	Class III
	Fascicular block without AV block or symptoms.
	Fascicular block with first-degree AV block without symptoms.
Hypersensitive carotid and neurocardiogenic syncope	**Class I**
	Recurrent syncope caused by carotid sinus stimulation; minimal carotid sinus pressure induces ventricular asystole of more than 3-s duration in the absence of any medication that depresses the sinus node or AV conduction.

AV, atrioventricular; *bpm*, beats per minute; *LV*, left ventricular.   *cont'd*

TABLE 14-1

INDICATIONS FOR PERMANENT PACING IN COMMONLY ENCOUNTERED CONDITIONS—cont'd

Disorder	Indication for Pacing
	Class IIa
	Recurrent syncope without clear, provocative events and with hypersensitive cardioinhibitory response.
	Class III
	A hyperactive cardioinhibitory response to carotid sinus stimulation in the absence of symptoms or in the presence of vague symptoms such as dizziness or lightheadedness.
	Recurrent syncope, lightheadedness, or dizziness in the absence of a hyperactive cardioinhibitory response.
	Situational vasovagal syncope in which avoidance behavior is effective.
Dilated cardiomyopathy	**Class I** indications for sinus node dysfunction or AV block as previously described.
	Class IIa
	Biventricular pacing in medically refractory, symptomatic New York Heart Association class III-IV heart failure with idiopathic dilated or ischemic cardiomyopathy, prolonged QRS interval ≥ 130 ms, LV end-diastolic diameter ≥ 55 mm, and ejection fraction ≤ 35%.
	Class III
	Asymptomatic dilated cardiomyopathy.
	Symptomatic dilated cardiomyopathy when patients are rendered asymptomatic by drug therapy.
	Symptomatic ischemic cardiomyopathy when the ischemia is amenable to intervention.

AV, atrioventricular; *bpm,* beats per minute; *LV,* left ventricular.

Asymptomatic patients with impaired AV conduction should be paced if there are periods of asystole lasting at least 3 seconds or a ventricular escape less than 40 bpm. The updated guidelines underscore the importance of cardiomegaly or left ventricular dysfunction in asymptomatic third-degree AV block with a class IIa indication.

3. **Conduction disturbance in myocardial infarction (MI).**

a. AV block and fascicular block complicating acute MI reflect a more extensive infarction and therefore portend a poor prognosis, despite the decreased incidence of this complication in the era of aggressive, early revascularization.

b. In 90% of people, the AV node is supplied by the AV nodal branch of the right coronary artery, with the left circumflex artery supplying the remainder. The bundle of His is fed by the right coronary artery with collateral flow from the left anterior descending artery and left circumflex artery. The right bundle and the left anterior fascicle are supplied almost solely by septal perforators of the left anterior descending artery and therefore are susceptible to ischemia during anterior MI. The left posterior fascicle enjoys relative protection because of its dual blood supply from branches of the right and left coronary arteries.

c. In inferior MI, AV block within the first 24 hours results from heightened vagal tone and usually responds to atropine. As edema subsequently develops at the AV node, progressive block may occur and is less responsive to atropine but typically resolves over 5 to 7 days. By contrast, left anterior descending artery occlusion in anterior MI causes necrosis of the septum and is associated with irreversible right bundle branch block, left anterior fascicular block, Mobitz type II, or complete heart block. In both types of MI, symptomatic bradycardia or advanced asymptomatic AV block may necessitate temporary transvenous pacing.

4. **Hypersensitive carotid sinus syndrome and neurocardiogenic syncope.** If carotid sinus stimulation produces recurrent syncope or if minimal carotid pressure induces more than 3 seconds of ventricular asystole in the absence of medications that suppresses the sinus node or AV conduction, then permanent pacing is considered a class I recommendation.

5. **Chronic heart failure.** Recent clinical trials support the use of biventricular pacing to provide synchronous contraction between the septum and ventricular free wall in patients with intraventricular conduction delay and dilated cardiomyopathy. In this more technically challenging procedure, a pacing wire is introduced into the coronary sinus to capture the left ventricular free wall, in addition to standard right atrial and ventricular leads. The Comparison of Medical Therapy, Pacing, and Defibrillation in Heart Failure (COMPANION) trial enrolled patients with ischemic or nonischemic New York Heart Association class III-IV heart failure, left ventricular ejection fraction of 35% or less, and a QRS interval greater than 120 milliseconds and randomized them to treatment with optimal medical therapy alone or medical therapy plus biventricular pacing with or without implantable cardioverter-defibrillator capability. Both pacing alone and pacing with implantable cardioverter-defibrillator therapy were associated with a 20% reduction in the combined primary endpoint of death or hospitalization.[3]

6. Among patients with pacemakers, a higher frequency of single-site right ventricular pacing has been associated with higher morbidity and mortality rates, suggesting that the benefits of AV synchronization and chronotropy may be mitigated by the ventricular dyssynchrony caused by single-site ventricular pacing.[4]

III. COMMON PACING MODES

Pacing modes are classified according to three- to five-letter codes. The first letter refers to the chamber paced (*A* for atrium, *V* for ventricle, *D* for dual or both chambers). The second letter refers to the chamber sensed and uses the same abbreviations as for pacing, with the addition of *O* to indicate that sensing is turned off. The third letter refers to the response of the pacemaker to a sensed signal: *I* for inhibit, *T* for trigger, or *D* for dual response of inhibiting or triggering for dual-chamber devices. A fourth letter (*R*), if present, signifies rate-adaptive pacing. These pacemakers incorporate sensors that monitor various physiologic parameters of metabolic demand (e.g., motion, minute ventilation, PO_2, central venous pH) and then adapt the pacing rate according to a clinician-programmed algorithm. The fifth letter in the code is added if antitachycardia pacing features are included, although most such features are now incorporated into automatic implantable cardioverter-defibrillators (*P,* antitachycardia pacing, *S,* shock, *D,* dual or both, *O,* neither).

The choice of a pacing mode is determined by many variables including the primary indication for pacing, exercise capacity, the need for AV synchrony, the responsiveness of the sinus node, and the need for mode switching. Table 14-2 outlines other common programmable features of pacemakers.

Many clinical trials have attempted to document clinical benefits of dual-chamber pacing and single-chamber pacing.[5] The recent Mode Selection Trial in Sinus Node Dysfunction (MOST) study found no difference in mortality or nonfatal stroke between DDDR and VVIR pacing in patients with sinus node dysfunction.[6] Dual-chamber pacing was associated with a lower incidence of new-onset and chronic atrial fibrillation, fewer symptoms of heart failure, and improved quality of life.

1. **DDD(R).** In DDD(R) mode, leads in the atrium and ventricle sense electrical events in both chambers and will either inhibit or trigger pacing depending on programmed timing cycles. Fig. 14-1 schematizes the timing cycle in a DDD(R) pacemaker.
a. If intrinsic atrial and ventricular activity are sensed before the lower rate limit (usually 60 bpm) has expired, both chambers will be inhibited. If no atrial activity occurs during a determined interval after ventricular activity (the VA interval), then atrial pacing occurs and another timing interval, called the atrioventricular interval (AVI), begins. If no ventricular activity is sensed by the end of the AVI, ventricular pacing is triggered.
b. Conversely, if ventricular activity is sensed before the end of the AVI, the ventricular pacing is inhibited. Ventricular events (either sensed or paced) start the post-VA refractory period (PVARP). Atrial events occurring during the PVARP are not sensed. P waves sensed after the PVARP inhibit atrial pacing.

14

BRADYCARDIA AND PACEMAKERS

TABLE 14-2

SOME COMMON PROGRAMMABLE FEATURES OF PACEMAKERS

Parameter	Description	Typical Variables
Mode	Programmed response from a pacemaker with or without intrinsic cardiac events.	DDD, DDI, VVI, AAI, DOO, VOO.
Lower rate limit	Rate at which pacemaker emits an output pulse without intrinsic cardiac activity.	30-150 bpm.
Ventricular refractory period	Interval of the pacemaker timing cycle following a sensed or paced ventricular event during which the ventricular sensing channel is totally or partially unresponsive to incoming signals.	150-500 ms.
Sensitivity	Ability to sense an intrinsic electrical signal, which depends on the amplitude, slew rate, and frequency of the signal.	Atrial: 0.18-8 mV. Ventricular: 1-4 mV.
Mode switch	Capability of a dual-chamber pacemaker to automatically switch from an atrial tracking mode to a non-atrial tracking mode when an atrial rhythm meets the criteria that the pacemaker determines to be pathologic. When the atrial rhythm meets the criteria for a physiologic rhythm, the mode switched back to an atrial tracking mode.	On or off; if on, the detection rates often are programmable for rates 120-190 bpm.
Atrioventricular interval	Period between the initiation of the paced or sensed atrial event and the delivery of a consecutive ventricular output pulse.	30-350 ms.
PVARP	Period after a paced or sensed ventricular event during which the atrial channel is refractory.	150-300 ms; in some devices, auto-PVARP adjusts with cycle length.
Pulse width	Duration over which the output is delivered.	0.05-1.9 ms.
Pulse amplitude	Magnitude of the voltage level reached during a pacemaker output pulse, usually expressed in volts.	0.5-8.1 V.
Circadian lower rate limit	Reduces the lower rate limit during sleeping hours.	

A, atrium; *D*, dual (both chambers); *I*, inhibit; *O*, off (sensing); *PVARP*, postventricular atrial refractory period; *V*, ventricle.

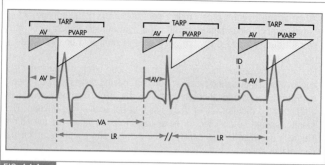

FIG. 14-1

Timing cycle of DDD pacemaker. *TARP*, total atrial refractory period. *(From Braunwald E et al, eds:* Braunwald's heart disease: a textbook of cardiovascular medicine, *6th ed, Philadelphia, 2001, WB Saunders.)*

14

BRADYCARDIA AND PACEMAKERS

c. This mode is indicated in patients with AV block. It has the advantage of maintaining AV synchrony and minimizes the incidence of the pacemaker syndrome but has a somewhat shortened lifespan because of its higher energy requirements. Newer rate-adaptive programming can prevent this mode from inappropriately tracking atrial arrhythmia.

2. **DDI(R).** Both atrium and ventricle are sensed, but the only response to a sensed event is inhibition. Unlike in the DDD mode, intrinsic atrial activity does not start the AVI timer, and so ventricular pacing is not triggered by intrinsic atrial depolarization. Ventricular pacing occurs only when the intrinsic ventricular rate is below a programmed rate or when the AVI expires after a paced atrial output. This mode may be useful in patients with frequent atrial tachyarrhythmias, which might be inappropriately tracked by DDD mode.

3. **VVI(R).** A single ventricular lead paces and senses only the ventricle. A sensed ventricular event inhibits pacemaker output. This mode is commonly used in patients with AV block and unorganized atrial rhythms such as atrial fibrillation. A major limitation is loss of AV synchrony and subsequent compromise of cardiac output.

4. **AAI.** A one-lead system that senses and paces only the atrium. Intrinsic atrial activity inhibits pacemaker output. This mode is suitable for patients with sinus node dysfunction who have intact AV conduction and are able to mount an appropriate heart rate response to exercise (chronotropically competent). The lack of backup ventricular pacing should AV block occur is a drawback, but the rate of progression of sinus node dysfunction to clinically significant AV nodal disease has been found to be less than 2% annually.

PEARLS AND PITFALLS

- When a single-ventricle pacemaker paces from the right ventricle, a left bundle branch block pattern results. If a right bundle branch block is present during a paced rhythm, lead placement should be evaluated immediately.
- Not all pacing spikes may be seen on a 12-lead electrocardiogram because of sampling intervals. In addition, pacing spikes may be seen in an inappropriate location on a rhythm strip. This may be a sensitivity artifact of the monitor rather than a sign of pacemaker dysfunction. The monitor should be checked to make sure the pacer filters are turned off. This will decrease the sensitivity of the monitor and eliminate artifactual pacemaker spikes.
- Patients with pacemakers undergoing surgery in which electrocautery is planned should have the mode reprogrammed to VOO or DOO mode, which paces the chambers in an asynchronous manner independent of intrinsic or ectopic electrical activity.
- Rates of infection of pacemaker systems are similar to those of other cardiovascular devices, about 4% annually. Infection may range from local inflammation of the pacemaker pocket to lead-associated endocarditis. Early infections are caused most commonly by *Staphylococcus aureus* and present with systemic signs and symptoms, whereas late infections are caused by more indolent organisms such as *Staphylococcus epidermidis* and tend to lack systemic signs. Treatment includes antibiotic therapy and extraction of the generator, pacemaker, and leads. The pacing system should be reimplanted on the contralateral chest wall after appropriate antibiotic therapy.[7]
- Pacemaker-mediated tachycardia or pacemaker reentrant tachycardia can occur in DDD mode when ventricular activity, usually a premature ventricular contraction, causes a retrograde P wave to be sensed by the pacemaker. The AVI timer begins, and a paced ventricular output may cause another retrograde P wave, setting up a reentrant circuit tachycardia at a rate equal to the maximum tracking rate. This complication is prevented by ensuring that the PVARP is sufficiently long to prevent sensing of retrograde P waves.
- The pacemaker syndrome refers to a constellation of symptoms and signs in response to ventricular pacing. The loss of AV synchrony in patients with a normally functioning pacemaker leads to atrial contraction against closed AV valves, mitral and tricuspid regurgitation, variable stroke volume, and elevated filling pressures. Symptoms include shortness of breath, dizziness from hypotension, fatigue, pulsations in the neck or abdomen, and cough. The incidence is up to 15% of patients with VVI pacemakers.
- Patients with profound bradycardia are at risk of dying from torsade de pointes due to the prolongation of the QT interval that accompanies the increased R-R interval from bradycardia.

REFERENCES

1. Gregoratos G et al: ACC/AHA guidelines for implantation of cardiac pacemakers and antiarrhythmia devices: executive summary. A report of the American College of Cardiology/American Heart Association Task Force on Practice Guidelines (Committee on Pacemaker Implantation), *Circulation* 97:1325, 1998. D
2. Gregoratos G et al: ACC/AHA/NASPE 2002 Guideline update for implantation of cardiac pacemakers and antiarrhythmia devices: summary article. A report of the American College of Cardiology/America Heart Association Task Force on Practice Guidelines (ACC/AHA/NASPE Committee to Update the 1998 Pacemaker Guidelines), *Circulation* 106:2145-2161, 2002. D
3. Bristow M et al: Cardiac resynchronization therapy with or without an implantable cardiac defibrillator in patients with advanced chronic heart failure, *N Engl J Med* 350:2140-2150, 2004. A
4. Wilkoff BL et al: Dual-chamber pacing or ventricular backup pacing in patients with an implantable defibrillator: the Dual Chamber and VVI Implantable Defibrillator (DAVID) Trial, *JAMA* 288:3115-3123, 2002. A
5. Gervasui L et al: Evidence base for pacemaker mode selection: from physiology to randomized trials, *Circulation* 109:443-451, 2004. C
6. Lamas GA et al: Ventricular pacing or dual-chamber pacing for sinus-node dysfunction, *N Engl J Med* 346:1854-1862, 2002. A
7. Darouiche R: Treatment of infections associated with surgical implants, *N Engl J Med* 350:1422-1429, 2004. C

14

BRADYCARDIA AND PACEMAKERS

Tachyarrhythmias and Implantable Cardioverter-Defibrillators

Jordan M. Prutkin, MD, MHS; and Ronald Berger, MD, PhD

15

FAST FACTS

- If there is difficulty distinguishing wide complex supraventricular tachycardia (SVT) from ventricular tachycardia (VT), treat as VT and follow the advanced cardiac life support algorithm.
- Hemodynamic stability cannot be used to distinguish SVT from VT.
- A history of structural heart disease is the best predictor of VT or SVT.
- Implantable cardioverter-defibrillators (ICDs) improve survival in primary and secondary prevention of sudden cardiac death.
- ICDs detect ventricular tachycardia or fibrillation on the basis of the ventricular rate (not the QRS width) and may deliver an electrical charge (1-36 J) or initiate rapid pacing to terminate these rhythms. Up to 30% of ICD shocks may be inappropriate.

I. SUPRAVENTRICULAR TACHYCARDIAS

1. There are many types of SVT, including sinus tachycardia, atrial fibrillation, atrial flutter, sinoatrial node reentrant tachycardia, multifocal atrial tachycardia, atrioventricular nodal reentrant tachycardia (AVNRT), atrioventricular reciprocating tachycardia (AVRT), and atrial tachycardia.
2. Patients with SVT and structural heart disease usually present in their 50s, whereas those with AVNRT or AVRT present in their 20s and 30s.[1] By far the most common SVT necessitating hospitalization is atrial fibrillation.
3. Symptoms of SVT include palpitations, fatigue, lightheadedness, chest discomfort, dyspnea, presyncope, and rarely syncope.
4. Regular and paroxysmal palpitations with sudden beginning and ending are most commonly AVNRT or AVRT. This is also suggested if palpitations cease with vagal maneuvers (e.g., Valsalva maneuver, carotid massage, facial immersion in cold water).
5. If the episodes occur several times per week, an ambulatory Holter may be useful to evaluate the rhythm. If they occur less frequently, event loop recorders can be used to capture the arrhythmia.
6. A narrow QRS is almost always an SVT (Fig. 15-1). If there is no P wave or evidence of atrial activity and the R-R interval is regular, it is most commonly AVNRT. This is also suggested by a pseudo–R wave in V1 and pseudo–S wave in leads II, III, and aVF.

7. If the patient is hemodynamically unstable, he or she should be cardioverted per the advanced cardiac life support guidelines. Adenosine is a useful diagnostic tool in evaluating stable, narrow complex, regular SVTs. First, 6 mg of intravenous adenosine is pushed rapidly with a quick normal saline flush. If this has no effect, 12 mg adenosine may be used next. If the rhythm stops with a P wave after the last QRS complex, this suggests AVNRT or AVRT. If the rhythm stops with the QRS complex, this suggests atrial tachycardia. If the rhythm continues, however, it may be that an inadequate dosage of adenosine was given. If there is continued atrial arrhythmia in the midst of adequate atrioventricular (AV) block, this suggests atrial fibrillation or flutter, excludes AVRT, and makes AVNRT very unlikely. Caution is advised when one is using adenosine in patients with severe asthma. Long-term treatment of AVNRT includes beta-blockers, nondihydropyridine calcium channel blockers, or digoxin, but the best long-term treatment is catheter ablation.

8. Determining whether wide QRS tachyarrhythmias are SVT with bundle branch block, SVT with antegrade accessory pathway conduction, or VT can be difficult (Fig. 15-2).

9. Wolff-Parkinson-White is a syndrome characterized by both preexcitation (delta waves) and tachycardia. The tachyarrhythmia typically is a narrow complex AVRT (orthodromic) due to antegrade conduction through the AV node and retrograde conduction through the accessory pathway. In this situation the delta waves at rest are not seen because conduction is through the AV node rather than the bypass tract.

a. Acute treatment for narrow complex orthodromic AVRT is adenosine.

b. Medical treatment for orthodromic AVRT includes beta-blockers, procainamide, or flecainide, although in practice catheter ablation definitively treats the accessory pathways.

c. Wide complex tachyarrhythmias and atrial fibrillation due to an accessory pathway (antidromic, conduction down the accessory pathway and reentrant through the AV node) should not be treated with beta-blockers, calcium channel blockers, adenosine, and digoxin because of the risk of slowing conduction through the AV node and speeding conduction down the bypass tract potentially, resulting in unstable arrhythmias.

d. If there is asymptomatic preexcitation without tachycardia, the prognosis is generally good. There is no indication for an electrophysiologic study (EPS) or catheter ablation in these patients because the positive predictive value of those who will become symptomatic is low. However, those with high-risk jobs such as school bus drivers, pilots, and scuba divers may undergo ablation.[1]

II. VENTRICULAR ARRHYTHMIAS AND ICDS

1. Several attempts have been made to improve the 5% survival rate from out-of-hospital cardiac arrest, including ICDs. Sudden cardiac death

15

TACHYARRHYTHMIAS AND ICDS

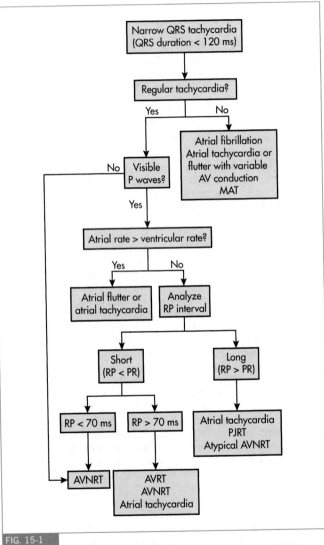

FIG. 15-1

Differential diagnosis for narrow QRS tachycardia. *AV*, atrioventricular; *AVNRT*, atrioventricular nodal reciprocating tachycardia; *AVRT*, atrioventricular reciprocating tachycardia; *MAT*, multifocal atrial tachycardia; *PJRT*, permanent form of junctional reciprocating tachycardia. *(From Gregoratos G et al: J Am Coll Cardiol 40:1703-1719, 2002.)*

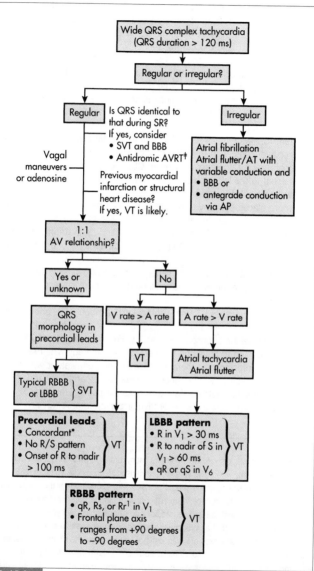

FIG. 15-2

See legend on the next page

occurs in approximately 400,000 people each year in the United States.[2] Those with coronary artery disease and left ventricular systolic dysfunction are at highest risk, with about 50% of deaths in those with congestive heart failure occurring suddenly.[2]

2. ICDs were introduced in the 1980s as a means of continuously monitoring ventricular rates. When the rate exceeds a programmed threshold, the device assumes that the patient has a malignant ventricular arrhythmia, and a shock is administered. In this way the ICD's detection of VT is based primarily on the ventricular rate rather than the width of the QRS complex on the surface electrocardiogram. Current ICD systems all have VVI pacing capability and may consist of one or two leads, with the latter configuration designed to allow dual-chamber pacing if necessary. Newer ICDs are available with a third lead connected to the left ventricular free wall through the coronary sinus to allow for biventricular pacing.

3. ICDs are placed similarly to pacemakers (see Chapter 14), with one or two electrodes for defibrillation and pacing. The pulse generator is connected to the lead in the right ventricle (and right atrium for two-lead systems). When the ICD fires, the circuit consists of a ventricular coil as one pole and the pulse generator and another coil in the right atrium as the other. The pulse generator typically is positioned on the patient's left side, allowing the maximum amount of current to traverse the heart.

4. The ICD distinguishes VT from ventricular fibrillation (VF), primarily on the basis of ventricular rates, although detection enhancements include electrogram features, onset, and stability. For example, most ICDs are programmed to have one to three zones of therapy. The device delivers the programmed therapy based on the heart rate it detects. Available therapies include antitachycardia pacing and low- and high-energy shock delivery. In antitachycardia pacing, the device initiates a short burst of rapid ventricular pacing in an effort to

---

Differential diagnosis for wide QRS complex tachycardia. A QRS conduction delay during sinus rhythm, when available for comparison, reduces the value of QRS morphology analysis. Adenosine should be used with caution when the diagnosis is unclear because it may produce VF in patients with coronary artery disease and atrial fibrillation with a rapid ventricular rate in preexcited tachycardias. *Concordant indicates that all precordial leads show either positive or negative deflections. Fusion complexes are diagnostic of VT. ‡In preexcited tachycardias, the QRS generally is wider (i.e., more preexcited) than sinus rhythm. A, atrial; AP, accessory pathway; AT, atrial tachycardia; AV, atrioventricular; AVRT, atrioventricular reciprocating tachycardia; BBB, bundle branch block; LBBB, left bundle branch block; RBBB, right bundle branch block; SR, sinus rhythm; SVT, supraventricular tachycardia; V, ventricular; VF, ventricular fibrillation; VT, ventricular tachycardia. (From Blomström-Lundquist C et al: J Am Coll Cardiol 42:1493-1531, 2003.)

interrupt the tachycardia by eliciting a wavefront that collides with that of the reentrant circuit. Shock may be delivered in the form of low-energy cardioversion or defibrillation. Most ICDs are capable of delivering 30 J or more to terminate unstable VT and VF. If the rhythm is VF, the device will provide a high-energy shock.

5. ICDs have a 98% success rate in terminating VF. Antitachycardia pacing can convert VT in 90% of cases and up to 98% with defibrillation.[1]

6. Complications of ICDs include pneumothorax, hematoma, infection, frequent shocks, acceleration of VT, oversensing and undersensing, lead malfunction, lead fractures or failure of insulation, a connection problem, magnetic interference, and psychological dysfunction.

7. Follow-up is necessary to monitor the implantation site, assess proper functioning of leads and the device, and detect arrhythmias. If the patient receives a single shock, he or she can be seen during a routine visit. If multiple shocks occur within 48 hours, the patient should be seen within 24 hours. All ICDs can be interrogated noninvasively to obtain the program describing what the device will do for a given abnormal heart rate. They also have the capacity to store electrograms to analyze the heart rhythm for which a patient received a shock.

III. INDICATIONS FOR ICDS

Current indications for ICDs are based on the 1998 practice guidelines and a 2002 update devised by the American College of Cardiology, the American Heart Association, and the North American Society of Pacing and Electrophysiology.[3] The indications follow the standard evidence-based tiered system: Class I indication means the procedure is generally agreed to be beneficial. Class IIa indications are those for which there is conflicting evidence or divergence of opinion, but the weight of evidence is in favor, and class IIb is similar to class IIa except that the efficacy of a procedure is less well established. This system is based on several randomized studies in primary and secondary prevention of sudden cardiac death (Table 15-1).

A. CLASS I

- Cardiac arrest caused by VT or VF that has an irreversible cause.
- Spontaneous sustained VT in the presence of structural heart disease.
- Syncope of unknown origin with hemodynamically important inducible VT or VF at EPS if drug therapy is ineffective, not tolerated, or not preferred.
- Nonsustained VT with coronary disease, prior myocardial infarction, left ventricular dysfunction, and inducible VF or sustained VT on EPS that is not suppressible by class I antiarrhythmic drugs.
- Spontaneous sustained VT in those without structural heart disease not amenable to other treatments.

B. CLASS IIA

- Ischemic cardiomyopathy with an ejection fraction less than or equal to 30% at least 1 month after myocardial infarction and 3 months after coronary artery revascularization surgery.

TABLE 15-1

SELECTED PRIMARY AND SECONDARY PREVENTION TRIALS OF ICD

	Control Group	Mean Left Ventricular Ejection Fraction	Average Follow-Up	Hazard Ratio (95% Confidence Interval)
PRIMARY PREVENTION				
Multicenter Automatic Defibrillator Implantation Trial[9]	Conventional	26%	27 mo	0.46 (0.26-0.82)
Multicenter Unsustained Tachycardia Trial[10]	Conventional	30%	39 mo	0.49 (0.35-0.69)
Coronary Artery Bypass Graft Patch Trial[4]	Conventional	27%	32 mo	1.07 (0.81-1.42)
Multicenter Automatic Defibrillator Implantation Trial II[11]	Conventional	23%	20 mo	0.65 (0.51-0.93)
SCD-HeFT[5]	Amiodarone or placebo	25%	3.8 yr	0.77 (0.62-0.96)
COMPANION[12]	Conventional	22%	16 mo	0.64 (0.48-0.86)
DEFINITE[13]	Conventional	21%	29 mo	0.65 (0.40-1.06)
SECONDARY PREVENTION				
Antiarrhythmics versus Implantable Defibrillators[6]	Amiodarone or sotalol	31%	1.5 yr	0.62 (0.47-0.81)
Cardiac Arrest Study Hamburg[7]	Amiodarone	45%	4.5 yr	0.77 (0.42-1.12)
Canadian Implantable Defibrillator Study[8]	Amiodarone	34%	3.0 yr	0.82 (0.61-1.10)

C. CLASS IIB

- Cardiac arrest presumed to be caused by VF when EPS is precluded by other medical conditions.
- Severe symptoms, such as syncope, attributable to ventricular tachyarrhythmias in patients awaiting cardiac transplantation.
- Long QT syndrome, hypertrophic cardiomyopathy, arrhythmogenic right ventricular dysplasia, and other inherited conditions with a risk for life-threatening ventricular tachyarrhythmias.
- Nonsustained VT with coronary artery disease, prior myocardial infarction, left ventricular dysfunction, and inducible sustained VT or VF at EPS.
- Recurrent syncope of undetermined origin in the presence of ventricular dysfunction and inducible ventricular arrhythmias at EPS when other causes of syncope have been excluded.
- Syncope of unexplained origin or family history of unexplained sudden cardiac death in association with typical or atypical right bundle branch block and ST elevations (Brugada's syndrome).
- Syncope in patients with advanced structural heart disease in whom thorough invasive and noninvasive investigations have failed to define a cause.

PEARLS AND PITFALLS

- Having an ICD implanted does not obviate external defibrillation. Because the device assesses the need for therapy on the basis of the heart rate, a patient may have symptomatic VT that is below the threshold for initiating automated therapy.
- ICDs are not indicated for patients with Wolff-Parkinson-White syndrome, VT caused by transient or reversible disorders, idiopathic VT curable by radiofrequency ablation, terminal illnesses, class IV refractory congestive heart failure in a patient who is not a transplant candidate, or significant psychiatric illness aggravated by ICD discharges.
- As demonstrated by the Coronary Artery Bypass Graft (CABG) Patch Trial, prophylactic ICD placement does not provide a mortality benefit even for high-risk patients with left ventricular dysfunction undergoing CABG if they have no history of symptomatic ventricular arrhythmias.[4]
- The guidelines probably will be changed to incorporate the results of three recent trials. The SCD-HeFT trial showed a 23% mortality reduction in those with ischemic or nonischemic New York Heart Association class II or III heart failure and ejection fraction of 35% or less.[6] The COMPANION study showed a 36% decrease in mortality in those with class III or IV ischemic or nonischemic cardiomyopathy and a wide QRS interval who received a biventricular pacemaker plus defibrillator compared with optimal medical therapy.[12] Finally, the DEFINITE study demonstrated a nonsignificant 35% mortality reduction in those with nonischemic cardiomyopathy, ejection fraction less than 36%, and frequent premature ventricular contractions or nonsustained VT.[13]
- Patients with known coronary disease who present with a wide complex tachycardia regardless of hemodynamics have VT until proven otherwise.

15

TACHYARRHYTHMIAS AND ICDS

- Adenosine, beta-blockers, digoxin, and calcium channel blockers are contraindicated in antidromic AVRT and atrial fibrillation associated with Wolff-Parkinson-White syndrome because of the risk of speeding conduction down the accessory pathway.

REFERENCES

1. Blomstrom-Lundqvist C et al: ACC/AHA/ESC guidelines for the management of patients with supraventricular arrhythmias: executive summary. A report of the American College of Cardiology/American Heart Association Task Force on Practice Guidelines and the European Society of Cardiology Committee for Practice Guidelines (Writing Committee to Develop Guidelines for the Management of Patients with Supraventricular Arrhythmias), *J Am Coll Cardiol* 42:1493-1531, 2003. D
2. Ezekowitz JA, Armstrong PW, McAlister FA: Implantable cardioverter defibrillators in primary and secondary prevention: a systematic review of randomized, controlled trials, *Ann Intern Med* 138:445-452, 2003. C
3. Gregoratos G et al: ACC/AHA/NASPE 2002 guideline update for implantation of cardiac pacemakers and antiarrhythmia devices: summary article. A report of the American College of Cardiology/American Heart Association Task Force on Practice Guidelines (ACC/AHA/NASPE Committee to Update the 1998 Pacemaker Guidelines), *J Am Coll Cardiol* 40:1703-1719, 2002. D
4. Bigger JT: Prophylactic use of implanted cardiac defibrillators in patients at high risk for ventricular arrhythmias after coronary artery bypass graft surgery. Coronary Artery Bypass Graft (CABG) Patch Trial Investigators, *N Engl J Med* 337:1569, 1997. A
5. Bardy GH et al: Amiodarone or an implantable cardioverter-defibrillator for congestive heart failure, *N Engl J Med* 352:225-237, 2005. A
6. Antiarrhythmics Versus Implantable Defibrillators (AVID) Investigators: A comparison of antiarrhythmic-drug therapy with implantable defibrillators in patients resuscitated from near-fatal ventricular arrhythmias, *N Engl J Med* 337:1576, 1997. A
7. Kuck KH et al: Randomized comparison of antiarrhythmic drug therapy with implantable defibrillators in patients resuscitated from cardiac arrest: the Cardiac Arrest Study Hamburg (CASH), *Circulation* 102:748-754, 2000. A
8. Connolly SJ et al: Canadian Implantable Defibrillator Study (CIDS): a randomized trial of the implantable cardioverter defibrillator against amiodarone, *Circulation* 101:1297-1302, 2000. A
9. Moss AJ et al: Improved survival with an implanted defibrillator in patients with coronary disease at high risk for ventricular arrhythmia. Multicenter Automatic Defibrillator Implantation Trial Investigators, *N Engl J Med* 335:1933, 1996. A
10. Buxton AE et al: A randomized study of the prevention of sudden death in patients with coronary artery disease. Multicenter Unsustained Tachycardia Trial Investigators, *N Engl J Med* 341:1882-1990, 1999. A
11. Moss AJ et al: Prophylactic implantation of a defibrillator in patients with myocardial infarction and reduced ejection fraction, *N Engl J Med* 346:877, 2002. A
12. Bristow MR et al: Cardiac-resynchronization therapy with or without an implantable defibrillator in advanced chronic heart failure, *N Engl J Med* 350:2140-2150, 2004. A
13. Kadish A et al: Prophylactic defibrillator implantation in patients with nonischemic dilated cardiomyopathy, *N Engl J Med* 350:2151-2158, 2004. A

Atrial Fibrillation

Rinky Bhatia, MD; Moeen Abedin, MD; and Hugh Calkins, MD

16

I. EPIDEMIOLOGY

A. DEFINITION

AF is an irregularly irregular supraventricular tachycardia characterized by disorganized atrial activation.

B. PREVALENCE

AF is the most common chronic rhythm disorder, affecting 5% of adults older than age 65.[1] The prevalence is increasing as the population ages. The presence of AF doubles the risk of cardiovascular mortality in patients with other cardiovascular disease.[2]

C. CLASSIFICATION

1. **Paroxysmal AF** is AF that starts and stops spontaneously.
2. **Persistent AF** is AF that necessitates electrical or pharmacologic cardioversion.
3. **Permanent AF** is AF that persists despite therapy or prompts a decision not to attempt to restore and maintain sinus rhythm.
4. **Lone AF** can be paroxysmal, persistent, or permanent. Lone AF is defined as AF occurring in patients younger than 65 years of age without underlying cardiovascular disease.

D. PATHOPHYSIOLOGY

AF is triggered by rapidly firing foci in the pulmonary veins and, less often, in the right atrium, superior vena cava, or coronary sinus.

1. Once triggered, AF is propagated by multiple migrating reentrant microwavelets, which lead to uncoordinated atrial contraction.
2. These wavelets rarely complete a circuit because of variation in conduction and refractoriness across the atrium, known as spatial heterogeneity.

3. An abnormal cardiac substrate allows AF to continue. AF begets AF by causing electrical remodeling; atrial ischemia and hibernation; structural remodeling; myocyte degeneration; and a dilated, hypocontractile atrium.

II. CLINICAL PRESENTATION

1. **Ambulatory monitoring of patients reveals that most episodes of AF are asymptomatic.**[3] The most common presenting symptom is fatigue. Other symptoms include chest pain, lightheadedness, and dyspnea.[3] Only 26% of patients hospitalized for AF complained of palpitations.[4]
2. Syncope is an uncommon manifestation of AF, but when present it is often associated with underlying sinus node dysfunction, aortic stenosis, hypertrophic cardiomyopathy, cerebrovascular disease, or an accessory atrioventricular (AV) pathway.[5]
3. Tachycardia can exacerbate other cardiac conditions such as coronary artery disease or congestive heart failure.
4. **The first step in evaluating patients with AF should be to determine hemodynamic stability.** Subsequent history taking should focus on symptoms, the pattern of AF (paroxysmal or persistent), the cause, underlying cardiac or extracardiac factors, and responses to previous treatments.
5. **Typical findings on examination** include an irregular pulse and irregular jugular venous pulsations. The examiner should also search for evidence of valvular disease or heart failure.

III. CAUSES

AF can be precipitated by cardiac or noncardiac causes.

1. **Cardiac causes** include hypertensive heart disease, cardiac surgery, valvular disease, acute myocardial infarction, myocarditis, and heart failure.[6] Between 30% and 60% of patients undergoing coronary artery bypass grafting or valve replacements experience self-limited postoperative AF.
2. **Noncardiac causes** of AF include hyperthyroidism (risk of AF is almost three times higher in patients with low thyroid-stimulating hormone),[7] pulmonary disease (PE), alcohol consumption, sepsis, sleep apnea, and medications (theophylline, adenosine, digitalis) (Box 16-1).

IV. DIAGNOSIS

1. **Electrocardiogram.** An irregularly irregular pulse is consistent with but not diagnostic of AF. An electrocardiogram is necessary to confirm the diagnosis. The key diagnostic electrocardiographic findings of AF are absence of P waves and irregularly irregular narrow QRS complexes. The atrial rate usually is 400 to 700 bpm. The ventricular rate depends on conduction through the AV node and usually is 120 to 180 bpm. Potential pitfalls include the following:

BOX 16-1

SECONDARY CAUSES OF ATRIAL FIBRILLATION

CONDITIONS LEADING TO INCREASED ATRIAL SIZE

Hypertensive heart disease (most common associated condition)*

Congestive heart failure (left ventricular systolic dysfunction)

Valvular heart disease

Acute pulmonary emboli

Atrial septal defect

CONDITIONS LEADING TO INCREASED ATRIAL IRRITABILITY

Binge alcohol consumption

Hyperadrenergic states (i.e., postoperative state, sepsis)

Thyrotoxicosis

Cardiac surgery

Theophylline

Myocarditis

*Data from Kannel WB et al: *N Engl J Med* 306:1018, 1982.

a. Sometimes F waves (fibrillatory waves) mimic P waves.
b. Extremely rapid ventricular response can appear to be regular.
c. It is important to distinguish AF from other conditions, such as sinus rhythm with frequent premature atrial contractions, sinus arrhythmia, multifocal atrial tachycardia, and atrial flutter.
d. The presence of a regular, narrow complex tachycardia at 150 bpm should raise suspicion for the presence of atrial flutter.
e. Preexisting bundle branch disease or aberrant ventricular conduction with rapid ventricular response can result in a wide complex tachycardia. It is important to differentiate this situation from ventricular tachycardia, which has significantly different clinical implications (see Chapter 15).[8]

2. **Holter monitoring** may identify paroxysmal AF or aid in assessing rate control.

3. **Echocardiography.**

a. Transthoracic echocardiography is helpful in identifying left atrial size, left ventricular (LV) hypertrophy, ejection fraction, valvular disease, pulmonary artery pressure estimate (pulmonary disease), and pericardial disease. Furthermore, transthoracic echocardiography is 39% to 63% sensitive in diagnosing left atrial thrombi.[9,10]
b. Transesophageal echocardiography (TEE) evaluates for thrombus in the left atrial appendage and helps guide cardioversion. TEE is 93% to 100% sensitive in diagnosing left atrial thrombi.

4. **Chest radiography** should be performed to evaluate for signs of heart failure or lung disease.

5. **Laboratory evaluation** should include thyroid-stimulating hormone and biomarkers if ischemia is suspected.

16

ATRIAL FIBRILLATION

V. MANAGEMENT (Fig. 16-1)

A. DETERMINING THE NEED FOR IMMEDIATE CARDIOVERSION

1. **Management begins with an assessment of hemodynamic stability. All patients with symptomatic hypotension caused by AF should be treated with immediate synchronized cardioversion.**
2. Patients with paroxysmal AF and a rapid ventricular response who have electrocardiographic evidence of acute myocardial infarction, angina, or heart failure that does not respond promptly to pharmacologic measures should also be cardioverted.[11]
3. Direct current (DC) cardioversion must be synchronized with intrinsic cardiac activity in order to avoid R-on-T-induced ventricular fibrillation.
4. Anterior-posterior positioning of paddles is associated with lower energy requirements and more successful cardioversion (87% vs. 76% with anterior-lateral alignment).
5. An initial energy of 200 J or greater is recommended for electrical cardioversion of AF. Biphasic defibrillation is more effective in terminating AF than monophasic waveforms.
6. The major risk of cardioversion is thromboembolism, which occurs in 1% to 7% of patients with AF lasting more than 48 hours who do not receive anticoagulation.
7. Should AF recur, antiarrhythmic therapy is recommended in conjunction with repeat cardioversion. Return of normal atrial contraction may be delayed by up to 1 week.

B. ESTABLISHING VENTRICULAR RATE CONTROL

The ventricular rate should be between 80 and 100 bpm during rest and activity (Table 16-1). The following are American College of Cardiology (ACC), American Heart Association (AHA), and ESP class I recommendations regarding rate control in AF:

1. Administer intravenous beta-blocker or calcium channel antagonists (verapamil, diltiazem) in the acute setting to slow the ventricular response to AF, exercising caution in patients with hypotension or heart failure.
2. **Beta-blockers** (esmolol, metoprolol, atenolol, propranolol) are the most effective drugs for rate control and should be used unless contraindications exist.
3. The presence of Wolff-Parkinson-White syndrome is a contraindication to beta-blocker and calcium channel blocker therapy because slowing AV node conduction can lead to ventricular fibrillation from rapid conduction via the accessory pathway. Catheter ablation should be recommended for patients with AF in the setting of Wolff-Parkinson-White syndrome.
4. Potential adverse effects of beta-blockers include hypotension, heart block, bradycardia, asthma, and heart failure (Table 16-1).
5. **Calcium channel blockers** are also effective for rate control but less effective than beta-blockers. Adverse effects include hypotension, heart block, and heart failure. For resistant patients, calcium channel blockers and beta-blockers can be used in combination (see Table 16-1).

6. **Amiodarone** should be considered in the acute setting for patients with rapid ventricular response refractory to beta-blocker or calcium channel blocker therapy or in patients with moderate to severe LV systolic dysfunction. Amiodarone should not be the first agent used for long-term rate control of AF because of its multiple toxicities.

7. **Digoxin** is the least effective drug for rate control of AF.

   a. Digoxin is not useful when there is increased sympathetic tone or decreased vagal input (i.e., during exercise) and should be avoided in physically active patients.

   b. Digoxin can be used in patients with a low ejection fraction or contraindications to beta-blockers or calcium channel blockers.

8. **Clinical variables influence which agent is used.**

   a. **Heart failure.** Negative inotropes, including beta-blockers and calcium channel blockers, may exacerbate decompensated heart failure and should be used with caution.

   b. **Hypotension.** Rapid ventricular response can shorten LV filling and cause hypotension, particularly in patients with structural heart disease and diastolic dysfunction. Slowing the ventricular response may improve hemodynamics by improving LV filling. Use of short-acting esmolol or intravenous amiodarone can be considered for these patients.

   c. **Acute AF** (i.e., in postoperative, septic, or other critically ill patients) commonly converts to sinus rhythm with establishment of rate control and treatment of the underlying condition.

C. ASSESSING THE NEED FOR STROKE PROPHYLAXIS

1. Based on the Framingham data, **AF increases the risk of stroke fivefold,** independent of heart failure and coronary artery disease. The overall incidence of stroke is 5% per year.[12]

2. Patients with AF and established risk factors should receive anticoagulation (warfarin) if no contraindications exist, targeting the international normalized ratio (INR) between 2 and 3.[11] Warfarin decreases the risk of stroke by two thirds in the following high-risk patients[13-19]:

- Those with valvular heart disease (most importantly mitral stenosis)
- Older adults (half of AF-associated stroke occurs in patients older than 75 years)
- Those with a history of transient ischemic attack or stroke
- Those with evidence of an ischemic event on brain computed tomography
- Those with a history of hypertension (especially systolic blood pressure greater than 160 mmHg)
- Those with heart failure or cardiomegaly (on chest film)
- Those with diabetes
- Those with coronary artery disease
- Those with atrial thrombi or spontaneous echo contrast in left atrial appendage seen on TEE

16

ATRIAL FIBRILLATION

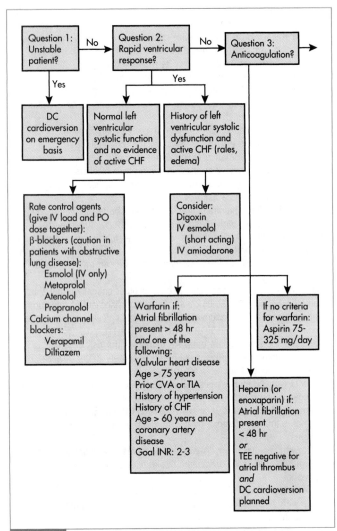

FIG. 16-1

Acute management of atrial fibrillation. *CHF,* congestive heart failure; *CVA,* cerebrovascular accident; *DC,* direct current; *INR,* international normalized ratio; *IV,* intravenous; *PO,* per os; *TEE,* transesophageal echocardiography; *TIA,* transient ischemic attack.

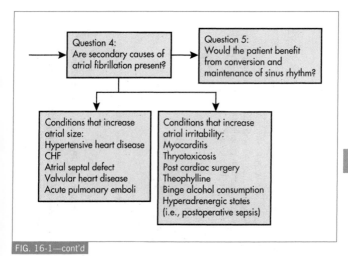

Question 4:
Are secondary causes of atrial fibrillation present?

Question 5:
Would the patient benefit from conversion and maintenance of sinus rhythm?

Conditions that increase atrial size:
Hypertensive heart disease
CHF
Atrial septal defect
Valvular heart disease
Acute pulmonary emboli

Conditions that increase atrial irritability:
Myocarditis
Thryotoxicosis
Post cardiac surgery
Theophylline
Binge alcohol consumption
Hyperadrenergic states
(i.e., postoperative sepsis)

FIG. 16-1—cont'd

16

ATRIAL FIBRILLATION

3. Patients between the ages 65 and 75 without any of these conditions may benefit more from warfarin than aspirin if no contraindications to anticoagulation exist.
4. In patients younger than 65 years old with *none* of these conditions, aspirin alone generally is sufficient. Aspirin is also acceptable in patients with contraindications to oral anticoagulation. Aspirin decreases the risk of stroke by one third.

D. RESTORING AND MAINTAINING SINUS RHYTHM

1. Rate and rhythm control in the treatment of AF have been compared in two recent clinical trials: Atrial Fibrillation Follow-up Investigation of Rhythm Management (AFFIRM)[20] and RACE.[21] These studies indicate that a strategy of rhythm control has no significant mortality benefit over rate control with anticoagulation among older adults with minimally symptomatic AF.
2. Elective cardioversion and, if necessary, antiarrhythmic therapy should be used to restore and maintain sinus rhythm in patients with disabling or otherwise unacceptable symptoms (ACC/AHA/ECS class I recommendation).[11]
3. **Circumferential pulmonary vein ablation** uses radiofrequency ablation to electrically isolate the pulmonary veins. It has been associated with improved survival (hazard ratio for death 0.46), 70% lower rates of AF recurrence, 55% reduction in major morbidities (heart failure, stroke, and transient ischemic attack), and improved quality of life. In addition, the maintenance of sinus rhythm in both ablation and antiarrhythmic

TABLE 16-1

PHARMACOLOGIC AGENTS AVAILABLE FOR VENTRICULAR RATE CONTROL

Drug	Starting Dosage	Maximum Dosage	Comments
β-Blockers			Do not attempt in patients with Wolff-Parkinson-White syndrome.
Esmolol	IV: 500 µg/kg/min over 1 min; increase by 50 µg/kg/min every 4 min; new bolus of 500 µg/kg every 4 min	200 µg/kg/min.	Effects wear off rapidly (within minutes) with drug discontinuation; because of rapid reversal, useful in patients with reactive airway disease whose tolerance of β-blockers is unknown.
Metoprolol	IV: load 5 mg over 1 min, repeat twice at 5-min intervals PO: start 50 mg bid	PO: 450 mg/day.	Metabolized by liver; available in once-a-day extended-release formulation (metoprolol succinate).
Atenolol	IV: 5 mg over 5 min, repeat after 10 min PO: start 50 mg qd	PO: 200 mg/day.	Excreted by kidney.
Propranolol	IV: 1-3 mg at 1 mg/min; can repeat after 2 min, then every 4 hr PO: start 10 mg tid or qid	PO: 640 mg/day.	Metabolized by liver; available in once-a-day extended-release formulation (Inderal LA).
Calcium channel blockers			Do not attempt in patients with Wolff-Parkinson-White syndrome.
Verapamil	IV: 2.5-10 mg over 2 min; can repeat 5-10 mg after 15-30 min PO: 80-120 mg tid or qid	IV: 20 mg. PO: 480 mg/day. PO: 360 mg.	Dosage adjustment needed for renal and hepatic insufficiency; consider starting bowel regimen; several once-a-day preparations available.

Diltiazem	IV: 20 mg over 2 min bolus, 5-15 mg/hr drip for 24 hr PO: start 30 mg qid		Hepatic metabolism and excretion; several once-a-day preparations available.
Others			
Digoxin	IV: 0.5-1 mg, 50% initially, then 25% 6 to 12 hr later twice PO: load 0.75-1.25 mg, then 0.05-0.25 mg/day	Check levels and electrocardiogram.	Primary metabolism via kidney; avoid serum levels > 2 ng/ml (stay at lower end of therapeutic range for women and older adults).
Amiodarone	IV: 150 mg IV bolus over 10 min, then 1 mg/min for 6 hr, then 0.5 mg/min for 18 hr PO: 800-1600 mg qd for 1-3 wk for load, divided bid or tid, maintenance at 200-400 mg/day		Monitor for thyroid, hepatic, and thyroid toxicity; amiodarone should not be used as the first agent for rate control in the ambulatory setting; IV amiodarone can be helpful as a second-line rate control agent in hospitalized patients.

IV, intravenous; *PO*, per os.

16

ATRIAL FIBRILLATION

groups was associated with significantly lower morbidity and mortality, challenging the results of AFFIRM and RACE.

E. ANTICOAGULATION BEFORE RESTORING SINUS RHYTHM

The ACC/AHA/ECS[11] class I recommendations for antithrombotic therapy to prevent ischemic stroke and systemic embolism in patients with AF undergoing cardioversion are as follows:

1. Administer anticoagulation therapy regardless of the method (electrical or pharmacologic) used to restore sinus rhythm.
2. Anticoagulate patients with AF lasting more than 48 hours or of unknown duration for at least 4 weeks before and after cardioversion (INR 2 to 3).
3. For patients who need immediate cardioversion:
   a. If not contraindicated, administer heparin concurrently with a weight-based intravenous bolus followed by a continuous infusion adjusted to prolong the activated partial thromboplastin time to 1.5 to 2 times the reference control value.
   b. Next, provide oral anticoagulation (INR 2 to 3) for a period of at least 4 weeks, as for patients undergoing elective cardioversion.
   c. Limited data from recent studies support the use of low molecular weight heparin for this indication.
4. Screening for the presence of thrombus in the left atrium or left atrial appendage with TEE is an alternative to routine pre-anticoagulation in candidates for cardioversion of AF. The risk of stroke is not different in patients who receive anticoagulation for 4 weeks than in those who undergo TEE-guided cardioversion.
5. **TEE-guided cardioversion does not eliminate the need for at least 4 weeks of anticoagulation after cardioversion** because the risk of thromboembolic events is higher in the 4 weeks immediately after conversion to sinus rhythm. The increased risk of stroke is believed to result from atrial stunning, which leads to atrial stasis and subsequent thrombus formation.
6. **Anticoagulation in chronic AF.** Although a number of risk stratification models are available for patients with chronic AF, the CHADS2 score is currently the best validated (Table 16-2).[22]

F. CHEMICAL CARDIOVERSION

1. **Ibutilide** is a class III antiarrhythmic used to facilitate DC cardioversion, particularly when DC cardioversion is initially unsuccessful. Ibutilide prolongs the QT interval and is associated with a 2% incidence of torsade de pointes; therefore it should not be used in patients with prolonged QT, LV hypertrophy, depressed LV function (ejection fraction less than 30%), hypokalemia, or hypomagnesemia. Patients need at least 4 hours of electrocardiographic monitoring after cardioversion to monitor for arrhythmias.
2. **Dofetilide** can also be used for cardioversion. Correct hypokalemia before use and adjust dosage for renal function. Adverse effects also include QT prolongation and torsade de pointes.

TABLE 16-2

CHADS2* AND ANTICOAGULATION IN ATRIAL FIBRILLATION

SCORE COMPOSITION

Heart failure: 1 point
Age >75: 1 point
Hypertension: 1 point
Diabetes mellitus: 1 point
Prior ischemic stroke: 2 points

Total Points	Event Rate per Year	Event Rate per Year with Warfarin
0	0.49	0.25
1	1.52	0.72
2	2.50	1.27
3	5.27	2.2
4	6.02	2.35
5 or 6	6.88	4.6

CHADS Score	Recommendation
0	Low risk of embolization and can be managed with aspirin
1-2	Intermediate risk of embolization
≥3	High risk of embolization and should be managed with warfarin in the absence of contraindications

*CHADS2 is an acronym for the 5 risk factors included in the scoring system: congestive heart failure, hypertension, age, diabetes, and stroke. The numeral 2 is added because a history of stroke merits 2 points. (It is the best predictor of embolism.)

G. MAINTAINING SINUS RHYTHM WITH ANTIARRHYTHMICS

1. The ACC/AHA/ESP class I recommendations for pharmacologic therapy to maintain sinus rhythm are as follows:
a. Base antiarrhythmic drug selection predominantly on patient safety.
b. Treat precipitating or reversible causes of AF before initiating antiarrhythmic drug therapy.
c. For patients with moderate to severe LV systolic dysfunction, the agent of choice is amiodarone.
d. For patients with ischemic heart disease with preserved LV systolic function, sotalol may be particularly useful because of its beta-blocker effect.
2. Antiarrhythmic drugs are organized by class as follows:
a. **Class IA agents** (quinidine, procainamide, disopyramide) can be used in patients without structural heart disease. Disopyramide may be used in AF precipitated by increased vagal tone. Adverse effects include torsade de pointes.
b. **Class IC agents** (flecainide and propafenone) are reserved for patients with normal systolic function and no underlying ischemic heart disease. Adverse effects include ventricular tachycardia, heart failure, hypotension, and enhanced AV nodal conduction leading to conversion to atrial flutter. Therefore flecainide should be used in conjunction with an AV nodal blocking agent.

   c. **Class III agents** include amiodarone, sotalol, and dofetilide.

      (1) **Amiodarone** is by far the most commonly prescribed antiarrhythmic agent and often is used to treat AF in patients with heart failure. Amiodarone has multiple adverse reactions, including pulmonary, thyroid, and hepatic toxicities, QT prolongation, hypotension, bradycardia, photosensitivity, neuropathy, optic neuritis, and skin discoloration. Evidence supporting the efficacy of amiodarone comes from the randomized Canadian Trial of Atrial Fibrillation (CTAF).[23] In CTAF, 69% of patients treated with amiodarone were in sinus rhythm, compared with 39% of patients treated with sotalol or propafenone at 1-year follow-up. Despite better rhythm control there was no significant difference in total mortality between the groups.

      (2) **Dofetilide** must be initiated at the hospital so that the patient can be observed for arrhythmias, specifically torsades. The DIAMOND-CHF[24] study randomized 1518 patients with LV ejection fractions below 35% to dofetilide or placebo (patients with glomerular filtration rate < 20 ml excluded). There was no significant difference in total mortality, but 12% of patients with AF in the dofetilide group converted to sinus rhythm, compared with 1% in the placebo group.

      (3) **Sotalol** often is used in patients with AF, coronary artery disease, and normal systolic function. Because of its arrhythmogenic potential, sotalol should not be given to patients with renal dysfunction, severe LV hypertrophy, prolonged QT intervals, bradycardia, or electrolyte abnormalities. Medications that impair AV conduction should be stopped or decreased before initiation of sotalol to lower the risk of bradycardia. The class III antiarrhythmic effect (action potential prolongation) appears at dosages of 120 to 160 mg twice daily.

H. OPTIONS FOR PERSISTENT, SYMPTOMATIC AF REFRACTORY TO MEDICAL THERAPY

1. **AV node ablation** with permanent pacemaker implantation is an option for patients with paroxysmal or persistent AF with rapid ventricular response refractory to antinodal or antiarrhythmic agents. This procedure is rarely performed because it does not eliminate AF or the need for anticoagulation, it renders the patient pacemaker dependent, and it causes ventricular dyssynchrony; however, patients with bradycardia-tachycardia syndrome can benefit from pacemaker insertion.

2. **Catheter ablation** has the potential to cure AF, with success rates of 60% to 85% in patients with paroxysmal AF and 40% to 70% in those with chronic AF.[25] Potential complications include pulmonary vein stenosis, stroke, tamponade, systemic embolism, and esophageal injury.

3. **Surgical ablation.** The Maze procedure occasionally is performed in conjunction with cardiac surgery for other indications. Criss-crossing

scars are placed in the atria in an attempt to prevent AF micro-reentry. Success rates are approximately 70% to 90%.

PEARLS AND PITFALLS

- Indications for hospital admission include rapid ventricular response greater than 150 bpm, heart failure (dyspnea, rales, elevated jugular venous pressure), neurologic symptoms, angina, syncope, and low blood pressure.

- Immediate anticoagulation with unfractionated heparin or low molecular weight heparin is not necessary. The annual risk of thromboembolic events in high-risk patients is 5% to 7%, making the daily risk 0.02%, which is low for the few days it takes to achieve a therapeutic INR. Warfarin-induced protein C and S inhibition (which occurs earlier than inhibition of the coagulation system) raises a theoretical concern for a prothrombic state in the first few days of warfarin therapy without heparin coverage; however, there is no clinical evidence demonstrating increased thrombotic events after initiation of warfarin without heparin.

- AF often occurs in critically ill patients because of increased sympathetic tone; however, secondary causes, such as pulmonary emboli, should be considered.

- Before elective DC cardioversion, make sure the patient has had therapeutic anticoagulation for 3 to 4 weeks (INR greater than 2, checked at least biweekly) or is currently therapeutically anticoagulated if TEE has demonstrated no evidence of an intracardiac clot.

- Cardioversion electrode pads should be placed in an anteroposterior orientation (front at T4 level just left of the sternum, back at same level).

- The initial setting for DC cardioversion is 100 J in the biphasic mode (200 J in the monophasic mode) with the defibrillator set in synchronized mode. If 100 J is unsuccessful, increase to 150 J, then 200 J.

- All patients must be anticoagulated after cardioversion because the risk of thromboembolic events is higher in the 4 weeks immediately after restoration of sinus rhythm.

16

ATRIAL FIBRILLATION

REFERENCES

1. Abedin Z, Conner R: *Interpretation of cardiac arrhythmias: self assessment approach,* Norwell, Mass, 2000, Kluwer. C
2. Kannel WB et al: Epidemiologic features of chronic atrial fibrillation, *N Engl J Med* 306:1018, 1982. C
3. Falk RH: Medical progress: atrial fibrillation, *N Engl J Med* 344:1067, 2001. C
4. Lip GYH, Tean KN, Dunn FG: Treatment of atrial fibrillation in a district general hospital, *Br Heart J* 71:92, 1994. B
5. Narayan SM, Cain ME, Smith JM: Atrial fibrillation, *Lancet* 350:943, 1997. C
6. Kannel WB et al: Coronary heart disease and atrial fibrillation: the Framingham study, *Am Heart J* 106:389, 1983. C
7. Sawin CT et al: Low serum thyrotropin concentrations as a risk factor for atrial fibrillation in older persons, *N Engl J Med* 331(19):1249-1252, 1994. B

8. Gupta AK, Thakur RK: Wide QRS tachycardia, *Med Clin North Am* 85:245, 2001. C

9. Manning WJ, Weintraub RM, Waksmonski CA, et al: Accuracy of transesophageal echocardiography for identifying left atrial thrombi. A prospective, intraoperative study, *Ann Intern Med* 123(11):817-822, 1995. B

10. Hwang JJ et al: Diagnostic accuracy of transesophageal echocardiography for detecting left atrial thrombi in patients with rheumatic heart disease having undergone mitral valve operations, *Am J Cardiol* 72(9):677-681, 1993. B

11. ACC/AHA/ESC guidelines for the management of patients with atrial fibrillation: executive summary, *Circulation* 104:2118, 2001. D

12. Wolf PA et al: Duration of atrial fibrillation and the imminence of stroke: the Framingham study, *Stroke* 14:664, 1983. C

13. Van Latum JC et al: Predictors of major vascular event in patient with a transient ischemic attack or minor ischemic stroke with non rheumatic atrial fibrillation. European Atrial Fibrillation Trial (EAFT) Study Group, *Stroke* 25:801, 1995. B

14. Hart RG et al: Factors associated with ischemic stroke during aspiring therapy in atrial fibrillation: analysis of 2012 participants in the SPAF I-III clinical trials, *Stroke* 30:1223, 1999. B

15. Stroke Prevention in Atrial Fibrillation Investigators: Stroke Prevention in Atrial Fibrillation study: final results, *Circulation* 84:527, 1991. A

16. Peterson P et al: Placebo-controlled randomized trial of warfarin and aspirin for prevention of thromboembolic complications in chronic atrial fibrillation: the Copenhagen AFASAK study, *Lancet* 28:175, 1989. A

17. Boston Area Anticoagulation Trial for Atrial Fibrillation Investigators: The effect of low dose warfarin on the risk of stroke in patients with nonrheumatic atrial fibrillation, *N Engl J Med* 323:1505, 1990. A

18. Stroke Prevention in Atrial Fibrillation Investigators: Warfarin versus aspirin for prevention of thromboembolism in atrial fibrillation: SPAF II study, *Lancet* 343:687, 1994. A

19. SPAF III Writing Committee for the Stroke Prevention in Atrial Fibrillation Investigators: Patients with nonvalvular atrial fibrillation at low risk of stroke during treatment with aspirin: SPAF III study, *JAMA* 279:1273, 1998. B

20. Atrial Fibrillation Follow-Up Investigation of Rhythm Management (AFFIRM) Investigators: A comparison of rate control with rhythm control in patients with atrial fibrillation, *N Engl J Med* 347:1825, 2002. A

21. vanGelder I et al: A comparison of rate control and rhythm control in patients with recurrent persistent atrial fibrillation, *N Engl J Med* 347:1834, 2002. A

22. Gage BF et al: Validation of clinical classification schemes for predicting stroke, *JAMA* 285:2864-2870, 2001. B

23. Roy D et al: Amiodarone to prevent recurrence of atrial fibrillation, *N Engl J Med* 342:913, 2000. A

24. Torp-Pedersen C et al: Dofetilide in patients with congestive heart failure and left ventricular dysfunction, *N Engl J Med* 341:857, 1999. A

25. Chen SA et al: Initiation of atrial fibrillation by ectopic beats originating from the pulmonary veins: electrophysiological characteristics, pharmacological responses and effects of radiofrequency ablation, *Circulation* 100:1879, 1999. B

Care of the Critically Ill

Franco D'Alessio, MD; and Henry E. Fessler, MD

FAST FACTS

- An intensivist-led multiprofessional intensive care unit (ICU) team decreases costs, length of stay, and mortality in critically ill patients.
- Critically ill patients with coagulopathy or on mechanical ventilation should receive gastrointestinal bleeding prophylaxis.
- All patients without coagulopathy should receive deep vein thrombosis prophylaxis.
- For all patients not in shock, the head of the bed should be elevated 30 to 45 degrees.
- Central venous catheters should be inserted using full barrier protection and removed as soon as they are no longer essential.
- Use of protocols, order sets, preprinted checklists, and structured rounds decreases errors and improves outcomes.
- Multiple organ dysfunction syndrome develops during 15% of all ICU admissions and is responsible for up to 80% of all ICU deaths.

17

Critical care medicine is unique among the subspecialties in that it seeks to treat patients with a wide variety of illnesses whose only commonality is the potential to develop multiorgan dysfunction and death. The goals of critical care medicine include resuscitating and stabilizing the patient, supporting failing organ systems, monitoring critical systems to prevent complications, addressing end-of-life issues, and recognizing futility. Many organ-specific ICU problems are covered in other chapters. This overview addresses issues common to ICU patients regardless of diagnosis.

I. EPIDEMIOLOGY

1. ICU care accounts for approximately 10% of all health care costs in the United States, an amount equal to 0.5% of the gross domestic product.[1]
2. Mortality in the ICU remains high, ranging in one series from 6.4% to 40% across ICUs, depending on severity of illness. Patients needing mechanical ventilation have mortality rates of 50% to 60%.[2]
3. Between 10% and 20% of ICU survivors die before discharge from the hospital. Determinants of post-ICU mortality include patient status before and during ICU stay and the decision to withhold life-sustaining treatments.[3]

II. ADMISSION CRITERIA AND PROGNOSTIC SCORING SYSTEMS

1. Although guidelines have been created for identifying patients who are likely to benefit from ICU care, individual institutions must tailor

admission criteria to both the patient population and available resources.

2. ICU care confers no benefit at the two extremes of disease severity. However, defining these groups can be difficult.[4] Clinical judgment as it relates to illness severity and prognosis are important decision-making tools.

3. The ICU admission decision process can be based on several models:

a. The *prioritization model* seeks to distinguish those who will benefit the most from admission from those who will not benefit at all.

b. The *diagnosis model* uses specific illnesses to determine ICU admission.

c. The *objective parameters model* uses predetermined criteria such as vital signs, laboratory values, and radiological tests to guide admission practices.

4. Advanced directives to forgo specific interventions (such as do-not-intubate) should not preclude ICU admission if other interventions available only in the ICU may be life saving. Conversely, a patient's vague wish that "everything" be done does not mandate ICU admission if an unavoidable death will only be briefly postponed.

5. There has been great interest in trying to predict outcomes in critically ill patients. Scoring systems initially were introduced in an attempt to prioritize ICU admissions (www.sfar.org/s/article.php3?id_article=60).

a. The Acute Physiological and Chronic Health Evaluation (APACHE II) tool is the most widely used illness scoring system and is based on age, comorbidities, and physiologic derangements occurring within the first 24 hours of admission (www.sfar.org/s/article.php3?id_article=60). APACHE scores are useful for comparing institutional performances and outcomes but should be used with caution for triaging ICU admissions.

b. The multiple-organ dysfunction score (Table 17-1) is an objective measure of the severity of organ dysfunction at the time of ICU admission and can quantify subsequent deterioration or improvement. The score correlates well with both mortality and length of ICU stay.[5]

6. For patients in the ICU, the need for continuing ICU care should be reassessed regularly.

III. ICU TEAM AND ROUNDS

1. An intensivist-led multidisciplinary approach to the management of critically ill patients has been shown to decrease costs, length of stay (LOS), and mortality.

2. The multidisciplinary team usually includes physicians, critical care nurses, pharmacists, respiratory therapists, nutritionists, and technicians. It is important to recognize the unique contribution made by each member of the team. For example, the presence of a pharmacist decreases adverse drug events, improves quality of care, and reduces costs.

TABLE 17-1

MULTIPLE-ORGAN DYSFUNCTION SCORE

Organ System	Score				
	0	1	2	3	4
Pao$_2$/Fio$_2$ ratio*	>300	226-300	151-225	76-150	≤75
Serum creatinine (mg/dl)	≤1.1	1.2-2.3	2.4-3.9	4.0-5.6	≥5.7
Serum bilirubin (mg/dl)	≤1.2	1.3-3.5	3.6-7	7.1-14	≥14.1
PAR†	≤10	10.1-15	15.1-20	20.1-30	>30
Platelet count‡	>120	81-120	51-80	21-50	≤20
GCS§	15	13-14	10-12	7-9	≤6

Predicted mortality: score of 0, <1%; 9-12, 25%; 13-16, 50%; 17-20, 75%; >20, 100%
*The Pao$_2$/Fio$_2$ ratio is calculated without reference to the use of mechanical ventilation or positive end-expiratory pressure.
†The pressure-adjusted heart rate (PAR) is calculated as the product of the heart rate (HR) multiplied by the ratio of the right atrial (central venous) pressure (RAP) to the mean arterial pressure (MAP): PAR = HR × RAP/MAP.
‡The platelet count is measured in platelets per milliliter × 10^3.
§The Glasgow Coma Score (GCS) should be calculated by the patient's nurse and is scored conservatively (for the patient receiving sedation or muscle relaxants, normal function is assumed unless there is evidence of intrinsically altered mentation).

3. ICU rounds serve not only to communicate the patient's current status and problems but also to establish specific management goals. The implementation of explicit, written daily goals is associated with a reduction in ICU LOS.[6]
4. Effective communication among the members of the ICU team is imperative. Communication failures can increase LOS, resource use, caregiver dissatisfaction, and risk of iatrogenesis. A system-based approach (Table 17-2) enhances communication and ensures a comprehensive evaluation of critical care patients during rounds.

IV. BASIC PRINCIPLES AND SAFETY IN THE ICU

1. Computerized or paper-based protocols for complex clinical ICU problems reduce unnecessary interclinician variability and improve patient outcomes.
a. Use of a nursing- and respiratory therapy–driven weaning protocol has been shown to decrease duration of mechanical ventilation.
b. Use of a sedation protocol that incorporates a sedation scale and regular, scheduled trials of sedation withdrawal decreases duration of mechanical ventilation.
c. Use of a protocol to prevent hyperglycemia reduces mortality in surgical patients and medical patients with acute myocardial infarction.
2. Critically ill patients are vulnerable during transportation. Intrahospital and interhospital transportation should include pretransport coordination and communication, trained transport personnel, transport equipment and medications, the patient's chart, continuous monitoring, and secure IV access.[7]

TABLE 17-2

SYSTEM-BASED APPROACH TO THE CRITICALLY ILL PATIENT

General	Set daily goals and formulate an action plan; communicate with members of the team.
	Review current medications, titrate, and adjust dosages (new renal or liver failure).
	Elevate head of bed; assess for decubitus ulcers.
	Communicate with and update patients and relatives.
Pulmonary	Assess for wheezes or crackles, spontaneous respiratory rate, frequency of secretion suctioning, and need for bronchodilator therapy.
	Review O_2 saturation, arterial blood gas, chest films, endotracheal tube position, and chest tube placement.
	Review ventilator settings, level of support, peak and plateau pressures, and auto-PEEP.
	Consider low tidal volume ventilation in patients with acute respiratory distress syndrome.
	Consider weaning trial if patient FIO_2 is <50%, PEEP is ≤5 with adequate sedation level.
	Consider early tracheostomy for patients in whom prolonged ventilation is anticipated.
Cardiovascular	Assess pulse, blood pressure, rhythm, extremity warmth, CVP, peripheral and sacral edema, and evidence of adequate perfusion (e.g., urine output, lactate).
	Evaluate and adjust preload (CVP, pulmonary artery occlusion pressure), afterload, cardiac output, and ischemia.
	Consider and titrate vasopressor, inotropic support, and antiarrhythmic therapy.
	Consider deep vein thrombosis prophylaxis.
Renal	Assess weight, net fluid balance, insensible fluid losses, urine output, blood urea nitrogen, creatinine, and electrolytes.
	Adjust renally excreted drugs.
	Consider early nephrology consultation if dialysis is anticipated.
	Consider N-acetylcysteine and hydration if radiocontrast agents will be administered.
Heme/ID	Assess temperature, bleeding sites, complete blood cell count with differential, and coagulation times.
	Minimize phlebotomy; establish transfusion needs.
	Recognize and treat acquired vitamin K deficiency in patients.
	Wash your hands before and after you examine patients.
	Examine site and determine duration of indwelling catheters. Can they be removed?
	Review cultures and antibiotic sensitivity data.

CVP, central venous pressure; *PEEP,* positive end-expiratory pressure.

TABLE 17-2

SYSTEM-BASED APPROACH TO THE CRITICALLY ILL PATIENT—cont'd

Gastrointestinal and nutritional	Assess for bowel sounds, distension, diarrhea, and constipation.
	Set goals for nutrition support; consider route, rate, and composition of nutritional support.
	Give gastrointestinal stress ulcer prophylaxis in patients on mechanical ventilation or those with coagulopathy.
	Consider the use of prokinetic and antiemetic agents.
Endocrine	Consider testing and treating relative adrenal insufficiency in patients with septic shock.
	Consider aggressive glycemic control with insulin in critically ill patients.
Neurologic	Assess neurologic status, sedation level, intracranial pressure, and occurrence of seizures.
	Titrate sedation and analgesic regimen to goal.
	Stop sedation once daily.
	Consider induction of hypothermia early after cardiac arrest.

17

CARE OF THE CRITICALLY ILL

3. Prevention of Complications.
a. Only patients who have a coagulopathy or who are undergoing mechanical ventilation are at significant risk for stress ulcer bleeding. In this population, H_2-receptor antagonists, sucralfate, or proton pump inhibitors can be used for acid suppression.
b. For critically ill patients who are not at high risk for bleeding, venous thromboembolism prophylaxis with unfractionated heparin or low molecular weight heparin is recommended. Intermittent compression devices with stockings can be used in patients at high risk of bleeding or who have other contraindications to heparin.
c. Nosocomial infections are 5 to 10 times more prevalent in the ICU and can significantly increase morbidity, LOS, and mortality. ICU nosocomial infections include catheter-related bloodstream infections, ventilator-associated pneumonia, urinary tract infections, and surgical or wound infections. Prevention requires a systematic approach to prevention, detection, and treatment.
   (1) All team members should be familiar with infection control policies including hand washing, use of isolation precautions, and maximal barrier precautions for the insertion of indwelling catheters.
   (2) Skin preparation with chlorhexidine reduces catheter-related bloodstream infections by half compared with povidone-iodine solution (see Chapters 2 and 58).
   (3) Elevating the head of the bed 30 to 45 degrees is an effective means of preventing ventilator-associated pneumonia (see Chapter 55).
d. Any new, unexplained fever in the critically ill patient merits a thorough clinical assessment before laboratory and imaging studies are ordered. The initial evaluation includes the following:

(1) Two sets of blood cultures (preferably from two different peripheral sites), urinalysis, and urine cultures. Additional blood cultures should be obtained if the suspicion of bacteremia or fungemia remains high.

(2) Examination of the intravascular catheters. If there is evidence of a tunnel infection, embolic phenomena, or sepsis, the catheter should be removed, the tip cultured, and a new catheter (if needed) inserted at a different site. In the presence of unexplained fever alone, central venous catheters may be exchanged over a wire, with the subcutaneous portion sent for quantitative culture. If the culture is positive, the new catheter should be removed unless the patient has defervesced (see Chapter 58).

(3) If ventilator-associated pneumonia is suspected on physical examination or radiographic evaluation, obtaining cultures from lower respiratory secretions is indicated. Quantitative bronchoscopic cultures have much better sensitivity and specificity than suctioned sputum because of the high prevalence of proximal airway colonization in intubated patients (see Chapter 55).

(4) If diarrhea (more than two loose stools) is present, *Clostridium difficile* toxin should be sent. Empiric treatment with metronidazole should be considered unless two assays are negative.

(5) Less common causes of fever include central nervous system infections and sinusitis (particularly in patients with nasogastric tubes).

V. ETHICAL ISSUES

One in five deaths in the United States occurs in an ICU. Recommendations to improve end-of-life care include the following[7]:

- A shared approach to end-of-life decision making involving the caregiver team and patient surrogates. Patients deserve to have their decisions guided by the judgment of their physicians and not merely receive a list of facts and options.
- Respect for patient autonomy and the intention to honor decisions to decline unwanted treatments should be conveyed to the family.
- The patient must be assured of a pain-free death. The patient must be given sufficient analgesia to alleviate pain and distress; if such analgesia hastens death, this double-effect should not detract from the primary aim to ensure comfort.

Recognition of futility is difficult for caregivers, patients, and families. Palliative care teams can be helpful in guiding families through this transition.

PEARLS AND PITFALLS

- Therapeutic decisions in the ICU often must be made in situations of diagnostic uncertainty and clinical instability.

- Phlebotomy from a critically ill patient for testing can average greater than or equal to 70 ml/day. The presence of an arterial catheter can further increase this amount by 30%.
- A neuromuscular blocking agent should never be used without appropriate sedation and analgesia and should be avoided, if possible, in patients on corticosteroids.
- The most valuable ICU monitor is an experienced, thoughtful nurse.
- ICU rounds at the bedside can improve outcomes. Questions that should be systematically raised include the following[8]:
  - Is the head of the bed elevated?
  - Is stress ulcer prophylaxis indicated?
  - Is deep vein thrombosis prophylaxis indicated?
  - Is pain well controlled and sedation well titrated?
  - Can the patient be weaned from mechanical ventilation?
- Pharmacokinetics often are altered in critical illness, and patients typically are on many medications. Drug-patient and drug-drug interactions are responsible for many complications and should be specifically considered in the differential diagnosis of new signs or organ dysfunctions.

17

CARE OF THE CRITICALLY ILL

REFERENCES

1. Halpern NA, Pastores SM, Greenstein RJ: Critical care medicine in the United States 1985-2000: an analysis of bed numbers, use, and costs, *Crit Care Med* 32(6):1254-1259, 2004. C
2. Knaus WA, Wagner DP, Zimmerman JE, et al: Variations in mortality and length of stay in intensive care units, *Ann Intern Med* 118:753-761, 1993. B
3. Azoulay E: Determinants of post–intensive care unit mortality: a prospective multicenter study, *Crit Care Med* 31(2):428-432, 2003. B
4. American College of Critical Care Medicine of the Society of Critical Care Medicine: Guidelines for ICU admission, discharge, and triage, *Crit Care Med* 27(3):633-638, 1999. B
5. Marshall JC, Cook DJ, Christou NV, et al: Multiple organ dysfunction score: a reliable descriptor of a complex clinical outcome, *Crit Care Med* 10:1638-1652, 1995. B
6. Pronovost P, Berenholtz S, Dorman T, et al: Improving the communication in the ICU using daily goals, *J Crit Care* 18(2):71-75, 2003. B
7. Warren J, Fromm RE Jr, Orr RA, et al: American College of Critical Care Medicine: guidelines for the inter- and intrahospital transport of critically ill patients, *Crit Care Med* 32(1):256-262, 2004. B
8. Thompson BT, Cox PN, Antonelli M, et al: Challenges in end-of-life care in the ICU: statement of the 5th International Consensus Conference in Critical Care: Brussels, Belgium, April 2003: executive summary, *Crit Care Med* 32(8):1781-1784, 2004. D

Acute Respiratory Failure

*Franco D'Alessio, MD; Kent R. Nilsson, Jr., MD, MA; Lara Wittine, MD;
and Landon S. King, MD*

> **FAST FACTS**
>
> - Respiratory failure can be divided into hypoxic respiratory failure ($PaO_2 < 60$ mmHg) and hypercapnic ventilatory failure ($PaCO_2 > 45$ mmHg with concurrent acidemia).
> - Initial evaluation of a patient in respiratory distress includes a focused history and physical exam, chest film, and arterial blood gas analysis. The goals of this initial evaluation are to determine the risk of impending respiratory failure, the type of respiratory failure (i.e., hypoxic or hypercarbic), and the specific cause.
> - For patients in extremis, ventilatory support should not be delayed.

Acute respiratory failure is one of the most time-sensitive situations in medicine because delay in diagnosis and treatment can result in significant morbidity and mortality. This chapter is meant to establish a framework for evaluating patients with respiratory failure. Clinical presentation, diagnosis, and management of the various disorders that may cause respiratory failure are addressed in subsequent chapters. Because of its prevalence and new insights into its management, adult respiratory distress syndrome (ARDS) is discussed in detail at the end of this chapter.

I. CLINICAL PRESENTATION

1. The presentation of respiratory distress varies widely and depends on both the underlying cause and the rapidity of onset (e.g., minutes to hours for a pulmonary embolism in contrast to days for a chronic obstructive pulmonary disease exacerbation). Signs and symptoms can be divided into those caused by hypoxemia or hypercarbia and those caused by the underlying disease process.
2. Symptoms of hypoxemia and hypercarbia.
a. Symptoms of hypoxemia vary but typically involve the central nervous system (confusion, agitation, and seizures), cardiovascular system (arrhythmias, hypotension, or hypertension), and respiratory system (dyspnea, tachypnea).
b. In contrast, hypercarbic respiratory failure presents predominantly with symptoms of somnolence, lethargy, dysarthria, and change in mental status. If respiratory acidosis is severe, myocardial depression can occur, which may lead to hypotension. Progressive hypoxemia and hypercarbia may blunt the sensation of dyspnea and can confound the clinical assessment of its severity.

   c. Because hypoxemia and hypercarbia often coexist, clinical presentation may reflect a combination of these symptoms.

3. Physical examination findings are nonspecific as to whether the primary derangement is hypoxia or hypercarbia. However, examination findings are extremely helpful in determining the underlying pathologic process (e.g., elevated jugular venous pressure and rales suggests congestive heart failure; prolonged expiration and wheezing suggest airway obstruction) and the degree of the patient's distress.

   a. Findings may include tachypnea, accessory muscle use, and paradoxical respirations.

   b. Inadequate cough, inability to protect the airway, use of accessory muscles, and pulsus paradoxus are all findings suggestive of impending respiratory failure. Often the simple question "Are you tiring out?" can be an astute diagnostic test for impending respiratory failure.

II. DIAGNOSTIC STUDIES

1. The arterial blood gas is the single most useful test to evaluate acid-base status and the degree of hypoxemia and hypercapnia. Hypoxemic respiratory failure is characterized by a Po_2 less than 60 mmHg; hypercapnic respiratory failure exists when there is acidosis (pH less than 7.34) and Pco_2 greater than 45 mmHg.

2. Once the patient has been evaluated and stabilized, a portable chest radiograph can provide insights into the cause of respiratory failure. Abnormalities include consolidations, diffuse alveolar infiltrates, effusions, and pneumothorax.

III. CAUSES OF RESPIRATORY FAILURE

A. HYPOXEMIC RESPIRATORY FAILURE

Hypoxemia (Pao_2 < 60 mmHg) usually is caused by one of five mechanisms: decreased Fio_2, hypoventilation, diffusion impairment (low D_{LCO}), ventilation-perfusion mismatch, and shunt. Careful analysis of the arterial blood gas and calculation of the A-a gradient (Box 18-1) can be useful in assessing the cause of hypoxemia.[1] See Fig. 18-1 for a diagnostic algorithm and Table 18-1 for details regarding the diagnosis and management of specific causes.

BOX 18-1

ALVEOLAR-ARTERIAL (A-a) OXYGEN GRADIENT EQUATION

A-a gradient = $[Fio_2\% \times (P_{ATM} - Pa_{H_2O}) - (Paco_2/R)] - Pao_2$.

At sea level on room air, this equation is:

   A-a gradient = $150 - (1.25 \times Paco_2) - Pao_2$.

Age-adjusted A-a gradient = $2.5 + (0.21 \times age)$.

Atmospheric pressure (P_{ATM}) is 760 mmHg at sea level; partial pressure of water vapor (Pa_{H_2O}) is 47 mmHg at sea level. The respiratory quotient (R) is approximately 0.8. Fio_2, fraction of inspired oxygen; $Paco_2$, arterial carbon dioxide pressure, used to approximate alveolar carbon dioxide pressure; Pao_2, alveolar oxygen pressure, equals $[Fio_2 \times (P_{ATM} - Pa_{H_2O}) - (Paco_2/R)]$; Pao_2, arterial oxygen pressure.

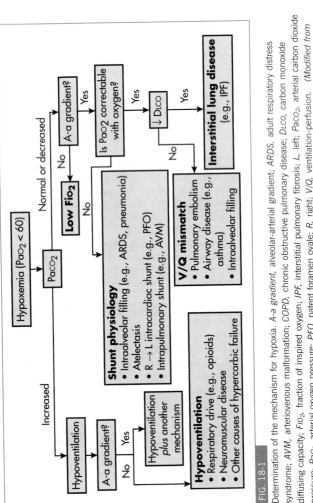

FIG. 18-1

Determination of the mechanism for hypoxia. *A-a gradient*, alveolar-arterial gradient; *ARDS*, adult respiratory distress syndrome; *AVM*, arteriovenous malformation; *COPD*, chronic obstructive pulmonary disease; *DLCO*, carbon monoxide diffusing capacity; *FIO2*, fraction of inspired oxygen; *IPF*, interstitial pulmonary fibrosis; *L*, left; *PaCO2*, arterial carbon dioxide pressure; *PaO2*, arterial oxygen pressure; *PFO*, patent foramen ovale; *R*, right; *V/Q*, ventilation-perfusion. *(Modified from Fauci AS et al:* Harrison's principles of internal medicine, *14th ed, New York, 1997, McGraw-Hill.)*

TABLE 18-1

DIFFERENTIAL DIAGNOSIS OF HYPOXEMIA

Cause of Hypoxemia	Mechanism of Hypoxemia	Associated Diseases	Comments
Decreased FiO_2	↓ Atmospheric pressure at high altitude or on airplanes.		Seldom clinically significant
Hypoventilation	↓ Alveolar O_2 tension. ↑ Alveolar CO_2 decreases alveolar O_2 concentration.	See Box 19-2	Should correct with a small amount of supplemental O_2
Diffusion impairment	↑ Time for O_2 to cross the alveolar-capillary membrane or loss of total alveolar-capillary surface area decreases O_2 delivery to hemoglobin.	Interstitial lung diseases	Desaturation with minimal exertion ↓ $DLCO$
Ventilation-perfusion mismatch	Altered ratio of ventilation to perfusion reduces efficiency of gas exchange and decreases O_2 delivery to hemoglobin.	Airway disease (asthma, chronic obstructive pulmonary disease, bronchitis, pneumonia) Interstitial lung disease Pulmonary vascular disease (pulmonary embolus, pulmonary hypertension)	Increased A-a gradient Normal or low PCO_2 PaO_2 corrects with supplemental O_2
Shunt	Mixed venous blood bypasses functional lung and lowers systemic O_2 tension.	Intrapulmonary alveolar disease (adult respiratory distress syndrome, atelectasis, pulmonary edema, pneumonia) Vascular disease (arteriovenous malformation, hepatopulmonary syndrome) Intracardiac (septal defects)	Increased A-a gradient Normal or mildly elevated PCO_2 PO_2 does not correct with supplemental O_2

A-a gradient, alveolar-arterial gradient; $DLCO$, carbon monoxide diffusing capacity; FiO_2, fraction of inspired oxygen; PaO_2, arterial oxygen pressure; PCO_2, partial pressure of carbon dioxide; PO_2, partial pressure of oxygen.

18

ACUTE RESPIRATORY FAILURE

B. HYPERCAPNIC RESPIRATORY FAILURE

1. Hypercapnia ($Paco_2 > 45$ mmHg and pH < 7.34) reflects either excessive CO_2 production or inadequate CO_2 elimination. Exercise, overfeeding, hyperthyroidism, burns, fever, and sepsis all increase CO_2 production by increasing the metabolic rate but rarely cause ventilatory failure. In contrast, decreased elimination of CO_2 reflects lack of ventilatory drive, a neuromuscular disorder, or conditions of increased respiratory compliance (Box 18-2).

2. Acute hypercapnic failure occurs only when the patient has concurrent acidemia, implying that the change in CO_2 was too rapid or too extreme for renal (metabolic) compensation. The pH indicates whether the hypercarbia is acute or chronic (see Chapter 71).

IV. MANAGEMENT

1. Acute management is aimed at providing respiratory support and correcting life-threatening gas exchange abnormalities in order to ensure adequate oxygenation and ventilation. Ultimately, treatment must be focused on managing the underlying cause of the respiratory failure.

2. For hypoxic respiratory failure, the mainstay of therapy is to provide supplemental O_2 using the simplest delivery system that maintains oxygenation with PaO_2 greater than 60 and O_2 saturation greater than 90%:

a. Nasal prongs usually increase FIO_2 by 3% to 4% for each 1 L of O_2 delivered.

b. Venturi masks allow more precise titration and delivery of supplemental oxygen than can be achieved with nasal cannula.

c. A properly fitting nonrebreather mask provides FIO_2 of about 80% to 90% through the use of a one-way valve that allows exhaled gases to exit the mask but prevents the entrainment of room air. If the valve is removed, the concentration of delivered O_2 is lower.

d. If these options are inadequate to improve oxygenation, then ventilatory support in the form of noninvasive positive-pressure ventilation or intubation with mechanical ventilation must be considered.

3. Management of hypercarbic respiratory failure depends on the underlying disorder. Noninvasive positive-pressure ventilation or intubation with mechanical ventilation can be used to correct life-threatening acidemia.

4. Ventilatory support.

a. Noninvasive positive-pressure ventilation is first-line therapy for hypercapnic respiratory failure in patients who can protect their airways, can handle their own secretions, and are hemodynamically stable. It can also be used in patients with hypoxic respiratory failure that is expected to be rapidly reversible with medical intervention (e.g., congestive heart failure) (see Chapter 19).

b. Indications for intubation and mechanical ventilation include noninvasive positive-pressure ventilation failure, apnea, hypoxemia

BOX 18-2

DIFFERENTIAL DIAGNOSIS OF HYPERCAPNIC RESPIRATORY FAILURE

↓ VENTILATORY DRIVE

Myxedema

Severe metabolic alkalosis

Multiple sclerosis

Sleep apnea, obstructive or central

Narcotic or benzodiazepine overdose

Central nervous system: medullary tumor, infarction, or other lesion

Encephalitis and postviral syndromes (e.g., Reye's syndrome)

NEUROMUSCULAR DISORDERS

Corticospinal Tracts and Anterior Horn Cells

Poliomyelitis

Amyotrophic lateral sclerosis

Tetanus

Trauma

Peripheral Nerve

Guillain-Barré syndrome

Diphtheria

Idiopathic or postzoster phrenic neuropathy

Porphyria

Disorders of Muscle

Muscular dystrophy

Periodic paralysis

Inflammatory (polymyositis, dermatomyositis)

Neuromuscular Junction

Myasthenia gravis

Cholinergic crisis

Botulism

Aminoglycoside toxicity

Tick paralysis

Metabolic Disorders

Hypercalcemia

Hypophosphatemia

CONDITIONS OF INCREASED COMPLIANCE

Obstructive lung disease

Massive obesity

Massive ascites

Kyphoscoliosis

Pneumothorax or pleural effusion

despite maximum supplementary O_2, upper airway obstruction, inability to clear secretions or protect the airway, severe respiratory acidosis, and progressive decline of the respiratory effort (see Chapter 19).

V. SPECIAL CASE: ADULT RESPIRATORY DISTRESS SYNDROME

A. EPIDEMIOLOGY AND ETIOLOGY

1. The cited incidence of ARDS (about 150,000 cases/year) probably is an underestimate in light of recent observations that about 20% of mechanically ventilated patients meet criteria for ARDS.[2]

2. Mortality from ARDS has improved but remains high despite lung protective strategies (36% to 40%). Most deaths are due either to the underlying cause (first 3 days) or to nosocomial infections or multiorgan dysfunction (more than 3 days), not simply progressive respiratory failure.[3]

3. The most common underlying causes associated with ARDS are sepsis (40%), severe trauma, aspiration, and massive transfusions (Box 18-3).

BOX 18-3

CAUSES OF INCREASED PERMEABILITY PULMONARY EDEMA (ADULT RESPIRATORY DISTRESS SYNDROME)

DIRECT PULMONARY INSULTS

Inhalation or Aspiration
Smoke
Toxic chemicals
Chlorine
Cocaine inhalation
Gastric acid
Oxygen toxicity
Water (near-drowning)
Numerous community or industrial chemical gas exposures

Drugs and Chemicals
Heroin and morphine
Salicylates
Bleomycin
Amiodarone
Methadone
Cocaine and amphetamines
Gemcitabine antineoplastic therapy
Tocolytic therapy
Numerous drugs and poisons

Infection
Viral (e.g., influenza)
Rickettsial
Bacterial (e.g., *Pneumococcus*)
Fungal
Tuberculosis
Protozoal (*Pneumocystis,* malaria)

Miscellaneous
Fat emboli
Amniotic fluid emboli
Air emboli
Pulmonary contusion
Radiologic contrast media

INDIRECT PULMONARY INSULTS
Sepsis
Shock
Multiple transfusions
Disseminated intravascular coagulation
Sickle cell crisis
Hyperthermia or hypothermia
Eclampsia
Bone marrow transplantation
Anaphylaxis
Diabetic ketoacidosis
Cardiopulmonary bypass
High altitude
Rapid lung reexpansion
Multisystem trauma
Neurogenic
Pancreatitis
Extreme physical exertion
Tumor lysis syndrome

Modified from Fraser RS: *Fraser and Pare's diagnosis of diseases of the chest*, 4th ed, Philadelphia, 1999, WB Saunders.

BOX 18-4

DEFINITION OF ADULT RESPIRATORY DISTRESS SYNDROME

Acute onset
PaO_2/FIO_2 ratio ≤200 (regardless of positive end-expiratory pressure levels)
Bilateral infiltrates seen on chest film
No clinical evidence of left atrial hypertension or pulmonary artery wedge pressure ≤18

Note: Acute lung injury is defined similarly except that the PaO_2/FIO_2 ratio is ≤300.
FIO_2, fraction of inspired oxygen; PaO_2, arterial oxygen pressure.
From Bernard GR, Artigas A, Brigham KL, et al: *Am J Respir Crit Care Med* 149:818-824, 1994.

B. DIAGNOSIS (Box 18-4)

C. MANAGEMENT

1. **Specific therapy.** The underlying cause of ARDS should be determined and treated aggressively (e.g., antibiotics for sepsis, corticosteroids for diffuse alveolar hemorrhage).

2. **Supportive therapy.**

a. **General measures.** If there is no contraindication, all patients should receive both deep vein thrombosis prophylaxis and stress ulcer prophylaxis (see Chapter 17). Patients should be adequately sedated because this facilitates ventilation and oxygenation.

b. **Fluid management.** The ARDS-net trial group is attempting to define optimal fluid management in patients with ARDS. Until these data are available, current recommendations are to attempt to maintain intravascular euvolemia. An empiric trial of diuretics can be attempted to improve oxygenation as long as it does not result in hypotension or renal compromise.

c. **Prone positioning.** Although prone positioning improves ventilation-perfusion matching both by increasing blood flow to better ventilated areas and by promoting reexpansion of collapsed lung units, it has not been shown to improve survival.[4]

d. **Ventilatory support.** The goal of mechanical ventilation in patients with ARDS is to provide adequate oxygenation without causing complications (e.g., ventilator-associated lung injury, barotrauma, oxygen toxicity, or hemodynamic instability). Several different ventilation strategies have been investigated, the most important of which are the following:

(1) Low tidal volume strategy. In patients with acute lung injury and ARDS, mechanical ventilation with low tidal volumes (6 ml/kg of predicted ideal body weight adjusted to maintain a plateau pressure of <30 cm of water) results in lower mortality than traditional ventilation (10 to 15 ml/kg).[5]

(2) High positive end-expiratory pressure strategy. In patients with acute lung injury and ARDS who receive mechanical ventilation with the low tidal volume strategy, clinical outcomes are similar regardless of whether low or high levels of positive end-expiratory pressure are used.[6]

(3) High-frequency oscillatory ventilation (HFOV). Recently, a randomized, controlled trial comparing HFOV with conventional ventilation (pressure control mode with a delivered tidal volume of 6 to 10 ml/kg) demonstrated that the use of HFOV leads to nonsustained improvements in the PaO_2/FIO_2 ratio and a trend toward lower mortality. HFOV is a safe and effective rescue therapy for patients with severe hypoxemic respiratory failure.[7]

e. **Inhaled vasodilators.** Inhaled nitric oxide (5 ppm) in patients with acute lung injury not caused by sepsis has been shown to improve oxygenation in the short term, but it has no significant impact on the duration of ventilatory support or mortality.[8]

f. **Exogenous surfactant.** Two multicenter, randomized, double-blind trials involving 448 patients with ARDS from various causes failed to show a mortality benefit for intratracheal doses of a recombinant surfactant protein C. Patients who received surfactant had a greater improvement in gas exchange during the 24-hour treatment period than patients who received standard therapy alone.[9]

g. **Corticosteroids.** Several prospective, placebo-controlled trials have shown no benefit from the use of high-dose corticosteroids early in the course of ARDS. However, one small study showed a possible role of steroids in the fibroproliferative phase of ARDS.[10] Larger randomized trials are ongoing.

PEARLS AND PITFALLS

- Cyanosis is not a reliable physical examination sign because it is observer dependent and requires more than 5 g/dl of desaturated hemoglobin.
- The sensation of dyspnea correlates poorly with the severity of respiratory failure.[11]
- Pulse oximetry depends on pulse-coordinated receipt of the light wavelengths of oxyhemoglobin transilluminated through the tissues. Readings may be inaccurate in the absence of an observed arterial waveform (e.g., with peripheral vascular disease, vasoconstriction, or interference from nail polish).
- Low SaO_2 out of proportion to PaO_2 suggests methemoglobinemia. Low PaO_2 out of proportion to high SaO_2 suggests carboxyhemoglobinemia. Four-channel co-oximetry confirms these diagnoses.
- Low central venous oxygen saturation caused by decreased cardiac output, sepsis, decreased oxygen carrying capacity, and hypermetabolism may contribute to hypoxemia.
- Insufficient delivery of oxygen to meet the metabolic demands of tissues can occur despite oxyhemoglobin saturations (SaO_2) greater than 90%. Arterial oxygen content depends on total hemoglobin, the percent hemoglobin saturation, and the amount of dissolved oxygen (arterial oxygen content = $[1.39 \times SaO_2 \times Hb] + [0.0031 \times PaO_2]$).

REFERENCES

1. Mellemgaard K: The alveolar-arterial oxygen difference: size and components of normal man, *Acta Physiol Scand* 67:10, 1966. B
2. Goss CH, Brower RG, Hudson LD, Rubenfeld GD: ARDS Network. Incidence of acute lung injury in the United States, *Crit Care Med* 31(6):1607-1611, 2003. B
3. Montgomery AB, Stager MA, Carrico CJ, et al: Causes of mortality in patients with the adult respiratory distress syndrome, *Am Rev Respir Dis* 132:485, 1985. B
4. Gattinoni L, Tognoni G, Pesenti A, et al: Effect of prone positioning on the survival of patients with acute respiratory failure, *N Engl J Med* 345:568, 2001. A

5. The Acute Respiratory Distress Syndrome Network: Ventilation with lower tidal volumes as compared with traditional tidal volumes for acute lung injury and the acute respiratory distress syndrome, *N Engl J Med* 342:1301, 2000. A

6. The National Heart, Lung, and Blood Institute ARDS Clinical Trials Network: Higher versus lower positive end-expiratory pressures in patients with the acute respiratory distress syndrome, *N Engl J Med* 351:327-336, 2004. A

7. Mehta S, Lapinsky SE, Hallet DC, et al: Prospective trial of high-frequency oscillation in adults with acute respiratory distress syndrome, *Crit Care Med* 29:1360, 2001. B

8. Taylor RW, Zimmerman JL, Dellinger RP, et al: Low-dose inhaled nitric oxide in patients with acute lung injury: a randomized controlled trial, *JAMA* 291(13):1603-1609, 2004. A

9. Spragg RG et al: Effect of recombinant surfactant protein C-based surfactant on the acute respiratory distress syndrome, *N Engl J Med* 351(9):884-892, 2004. A

10. Meduri GU, Headley S, Golden E, et al: Effect of prolonged methyl-prednisolone therapy in unresolving acute respiratory distress syndrome, *JAMA* 280:159, 1998. A

11. Wasserman K: Exercise testing in the dyspneic patient. The chairman's postconference reflections, *Am Rev Respir Dis* 129(Suppl):1-2, 1984.

18

ACUTE RESPIRATORY FAILURE

Invasive and Noninvasive Ventilation

Matthew Pipeling, MD; David N. Hager, MD; and Landon S. King, MD

FAST FACTS

- Reasons for intubation and mechanical ventilation include inadequate ventilation or oxygenation and airway protection.
- Typical initial settings for assist-control ventilation are a tidal volume (V_t) of 6 to 10 ml/kg predicted body weight, respiratory rate (RR) of 10 to 15 breaths/min, positive end-expiratory pressure (PEEP) of 5 cm H_2O (unless predominantly unilateral disease or elevated intracranial pressure), and fraction of inspired oxygen (FIO_2) of 1 (100% O_2; should be quickly titrated down as appropriate).
- Arterial blood gases should be checked 15 minutes after initiation of mechanical ventilation and settings adjusted accordingly.
- In mechanically ventilated patients, respiratory acidosis (elevated $PaCO_2$) may be corrected by increasing V_t or RR to increase the alveolar ventilation.
- Oxygenation may be improved by an increase in FIO_2 or PEEP.
- Hypotension may result from excessive PEEP, especially in the patient with volume depletion.

Ventilatory support is a life-sustaining therapy for the critically ill patient that has changed markedly since the introduction of the iron lung in 1928. Despite advances in technology, the goals of therapy remain to reduce the work of breathing, improve oxygenation, and correct progressive respiratory acidosis. New therapies, such as high-frequency oscillatory ventilation, have further refined our ability to meet these goals. This chapter provides an approach to both invasive and noninvasive ventilation in this continuously evolving field.

I. EPIDEMIOLOGY

The need for mechanical ventilation is one of the most common reasons for admission to the intensive care unit. In one study of patients who needed mechanical ventilation, 66% had acute respiratory failure, 15% were in a coma, 13% had chronic obstructive pulmonary disease (COPD), and 5% had neuromuscular weakness.[1]

II. CLINICAL PRESENTATION

1. The decision to initiate mechanical ventilation often is based on the patient's overall condition rather than on clearly defined parameters.

Indications for intubation include hypercarbic respiratory failure, hypoxemia, and an inability to protect the airway.

2. Clinical signs indicating that mechanical ventilation may be necessary include use of accessory muscles of breathing, inability to speak in full sentences, rapid shallow breathing, hypoxemia refractory to supplemental oxygen, and altered mental status.

3. For additional discussion, see Chapter 18.

III. INTUBATION

1. Endotracheal tube (ETT) placement is one of the most complication-ridden aspects of mechanical ventilation. Complications include esophageal intubation, aspiration, laryngeal damage, pneumothorax, and death.

2. Immediately after intubation, ETT position should be evaluated by auscultation of both lungs and end-tidal CO_2 measurement. The ETT should be secured and note should be made of the ETT length at the teeth.

3. Chest radiography should be performed as soon as possible to ensure proper tube position (about 2 to 4 cm above the carina).

IV. MODES OF VENTILATION

A. TRADITIONAL MODES OF INVASIVE VENTILATION (Table 19-1)

1. Clinical judgment and familiarity play prominent roles in the selection of a ventilation mode.[2,3] Box 19-1 outlines parameters involved in traditional modes of ventilation.

2. Assist-control ventilation (ACV).

a. In ACV, the clinician sets a baseline RR and V_t, thereby establishing a minimum minute ventilation (V_E). Additional inspiratory efforts initiated by the patient result in delivery of the full programmed V_t.

b. Advantages of ACV include full respiratory support and a guaranteed V_E.

c. The main disadvantage of ACV is in patients breathing at a rate above the set RR because each breath will trigger a full V_t. This can lead to respiratory alkalosis or, in patients with airway obstruction, breath-stacking and hyperinflation. Complications of hyperinflation include barotrauma, pneumothorax, and auto-PEEP, which can cause hypotension through decreased venous return.

3. Synchronized intermittent mandatory ventilation (SIMV).

a. In SIMV, just as in ACV, the clinician determines a baseline RR and V_t to determine a baseline V_E. However, unlike in ACV, a patient-initiated breath results in a V_t that depends on the patient's effort.

b. A potential advantage of SIMV is that breaths over the SIMV set rate will be at a variable, often lower V_t. This limits the risk of respiratory alkalosis, hyperinflation, and auto-PEEP.

c. A disadvantage is that the work of breathing may increase. Although this mode may be useful for the purpose of respiratory muscle exercise,

TABLE 19-1

GUIDELINES FOR INITIAL VENTILATOR SETTINGS FOR VARIOUS CLINICAL INDICATIONS

Clinical Setting	Clinical Objectives	Tidal Volume (ml/kg)	Target pH/PacO$_2$	Target Pao$_2$	Positive End-Expiratory Pressure (cm H$_2$O)
Routine (e.g., postoperative, drug overdose)	Prevent atelectasis	7-10	Normal	Normal	0-5
Obstructive lung disease (e.g., chronic obstructive pulmonary disease, asthma)	Unload ventilatory muscles, prevent hyperinflation	5-7	Permissive hypercapnia	Normal	0-5 or more if auto-positive end-expiratory pressure present
Acute lung injury (e.g., acute respiratory distress syndrome)	Prevent further lung injury, support oxygenation	5-7	Permissive hypercapnia	If severe, may tolerate 50-60 mmHg	Usually 8-15
Focal or unilateral pulmonary disease (e.g., lobar pneumonia)	Avoid barotrauma, support oxygenation	7-10	Normal	Normal	Avoid or use cautiously
Acute brain injury (e.g., head trauma)	Maintain cerebral perfusion pressure	7-10	Normal or respiratory alkalosis	Normal	Avoid

Modified from Albert R, Spiro S, Jett J: *Comprehensive respiratory medicine*, St Louis, 1999, Mosby.

> ### BOX 19-1
> #### PARAMETERS OF TRADITIONAL VENTILATION
>
> Minute ventilation (V_E) = Respiratory rate (RR) × Tidal volume (V_t).
>
> V_E = Alveolar ventilation (V_A)* + Dead space ventilation (V_D).
>
> Positive end-expiratory pressure (PEEP)† minimizes atelectasis and decreases intrapulmonary shunting.
>
> Plateau pressure (P_{plat}) is a static pressure measured at end-inspiration and is related to respiratory system compliance (C_{RS}) = $V_t/(P_{plat} - PEEP)$. See Fig. 19-1.
>
> Peak airway pressure (P_{pk}) depends on C_{RS}, V_t, and airway resistance, (R_{aw}) = $(P_{pk} - P_{plat})$/Inspiratory flow rate. See Figure 19-1.

*$Paco_2$ is inversely proportional to V_A.
†Oxygenation may be improved by increasing Fio_2 or PEEP.

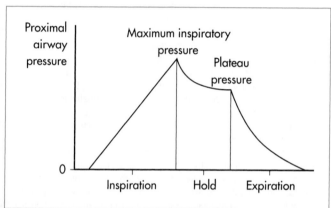

FIG. 19-1
Relationship of peak airway pressure and plateau pressure to the ventilatory cycle. *(From Albert R, Spiro S, Jett J: Comprehensive respiratory medicine, St Louis, 1999, Mosby.)*

adding pressure support or changing to ACV is appropriate in the fatiguing patient.

4. Pressure support ventilation (PSV).
   a. In PSV, the clinician sets the peak airway pressure, and the patient's efforts determine the flow rates, RR, and V_t. Positive pressure delivered by the ventilator reduces the work of breathing. The amount of pressure support should be titrated to patient comfort, as evidenced by RR and V_t.
   b. PSV offers the advantage of patient comfort in alert patients because PSV allows for natural variance in RR and V_t.

c. A disadvantage of PSV is that there is no guaranteed ventilation. Therefore if the patient stops breathing for any reason (e.g., fatigue), ventilation ceases. Apnea alarms and SIMV set at a low backup rate (RR of 6 to 8) can be used as precautions to avoid this problem.

B. NONTRADITIONAL MODES OF INVASIVE VENTILATION

1. High-frequency oscillatory ventilation (HFOV).[4,5]

a. HFOV is a nontraditional mode of ventilation that is increasingly used to treat refractory hypoxemia, particularly when it is associated with acute lung injury. HFOV uses extremely high RR (about 180 to 300 breaths/min), with V_ts that are presumed to be low but have not yet been well defined. Gas exchange is poorly understood but believed to take place via a variety of mechanisms including both Pendeluft and direct bulk flow, longitudinal dispersion, and facilitated diffusion. By oscillating around a set mean airway pressure, HFOV lowers peak airway pressure, recruits atelectatic alveoli, and prevents hysteresis-associated lung injury. A single randomized trial in adults, powered only for equivalence, did not reveal a mortality benefit of HFOV over conventional ventilation. However, there was a trend toward improved survival in the HFOV group (37% vs. 52%).[6]

b. Disadvantages of HFOV include the risk of dynamic hyperinflation and hemodynamic compromise. In addition, HFOV renders the physical examination virtually useless as a diagnostic tool. Finally, the effects of HFOV on hemodynamics have not been fully defined.

c. For a patient to be on HFOV, heavy sedation and often paralysis are necessary. Oxygenation is improved by increasing the mean airway pressure (mPAW), and ventilation is improved either increasing the pressure amplitude of oscillation (ΔP) or decreasing the frequency.

2. Inverse ratio ventilation involves prolonging the inspiratory time to generate an inspiratory to expiratory ratio of 1 or more, which increases mPAW to improve oxygenation. Patients on inverse ratio ventilation need heavy sedation. No studies demonstrate the benefit of inverse ratio ventilation.

3. Airway pressure release ventilation involves the application of continuous positive airway pressure with regular release of this pressure at a defined RR to permit ventilation. Patients may also breathe spontaneously at any point in the ventilatory cycle. Airway pressure release ventilation results in lower airway pressures and may improve hemodynamics.

4. Prone positioning of a mechanically ventilated patient may improve oxygenation via increased functional residual capacity, improved ventilation-perfusion matching, or reduction of compressive effects. However, studies have not revealed a mortality benefit.[7]

C. NONINVASIVE POSITIVE-PRESSURE VENTILATION

1. Noninvasive positive-pressure ventilation (NPPV) is the delivery of positive-pressure mechanical ventilation via a mask applied to the nose, mouth, or both instead of via invasive methods such as an ETT

or tracheostomy. Bilevel positive airway pressure is one commonly used method of NPPV in which expiratory positive airway pressure, analogous to PEEP, is used to improve oxygenation, and inspiratory positive airway pressure, analogous to pressure support, is used to improve ventilation.

2. Contraindications to NPPV include agitation, lack of cooperation, severe facial deformity or trauma, hemodynamic instability, copious secretions, or an inability to protect airway.

3. NPPV has been shown to reduce the need for intubation in a number of clinical settings including acute exacerbations of COPD, cardiogenic pulmonary edema, and immunocompromised patients with acute respiratory failure.[8] A recent meta-analysis of NPPV in acute exacerbations of COPD showed that NPPV significantly reduced mortality and the need for intubation (relative risk 0.52 and 0.41, respectively).[9] It does not prevent reintubation in patients who develop postextubation respiratory distress.[10]

4. Typical initial settings are inspiratory positive airway pressure of 10 cm H_2O and expiratory positive airway pressure of 5 cm H_2O.

V. MANAGEMENT OF THE VENTILATED PATIENT

A. SEDATION AND PARALYSIS

1. Because both intubation and mechanical ventilation are unpleasant and typically associated with agitation and anxiety, most mechanically ventilated patients need some sedation and analgesia. Combination therapy with a narcotic (e.g., fentanyl) and a benzodiazepine (e.g., midazolam) is a commonly used strategy. A daily sedative-free interval decreases length of mechanical ventilation and intensive care unit stay.[11]

2. Most mechanically ventilated patients are managed adequately without paralytic agents. However, continuous paralysis sometimes is necessary to effectively ventilate and oxygenate patients under certain situations such as HFOV. Continuous paralysis usually is maintained with nondepolarizing neuromuscular blocking agents (e.g., vecuronium) and is monitored by the response to a "train of four" stimulus to a peripheral nerve.[12]

3. Paralyzed patients must be heavily sedated and need venous thromboembolism prophylaxis.

4. Corticosteroids should be avoided in patients paralyzed with nondepolarizing neuromuscular blocking agents because their use is associated with a higher incidence of critical illness myopathy.[13]

B. WEANING

1. Before any attempt is made to wean a patient from ventilatory support, it is important to ensure that there has been resolution or improvement in the process that caused respiratory failure necessitating mechanical ventilation, discontinuation of paralytics and reduction or elimination of sedatives, hemodynamic stability, and correction of major electrolyte and metabolic disorders.[14]

19

INVASIVE AND NONINVASIVE VENTILATION

2. In addition, adequate gas exchange, defined by a PaO_2 of at least 60 mmHg with an FIO_2 of 0.4 or less and a PEEP of 5 cm H_2O or less or PaO_2/FIO_2 of at least 200 mmHg, must be achieved.

3. Ventilatory capacity can help predict successful weaning.[15]

a. A maximal inspiratory pressure less than −20 cm H_2O predicts successful extubation only about 60% of the time. More importantly, a maximal inspiratory pressure greater than −20 cm H_2O predicts failure 100% of the time.

b. The rapid shallow breathing index (RR/V_t [in liters]) is a better predictor of successful extubation than is maximal inspiratory pressure. A rapid shallow breathing index less than 105 breaths/min/L predicts a 78% success rate, and a rapid shallow breathing index of 105 breaths/min/L or more predicts a 95% failure rate.

4. Once a patient is deemed appropriate for weaning, withdrawal of ventilatory support should be pursued aggressively, although some patients will need a prolonged wean.[16] This can be accomplished by performing spontaneous breathing trials. Spontaneous breathing trials usually are performed via T-piece with or without the addition of continuous positive airway pressure. For patients who fail rapid withdrawal of ventilatory support, daily spontaneous breathing trials decrease the duration of intubation and intensive care unit stay.[17]

5. Factors that may contribute to difficulty to wean from mechanical ventilation include volume overload, metabolic and electrolyte abnormalities, poor respiratory center output from sedation or intrinsic central depression, peripheral neuromuscular disorder, overfeeding with compensatory hyperventilation, and poor cardiac function.

C. TROUBLESHOOTING: HYPOXEMIA

Evaluation of new-onset hypoxemia or respiratory distress in a mechanically ventilated patient requires a careful, systematic approach to assess for the cause and to direct therapy. Fig. 19-2 outlines such an approach.

VI. COMPLICATIONS OF MECHANICAL VENTILATION

1. Oxygen toxicity. Prolonged exposure to high concentrations of oxygen can cause a number of toxic effects including absorption atelectasis, acute tracheobronchitis, and acute parenchymal lung injury. Although observational studies suggest that the mechanism of damage may be related to increased free radical production, there is no clear threshold FIO_2 at which toxicity develops. In fact, data suggest that patients with acute lung injury may exhibit resistance to prolonged oxygen exposure. However, it is generally prudent to minimize the FIO_2 to maintain a PaO_2 of 60 mmHg.[18,19]

2. Ventilator-associated pneumonia is a nosocomial pneumonia developing in a patient 48 hours after initiation of mechanical ventilation. Diagnosis can be difficult and may entail bronchoscopic sampling of the

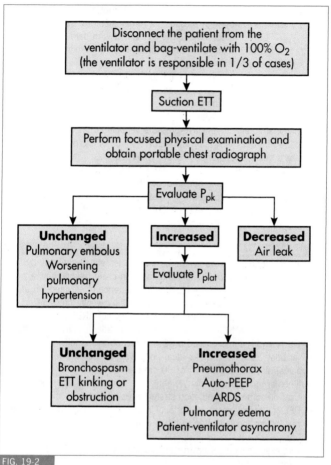

FIG. 19-2

Evaluation of the acutely hypoxemic patient on mechanical ventilation. *ARDS,* acute respiratory distress syndrome; *ETT,* endotracheal tube; *PEEP,* positive end-expiratory pressure; *P_{pk},* peak airway pressure; *P_{plat},* plateau pressure.

lower airways with quantitative cultures. Ventilator-associated pneumonia is associated with mortality rates of 24% to 50%.[20]

3. Mechanical ventilation at high V_t and P_{plat} is increasingly recognized as a cause of lung injury. These injuries have been classified as barotrauma and volutrauma, although they probably represent a continuum of pressure-induced lung injury.

a. *Barotrauma*[21] traditionally has referred to the rupture of small airways and alveolar walls by high pressure. It remains controversial if elevated P_{pk}, P_{plat}, PEEP, or a combination is associated with barotrauma. The extravasation of air can result in pneumothorax, pneumomediastinum, or subcutaneous emphysema.

b. *Volutrauma*,[22] also known as ventilator-associated lung injury, is felt to result from overdistension of airspaces rather than actual rupture and results in pulmonary edema, diffuse alveolar damage, and epithelial and microvascular permeability.

4. Hemodynamic effects. Positive-pressure ventilation has two opposing effects on hemodynamics. The increased intrathoracic pressure causes a decrease in venous return, which can result in decreased preload. At the same time, it decreases left ventricular afterload. The net effect on cardiac output depends on the patient. In general, the effects of positive-pressure ventilation on preload predominate in hypovolemic patients, whereas the effects on afterload predominate in patients with systolic dysfunction (ejection fraction <30%).

VII. SPECIAL SITUATIONS

1. Acute respiratory distress syndrome (ARDS) is defined clinically by the presence of bilateral pulmonary infiltrates on chest radiography, a PaO_2/FIO_2 less than 300 mmHg, and no evidence of elevated left atrial pressure (i.e., if measured, pulmonary capillary wedge pressure <18 mmHg). The presentation and pathophysiology of ARDS are discussed in Chapter 18. With respect to ventilation in patients with ARDS, the ARDS Network demonstrated a 22% reduction in mortality by using lower tidal volumes (6 ml/kg ideal body weight), permissive hypercapnia, and a goal P_{plat} of 30 cm H_2O or less.[23] Box 19-2 outlines an approach to low V_t ventilation. There is no difference in clinical outcomes in ventilation strategies using higher or lower levels of PEEP.[24] Improvement in mortality with low V_t ventilation is proposed to result from the reduction in inflammation induced by lung stretch injury.

2. Severe exacerbations of obstructive disease (asthma, COPD) pose a unique set of dangers because these patients are at risk of hyperinflation and auto-PEEP caused by increased RR and slowly emptying lungs. Auto-PEEP can have adverse effects with respect to pressure-induced lung injury and cardiac output. Using high inspiratory flow rates to maximize expiratory time can minimize the risk or severity of auto-PEEP. Permissive hypercapnia often is appropriate in these patients.

PEARLS AND PITFALLS

- With auto-PEEP–induced hypotension, disconnecting the ETT from the ventilator will quickly decrease intrathoracic pressure and restore the blood pressure.

BOX 19-2

PROTOCOL FOR LOW V$_t$ VENTILATION IN ACUTE LUNG INJURY

Step 1: Calculate PBW:

Male PBW (kg) = (Height [inches] − 60) × 2.3 + 50.

Female PBW (kg) = (Height [inches] − 60) × 2.3 + 45.5.

Step 2: Decrease V$_t$ by 1 ml/kg PBW every 2 hr until V$_t$ is 6 ml/kg PBW.

If P$_{plat}$ > 30 cm H$_2$O, decrease V$_t$ by 1 ml/kg PBW to minimum of 4 ml/kg PBW to achieve P$_{plat}$ ≤ 30 cm H$_2$O.

If P$_{plat}$ < 25 cm H$_2$O and V$_t$ < 6 ml/kg PBW, increase V$_t$ by 1 ml/kg PBW to goal of 6 ml/kg PBW or until P$_{plat}$ > 25 cm H$_2$O.

If severe dyspnea (i.e., "double-breathing") is present with V$_t$ ≥ 7 mL/kg PBW but P$_{plat}$ > 30 cm H$_2$O, additional sedation may be necessary.

Step 3: Maintain oxygenation (goal PaO$_2$ of 55-80 mmHg or SaO$_2$ of 88-95%). The following is a guide for potential FiO$_2$-PEEP combinations:

FiO$_2$	0.3	0.4	0.4	0.5	0.5	0.6	0.7	0.7	0.7	0.8	0.9	0.9	0.9	1.0
PEEP (cm H$_2$O)	5	5	8	8	10	10	10	12	14	14	14	16	18	18-24

PBW, predicted body weight.

19

- When a patient is fighting the ventilator, increasing sedation may be necessary, but the potential causes of agitation should always be evaluated carefully.
- Because of decreased compliance of the chest wall, morbidly obese patients are at high risk of barotrauma when undergoing volume-cycled positive-pressure ventilation. Positioning the patient in a semi-upright position takes advantage of gravity and may decrease airway pressures.

REFERENCES

1. Esteban A et al: How is mechanical ventilation employed in the intensive care unit? An international utilization review, *Am J Respir Crit Care Med* 161:1450-1458, 2000. C
2. Groeger JS et al: Assist control versus synchronized intermittent mandatory ventilation during acute respiratory failure, *Crit Care Med* 17:607-612, 1989. B
3. Tobin MJ: Mechanical ventilation, *N Engl J Med* 330:1056-1061, 1994. C
4. Mehta S et al: High-frequency oscillatory ventilation in adults: the Toronto experience, *Chest* 126:518-527, 2004. B
5. Krishnan JA, Brower RG: High-frequency ventilation for acute lung injury and ARDS, *Chest* 118:795-807, 2000. C
6. Derdak S et al: High-frequency oscillatory ventilation for acute respiratory syndrome in adults: a randomized, controlled trial, *Am J Respir Crit Care Med* 166:801-808, 2002. A
7. Gattinoni L et al: Effect of prone positioning on the survival of patients with acute respiratory failure, *N Engl J Med* 345:568-573, 2001. A

INVASIVE AND NONINVASIVE VENTILATION

8. Liesching T et al: Acute applications of noninvasive positive pressure ventilation, *Chest* 124:699-713, 2003. C

9. Ram F et al: Non-invasive positive pressure ventilation for treatment of respiratory failure due to exacerbations of chronic obstructive pulmonary disease (Cochrane review). In *The Cochrane library,* Issue 3. Chichester, UK, 2004, Wiley. C

10. Esteban A et al: Noninvasive positive-pressure ventilation for respiratory failure after extubation, *N Engl J Med* 350:2452-2460, 2004. A

11. Hogarth DK, Hall J: Management of sedation in mechanically ventilated patients, *Curr Opin Crit Care* 10:40-46, 2004. C

12. Kleinpell R et al: Use of peripheral nerve stimulators to monitor patients with neuromuscular blockade in the ICU, *Am J Crit Care* 5:449-454, 1996. B

13. Leatherman JW et al: Muscle weakness in mechanically ventilated patients with severe asthma, *Am J Respir Crit Care Med* 153(5):1686-1690, 1996. B

14. Lessard MR, Brochard LJ: Weaning from ventilatory support, *Clin Chest Med* 17:475-489, 1996. C

15. Yang K, Tobin MJ: A prospective study of indexes predicting the outcome of weaning from mechanical ventilation, *N Engl J Med* 324:1445-1450, 1991. B

16. Esteban A et al: A comparison of four methods of weaning patients from mechanical ventilation, *N Engl J Med* 332:345-350, 1995. A

17. Ely EW et al: Effect on the duration of mechanical ventilation of identifying patients capable of breathing spontaneously, *N Engl J Med* 335:1864-1869, 1996. A

18. Davis WB et al: Pulmonary oxygen toxicity. Early reversible changes in human alveolar structures induced by hyperoxia, *N Engl J Med* 309:878-883, 1983. B

19. Capellier G et al: Oxygen tolerance in patients with acute respiratory failure, *Intensive Care Med* 24:422-428, 1998. B

20. Chastre J, Fagon JY: Ventilator-associated pneumonia, *Am J Respir Crit Care Med* 165:867-903, 2002. C

21. Anzueto A et al: Incidence, risk factors and outcome of barotrauma in mechanically ventilated patients, *Intensive Care Med* 30:612-619, 2004. B

22. Sandur S, Stoller JK: Pulmonary complications of mechanical ventilation, *Clin Chest Med* 20:223-247, 1999. C

23. The Acute Respiratory Distress Syndrome Network: Ventilation with lower tidal volumes as compared with traditional tidal volumes for acute lung injury and the acute respiratory distress syndrome, *N Engl J Med* 342:1301-1308, 2000. A

24. The National Heart, Lung, and Blood Institute ARDS Clinical Trials Network: Higher versus lower positive end-expiratory pressures in patients with the acute respiratory distress syndrome, *N Engl J Med* 351:327-336, 2004. A

Hypotension and Shock

R. Scott Stephens, MD; Saptarsi Haldar, MD;
and Charles M. Wiener, MD

FAST FACTS

- Shock is a clinical diagnosis defined by inadequate end organ perfusion in the setting of hemodynamic instability.
- The fundamental hemodynamic derangement (hypovolemic, cardiogenic, or distributive) should be identified before therapy is initiated.
- Hypovolemic shock may be caused by active hemorrhage without overt evidence of bleeding.
- If hypotension has a cardiogenic cause, consider cardiac and extramyocardial disease (e.g., tamponade, tension pneumothorax, pulmonary embolism).
- Distributive shock may result from systemic inflammatory states (e.g., sepsis) or from vasoactive medications (e.g., calcium channel blockers).
- Definitive treatment is directed at reversing the underlying insult. Goals of supportive therapy include the maintenance of end organ perfusion.
- For refractory hypotension, consider the following possibilities: an overwhelming systemic inflammatory state, adrenal insufficiency, a mixed physiologic condition (e.g., sepsis and congestive heart failure), and neurogenic shock.

Hypotension may fall anywhere on a physiologic spectrum that ranges from asymptomatic hypotension to irreversible organ damage. Shock is a clinical diagnosis, generally defined as evidence of organ hypoperfusion in the setting of hemodynamic instability. Overall, roughly 50% of all patients who develop shock will die. Early diagnosis and therapy are essential to maintain or restore perfusion of end organs, correct the underlying pathophysiologic derangement, and prevent the development of irreversible end organ dysfunction and death. This chapter provides a framework for approaching and managing shock.

I. GENERAL PRINCIPLES

A. PHYSIOLOGY OF SHOCK

1. One of the key determinants of end organ perfusion is the pressure gradient across the vascular bed. It can be modeled as

$$80(MAP - CVP) = CO \times SVR$$

where MAP = mean arterial pressure, CVP = central venous pressure, CO = cardiac output, and SVR = systemic vascular resistance. Cardiac output is the product of heart rate (HR) and stroke volume (SV; CO = HR × SV), and SVR is determined by the resistance of the arteriolar bed.

2. According to this model, shock can be categorized into three fundamental physiologic derangements: hypovolemic shock (low SV secondary to low ventricular end-diastolic pressure), cardiogenic shock (low SV secondary to pump failure), and distributive shock (inappropriately low systemic vascular resistance). Table 20-1 summarizes the physiologic derangements that cause shock.

TABLE 20-1

DETERMINING THE CAUSE OF SHOCK USING PULMONARY ARTERY CATHETERIZATION

Diagnosis	PCWP	CO	Comments
Hypovolemic shock	↑↑	↓↓	
Cardiogenic shock			
Myocardial dysfunction	↑↑	↓↓	Massive myocardial infarction (>40% LV), severe cardiomyopathy, or myocarditis.
Mechanical defect			
Acute ventricular septal defect	↑	LVCO ↓↓ and RVCO > LVCO	Predominant shunt is left → right. Pulmonary blood flow > system blood flow. O₂ step-up occurs at RV level.
Acute mitral regurgitation	↑↑	Forward CO ↓↓	V waves in PCWP tracing.
Right ventricular infarction	Normal or ↓	↓↓	Elevated RA and RV filling pressures with low or normal PCWP.
Obstructive (extracardiac)			
Pericardial tamponade	↑	↓ or ↓↓	RA mean, RV end-diastolic, and PCWP mean pressures are elevated and within 5 mmHg of one another.
Massive pulmonary embolism	Normal or ↓	↓↓	Usual finding is elevated right-sided pressures.
Distributive shock	↓ or normal	↑ or normal	In severe septic shock, CO may decrease.

Data from Parrillo JE, Ayres SM, eds: *Major issues in critical care medicine*, Baltimore, 1984, Williams & Wilkins.

CO, cardiac output; *LV*, left ventricular; *LVCO*, left ventricular cardiac output; *PCWP*, pulmonary capillary wedge pressure; *RA*, right atrial; *RV*, right ventricular; *RVCO*, right ventricular cardiac output.

3. The model also lends insight to a key concept: vasomotor autoregulation. The arterial supply of each organ bed can differentially regulate its resistance to maintain constant flow over a range of systemic pressures, allowing the selective perfusion of one organ (e.g., the brain) over another (e.g., skeletal muscle) during low-pressure states. During chronic hypertension organ beds adjust their effective flow. Thus a patient who has had a systolic blood pressure of 190 mmHg for months may acutely hypoperfuse the brain at a "normal" systolic blood pressure.

B. CLINICAL PRESENTATION

1. The symptoms of hypotension are protean and include nonspecific symptoms such as dizziness, weakness, and nausea. Symptoms may not correlate with the degree of hypotension or with the patient's clinical stability. Therefore the absence of symptoms should not completely reassure the clinician in the face of marked hypotension.
2. Physical examination should focus on the following:
   a. **Assessing circulation and volume status.** Physical examination findings suggestive of ineffective circulation include altered mental status, decreased urine output, cool extremities, and delayed capillary refill.
   b. **Distinguishing between hypovolemic, cardiogenic, and distributive shock.** Examination of the circulatory system is essential in classifying the type of shock. In particular, examination of the jugular venous pressure can help distinguish ineffective forward flow (elevated jugular venous pressure) from decreased preload (low jugular venous pressure).
   c. **Determining the primary physiologic insult.** Although the causes of shock are numerous, a prompt physical examination of each of the major organ systems may help identify the underlying pathophysiologic derangement (e.g., new apical murmur in acute mitral regurgitation). See Table 20-2.

C. DIAGNOSIS

1. In many cases the history and the events preceding shock indicate the most likely diagnosis. Physical findings can corroborate the cause suspected on the basis of history.
2. The degree of shock and evidence of multiorgan system dysfunction should be ascertained through physical examination and laboratory analysis (Table 20-3).
3. See Fig. 20-1 for an approach to the evaluation and management of shock.
4. A differential diagnosis is provided in Box 20-1.

D. GENERAL MANAGEMENT STRATEGIES (see Fig. 20-1)

1. The airway and proper oxygenation must be maintained. If indicated, endotracheal intubation or mechanical ventilation should be instituted without delay.
2. With few exceptions (e.g., decompensated chronic pulmonary hypertension, cardiogenic shock with pulmonary edema), fluid

20

HYPOTENSION AND SHOCK

resuscitation is the cornerstone of therapy for hypotension and shock. Both colloid and crystalloid solutions have been used for rapid volume resuscitation. A recent randomized controlled trial of almost 7000 patients who needed volume resuscitation demonstrated equivalency between 4% albumin and saline. Although additional subgroup analysis suggests benefits of colloid in certain patient populations, this has yet to be proven prospectively.[1]

3. Whether a patient will respond to fluid challenge is best predicted by dynamic parameters such as the expiratory decrease in arterial systolic pressure (Δdown) in intubated patients, the respiratory change in pulse pressure (ΔPP), and the inspiratory decrease in right atrial pressure (ΔRAP). Values for Δdown greater than 5 mmHg, ΔPP greater than

TABLE 20-2

KEY FINDINGS ON PHYSICAL EXAMINATION OF THE PATIENT IN SHOCK

System	Finding	Associated Conditions
HEENT	Dry mucous membranes	Dehydration
Neck	↑ JVP	Tamponade, constrictive pericarditis (Kussmaul's sign), right ventricular infarction, pulmonary embolism
	Flat JVP	Hypovolemia
	Stridor	Anaphylaxis, airway obstruction
Cardiovascular	Bradyarrhythmia or tachyarrhythmia	Unstable rhythm
	Left-right ventricular heave, S_3	Ventricular failure
	Pulsus paradoxus	Tamponade, respiratory distress
	New murmur	Acute or decompensated valvular lesion
Lungs	Tachypnea	Early sepsis, pulmonary embolism
	Absent breath sounds	Tension pneumothorax, pleural effusion, esophageal or mainstem bronchus intubation
	Wheezing	Anaphylaxis, obstructive physiology (e.g., asthma)
Abdomen	Tense, distended	Abdominal catastrophe, ascites, peritonitis
	Pulsatile mass	Ruptured abdominal aortic aneurysm
Rectal	Bright red blood or melena	Gastrointestinal hemorrhage
	Diminished tone	Spinal cord injury
Extremities	Cool, clammy skin	Shock with compensatory vasoconstriction
	Peripheral edema	Right heart failure
	Asymmetric edema	Deep vein thrombosis
Neurologic	Agitation, delirium	Poor cerebral perfusion
	Meningeal signs	Meningitis

HEENT, head, eyes, ears, nose, and throat; *JVP,* jugular venous pressure.

TABLE 20-3

ORGAN SYSTEM DYSFUNCTION IN SHOCK

Organ System	Manifestation
Central nervous system	Encephalopathy (ischemic or septic), cortical necrosis
Heart	Tachycardia, bradycardia, supraventricular tachycardia, ventricular ectopy, myocardial ischemia, myocardial depression
Pulmonary	Acute respiratory failure caused by hypoperfusion of the diaphragm, adult respiratory distress syndrome
Kidney	Prerenal failure, acute tubular necrosis
Gastrointestinal	Ileus, erosive gastritis, pancreatitis, acalculous cholecystitis, colonic submucosal hemorrhage, transluminal translocation of bacteria and endotoxin
Liver	Ischemic hepatitis ("shock liver")
Hematologic	Disseminated intravascular coagulation, dilutional thrombocytopenia
Metabolic	Hyperglycemia, glycogenolysis, gluconeogenesis, hypoglycemia (late), hypertriglyceridemia
Immune system	Gut barrier function depression, cellular immune depression, humoral immune depression

Data from Goldman L, Bennet JC: *Cecil textbook of medicine,* 21st ed, Philadelphia, 2000, WB Saunders.

13%, and ΔRAP greater than 1 mmHg have all been found to correlate with responsiveness to fluid infusion. In contrast, static parameters such as central venous pressure, right atrial pressure, and pulmonary artery occlusion pressure have not been shown consistently to predict fluid responsiveness.[2]

II. CAUSES, PATHOPHYSIOLOGY, AND SPECIFIC TREATMENTS

A. HYPOVOLEMIC AND HEMORRHAGIC SHOCK

1. The fundamental insult in hemorrhage and hypovolemia is loss of cardiac filling pressure secondary to inadequate venous return. The body attempts to compensate by increasing venous tone to augment preload, heart rate and contractility to augment cardiac output, and arteriolar tone to augment systemic pressure. If hypovolemia persists, however, the heart cannot fill in diastole, leading to loss of cardiac output, organ ischemia, pulseless electrical activity, and death.
2. The differential diagnosis for hypovolemic shock is listed in Box 20-1. Because hemorrhage is the most common cause of hypovolemic shock, the following discussion focuses on its diagnosis and management.
3. Among medical patients, common sources of hemorrhage include the gastrointestinal tract and retroperitoneal, thoracic, abdominal, or femoral bleeding after percutaneous instrumentation. Significant volumes of blood can accumulate in these spaces without obvious examination findings; computed tomography scans can be useful for diagnosis. Bleeding may be overt or occult, and the search for a source should be

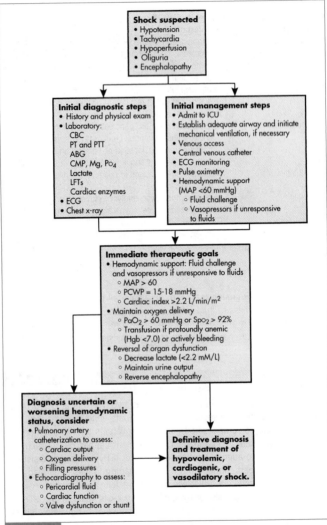

Shock suspected
- Hypotension
- Tachycardia
- Hypoperfusion
- Oliguria
- Encephalopathy

Initial diagnostic steps
- History and physical exam
- Laboratory:
  - CBC
  - PT and PTT
  - ABG
  - CMP, Mg, PO_4
  - Lactate
  - LFTs
  - Cardiac enzymes
- ECG
- Chest x-ray

Initial management steps
- Admit to ICU
- Establish adequate airway and initiate mechanical ventilation, if necessary
- Venous access
- Central venous catheter
- ECG monitoring
- Pulse oximetry
- Hemodynamic support (MAP <60 mmHg)
  - Fluid challenge
  - Vasopressors if unresponsive to fluids

Immediate therapeutic goals
- Hemodynamic support: Fluid challenge and vasopressors if unresponsive to fluids
  - MAP > 60
  - PCWP = 15-18 mmHg
  - Cardiac index >2.2 L/min/m^2
- Maintain oxygen delivery
  - PaO_2 > 60 mmHg or SpO_2 > 92%
  - Transfusion if profoundly anemic (Hgb <7.0) or actively bleeding
- Reversal of organ dysfunction
  - Decrease lactate (<2.2 mM/L)
  - Maintain urine output
  - Reverse encephalopathy

Diagnosis uncertain or worsening hemodynamic status, consider
- Pulmonary artery catheterization to assess:
  - Cardiac output
  - Oxygen delivery
  - Filling pressures
- Echocardiography to assess:
  - Pericardial fluid
  - Cardiac function
  - Valve dysfunction or shunt

Definitive diagnosis and treatment of hypovolemic, cardiogenic, or vasodilatory shock.

FIG. 20-1

Management of hypotension and shock. *ABG,* arterial blood gas; *CBC,* complete blood cell count; *CMP, comprehensive metabolic panel; ECG,* electrocardiogram; *Hgb,* hemoglobin; *ICU,* intensive care unit; *LFTs,* liver function tests; *MAP,* mean arterial pressure; *PCWP,* pulmonary capillary wedge pressure; *PT,* prothrombin time; *PTT,* partial thromboplastin time. (*Modified from Goldman L, Bennett JC:* Cecil textbook of medicine, *21st ed, Philadelphia, 2000, WB Saunders.*)

BOX 20-1

DIFFERENTIAL DIAGNOSIS OF SHOCK BY CLASSIFICATION

HYPOVOLEMIC SHOCK

Venodilation: sepsis, anaphylaxis, toxins

Hemorrhagic: gastrointestinal, retroperitoneal

Fluid loss

    External: vomiting, diarrhea

    Interstitial fluid redistribution: thermal injury, anaphylaxis

CARDIOGENIC

Myopathic

Myocardial infarction

Myocarditis

Cardiomyopathy

Sepsis

Pharmacologic (e.g., β-blockers)

Mechanical

Valvular (stenosis or regurgitant)

Ventricular septal defect

Hypertrophic obstructive cardiomyopathy

Arrhythmic

Bradyarrhythmia or tachyarrhythmia

Obstructive (Extracardiac)

Decreased preload

    Venous obstruction (e.g., superior vena cava syndrome)

    ↑ Intrathoracic pressure: tension pneumothorax, mechanical ventilation, asthma

    ↓ Cardiac compliance: tamponade, constrictive pericarditis

Increased ventricular afterload

    Right ventricle: pulmonary embolism, pulmonary hypertension

    Left ventricle: aortic dissection

DISTRIBUTIVE

Septic (bacterial, fungal, viral)

Toxic shock syndrome

Anaphylactic

Neurogenic

Adrenal crisis

Thyroid storm

Toxic (e.g., nitroprusside)

Data from Goldman L, Bennett JC: *Cecil textbook of medicine,* 21st ed, Philadelphia, 2000, WB Saunders.

aggressive. The absence of tachycardia does not rule out significant hemorrhage.[3] A loss of whole blood does not change the proportions of plasma and red cells, so a decrease in hematocrit may not be evident for up to 12 hours.[4]

4. Initial resuscitative efforts should focus on rapid intravascular volume expansion. Because the infusion rate through a catheter is proportional to the cross-sectional radius and inversely proportional to the length,

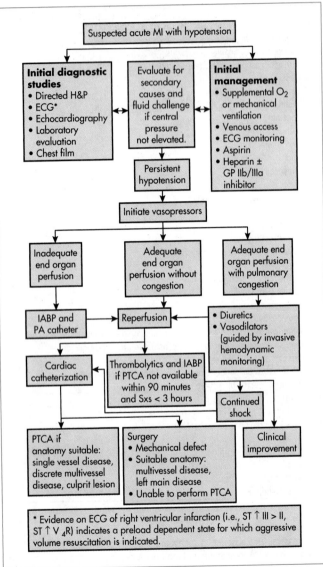

Suspected acute MI with hypotension

Initial diagnostic studies
- Directed H&P
- ECG*
- Echocardiography
- Laboratory evaluation
- Chest film

Evaluate for secondary causes and fluid challenge if central pressure not elevated.

Initial management
- Supplemental O_2 or mechanical ventilation
- Venous access
- ECG monitoring
- Aspirin
- Heparin ± GP IIb/IIIa inhibitor

Persistent hypotension

Initiate vasopressors

Inadequate end organ perfusion

Adequate end organ perfusion without congestion

Adequate end organ perfusion with pulmonary congestion

IABP and PA catheter

Reperfusion

- Diuretics
- Vasodilators (guided by invasive hemodynamic monitoring)

Cardiac catheterization

Thrombolytics and IABP if PTCA not available within 90 minutes and Sxs < 3 hours

Continued shock

PTCA if anatomy suitable: single vessel disease, discrete multivessel disease, culprit lesion

Surgery
- Mechanical defect
- Suitable anatomy: multivessel disease, left main disease
- Unable to perform PTCA

Clinical improvement

* Evidence on ECG of right ventricular infarction (i.e., ST ↑ III > II, ST ↑ V$_4$R) indicates a preload dependent state for which aggressive volume resuscitation is indicated.

FIG. 20-2   *See legend on the opposite page*

the ideal catheter is wide and short. Either two large-bore peripheral intravenous lines or a large-bore central venous catheter such as a percutaneous introducer sheath is acceptable; because of its length, a triple-lumen central venous catheter is not as useful.

5. Definitive treatment includes obtaining hemostasis, which may entail surgical intervention.

B. CARDIOGENIC SHOCK

1. Cardiogenic shock is clinically defined as low cardiac output and evidence of tissue hypoxia in the presence of adequate intravascular volume. Cardiogenic shock complicates the course of 5% to 10% of patients with acute myocardial infarction, and mortality ranges from 50% to 80%.[5,6] The pathophysiology and management of myocardial infarction are discussed in detail elsewhere, but several key points are presented here.

2. The primary defect in cardiogenic shock is the inability of the heart to maintain cardiac output, which is the product of stroke volume and heart rate. Therefore cardiogenic shock is caused by disorders that either decrease heart rate (e.g., bradyarrhythmias) or lower stroke volume (e.g., tachyarrhythmias, disorders of myocardial contractility, or mechanical abnormalities of the intracardiac or extracardiac structures). The remainder of this discussion focuses on cardiogenic shock arising from myocardial infarction.

3. Cardiac causes. Massive myocardial infarction leading to systolic and diastolic dysfunction is the most common cause of cardiogenic shock. Compensatory increases in heart rate increase myocardial oxygen demand, worsening the ischemic insult. Classically, SVR is thought to increase in the face of decreased cardiac output. This paradigm has been challenged recently because studies of patients in cardiogenic shock have revealed that SVR often is low even in the presence of vasopressors.

4. Management (Fig. 20-2).

a. Prompt reperfusion is critical. The SHOCK Trial randomized 302 patients with cardiogenic shock to emergent revascularization or initial medical stabilization. At 6 months, there was a 13% absolute reduction in mortality in the group undergoing revascularization.[7] Percutaneous coronary intervention is preferred if possible.[8]

Management of cardiogenic shock caused by MI. *ECG*, electrocardiogram; *GP*, glycoprotein; *H&P*, history and physical examination; *IABP*, intraaortic balloon pump; *MI*, myocardial infarction; *PA*, pulmonary artery; *PTCA*, percutaneous transluminal coronary angioplasty. *(Modified from Goldman L, Bennett JC: Cecil textbook of medicine, 21st ed, Philadelphia, 2000, WB Saunders; and Hollenberg SM et al: Ann Intern Med 131:47, 1999.)*

20

HYPOTENSION AND SHOCK

b. Initial management of left ventricular infarction with shock should include fluid resuscitation unless pulmonary edema is present. Intra-aortic balloon counterpulsation reduces supply-demand mismatch and may have a mortality benefit.[9] In contrast to vasopressors and inotropic agents, intraaortic balloon counterpulsation therapy increases cardiac output, improves coronary blood flow, and does not cause an increase in oxygen demand.

C. DISTRIBUTIVE SHOCK

1. Definition. Distributive shock results from an uncoupling of the tone and permeability of the resistance vessel bed. This is the result of an inciting event that causes the blood vessels to have inappropriately low SVR, leading to maldistribution of blood volume.

2. Causes. Although sepsis is the most common cause of distributive shock, many conditions (e.g., pancreatitis) can cause systemic inflammation similar to that seen in sepsis. Importantly, any form of long-lasting shock can lead to inappropriate vasodilation and distributive shock. A list of causes of distributive shock appears in Box 20-1.

3. Treatment. Because the hypotension is caused by vasodilation and increased vascular permeability leading to functional decrease in intravascular volume, therapy should begin with rapid infusion of volume in the form of crystalloid. Volume deficits may be impressive: 10 L or more may be necessary. Treatment should be expeditious because early resuscitation and treatment with the goal of hemodynamic optimization confer a mortality benefit.[10] Functional adrenal insufficiency contributing to the loss of vascular tone may be treated with corticosteroids.[11]

III. INOTROPES AND VASOPRESSORS

1. If patients with adequate intravascular volume remain hypotensive to the point of inadequate tissue perfusion, support with inotropes or vasopressors may be necessary. All vasopressors and inotropes should be given through a central line with invasive blood pressure monitoring. Choice of agent depends on the underlying cause of shock and the corresponding pathophysiology. Dosages, indications, and an overview of the pharmacologic effects of each medication are listed in Table 20-4.

2. Cardiogenic shock represents pump failure. Therefore the goal of inotropic therapy is to improve cardiac output. Three agents—dobutamine, milrinone, and dopamine—are commonly used. It is important to understand the pharmacology and attendant complications for each of these agents.

a. Dobutamine. Dobutamine, a selective beta-1 agonist, increases contractility and cardiac output. Because it has peripheral vasodilatory properties, it can worsen hypotension and should be used with caution if systolic blood pressure is less than 80 mmHg. Its inotropic

TABLE 20-4
INOTROPES AND VASOPRESSORS

Agent	Usual Dosage	Chronotropy*	Inotropy	Vasoconstriction	Vasodilatation	Dopaminergic	Hemodynamic Response
Dobutamine	2.5-10 μg/kg/min	1-2+	3-4+	0	2+	0	↑ Cardiac contractility ↓ Systemic pressure
Milrinone	0.25-1 μg/kg/min	1+	3+	0	2+	0	↑ Cardiac contractility ↓ Systemic pressure
Dopamine	1-4 μg/kg/min	1+	1+	0	1+	4+	↑ Cardiac contractility
	5-10 μg/kg/min	2+	2+	2+	0	2+	↑ Cardiac contractility
	10-25 μg/kg/min	2+	3+	3+	0	2+	↑ Systemic pressure
Norepinephrine	1-30 μg/kg/min	1+	2+	4+	0	0	↑ Heart rate ↑ Systemic pressure
Epinephrine	1-10 μg/kg/min	4+	4+	4+	3+	0	↑ Systemic pressure ↑ Cardiac contractility
Phenylephrine	40-180 μg/kg/min	0	0	3+	0	0	↑ Systemic pressure
Vasopressin	0.01-0.04 U/min	—	?	?+	?	0	↑ Systemic pressure

Modified from Holmes CL, Walley KR: *Curr Opin Crit Care* 10:442-448, 2004. Data on relative potency among these agents from Parrillo JE, Ayres SM, eds: *Major issues in critical care medicine*, Baltimore, 1984, Williams & Wilkins. Vasopressin is not included because its relative potency has not been established (Holmes et al 2004).
*The 0 to 4+ scoring system is an arbitrary system to allow comparison.

HYPOTENSION AND SHOCK

properties can increase myocardial O_2 demand, inducing or worsening ischemia.

b. Milrinone. Milrinone is a phosphodiesterase inhibitor whose effects are similar to those of adrenergic agonists as it acts downstream of the beta-adrenergic receptor. Therefore it is an ideal inotrope in patients who have received beta-blockers. Milrinone has peripheral vasodilatory properties but does not tend to increase myocardial O_2 consumption.[12]

c. Dopamine. The effects of dopamine are dose dependent. At low to medium dosages, dopamine acts on beta-1 receptors and increases cardiac output. At higher dosages, dopamine activates alpha-adrenergic receptors, producing peripheral vasoconstriction. For patients with systolic pressures less than 80 mmHg, dopamine, with its combined inotropic and vasopressor effects, may be an option. However, it has the potential to induce supraventricular tachycardias and worsen myocardial ischemia.

3. Distributive shock. Because the fundamental derangement is low systemic resistance, pressor therapy should seek to augment blood pressure through peripheral vasoconstriction. Agents commonly used are dopamine, phenylephrine, norepinephrine, and vasopressin. There is little evidence to guide initial choice of pressor, and no randomized prospective studies have demonstrated their benefit in patients with septic shock.

a. Dopamine. Dopamine often is avoided as a first-line agent in distributive shock because of its potential to induce arrhythmias.

b. Phenylephrine. This agent has pure alpha-adrenergic agonist activity, conferring vasoconstrictive properties with minimal inotropy or chronotropy. The resultant increase in SVR raises the mean arterial pressure. Because of its tendency to increase afterload, however, it is relatively contraindicated in patients with known coronary artery disease.

c. Norepinephrine. This drug has both alpha- and beta-adrenergic activity, resulting in extremely potent vasoconstriction and an increase in cardiac output. Therefore it does have arrhythmogenic potential. Observational studies suggest that, compared with patients treated with dopamine, patients treated with norepinephrine have better hemodynamics and lower mortality.[13,14]

d. Vasopressin. Otherwise known as antidiuretic hormone, vasopressin is a potent vasoconstrictor that has been shown to be deficient in certain distributive shock states (e.g., sepsis).[15,16] It is important to note that vasopressin is not a pressor in the traditional sense because the goal of therapy is replacement. Therefore it should not be titrated. Trials using vasopressin replacement therapy have demonstrated a decrease in catecholamine pressor needs and an increase in urine output and creatinine clearance. High dosages of vasopressin carry a risk of coronary vasospasm and impaired splanchnic perfusion.

PEARLS AND PITFALLS

- Patients who have large myocardial infarctions and are in cardiogenic shock might be expected to have high end-diastolic pressures. In up to 25% of Killip class IV myocardial infarctions, however, patients have low filling pressures and need volume resuscitation.
- The five main causes of refractory hypotension are inadequate volume resuscitation, adrenal insufficiency, vasoactive drug toxicity, neurogenic shock, and mixed states.
- Any patient receiving long-term steroid therapy should be assumed to be adrenally insufficient, and "stress dose" steroids should be instituted without delay. Bacteremia, coagulopathy, and acquired immunodeficiency syndrome are conditions that commonly predispose patients to adrenal hemorrhage and adrenalitis.
- The thoracic spinal cord has sympathetic efferents that can augment chronotropy, inotropy, and vasomotor tone. High spinal anesthesia, spinal cord trauma, and malignancy, ischemia, or infection at a thoracic level can disrupt sympathetic autoregulation.
- Organs that usually compensate for hypotension may themselves be diseased, creating a mixed state. For example, a patient with heart failure who becomes septic cannot increase cardiac output in response to the distributive shock. These situations can be extremely difficult to treat and often necessitate invasive hemodynamic monitoring in order to guide therapy.
- Vasopressors should be titrated to increase blood pressure with the goal of increasing end organ perfusion. Because systemic vascular resistance is derived from the cardiac output and perfusion pressure formula, it is not measured directly and should not be used to titrate vasoactive agents.

20

HYPOTENSION AND SHOCK

REFERENCES

1. SAFE Study Investigators: A comparison of albumin and saline for fluid resuscitation in the intensive care unit, *N Engl J Med* 350:2247-2256, 2004. A
2. Michard F, Teboul JL: Predicting fluid responsiveness in ICU patients: a critical analysis of the evidence, *Chest* 121:2000, 2002. C
3. Victorino G et al: Does tachycardia correlate with hypotension after trauma? *J Am Coll Surg* 196:679, 2003. B
4. Ebert RV et al: Response of normal subjects to acute blood loss, *Arch Intern Med* 68:687, 1941. B
5. Forrester JS et al: Medical therapy of acute myocardial infarction by application of hemodynamic subsets (second of two parts), *N Engl J Med* 295:1404, 1976. C
6. Hochman JS et al: Current spectrum of cardiogenic shock and effect of early revascularization on mortality. Results of an international registry. SHOCK Registry Investigators, *Circulation* 91:873, 1995. B
7. Hochman JS et al: Early revascularization in acute myocardial infarction complicated by cardiogenic shock. SHOCK Investigators. Should we emergently revascularize occluded coronaries for cardiogenic shock? *N Engl J Med* 341(9):625-634, 1999. A

8. Hollenberg SM et al: Cardiogenic shock, *Ann Intern Med* 131:47, 1999. C

9. Ferguson JJ III et al: The current practice of intra-aortic balloon counterpulsation: results from the Benchmark Registry, *J Am Coll Cardiol* 38(5):1456, 2001. B

10. Rivers E et al: Early goal-directed therapy in the treatment of severe sepsis and septic shock, *N Engl J Med* 345:1368, 2001. A

11. Annane D et al: Effect of treatment with low doses of hydrocortisone and fludrocortisone on mortality in patients with septic shock, *JAMA* 288(7):862, 2002. A

12. Felker GM et al: Heart failure etiology and response to milrinone in decompensated heart failure. Results from the OPTIME-CHF study, *J Am Coll Cardiol* 41:997-1003, 2003. B

13. Martin C et al: Norepinephrine or dopamine for the treatment of hyperdynamic septic shock? *Chest* 103(6):1826, 1993. A

14. Martin C et al: Effect of norepinephrine on the outcome of septic shock, *Crit Care Med* 28(8):2758, 2000. B

15. Holmes CL et al: Physiology of vasopressin relevant to the management of septic shock, *Chest* 120:989-1002, 2001. C

16. Patel BM et al: Beneficial effects of short-term vasopressin infusion during severe septic shock, *Anesthesiology* 96:576-582, 2002. A

Sepsis

Nisa Maruthur, MD; Sarah Noonberg, MD, PhD;
and Trish M. Perl, MD, MS

FAST FACTS

- Sepsis is a syndrome consisting of the combination of a systemic inflammatory response and the presence of infection.
- Cultures from all potential sources should be obtained before administration of antibiotics.
- Risk factors for poor outcome in sepsis include hypothermia, leukopenia, low arterial pH, shock, multiorgan dysfunction, age greater than 40 years, and medical comorbidities.[1,2]
- Coagulase-negative *Staphylococcus* infection is associated with the lowest mortality rate (15% to 20%), and candidal, enterococcal, and pseudomonal infections are associated with the highest mortality rates (30% to 40%) in sepsis.[3]
- Urosepsis confers a lower mortality rate than do intraabdominal, pulmonary, and unidentified sites of infection.[4]
- Patients with septic shock often have fluid deficits of 6 to 10 L and need aggressive fluid resuscitation.[5]
- The cornerstones of therapy for sepsis are volume resuscitation, early antibiotic therapy, hemodynamic support with vasopressors as necessary, and glycemic control. Therapy with steroids or activated protein C may be indicated in certain clinical situations.

21

I. EPIDEMIOLOGY

1. Sepsis is a clinical syndrome arising from an overwhelming systemic inflammatory and procoagulant response to infection that causes widespread tissue injury. The clinical continuum of disease is as follows: systemic inflammatory response syndrome → sepsis → severe sepsis → septic shock → multisystem organ failure → death[6,7] (Table 21-1).
2. A recent retrospective review of 750 million hospital admissions from 1979 to 2000 showed that whereas in-hospital mortality has decreased from 28% to 18%, there has been an 8.7% annualized increase in the incidence of sepsis. This increase may result partly from the increasing use of enhanced chemotherapeutic regimens and the acquired immunodeficiency syndrome epidemic, both of which have increased the number of immunocompromised patients.
3. The incidence of sepsis is increased in men and nonwhites.[8]

II. PRESENTATION

1. The symptoms of sepsis are symptoms of both the infection and the host's response. They may include fever, chills, disorientation,

TABLE 21-1

DEFINITIONS OF THE DIFFERENT STAGES IN SEPSIS

Term	Definition
Bacteremia	Presence of viable bacteria in the blood
Systemic inflammatory response syndrome	Severe inflammatory response characterized by two or more of the following: temperature $> 38°$ C or $< 36°$ C, heart rate > 90 beats/min, respiratory rate > 20 breaths/min or $PaCO_2 < 32$ mmHg, white blood cell count $> 12,000/mm^3$ or $< 4000/mm^3$, or $> 10\%$ bands
Sepsis	Presence of systemic inflammatory response syndrome with definitive evidence of infection
Severe sepsis	Sepsis associated with organ dysfunction, hypoperfusion, or hypotension (systolic blood pressure < 90 mmHg or > 40 mmHg decrease from baseline systolic blood pressure)
Septic shock	Sepsis with hypotension despite adequate fluid resuscitation and perfusion abnormalities that may include oliguria, altered mental status, or lactic acidosis
Multiple-organ dysfunction syndrome	Presence of altered organ function in an acutely ill patient such that homeostasis cannot be maintained without intervention

Data from Bone RC et al: *Chest* 101:1644, 1992.

confusion, abdominal pain, nausea, vomiting, diarrhea, dyspnea, cough productive of sputum, dysuria, and flank pain.
2. Patients with sepsis often are first identified because of changes in vital signs in the setting of suspected infection. Vital sign abnormalities include hyperventilation, tachycardia, hypotension, fever, and hypothermia. Physical examination findings often suggest a source of infection.
3. Abnormal laboratory findings include an acute respiratory alkalosis on arterial blood gas analysis, an increase in serum lactate, hyperglycemia or hypoglycemia, leukocytosis or leukopenia, and values consistent with organ dysfunction such as an elevated serum creatinine.
4. Imaging studies can reveal a source of infection such as infiltrate on chest radiography or abscess on computed tomography.

III. CAUSES

In an epidemiologic study of episodes of severe sepsis at eight academic medical centers, 40% involved gram-negative bacteria, 31% involved gram-positive bacteria, 16% had polymicrobial involvement, and 6% involved fungi.[9] Community-acquired methicillin-resistant *Staphylococcus aureus* infections should be considered, especially in patients who have received antibiotics in the past 3 months, reside in nursing homes, or have an indwelling Foley catheter.[10]

IV. DIAGNOSIS

1. The diagnosis of sepsis should be considered in any patient exhibiting the cardinal signs of systemic inflammation. Unfortunately, because sepsis is a clinical syndrome rather than a specific disease entity, no single marker or gold standard for diagnosis exists (see Table 21-1).

2. Many patients who appear septic do not have documented infection, and many disease states can mimic the appearance of sepsis. The differential diagnosis of sepsis includes pancreatitis, hypothermia, drug toxicity, azathioprine hypersensitivity, cardiogenic shock, and cardiac tamponade.

3. Because sepsis results from infection, a thorough search for an infectious source is the first step in diagnosis (Box 21-1).

4. A history and physical examination should be focused and expedited. Knowledge of the patient's medical history may reveal the presence of prostheses or grafts, which can be a hidden source of infection. A full skin examination, especially of the sacrum, may reveal unexpected decubitus ulcers.

5. Cultures should be obtained from all potential sources.

a. Blood from peripheral sites and all central lines should be collected in a sterile fashion for aerobic and anaerobic culture before initiation of antibiotic therapy.

b. The urinary tract, especially in elderly and immunocompromised patients, is a common and often asymptomatic source of infection. Urinary tract infection may manifest solely with mental status changes in older adults.

c. The utility of sputum Gram stain and culture is controversial, but they may be valuable for patients who are able to produce an adequate sample. Suctioning of sputum from patients receiving mechanical ventilation may provide clues to diagnosis, but results must be interpreted with caution because of the frequent colonization of the respiratory tract in intubated patients.

BOX 21-1

DIAGNOSTIC STUDIES USEFUL IN DETERMINING THE CAUSE OF SEPSIS

History and physical examination

Blood cultures (central line, peripheral)

Sputum Gram stain, cultures

Paracentesis if appropriate

Lumbar puncture if appropriate

Radiographic studies: chest radiograph and computed tomography of chest, abdomen, pelvis

Evaluation for foreign bodies (hemodialysis catheter, fistulas, prosthetic joints)

Skin examination (decubitus ulcers, perirectal abscess, rash)

Urinalysis and urine culture

21

SEPSIS

d. Despite thorough evaluation, no source of infection is documented in approximately 20% to 30% of patients who appear clinically septic.[9]
6. Blood pH and lactate determinations remain the standard means of assessing regional or global tissue hypoxia and the presence of anaerobic metabolism.
7. Occasionally, pulmonary artery (Swan-Ganz) catheters can help to distinguish septic shock from cardiogenic shock when the diagnosis is in doubt, but their routine use in the diagnosis and management of sepsis is controversial (see supplemental PDA Chapter 1).

V. RISK STRATIFICATION, PROGNOSIS, AND MORTALITY

1. Although studies have identified risk factors for adverse outcomes, there is no generally accepted risk stratification system for sepsis.[1,2] Risk factors can be broadly grouped into host, microbial, and environmental factors[11] (Box 21-2). Levels of inflammatory mediators, such as interleukin-6 and tumor necrosis factor, are not useful as prognostic markers, but they may have value in predicting response to upcoming therapies.
2. The natural history of sepsis was studied in a population of 3708 patients admitted to a single tertiary care center. On admission, 68% of patients met American College of Chest Physicians/Society of Critical Care Medicine (ACCP/SCCM) criteria for systemic inflammatory response syndrome. Among these patients, sepsis developed in 26%, severe sepsis in 18%, and septic shock in 4%. The prognostic value of these definitions is reflected in the stepwise progression in mortality (Table 21-2).[12]
3. Coagulase-negative *Staphylococcus* infection is associated with the lowest mortality rate (15% to 20%), and candidal, enterococcal, and

BOX 21-2
RISK FACTORS FOR POOR OUTCOMES IN SEPSIS
HOST FACTORS
Hypothermia (temperature < 35.5°C)
Leukopenia (WBC < 4000/mm³)
Arterial blood pH < 7.33
Shock
Multiorgan dysfunction (renal failure, respiratory failure, cardiac failure)
Age > 40 years
Medical comorbidities
CONTROVERSIAL RISK FACTORS
Serum cortisol level
RISK FACTORS UNDER STUDY
Genetic polymorphisms (in genes encoding TNF-α, IL-1, IL-6)

Modified from Kreger BE et al: *Am J Med* 68:344, 1980; Brun-Buisson C et al: *JAMA* 274:968, 1995; and Annane D et al: *JAMA* 283:1038, 2000.

TABLE 21-2

MORTALITY AMONG PATIENTS WITH SEPSIS

Severity of Disease	Mortality (%)
Systemic inflammatory response syndrome	7
Sepsis	16
Severe sepsis	20
Septic shock	46

Data from Rangel-Frausto MS et al: *JAMA* 273:117, 1995.

pseudomonal infections are associated with the highest mortality rates (30% to 40%) in sepsis.

4. Early recognition and prompt treatment of infection with adequate antibiotics have been shown to positively affect outcome.[13] One study involving 2124 patients with gram-negative bloodstream infections revealed that the mortality rate nearly doubled (18% vs. 34%) when antibiotics did not cover the identified pathogens.[14] The importance of the vigilant review of culture data was underscored in a recent international sepsis trial of an anti–tumor necrosis factor monoclonal antibody; inadequate antibiotic coverage was documented in 6% of cases.[15]

5. Despite recent advances in the treatment of patients with the human immunodeficiency virus (HIV), pyogenic infections and sepsis remain common. Reasons for this association are unclear but may be a result of several factors. First, patients with HIV often are neutropenic because of either primary HIV infection or antiretroviral therapy–induced bone marrow suppression. Even when neutrophil counts are normal, neutrophil function may be suboptimal because of decreased chemotaxis and lower levels of cytokine production. Second, anticapsular antibodies may be low. Finally, the use of long-term antibiotic prophylaxis may lead to colonization with multidrug-resistant organisms. Consequently, HIV-infected patients are more likely to progress to sepsis from routine infections, and they have a higher mortality rate than HIV-negative patients.[16] Contrary to prior reports, one study has suggested that bacterial pathogens are now more common than opportunistic pathogens in HIV-infected patients who are in intensive care units (ICUs). Mortality was not associated with CD4 count, but it was associated with neutropenia and severity of sepsis.[17]

VI. MANAGEMENT

A. ANTIBIOTIC COVERAGE

1. Empiric broad-spectrum antibiotic coverage should be initiated early; the choice of agent should be determined by the suspected site or source of infection and local resistance patterns.

2. Patients with hospital-acquired sepsis should receive adequate coverage for pseudomonal and methicillin-resistant *Staphylococcus aureus* infections.

3. Once the causative organism and its sensitivities are known, antibiotic coverage should be narrowed to reduce the growing problem of multidrug-resistant pathogens.

4. Lack of clinical response should prompt a search for a persistent source of infection, second site of infection, resistant organism, or unsuspected organism.

5. Source control of infection should be considered for all cases of sepsis. Examples include drainage of an abscess or removal of an infected vascular catheter.[18]

B. SUPPORTIVE CARE: HEMODYNAMICS

1. Box 21-3 lists tools and methods for hemodynamic stabilization and monitoring in patients with sepsis.

2. A recent randomized, controlled study showed that early (during the first 6 hours of resuscitation) goal-directed hemodynamic support significantly decreases mortality.[19]

3. Most patients need fluid resuscitation to maintain preload because of the increased vascular permeability, increased venous capacitance, and substantial insensible losses associated with sepsis.[20] Although colloid solutions may increase intravascular oncotic pressure, they have not been shown to lower mortality more than crystalloid solutions. A recent multicenter, randomized, double-blind trial showed that the use of 4% albumin or normal saline for fluid resuscitation in ICU patients resulted in similar outcomes at 28 days. However, the study suggested a possible benefit with the use of 4% albumin in septic patients.[21]

4. Fluid challenges with 500 to 1000 ml normal saline given over no more than 30 minutes should be given to septic patients. The determination of the need for further fluids should be based on urine output, blood pressure, and evidence of volume overload.[22]

BOX 21-3
HEMODYNAMIC STABILIZATION AND TOOLS RECOMMENDED FOR HEMODYNAMIC MONITORING IN SEPSIS
MONITORING TOOLS
Stable, adequate intravenous access, probably central venous catheter
Arterial line for blood pressure and arterial blood gas monitoring
Urinary catheter to monitor urine output
Swan-Ganz catheter (controversial; see supplemental PDA Chapter 1)
STABILIZATION METHODS
Infuse normal saline boluses (250-500 ml) over 5-10 min and reassess hemodynamics after each bolus.
Administer vasopressors as needed, with the goal of maintaining systemic vascular resistance; the appropriate initial choice for patients with adequate fluid resuscitation is norepinephrine or dopamine.

Modified from Levy MM, Fink MP, Marshall JC, et al: *Crit Care Med* 31(4):1250-1256, 2003.

5. Patients who remain hypotensive despite adequate fluid resuscitation are in septic shock and need vasopressor therapy. Intensive care monitoring is essential, and all patients should have central venous access and indwelling arterial catheters to allow the administration and titration of vasopressors. Although there is ongoing debate about the optimal first pressor to use in sepsis, the systemic vascular resistance is the primary determinant of blood pressure that is altered; therefore dopamine and norepinephrine are logical first-choice agents (see Chapter 20).[23]

C. SUPPORTIVE CARE OF ORGAN SYSTEMS IN SEPSIS

All organ systems are at risk of failure in sepsis (Table 21-3), and supportive care should be tailored to each patient's needs. Indexes to monitor in sepsis include both global (e.g., mean arterial pressure, urine output, and mixed venous oxygen saturation) and regional (e.g., cardiac enzymes, serum creatinine, and liver function tests) measurements of hypoperfusion. Specifically, there has been a recent focus on splanchnic circulation compromise (manifested by mucosal ulceration, ileus, and malabsorption) as an important indicator of regional hypoperfusion. The

21

SEPSIS

TABLE 21-3
EFFECTS OF SEPSIS ON VARIOUS ORGAN SYSTEMS

System	Effects
Pulmonary	Increased microvascular permeability leads to deposition of protein-rich edema within the lungs and ventilation-perfusion mismatches.
	Decreased lung compliance from acute respiratory distress syndrome.
Cardiovascular	Hyperdynamic state increases myocardial O_2 demand.
	Loss of vasomotor regulation leads to inability to direct blood to core organs.
	Hypotension leads to tissue hypoperfusion and hypoxia.
Neurologic	Inadequate oxygen delivery leads to agitation and delirium.
	Decreased responsiveness leads to inability to protect the airway.
Gastrointestinal	Compromised barrier function of the gut leads to bacterial translocation and release of additional systemic endotoxin.
	Ineffective hepatic clearance of enteric bacterial byproducts perpetuates systemic inflammation.
	Inability to eat leads to nutritional deficiencies.
Hematologic	Bone marrow suppression and thrombocytopenia are common.
	Severe sepsis and shock can lead to disseminated intravascular coagulation.
	Altered red blood cell deformability leads to capillary occlusion and thrombosis.
Renal	Hypoperfusion and ischemic tubular necrosis lead to oliguria and ARF.
	Use of intravenous contrast dye and aminoglycosides contributes to ARF.

ARF, acute renal failure.

use of gastric tonometry to measure intramucosal P_{CO_2} is under study as a measure of regional hypoperfusion.

1. **Pulmonary.** In many patients, acute respiratory failure develops; this is often a result of increased minute ventilatory demand, pulmonary edema, respiratory muscle fatigue, and the acute respiratory distress syndrome (see Chapter 18).

2. **Renal.** Oliguria and acute renal failure often accompany sepsis, although less than 5% of patients need dialysis.[27] Most surviving patients ultimately recover renal function.

3. **Hematologic.** Given the alterations that occur in the coagulation cascade during sepsis, several trials have attempted to address whether modification of these perturbations improves outcomes. In the PROWESS trial, recombinant activated protein C was shown to be the first sepsis-specific therapy to have proven benefit. This large, randomized controlled trial demonstrated a relative risk reduction of 19.4% in 28-day mortality with the use of recombinant activated protein C therapy. A clear trend toward an increased risk of bleeding was demonstrated in the treated patients, but it did not reach statistical significance.[24] Subgroup analyses of the PROWESS data suggest that the use of activated protein C may be especially beneficial in older adults, those with multiple-organ dysfunction, males, Caucasians, and patients with chronic obstructive pulmonary disease, lung infection, gram-positive bacterial infection, overt disseminated intravascular coagulation, or a high risk of mortality. However, additional studies are necessary in order to determine the actual usefulness of activated protein C in the various subgroups.[25-27] Activated protein C is currently licensed by the U.S. Food and Drug Administration for use in adult patients with sepsis and an APACHE II score of at least 25 on admission.[28] The risk of bleeding associated with activated protein C must be weighed against its associated benefits.[29]

4. **Endocrine.**

   a. Intensive insulin therapy to maintain blood glucose between 80 and 110 mg/dl (as compared with 180 to 200 mg/dl) has been shown to reduce mortality and morbidity and is discussed in greater detail in Chapter 25.[30]

   b. Accumulating evidence of the inflammatory pathogenesis of sepsis and the demonstration of adrenal insufficiency in significant numbers of patients with sepsis provides a solid scientific basis for steroid replacement therapy. In 2002, in a large randomized clinical trial, 300 patients with refractory septic shock were assigned to receive either placebo or hydrocortisone 50 mg intravenously every 6 hours and oral fludrocortisone 50 μg daily for 7 days.[31] Patients were given adrenocorticotropic hormone (250 μg) stimulation testing and classified as having relative adrenal insufficiency if the total serum cortisol levels rose less than 9 μg/dl. In this subgroup, there was a 10% absolute risk reduction in death at 28 days as compared with placebo (63% vs.

53%). In a recent study, it was found that free cortisol in critically ill patients was unchanged. The benefit of steroid therapy may result from the presence of steroid resistance in critically ill patients, but the true mechanism of benefit is unclear.[32]

PEARLS AND PITFALLS

- Sepsis should be considered in all patients at risk for infection who present with tachypnea, tachycardia, and acute respiratory alkalosis.
- Urinary tract infections are a common cause of sepsis and can be asymptomatic.
- Sinus infections are a common source of infection, especially in patients with nasogastric tubes.
- Patients with sepsis often are 6 to 10 L volume depleted and need aggressive volume resuscitation. Pressor support with inadequate volume resuscitation increases the risk of digital necrosis.
- Broad-spectrum antibiotics should be initiated early, and the spectrum of antibiotic coverage should be narrowed once culture data are available.

REFERENCES

1. Kreger BE et al: Gram-negative bacteremia. IV. Re-evaluation of clinical features and treatment in 612 patients, *Am J Med* 68:344, 1980. B
2. Brun-Buisson C et al: Incidence, risk factors, and outcome of severe sepsis and septic shock in adults: a multicenter prospective study in intensive care units, *JAMA* 274:968, 1995. A
3. Rangel-Frausto MS: The epidemiology of bacterial sepsis, *Infect Dis Clin North Am* 13:299, 1999. C
4. Krieger JN et al: Urinary tract etiology of bloodstream infections in hospitalized patients, *J Infect Dis* 148:57, 1983. C
5. Task Force of the American College of Critical Care Medicine, Society of Critical Care Medicine: Practice parameters for hemodynamic support of sepsis in adult patients in sepsis, *Crit Care Med* 27(3):639-660, 1999. D
6. Levy MM et al: 2001 SCCM/ESICM/ACCP/ATS/SIS International Sepsis Definitions Conference, *Crit Care Med* 31(4):1250-1256, 2003. D
7. Bone RC et al: Definitions for sepsis and organ failure and guidelines for the use of innovative therapies in sepsis. ACCP/SCCM Consensus Conference Committee, *Chest* 101:1644, 1992. D
8. Martin GS et al: The epidemiology of sepsis in the United States from 1979 through 2000, *N Engl J Med* 348:1546-1554, 2003. C
9. Sands KE et al: Epidemiology of sepsis syndrome in 8 academic medical centers. Academic Medical Center Consortium Sepsis Project Working Group, *JAMA* 278(3):234-240, 1997. C
10. Rezende NA et al: Risk factors for methicillin-resistance among patients with *Staphylococcus aureus* bacteremia at the time of hospital admission, *Am J Med Sci* 323(3):117-123, 2002. B
11. Annane D et al: A 3-level prognostic classification in septic shock based on cortisol levels and cortisol response to corticotropin, *JAMA* 283:1038, 2000. B
12. Rangel-Frausto MS et al: The natural history of the systemic inflammatory response syndrome (SIRS): a prospective study, *JAMA* 273:117, 1995. B
13. Pittet D: Nosocomial bloodstream infections. In Wenzel RP et al, eds: *Prevention and control of nosocomial infections,* Baltimore, 1993, Williams & Wilkins. C

21

SEPSIS

14. Leibovici L et al: Monotherapy versus beta-lactam aminoglycoside combination treatment for gram-negative bacteremia: a prospective, observational study, *Antimicrob Agents Chemother* 41:1127, 1997. A

15. Sprung CL et al: International sepsis trial (Intersept): role and impact of a clinical evaluation committee, *Crit Care Med* 24:1441, 1996. A

16. Proctor RA: Bacterial sepsis in patients with acquired immunodeficiency syndrome, *Crit Care Med* 29:683, 2001. B

17. Rosenberg AL et al: The importance of bacterial sepsis in intensive care unit patients with acquired immunodeficiency syndrome: implications for future care in the age of increasing antiretroviral resistance, *Crit Care Med* 29:548, 2001. C

18. Jimenez MF, Marshall JC: Source control in the management of sepsis, *Intensive Care Med* 27:S49-S62, 2001. C

19. Rivers E et al: Early goal-directed therapy in the treatment of severe sepsis and septic shock, *N Engl J Med* 345(19):1368-1377, 2001. A

20. Rackow EC, Atiz ME: Mechanisms and management of septic shock, *Crit Care Clin* 9(2):219-237, 1993. C

21. Finfer S et al: A comparison of albumin and saline for fluid resuscitation in the intensive care unit, *N Engl J Med* 350:2247-2256, 2004. A

22. Dellinger RP et al: Surviving Sepsis Campaign guidelines for management of severe sepsis and septic shock, *Crit Care Med* 32(3):858-873, 2004. D

23. Task Force of the American College of Critical Care Medicine, Society of Critical Care Medicine: Practice parameters for hemodynamic support of sepsis in adult patients, *Crit Care Med* 27:639, 1999. D

24. Bernard GR et al: Efficacy and safety of recombinant human activated protein C for severe sepsis, *N Engl J Med* 344:699, 2001. A

25. Dhainaut J, Laterre P: Drotrecogin alfa (activated) in the treatment of severe sepsis patients with multiple-organ dysfunction: data from the PROWESS trial, *Intensive Care Med* 29:894-903, 2003. A

26. Ely EW, Laterre P: Drotrecogin alfa (activated) administration across clinically important subgroups of patients with severe sepsis, *Crit Care Med* 31:12-19, 2003. C

27. Ely EW, Angus DC: Drotrecogin alfa (activated) treatment of older patients with severe sepsis, *Clin Infect Dis* 37:187-195, 2003. C

28. Knaus WA, Draper EA: APACHE II: a severity of disease classification system, *Crit Care Med* 13(10):818-829, 1985. C

29. Warren HS, Suffredini AF: Risks and benefits of activated protein C treatment for severe sepsis, *N Engl J Med* 347(13):1027-1030, 2002. D

30. van den Berghe G et al: Intensive insulin therapy in critically ill patients, *N Engl J Med* 345:1359, 2001. A

31. Annane D et al: Effect of treatment with low doses of hydrocortisone and fludrocortisone on mortality in patients with septic shock, *JAMA* 288:862, 2002. A

32. Hamrahian A et al: Measurements of serum free cortisol in critically ill patients, *N Engl J Med* 350:1629, 2004. B

Inpatient Dermatology

Laura Y. McGirt, MD; Rebecca A. Kazin, MD;
Keliegh S. Culpepper, MD; and Karen Scully, MD

FAST FACTS

- Many common systemic illnesses may have accompanying cutaneous manifestations (Table 22-1).
- The incidence of cutaneous drug reactions is 1% to 3%, and for certain drugs it approaches 10%.[1]
- Cutaneous metastases occur in 10% of patients with metastatic cancer.[2]
- Rapidly progressive skin changes, especially when associated with worsening clinical condition, always warrant a dermatology consultation.

22

Although the skin is the most accessible of the human organ systems, it can be the most overlooked aspect of the physical examination. Cutaneous abnormalities not only can indicate pathological processes solely involving the skin but also can be the presenting manifestation of systemic diseases. It is important to evaluate any dermatologic findings your patients exhibit to aid in diagnoses and quickly and accurately identify emergent situations. This chapter presents commonly encountered dermatoses and the dermatologic conditions that warrant immediate intervention.

Infection and Infestation

I. TOXIC SHOCK

A. EPIDEMIOLOGY AND ETIOLOGY

Toxic shock syndrome is a rapidly progressing condition caused by the production of the toxic shock syndrome toxin (TSST-1) enterotoxin by *Staphylococcus aureus*. Approximately half of reported cases are found to be associated with menstruation and tampon use, and the other half are associated with surgical procedures, wounds, burns, and infections. Of note, streptococcal species are known to cause gangrenous myositis and necrotizing fasciitis, a condition called streptococcal toxic shock syndrome.

B. CLINICAL PRESENTATION

Please see Box 22-1.

C. DIAGNOSIS

Please see Box 22-1.[3]

1. Differential diagnosis includes Rocky Mountain spotted fever, meningococcal encephalitis, streptococcal toxic shock, leptospirosis, dengue fever, and typhoid fever.
2. Blood and wound cultures and serologies are helpful in determining the causative agent. Notably, if *Streptococcus* is cultured from the blood or

TABLE 22-1

COMMON CUTANEOUS MANIFESTATIONS OF INTERNAL DISEASE

Disease	Cutaneous Manifestations
Hepatitis C	Porphyria cutanea tarda, erythema nodosum, leukocytoclastic vasculitis (Plate 1), cryoglobulinemia, polyarteritis nodosa, possibly lichen planus
Hepatitis B	Polyarteritis nodosa, leukocytoclastic vasculitis (Plate 1), cryoglobulinemia, serum sickness reaction with urticaria
Chronic liver disease	Striae, telangiectasia, gynecomastia (men), acne, localized scleroderma
Renal failure	Pseudoporphyria, calcinosis cutis, calciphylaxis (Plate 2), pruritus, perforating disorders
Diabetes	Acanthosis nigricans, diabetic bullae, necrobiosis lipoidica diabeticorum (Plate 3), eruptive xanthoma, widespread granuloma annulare

BOX 22-1

CLINICAL CRITERIA FOR DIAGNOSIS OF TOXIC SHOCK SYNDROME

Fever: temperature > 38.9° C

Hypotension: systolic blood pressure ≤ 90 mmHg or orthostatic drop in diastolic blood pressure ≥ 15 mmHg

Rash: diffuse macular erythroderma

Desquamation: 1-2 weeks after onset, especially palms and soles

Multisystem involvement: ≥ 3 of the following organ systems:

Gastrointestinal: vomiting or diarrhea

Musculoskeletal: severe myalgias, or creatine kinase more than twice upper limit of normal

Hematologic: thrombocytopenia

Hepatic: transaminases or bilirubin more than twice upper limit of normal

Renal: blood urea nitrogen or creatinine more than twice upper limit of normal, or pyuria

Mucous membranes: hyperemia

Central nervous system: altered mental status

wound, a surgical consultation is necessary immediately to evaluate the need for debridement or amputation.

D. MANAGEMENT

1. The initial management of toxic shock syndrome is mainly supportive. Intravenous fluids and pressors may be necessary in the setting of severe hypotension. Most importantly, the source of the infection (e.g., a tampon) should be removed, if possible.

2. Antibiotics have not been clearly shown to alter the course, but it is recommended to use clindamycin (decrease synthesis of TSST-1) in addition to oxacillin. It may be prudent to treat patients at risk for methicillin-resistant *S. aureus* with vancomycin in lieu of oxacillin.

3. In one small study, high-dose corticosteroids (methylprednisolone 10 to 30 mg/kg/day) reduced the severity and duration of symptoms but did not reduce mortality.[4]

II. HERPES ZOSTER

A. EPIDEMIOLOGY AND ETIOLOGY

Herpes zoster is a common dermatologic condition that has a lifetime incidence of about 15%. It is most common in the immunocompromised or those with immunologic senescence (e.g., older adults). Herpes zoster results from reactivation of the varicella-zoster virus in a nerve ganglion. It spreads along the sensory nerve and thus has a dermatomal distribution.

B. CLINICAL PRESENTATION

Herpes zoster usually begins with pain or paresthesia and can mimic internal causes of pain such as a myocardial infarction and gastrointestinal pain. After a few days, vesicles appear. These are grouped vesicles on an erythematous base, and they may coalesce into larger vesicles. After several days they may turn into pustules that become crusted over. The hallmark of zoster is its dermatomal distribution. The most common sites are the face and the lower thoracic and lumbar regions (Plate 4).

C. DIAGNOSIS

Herpes zoster is a clinical diagnosis, but a Tzanck smear of a scraping from the base of a vesicle showing giant cells (multinucleated keratinocytes) may be helpful. It is important to note that the presence of multinucleated keratinocytes alone does not establish a diagnosis of herpes zoster because a positive Tzanck smear is also seen with herpes simplex infections. A culture or direct fluorescent antibody test from the vesicle base is necessary to differentiate between varicella-zoster and herpes simplex.

D. MANAGEMENT

1. Treatment should be initiated immediately with either valacyclovir or famciclovir.
2. In addition to treating the infection, these agents have been shown to reduce both pain and the incidence of postherpetic neuralgia (PHN), which can persist for weeks to years after infection.[5] Other first-line agents for PHN include gabapentin and lidocaine patch (5%), whereas opioid analgesics and tricyclic antidepressants are considered second-line therapy.[6] The benefit of systemic steroids in preventing PHN is controversial, and currently they are not recommended.[7]
3. Herpes zoster is contagious to those who have not been exposed to the varicella virus, and patients should be placed on contact precautions. Once the lesions are crusted over, the virus is no longer contagious.
4. Vesicles on the tip of the nose suggest a V_1 dermatomal distribution. Given the attendant morbidities associated with zoster ophthalmicus, an ophthalmology consultation is necessary.

22

INPATIENT DERMATOLOGY

5. Patients who have more than 25 vesicles outside the primary affected dermatome may have disseminated zoster. Such patients generally are immunocompromised and warrant investigation for HIV or an underlying malignancy. These patients may also be at risk for visceral involvement and need intravenous treatment with acyclovir. Patients with disseminated zoster should be placed on both contact and airborne isolation.

III. SCABIES

A. EPIDEMIOLOGY AND ETIOLOGY

Scabies is a highly contagious infestation of the skin caused by the *Sarcoptes scabiei* mite. Transmission is human to human and requires close physical contact.

B. CLINICAL PRESENTATION

Please see Table 22-2.

C. DIAGNOSIS

1. Diagnosis often is difficult in common scabies. Skin scrapings are evaluated in mineral oil under the microscope. Identification of mites, ova, or feces is diagnostic (Plate 5).
2. Norwegian or crusted scabies is easy to diagnose because of the large number of mites and distinctive clinical appearance (Plate 6).

TABLE 22-2

FEATURES OF COMMON SCABIES AND NORWEGIAN SCABIES

	Common Scabies (Plate 5)	Norwegian Scabies (Plate 6)
Host	Immunocompetent adults, nursing home residents, or mentally debilitated patients	Immunocompromised (human immunodeficiency virus, organ transplant, or malignancy), mentally or physically debilitated patients
Average number of mites per host	10	Thousands
Most common lesion sites	Burrows or inflammatory papules may occur on palms and soles, wrists, ankles, web spaces, penis, areolae, axillae, and waistline	Sandy hyperkeratosis over entire body; often misdiagnosed as psoriasis
Pruritus	Mild to severe	Not present, or patients are unable to complain or scratch
Ease of transmission	Close personal contacts	Highly contagious via skin and fomite contact
Treatment	Permethrin, topical steroids, antihistamines	Permethrin; may need multiple treatments; consider ivermectin

D. MANAGEMENT

Please see Table 22-2.

1. Nursing and support staff and household contacts should be treated. Family members and friends not living in the patient's household may be affected and should be contacted. If the patient lives in a chronic care facility, the institution should be notified that the patient has scabies. All linens must be changed after the first treatment.
2. Patients with common scabies must be placed on contact precautions until 24 hours after the first treatment of permethrin, and patients with Norwegian scabies must have contact precautions maintained until 24 hours after the second treatment.[8]
3. After the first treatment with a topical scabicide the patient may be given oral antihistamines, and a midpotency topical steroid such as triamcinolone 0.1% cream may be applied twice a day to help with pruritus. Oral antibiotics may be necessary to treat any secondary infection from scratching. Pruritus may persist weeks to months after the scabies infestation has been appropriately treated. If all affected contacts are not appropriately treated, reinfection with the mite may occur.

Drug Reactions

I. MORBILLIFORM DRUG ERUPTION

A. BACKGROUND AND CLINICAL PRESENTATION

1. Morbilliform drug eruption is the most common drug-induced eruption. Its resemblance to measles accounts for its name.
2. Erythematous macules and papules are present on the upper trunk and extremities (Plate 7) and may involve the palms and soles. They blanch with pressure and may become confluent.
3. Pruritus and fever are features, and in contrast to more severe drug reactions, skin pain is not present. The eruption develops within 7 to 14 days of beginning a medication and may persist for up to 2 weeks after the medication is discontinued. It does not progress to a more serious reaction.

B. DIAGNOSIS AND MANAGEMENT

1. The differential diagnosis includes measles, viral exanthem, folliculitis, miliaria, disseminated candidiasis, graft versus host disease, and Rocky Mountain spotted fever.
2. Class II or III topical steroids and oral antihistamines are helpful. The best course of action with respect to the offending drug is to discontinue it.

II. ERYTHEMA MULTIFORME, STEVENS-JOHNSON SYNDROME, AND TOXIC EPIDERMAL NECROLYSIS

A. EPIDEMIOLOGY AND ETIOLOGY

Erythema multiforme (EM), Stevens-Johnson syndrome (SJS), and toxic epidermal necrolysis (TEN) are three similar clinical disorders with varying

BOX 22-2

SOME CAUSES OF ERYTHEMA MULTIFORME AND STEVENS-JOHNSON SYNDROME

MEDICATIONS

Sulfonamides

Penicillin

Nonsteroidal antiinflammatory drugs

Phenytoin

Allopurinol

Other antibiotics

INFECTIONS

Herpes simplex virus

Mycoplasma pneumonia

Hepatitis C

Histoplasmosis

Epstein-Barr virus

Adenovirus

symptoms that potentially exist on the same spectrum. Differentiating these disorders can be difficult in severe cases, and the dermatology literature is fraught with controversy regarding the exact classification of SJS and TEN. Numerous medications or infections, some of which are listed in Box 22-2, are known to cause SJS and TEN.

B. CLINICAL PRESENTATION

1. The mild form (EM minor) has localized cutaneous involvement that is usually acral. The patient has erythematous, annular or targetoid macules that may itch. Mucous membrane involvement is limited to one site, often the mouth. The eruption is self-limited. Although this minor form may be drug related, patients who have recurrent episodes usually have a history of recurrent herpes simplex virus infections. The herpes simplex virus outbreak predates or is concurrent with the eruption.

2. SJS (also called EM major) is the more severe form. Erythematous targetoid macules and patches can form bullae (Plate 8) and may coalesce, leading to widespread cutaneous involvement (Plate 9). Patients may complain of pain or burning. Subsequently the skin sloughs. Gentle pressure on a bulla or erythematous skin may cause sloughing (Nikolsky's sign). In contrast to EM minor, SJS affects two or more mucous membrane areas (eyes, mouth, or genitalia).

3. TEN is a rapidly progressive, widespread eruption with erythematous macules that develop vesicles and bullae. The lesions coalesce, and the skin sloughs in large sheets (Plate 10). Patients may complain of burning or pain of skin and mucosal sites before clinical involvement. Mucous membranes of the mouth, eyes, and anogenital area become denuded and have hemorrhagic crusting. Any part of the respiratory

tree may be involved. Nikolsky's sign is present. Microscopic examination reveals full-thickness epidermal necrosis.

C. DIAGNOSIS

As the name *multiforme* implies, the clinical presentation varies. If this diagnosis is considered, biopsy and dermatology consultation may be valuable. TEN usually is induced by medication. Common offenders are the same as for SJS, but TEN has also been associated with dozens of other medications. Information about any nonprescription medications and supplements the patient is taking (e.g., ibuprofen) must be elicited.

D. MANAGEMENT

1. EM minor is self-limited. Suppressive treatment of herpes simplex virus infection with antiviral medications may prevent future outbreaks. Topical steroids may relieve local symptoms. Viscous lidocaine can alleviate discomfort from oral erosions.
2. Treatment of SJS includes identification and treatment of the underlying infection or discontinuation of a suspected medication.
3. In the case of TEN, the causative drug should be discontinued as soon as possible. Early discontinuation improves survival.[9] Potential underlying infection should be treated. Dermatology, ophthalmology, and nutrition consultation should be sought. Oxygenation and respiratory status are monitored, and a low threshold to transfer the patient to the intensive care unit or burn unit is appropriate. If a large body surface area (i.e., > 30%) is involved, transfer to a burn unit should be considered early because delay in such a transfer is associated with higher mortality.[10]
4. Prophylactic antibiotic treatment should be instituted, and high-risk sensitizers (e.g., sulfa-based drugs) should be avoided. Sputum, blood, urine, and skin specimens should be cultured regularly.
5. Prompt treatment with intravenous immunoglobulin may be of benefit.[11,12]
6. The use of central lines should be avoided, if possible.
7. Wounds may be dressed with silver-coated dressings (e.g., Acticoat) or a nonstick wound dressing (e.g., Xeroform gauze). Any skin debridement should be postponed until disease progression has stopped.

III. HYPERSENSITIVITY SYNDROME

A. EPIDEMIOLOGY AND ETIOLOGY

This syndrome is also called drug rash with eosinophilia and systemic symptoms (DRESS). Common causal agents include anticonvulsants such as phenytoin, carbamazepine, and phenobarbital, as well as sulfonamides and allopurinol.

B. CLINICAL PRESENTATION

1. This syndrome is defined by a very severe and characteristic drug reaction that leads to a diffuse papulopustular, erythematous skin rash that can become exfoliative. Systemic involvement includes

lymphadenopathy and fever and can affect the liver, lungs, heart, and kidneys.

2. The classic finding of eosinophilia is found in about 90% of cases, and monocytes are elevated in about 40%.

C. DIAGNOSIS AND MANAGEMENT

1. The combination of clinical symptoms, eosinophilia, and use of a potential offending agent should lead to a high suspicion for DRESS. It is imperative that the suspect medication be removed promptly because there is a 10% mortality associated with this syndrome.[13]

2. Initial therapy consists of supportive care for specific systemic dysfunction, the maintenance of a warm environmental temperature, and the use of antiseptics and topical corticosteroids. Systemic corticosteroids (0.5 to 1 mg/kg) have been shown to improve symptoms and laboratory values but are currently recommended only in patients with life-threatening visceral involvement.[14] Further studies are necessary to fully evaluate the effect of systemic corticosteroids on the course of the disease.

3. There is a high risk of cross-reactivity between the three anticonvulsant medications listed, and all must be avoided if any one precipitated the reaction.

Miscellaneous

I. CALCIPHYLAXIS

A. EPIDEMIOLOGY AND ETIOLOGY

Calciphylaxis is a painful retiform purpura with histological evidence of calcium deposition in small and medium-sized cutaneous vessels and superficial vascular thrombosis. Although it is rare, its incidence has been increasing lately as a result of the use of calcium and vitamin D analogs to treat hyperparathyroidism. It occurs most often in patients on dialysis (hemodialysis more commonly than peritoneal) who have secondary hyperparathyroidism. Calciphylaxis has also been reported in patients with a decrease in functional protein C, primary hyperparathyroidism in the absence of renal disease, and metastatic breast cancer.

B. CLINICAL PRESENTATION

1. Tender induration of the skin progresses to ulcers and eschars, which may become very large (Plate 2). The surrounding skin may appear livedoid. Occasionally, calcification is seen on plain film x-ray examination.

2. Calciphylaxis usually affects the abdomen or legs.

C. DIAGNOSIS

1. The differential diagnosis includes hyperoxaluria, vasculitis, anticoagulant-induced skin necrosis, disseminated intravascular coagulation, antiphospholipid antibody syndrome, cholesterol emboli (Plate 11), and deep fungal infection.

2. A skin biopsy is necessary to identify calcium deposition within the vessels.

D. MANAGEMENT

1. Patients with calciphylaxis generally have a poor prognosis and commonly die from sepsis. A dermatology consultation is necessary to evaluate the need for biopsy.
2. Calcium and phosphate imbalance should be corrected, with a calcium phosphate product goal of less than 72. Subtotal parathyroidectomy may be beneficial[15] and should be considered. Hyperbaric oxygen treatment has been used for patients without underlying hyperparathyroidism.[16]
3. If the functional protein C level is abnormal, a hematology consultation should be considered.

II. CHOLESTEROL EMBOLI

A. EPIDEMIOLOGY AND ETIOLOGY

Cholesterol emboli are the result of unstable atherosclerotic plaques that embolize to skin and other organs. In addition to mechanical disruption, thrombolytic agents and anticoagulants can destabilize plaques, which then embolize.

B. CLINICAL PRESENTATION

1. Patients usually have a history of atherosclerotic disease. A common scenario is the discovery of purpuric lesions on the legs and feet after cardiac catheterization (Plate 11).
2. Livedo reticularis (Plate 12) is the presenting finding in 50% of patients[17] and may be elicited by having the patient stand.[18] Lesions may progress to ulceration and gangrene.

C. DIAGNOSIS

1. The differential diagnosis includes vasculitis, septic bacterial emboli from an infected aneurysm or endocarditis, and periarteritis nodosa.
2. There is no specific test to diagnose cholesterol embolization, and biopsy is not indicated in the appropriate clinical context. Laboratory abnormalities that can be seen include elevated erythrocyte sedimentation rates, leukocytosis, eosinophilia, and hypocomplementemia.

D. MANAGEMENT

1. The patient should be evaluated for manifestations of systemic embolization (neural, renal, gastrointestinal, and ocular). Hypertension and hyperlipidemia should be controlled.
2. The use of anticoagulants is controversial because they may cause cholesterol emboli. Oral corticosteroids may be of benefit.[19] Aggressive local wound care is necessary for skin ulcers.

III. ERYTHRODERMA

A. EPIDEMIOLOGY AND ETIOLOGY

Erythroderma is a cutaneous reaction pattern common to many skin conditions (Box 22-3), although often the underlying cause is not found. Most cases of erythroderma are subacute. Acute onset of erythroderma

22

INPATIENT DERMATOLOGY

> **BOX 22-3**
>
> **SOME CAUSES OF ERYTHRODERMA**
>
> Drug reaction
> Cutaneous T cell lymphoma or Sézary syndrome
> Atopic dermatitis
> Paraneoplastic erythroderma
> Psoriasis
> Seborrheic dermatitis
> Ichthyosis
> Contact dermatitis
> Dermatomyositis

should prompt consideration of scarlet fever, toxic epidermal necrolysis, scalded skin syndrome (staphylococcus or streptococcus associated), sunburn, graft versus host disease, or drug reaction.

B. CLINICAL PRESENTATION

1. Patients have erythema of more than 90% of their skin. Scaling, weeping, and fissuring may be present. Honey-colored crusting may indicate secondary impetiginization.
2. Erythroderma increases cardiac output, and this may exacerbate underlying cardiac disease. Patients may be hypothermic or have electrolyte abnormalities. Discomfort may limit mobility.
3. If the onset of erythroderma is acute, scale often is found on the skin.

C. DIAGNOSIS

The history may reveal a preexisting condition, such as psoriasis (Plate 13), or a causative medication. A dermatology consultation is necessary to evaluate the need for biopsy and treatment.

D. MANAGEMENT

1. Treatment is tailored to the underlying condition. Antibiotic treatment of bacterial superinfection should be administered. Hypothermia and fluid-electrolyte imbalance should be corrected.
2. Patients at risk for cardiac compromise should be evaluated. Midpotency topical steroids may alleviate symptoms, but definitive diagnosis is necessary to target the appropriate treatment.

PEARLS AND PITFALLS

- Although cultures and a Tzanck preparation to look for multinucleated giant cells are helpful for the diagnosis of herpes zoster, this approach generally is not necessary if the clinical appearance is obvious. Therefore treatment may be initiated on the basis of clinical appearance alone.
- Because allopurinol is renally cleared, changes in renal function can lead to supratherapeutic levels that precipitate a hypersensitivity reaction.
- Nephrogenic fibrosing dermopathy is a scleroderma-like cutaneous disorder that was originally described in 2000.[20] Although the cause of

> **BOX 22-4**
>
> **COMMON CAUSES OF LIVEDO RETICULARIS**
>
> Cutis marmorata (physiological livedo)
> Polyarteritis nodosa
> Connective tissue disease-associated vasculitis
> Antiphospholipid antibody syndrome
> Sneddon's syndrome
> Calciphylaxis
> Hyperoxaluria
> Cholesterol emboli
> Disseminated intravascular coagulation

this disease is unknown, it has been identified only in patients with acute or chronic renal insufficiency. The lesions range from skin-colored to erythematous papules that coalesce into plaques and may develop a *peau d'orange* texture. Bullae and nodules may also be present. The involved skin eventually becomes thickened and woody (Plate 14).[20-22] The lesions often are symmetric and classically found on the extremities and trunk. The face, palms, and soles typically are spared. Contractures can develop within days of initial presentation. They can be devastating, leaving patients wheelchair bound secondary to plantar flexion.

- Livedo reticularis (Plate 12) is a clinical finding that has myriad underlying causes (Box 22-4), some of which represent medical emergencies, such as disseminated intravascular coagulation.[23]
- Erythema ab igne mimics livedo reticularis. Chronic thermal damage to the skin produces a marbled pigmentation. Radiators and heating pads are common causes.
- Useful Web sites include www.dermatlas.com and www.telemedicine.org/stamfor1.htm.

REFERENCES

1. Svensson CK, Cowen EW, Gaspari AA: Cutaneous drug reactions, *Pharmacol Rev* 53(3):357, 2001. B
2. Lookingbill D, Spangler N, Helm KF: Cutaneous metastases in patients with metastatic carcinoma: a retrospective study of 4020 patients, *J Am Acad Dermatol* 29:228, 1993. B
3. Data from CDC: Case definitions for public health surveillance, *MMWR Morb Mortal Wkly Rep* 39(RR-13):1, 1990. D
4. Todd JK, Ressman M, Caston SA, Todd BH, Wiesenthal AM: Corticosteroid therapy for patients with toxic shock syndrome, *JAMA* 252(24):3399-3402, 1984. B
5. Tyring SK et al: Antiviral therapy for herpes zoster: randomized, controlled clinical trial of valacyclovir and famciclovir therapy in immunocompetent patients 50 years and older, *Arch Fam Med* 9:863, 2000. A
6. Dworkin RH, Schmader KE: Treatment and prevention of postherpetic neuralgia, *Clin Infect Dis* 36:877-882, 2003. C

7. Whitley RJ et al: Acyclovir with and without prednisone for the treatment of herpes zoster: a randomized, placebo-controlled trial. The National Institute of Allergy and Infectious Diseases Collaborative Antiviral Study Group, *Ann Intern Med* 125:376, 1996. B

8. Obasanjo OO et al: An outbreak of scabies in a teaching hospital: lessons learned, *Infect Control Hosp Epidemiol* 22(1):13, 2001. B

9. Garcia-Duval I et al: Toxic epidermal necrolysis and Stevens-Johnson syndrome: does early withdrawal of causative drugs decrease the risk of death? *Arch Dermatol* 136:323, 2000. B

10. McGee T, Munster A: Toxic epidermal necrolysis syndrome: mortality rate reduced with early referral to regional burn center, *Plast Reconstr Surg* 102(4):1018, 1998. B

11. Viard I et al: Inhibition of toxic epidermal necrolysis by blockade of CD95 with human intravenous immunoglobulin, *Science* 282:490, 1998. B

12. Stella M et al: Toxic epidermal necrolysis treated with intravenous high-dose immunoglobulins: our experience, *Dermatology* 203:45, 2001. B

13. Callot V, Roujeau JC, Bagot M, et al: Drug-induced pseudolymphoma and hypersensitivity syndrome. Two different clinical entities, *Arch Dermatol* 132:1315-1321, 1996. C

14. Ghislain PD, Roujeau JC: Treatment of severe drug reactions: Stevens-Johnson syndrome, toxic epidermal necrolysis and hypersensitivity syndrome, *Dermatol Online J* 8(1):5, 2002. C

15. Girotto JA et al: Parathyroidectomy promotes wound healing and prolongs survival in patients with calciphylaxis from secondary hyperparathyroidism, *Surgery* 130(4):645, 2001. B

16. Podymow T, Wherrett C, Burns KD: Hyperbaric oxygen in the treatment of calciphylaxis: a case series, *Nephrol Dial Transplant* 16 (11):2176, 2001. B

17. Falanga V, Fine MJ, Kapoor WN: The cutaneous manifestations of cholesterol crystal embolization, *Arch Dermatol* 122(10):1194, 1986. B

18. Sheehan MG, Condemi JJ, Rosenfeld SI: Position dependent livedo reticularis in cholesterol emboli syndrome, *J Rheumatol* 20(11):1973, 1993. B

19. Mann SJ, Sos TA: Treatment of atheroembolization with corticosteroids, *Am J Hypertens* 4(8 Pt 1):831, 2001. B

20. Cowper SE, Robin HS, Steinberg SM, et al: Scleromyxedema-like cutaneous diseases in renal-dialysis patients, *Lancet* 356:1000-1001, 2000. B

21. Cowper SE, Su LD, Bhawan J, Robin HS, LeBoit PE: Nephrogenic fibrosing dermopathy, *Am J Dermatopathol* 23(5): 383-393, 2001. B

22. Cowper SE: Nephrogenic fibrosing dermopathy: the first 6 years, *Curr Opin Rheumatol* 15:785-790, 2003. C

23. Fleischer AB, Resnick SD: Livedo reticularis, *Dermatol Clin* 8:347, 1990. C

Dermatologic Disorders in Human Immunodeficiency Virus

Anandi N. Sheth, MD; and Ciro Martins, MD

FAST FACTS

- Acquired immunodeficiency syndrome (AIDS)-defining conditions of the skin include disseminated fungal infections, Kaposi's sarcoma (KS), disseminated mycobacteria, and chronic ulcerating herpes simplex.[1]
- Dermatologic conditions may be a patient's first manifestation of human immunodeficiency virus (HIV) infection.
- Multiple dermatologic conditions (including infections) may exist in one patient.
- More than 80% of HIV-positive people will have at least one dermatologic problem that necessitates medical attention during the course of their HIV infection.
- Although antiretroviral therapy reduces many dermatologic diseases, adverse cutaneous drug reactions are very common.

23

Cutaneous disorders affect more than 80% of patients with HIV and are especially common as the CD4 count decreases.[2] Since the beginning of the highly active antiretroviral therapy (HAART) era, there has been an increase in the incidence of inflammatory skin disorders as compared with infections and neoplasms. It has also been observed that certain skin conditions tend to flare up as the CD4 counts start to increase as part of the immunologic reconstitution syndrome. Whereas some dermatologic conditions are nearly exclusive to HIV-infected people (e.g., KS), others are seen with greater frequency or severity in patients with HIV (e.g., seborrheic dermatitis). This chapter describes some of the more common dermatologic disorders seen in patients with HIV.

I. INFECTIOUS

A. BACILLARY ANGIOMATOSIS (Plate 18)

1. **Epidemiology and etiology.** Bacillary angiomatosis (BA) is a common dermatologic disorder affecting patients with a CD4 count of less than 100 cells/mm³. It is caused by *Bartonella henselae* or *quintana* (fastidious pleomorphic gram-negative bacilli). *B. henselae* is commonly associated with lymph node, splenic, and liver infection, whereas *B. quintana* often causes bone or soft tissue involvement.
2. **Clinical presentation.** BA lesions are firm, nonblanching, red or purple papules that expand into vascular nodules or pedunculated masses; they may bleed extensively with trauma.

3. **Diagnosis.** The differential diagnosis includes hemangioma, KS, pyogenic granuloma, and dermatofibroma. Diagnosis is made by biopsy with identification of the organism. Serologic testing is available, with high immunoglobulin G titers suggesting acute infection. Polymerase chain reaction (PCR) is also available for blood or tissue samples.

4. **Treatment.** Treatment is with either erythromycin or doxycycline with or without rifampin for more than 3 months.[3]

B. DISSEMINATED, DEEP, OR SYSTEMIC FUNGAL INFECTION

1. **Epidemiology and etiology.** Dermatologic manifestations occur in 10% of patients with disseminated cryptococcosis and histoplasmosis. Causes of dermatologic lesions from disseminated fungal infection are stated later in this chapter. Superficial fungal infections are also more common and severe in HIV-infected patients (Table 23-1).

TABLE 23-1

SUPERFICIAL FUNGAL INFECTIONS

Form	Cause	Presentation	Treatment
DERMATOPHYTES			
Tinea corporis	*Trichophyton Microsporum Epidermophyton* species (seen with potassium hydroxide prep)	"Ringworm": circular, red, scaly with central clearing on the body	Topical antifungal cream for 2-4 wk (e.g., Clotrimazole 1% ketoconazole 2%, miconazole 2%, Terbinafine 1%); oral therapy for severe or refractory disease
Tinea cruris		"Jock itch": red, scaly, well-demarcated lesion in groin	
Tinea pedis		"Athlete's foot": pruritus, scaly lesions between the fingers or toes	
Onychomycosis		Discoloration of the nail bed with thickening of the nail	Terbinafine 240 mg/d for 2-3 mo or itraconazole 400 mg/d for 1 wk per month for 2-3 mo
Tinea capitis		Scaly patch on the scalp, alopecia common	Griseofulvin 250-500 mg for 6-8 wk or Terbinafine 250 mg for 2-4 wk
OTHER			
Cutaneous candidiasis	*Candida* species	Moist, red, scaling rash with satellite lesions	Topical ketoconazole, miconazole, clotrimazole, or nystatin
Tinea versicolor	*Malassezia furfur*	Multiple white to reddish-brown lesions with fine scale over the chest, back, abdomen, and extremities	Selenium sulfide lotion or topical azole

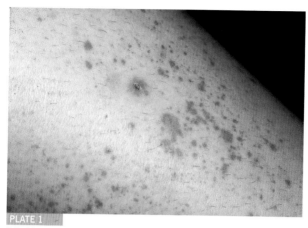

PLATE 1

Palpable purpura is the clinical correlate to small vessel vasculitis. The legs are a common location for this condition.

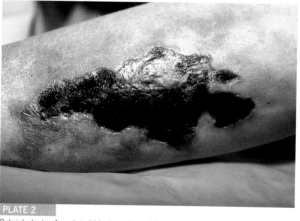

PLATE 2

Calciphylaxis. Angulated black eschar with surrounding livedo. Note the bullous change at the inferior edge of the eschar. Cholesterol emboli may have a similar eschar and often involve the digits.

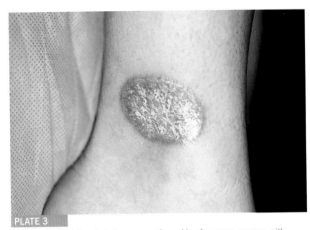

PLATE 3

Necrobiosis lipoidica diabeticorum on the ankle of a young woman with type 1 diabetes. Beneath the scale the skin has a yellowish hue and telangiectasia.

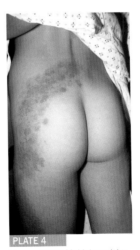

PLATE 4

Herpes zoster. Multiple vesicles are present singly and in clusters in a dermatomal distribution. *(Courtesy Bernard Cohen, MD, Dermatlas.com.)*

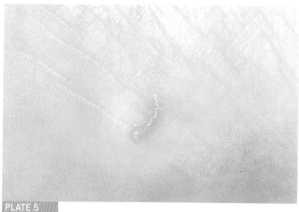

PLATE 5

Scabies burrow. Note the elevated ridge of skin, with mild surrounding erythema. A gray speck (scabies mite) may sometimes be observed at one end of the burrow. *(From White G, Cox N: Diseases of the skin: a color atlas and text, London, 2000, Mosby.)*

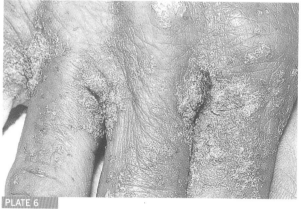

PLATE 6

Crusted scabies. The hyperkeratosis of the skin appears as a fine, sandy thickening, and scrapings demonstrate countless mites. *(From White G, Cox N: Diseases of the skin: a color atlas and text, London, 2000, Mosby.)*

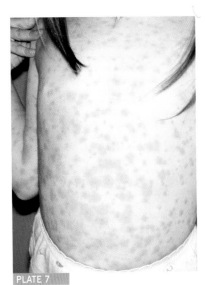

PLATE 7

Morbilliform eruption caused by amoxicillin and clavulanate potassium. *(Courtesy Bernard Cohen, MD, Dermatlas.com.)*

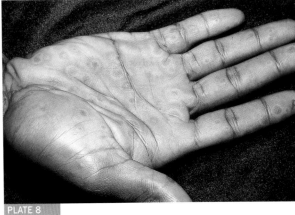

PLATE 8

Erythema multiforme. The classic lesions are erythematous targetoid lesions on the palms and soles. *(From Johns Hopkins Dermatology Residents Teaching Set.)*

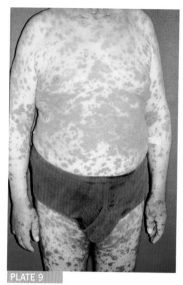

PLATE 9

Erythema multiforme. Diffuse truncal involvement. *(From Johns Hopkins Dermatology Residents Teaching Set.)*

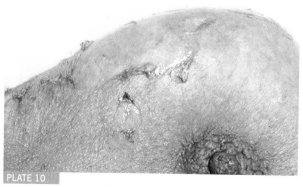

PLATE 10

Toxic epidermal necrolysis. The skin is erythematous and easily denuded.

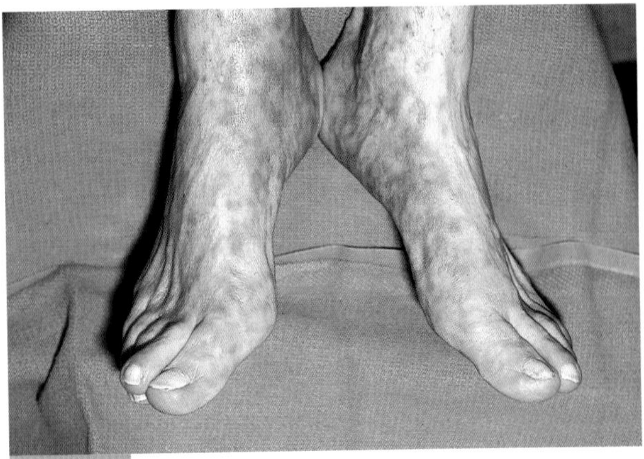

PLATE 11

Cholesterol emboli. Livedo is present on the distal extremities. In some patients, these areas progress to necrosis.

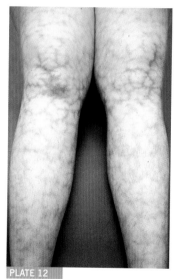

PLATE 12

Livedo reticularis. The classic fishnet
pattern is demonstrated.

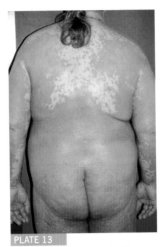

PLATE 13

Erythroderma from psoriasis. Clues in the clinical history (this patient had a history of classic plaque psoriasis) and examination may point to the correct diagnosis, but a biopsy often is necessary to make a definitive diagnosis.

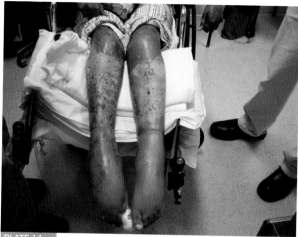

PLATE 14
Nephrogenic fibrosing dermopathy.

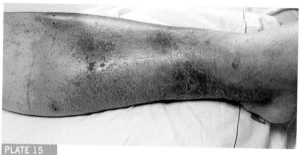

PLATE 15
Stasis dermatitis. Erythema of the lower extremity may mimic cellulitis, but chronic stasis changes (edema, varicosities, speckled brown discoloration of the skin from hemosiderin) usually are present in both lower extremities. (*Courtesy Bernard Cohen, MD, Dermatlas.com.*)

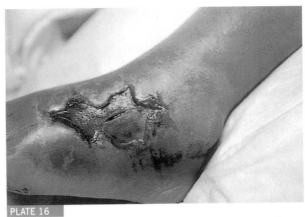

PLATE 16

Necrotizing fasciitis in a later stage with skin necrosis. In early stages the patient may have only pain, swelling, and erythema. *(From White G, Cox N: Diseases of the skin: a color atlas and text, London, 2000, Mosby.)*

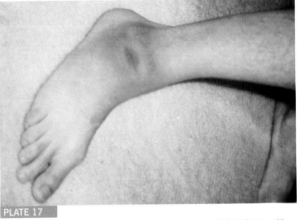

PLATE 17

Brown recluse spider bite. Early changes include a targetoid erythema with mild swelling of the joint.

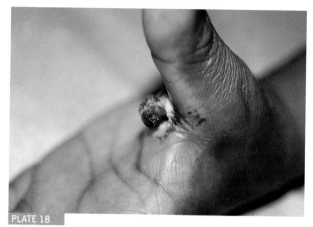

PLATE 18

Bacillary angiomatosis.

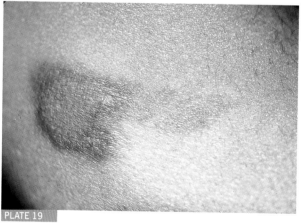

PLATE 19

Kaposi's sarcoma on the leg. The lesion is reddish-brown because of its vascular nature and accompanying hemosiderin deposition.

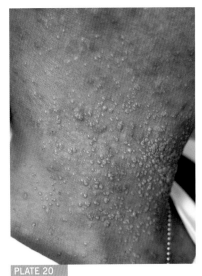

PLATE 20
Molluscum contagiosum.

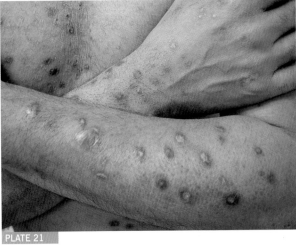

PLATE 21
Prurigo nodules on a patient infected with human immunodeficiency virus.
(Image courtesy of David Kouba, MD, PhD.)

2. **Clinical presentation**. Fungal infections that disseminate may have dermatologic involvement as their primary manifestation (*Sporothrix schenkii*) or in addition to other organ involvement (*Cryptococcus neoformans, Coccidioides immitis, Histoplasma capsulatum, Penicillium marneffei*). Various types of lesions can be seen, including erythematous or umbilicated papules, nodules, pustules, and vesicles. Lesions are found most often on the face, neck, and scalp but can be seen in other locations. Skin lesions may precede other organ signs or symptoms by weeks in disseminated cryptococcosis, thus allowing for earlier treatment and diagnosis if recognized.

3. **Diagnosis**. Skin biopsy with methenamine silver stain or periodic acid stain diatase (PASD) stains shows encapsulated budding yeast with culture of biopsy specimen positive for *C. neoformans* in cryptococcosis or intracellular budding yeast in histoplasmosis. Serum cryptococcal antigen usually is positive in disseminated cryptococcosis, and urine histoplasma antigen is a sensitive test for rapid diagnosis of histoplasmosis.

4. **Treatment**. Treatment of cryptococcosis is addressed in Chapter 49 and histoplasmosis in Chapter 61. Of note, all are treated systemically, not topically.

C. FOLLICULITIS

1. **Epidemiology and etiology.** Bacterial (mainly *S. aureus*) causes are most common, but HIV-infected patients also may have gram-negative and fungal causes, as well as noninfectious eosinophilic folliculitis. Methicillin-resistant *Staphylococcus aureus* has been reported recently as an emerging and important cause of community-acquired skin and soft tissue infections, especially in HIV-infected patients.

2. **Clinical presentation.** Patients present with papules and pustules, often pruritic, over the face, trunk, and extremities.

3. **Diagnosis.** The diagnosis is based on clinical presentation, with subsequent Gram stain of the pus often revealing the infectious agent. Eosinophilic folliculitis is recognized by peripheral blood eosinophilia and eosinophilic inflammation of the hair follicle.

4. **Treatment.** Treatment is against the offending agent (systemic antibiotics for bacterial causes, topical antifungal creams for fungal causes, or topical corticosteroids with or without phototherapy for eosinophilic folliculitis). Community-acquired methicillin-resistant *Staphylococcus aureus* skin infections often are susceptible to clindamycin.[4] See Chapter 60 for details on skin and soft tissue infections.

D. HERPES VIRUS INFECTIONS

Please see Chapter 22.

E. KAPOSI'S SARCOMA (Plate 19)

1. **Epidemiology and etiology.** KS is caused by human herpes virus 8 (HHV-8) infection, probably a sexually transmitted virus seen primarily in men. Risk factors for HHV-8 seropositivity include history of

23

DERMATOLOGIC DISORDERS IN HIV

sexually transmitted disease and high number of male sexual partners. The incidence has significantly decreased since the advent of HAART.

2. **Clinical presentation**. KS lesions usually are painless, nonpruritic violaceous to brownish-red macules, patches, plaques, nodules, and tumors with a round to oval shape and a tendency for symmetric distribution. The lesions are more commonly seen over the lower extremities, face, oral mucosa, and genitalia. Extracutaneous spread is common, especially to the lymphatic, gastrointestinal, and respiratory tracts.

3. **Diagnosis**. The differential diagnosis includes BA, hemangioma, pyogenic granuloma, nevus, hematoma, and B-cell lymphoma. Skin biopsy is diagnostic and reveals proliferation of atypical spindle cells and hemosiderin-laden macrophages.[5] If the patient has other symptoms, further imaging or diagnostic testing should be done to evaluate for extracutaneous involvement.

4. **Prognosis and treatment**. Good prognostic indicators are lesions confined to the skin, higher CD4 count (more than 150 cells/mm^3), and no systemic symptoms.[6] Although KS has no known cure, a variety of treatments exist for cutaneous and systemic disease. Treatment is indicated only when there is symptomatic systemic involvement, rapid progression of cutaneous lesions, impairment of a vital function caused by a KS lesion, and significant impairment of the patient's quality of life. For patients with few skin lesions and no symptomatic visceral involvement, treatment is palliative and includes cryotherapy, surgical excision, intralesional injections of vinblastine, topical 9-cis retinoic acid gel, and radiation therapy. Systemic chemotherapy is warranted for higher tumor burden (> 25 skin lesions) and symptomatic systemic involvement. This generally includes liposomal anthracyclines or paclitaxel. Successful HAART is associated with disappearance or decrease in number of lesions and improved survival in patients with KS. Although antivirals against HHV-8 exist, they have not been shown to be beneficial.

F. **MOLLUSCUM CONTAGIOSUM (Plate 20)**

1. **Epidemiology and etiology.** Molluscum contagiosum is caused by the poxvirus and has a prevalence of more than 18% in HIV-positive patients. Patients often have multiple or larger lesions when CD4 count falls.

2. **Clinical presentation.** Lesions are characteristically small, pearly, flesh-colored papules with central umbilication; they occur anywhere on the body except palms and soles, but most commonly they appear on the face, neck, and genitals.

3. **Diagnosis**. Differential diagnosis includes disseminated cryptococcosis or histoplasmosis. Diagnosis is generally clinical but may be confirmed by Tzanck smear or biopsy showing intraepidermal molluscum bodies.

4. **Treatment**. The lesions generally disappear with appropriate antiretroviral therapy. Curettage, topical retinoids, cryotherapy, and cauterization are other therapeutic options.

II. NONINFECTIOUS

A. APHTHOUS ULCER

1. **Epidemiology and etiology.** Recurrent aphthous stomatitis is the most common disorder of the oral mucosa seen in both HIV-positive and HIV-negative people. However, HIV patients have larger, more frequent, and more painful lesions. The cause is unknown.
2. **Clinical presentation.** Aphthous ulcers are painful, round, clearly defined ulcers with a grayish base that commonly appear in the oral cavity of both immunocompetent and immunocompromised people. In advanced HIV, aphthous ulcers may occur more often or become larger. They may cause severe odynophagia, leading to decreased oral intake and subsequent weight loss.
3. **Diagnosis.** The differential diagnosis includes cytomegalovirus, herpes simplex virus, Behçet's disease, and drug-related ulcers. The diagnosis is based on clinical findings and viral culture to rule out the aforementioned causes if suspected. Biopsy may be helpful to rule out other infectious or vasculitic processes.
4. **Treatment.** For mild cases, symptomatic relief is possible with viscous lidocaine solution. For chronic cases, oral corticosteroids or intralesional steroid injections are indicated. Thalidomide has been effective in severe, refractory cases in experimental settings.[7]

B. PRURIGO NODULARIS (Plate 21)

1. **Epidemiology and etiology.** Prurigo nodularis is a disease of unknown origin associated with repetitive trauma to the skin by scratching or rubbing. It is more prevalent in HIV-positive patients but can also be seen with other cutaneous and systemic disorders or as an isolated condition in HIV-negative people.
2. **Clinical presentation.** Lesions consist of hyperpigmented, hyperkeratotic papules and nodules, with or without excoriation and crusting, often seen with other signs of scratching, in easily reachable areas of the body. Severe, intractable pruritus results in skin trauma and lichenification, which results in further pruritus and scratching, creating a vicious cycle that results in prurigo nodularis lesions.
3. **Diagnosis.** Evaluation should exclude other primary skin diseases and alternative causes of pruritus (e.g., renal insufficiency, cholestasis, thyroid disease, polycythemia vera, lymphoma). Biopsy shows epidermal hyperplasia.
4. **Treatment.** Topical or intralesional corticosteroids, capsaicin and doxepin creams, excision, and cryotherapy are potential treatment options but are often unsuccessful. Oral antihistamines at night help prevent nighttime excoriation. Phototherapy has also shown to be of benefit.[8]

23

DERMATOLOGIC DISORDERS IN HIV

C. DRUG ERUPTION
Please see Chapter 22.

D. LIPODYSTROPHY

1. **Epidemiology and etiology.** Lipodystrophy results from redistribution of body fat. Studies show that more than 15% of patients on protease inhibitor–containing antiretroviral regimens develop evidence of lipodystrophy, irrespective of which protease inhibitor was used.[9] Mean onset of symptoms is 6 to 12 months after initiation of therapy.

2. **Clinical presentation.** Typical findings include loss of subcutaneous fat from face, arms, and legs, often with concomitant deposition of fat in the neck, upper back, and visceral abdomen. Patients may have associated insulin resistance and dyslipidemia.

3. **Diagnosis.** Diagnosis is based on history and clinical examination.

4. **Treatment.** No specific pharmacologic therapy is available for abnormal fat distribution. Recombinant human growth hormone has been studied with some evidence of reduction in visceral fat deposition, but use is currently not recommended because of its adverse effects on glucose metabolism.[10] Surgical procedures including liposuction and autologous fat transplantation from areas of fat accumulation to areas of fat loss may be considered, although fat donor sites usually are not available in these patients, and fat may reaccumulate quickly after surgical intervention.[11] Switching to a non–protease inhibitor–based therapy showed minimal improvement in glucose intolerance and dyslipidemia, but studies showed no improvement in abnormal fat distribution.[12]

PEARLS AND PITFALLS

- Reactivation herpes zoster is seen in 25% of patients with HIV infection, often with frequent recurrences and atypical lesions.[13] Patients often develop herpes zoster months after initiation of HAART during immune reconstitution.
- Seborrheic dermatitis is extremely common in HIV-infected patients, who often have more severe and extensive involvement. Treatment is with mild-potency topical steroids and tar-based, zinc pyrithione, or ketoconazole shampoo.
- Because multiple infections may occur simultaneously in immunocompromised patients, it is imperative to send biopsy specimens for all appropriate cultures (i.e., bacterial, fungal, mycobacterial, pneumonia, and viral).
- Any culture positive for *Cryptococcus* mandates a lumbar puncture to evaluate for meningeal involvement.
- Cutaneous drug eruptions occur more commonly in HIV-infected people than in the general population.
- Several drugs used in patients with HIV, notably sulfonamides, dapsone, abacavir, amprenavir, and nonnucleoside reverse transcriptase inhibitors (particularly nevirapine), are associated with hypersensitivity syndrome.[14]

- Abacavir hypersensitivity has been associated with severe, life-threatening reaction. Patients with a history of abacavir hypersensitivity should never be rechallenged.

REFERENCES

1. Centers for Disease Control and Prevention: Revised classification system for HIV infection and expanded surveillance case definition for AIDS among adolescents and adults, *MMWR* 41:1, 1992. D
2. Coopman SA et al: Cutaneous disease and drug reactions in HIV infection, *NEJM* 328:1670-1674, 1993. B
3. Koehler JE, Tappero JW: Bacillary angiomatosis and bacillary peliosis in patients infected with human immunodeficiency virus, *Clin Infect Dis* 17(4):612-624, 1993. C
4. Marcinak JF, Frank AL: Treatment of community-acquired methicillin-resistant *Staphylococcus aureus* in children, *Curr Opin Infect Dis* 16(3):265-269, 2003. C
5. Garman ME, Tyring SK: The cutaneous manifestations of HIV infection, *Dermatol Clin* 20(2):193-208, 2002. C
6. Krown SE, Testa MA, Huang J: AIDS-related Kaposi's sarcoma: prospective validation of the AIDS Clinical Trials Group staging classification, *J Clin Oncol* 15(9):3085-3092, 1997. B
7. Aweeka F et al: Pharmacokinetics and pharmacodynamics of thalidomide in HIV patients treated for oral aphthous ulcers, *J Clin Pharmacol* 41(10): 1091-1097, 2001. B
8. Lim HW et al: UVB phototherapy is an effective treatment of pruritus in patients infected with HIV, *J Am Acad Dermatol* 37:414-417, 1997. B
9. Martinez E et al: Risk of lipodystrophy in HIV-1–infected patients treated with protease inhibitors: a prospective cohort study, *Lancet* 357:592-598, 2001. B
10. Schwarz JM et al: Effects of recombinant human growth hormone on hepatic lipid and carbohydrate metabolism in HIV-infected patients with fat accumulation, *J Clin Endocrinol Metab* 87:942-945, 2002. B
11. Ponce-de-Leon S et al: Liposuction for protease-inhibitor–associated lipodystrophy, *Lancet* 353:1244, 1999. B
12. Martinez E et al: Impact of switching from human immunodeficiency virus type 1 protease inhibitors to efavirenz in successfully treated adults with lipodystrophy, *Clin Infect Dis* 31(5):1266-1273, 2001. B
13. Glesby MJ, Moore RD, Chaisson RE: Clinical spectrum of herpes zoster in adults infected with human immunodeficiency virus, *Clin Infect Dis* 21:370-375, 1995. B
14. Carr A, Cooper DA: Adverse effects of antiretroviral therapy, *Lancet* 356:1423-1430, 2000. C

23

DERMATOLOGIC DISORDERS IN HIV

Management of Chronic Wounds

Amanda M. Clark, RN, BSN, CWCN

FAST FACTS

- In patients with normal healing, wounds should heal in 4 to 6 weeks. Wounds that do not heal in that time may warrant the intervention of a specialist.
- Chronic wounds often have an underlying cause, such as pressure, vascular disease, infection, autoimmune disease, or diabetes.[1] Management of chronic wounds requires attention to the primary problem or cause of the wound, appropriate medical and surgical management, and local wound care.

I. EPIDEMIOLOGY

Most chronic wounds are a result of pressure, venous stasis, arterial insufficiency, or diabetic neuropathic changes.

1. Pressure ulcers are a serious complication of chronic illness and hospitalization with an incidence in acute care settings of approximately 7%.[2] Most of these ulcers develop on the sacrum and coccyx within a 5-day length of stay. Critical care patients are even more susceptible, with a 41% prevalence rate.
2. Venous stasis ulcers account for 70% to 90% of all lower extremity ulcers. An estimated 1% of the population has venous stasis ulcers.[3] These ulcers can remain for months to years, and after they heal they have a high rate of recurrence.
3. Of the 7.5 million U.S. residents who have diabetes, 30% have peripheral vascular disease and 15% have lower extremity ulcers.[4] These wounds do not heal unless arterial flow is restored to the affected limb.
4. Foot ulcers develop in 15% of patients with diabetes. Diabetic foot wounds account for 50% of all nontraumatic amputations in the United States.[5]

II. PRESENTATION AND BASIC WOUND ASSESSMENT

A. HISTORY

1. In wound assessment, the onset, duration, and degree of pain must be determined.
2. In addition, comorbidities affecting wound healing must be determined. Such comorbidities include diabetes, venous or arterial insufficiency, autoimmune disease, malnutrition, or incontinence.

B. PHYSICAL EXAMINATION

Physical examination of the wound should focus on its appearance and the number of layers of skin that are involved.

1. **Appearance.** The following macroscopic indexes apply to all wounds, regardless of origin:

a. Color (red-yellow-black system).[6] If more than one color is present, treatment is guided by the least healthy color.

    (1) Red wound base. Granulation tissue is described as beefy red and shiny. It is characteristic of healthy wound healing.[7]

    (2) Yellow wound base. The yellow wound base is composed of devitalized tissue, fibrin slough, or purulent exudate. The color may vary from creamy white to brown.

    (3) Black wound base. The black wound base is necrotic and may be either moist or dry. Dry eschar suggests ischemia.

b. Exudate. Attention should be paid to volume, color, odor, and consistency.

c. Size, depth, and location. In assessing the size of an ulcer, it is crucial to determine both the extent and direction of sinus tracts (if present) and whether the wound is undermined (destruction of tissue under wound margins, which creates a shelf).

d. Surrounding skin. The surrounding skin must be evaluated for the presence of induration, fluctuance (may signal deeper tissue damage), maceration (may indicate failure of dressing to absorb exudate), or erythema.

e. Presence of edema. Edema may be associated with venous insufficiency, inflammation, or infection.

2. **Partial- versus full-thickness ulcers.** This refers only to the level of skin injured, not to the type of tissue in the wound bed.

a. Partial thickness. Tissue loss is confined to the epidermis and part of the dermis. Healing occurs by epithelialization.

b. Full thickness. Tissue loss extends below the dermis and may include subcutaneous tissue, muscle, and bone. Healing occurs through the healing cascade and includes scar formation.[7]

III. CAUSES

A. PRESSURE ULCERS

1. Definition: "A pressure ulcer is any lesion caused by unrelieved pressure resulting in damage of underlying tissue. Pressure ulcers usually occur over bony prominences and are graded or staged to classify the degree of tissue damage observed."[8]

2. Pressure ulcer staging (see Fig. 24-1).

a. A pressure ulcer cannot be staged accurately until the necrotic tissue is removed.

b. Pressure ulcers cannot be "reverse staged" because the stages are based on layers of tissue damage that can never be regenerated; for example, a stage IV ulcer will never heal to become a stage III because the wound fills with granulation tissue (not the original tissue layers).

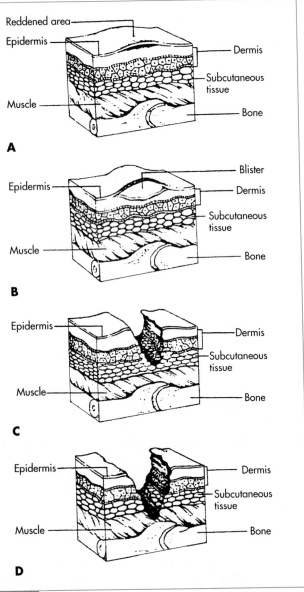

A

B

C

D

FIG. 24-1

See legend on the opposite page

B. LOWER EXTREMITY ULCERS

The majority of lower extremity ulcers are caused by venous stasis, arterial insufficiency, and diabetic neuropathic changes. See Table 24-1 for details.

IV. DIAGNOSIS

See Tables 24-1 and 24-2 for the characteristic and diagnostic features of each type of wound.

V. TREATMENT

In managing a chronic wound, treatment options include topical therapy and more aggressive debridement strategies such as pulsatile lavage, sharp instrument debridement, and surgical debridement. The remainder of this chapter focuses on topical therapy. Wound care specialists and surgeons should be consulted as clinically indicated for more aggressive debridement strategies. Antibiotics should be used only when clinical wound infection is present and should be administered systemically. Topical antimicrobials are not advocated for chronic wounds.[9]

A. GOALS OF TOPICAL THERAPY

Topical therapy promotes wound healing by creating an environment conducive to healing and by eliminating factors that lead to additional tissue injury.[10]

1. Wound healing is promoted by the following:
a. Protecting the healing wound from trauma and bacterial invasion.
b. Providing thermal insulation to maintain normal tissue temperature, which improves blood flow to the wound and enhances epidermal migration.
c. Maintaining a moist wound surface.
d. Removing necrotic tissue and foreign bodies, which prolong the inflammatory process and act as media for bacterial growth.
2. Additional tissue damage is prevented by the following:
a. Identifying and eliminating infection (see Chapter 60).
b. Obliterating dead space, which can lead to abscess and sinus tract formation.

Staging of pressure ulcers. **A**, Stage I: Nonblanching erythema of intact skin. **B**, Stage II: Partial-thickness skin loss involving the epidermis, dermis, or both. **C**, Stage III: Full-thickness skin loss involving damage or necrosis to subcutaneous tissue, which may extend down to underlying fascia. **D**, Stage IV: Full-thickness skin loss with extensive destruction, tissue necrosis, or damage to muscle or bone. *(Drawings from Hess CT: Wound care: nurse's clinical guide, Springhouse, Pa, 1995, Springhouse. Text from National Pressure Ulcer Advisory Panel Consensus Conference 1998: Staging of pressure ulcers.)*

TABLE 24-1

QUICK ASSESSMENT OF LEG ULCERS

	Venous Insufficiency (Stasis)	Arterial Insufficiency	Peripheral Neuropathy
Risk factors	Previous deep venous thrombosis, congestive heart failure, obesity, vascular ulcers, traumatic injury, orthopedic procedures	Peripheral vascular disease, diabetes, smoking, dyslipidemia, hypertension, anemia, surgical or traumatic injury to extremity	Diabetes, spinal cord injury, Hansen's disease (leprosy)
Symptoms	Pain reduced by elevation	Increased pain with activity or elevation	Paresthesias Relief of pain with ambulation
Location	Medial aspect of lower leg and ankle Superior to medial malleolus	Toe tips or web spaces Phalangeal heads around lateral malleolus Areas exposed to pressure or repetitive trauma	Plantar aspect of foot Metatarsal heads Heels Altered pressure points and sites of painless trauma or repetitive stress
APPEARANCE			
Color	Ruddy	Pale or pallid on elevation; dependent rubor	Normal skin tones
Surrounding skin	Venous dermatitis Hyperpigmentation	Shiny, taut, thin, dry, hair loss on lower extremities Atrophy of subcutaneous tissue	Trophic skin changes, fissuring and callus formation
Depth	Shallow	Deep	Variable
Wound margins	Irregular	Even	Well defined
Exudate	Moderate or heavy	Minimal	Variable
Edema	Pitting or nonpitting Possible induration or cellulitis	Variable	Cellulitis Erythema and induration common

Skin temperature	Normal to warm	Cold	Warm
Granulation tissue	Often present	Rarely present	Often present
Infection	Less common	Common	Common
		Necrosis, eschar, gangrene possible	Necrotic tissue variable, gangrene uncommon
EVIDENCE OF PERFUSION			
Peripheral pulses	Present and palpable	Absent or diminished	Present and palpable
Capillary refill	Normal (< 3 s)	Delayed (> 3 s) ankle-brachial index < 0.8	Normal (< 3 s)
Pain	Minimal unless infected or desiccated	Intermittent claudication, resting, positional, nocturnal	Diminished sensitivity to touch; reduced response to pinprick (usually painless)
Treatment	Measures to improve venous return: surgical obliteration of damaged veins, elevation of legs, compression therapy to provide > 30 mmHg compression at ankle. Topical therapy (see Table 24-2)	Measures to improve tissue perfusion: revascularization if possible, medications to improve red blood cell transit through narrowed vessels, lifestyle changes (e.g., no tobacco, no caffeine, avoidance of cold), hydration, measures to prevent trauma to tissues (appropriate footwear at all times). Topical therapy (see Table 24-2)	Measures to eliminate trauma: pressure relief for heel ulcers, "offloading" for plantar ulcers (bedrest, contact casting, or orthopedic shoes), appropriate footwear. Tight glucose control. Aggressive infection control. Topical therapy (see Table 24-2)

Modified from WOCN: Clinical fact sheet. Quick assessment of leg ulcers: www.wocn.org.

MANAGEMENT OF CHRONIC WOUNDS

TABLE 24-2

GUIDELINES FOR TOPICAL THERAPY

	Red	Yellow	Black
Appearance	Red or pink wound with or without granulation tissue.	Soft necrotic tissue, slough, or thick, tenacious exudate from creamy ivory to yellow green. Pus, fibrous material, and cellular components may be present.	Black, gray, or brown adherent necrotic tissue (eschar). Pus, fibrous material, and cellular components may be present.
Goal	Protection (debridement not necessary).	Cleansing (debridement appropriate).	Elimination of necrotic tissue. Debridement. Debridement depends on location and type of eschar.
Wound cleansing	Atraumatic, gentle cleansing.	Aggressive wound cleansing.	
Shallow wound, stage I or II	Dry Wound For fragile skin: Nonadherent, impregnated dressing appropriate for fragile skin (i.e., Xeroform, Adaptic, Vaseline gauze); change BID and PRN; may cover with secondary dressing. Transparent film or hydrocolloid dressing (change as recommended by manufacturer, usually q3-4d and PRN); may first apply a thin layer of hydrogel over wound surface for added moisture; not recommended for fragile skin. Solid hydrogel sheet: Cut to fit wound, apply cover dressing, change QOD and PRN.	Dry Wound Hydrocolloid dressing: Change q3-5d and PRN; may first apply a thin layer of hydrogel over wound surface; not recommended on fragile skin. Enzymatic debridement cream: Apply to necrotic wound bed and cover with saline gauze; expect increased drainage.	Tips of Extremity (Fingers or Toes) Keep dry, open to air; allow to autolyse; monitor for signs of infection. Heels Relieve pressure to area and monitor changes. If dry, hard, black eschar is present without drainage or erythema, leave dry. If open, moist, or draining, hydrocolloid q2-3d or hydrogel impregnated gauze QD. Other Areas If unsure of depth, sharp debridement as soon as possible to minimize infection risk.

Moist Wound
Hydrocolloid: Change q3-5d and PRN.
Polyurethane foam: Apply to wound and secure with wrap bandage; change q2-5d and PRN.

Moist Wound
Calcium alginate or Hydrofiber: change q1-3d or when strikethrough to secondary dressing occurs.
Enzymatic debriding cream: Apply to necrotic wound base and cover with gauze; expect increased drainage.
Hydrocolloid: Change q2-5d and PRN; limited absorptive capacity.

Enzymatic debriding cream: Apply to necrotic base and cover with gauze; expect increased drainage.
Superficial eschar: Film or hydrocolloid dressing over area may accelerate autolysis; change q1-2d to monitor eschar deterioration.

Moderately to Heavily Exudative Wound
Calcium alginate or Hydrofiber: change q1-3d and PRN for strikethrough to secondary dressing.
Foam: Secure with wrap and change q2-5d and PRN.

Dry Wound
Hydrogel-impregnated gauze with secondary dressing QD; may change q3d if secondary dressing is thin film or hydrocolloid.

Dry Wound
Hydrogel-impregnated gauze with secondary dressing QD; may change q3d if secondary dressing is thin film or hydrocolloid.
Enzymatic debriding cream: Apply to necrotic wound and cover with gauze packing; expect increased drainage.
Moist Wound
Calcium alginate or Hydrofiber: change q1-3d or PRN for strikethrough to secondary dressing.

Deep wound, stage III or IV

Moist Wound
Calcium alginate or Hydrofiber packing; change q1-3d and PRN for strikethrough to secondary dressing.
Negative-pressure system.

Modified from Johns Hopkins Hospital: *Management of a patient requiring wound care.* Appendix B. Guidelines for wound management, 2004.

24

MANAGEMENT OF CHRONIC WOUNDS

   c. Absorbing excess exudates, thereby protecting surrounding skin from maceration.

B. GUIDELINES FOR TOPICAL THERAPY

1. Topical therapy is a continually changing field, and new products are introduced regularly. Table 24-2 gives examples of some commonly used product categories.
2. Advanced wound care products increase patient comfort, reduce costs, and minimize nursing hours needed. Saline gauze dressing can also be used but must be changed frequently enough to prevent drying of the wound and to absorb drainage.

PEARLS AND PITFALLS

- A fever workup in a hospitalized patient should include a thorough examination of all decubitus ulcers. Sinus tracts and abscesses arising from decubitus ulcers are occult sources of fever that are easily overlooked.
- Patients with pressure ulcers are susceptible to nosocomial infections.[11]
- Nutritional status is a good indicator of wound healing potential.[12]
- All chronic wounds are contaminated, although not all are infected. A positive wound culture does not necessarily indicate infection, and a colonized wound can heal.[9]
- Tissue biopsy is the gold standard for determining whether a wound is infected.[13] Bone biopsy with histologic examination is the gold standard for diagnosing osteomyelitis.[14]
- A positive probe to bone is consistent with osteomyelitis with a specificity of 85% in diabetic patients. When a positive probe is combined with an abnormal plain film, no further testing is necessary.[15]
- Stable eschar on an extremity should not be debrided if poor vascular supply is suspected, as in diabetes or arterial disease. The goal of topical therapy is to keep the wound dry and prevent infection.

REFERENCES

1. Kane D, Krasner D: Wound healing and wound management. In Krasner D, Kane D, eds: *Chronic wound care,* 2nd ed, Wayne, Pa, 1997, Health Management Publications. C
2. Whittington K, Patrick M, Roberts J: A national study of pressure ulcer prevalence and incidence in acute care hospitals, *J Wound Ostomy Continence Nurs* 27:209, 2000. B
3. Baker SR et al: Epidemiology of chronic venous ulcers, *Br J Surg* 78:864, 1991. C
4. Levin ME: The diabetic foot: pathophysiology, evaluation, treatment. In Levin ME, O'Neal LW, eds: *The diabetic foot,* 4th ed, St Louis, 1988, Mosby. C
5. Pecoraro RE, Reiber GE, Burgess EM: Pathways to diabetic limb amputation: basis for prevention, *Diabetes Care* 13:513, 1990. C
6. Cuzzell J: The new RYB color code, *Am J Nurs* 88:1342, 1988. C
7. Cooper DM: Wound assessment and evaluation of healing. In Bryant RA, ed: *Acute and chronic wounds: nursing management,* St Louis, 1992, Mosby. C

8. Agency for Health Care Policy and Research: *Treatment of pressure ulcers* (Clinical Practice Guideline No. 15), Rockville, Md, 1994, AHCPR Public Health Service, U.S. Department of Health and Human Services; AHCPR Pub. No. 95-0652. D

9. Gilchrist B: Infection and culturing. In Krasner D, Kane D, eds: *Chronic wound care,* 2nd ed, Wayne, Pa, 1997, Health Management Publications. C

10. Doughty DB: Principles of wound healing and wound management. In Bryant RA, ed: *Acute and chronic wounds: nursing management,* St Louis, 1992, Mosby. C

11. Allman RM et al: Pressure ulcers, hospital complications, and disease severity: impact on hospital costs and length of stay, *Adv Wound Care* 12:22, 1999. B

12. Collins N: Assessment and treatment of involuntary weight loss and protein-calorie malnutrition, *Adv Skin Wound Care* 13(suppl):4-10, 2000. C

13. Mureebe LM, Morris DK: Wound infection: a physician's perspective, *Ostomy Wound Manage* 44:56, 1998. C

14. Bonham P: A critical review of the literature. Part II. Antibiotic treatment of osteomyelitis in patients with diabetes and foot ulcers, *J Wound Ostomy Continence Nurs* 28:141-149, 2001. C

15. Snyder RJ, Cohen MM, Sun G, Livingston J: Osteomyelitis in the diabetic patient: diagnosis and treatment. Part 2. Medical, surgical, and alternative treatments, *Ostomy Wound Manage* 47:24-41, 2001. C

MANAGEMENT OF CHRONIC WOUNDS

Inpatient Management of Endocrinologic Disorders

Lauren Averett, MD; and Roberto Salvatori, MD

FAST FACTS

- Diabetes mellitus is the fourth most common condition in all hospitalized patients.
- Goals for maximum blood sugar (BS) should be less than 110 mg/dl in the intensive care unit (ICU) and less than 180 mg/dl (with preprandial BS < 110 mg/dl) in the non-ICU setting.
- Type 1 diabetics need insulin therapy at all times, even when fasting, to prevent ketosis.
- Intravenous insulin is the treatment of choice for persistent hyperglycemia, which is defined as a serum glucose greater than 350 mg/dl for more than 6 hours.
- Treatment of nonthyroidal illness syndrome (NTIS) with thyroid hormone supplementation is not currently recommended.

I. INPATIENT DIABETES MANAGEMENT

Diabetics are admitted to the hospital six times more often than nondiabetics,[1] and their hospitalizations are complicated by greater morbidity and lengths of stay 1 to 3 days longer.[2] Prospective randomized controlled trials have demonstrated lower morbidity and mortality rates in patients with tight glycemic control during their hospitalizations.[3] The benefits of tight glycemic control included lower rates of inpatient mortality, bloodstream infections, acute renal failure, transfusion, and critical illness polyneuropathy, thereby prompting the American College of Endocrinology to publish its first position paper addressing guidelines for inpatient management in 2004.[4] However, although randomized controlled trials have suggested goals for maximum blood glucose levels, rigorous studies have not yet been undertaken to compare interventions meant to achieve these goals. Therefore recommendations for maintaining euglycemia are based primarily on expert opinion.

A. HYPERGLYCEMIA

1. Hyperglycemia is an independent marker of poor inpatient outcomes in a variety of clinical settings, including acute coronary syndromes, cardiac surgery, stroke, and labor and delivery.
2. **Goals for maximum BS should be less than 110 mg/dl in the ICU and less than 180 mg/dl (with preprandial BS < 110 mg/dl) in the non-ICU setting.**

3. Achieving glycemic control requires accurate anticipation of future blood glucose levels, which can be challenging in the inpatient setting. Factors affecting BS in the inpatient setting include the following:

a. Decreased carbohydrate intake: fasting, nausea and vomiting, and calorie-restricted diet (particularly in patients not adherent to a diabetic diet at home).

b. Increased carbohydrate intake: total parenteral nutrition, tube feeds, and dextrose-containing intravenous (IV) fluids.

c. Medications: corticosteroids, gatifloxacin, atypical antipsychotics, protease inhibitors, thiazide diuretics, niacin, lithium, rifampin, phenytoin, and IV medications mixed in dextrose-containing solutions.

4. Treatment of hyperglycemia for patients in the ICU.

a. For patients in the ICU, intensive insulin therapy is recommended, with a goal BS of less than 110 mg/dl. This may be achieved by either IV insulin therapy or subcutaneous insulin. Box 25-1 and Table 25-1 review the indications for and management of insulin drips.

b. When subcutaneous insulin is used, a basal dose of long-acting insulin (e.g., insulin glargine every evening or neutral protamine Hagedorn twice daily) should be given in addition to short-acting insulin, which can be given before meals and at bedtime or every 6 hours according to a sliding scale (Tables 25-2 and 25-3) that adjusts for caloric intake and breakthrough hyperglycemia.

c. **Sliding scale insulin alone is not recommended because of high rates of hyperglycemia and hypoglycemia.**

5. **Diet.** Where appropriate, patients should be on an American Diabetes Association calorie-restricted diet (generally 25 to 35 kcal/kg and 1 to 1.5 g/kg of protein). Nutrition consultation often aids in patient education. Finally, diet should be further modified based on a patient's comorbidities.

a. Dyslipidemia. Limit saturated fatty acids and *trans*-unsaturated fatty acids to less than 10% or, preferably, less than 7% of total energy intake.

25

MANAGEMENT OF ENDOCRINOLOGIC DISORDERS

BOX 25-1

INDICATIONS FOR AN INTRAVENOUS INSULIN DRIP

Critical illness

Prolonged fasting in insulin-deficient patients (e.g., type 1 diabetics)

Perioperative period

After organ transplant

Total parenteral nutrition

Hyperglycemia exacerbated by high-dose glucocorticoid therapy

Stroke

Labor and delivery

A dose-finding strategy before conversion to subcutaneous insulin therapy

Other illnesses requiring prompt glucose control (e.g., acute myocardial infarction)

TABLE 25-1

MANAGEMENT OF IV INSULIN DRIPS IN PATIENTS WITH HYPERGLYCEMIA*

Initiation	BS $\leq$ 140 mg/dl: Do not begin drip.
	BS 141-220 mg/dl: 2 U IV bolus, then initiate drip at 2 U/hr.
	BS > 220 mg/dl: 4 U IV bolus, then initiate drip at 4 U/hr.
	Goal: Maintain blood glucose between 100 and 140 mg/dl.
Monitoring	Check BS qh after initiation of drip, after any changes to drip, if BS is changing > 50 mg/dl/hr, or if BS is < 60 mg/dl or > 120 mg/dl.
	After 3 consecutive measurements between 100 and 140 mg/dl, BS may be checked q2h. If the insulin drip rate remains constant for 12 hr, BS monitoring may be reduced to q4h.
	Check BS 4 hr after discontinuation of insulin drip.
	Monitor K^+ at least q12h (low K^+ increases insulin resistance, and insulin may rapidly lower K^+).
Dosage adjustments	Titrate insulin drip in increments of 0-4 U/hr to obtain goal BS between 100 and 140 mg/dl (rate of BS change should not exceed 25 mg/dl/hr).
	Consider factors affecting blood sugar before making any adjustment (e.g., did the patient just receive a medication given with juice or in D5?).
Hypoglycemia	BS 41-60 mg/dl: Give 12.5 g D50 IV push and decrease insulin drip by 50%.
	BS < 40 mg/dl: Give 25 g D50 IV push and discontinue insulin drip.
	Restart drip (with or without bolus) after 2 consecutive BS > 140 mg/dl.

Modified from the Johns Hopkins Hospital *Medical Nursing Service Standards of Care Manual*, Baltimore, 2003.

BS, blood sugar; *D50*, 50% dextrose; *IV*, intravenous.

*This table addresses the use of insulin drips in patients without diabetic ketoacidosis or hyperglycemic hyperosmolar syndrome.

---

b. Hypertension. Limit sodium intake to 2.4 g or sodium chloride to 6 g/d.

c. Microalbuminuria. Limit protein to 0.8 to 1 g/kg/d.

6. **BS monitoring: before meals and at bedtime (if eating) or every 6 hours (if not eating).** After 48 hours, the clinician may consider decreasing frequency of monitoring to twice daily if the patient is taking only oral agents or daily insulin and has remained euglycemic on a stable regimen.

7. **Medications.**

a. If a patient is not eating or is moderately ill:

   (1) Discontinue sulfonylureas (increased risk of hypoglycemia), metformin (risk of lactic acidosis if renal failure develops), and alpha-glucosidase inhibitors (require oral intake to function).

   (2) Thiazolidinediones may be continued at their usual dosage in patients with normal cardiac function.

TABLE 25-2

PHARMACOKINETICS OF INSULIN PREPARATIONS[5]

Insulin Preparation	Onset of Action	Peak Action	Duration of Action
Lispro/Aspart (Humalog, Novalog)	5-15 min	1-2 hr	4-6 hr
Human Regular (Novolin R, Humulin R)	30-60 min	2-4 hr	6-10 hr
Human neutral protamine Hagedorn/Lente	1-2 hr	4-8 hr	10-20 hr
Ultralente (Humulin U)	2-4 hr	Unpredictable	16-20 hr
Glargine (Lantus)	1-2 hr	Flat	24 hr

TABLE 25-3

SLIDING SCALE INSULIN (REGULAR INSULIN)*

Blood Sugar Level (mg/dl)	Low-Dose Insulin Coverage	Medium-Dose Insulin Coverage	High-Dose Insulin Coverage	Comments
≤ 60	Notify physician	Notify physician	Notify physician	Give 15 g fast-acting carbohydrate or 1 ampule 50% dextrose, recheck in 15-30 min.
61-139	0 U	0 U	0 U	
140-180	3 U	4 U	5 U	
181-280	6 U	8 U	10 U	
281-400	9 U	12 U	15 U	If patient needs this dosage twice in 24 hr, consider moving to next higher scale, individualizing scale, or adding NPH or insulin drip.
> 400	Notify physician	Notify physician	Notify physician	Consider higher scale, NPH, or insulin drip.

Modified from the Johns Hopkins Hospital *Medical Nursing Service Standards of Care Manual*, Baltimore, 2003.

NPH, neutral protamine Hagedorn.

*Insulin needs may vary greatly, particularly in patients with type 2 diabetes and insulin resistance.

(3) Use short-acting insulin sliding scale for the first 24 to 48 hours to assess the patient's insulin requirements. Once the patient's 24-hour insulin requirement has been determined, give one third to one half of this amount as a long-acting agent (e.g., neutral protamine Hagedorn in divided twice-daily dosing with two thirds given in the morning and one third at night).

b. If a patient is eating and is stable:

(1) Administer sulfonylureas at 25% to 50% of usual dosage. This may be increased to 100% of home dosage in stable patients to evaluate adequacy of the patient's anticipated outpatient regimen.

Because these agents can induce hypoglycemia, dosages should be increased gradually.

(2) Continue alpha-glucosidase inhibitors and thiazolidinediones at patient's usual dosage.

(3) **Metformin should be avoided in any patient who may need IV contrast for radiographic studies or is at risk for dehydration or renal failure.**

(4) Use sliding scale insulin before meals and at bedtime for breakthrough hyperglycemia.

(5) 24-hour insulin needs should be assessed daily, and oral agents should be adjusted accordingly. Alternatively, half of the patient's daily insulin should be administered as a long-acting insulin.

8. Type 1 diabetics will need some insulin at all times, regardless of whether they are eating.

a. Insulin may be decreased or held if the patient is not able to eat for part of the day (e.g., for a procedure that will be completed in the morning). However, any patient with decreased oral intake for a longer period of time should receive insulin and glucose-containing IV fluids. Insulin may be given subcutaneously or via IV drip.

9. As discharge nears, begin patient education on how to take diabetic medications, monitor blood glucose (preferably on the glucometer the patient will be using at home), and recognize and treat hypoglycemia.

B. HYPOGLYCEMIA

1. Monitoring.

a. Tight glycemic control in the inpatient setting can be performed only where appropriate monitoring is available. Even a few minutes of severe hypoglycemia (e.g., blood glucose < 50 mg/dl) can cause arrhythmias, seizures, and other cognitive defects. Therefore all diabetic regimens must first minimize the risk of hypoglycemia through frequent monitoring or slightly higher glucose levels.

b. Although insulin infusions can be administered safely and with superior outcomes to sliding scale insulin, they entail frequent blood glucose monitoring, particularly in the first hours after they are initiated.

2. Risk factors for hypoglycemia include decreased oral intake, renal insufficiency, liver disease, infection, pregnancy, cancer, burns, and adrenal insufficiency.

3. Risk factors for hypoglycemic unawareness include beta blockade, sedation, advanced age, and long history of diabetes or evidence of diabetic neuropathy.

4. **Treatment of hypoglycemia** (BS < 60 mg/dl). Give 15 g of fast-acting carbohydrate (4 oz fruit juice or nondiet soda). If the patient is not eating or obtunded, give 25 ml (1 ampule) of 50% dextrose IV push. Recheck BS in 15 minutes and repeat glucose administration if BS is less than 80 mg/dl.[6] Repeat BS 60 minutes after the last glucose administration because glucose levels begin to fall about 1 hour after glucose ingestion.

C. MODIFICATION OF COMORBID RISK FACTORS

Where appropriate, hospitalization should also be used to assess the patient's overall diabetic care and to identify comorbidities that place diabetics at additional risk. If not recently performed, diabetic patients should have measurements of hemoglobin A_{1c} (goal < 7), fasting lipid panel (goal low-density lipoprotein < 100), creatinine, and an assay for microalbuminuria (which, if positive, is an indication for use of an angiotensin-converting enzyme inhibitor or angiotensin II receptor blocker [ARB]). Blood pressure should be controlled at less than 130/80, and patients should be counseled on nutrition, exercise, and smoking cessation.

II. STEROIDS IN THE CRITICALLY ILL (See Chapter 26)

1. Treatment with corticosteroids is indicated in critically ill patients with evidence of adrenal insufficiency, particularly in the setting of septic shock. Otherwise, the role of corticosteroids in critical illness remains controversial.
2. A meta-analysis of steroids in septic shock demonstrated that patients who have vasopressor-dependent septic shock for 2 to 72 hours benefit from 5 to 7 days of physiologic hydrocortisone, followed by a 5- to 7-day taper. The same analysis did not show significant enough mortality differences between responders and nonresponders to a corticotrophin stimulation test to preclude treating responders in septic shock with corticosteroids.[7]

III. NONTHYROIDAL ILLNESS SYNDROME

1. Low serum concentrations of T_3 are commonly seen in patients with mild illness, followed by decreases in T_4 and thyroid-stimulating hormone as the severity of illness increases.
2. Decreases in T_3 are thought to be adaptive (particularly in response to carbohydrate deprivation) and are attributed to decreased activity of 5′-monodeiodinase type 1, which converts T_4 to T_3 (Box 25-2). Decreases

---

BOX 25-2

FACTORS CONTRIBUTING TO ALTERED THYROID HORMONE METABOLISM AND ACTION IN NONTHYROIDAL ILLNESS SYNDROME

Reduced serum thyroid hormone binding proteins
Reduced type 1 5′-deiodinase activity
Increased type 3 5′-deiodinase activity
Inhibition of thyroid-releasing hormone and thyroid-stimulating hormone (e.g., caused by dopamine, glucocorticoids, and leptin)
Cytokine action on hypothalamus, pituitary, and thyroid
Limited availability of thyroid receptor coactivators
Altered thyroid hormone receptor expression
Reduced thyroid-stimulating hormone bioactivity caused by altered glycosylation

TABLE 25-4

MAJOR SIDE EFFECTS OF CORTICOSTEROIDS

Organ System	Side Effect	Recommended Screening and Prophylaxis
Cardiovascular	Accelerated atherosclerosis (caused by elevations in lipoproteins or blood glucose) Elevated blood pressure Elevated risk of ventricular rupture in acute myocardial infarction	Check fasting lipid panel and treat dyslipidemias; monitor for and treat hyperglycemia. Monitor blood pressure.
Central nervous system	Hypomania Memory impairment Akathisia, insomnia, depression	
Diabetes	Increased gluconeogenesis, suppressed insulin secretion, increased insulin resistance from steroid-induced weight gain	Adjust diabetic therapy.
GI	Gastritis, ulceration, GI bleeding Pancreatitis Visceral rupture Masking of serious GI disease	Damage to GI mucosa results from the combination of steroids with nonsteroidal antiinflammatory drugs. Consider GI prophylaxis with a proton pump inhibitor in patients taking both drugs (e.g., patients with rheumatoid arthritis). Maintain a low threshold of suspicion for intraabdominal processes in patients on chronic steroid therapy.
Reproductive	Menstrual irregularities Decreased fertility in males and females	
Infection	TB *Pneumocystis carinii* pneumonia Pneumonia, influenza	Patients at risk for TB should have initial screening with chest film and PPD (≥ 5 mm considered positive). Patients with evidence of active or latent TB should receive treatment. Chest film should be repeated annually while patient is on corticosteroids.

	Prophylaxis with low-dose trimethoprim-sulfamethoxazole is recommended in all patients who will be on large dosages of chronic steroids (e.g., > 20 mg prednisone) without a contraindication.[10] CD4 ≤ 200 while on immunosuppressive therapy indicates increased risk of *Pneumocystis carinii* pneumonia.[11] Vaccinate patient.
Musculoskeletal	Osteoporosis (bone loss occurs in 50% of patients on steroids because of decreased formation, increased resorption, increased urinary calcium excretion, decreased intestinal calcium resorption, and decreased testosterone and estrogen levels)
	1. DEXA scan at initiation of therapy in subjects already at risk and then every 6-12 mo.
	2. Supplementation with calcium 1500 mg/d and vitamin D 400-800 IU/d.
	Osteonecrosis (femoral head > knee, shoulder), higher risk in systemic lupus erythematosus
	3. Bisphosphonates in all patients at risk for osteoporosis, history of fracture, bone thinning on DEXA scan, or anticipation of > 3 mo steroid therapy (caution in women of childbearing age).
	Myopathy
	4. Weight-bearing exercise.
	May be associated with higher initial dosage of corticosteroids.
Ophthalmic	Cataracts (occur in posterior subcapsular location, bilateral)
	Screening by ophthalmologist at routine intervals. Cataracts may stabilize with dosage reduction.
	Glaucoma	More common with steroid eyedrops, usually occur in patients with family history of glaucoma.
Pregnancy	Increased incidence of cleft palate
Skin and soft tissue	Skin thinning and purpura
	Cushingoid features (moon facies, truncal obesity, buffalo hump, weight gain)
	Fluid retention	Monitor volume status in sensitive patients (i.e., those with renal disease or heart failure).

DEXA, dual-energy x-ray absorptiometry; *GI,* gastrointestinal; *PPD,* purified protein derivative; *TB,* tuberculosis.

MANAGEMENT OF ENDOCRINOLOGIC DISORDERS

25

in total T_4 are seen in up to 50% of patients in the ICU and are associated with higher mortality rates.

3. Despite its association with higher mortality rates, treatment of NTIS with thyroxine supplementation is not currently recommended because there is no evidence that thyroid hormone supplementation in nonthyroidal illness decreases mortality.

4. Only 1% to 2% of hospitalized patients have a primary thyroid disorder. See Chapter 28 for the diagnosis of primary thyroid illness in patients with NTIS.[8,9]

IV. LONG-TERM MANAGEMENT WITH CORTICOSTEROIDS

1. Corticosteroids are a mainstay of treatment for many autoimmune and inflammatory diseases. Although they can provide tremendous benefit, they can also have significant adverse effects when used at high dosages for extended periods of time.

2. Side effects from corticosteroids are both dose-related and cumulative. Therefore patients should be kept on the smallest dosage possible for the shortest possible period of time. Prednisone 5 mg daily is considered a physiologic dosage of corticosteroids.

3. Patients should be educated about the risks associated with corticosteroids, and appropriate prophylaxis and screening should be used to minimize these risks. Major side effects of corticosteroids are reviewed in Table 25-4.

4. Patients on chronic corticosteroids will need significantly higher dosages during periods of acute illness or extreme physical stress. See Chapter 26 for appropriate dosing.

PEARLS AND PITFALLS

- Prophylaxis with low-dose trimethoprim-sulfamethoxazole is recommended in all patients who will be on chronic high-dose steroids without a contraindication.
- Metformin generally should be avoided in hospitalized patients, particularly in those who are at risk for renal failure or dehydration or who may need intravenous contrast dye.
- Thiazolidinediones are contraindicated in patients with symptomatic heart failure and should be used with caution in patients with underlying cardiovascular disease because they may cause fluid retention and precipitate decompensated heart failure.
- Consider hypoglycemia in all patients with altered mental status, particularly if they are on medications to reduce their blood glucose.
- Glargine insulin cannot be mixed in the same syringe with any other insulin.
- When administered intravenously, the dosage of thyroxine should be reduced to 70% of the oral dosage.
- Low serum total T_3 in critically ill patients predicts poor outcome.[12]
- Carafate reduces the absorption of L-thyroxine.

REFERENCES

1. Moss SE, Klein R, Klein BE: Risk factors for hospitalization in people with diabetes, *Arch Intern Med* 159:2053, 1999. B
2. Roman SH, Harris MI: Management of diabetes mellitus from a public health perspective, *Endocrinol Metab Clin North Am* 26:443, 1997. C
3. van den Berghe G et al: Intensive insulin therapy in critically ill patients, *N Engl J Med* 345:1359, 2001. A
4. Garber AJ et al: American College of Endocrinology position statement on inpatient diabetes and metabolic control, *Endocr Pract* 10(Suppl 2):4, 2004. D
5. Mudaliar S, Edelman SV: Insulin therapy in type 2 diabetics, *Endocrinol Metab Clin North Am* 30:935, 2001. C
6. Trence DL et al: The rationale and management of hyperglycemia for inpatients with cardiovascular disease: time for change, *J Clin Endocrinol Metab* 88:2430, 2003. C
7. Minneci P et al: Meta-analysis: the effect of steroids on survival and shock during sepsis depends on the dose, *Ann Intern Med* 141:47, 2004. C
8. Spencer CA et al: Application of a new chemiluminometric thyrotropin assay to subnormal measurement, *J Clin Endocrinol Metab* 70:453, 1990. B
9. Spencer CA et al: Specificity of sensitive assays of thyrotropin (TSH) used to screen for thyroid disease in hospitalized patients, *Clin Chem* 33:1391, 1987. B
10. Klein NC, Go CH, Cunha BA: Infections associated with steroid use, *Infect Dis Clin North Am* 15:423, 2001. C
11. Gluck T et al: *Pneumocystis carinii* pneumonia as a complication of immunosuppressive therapy, *Infection* 28:227, 2000. B
12. Jarek MJ et al: Endocrine profiles for outcome prediction from the intensive care unit, *Crit Care Med* 21:543, 1993. B

25

MANAGEMENT OF ENDOCRINOLOGIC DISORDERS

Adrenal Insufficiency

Ann Reed, MD; Assil Saleh, MD; and Roberto Salvatori, MD

FAST FACTS

- Addison's disease, or primary adrenal insufficiency (AI), is caused by destruction of the adrenal glands. Secondary AI is caused by lack of secretion of adrenocorticotropic hormone (ACTH) by the pituitary gland. The two diseases are quite different: In primary AI both glucocorticoid and mineralocorticoid hormones are missing, whereas in secondary AI mineralocorticoid production is maintained.
- Primary AI is now most commonly caused by autoimmune adrenal destruction.[1,2] At least 90% of glandular function must be disrupted before clinical AI becomes evident.
- Signs and symptoms of AI may be nonspecific and difficult to recognize, yet AI is potentially fatal if unrecognized and untreated. Death usually results from hypotension or cardiac arrhythmia caused by hyperkalemia.
- AI is suspected on the basis of nonspecific symptoms (e.g., weight loss, fatigue, nausea, vomiting, depression) and more specific findings (e.g., hypotension, hypoglycemia, hyponatremia, in primary AI, hyperkalemia, hyperpigmentation).
- Glucocorticoid replacement is the mainstay of AI therapy. The goal is to use the smallest dosage needed to relieve symptoms yet avoid steroid-related complications (e.g., weight gain, osteoporosis, glucose intolerance).
- Up to 40% of critically ill patients in intensive care unit (ICU) settings were thought to have AI, but recently it was demonstrated that their serum free cortisol levels may be normal. Using free cortisol measurement, it is likely that the prevalence of AI in patients in the ICU will be found to be lower.[3]

I. EPIDEMIOLOGY

1. In 1855, Thomas Addison first reported a condition caused by "failure of the suprarenal glands" and characterized by "languor, debility, and remarkable feebleness of the heart," a disorder now recognized as AI.[4]
2. AI may be primary (in conditions of direct destruction of the adrenal glands, such as Addison's disease, or caused by medications that interfere with steroid synthesis, such as ketoconazole) or secondary (caused by derangement of the hypothalamic-pituitary-adrenal [HPA] axis, as occurs with long-term use of exogenous steroids or in patients with hypopituitarism of different origins) (Box 26-1). The acute presentation of AI is a medical emergency necessitating urgent diagnosis and therapy.[5,6]

BOX 26-1

CAUSES OF ADRENAL INSUFFICIENCY

PRIMARY ADRENAL INSUFFICIENCY

Autoimmune

Autoimmune adrenalitis (isolated or as part of type I and type II autoimmune polyglandular disease).

Infection

Tuberculosis.

Fungal infections (e.g., histoplasmosis, cryptococcosis, blastomycosis).

Human immunodeficiency virus related (e.g., cytomegalovirus, *Mycobacterium avium-intracellulare, Cryptococcus, Toxoplasma,* Kaposi's sarcoma).

Adrenal Hemorrhage

Waterhouse-Friderichsen syndrome.

Lupus anticoagulant, antiphospholipid antibodies.

Idiopathic thrombocytopenic purpura, heparin-induced thrombocytopenia.

Iatrogenic (e.g., anticoagulation).

Metastatic Disease

Particularly lung, breast, kidney, lymphoma, malignant melanoma.

Infiltrative disease (e.g., hemochromatosis, amyloidosis).

Drugs

Ketoconazole, etomidate, aminoglutethimide, metyrapone, mitotane (reduce steroid synthesis).

In patients on steroid replacement, rifampin, diphenylhydantoin, or phenobarbital can increase steroid catabolism and cause increased steroid needs.

Genetic

Adrenoleukodystrophy and the milder variant adrenomyeloneuropathy (both inherited as an X-linked recessive trait).

SECONDARY ADRENAL INSUFFICIENCY

Cessation of prior glucocorticoid therapy.

Pituitary and hypothalamic disorders: infiltrative tumor (adenoma, craniopharyngioma), sarcoidosis, histiocytosis X, lymphocytic hypophysitis, hemorrhage.

Empty sella syndrome.

Postpartum pituitary necrosis (Sheehan's syndrome).

Postsurgical head trauma (after transsphenoidal pituitary surgery or after removal of functioning adrenal adenoma).

Megestrol use.

Modified from Oelkers W: *N Engl J Med* 335:1206, 1996; and Werbel SS, Ober KP: *Endocrinol Metab Clin North Am* 22:303, 1993.

3. Although tuberculosis remains the most common cause of primary AI in developing nations, **autoimmune destruction of the adrenal glands has now become the leading cause of primary AI in Western countries.**[2]
4. In males, an often unrecognized cause of primary AI is adrenoleukodystrophy or the milder variant adrenomyeloneuropathy

(both inherited as an X-linked recessive trait), caused by accumulation of very long fatty acids in the adrenal cortex and central nervous system.

5. Currently, Addison's disease (primary AI) has an incidence of about 5 to 6 cases per million people per year and a prevalence of 35 to 60 cases per million in Western countries.[7,8] In adults the mean age at diagnosis is 40.[9]

6. Autoimmune AI may occur alone or in conjunction with other endocrinopathies. Two types of polyglandular failure syndromes exist: type 1, usually occurring in childhood and often associated with hypoparathyroidism and mucocutaneous candidiasis, and type 2, which occurs in adulthood and is associated with insulin-dependent diabetes mellitus, autoimmune thyroid disease, alopecia areata, and vitiligo.[10,11] **In one series, nearly half of patients with Addison's disease were found to have another autoimmune condition.**[12]

7. AI has been described as "the unforgiving master of nonspecificity and disguise" because of its multitude of possible clinical presentations.[13]

II. PATHOPHYSIOLOGY AND ETIOLOGY

1. The HPA axis is integral to a diverse range of body functions and is crucial for maintaining homeostasis.

2. Destruction of adrenal cortical tissue results in primary AI, which becomes clinically apparent when more than 90% of glandular function is lost.[14] In autoimmune adrenalitis, this destruction is caused by cytotoxic lymphocytes, which generally spare the adrenal medulla.[2]

3. The principal hormone of the HPA axis, cortisol, is produced in a circadian and highly regulated fashion. The highest serum concentration occurs between 6 and 8 AM, and nadir occurs around 11 PM. Fig. 26-1 depicts the regulation of cortisol secretion and lists the major effects of cortisol on the body.

4. Only about 10% of circulating cortisol is free and physiologically active. The remaining 90% is bound to cortisol-binding globulin and albumin and thus is affected by changes that alter plasma levels of these proteins, such as estrogen therapy and chronic illness.[3,15] Inadequate cortisol is a source of significant morbidity and mortality, particularly in critically ill patients, and complete absence of cortisol production is lethal.[14]

III. CLINICAL PRESENTATION AND DIAGNOSIS

1. AI may manifest in varying degrees of severity along a broad clinical continuum, ranging from mild constitutional symptoms elicited only with stress to frank hemodynamic collapse. In general, primary AI is more dramatic and more dangerous than secondary AI. Major clinical features of AI are listed in Box 26-2.

2. **Patients taking supraphysiologic dosages of exogenous steroids (prednisone equivalent of 5 to 7.5 mg a day) for more than 3 weeks are at risk for secondary AI.** After steroids are discontinued, ACTH may

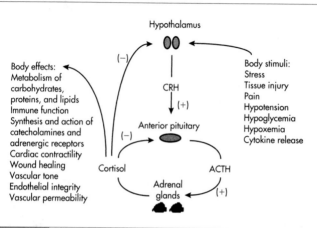

FIG. 26-1

Hypothalamic-pituitary-adrenal axis. Corticotropin-releasing hormone (CRH) and arginine vasopressin are produced by the hypothalamus in response to a variety of stimuli. CRH induces the anterior pituitary to release adrenocorticotropin (ACTH), which triggers cortisol secretion from the adrenal glands. Cortisol exerts a negative feedback effect on the anterior pituitary and hypothalamus, inhibiting release of CRH and ACTH and thereby regulating its own secretion.

take 5 to 8 months to recover, with endogenous steroid production taking up to 1 year to normalize.[6,16]

3. **Definitive diagnosis of suspected AI consists of two steps: ascertaining whether cortisol production is adequate and localizing the culprit anatomic lesion.** The methods are presented in Fig. 26-2.

4. In nonstressed patients, a morning cortisol less than 3 μg/dl is virtually diagnostic of AI, and a value greater than 18 μg/dl rules the diagnosis out. Patients who fall in the middle need some form of dynamic testing. The two gold standard tests are difficult to perform because of fading expertise and possible danger (insulin-induced hypoglycemia) or intermittent drug shortage (metyrapone). Therefore ACTH stimulation testing is used with increasing frequency. It is important to understand that this test relies on the presence of destruction or atrophy of the adrenal cortex. **If secondary AI is new (< 1 month), it is possible for the ACTH stimulation test to give a false negative result.**

5. A high-dose (250 μg) or low-dose (1 μg) ACTH stimulation test may be used to determine adrenal function in patients with morning cortisol levels in the indeterminate range. Cortisol should be drawn at baseline and then at 30 minutes (1 μg) or 30 to 60 minutes (250 μg) after ACTH administration. **The 1-μg test may be more sensitive in the**

BOX 26-2

CLINICAL FEATURES OF ADRENAL INSUFFICIENCY

PRIMARY ADRENAL INSUFFICIENCY

Hyperpigmentation

Hyperkalemia

Vitiligo

Autoimmune thyroid disease

Central nervous system symptoms in adrenomyeloneuropathy (e.g., spastic paralysis)

SECONDARY ADRENAL INSUFFICIENCY

Pallor without significant anemia

Amenorrhea, diminished libido, impotence

Reduced axillary and pubic hair

Small testes

Secondary hypothyroidism

Prepubertal growth deficit, delayed puberty

Headache, visual changes

BOTH PRIMARY AND SECONDARY ADRENAL INSUFFICIENCY

Fatigue, weakness

Depression, apathy, confusion

Anorexia, weight loss

Dizziness, orthostatic hypotension

Nausea, vomiting, diarrhea

Hypoglycemia, hyponatremia*

Mild normocytic anemia, lymphocytosis, eosinophilia

ACUTE ADRENAL CRISIS

Dehydration, hypotension, shock (out of proportion to severity of current illness)

Abdominal pain (mimicking acute abdomen)

Unexplained hypoglycemia

Unexplained fever

Electrolyte derangements

From Oelkers W: *N Engl J Med* 335:1206, 1996; and Zaloga GP, Marik P: *Crit Care Clin* 17:25, 2001.

*Hyponatremia in primary adrenal insufficiency is a consequence of aldosterone deficiency and resultant sodium wasting; in secondary adrenal insufficiency it is a consequence of cortisol deficiency, vasopressin release, and water retention.[11]

diagnosis of secondary AI,[6] but the second cortisol level must be drawn at 30 minutes to avoid false-positive test results[17] (Fig. 26-3). Normal response is considered a cortisol peak greater than 20 µg/dl (high-dose test) or above 18.1 µg/dl (low-dose test).

6. Dexamethasone does not cross-react with the cortisol assay. Therefore patients can undergo an ACTH stimulation test while on dexamethasone. However, it is important to note that the pre-ACTH value will be low in patients taking dexamethasone, and it is the

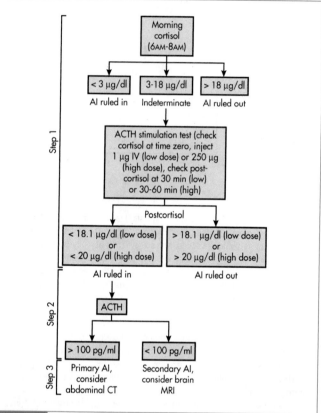

Step 1

Morning cortisol (6AM-8AM)

< 3 µg/dl — AI ruled in

3-18 µg/dl — Indeterminate

> 18 µg/dl — AI ruled out

ACTH stimulation test (check cortisol at time zero, inject 1 µg IV (low dose) or 250 µg (high dose), check post-cortisol at 30 min (low) or 30-60 min (high)

Postcortisol

< 18.1 µg/dl (low dose) or < 20 µg/dl (high dose) — AI ruled in

> 18.1 µg/dl (low dose) or > 20 µg/dl (high dose) — AI ruled out

Step 2

ACTH

Step 3

> 100 pg/ml — Primary AI, consider abdominal CT

< 100 pg/ml — Secondary AI, consider brain MRI

FIG. 26-2

Diagnostic evaluation of adrenal insufficiency (AI). *ACTH*, adrenocorticotropic hormone; *CT*, computed tomography; *IV*, intravenously; *MRI*, magnetic resonance imaging.

26

ADRENAL INSUFFICIENCY

    stimulated value that must be interpreted because dexamethasone will still suppress endogenous cortisol production.

7. **After AI is diagnosed, the physician must determine its cause. If AI is primary, ACTH is frankly elevated (more than 100 pg/ml).** Low or inappropriately normal plasma ACTH indicates secondary AI. Brain magnetic resonance imaging (secondary AI) or abdominal computed tomography (primary AI) may be indicated.

8. **AI has been a topic of debate in the ICU setting.**

a. A recent randomized controlled study of 300 patients with septic shock found that patients with relative AI (defined as failure to increase

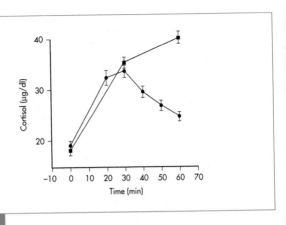

FIG. 26-3

Low- and high-dose cosyntropin stimulation tests. Plasma cortisol levels before and after high-dose (*squares*, 250 μg) and low-dose (*circles*, 0.5 μg/m^2) cosyntropin stimulation tests. In the low-dose test, cortisol level falls abruptly 30 minutes after cosyntropin administration, illustrating the need to measure the stimulated value at exactly 30 minutes. The stimulated cortisol value can be measured at 30 or 60 minutes when the high-dose regimen is used. (*Data from Mayenknecht J et al: J Clin Endocrinol Metab 83:1558, 1998.*)

cortisol level 9 μg/dl after injection of 250 μg cosyntropin) had significantly lower mortality than controls when treated with hydrocortisone 50 mg intravenously (IV) every 6 hours and 50 μg fludrocortisone orally each day for 7 days without an increase in complication rate.[18]

b. A meta-analysis of 13 randomized controlled studies suggested that lower-dose steroids (200 to 300 mg of hydrocortisone equivalent per day) may have some benefit in septic shock, but higher dosages are detrimental.[19] However, the benefits seen with lower dosages of steroids in this study were seen regardless of whether the patient was adrenal insufficient, suggesting that steroids were helpful for reasons other than AI.

c. Most importantly, it has recently been demonstrated that free serum cortisol often is normal in patients in the ICU who have low total serum cortisol, probably because of a reduction of binding proteins.[3]

9. **AI is much more common in HIV-positive patients than in the general population.** Prevalence estimates have ranged from 5% to 20%.[20-22] This is particularly the case for patients who have disseminated opportunistic infections, such as *Mycobacterium avium-intracellulare* infection, tuberculosis, histoplasmosis, or cytomegalovirus infection, and appear to be responding inadequately to standard therapies.[23]

10. Isolated hypoaldosteronism can mimic the electrolyte and volume abnormalities of primary AI, yet cortisol secretion is unaffected.

IV. MANAGEMENT
A. MANAGEMENT OF SYMPTOMATIC CHRONIC AI

1. Glucocorticoid replacement is indicated for all patients with AI. **The goal is to use the smallest dosage needed to relieve symptoms yet avoid steroid-related complications** (e.g., weight gain and osteoporosis). Hydrocortisone 10 to 15 mg per os (PO) every morning and 2.5 to 5 mg PO every evening typically is adequate. Table 2 in Part III, Comparative Pharmacology and Dosing Tables, lists alternative glucocorticoid preparations.

2. **Mineralocorticoid replacement (fludrocortisone 50 to 200 μg PO daily) should be included for patients with primary AI only.** Salt and fluid intake should be encouraged, and blood pressure, serum potassium level, and plasma renin level should be followed. Plasma renin should be maintained in the upper-normal range.

3. Androgen replacement in women (dehydroepiandrosterone 25 to 50 mg PO daily) may be necessary to reduce malaise and sexual dysfunction.

4. If a febrile illness or injury occurs in a patient being treated for AI, the glucocorticoid dosage should be increased by two to three times during the event. If the patient is also being treated with mineralocorticoids or androgens, the dosages of these agents should be maintained and not increased.

5. **Suggested supplementation for surgical procedures** (supplement on call to operating room and continue postoperatively with intermittent or continuous IV dose).

a. For most radiographic studies and minor procedures under local anesthesia, no supplementation is necessary.

b. For minor operations such as herniorrhaphy, administer hydrocortisone 25 mg IV with the induction of anesthesia, then resume usual oral doses.

c. For moderate surgeries such as cholecystectomy or joint replacement, hydrocortisone 50 to 75 mg IV per day (in three divided doses) should be given on call to the operating room and continued for 1 to 2 days postoperatively.

d. For major procedures such as coronary bypass, hydrocortisone 100 to 150 mg IV per day (in three divided doses) for 2 to 3 days should be given. Taper as stress resolves.

6. Emergency precautions.

a. Supplementary ampules of glucocorticoid for self-injection (e.g., hydrocortisone 100 mg or dexamethasone 4 mg intramuscularly) in case of vomiting should be given to all patients.

b. All patients should wear a Medic-Alert or similar warning bracelet.

7. In patients with both hypothyroidism and hypoadrenalism, cortisol should be replaced first because thyroid hormone can accelerate cortisol catabolism and precipitate adrenal crisis.

ADRENAL INSUFFICIENCY 26

B. EMERGENCY MANAGEMENT OF ACUTE AI (ADRENAL CRISIS)

1. Establish large-bore intravenous access.
2. Order and send for immediate assessment a basic metabolic panel and routine plasma cortisol and ACTH levels. Continue therapy while laboratory work is being processed.
3. Infuse 2 to 3 L of 5% dextrose in normal saline as rapidly as can be safely administered.
4. Administer hydrocortisone 50 mg every 8 hours IV. Alternatively, give one dose of dexamethasone 4 mg IV, perform ACTH stimulation test, then switch to hydrocortisone 50 mg every 8 hours IV.
5. Taper steroids as rapidly as conditions permit.
6. Identify and treat triggers.

PEARLS AND PITFALLS

- Drugs such as ketoconazole can interfere with steroid synthesis and cause primary AI. Fluconazole, a more commonly used antifungal, does not have the same side effect.[24]
- Patients on steroids for longer than 3 weeks at dosages of prednisone equivalent 5 to 7.5 mg/day are at risk for secondary AI. It can take up to a year for the adrenal axis to recover after long exogenous steroid use.
- ACTH stimulation tests may be performed on patients being treated with dexamethasone, but the prestimulation cortisol is not interpretable. The stimulated value must be drawn at 30 minutes if the low-dose ($1\ \mu g$) test is used.
- In patients with both hypothyroidism and hypoadrenalism, steroids should be replaced first.

REFERENCES

1. Kasperlik-Zaluska AA et al: Association of Addison's disease with autoimmune disorders: a long-term observation of 180 patients, *Postgrad Med J* 67:984, 1991. A
2. Oelkers W: Adrenal insufficiency, *N Engl J Med* 335:1206, 1996. B
3. Hamrahian AH, Oseni TS, Arafah BM: Measurements of serum free cortisol in critically ill patients, *N Engl J Med* 350(16):1629, 2004. A
4. Addison T: *On the constitutional and local effects of diseases of the supra-renal capsules,* London, 1855, Samuel Highley. B
5. Sonino N: The use of ketoconazole as an inhibitor of steroid production, *N Engl J Med* 317(13):812, 1997. C
6. Cooper MS, Stewart PM: Corticosteroid insufficiency in acutely ill patients, *N Engl J Med* 2003; 348(8):727, 2003. C
7. Kong MF, Jeffcoate W: Eighty-six cases of Addison's disease, *Clin Endocrinol (Oxf)* 41:757, 1994. B
8. Willis AC, Vince FP: The prevalence of Addison's disease in Coventry, UK, *Postgrad Med J* 73:286, 1997. B
9. Oelkers W, Diederich S, Bahr V: [Diagnosis of adrenal cortex insufficiency], *Dtsch Med Wochenschr* 119:555, 1994. C
10. Ahonen P et al: Clinical variation of autoimmune polyendocrinopathy-candidiasis-ectodermal dystrophy (APECED) in a series of 68 patients, *N Engl J Med* 322:1829, 1990. B

11. Betterle C et al: Type 2 polyglandular autoimmune disease (Schmidt's syndrome), *J Pediatr Endocrinol Metab* 9(suppl 1):113, 1996. B
12. Zelissen PM, Bast EJ, Croughs RJ: Associated autoimmunity in Addison's disease, *J Autoimmun* 8:121, 1995. B
13. Brosnan CM, Gowing NF: Addison's disease, *BMJ* 312:1085, 1996. B
14. Zaloga GP, Marik P: Hypothalamic-pituitary-adrenal insufficiency, *Crit Care Clin* 17:25, 2001. B
15. Grinspoon SK, Biller BM: Clinical review 62: laboratory assessment of adrenal insufficiency, *J Clin Endocrinol Metab* 79:923, 1994. A
16. Graber AL et al: Natural history of pituitary-adrenal recovery following long-term suppression with corticosteroids, *J Clin Endocrinol Metab* 25:11, 1965. B
17. Mayenknecht J et al: Comparison of low and high dose corticotrophin stimulation tests in patients with pituitary disease, *J Clin Endocrinol Metab* 83:1558, 1998. B
18. Annane D et al: Effect of treatment with low doses of hydrocortisone and fludrocortisone on mortality in patients with septic shock, *JAMA* 288:862, 2002. A
19. Minneci PC et al: Meta-analysis: the effect of steroids on survival and shock during sepsis depends on the dose, *Ann Intern Med* 141:47, 2004. C
20. Dobs AS et al: Endocrine disorders in men infected with human immunodeficiency virus, *Am J Med* 84:611, 1988. B
21. Findling JW et al: Longitudinal evaluation of adrenocortical function in patients infected with the human immunodeficiency virus, *J Clin Endocrinol Metab* 79:1091, 1994. A
22. Raffi F et al: Endocrine function in 98 HIV-infected patients: a prospective study, *AIDS* 5:729, 1991. A
23. Eledrisi MS, Verghese AC: Adrenal insufficiency in HIV infection: a review and recommendations, *Am J Med Sci* 321:137, 2001. B
24. Magill SS et al: Impact of fluconazole prophylaxis on cortisol levels in critically ill surgical patients, *Antimicrob Agents Chemother* 48(7):2471, 2004. B

26

ADRENAL INSUFFICIENCY

Diabetic Ketoacidosis and Hyperosmolar Hyperglycemic State

Rita Rastogi, MD; Gregory O. Clark, MD;
and Christopher D. Saudek, MD

FAST FACTS

- Diabetic ketoacidosis (DKA) is defined by the triad of hyperglycemia (> 250 mg/dl), acidemia (arterial pH 7.3 or less; serum bicarbonate 18 mEq/L or less), and ketonemia.
- Hyperosmolar hyperglycemic state (HHS) consists of severe hyperglycemia (> 600 mg/dl); hyperosmolarity (330 mOsm/kg or more); and, when osmolarity is greater than approximately 340 mOsm/kg, altered mental status.
- Mortality rates are 2% to 14% for DKA and approximately 10% to 50% for HHS.
- Infection is the most common precipitant of DKA and HHS. Nonadherence to insulin therapy is the most common precipitant of DKA and HHS in urban African Americans.[1]
- Volume depletion is the rate-limiting step in the development of HHS. Severe hyperglycemia develops when fluid intake fails to compensate for fluids lost through osmotic diuresis.
- Treatment of DKA and HHS includes administration of intravenous (IV) fluid to correct dehydration and hyperosmolarity, administration of insulin to reverse hyperglycemia and ketoacidosis (in DKA), correction of electrolyte abnormalities, identification of precipitants, and frequent patient monitoring. Complications of treatment include hypoglycemia; hypokalemia; and, rarely, cerebral edema.
- The diagnosis and treatment of DKA and HHS outlined in this chapter are based on American Diabetes Association recommendations.[2]

Diabetic Ketoacidosis

I. CLINICAL PRESENTATION

1. **Symptoms.** Acute hyperglycemia is accompanied by polyuria, polydipsia, weight loss, dehydration, weakness, and fatigue. Patients with acidosis complain of nausea, vomiting, "air hunger," abdominal pain, and fatigue. The neurologic manifestations include stupor, coma, and seizures (although these are more common in HHS).

2. **Physical examination** reveals evidence of dehydration, including poor skin turgor, dry mucous membranes, absence of axillary sweat, tachycardia, and orthostatic hypotension. Signs of ketoacidosis include Kussmaul respirations (rapid and deep breathing as respiratory compensation for metabolic acidosis), fruity breath odor (an indication of ketonemia), emesis and abdominal guarding (common), and guaiac-positive stools resulting from hemorrhagic gastritis. **Altered mental status should be noted because it identifies those at highest risk for a bad outcome.**

II. DIAGNOSIS

1. DKA is defined by the triad of hyperglycemia (blood glucose > 250 mg/dl), ketonemia or ketonuria, and acidemia (pH $\leq$ 7.3; serum bicarbonate $\leq$ 18 mEq/L). It usually occurs in patients with type 1 diabetes mellitus but can occur in those with type 2 diabetes. DKA usually develops rapidly, often in less than 24 hours.
2. Perform a thorough physical examination looking for evidence of an underlying precipitant (e.g., cellulitis, pancreatitis, apprendicitis, heart failure) (Box 27-1).
a. **An arterial blood gas** (ABG) must be drawn to assess acidosis and respiratory compensation. At the same time, obtain a venous blood gas (VBG), and assess how it correlates with the ABG. From there on, only VBGs are needed to follow the serum pH and CO_2 levels.
b. **Serum and urine ketones** should be quantified to identify ketosis as cause of acidosis.
c. **Further laboratory analysis should include complete serum chemistries, including transaminases, amylase, lipase, cardiac enzymes, lactate, serum volatile screen, plasma osmolality, and toxicology screen.**
d. **Complete blood cell count with differential.** The white blood cell count often is markedly elevated, even in the absence of infection, and is proportional to the degree of ketonemia.
e. **Urinalysis** should be completed, particularly to rule out urinary tract infection. Note that the presence of urine ketones is not diagnostic of DKA because they may occur without acidosis in normal fasting. Also, captopril and other sulfhydryl drugs can cause a false positive ketone test with the nitroprusside reagent.
f. Cultures of blood, urine, or sputum should be obtained.
g. Amylase (and less often lipase) levels may be elevated by nonpancreatic sources. Transaminitis may be observed in DKA and resolves with treatment.
h. Chest radiography should be performed if clinically indicated. An electrocardiogram should be evaluated for evidence of ischemia and electrolyte abnormalities. Calculate the corrected serum sodium level.
3. **Serum sodium** levels normally are low in the presence of hyperglycemia because the osmolar load of extracellular glucose causes a shift of free

> **BOX 27-1**
>
> **COMMON PRECIPITANTS OF DIABETIC KETOACIDOSIS[5]**
>
> | | |
> |---|---|
> | New-onset diabetes | Sympathomimetic agents |
> | Pregnancy | Phenytoin |
> | Infection | Estrogens |
> | Inadequate insulin delivery | Nicotinic acid |
> | Nonadherence to therapy | Danazol |
> | Insulin pump failure | Diazoxide |
> | Surgery | Growth hormone |
> | Critical illness | Pentamidine |
> | Trauma | Gatifloxacin |
> | Myocardial infarction | Tacrolimus |
> | Stroke | Indomethacin |
> | Pancreatitis | Thyroid hormone |
> | Medications | Chlorpromazine |
> | Corticosteroids | Salicylates |
> | High-dose thiazides | |

water out of the cells. The "corrected" serum sodium is calculated by adding 1.6 mEq/L to the measured Na^+ for each 100 mg/dl glucose above 100 mg/dl. **An elevated "corrected" serum sodium reflects the severity of dehydration.**

4. Serum potassium is shifted extracellularly by acidosis, passive diffusion with water, and insulin deficiency itself. Hyperkalemia may exist despite total body potassium depletion. Conversely, insulin administration shifts potassium into cells, causing a predictable drop in serum potassium and significant risk of hypokalemia.

5. The anion gap and serum osmolality should be calculated to assess acid-base status and hydration; the anion gap is calculated as $Na^+ - (Cl^- + HCO_3^-)$ (mEq/L). (Do not use the calculated serum sodium values. Calculate the anion gap using the values on the serum chemistry panel.) As a "rule of thumb," a normal anion gap in a particular patient is the serum albumin level multiplied by 3 (serum albumin × 3). See Chapter 71 for further discussion.

   a. Nongap metabolic acidosis (secondary to urinary loss of ketoacids, which serve as precursors to bicarbonate generation) is common on presentation in DKA in patients with intact renal function and often is the major acid-base abnormality after ketosis has resolved.

   b. Other tests (e.g., blood lactate concentration and drug concentration levels) can help distinguish DKA from other causes of high–anion gap metabolic acidosis including lactic acidosis, chronic renal failure, and ingestion of ethanol, salicylates, methanol, and ethylene glycol.

6. **Calculated osmolality** should be compared with measured osmolality to exclude the presence of unmeasured osmoles such as ethanol or

methanol. Serum osmolality = 2[Na$^+$ (mEq/L)] + [Glucose (mg/dl)/18] + [Blood urea nitrogen (mg/dl)/2.8]. Because urea is freely permeable across cell walls and may not contribute to effective serum osmolarity, some authorities omit it from the calculation. Note that serum osmolarity is affected predominantly by serum sodium concentration. If serum sodium is appropriately diluted in hyperglycemia, the effective osmolarity is normalized; however, a high serum sodium in the setting of hyperglycemia indicates severe dehydration and hyperosmolarity.

7. **During therapy:**
a. **Blood glucose should be checked hourly while IV insulin is titrated.**
b. **Electrolytes, blood urea nitrogen, and creatinine should be checked every 2 to 4 hours until stable, with special attention to serum potassium.**
c. **Acidosis should be monitored by venous pH measurement every 2 hours.**
8. Monitoring serum ketones can be misleading during DKA treatment because correction of acidosis shifts redox equilibrium from beta-hydroxy butyrate toward acetoacetate. Because the latter is measured by most bedside assessments, ketonemia may appear to increase as total ketosis actually decreases.

III. RISK STRATIFICATION AND PROGNOSIS

Depending on the severity of the disease, the patient can be monitored and treated in the emergency department, but patients often have to be admitted to the general medicine floor or intensive care unit. Table 27-1 **outlines a method for risk stratifying patients.**

IV. MANAGEMENT

A. FLUID MANAGEMENT

1. Fluid deficits average 6 L in DKA.
2. The corrected serum sodium should be determined upon admission. The management of DKA should begin with fluid resuscitation, regardless of the degree of hyperosmolarity.
3. Give 1 L or 15 to 20 ml/kg of normal saline (0.9% NaCl) over 1 hour to restore intravascular volume and renal perfusion. Continue normal saline at this rate until blood pressure and organ perfusion are restored (as evidenced by urine output and physical examination).
4. More conservative rehydration may be necessary in the presence of cardiac or renal compromise. Additionally, fluid deficits should be replaced at a slower rate (i.e., over 48 hours) in patients younger than 20 years because of the increased risk of cerebral edema.
5. If the corrected serum sodium level is normal to high (indicating more severe dehydration), switch to half normal saline (0.45% NaCl) at a rate of 4 to 14 ml/kg/hr after initial fluid resuscitation is achieved.

27

DKA AND HYPEROSMOLAR HYPERGLYCEMIC STATE

TABLE 27-1

RISK STRATIFICATION OF PATIENTS WITH DKA

Severity	Plasma Glucose (mg/dl)	Arterial pH	Serum Bicarbonate (mEq/L)	Anion Gap (mEq/L)
Mild	> 250	7.25-7.3	15-18	> 10
Moderate	> 250	7-7.24	10-14	> 12
Severe	> 250	< 7	< 10	> 12

If the corrected serum sodium is low (indicating more normal serum osmolarity), continue normal saline at a rate of 4 to 14 ml/kg/hr.

6. Change the IV fluid to 5% dextrose with 0.45% NaCl when the serum glucose concentration falls below 250 mg/dl (or 300 mg/dl in HHS) to maintain the glucose level between 150 and 200 mg/dl (or 250-300 mg/dl in HHS) until DKA resolves.

7. **Cerebral edema.** Serum osmolality should not decrease more than 3 mOsm/kg/hr. If cerebral edema does develop, mannitol has been shown to have beneficial effects in some case reports and should be given 0.25 to 1.0 g/kg over 20 minutes. Mannitol infusion can be repeated in 2 hours if necessary. Alternatively, the clinician can use hypertonic saline (3%) at 5 to 10 ml/kg over 30 minutes.[3]

B. INSULIN ADMINISTRATION

1. **Check the serum potassium before administering insulin. Hypokalemia (K^+ < 3.3 mEq/L) should be corrected before IV insulin administration.**

2. **Administer regular insulin 0.15 U/kg as an IV bolus (about 10 U on average).** Although there are no compelling data to support this step in management, an initial insulin bolus is helpful because there is often a delay in initiation of the insulin drip.

3. **Infuse at 0.1 U/kg/hr (about 7 U/hr).**

4. **Check glucose hourly.** Double the insulin infusion hourly until the glucose level falls by about 50 to 100 mg/dl/hr.

5. **When the glucose level reaches 250 mg/dl (or 300 mg/dl in HHS), adjust the insulin infusion to maintain serum glucose between 150 and 200 mg/dl until acidosis has resolved (bicarbonate > 18 mEq/L, venous pH > 7.3, anion gap < 12, and serum osmolality < 315 mOsm/kg in HHS).** Once acidosis has resolved, administer short-acting insulin subcutaneously and continue IV insulin for an additional 1 to 2 hours. Intravenous insulin has a half-life of about 6 minutes, and if it is discontinued before subcutaneous insulin has taken effect, ketoacidosis may recur. Therefore, under no circumstances should the insulin drip be discontinued unless subcutaneous insulin has already been administered. If patient remains on a nothing by mouth status despite resolution of DKA, IV insulin administration may continue. Alternatively,

regular insulin can be administered subcutaneously every 4 hours on the basis of blood glucose levels while the patient is taking nothing by mouth.

6. When DKA has resolved and the patient is able to drink, previous subcutaneous insulin regimens may be resumed. **Patients with newly diagnosed type 1 diabetes may need a total insulin dosage of 0.6 to 0.7 U/kg/day as a multidose regimen of short-acting and longer-acting insulin.** Patients with type 2 diabetes who presented with DKA may respond to oral agents only after resolution of DKA. Dosages should be modified based on subsequent glucose levels.

C. ELECTROLYTE MONITORING AND REPLACEMENT

1. **Potassium.** Serum potassium levels can be low, normal, or high, yet total body deficits average 3 to 5 mEq/kg in DKA. Hypokalemia may cause cardiac arrhythmias that can be fatal in DKA. Keep in mind that serum potassium levels fall during treatment with insulin, bicarbonate, or IV fluid.

a. If K^+ level is less than 3.3 mEq/L, administer 40 mEq K^+ hourly until K^+ level is 3.3 mEq/L or higher before commencing insulin therapy.

b. If K^+ is 3.3 to 5.5 mEq/L, administer 20 to 30 mEq K^+ per liter of IV fluid in anticipation of falling K^+ during treatment. Goal serum K^+ is 4 to 5 mEq/L.

c. If K^+ is 5.5 mEq/L or higher, withhold potassium but monitor K^+ every 2 hours.

d. Appropriate K^+ supplementation dosages may be lower in the presence of renal compromise.

2. **Bicarbonate.** Bicarbonate administration should be considered only in cases of life-threatening acidosis. Its use is controversial even when the pH is 6.9 to 7.1. Studies have been inconclusive in patients with a pH below 6.9, but the American Diabetes Association recommends treatment with sodium bicarbonate as follows.

a. When pH is less than 6.9, 100 mmol $NaHCO_3$ over 2 hours.

b. When pH is 6.9 to 7, 50 mmol $NaHCO_3$ over 1 hour.

c. Repeat every 2 hours until pH is greater than 7.

d. Monitor K^+ (bicarbonate therapy lowers serum K^+).

3. In patients younger than 20 years, bicarbonate should be given only if pH is less than 7 after 1 hour of hydration. Give 1 to 2 mEq/kg in half normal saline over 1 hour.

4. **Phosphate.** DKA depletes total body phosphate, and serum phosphate levels decrease with insulin therapy. Treatment with phosphate may cause hypocalcemia and has not been shown to affect clinical outcome in DKA. In certain circumstances, however, phosphate supplementation is important for preventing cardiac and skeletal muscle weakness. When the serum phosphate level is less than 1 mg/dl or when the patient has cardiac dysfunction, anemia, or respiratory depression, potassium phosphate can be given at 20 to 30 mEq per liter of replacement fluid.[4]

27

DKA AND HYPEROSMOLAR HYPERGLYCEMIC STATE

5. **Magnesium.** Magnesium often is depleted in DKA and can make treatment of hypokalemia difficult if not supplemented in parallel. The goal magnesium level should be greater than 2.0 mg/dl.

Hyperosmolar Hyperglycemic State[2,5]

I. EPIDEMIOLOGY

1. HHS is defined by plasma glucose concentration greater than 600 mg/dl (often to > 1000 mg/dl), total serum osmolality greater than 330 mOsm/kg, and the absence of severe ketoacidosis.
2. Approximately 50% of patients have a high anion gap metabolic acidosis consistent with mild ketonemia or ketonuria, but serum pH usually is greater than 7.3, and serum bicarbonate is greater than 18 mEq/L.
3. HHS usually develops among patients with type 2 diabetes mellitus (insulin resistance) and occurs more often in those older than 65 years.
4. **Although DKA and HHS are distinct clinical entities, in practice they often overlap, with varying degrees of hyperosmolarity and acidosis at the time of presentation.** It is also clear that just as DKA occurs in type 2 diabetes, hyperosmolarity can occur in type 1 diabetes.
5. Common precipitating factors in the development of HHS include impaired thirst (in older adults and after stroke), conditions that can cause dehydration (dialysis, excessive diuresis, burns), infection, surgery, pregnancy, critical illness, and medications (similar to those shown in Box 27-1).

II. CLINICAL PRESENTATION

1. The clinical presentation of HHS is similar to that of DKA except that the signs and symptoms of severe acidosis are not present, and neurologic manifestations can be more severe because hyperosmolarity is present to a greater degree. Mental obtundation and coma are more common, but by no means are they universal findings. Focal neurologic deficits, such as hemiparesis, hemianopsia, and seizures occasionally are the predominant symptoms at presentation in HHS.
2. **The commonly used term "hyperosmolar nonketotic coma" is misleading because mild ketosis can exist and coma is unusual. HHS develops more slowly than DKA, with polyuria, polydipsia, and weight loss often preceding admission by several days.**

III. DIAGNOSIS

1. The diagnosis of HHS is similar to that of DKA. Laboratory examination usually reveals the following:
a. Plasma glucose greater than 600 mg/dl.
b. Serum osmolality greater than 330 mOsm/kg, with high corrected serum sodium (not appropriately diluted for hyperglycemia).
c. Arterial pH greater than 7.3 and serum bicarbonate greater than 18 mEq/L.

d. Possible mild ketonuria or ketonemia.
2. Sometimes DKA and HHS overlap, and patients develop ketosis, acidosis, and hyperosmolality.

IV. RISK STRATIFICATION AND PROGNOSIS

Mortality rates in HHS are much higher than in DKA and have been reported to range from 10% to 50%. The severity of mental status changes is related to the degree of hyperosmolarity. Stupor and coma typically are present when osmolality is greater than 350 mOsm/kg H_2O.[2]

V. MANAGEMENT

1. Fluid deficits average 9 L in HHS.
2. Total body potassium deficits average 4 to 6 mEq/kg in HHS.
3. Fluid, insulin, and electrolyte management are similar to those of DKA. A bolus of 0.9% NaCl should be administered in hypovolemic shock and when the corrected serum sodium is low; 0.45% NaCl should be given when the corrected serum sodium is normal or high.
4. When the glucose level reaches 300 mg/dl, adjust the insulin infusion to maintain the glucose level between 250 and 300 mg/dl until serum osmolality is less than 315 mOsm/kg and mental status is normal.

PEARLS AND PITFALLS

- Administer bicarbonate only when serum pH is less than 7.0 in DKA.
- Hypoglycemia can complicate aggressive treatment of DKA and HHS. Add dextrose 5% to rehydration fluid as plasma glucose improves to about 250 mg/dl in DKA and about 300 mg/dl in HHS. Adjust insulin administration to maintain mild hyperglycemia until DKA or HHS has resolved.
- Hyperglycemia and ketoacidosis can recur if intravenous administration of insulin is stopped before subcutaneous administration is started. Give regular insulin subcutaneously for 1 to 2 hours before stopping IV insulin administration.
- Cerebral edema is rare but often fatal and occurs during treatment of both DKA and HHS, most commonly in children. It may be prevented by avoidance of early and excessive use of hypotonic saline and a gradual resolution of serum hyperosmolarity. Mental status should be monitored frequently because cerebral edema may develop rapidly. Diagnosis is confirmed by computed tomography scan of the brain.
- Patients should be advised before hospital discharge never to discontinue insulin therapy unless told by a physician.

REFERENCES

1. Umpierrez GE et al: Hyperglycemic crises in urban blacks, *Arch Intern Med* 157(6):669, 1997. B
2. American Diabetes Association: Hyperglycemic crises in diabetes, *Diabetes Care* 27(Suppl 1):S94-S102, 2004.

27

DKA AND HYPEROSMOLAR HYPERGLYCEMIC STATE

3. Dunger DB et al: ESPE/LWPES consensus statement on diabetic ketoacidosis in children and adolescents, *Arch Dis Child* 89:188, 2004. D
4. Fisher JN, Kitabchi AE: A randomized study of phosphate therapy in the treatment of diabetic ketoacidosis, *J Clin Endocrinol Metab* 57(1):177, 1983. A
5. Ennis ED, Stahl EJ, Kreisberg RA: The hyperosmolar hyperglycemic syndrome, *Diabetes Rev* 2:115, 1994. C

Thyroid Disorders

Amin Sabet, MD; Gail V. Berkenblit, MD, PhD; and Matthew Kim, MD

28

Hypothyroidism

I. EPIDEMIOLOGY

1. Thyroid disease is more common among women, older adults, patients with autoimmune disorders, and patients with a strong family history of thyroid dysfunction.
2. Hypothyroidism may be detected in 5% to 8% of randomly screened populations.
3. Primary hypothyroidism, caused by failure of the gland itself, accounts for 99% of all cases of hypothyroidism. Secondary or central hypothyroidism, caused by failure of the hypothalamus or pituitary gland, accounts for less than 1% of all cases of hypothyroidism. Specific causes of hypothyroidism are listed in Table 28-2.

TABLE 28-1

AMIODARONE-INDUCED THYROID DYSFUNCTION

	Hypothyroidism	Type I Thyrotoxicosis	Type II Thyrotoxicosis
Incidence	Up to 25% in iodine-sufficient regions[2]	Develops in 2% to 23% of patients treated with amiodarone[1-3]	May coexist with type I
	Patients with preexisting autoimmune thyroid conditions at higher risk	Commonly seen in iodine-deficient regions, particularly in patients with preexisting nodular goiter	
Mechanism	Decreased peripheral conversion of thyroxine to triiodothyronine	Excessive thyroid hormone synthesis and release in response to iodine load (the Jod-Basedow phenomenon)	Drug-induced destructive thyroiditis with release of stored hormone
	Decreased thyroid hormone secretion in the setting of iodine excess (Wolff-Chaikoff effect)		
Diagnosis			
Thyroid antibodies	Often present	Often present	Generally absent
Iodine-123 uptake values	Usually low in iodine-sufficient regions	Low in iodine-sufficient regions	Low
Color Doppler ultrasonography	Variable findings	May reveal hypervascularity[4]	Reduced blood flow[4]
Therapy	Thyroid hormone replacement	High dosages of methimazole or propylthiouracil	Corticosteroids, iopanoic acid
		Possibly potassium perchlorate to block further iodine uptake	

Modified from Pierce et al: *N Engl J Med* 348:2646, 2003.

TABLE 28-2

CAUSES OF HYPOTHYROIDISM

Cause	Mechanism	Thyroid Examination
Hashimoto's disease	Autoimmune destruction	Firm, bosselated gland with pyramidal lobe
Ablation or resection	Removal of functioning thyroid tissue	Atrophic or cervical scar
Central hypothyroidism	Pituitary or hypothalamic failure	Atrophic
Iodine deficiency	Low substrate for iodination	Goiter
Lithium	Decreased thyroid hormone synthesis	Goiter
Amiodarone	Wolff-Chaikoff effect thyroiditis	Goiter or normal
Peripheral resistance	Rare genetic defect in triiodothyronine nuclear receptor	Normal

4. The three most common underlying causes of primary hypothyroidism in the United States are autoimmune thyroiditis (also known as Hashimoto's thyroiditis); postablative hypothyroidism, which develops after radioactive iodine treatment for hyperthyroidism; and postsurgical hypothyroidism, which develops after resection of a critical mass of thyroid tissue.

II. CLINICAL PRESENTATION

1. Symptoms associated with hypothyroidism may include fatigue, weight gain, cold intolerance, hoarseness, constipation, dry skin, arthralgias, and myalgias.

2. Physical findings may include bradycardia, cool dry skin, brittle hair and nails, macroglossia, and delayed terminal relaxation of deep tendon reflexes.

3. Triiodothyronine (T_3) increases cardiac inotropy and chronotropy while decreasing peripheral vascular tone. A relative deficiency of T_3 may explain the high systemic vascular resistance that characterizes hypothyroid heart failure.[1] Pericardial effusions and ascites may complicate congestive heart failure.

4. Laboratory tests may reveal evidence of hyponatremia, macrocytic anemia, elevated creatine phosphokinase levels, elevated prolactin levels, and abnormal liver function test results. In the Colorado Thyroid Disease Prevalence Study, cholesterol levels were observed to rise in direct proportion to TSH levels in subjects with detectable hypothyroidism.[5]

5. Severe hypothyroidism may culminate in myxedema coma, a condition characterized by hypothermia, hypotension, bradycardia, and altered mental status. Risk factors for the development of myxedema coma may include old age, poor access to health care, and long-standing

thyroid dysfunction. Acute cases have been reported to occur after thyroid resection.

6. Autoimmune thyroiditis may be associated with other autoimmune disorders including pernicious anemia, myasthenia gravis, and vitiligo.

7. **Polyglandular autoimmune syndrome type II** (also known as Schmidt's syndrome) is an endocrinopathy characterized by autoimmune thyroiditis and autoimmune adrenalitis.

a. Hypoparathyroidism, type 1 diabetes mellitus, and primary ovarian failure may also be seen.

b. Schmidt's syndrome should always be considered in patients presenting with primary hypothyroidism associated with weight loss or salt cravings.

c. Pretreatment with glucocorticoids may be crucial in this setting, as levothyroxine replacement may increase cortisol metabolism and precipitate an adrenal crisis.

III. DIAGNOSIS

A. NONTHYROIDAL ILLNESS

1. When thyroid function tests are checked in the setting of severe nonthyroidal illness, secondary changes in TSH and thyroid hormone levels that reflect the impact of illness itself may yield results that appear to be consistent with primary thyroid dysfunction.[6] Fig. 28-1 depicts the thyroid hormone changes observed in nonthyroidal illness.

2. A study of 1580 patients in a large urban hospital demonstrated the extent to which thyroid function tests may be disrupted by the effects of nonthyroidal illness.[7,8] Abnormal TSH levels were observed in 17% of tested patients. Among these patients, only 24% with measured TSH levels less than 0.1 mIU/ml had underlying hyperthyroidism or thyrotoxicosis, and only 14% with measured TSH levels greater than 7 mIU/ml had underlying primary hypothyroidism.

3. Given these findings, clinical correlation is important when thyroid function tests are checked in severely ill patients. The presence of a goiter, history of pituitary disease, history of radioactive iodine treatment, or findings consistent with prior thyroid surgery may help to establish a correct diagnosis. For patients without any findings consistent with underlying thyroid dysfunction, retesting 6 to 8 weeks after recovery may be recommended.

B. HYPOTHYROIDISM

1. **A suspected diagnosis of primary hypothyroidism may be confirmed when thyroid function tests reveal an elevated TSH level in conjunction with a low T_4 level** (Table 28-3). T_4 exhibits a log-linear relationship with TSH, such that twofold changes in T_4 levels result in fiftyfold changes in TSH levels.

2. According to current guidelines, a screening TSH level should be checked in all women older than 60 years and in any patient presenting with dementia, an elevated cholesterol level, an autoimmune disorder, or a strong family history of thyroid dysfunction.[9,10] Periodic

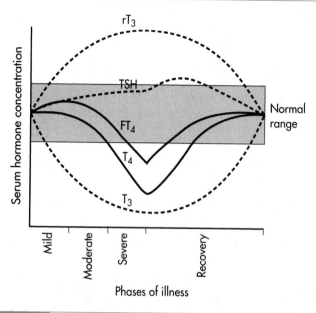

FIG. 28-1

Thyroid hormone levels and severity of nonthyroidal illness. Thyroid hormone levels change with course and severity of nonthyroidal illness. *FT₄,* free thyroxine; *rT₃,* reverse triiodothyronine; *T₃,* triiodothyronine; *T₄,* thyroxine; *TSH,* thyroid-stimulating hormone. *(From Moore WT, Eastman R: Diagnostic endocrinology, 2nd ed, St Louis, 1996, Mosby.)*

28

THYROID DISORDERS

TABLE 28-3

DIAGNOSTIC TESTS IN THYROID DISEASE

Diagnosis	Thyroid-Stimulating Hormone	Free Thyroxine
HYPOTHYROIDISM		
Overt	High	Low
Subclinical	High	Normal
Euthyroid	Normal	Normal
HYPERTHYROIDISM		
Subclinical	Low	Normal
Overt	Low	High

Normal values for thyroid-stimulating hormone are 0.5 to 5 mIU/L. Normal values for free thyroxine are 0.9 to 1.9 ng/dl.

screening of patients taking lithium or amiodarone also is recommended.

3. Total T_4 levels may be affected by changes in binding protein levels and affinities. Free T_4 assays, which measure the unbound fraction of thyroxine present in the bloodstream, may provide a more direct assessment of thyroid function. The T_3 resin uptake and derived free thyroxine index tests have been largely supplanted by free T_4 assays.

4. Secondary or central hypothyroidism, caused by failure of the hypothalamus or pituitary gland, is characterized by a reproducibly low free T_4 level. TSH measurement is considered unreliable in this setting because normal levels may not always reflect an adequate level of function.

5. Detection of antithyroid antibodies may support a suspected diagnosis of underlying autoimmune thyroiditis. Antithyroid peroxidase antibodies (also known as antimicrosomal antibodies) are more likely than antithyroglobulin antibodies to be positive in cases of autoimmune thyroiditis. Elevated antithyroid antibody titers may be associated with a greater likelihood of progression to overt hypothyroidism in the setting of subclinical hypothyroidism, characterized by elevated TSH levels with a normal total or free T_4 level.

IV. MANAGEMENT

1. Despite findings indicating that low T_4 levels correlate with an adverse prognosis in hospitalized patients and that low T_3 levels are a strong independent predictor of death in cardiac patients,[11] no studies to date have been able to demonstrate a mortality benefit from thyroid hormone supplementation in the setting of nonthyroidal illness.

2. The usual daily replacement dosage of levothyroxine for most adult patients may be estimated as 1.7 μg/kg lean body weight. Older adults may need only 1 μg/kg lean body weight because of decreased thyroid hormone clearance. **Levothyroxine may be started at a full replacement dosage in patients younger than age 50 without evidence of heart disease.** For patients with known or suspected heart disease, treatment should be started at a dosage of 12.5 to 25 μg daily and increased gradually by 12.5 to 25 μg increments at 4-week intervals on the basis of TSH levels.

3. In cases of myxedema coma, treatment should begin with intravenous administration of levothyroxine (500-μg bolus followed by 1.5 to 2 μg/kg/day) alone or with T_3 (10 μg IV every 8 hours). Supportive measures and treatment of comorbid conditions are crucial. Glucocorticoids should be administered in stress doses after a cosyntropin stimulation test has been performed to check for evidence of concomitant adrenal insufficiency.

4. **Whether patients with subclinical hypothyroidism should be treated remains controversial.**[12,13] Many experts advocate treating patients with potentially referable symptoms or significant hypercholesterolemia.

Thyrotoxicosis

I. DEFINITIONS AND EPIDEMIOLOGY

1. Thyrotoxicosis is a clinical syndrome characterized by exposure to excessive amounts of thyroid hormone. Hyperthyroidism is more narrowly defined as thyrotoxicosis caused by the excessive production and secretion of endogenous thyroid hormone by functional thyroid tissue. Specific causes of thyrotoxicosis and hyperthyroidism are listed in Table 28-4.

2. Hyperthyroidism may be detected in 2% of women and 0.2% of men. **The most common underlying causes of hyperthyroidism are Graves disease, toxic adenoma, and toxic multinodular goiter.**

3. Graves disease may present at any age, with a peak incidence in the third and fourth decades of life. A strong family history of thyroid dysfunction is typical.

4. Toxic adenomas may present at any age, although they tend to be more common in younger individuals. Toxic multinodular goiters typically present in older adults with histories of nodular thyroid disease.

5. Nonhyperthyroid disorders that may present with evidence of thyrotoxicosis include iatrogenic thyrotoxicosis, subacute thyroiditis, silent thyroiditis, and thyrotoxicosis factitia.

28

THYROID DISORDERS

TABLE 28-4
CAUSES OF THYROTOXICOSIS

Cause	Mechanism	Thyroid Examination
Graves disease	Stimulatory anti–TSH receptor antibodies	Diffuse goiter
Toxic multinodular goiter	Activating mutations of TSH receptor or Gs-α gene	Nodules
Subacute thyroiditis	Destruction that releases stored hormone	Minimal goiter
de Quervain's	Postviral	Tender
Painless	Autoimmune	Nontender
Computed tomography dye or amiodarone	Iodine surplus (Jod-Basedow) or toxic thyroiditis	Nodular or diffuse goiter or normal
Hydatiform mole	Human chorionic gonadotropin cross-activation of TSH receptors	Minimal goiter
Pituitary tumor	TSH overproduction	Minimal goiter
Struma ovarii	Ectopic thyroid tissue in ovarian tumor	Normal
Exogenous thyrotoxicosis		Normal
Iatrogenic	Oversupplementation of thyroxine	
Factitious	Surreptitious ingestion of thyroxine	

TSH, thyroid-stimulating hormone.

6. Postpartum thyroiditis is a type of silent thyroiditis that develops 2 to 6 months after delivery. It may occur in 5% of women.

II. CLINICAL PRESENTATION

1. Symptoms associated with thyrotoxicosis include fatigue, heat intolerance, weight loss, palpitations, exercise impairment, hyperdefecation, hair loss, diaphoresis, oligomenorrhea, anxiety, irritability, and tremulousness. Patients with mild to moderate thyroid eye disease (also know as Graves ophthalmopathy) may also complain of excessive redness, watering of the eyes, or irritation with a foreign body sensation. Patients with severe thyroid eye disease may report episodic blurring of vision or diplopia.

2. **Classic symptoms generally decrease with advancing age, making diagnosis more difficult.** Older patients may present with an apathetic form of hyperthyroidism characterized predominantly by marked weight loss and cardiovascular complications including atrial fibrillation and congestive heart failure.[14]

3. **Physical findings may include tachycardia; a widened pulse pressure; a fixed stare; lid lag; warm, moist skin; proximal muscle weakness; a resting tremor; and hyperreflexia.** A palpable goiter may be detected in 95% of patients with hyperthyroidism, although 50% of patients with the apathetic form may not have an enlarged thyroid gland. Hyperthyroidism may be detected in 5% of patients presenting with new-onset atrial fibrillation.[15]

4. Patients with underlying Graves disease may also present with proptosis, periorbital edema, ophthalmoplegia, an audible bruit or palpable thrill over the thyroid gland, or (rarely) clubbing of the terminal phalanges, known as thyroid acropachy. Infiltrative dermopathy, a condition characterized by hyperpigmented nonpitting induration of the skin that often develops in pretibial areas, may be seen in 5% to 10% of patients with underlying Graves disease.

5. Laboratory tests may reveal evidence of hypercalcemia, elevated alkaline phosphatase levels, anemia, and mild granulocytopenia. Low bone mineral density measurements may be noted on dual-energy x-ray absorptiometry scanning.

6. Hyperthyroidism coupled with an increased sensitivity to the effects of thyroid hormone may precipitate a life-threatening condition known as thyroid storm. This clinical syndrome is characterized by a constellation of findings including hyperthermia, delirium, tachyarrhythmias, and high-output cardiac failure. It may be triggered by physiologic stress, trauma, surgery, the onset of acute illness, or exposure to an iodine load. Thyroid hormone levels may only be mildly to moderately elevated.[16]

III. DIAGNOSIS

1. A suspected diagnosis of thyrotoxicosis may be confirmed when thyroid function tests reveal a low TSH level in conjunction with an elevated T_4 level (see Table 28-3).

2. It should be noted that 5% to 10% of patients with hyperthyroidism may have elevated T_3 levels with normal T_4 levels. Therefore T_3 measurement may be important when a diagnosis of hyperthyroidism is suspected but the T_4 level falls within the normal range.

3. In rare cases of hyperthyroidism caused by increased secretion of TSH from a pituitary adenoma, TSH levels may be elevated or normal.

4. Measurement of radioiodine uptake may help to distinguish between hyperthyroid and nonhyperthyroid states. Elevated thyroid hormone production in hyperthyroid states usually is associated with increased radioiodine uptake after 6 to 24 hours. Low thyroid hormone production, caused by inflammation and destruction of thyroid tissue in the setting of thyroiditis, usually is associated with low or absent radioiodine uptake in the same interval. Radioiodine uptake may also be low when intake of supraphysiologic dosages of thyroid hormone suppresses TSH levels, effectively shutting down endogenous production of thyroid hormone.

5. Whereas thyroglobulin levels may be normal or elevated in cases of nonhyperthyroid thyrotoxicosis caused by thyroiditis, they are usually low or undetectable in cases of nonhyperthyroid thyrotoxicosis caused by intake of supraphysiologic dosages of thyroid hormone.

6. Although thyroid-stimulating immunoglobulin (also known as anti-TSH receptor antibody) titers often are noted to be elevated in cases of Graves disease, elevated titers in themselves are not considered diagnostic. Quantitative thyroid-stimulating immunoglobulin titers may also function as an index of activity that can be used to monitor the status of thyroid eye disease.

IV. MANAGEMENT

1. Whereas mild cases of Graves disease may resolve spontaneously over time, moderate to severe cases usually necessitate treatment with antithyroid medications, radioiodine ablation therapy, or subtotal thyroidectomy procedures.

a. Antithyroid medications inhibit the production of thyroid hormone. When titrated to therapeutic dosages, they can effectively restore a patient to a euthyroid state over the course of 4 to 12 weeks. Prolonged therapy may be necessary, carrying the attendant risks of rare but problematic side effects.

b. Radioiodine ablation therapy delivers a targeted dose of iodine-131 that is taken up and concentrated by hyperfunctioning thyroid tissue. It is a safe and effective form of treatment that can restore a patient to a euthyroid state over the course of 3 to 6 months. There is a significant risk of postablative hypothyroidism after administration of a therapeutic dose of radioiodine.

c. Subtotal thyroidectomy procedures usually are performed only in special circumstances when severe complications mandate urgent treatment or when limiting side effects or patient preferences preclude the use of antithyroid medications or radioiodine.

2. Beta-blockers may help to control symptoms of thyrotoxicosis, including palpitations, tremulousness, and anxiety. Although propranolol offers the theoretical advantage of helping to control thyrotoxicosis by inhibiting the peripheral conversion of T_4 to T_3, it must be taken frequently. Alternative beta-blockers such as atenolol and metoprolol, dosed in daily or twice-daily increments, are commonly used in practice.

3. Propylthiouracil and methimazole are antithyroid medications that inhibit thyroid hormone production. Propylthiouracil also inhibits the peripheral conversion of T_4 to T_3. Therefore it may offer advantages in the treatment of thyroid storm or severe hyperthyroidism. Mild to moderate hyperthyroidism can be treated with propylthiouracil (50 to 200 mg every 8 hours) or methimazole (5 to 40 mg daily). Methimazole allows for daily dosing that may increase compliance with therapy. Side effects associated with antithyroid medications include allergic dermatitis, hepatotoxicity, arthritis, and vasculitis. Agranulocytosis, often preceded by the onset of a sore throat and fever, is a side effect that develops in about 0.5% of patients. **Detection of reduced granulocyte counts should prompt immediate discontinuation of antithyroid medications.**

4. Adjunctive therapies may be used to treat thyroid storm or severe hyperthyroidism (Box 28-1).

a. Iodine, administered in the form of Lugol's solution or saturated solution of potassium iodide, may help to block the release of thyroid hormone. Pretreatment with methimazole or propylthiouracil may help to curtail increased thyroid hormone synthesis that may be triggered by iodine administration.

b. Systemic glucocorticoids administered in stress doses may decrease peripheral conversion of T_4 to T_3.

c. Acetaminophen should be used as an antipyretic because aspirin may exacerbate thyrotoxicosis by displacing thyroid hormone from binding proteins.

5. Symptoms of thyrotoxicosis that develop in the setting of subacute thyroiditis and silent thyroiditis usually can be managed with limited

---

BOX 28-1

ACUTE MANAGEMENT OF THYROID STORM

Propranolol 60-80 mg per os q4h

Methimazole 30 mg q6h or propylthiouracil 250 mg per os q4h

Lugol's iodine solution or saturated solution of potassium iodide 10 gtt per os q8h

Hydrocortisone 100 mg intravenously q8h

Cooling blanket and other supportive measures

courses of beta-blockers. Serial thyroid function tests should be monitored over time to check for evidence of primary hypothyroidism.
6. Consider treating subclinical hyperthyroidism characterized by a low or suppressed TSH level with normal T_4 and T_3 levels. Decreased bone mineral density and an increased risk of developing atrial fibrillation have been reported as complications of this disorder.[17-19]

Structural Thyroid Disorders

I. EPIDEMIOLOGY

1. Structural thyroid disorders include thyroid nodules and nontoxic goiter. Nontoxic goiter can be classified as either simple or multinodular.
2. Palpable thyroid nodules may be detected in approximately 4% to 10% of the population. The prevalence of thyroid nodules in postmortem examination is closer to 50%.[20] Thyroid nodules are common incidental findings on radiologic studies.
3. Among patients with known thyroid nodules, the incidence of cancer is higher in children and adults younger than 30 or older than 60 years of age.
4. Patients with a history of head and neck radiation are at a higher risk of developing thyroid cancer.
5. Conditions that may be associated with the development of a nontoxic goiter include iodine deficiency, exposure to dietary goitrogens, thyroiditis, and congenital defects in thyroid hormone production.

II. CLINICAL PRESENTATION

1. On discovery of a thyroid nodule, patients should be asked about any history of head or neck radiation exposure used to treat enlarged tonsils, adenoids, or skin conditions.
2. Compressive symptoms caused by expansive growth or substernal extension of a goiter may include variable proximal dysphagia, hoarseness, exertional dyspnea, chronic cough, and a sensation of choking noted when lying recumbent in certain positions.
3. Patients with compressive symptoms caused by expansive growth of a goiter may have noted visible or palpable enlargement of the thyroid gland for many years. Patients with similar symptoms caused by substernal extension of a goiter may be unaware of their condition.
4. The presence of a goiter with substernal extension may be suggested by an inability to palpate the inferior border of a lobe of the thyroid gland.
5. Tracheal deviation or distended neck veins may be present in patients with substernal extension of a goiter. An exacerbation of compressive symptoms or development of facial plethora that occurs when the arms are extended above the head for 30 seconds to restrict the thoracic inlet is a finding known as Pemberton's sign.

28

THYROID DISORDERS

III. DIAGNOSIS

1. The TSH level should be checked in any patient presenting with a thyroid nodule or goiter. Detection of underlying thyrotoxicosis may suggest the presence of a toxic adenoma or toxic multinodular goiter.
2. Ultrasonography is the imaging modality of choice in evaluating the dimensions and distribution of thyroid nodules.
3. In a patient with a thyroid nodule and low TSH level, a radionuclide thyroid scan can be performed to determine whether the nodule is hyperfunctional. Nodules that are hyperfunctional do not warrant biopsy.

IV. MANAGEMENT

1. Fig. 28-2 depicts an algorithm for the management of thyroid nodules.[20]
2. The efficacy of using levothyroxine to suppress TSH levels in an effort to reduce the size of a solitary thyroid nodule has not been clearly established. Furthermore, this therapy increases the risk of iatrogenic thyrotoxicosis with the attendant risks of atrial arrhythmias and decreased bone mineral density. For this reason, the patient's risk factors should be considered before suppressive therapy is instituted.
3. Asymptomatic nontoxic goiters do not warrant treatment.
4. Symptomatic nontoxic goiters may be treated with levothyroxine suppression therapy or surgery.

PEARLS AND PITFALLS

- The diagnosis of thyroid dysfunction in hospitalized patients is fraught with pitfalls. Dopamine, systemic glucocorticoids, and octreotide all inhibit pituitary release of TSH and result in low TSH levels, independent of metabolic status. Diagnosis is further complicated by the effects of nonthyroidal illness on the hypothalamic-pituitary-thyroid axis.
- Treatment with interferon-alfa and interleukin-2 may be associated with a form of autoimmune thyroiditis. This may lead to transient thyrotoxicosis but more often leads to the development of primary hypothyroidism.
- Commonly used assays for free T_4 may be affected by endogenous antibodies to T_4, abnormal binding proteins, or illness.[21] Therefore a free T_4 level found to be inconsistent with the clinical state and TSH level should be reevaluated by quantitation of T_4 in a dialysate or ultrafiltrate of serum, which is the most accurate and direct determination of free T_4.
- Concurrent medications may affect levothyroxine uptake by decreasing absorption (iron, bile acid sequestrants, antacids) or altering metabolism (rifampin, many antiepileptic drugs).
- Patients with a rapidly growing solid thyroid mass should be referred for surgery even if a fine-needle aspiration biopsy does not reveal malignancy.

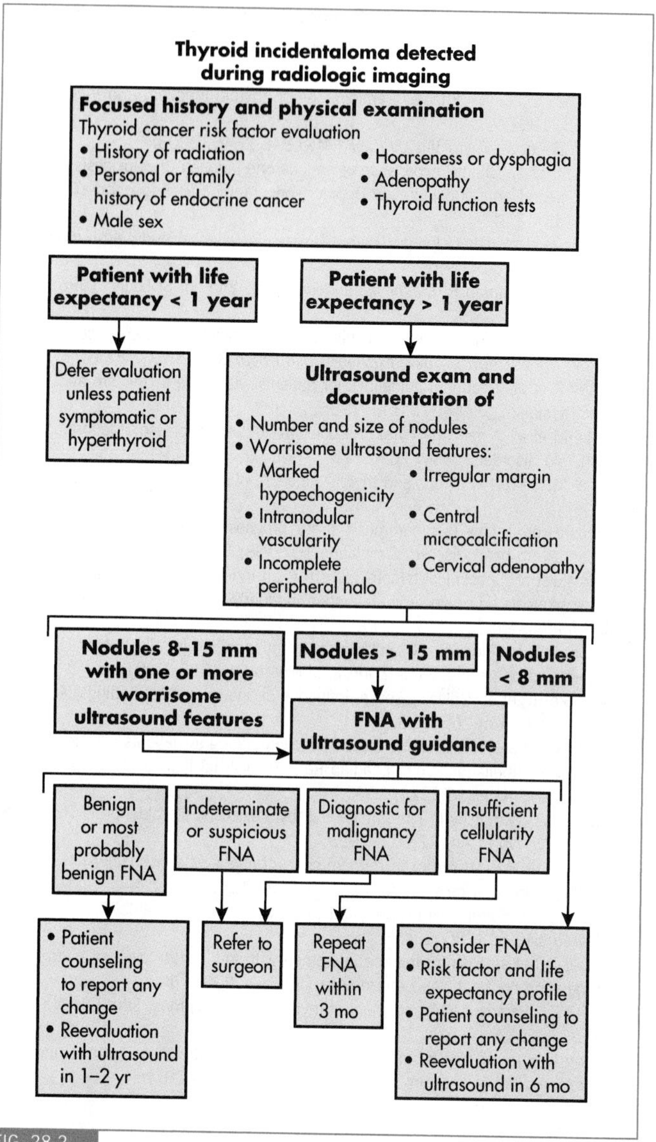

FIG. 28-2

Algorithm for the management of thyroid nodules detected incidentally during radiologic imaging. *FNA*, fine-needle aspiration. *(From Silver RJ, Parangi S: Surg Clin North Am 84:907, 2004.)*

REFERENCES

1. Klein I, Ojamaa K: Thyroid hormone and the cardiovascular system, *N Engl J Med* 344:501, 2001. C
2. Haraj KJ, Licata AA: Effects of amiodarone on thyroid function, *Ann Intern Med* 126:63, 1997. C
3. Pearce EN et al: Thyroiditis, *N Engl J Med* 348:2646, 2003. C
4. Eaton SE et al: Clinical experience of amiodarone-induced thyrotoxicosis over a 3-year period: role of colour-flow Doppler sonography, *Clin Endocrinol (Oxf)* 56:33, 2002. B
5. Canaris G et al: The Colorado Thyroid Disease Prevalence Study, *Arch Intern Med* 160:526, 2000. B
6. Moore WT, Eastman R: *Diagnostic endocrinology,* 2nd ed, St Louis, 1996, Mosby. C
7. Spencer C et al: Specificity of sensitive assays of thyrotropin used to screen for thyroid disease in hospitalized patients, *Clin Chem* 33:1391, 1987. B
8. Singer P et al: Treatment guidelines for patients with hyperthyroidism and hypothyroidism, *JAMA* 273:808, 1995. D
9. Surks M et al: American Thyroid Association guidelines for use of laboratory tests in thyroid disorders, *JAMA* 263:1529, 1990. D
10. Surks M, Sievert R: Drugs and thyroid function, *N Engl J Med* 333:1688, 1995. C
11. Iervasi G et al: Low-T_3 syndrome: a strong prognostic predictor of death in patients with heart disease, *Circulation* 107:708, 2003. B
12. Hak AE et al: Subclinical hypothyroidism is an independent risk factor for atherosclerosis and myocardial infarction in elderly women: the Rotterdam Study, *Ann Intern Med* 132:270, 2000. B
13. McDermott M, Ridgway EC: Subclinical hypothyroidism is mild thyroid failure and should be treated, *J Clin Endocrinol Metab* 86:4585, 2001. C
14. Nordyke RF et al: Graves disease: influence of age on clinical findings, *Arch Intern Med* 148:626, 1988. B
15. Kahn AD et al: How useful is thyroid function testing in patients with recent onset atrial fibrillation? The Canadian Registry of Atrial Fibrillation Investigators, *Arch Intern Med* 156:2221, 1996. B
16. Burch HB, Wartofsky L: Life-threatening thyrotoxicosis: thyroid storm, *Endocrinol Metab Clin North Am* 22:263, 1993. C
17. Sawin C et al: Low serum thyrotropin concentrations as a risk factor for atrial fibrillation in older persons, *N Engl J Med* 331:1249, 1994. B
18. Auer J et al: Subclinical hyperthyroidism as a risk factor for atrial fibrillation, *Am Heart J* 142:838, 2001. B
19. Bauer DC et al: Risk for fracture in women with low serum levels of thyroid-stimulating hormone, *Ann Intern Med* 134:561, 2001. B
20. Silver RJ, Parangi S: Management of thyroid incidentalomas, *Surg Clin North Am* 84:907, 2004. C
21. Wang R et al: Accuracy of free thyroxine measurements across natural ranges of thyroxine binding to serum proteins, *Thyroid* 10:31, 2000. B

Disorders of Calcium Homeostasis

Rachel Derr, MD; and Suzanne Jan de Beur, MD

FAST FACTS

- Hyperparathyroidism is the most common cause of hypercalcemia in the outpatient setting and is often asymptomatic. In the inpatient setting, the most common cause of hypercalcemia is malignancy, which usually is already in an advanced stage.
- Vitamin D deficiency is the most common cause of hypocalcemia. Renal failure and older age are risk factors for vitamin D deficiency. In the inpatient setting, hypocalcemia often is associated with hypomagnesemia and with critical illnesses such as sepsis and acute pancreatitis.
- Corrected serum calcium = measured calcium + 0.8(4 − albumin).
- Symptomatic moderate hypercalcemia (more than 12 mg/dl) and severe hypercalcemia (> 14 mg/dl) must be treated immediately and aggressively. Volume resuscitate with normal saline, promote calcium excretion with loop diuretics once the patient is euvolemic, and halt osteoclastic bone resorption with calcitonin and bisphosphonates.
- Symptomatic hypocalcemia should be treated with continuous intravenous calcium gluconate and calcitriol. Asymptomatic hypocalcemia is treated with oral calcium (often calcium carbonate) and vitamin D.

Calcium and phosphate homeostasis is controlled by parathyroid hormone (PTH), 25-dihydroxy-vitamin D (calcitriol), and to a lesser extent calcitonin. The actions of these hormones influence bone formation and resorption, intestinal absorption, and renal excretion of calcium and phosphate.

I. DISEASES RESULTING IN HYPERCALCEMIA

A. EPIDEMIOLOGY

1. Although the normal range may vary depending on the laboratory, **hypercalcemia is defined as a calcium level above 10.5 mg/dl** (2.5 mmol/L).
2. The physiologically active form of calcium is ionized calcium. Normal ionized calcium is 4 to 5.6 mg/dl (1 to 1.4 mmol/L). An elevated ionized calcium despite a normal total calcium level is characteristic of metabolic acidosis.

3. The most common cause of hypercalcemia in ambulatory patients is primary hyperparathyroidism, accounting for more than 90% of cases. Malignancy is the most common cause in hospitalized patients, accounting for more than 50% of cases of hypercalcemia in the hospital. Hypercalcemia secondary to malignancy usually presents in the context of advanced, clinically obvious disease.

4. The prevalence of primary hyperparathyroidism is approximately 100 per 100,000 people, but the incidence has declined in recent years for unclear reasons.[1] Primary hyperparathyroidism most commonly presents in the fifth and sixth decades, and it is two to three times more common in women than in men.[2]

B. CLINICAL PRESENTATION

1. **Renal.** Nephrolithiasis caused by hypercalciuria is present in up to 20% of patients with primary hyperparathyroidism. Hypercalcemia may lead to nephrogenic diabetes insipidus, leading to polyuria and dehydration. Hypercalcemia also causes renal vasoconstriction, which can cause a reversible decrease in the glomerular filtration rate. Additionally, long-standing disease can also lead to calcification of the renal tubules, called nephrocalcinosis, which can compromise renal function.

2. **Musculoskeletal.** Increased osteoclast activity induced by excessive PTH can cause osteopenia or osteoporosis, bone cysts (osteitis fibrosa cystica), fibrous nodules, bone pain, and fractures. Diffuse myalgias and generalized fatigue are also common.

3. **GI.** Constipation, vague abdominal pain, and anorexia are common complaints of hypercalcemic patients. Acute pancreatitis and peptic ulcer disease are rare manifestations of severe hypercalcemia.

4. **Neurologic and cognitive.** Mild hypercalcemia can lead to anxiety, depression, and decreased cognitive function. Dramatic changes in mental status, hallucinations, and coma can result from severe hypercalcemia.

5. **Most common presentation.** Since the introduction of routine biochemical screening in the 1970s, most cases of hypercalcemia are now diagnosed incidentally. Upon questioning, "asymptomatic" patients often complain of symptoms such as fatigue, weakness, vague abdominal pain, anorexia, and depression.[3]

6. **Findings.** There are few specific findings of hypercalcemia on physical examination; rather, most findings are related to the underlying cause. Band keratopathy (subepithelial calcium phosphate deposits in the cornea) is a rare finding that can be detected by slit lamp examination. A short QT interval on the electrocardiogram is common in severe hypercalcemia. Radiographs may show nephrocalcinosis and cortical bone erosion.

C. ETIOLOGY AND DIAGNOSIS

1. Common causes of hypercalcemia and their effects on laboratory studies are presented in Table 29-1.

2. Medications are another common cause of hypercalcemia. Thiazides often lead to elevated calcium levels by unmasking primary

hyperparathyroidism; the thiazide should be discontinued and the calcium level remeasured before further workup is done. Additionally, persistently elevated calcium levels are seen in a small portion of patients on chronic lithium therapy.[6] Intoxication with vitamin A, calcium-containing antacids (milk-alkali syndrome), or calcium supplements also result in hypercalcemia.

3. Less common causes include states of increased bone turnover such as Paget's disease paired with immobilization. Endocrinopathies, including hyperthyroidism, adrenal insufficiency, pheochromocytoma, and acromegaly, should also be considered in the differential diagnosis.

4. **The first step in the evaluation of hypercalcemia is to establish whether the process is PTH dependent** (Fig. 29-1). A low intact PTH suggests a PTH-independent process such as malignancy, states of vitamin D excess including granulomatous diseases, and other endocrinopathies. A high intact PTH suggests a PTH-dependent process. If the intact PTH is high, check a 24-hour urine calcium to differentiate between familial hypocalciuric hypercalcemia and hyperparathyroidism.

D. RISK AND PROGNOSIS

1. Hypercalcemia has been associated with an increased mortality rate, probably caused by cardiovascular disease and malignancy.[7,8] **Hypercalcemia associated with malignancy usually correlates with advanced disease and carries a poor prognosis.**

2. Approximately 30% of patients with asymptomatic hyperparathyroidism develop symptomatic hypercalcemia over a 10-year period. One-fifth of patients develop a decrease in bone density (of $> 10\%$) at one or more sites.[9]

E. MANAGEMENT

1. **Severe hypercalcemia and symptomatic moderate hypercalcemia must be treated aggressively and immediately. Multiple agents usually are used concurrently for greater efficacy** (Table 29-2).

2. Mild or asymptomatic hypercalcemia can be managed in the outpatient setting. Identify the underlying cause. Discontinue calcium supplements. Stop any other medication that can be contributing and recheck the calcium level in a couple of weeks. Encourage oral hydration, high salt intake, physical activity, and avoidance of immobilization.

3. According to the 2002 National Institutes of Health Consensus Development Conference, **patients with asymptomatic primary hyperparathyroidism should be referred to an experienced surgeon for parathyroidectomy if one of the following criteria is met:** serum calcium 1 mg/dl above the upper limit of normal, 24-hour urine calcium above 400 mg, creatinine clearance reduced by 30%, dual-energy x-ray absorptiometry scan t-score less than −2.5 at any site, or age younger than 50 years.[11]

Text continued on p. 343

29

DISORDERS OF CALCIUM HOMEOSTASIS

TABLE 29-1

CAUSES OF HYPERCALCEMIA AND ASSOCIATED LABORATORY FINDINGS

Diagnosis	Plasma					Urine		Comments
	Ca^{2+}	PO_4	PTH	25(OH)VitD	1,25(OH)$_2$VitD	Ca^{2+}	PO_4*	
Primary hyperparathyroidism	↑	N/↓	↑	N	N/↑	↑	↓	Parathyroid adenoma = 80%; diffuse hyperplasia = 15-20%, half of which are related to MEN syndrome type I or type IIa; carcinoma < 1%.
Tertiary hyperparathyroidism	↑	N/↓	↑	N	N/↑	↑	↓	Autonomously functioning parathyroid gland on the background of secondary hyperparathyroidism, usually associated with renal dysfunction.
Malignancy Osteolysis	↑	N/↑	↓	N	N	↑↑	↑	Solid tumors that metastasize to bone, such as breast cancer and non–small cell lung cancer, and multiple myeloma stimulate osteoclasts via cytokines to resorb bone. Alkaline phosphatase is high.[4]
PTH-rp	↑	N/↓	↓	N	N	↑↑	↓	80% of cases of solid tumors associated with hypercalcemia have elevated levels of PTH-rp, a protein with homology to PTH that normally functions in growth and development. Squamous cell cancers, breast, and renal cell cancers commonly secrete PTH-rp.

Calcitriol-producing	↑	N/↑	→	N/↓	↑	↑	↑	Seen in Hodgkin's and non-Hodgkin's lymphoma.
Granulomatous disease	↑	N/↑	→	N/↓	↑↑	↑↑	↑	Increased calcitriol production by activated macrophages in granulomas. Hypercalcemia occurs in as many as 10% of patients with sarcoidosis[5] and can also be seen in tuberculosis and fungal infections.
Vitamin D intoxication	↑	N/↑	→	↑↑	N	↑↑	↑	Overdose of vitamin D supplements. Hypercalcemia can be prolonged because of the storage of vitamin D in fat.
Familial hypocalciuric hypercalcemia	↑	N	N/↑	N	N	↓↓	N/↓	Autosomal dominant syndrome in which hypercalcemia presents in first decade and is usually mild and benign. Generally, no treatment is necessary.

Modified from Moore WT, Eastman RC: *Diagnostic endocrinology,* 2nd ed, St Louis, 1996, Mosby.

Ca^{2+}, calcium; *MEN,* multiple endocrine neoplasia; PO_4, phosphate; *PTH,* parathyroid hormone; *PTH-rp,* parathyroid hormone-related protein; $1,25(OH)_2VitD$, 1,25-dihydroxyvitamin D (calcitriol); *25(OH)VitD,* 25-hydroxyvitamin D (calcidiol).

*Urine phosphate is measured by the ratio of the renal threshold for phosphorus (6) divided by the glomerular filtration rate.

29

DISORDERS OF CALCIUM HOMEOSTASIS

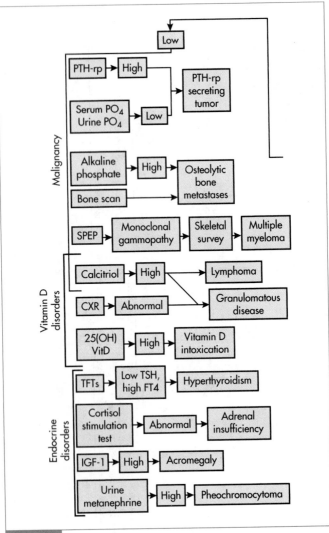

FIG. 29-1

Diagnostic algorithm for evaluating hypercalcemia. *Ca²⁺*, calcium; *CXR*, chest radiograph; *FT4*, free thyroxine; *iCa²⁺*, ionized calcium; *IGF-1*, insulin growth factor 1; *iPTH*, intact parathyroid hormone; *MEN*, multiple endocrine neoplasia; *PO₄*, phosphate; *PTH-rp*, parathyroid hormone–related protein; *SPEP*, serum protein electrophoresis; *TFTs*, thyroid function tests; *TSH*, thyroid-stimulating hormone; *25(OH)VitD*, 25-hydroxyvitamin D.

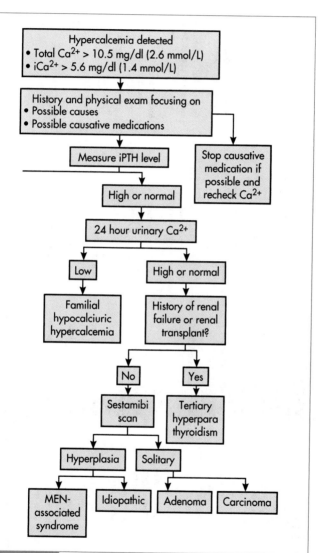

FIG. 29-1—cont'd

TABLE 29-2

PHARMACOLOGIC OPTIONS FOR TREATING HYPERCALCEMIA

Treatment Agent	Mechanism	Indication	Dosing	Onset of Action	Cautions
Normal saline	Enhances glomerular filtration and thus excretion of calcium	All cases of severe hypercalcemia or symptomatic moderate hypercalcemia	Start with 200-300 ml/hr to achieve urine output of 100-150 ml/hr. Hydrate with 2-4 L for 1-3 d.	Within hours	Monitor carefully in patients with heart failure and renal failure patients.
Furosemide (Lasix)	Inhibits calcium resorption in the distal renal tubule	With hydration once the patient is euvolemic	Low dosages of 10-20 mg IV.	Within hours	Dehydration, hypokalemia, hypomagnesemia.
Calcitonin (Calcimar or Miacalcin)	Decreases bone resorption, increases renal calcium excretion	Once the patient is euvolemic	4-8 IU/kg intramuscularly or subcutaneously q6h. Nasal calcitonin is not effective.	Within hours	Tachyphylaxis develops after a couple of days.
Bisphosphonates* Zoledronate (Zometa) Pamidronate (Aredia)	Decreases bone resorption by inhibiting osteoclasts	Preferred in malignancy-related hypercalcemia	Zoledronate 4 mg IV over 15 min, pamidronate 60-90 mg IV over 4 hr.	Within 2-4 d	Rare nephrotoxicity, hypocalcemia, rebound hypercalcemia in hyperparathyroidism.
Glucocorticoids	Inhibits 25-hydroxy-vitamin D conversion to calcitriol	Effective in cases of vitamin D intoxication, granulomatous diseases, and hematologic malignancies	Hydrocortisone 200 mg intravenously for 3 d.	2-5 d	Immunosuppression, myopathy.
Gallium nitrate (Ganite)	Inhibits osteoclastic bone resorption	Second-line agent but can be particularly effective in cases of PTH-rp-mediated hypercalcemia	100-200 mg IV continuously for 5 d.	2-5 d	Renal toxicity.

Modified from Carroll M, Schade D: *Am Fam Physician* 67(9):1959-1966, 2003.

IV, intravenously; *PTH-rp*, parathyroid hormone-related protein.

*... of ... and ... considered to because of its greater potency and shorter time of administration.[10]

II. DISEASES RESULTING IN HYPOCALCEMIA

A. EPIDEMIOLOGY

1. **A calcium level below 8 mg/dl (2 mmol/L) constitutes hypocalcemia. However,** total levels cannot be interpreted without the concurrent measurement of albumin, which is the major calcium binding protein. Therefore hypoalbuminemia artificially lowers total calcium levels and must be taken into consideration: Corrected calcium = Measured + (0.8[4 − albumin]). Alternatively, the unbound or ionized calcium level can be used to diagnose hypocalcemia.

2. **The most common cause of hypocalcemia is vitamin D deficiency, which is very prevalent in the general population.**[12,13]

3. Hypoparathyroidism is a less common cause of hypocalcemia. The most common cause of acute or chronic hypoparathyroidism is injury to or removal of the parathyroid glands during neck surgery.

B. CLINICAL PRESENTATION

1. The clinical presentation depends on the calcium level and the acuity of the hypocalcemia. Paresthesias are the typical early manifestation of hypocalcemia. Hypocalcemia from chronic hypoparathyroidism may be so gradual that the only symptom is visual impairment from cataracts years later. Few patients with hypocalcemia from renal failure are symptomatic.

a. **Neuromuscular.** Perioral paresthesia, tingling of the hands and feet, and spontaneous or latent tetany are predominant symptoms of hypocalcemia. **In severe or acute hypocalcemia, seizures or laryngeal spasm may occur.** Long-standing hypocalcemia associated with hyperphosphatemia can lead to extrapyramidal movement disorders secondary to basal ganglia calcification.

b. **Psychiatric.** Irritability, depression, and, in severe cases, psychosis can result from hypocalcemia.

c. **Cardiac.** Hypocalcemia has been associated with decreased myocardial contractility and may lead to congestive heart failure.

2. Physical examination and diagnosis.

a. Chronic hypocalcemia can lead to cataracts, dental abnormalities, dry and hyperpigmented skin, brittle hair, and nails with transverse grooves. When associated with hypophosphatemia, chronic hypocalcemia can also result in defects in the mineralization of new bone (osteomalacia).

b. Chvostek's sign and Trousseau's sign are very useful in diagnosing hypocalcemia. Chvostek's sign is the contraction of the ipsilateral facial muscles elicited by tapping the facial nerve just anterior to the ear. Trousseau's sign is carpal spasm 3 minutes after inflation of the blood pressure cuff 10 mmHg above the systolic blood pressure.

c. The electrocardiogram may show a prolonged QT interval.

C. ETIOLOGY AND DIAGNOSIS

1. Common causes of hypocalcemia and their effects on laboratory studies are presented in Table 29-3. Hypocalcemia often is associated with

29

DISORDERS OF CALCIUM HOMEOSTASIS

TABLE 29-3

CAUSES OF HYPOCALCEMIA

Diagnosis	Plasma Ca^{2+}	Plasma PO$_4$	Plasma PTH	Plasma 25(OH)VitD	Plasma 1,25(OH)$_2$VitD	Urine Ca^{2+}	Urine PO$_4$	Comments
Renal disease	↓	↑	↑↑	N	↓	↓	↓↓	Poor activity of renal 25(OH)VitD-1α-hydroxylase, decreased renal phosphate excretion, excessive loss of 25(OH)VitD in nephrotic syndrome.
Vitamin D deficiency	↓	N/↓	↑↑	↓↓	N/↓	↓	↓↓	Inadequate dietary intake of vitamin D. Malabsorption of vitamin D. Lack of sun exposure. Decreased hepatic synthesis of 25(OH) vitamin D. Increased hepatic catabolism of 25(OH)VitD by medications (e.g., anticonvulsants) that increase cytochrome P-450 enzymes.
Vitamin D–dependent rickets								
Type I	↓	N/↓	↑↑	N	↓	↓↓	↓	Rare disorder of deficient activity of renal 25(OH)VitD-1α-hydroxylase.
Type II	↓	N/↓	↑↑	N	↑↑	↓↓	↓	Rare disorder of end organ resistance to 1,25(OH)$_2$VitD secondary to a mutation in the vitamin D receptor.
Hypoparathyroidism	↓	↑	N/↓	N	↓	↑	N/↓	Surgical, idiopathic, or related to polyglandular autoimmune syndrome type I. Also can be secondary to low magnesium levels, which induce PTH resistance or deficiency.
Pseudohypoparathyroidism	↓	↑	↑↑	N	↓	↑	N/↓	Peripheral end organ resistance to PTH.

Modified from Moore WT, Eastman RC: *Diagnostic endocrinology*, 2nd ed, St Louis, 1996, Mosby.
AHO, Albright's hereditary osteodystrophy; *Ca^{2+}*, calcium; *N*, normal; *PO$_4$*, phosphate; *PTH*, parathyroid hormone; *25(OH)VitD*, 25 hydroxyvitamin D (calcidiol); *1,25(OH)$_2$VitD*, ... *dihydroxyvitamin D (calcitriol)*.

critical illnesses such as acute pancreatitis and sepsis, in which the degree of hypocalcemia correlates with the severity of illness.

2. Increased intravascular binding of ionized calcium can lead to symptomatic hypocalcemia. This can occur with multiple blood transfusions, which contain excess citrate (a calcium chelator), and acute respiratory alkalosis, which increases the binding of calcium to albumin in serum.

3. When evaluating hypocalcemia (Fig. 29-2), first check the serum phosphorus. Low phosphorus is associated with low levels of vitamin D. If phosphorus is normal or high, check the intact PTH, which is low in hypoparathyroidism and high in renal disease and pseudohypoparathyroidism.

D. RISK AND PROGNOSIS

1. Chronic hypocalcemia in patients with end-stage renal disease is associated with excess mortality (relative risk = 2.1) and the development of new and recurrent ischemic heart disease and cardiac failure.[14]

2. Vitamin D deficiency–related hypocalcemia is associated with osteopenia and osteoporosis. Older women with vitamin D deficiency have a twofold increase in the risk of hip fracture.[15]

E. MANAGEMENT

1. **Acute, symptomatic hypocalcemia.**
a. **Treat with 1 to 2 g of intravenous calcium gluconate over 10 to 20 minutes followed by a slow infusion of calcium at 0.5 to 1.5 mg/kg/hour.** Calcium gluconate usually is preferred over calcium chloride because it is less likely to cause tissue necrosis if extravasated.
b. Increase gastrointestinal absorption of calcium with calcitriol. Start at 0.25 μg twice a day and titrate up after a couple of doses. Always replete the magnesium if low.

2. **Chronic hypocalcemia associated with hypoparathyroidism** should be treated with oral calcium, usually calcium carbonate 1000 mg three to four times per day, and calcitriol 0.25 μg three times per day to maintain serum calcium in low-normal range (8 to 8.5 mg/dl). Higher values run the risk of hypercalciuria because these patients lack the PTH-mediated renal tubular calcium reabsorption. Although not approved by the U.S. Food and Drug Administration, synthetic PTH, administered subcutaneously twice a day, reduces calcium levels without causing hypercalciuria and may be helpful in cases of refractory hypoparathyroidism.[16]

3. **Chronic hypocalcemia associated with vitamin D deficiency** and hypophosphatemia should be treated with oral calcium supplementation and vitamin D.
a. Ergocalciferol (vitamin D_2) is given once weekly as 50,000 IU orally or parenterally until replete. It is a low-cost agent but is metabolized by the liver and kidneys and has a slow onset and long duration of action.

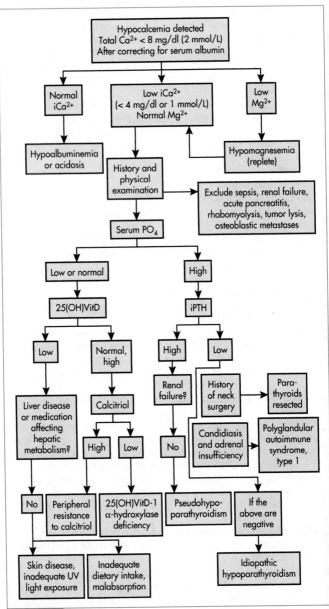

FIG. 29-2

See legend on the opposite page

b. Calcidiol (25-hydroxyvitamin D) is available in capsules of 20 and 50 μg. Its action is more rapid and not as prolonged as that of ergocalciferol.

c. Calcitriol (1,25-dihydroxyvitamin D) has the most rapid onset (within hours) and a shorter duration of action (half-life 4 to 6 hours) and does not require endogenous activation.

4. **Chronic hypocalcemia associated with renal insufficiency** and hyperphosphatemia is treated with vitamin D supplementation. Oral phosphate binders should be given to impair phosphate absorption. Calcium carbonate usually is given as well. Calcitriol or another vitamin D analog is necessary to treat the secondary hyperparathyroidism associated with renal failure. The recently introduced medication cinacalcet is a calcimimetic agent for secondary hyperparathyroidism in patients with renal disorders. It has been shown to lower parathyroid levels and improve calcium-phosphate homeostasis in comparison to placebo.[17]

PEARLS AND PITFALLS

- Patients with hypercalcemia may present with "stones, bones, moans, abdominal groans, and psychiatric overtones."
- Hypocalcemia is reliably tested for with Trousseau's and Chvostek's signs.
- Trousseau's sign is not negative unless the blood pressure cuff has been inflated 10 mmHg above the systolic blood pressure for a full 3 minutes.
- Chvostek's sign is positive in up to 10% of the general population.
- Always identify the underlying cause of hypercalcemia or hypocalcemia.
- Severely hypercalcemic patients are volume depleted; they must be well hydrated before a loop diuretic is administered.
- Severely hypocalcemic patients should be treated with a calcium gluconate drip rather than with repeated intravenous boluses, which raise calcium levels for only a few hours. High dosages of calcitriol also should be used.
- The dietary intake of calcium and vitamin D is inadequate in most sick and older adults. Achieving an adequate daily intake of vitamin D (800 to 1000 IU) and elemental calcium (1000 to 1500 mg) with the help of dietary supplementation reduces bone loss and nonvertebral fracture risk in men and women older than 65.[18]

29

DISORDERS OF CALCIUM HOMEOSTASIS

Diagnostic algorithm for evaluating hypocalcemia. Ca^{2+}, calcium; iCa^{2+}, ionized calcium; *iPTH*, intact parathyroid hormone; Mg^{2+}, magnesium; PO_4, phosphate; *25(OH)VitD*, 25-hydroxyvitamin D.

REFERENCES

1. Wermers RA, Khosla S, Atkinson EJ, Hodgson SF, O'Fallon WM, Melton LJ: The rise and fall of primary hyperparathyroidism: a population-based study in Rochester, Minnesota, 1965-1992, *Ann Intern Med* 126:6 433-440, 1997. B

2. Heath HWI, Hodgson SF, Kennedy MA: Primary hyperparathyroidism: incidence, morbidity and potential economic impact in a community, *N Engl J Med* 302:189-193, 1980. B

3. Bilezikian JP, Silverberg SJ: Clinical practice: asymptomatic primary hyperparathyroidism, *N Engl J Med* 350(17):1746-1751, 2004. C

4. Roodman GD: Mechanisms of bone metastasis, *N Engl J Med* 350(16):1655-1664, 2004. C

5. Sharma OP: Vitamin D, calcium and sarcoidosis, *Chest* 109:535-539, 1996. C

6. Bendz H, Sjodin I, Toss G, Berglund K: Hyperparathyroidism and long-term lithium therapy: a cross-sectional study and the effect of lithium withdrawal, *J Intern Med* 240(6):357-365, 1996. B

7. Leifsson BG, Ahren B: Serum calcium and survival in a large health screening program, *J Clin Endocrinol Metab* 81(6):2149-2153, 1996. B

8. Lundgren E, Lind L, Palmer M, Jakobsson S, Ljunghall S, Rastad J: Increased cardiovascular mortality and normalized serum calcium in patients with mild hypercalcemia followed up for 25 years, *Surgery* 130(6):978-985, 2001. B

9. Silverberg SJ, Shane E, Jacobs TP, Siris E, Bilezikian JP: A 10-year prospective study of primary hyperparathyroidism with or without parathyroid surgery, *N Engl J Med* 341(17):1249-1255, 1999. B

10. Major P, Lortholary A, Hon J, et al: Zoledronic acid is superior to pamidronate in the treatment of hypercalcemia of malignancy: a pooled analysis of two randomized, controlled clinical trials, *J Clin Oncol* 19:558, 2001. A

11. Bilezikian JP et al: Summary statement from a workshop on asymptomatic primary hyperparathyroidism: a perspective for the 21st century, *J Clin Endocrinol Metab* 87(12):5353-5361, 2002. D

12. Harris SS, Soteriades E, Coolidge JA, Mudgal S, Dawson-Hughes B: Vitamin D insufficiency and hyperparathyroidism in a low income, multiracial, elderly population, *J Clin Endocrinol Metab* 85(11):4125-4130, 2000. B

13. Thomas M et al: Hypovitaminosis D in medical inpatients, *N Engl J Med* 338:777-783, 1998. B

14. Foley RN, Parfrey PS, Harnett JD, et al: Hypocalcemia, morbidity, and mortality in end-stage renal disease, *Am J Nephrol* 16(5):386-393, 1996. B

15. Cummings SR, Browner WS, Bauer D, et al: Endogenous hormones and the risk of hip and vertebral fractures among older women, *N Engl J Med* 339:733-738, 1998. B

16. Winer KK, Ko CW, Reynolds JC, et al: Long-term treatment of hypoparathyroidism: a randomized controlled study comparing parathyroid hormone-(1-34) versus calcitriol and calcium, *J Clin Endocrinol Metab* 88(9):4214-4220, 2003. A

17. Block G et al: Cinacalcet for secondary hyperparathyroidism in patients receiving hemodialysis, *N Engl J Med* 350:1516-1525, 2004. A

18. Dawson-Hughes B, Harris S, Krall E, Dallal G: Effect of calcium and vitamin D supplementation on bone density in men and women 65 years of age or older, *N Engl J Med* 337:670-676, 1997. A

Approach to Abdominal Pain

Jonathan M. Gerber, MD; Vandana R. Long, MD;
and Francis Giardiello, MD

> **FAST FACTS**
>
> - Generate a differential diagnosis on the basis of the location of the patient's pain (Table 30-1).
> - Determine within minutes whether the abdominal pain represents an emergent, urgent, low-risk, or chronic condition and act accordingly.
> - Maintain a low threshold for ordering imaging and obtaining early surgical consultation for immunocompromised, elderly, mentally ill, and intoxicated patients.
> - All women of childbearing age with abdominal pain should have a pregnancy test, and most should have a pelvic examination.
> - Early diagnosis and treatment can dramatically reduce morbidity and mortality in many abdominal conditions.

30

I. GENERAL APPROACH TO ABDOMINAL PAIN

A. HISTORY

1. Appropriate evaluation of abdominal pain includes a thorough and systematic evaluation. The type of pain and symptoms should guide the differential diagnosis and initial management.
2. **Description.** The clinician should determine the duration, rapidity of onset, character (severity, constancy, quality), site (Table 30-1), radiation, aggravating and relieving factors (change of position, stress, association with meals or menstrual cycle), and associated symptoms. The review of systems should address nausea, vomiting, diarrhea, constipation, hematemesis, melena, hematochezia, dysphagia, odynophagia, changes in appetite, early satiety, weight loss, jaundice, pruritus, flatulence, dysuria, hematuria, vaginal or penile discharge, menses, fevers and chills, diaphoresis, trauma, skin, joint, or ocular symptoms.
3. **Types of pain**
   a. **Visceral pain is dull and poorly localized.** The site of perceived pain corresponds to the dermatomal level at which visceral afferents enter the spinal cord (often perceived as periumbilical because of the bilateral midline innervation of the gastrointestinal tract).
   b. **Parietal pain is sharp and well-demarcated pain,** reflecting the somatic innervation overlying areas of inflammation.
   c. **Referred pain** occurs in an area distant from the site of disturbance. It is perceived as superficial, aching pain in somatic distributions whose afferents enter the spinal cord at or near the same level as affected visceral afferents.

TABLE 30-1

ABDOMINAL PAIN BY LOCATION*

Right Upper Abdomen	Middle Upper Abdomen	Left Upper Abdomen
Choledocholithiasis	Gastroesophageal reflux disease	Splenic rupture
Acute cholecystitis	Esophagitis	Splenic infarct
Cholangitis	Hiatal hernia	Pancreatitis
Hepatitis	Gastritis	Pneumonia
Hepatic congestion	Pancreatitis	Myocardial infarction
Pneumonia	Peptic ulcer (gastric, duodenal)	Gastric ulcer
Myocardial infarction	Gastric outlet obstruction	Pyelonephritis
Appendicitis	Choledocholithiasis	
Pyelonephritis	Superior mesenteric artery syndrome	
	Myocardial infarction	
	Appendicitis	
	Aortic aneurysm	
	Aortic dissection	

	Middle Abdomen	
	Bowel obstruction	
	Gastroenteritis	
	Irritable bowel syndrome	
	Malabsorption	
	Bowel perforation	
	Peritonitis	
	Mesenteric ischemia	

Right Lower Abdomen	Middle Lower Abdomen	Left Lower Abdomen
Appendicitis	Endometriosis	Diverticulitis
Typhlitis	Endometritis	Ureteral colic
Mesenteric adenitis	Pelvic inflammatory disease	Pyelonephritis
Ureteral colic	Ectopic pregnancy	Inflammatory bowel disease
Pyelonephritis	Ovarian cyst rupture	Pelvic inflammatory disease
Inflammatory bowel disease	Bladder distension	Ectopic pregnancy
Diverticulitis	Cystitis	Ruptured ovarian cyst
Pelvic inflammatory disease	Strangulated hernia	Mittelschmerz
Ectopic pregnancy		Strangulated hernia
Ruptured ovarian cyst		
Mittelschmerz		
Strangulated hernia		

*This is a general guide to abdominal pain by location. Each box represents a region of the abdomen and common causes of pain in that location. These lists are not all inclusive, and the areas where pain is perceived overlap.

4. **Past medical history.** Queries should include prior abdominal surgeries, hernias, malignancy, immunocompromise, peripheral vascular disease, coagulopathy, thromboembolic disease, diabetes mellitus, history of sexually transmitted diseases, and medications.

B. PHYSICAL EXAMINATION

1. **General inspection** provides an assessment of the patient's level of distress and may assist in diagnosis (patients will be immobile in peritonitis, writhing in pain in renal colic). When accompanied by abdominal pain, new-onset jaundice usually indicates biliary obstruction.

2. **Vital signs** should be repeated frequently in ill-appearing and distressed patients. Because patients may have limited oral intake or hemorrhage, orthostatic vital signs and volume status should be assessed.

a. **Abdominal examination** should include inspection, auscultation, palpation, and percussion. Inspect surgical scars, distension, masses, distended veins (caput medusae), visible peristalsis, ecchymosis (Cullen's sign, periumbilical ecchymosis; Grey Turner's sign, flank discoloration), and hernias.

b. **Palpation.** Look for guarding, rigidity, tenderness, rebound, masses (pulsatile in aortic aneurysm), organomegaly, pulsatile liver, bladder distension, costovertebral angle tenderness, Murphy's sign in cholecystitis (arrest of inspiration with right upper quadrant palpation), shifting dullness.

3. **Rectal examination** should be performed, including an assessment for gross and occult blood.

4. **Women who are sexually active and of reproductive age should undergo pelvic examination** with special attention to discharge, cervical motion tenderness, ovarian masses, and cysts. Men should have a testicular examination. All patients complaining of lower abdominal or groin pain should be examined for hernias.

C. DIAGNOSTIC TESTING

1. **Laboratory testing** should include a complete blood cell count with differential, urinalysis and urine culture, and liver and renal function tests in most patients. Patients with suspected bleeding or potential surgical conditions should have coagulation studies and a blood type and screen (or crossmatch). All women of childbearing age should have a pregnancy test.

2. **Electrocardiogram.** An electrocardiogram should be performed on most patients, especially those with nausea, cardiovascular risk factors, or unstable vital signs, to evaluate for occult coronary ischemia or myocardial infarction.

3. **Plain film radiography.** Chest films and upright abdominal films should be obtained to rule out pneumonia and free air (in patients with suspected perforation). Abdominal plain films can reveal bowel dilation, cecal diameter, or air-fluid levels indicating obstruction. Thumbprinting

or pneumatosis intestinalis (air in the bowel wall) suggests bowel ischemia or infarction.

4. **Ultrasound** is the imaging modality of choice in evaluating pelvic pain in women and right upper quadrant pain. It is also useful for marking fluid collections for possible bedside aspiration.

5. **Computed tomography** (CT) assesses for a wide differential, including aortic aneurysm, intestinal ischemia, diverticulitis, appendicitis, inflammatory bowel disease (IBD), bowel obstruction, pancreatic disease, renal stones, neoplasm, and intraabdominal abscess. CT is inferior to magnetic resonance imaging (MRI) and ultrasound in imaging of hepatobiliary and pelvic diseases.

6. **MRI.** Magnetic resonance cholangiopancreatography is useful in patients with hepatobiliary or pancreatic disease. Magnetic resonance angiography and venography are helpful in cases of suspected vascular disease. MRI is a good alternative to CT in patients with contrast allergy or renal impairment. Unfortunately, MRI is limited by lengthy imaging times, cost, and low availability.

D. INITIAL MANAGEMENT

Within minutes, determine whether the patient's abdominal pain signifies an emergency or a low-risk or chronic process. Withhold narcotic analgesics until an initial assessment can be made.

1. Establish intravenous (IV) access (ideally two large-bore peripheral lines for any unstable patient).

2. Initiate nothing by mouth (NPO) status until the patient proves stable.

3. Provide supportive care, including fluid and electrolyte management as volume status dictates (use caution in older adults or patients with a history of congestive heart failure).

4. Place a nasogastric (NG) tube if there is bleeding, obstruction, or significant nausea or vomiting.

5. Place a Foley catheter in unstable patients to monitor volume status.

6. Initiate cardiac monitoring of any potentially unstable patients.

7. Provide supplemental oxygen as needed.

8. Order appropriate diagnostic workup and consultations.

9. Administer early antibiotics if indicated.

II. ABDOMINAL EMERGENCIES

1. Bowel perforation.

a. **Clinical presentation.** Patients may have a history of peptic ulcer disease, IBD, diverticulitis, abdominal surgery, trauma, or recent endoscopic procedures. Pain may be localized or diffuse, depending on the extent of inflammation. Fever, rebound tenderness, guarding, a rigid abdomen, and absent bowel sounds in a motionless patient suggest peritonitis.

b. **Diagnosis.** An upright or a left lateral decubitus film can reveal free air. Radiographic examination is only 38%[1] sensitive in diagnosing free air. If perforation is suspected but no free air is visible on plain film, a CT scan should be obtained.

c. **Management.** Emergent surgical consultation should be pursued, and the patient should remain NPO. Supportive therapy should include IV fluids, antibiotics, and analgesics.

2. Ruptured ectopic pregnancy.

a. **Clinical presentation.** Suggestive features include abdominal pain, a history of amenorrhea, and acute vaginal bleeding in a woman of reproductive age. Intrauterine devices, history of pelvic inflammatory disease, and prior tubal pregnancy all predispose to ectopic pregnancy. Patients often are asymptomatic before rupture. Guarding, rigidity, and hypotension are common after rupture. Adnexal tenderness, mass, and uterine enlargement may be found on pelvic examination.

b. **Diagnosis.** The diagnosis is confirmed by serum beta–human chorionic gonadotropin (β-hCG) level greater than 1500 IU/L and an empty uterus by transvaginal ultrasound (note that the presence of intrauterine pregnancy does not preclude an ectopic twin, especially in patients who have undergone in vitro fertilization). The differential diagnosis includes ruptured hemorrhagic ovarian cyst if β-hCG is negative.

c. **Management.** Rupture is associated with high mortality; therefore, emergent gynecologic consultation is indicated if rupture is suspected. Stable, unruptured cases can be managed with methotrexate.[2]

3. Ruptured abdominal aortic aneurysm.

a. **Clinical presentation.** Patients with a history of vascular disease, tobacco use (fivefold increased risk[3]), and positive family history (fourfold increased risk[4]) are more likely to have an aortic aneurysm. Pain is initially throbbing and pulsatile in the epigastric or lumbar region, becoming steady and continuous after rupture. Pain may radiate to the back, groin, or testes. On examination, a pulsatile mass above the umbilicus and hypotension are common.

b. **Diagnosis.** Patients should be observed closely if rupture is suspected. Aneurysms with diameter greater than 5.5 cm or growth by more than 0.5 cm diameter in 6 months are more likely to rupture; those less than 4 cm in diameter are unlikely to rupture.[5] Ultrasound is almost 100% sensitive but can be limited by obesity or overlying bowel gas.[6] A CT scan should be performed if ultrasound is nondiagnostic.

c. **Management.** Emergent surgical consultation is mandatory. Mortality exceeds 50%. Supportive care includes fluid resuscitation and correction of any coagulopathy with vitamin K and fresh frozen plasma. Controversy exists regarding the use of β-blockers in nonhypotensive patients. Present data do not support a mortality benefit from β-blockers. If hypertension control is necessary, a short-acting IV agent is recommended.

4. Bowel obstruction.

a. **Clinical presentation.** Anorexia, nausea, vomiting (especially with more proximal obstruction), colicky abdominal pain, constipation or diarrhea, and obstipation are common symptoms.

      (1) Patients may have a history of hernia, abdominal surgery (adhesions), IBD, cancer, prior obstruction, unintentional weight loss, trauma, or impaired coagulation (hematoma).

      (2) On physical examination the abdomen is distended, and bowel sounds may be absent or high pitched and "tinkling," as in small bowel obstruction. A mass may be palpable on abdominal or rectal examination. A strangulated (irreducible, tender, swollen, erythematous) hernia may be present. If the patient is febrile or has signs of peritonitis, the possibility of bowel perforation, strangulation, or necrosis should be considered.

  b. **Diagnosis.** Abdominal radiograph examination can help differentiate large bowel obstruction (haustra do not cross the lumen) and small bowel obstruction (valvulae conniventes cross the entire lumen). In small bowel obstruction, plain films show central gas shadows, gas absent in the large bowel, air-fluid levels, and bowel distension proximal to the obstruction. Cecal diameter greater than 10 cm raises concern for bowel necrosis and perforation and should prompt consideration of bowel decompression or surgical intervention. If suspicion is high for obstruction, x-ray examination should be followed by an abdominal CT scan. The radiograph is 77% sensitive and 50% specific for bowel obstruction, whereas CT is 93% sensitive and 100% specific. The level of obstruction can be accurately predicted by CT scan in 93% of cases, compared with only 60% of patients by plain film. The cause of obstruction can be determined 87% of the time with CT, compared with only 7% with plain film.[7]

  c. **Management.** Patients should be maintained NPO and treated with NG tube decompression and aggressive IV fluid and electrolyte resuscitation. Early surgical consultation should be obtained. Evidence of strangulation, necrosis, or complete (especially colonic) or closed-loop obstruction constitutes a surgical emergency. Mortality markedly increases once bowel necroses. Emergent surgery is critical to salvage at-risk bowel and resect necrotic bowel. Partial obstruction is much more likely to be amenable to nonoperative management than complete obstruction. Surgery should be considered if partial obstruction does not improve within 24 hours of observation.

  d. **Causes of obstruction** include incarcerated hernia, adhesions, stricture (caused by radiation, ischemia, IBD, or other causes), neoplasm, volvulus, intussusception, trauma or hematoma, gallstone ileus, and bezoar. Specific treatment should be directed at the underlying cause. Note that colonic pseudoobstruction, or Ogilvie's syndrome, is a functional bowel obstruction. Neostigmine therapy should be considered in these cases.

  5. Toxic megacolon.

  a. **Clinical presentation.** Patients with IBD, infection with Clostridium difficile or other infectious colitis, ischemic colitis, diverticulitis, colon cancer, and the human immunodeficiency virus are at risk. Patients often have at least 1 week of abdominal pain caused by one of the aforementioned conditions, followed by bloody diarrhea, severe pain, and distension. Patients appear ill and often are hypotensive with fever and signs of peritonitis (abdominal tenderness, guarding, rebound).

b. **Diagnosis.** The diagnosis is established by colonic dilation of more than 6 cm on imaging; three of the following: fever, tachycardia, leukocytosis, and anemia; and dehydration, mental status changes, hypotension, or electrolyte disturbances.[8] A stool sample should be sent for Gram stain, cultures, fecal leukocytes, and C. difficile toxin.

c. **Management.** The patient should be kept NPO, and an NG tube should be inserted for decompression. Daily abdominal films should be obtained. Therapy includes IV fluids, electrolyte repletion, and broad-spectrum antibiotics (including metronidazole or oral vancomycin to cover for C. difficile). Avoid antimotility agents and narcotics because they may increase the risk of perforation. Immediate surgical consultation should be obtained. Colectomy is indicated if signs of perforation are present or symptoms persist beyond 48 hours with conservative management.

6. Appendicitis.

a. **Clinical presentation.** Abdominal pain initially is central, dull, and crampy. It later migrates to the right lower quadrant (RLQ) and changes in character to sharp pain exacerbated by movement (peritonitis). Associated symptoms include nausea, anorexia, and fever. Resolution of pain followed by the onset of peritoneal signs implies perforation. Physical examination reveals RLQ tenderness and guarding with palpation at McBurney's point and RLQ pain with left lower quadrant (LLQ) palpation (Rovsing's sign), RLQ pain with extension of the right hip (iliopsoas sign), and RLQ pain with internal rotation of the hip (obturator sign). Rectal examination may elicit tenderness if the inflamed appendix is adjacent to the rectum.

b. **Diagnosis.** The white blood cell count often is elevated. CT scan may reveal thickening of the appendiceal wall (> 2 mm), appendicolith, phlegmon, abscess, free fluid, or fat stranding in the RLQ. The CT scan is 96% to 98% sensitive and 83% to 89% specific for appendicitis.[9] Plain films usually are not helpful. The appendix is visualized by ultrasound in only one third of cases. If it is visualized, however, a diameter of more than 6 mm suggests appendicitis.[10]

c. **Management.** Obtain immediate surgical consultation for appendectomy. Patients should be kept NPO and receive IV antibiotics and fluids. Stable patients or poor surgical candidates may be managed nonoperatively, with antibiotics and supportive care alone, but up to 40% ultimately need appendectomy.[11] Select cases of contained perforation with localized abscess may be treated initially with antibiotics and percutaneous (radiology-guided) aspiration, followed by delayed appendectomy (at 6 weeks).

7. Ovarian torsion.

30

APPROACH TO ABDOMINAL PAIN

a. **Clinical presentation.** Premenopausal women (especially those younger than age 30) present with sudden onset of sharp, severe lower abdominal or pelvic pain on the side of the affected ovary and possible radiation to the back, flank, or ipsilateral groin or thigh. Associated nausea and vomiting may be present. Straining, exercise, or sexual intercourse may precipitate onset. Incidence is higher in pregnancy and after ovulation induction. Pain generally is constant and worsens as ischemia progresses to infarction, but repeated torsion and de-torsion may result in intermittent symptoms. Ovarian enlargement (particularly if > 6 cm), often caused by cyst, tumor, or abscess, predisposes to torsion. The right side is more commonly involved. A tender, adnexal mass may be palpable on the affected side on pelvic examination. Fever may be present. Infarction may result in peritonitis and hemodynamic compromise.

b. **Diagnosis.** Leukocytosis may be present. A positive β-hCG does not exclude torsion. Transvaginal color Doppler ultrasound establishes the diagnosis in most cases (87% accuracy) and may suggest viability.[12]

c. **Management.** Immediate gynecologic consultation should be obtained, with emergency surgery to resolve torsion and salvage the involved ovary (if still viable).

III. URGENT ABDOMINAL CONDITIONS

1. Cholecystitis and cholangitis (see Chapter 32).
2. Pancreatitis (see Chapter 31).
3. Hepatitis (see Chapters 33 and 34).
4. Diverticulitis.
a. **Clinical presentation.** Patients report LLQ pain (rarely RLQ pain), often with a history of similar symptoms in the past. Nausea, vomiting, and altered bowel habits are common. On examination, LLQ tenderness and occasionally a palpable mass are present. A toxic appearance, with localized or diffuse rebound tenderness and guarding, suggests perforation.
b. **Diagnosis.** A leukocytosis usually is present. Free air on plain film indicates perforation. CT scan may demonstrate focal thickening, fluid collection, perforation, fistula, or obstruction.
c. **Management.** Initial treatment includes oral antibiotics and a clear liquid diet. If no improvement occurs, a trial of NPO status and IV antibiotics should be instituted. Surgical consultation is indicated for perforation, abscess, obstruction, or fistula.
5. Mesenteric ischemia.
a. **Clinical presentation.** Underlying hypercoagulable states, potential embolic sources (atrial fibrillation or endocarditis), or vascular disease (including atherosclerosis and vasculitides) may be present. Postprandial pain suggests abdominal angina. Infarction is heralded by the onset of constant, severe pain. Patients typically experience diffuse abdominal pain, often out of proportion to physical findings. As

ischemia progresses to infarction (with resultant peritonitis), abdominal distension, occult or gross blood in the stool, rebound tenderness, guarding, or absent bowel sounds may be found on examination.

b. **Diagnosis.** Patients may have a leukocytosis with a left shift, metabolic acidosis (lactic acid), and elevated levels of amylase, lactate dehydrogenase, or creatine kinase with persistent ischemia. Plain films may reveal ileus, bowel wall thickening, or pneumatosis intestinalis. CT has a sensitivity of 64% and a specificity of 92% for bowel ischemia.[13] Mesenteric angiography remains the gold standard, but CT angiography and magnetic resonance angiography (plus magnetic resonance venography in thrombotic disease) are emerging as noninvasive alternatives.

c. **Management.** Therapy is supportive, with correction of metabolic acidosis, antibiotics, IV fluids, and insertion of an NG tube for decompression. Anticoagulation with IV heparin should be initiated unless bleeding or infarction is present or surgery is imminent. Early surgical consultation should be obtained, given the risk of bowel necrosis, which represents an emergency necessitating immediate resection. Interventional radiology may offer additional options, including catheter-guided thrombolysis, embolectomy, angioplasty, and stent placement.

6. Peptic ulcer disease and gastritis.

a. **Clinical presentation.** Typically, patients have epigastric or left upper quadrant pain that improves (duodenal ulcers) or worsens (gastric ulcers) with eating. Anorexia, nausea, and vomiting are more common with gastric ulcers. Epigastric tenderness may be present on physical examination. Rectal examination may reveal gross or occult blood. Peritonitis implies perforation and may portend hemodynamic compromise. Obstruction may occur with gastric outlet ulcers. Significant upper or lower gastrointestinal bleeding may be present chronically or acutely. Patients may present in extremis if bleeding is severe.

b. **Diagnosis.** If signs of peritonitis are present, an upright plain film or a CT scan is necessary immediately to rule out perforation. Otherwise, esophagogastroduodenoscopy with biopsy (with Diff-Quik staining for Helicobacter pylori) should be pursued. Complete blood count, coagulation tests, routine chemistries, and type and cross should be sent if bleeding is present.

c. **Management.** An H_2 blocker or oral proton pump inhibitor is administered in chronic or stable cases. In cases of hemorrhage see Chapter 37. If peritonitis is present, emergent surgical consultation should be obtained. If present, *H. pylori* should be eradicated. Malignancy should be ruled out via biopsy of gastric ulcers.

IV. LOW-RISK AND CHRONIC CONDITIONS

1. **Abdominal wall pain.** Presentation depends on the specific cause. Notable causes include hernias, trauma or surgery, muscle strains and

30

APPROACH TO ABDOMINAL PAIN

tears, cutaneous nerve root impingement, slipping rib syndrome, and myofascial irritation. Abdominal wall pain may also be secondary to thoracic nerve radiculopathy (T7 to T12), including herpes zoster. Hernias (of which inguinal hernias are the most common, with a male to female predominance of 10:1) are predisposed by straining, pregnancy, obesity, prior surgery, and ascites. Most patients appear well. Pain typically is well localized and related to position or activity but not meals or bowel movements. Carnett's sign (increased tenderness with tensing of the abdominal musculature) is suggestive but not diagnostic of abdominal wall pain.[14] Discrete areas of focal tenderness may be present. Hernias, incisional scars, or trauma may be evident. Hooking the inferior (floating) ribs and pulling anteriorly may elicit pain (and occasionally a click) in slipping rib syndrome. Injection of local anesthetic into a trigger point (provided structural disease has been ruled out) may be both diagnostic and therapeutic. With the exception of strangulated hernia, which constitutes a surgical emergency, most conditions are not life threatening. Patient reassurance is a staple of therapy.

2. **Nephrolithiasis** (see Chapter 70).
3. **Pyelonephritis** (see Chapter 59).
4. **Pelvic inflammatory disease** (see supplemental PDA Chapter 7).
5. **IBD** (see Chapter 38).
6. **Biliary colic** (see Chapter 32).
7. **Gastroenteritis** (see Chapter 39).
8. **Irritable bowel syndrome (IBS).** The onset of IBS usually is in the late teens to early twenties. Patients may have mood or anxiety disorders. Symptoms include crampy abdominal pain, bloating, sensation of incomplete evacuation, diarrhea or constipation, mucus production, urgency, and pain relieved by defecation. IBS is a diagnosis of exclusion, so structural and metabolic abnormalities should be ruled out before the diagnosis of IBS is established.[15] Diagnostic criteria include abdominal pain for at least 12 weeks out of the year (need not be consecutive) and two of three of the following symptoms: pain relieved by defecation, change in stool frequency, and change in stool appearance. Treatment includes symptom control with dietary modification (i.e., increase in fiber and avoidance of foods that precipitate or aggravate symptoms), stress management, and medications (anticholinergics, antidepressants, antidiarrheals, or serotonin agonists or antagonists), depending on symptoms.
9. **Endometriosis** affects premenopausal women with growth of endometrial tissue outside the uterus. Many, if not most, women are asymptomatic. Presenting symptoms are most commonly pelvic pain and infertility. Pain typically is worse with menses (dysmenorrhea) and intercourse (dyspareunia). Abnormal uterine bleeding may be present as well. Rectal implants may cause pain and hematochezia. Tender nodules in the cul-de-sac or along the uterosacral ligaments may be

palpable on pelvic examination. Manipulation of the uterus may be painful and tender, and adnexal masses may be present. Rarely, implants may be seen outside the abdomen or pelvis manifesting with pain or bleeding. Laparoscopy, with or without biopsy, is the diagnostic modality of choice. However, the diagnosis often is presumed based on consistent history and physical findings and confirmed by response to empiric therapy. Serum CA-125 often is elevated, but it is not specific for endometriosis. Imaging generally is not useful. Treatment is aimed at controlling pain and achieving fertility. Pain may be managed with nonsteroidal antiinflammatory drugs, hormonal therapy, or surgery. Total hysterectomy with bilateral salpingo-oophorectomy is curative with regard to pain in women in whom fertility is not desired.[16]

V. UNUSUAL CAUSES OF ABDOMINAL PAIN

1. **Lead poisoning.** Patients have diffuse and poorly localized pain, with a rigid abdomen. They may also have mental status changes, peripheral neuropathy, and anemia. Diagnosis is confirmed by serum lead level. Treatment consists of chelation therapy.

2. **Porphyria.** Presenting symptoms include colicky abdominal pain, vomiting and diarrhea or constipation, proximal myalgias, peripheral neuropathy, mental status changes, and diaphoresis. Patients often have an ileus, with abdominal distension. Treatment with Hemin (a heme oxygenase substrate analog) may be considered. Therapy is otherwise supportive. Exacerbating agents should be avoided.

3. **Familial Mediterranean fever** is an autosomal recessive disorder characterized by recurrent and severe episodes of abdominal pain (peritonitis) and fever in patients of Mediterranean background. Genetic testing is available for diagnosis. Colchicine is used for treatment or prophylaxis.

4. **Angioneurotic edema.** Severe episodic abdominal pain is caused by C1 esterase inhibitor deficiency. The C4 and C2 levels and C1 inhibitor activity are low. Treatment is supportive and symptomatic. Attenuated androgens may be effective. Transfusion with C1 inhibitor concentrate may also be useful; however, this is currently available only for research.

5. **Sphincter of Oddi dysfunction.** Spasm or stricture of the sphincter of Oddi results in elevated common bile duct pressure. Patients present with symptoms of biliary colic. Liver function tests reveal cholestasis, and right upper quadrant ultrasound shows ductal dilation. Endoscopic sphincterotomy often is effective.

6. **Eosinophilic gastroenteritis.** An eosinophilic infiltrate is present in the mucosa, muscularis, or serosa. Patients present with abdominal pain, diarrhea, nausea or vomiting, fever, malabsorption, and peripheral eosinophilia. Corticosteroids are the mainstay of treatment.

7. **Mesenteric adenitis** may present with abdominal pain or tenderness (generally RLQ, caused by enlarged lymph nodes), fever, nausea, and

acute diarrhea and often is misdiagnosed as appendicitis. Mesenteric adenitis often is caused by viral infection but may be secondary to bacterial gastroenteritis and may be associated with streptococcal pharyngitis. Joint and skin abnormalities (erythema nodosum and multiforme) may be present when infection is caused by *Yersinia* spp. The course generally is self-limited, and care is supportive.

8. **Collagenous and lymphocytic colitis.** Symptoms include crampy abdominal pain and watery diarrhea, with a predominance in middle-aged women. The diagnosis is confirmed by colonoscopy with biopsy. Treatment includes antidiarrheal agents, salicylates, and removal of any offending agents (especially nonsteroidal antiinflammatory drugs). Steroids (or other immunosuppressants) and, rarely, surgery may be necessary. Collagenous colitis often is confused with IBS.

9. **Typhlitis** (necrotizing enterocolitis) manifests as fever, RLQ pain, and tenderness in neutropenic patients; it is often misdiagnosed as appendicitis. Treatment consists of broad-spectrum antibiotics. Surgery may be necessary if peritonitis, perforation, or bleeding is present or further deterioration occurs despite appropriate nonoperative management.

10. **Graft versus host disease.** Patients may present with abdominal pain and diarrhea after bone marrow transplantation. The diagnosis is established by endoscopy with biopsy (see supplemental PDA Chapter 5).

11. **Budd-Chiari syndrome.** Hepatic vein thrombosis presents with abdominal pain, ascites, hepatomegaly, and liver failure. See Chapter 33 for more details.

PEARLS AND PITFALLS

- Consider extra-abdominal or systemic causes of abdominal pain such as esophageal spasm or rupture, myocardial ischemia, pericarditis, pneumonia, uremia, diabetic ketoacidosis, hyperparathyroidism, vasculitis, sickle cell anemia, toxins, trauma, and herpes zoster.
- Many low-risk or chronic conditions may progress to emergencies, especially late in the course or if inadequately treated.
- Expect concomitant coronary artery disease in patients with abdominal vascular disease.
- Hematoma may simulate a mass (and cause obstruction) in coagulopathic patients.
- Cervical motion tenderness denotes peritonitis and is not specific for pelvic inflammatory disease.
- Medications used for other conditions may cause or complicate abdominal disorders. For example, the medications used to treat the human immunodeficiency virus and acquired immunodeficiency syndrome can cause pancreatitis and renal stones. Steroids place patients at greater risk of gastritis, peptic ulcer disease, pancreatitis, and bowel perforation. Steroids may also mask the symptoms of many

intraabdominal conditions. Aspirin and nonsteroidal antiinflammatory drugs may cause gastritis or peptic ulcer disease and gastrointestinal bleeding.

- A diagnostic paracentesis (with specimens sent for cell count and differential, Gram stain, culture, and albumin) should be performed in all patients with ascites and abdominal pain to rule out spontaneous bacterial peritonitis (see Chapter 36).

REFERENCES

1. Stapakis JC, Thickman D: Diagnosis of pneumoperitoneum: abdominal CT scan versus upright chest film, *J Comput Assist Tomography* 16:713, 1992. B
2. Lipscomb GH, McCord ML, Stovall TG, Huff G, Portera SG, Ling FW: Predictors of success of methotrexate treatment in women with tubal ectopic pregnancies, *N Engl J Med* 341:1974-1978, 1999. B
3. Lederle FA, Johnson GR, Wilson SE, et al: Prevalence and associations of abdominal aortic aneurysm detected through screening. Aneurysm Detection and Management (ADAM) Veterans Affairs Cooperative Study Group, *Ann Intern Med* 126:441-449, 1997. B
4. Salo JA et al: Familial occurrence of abdominal aortic aneurysm, *Ann Intern Med* 130:637, 1999. B
5. Powell JT, Greenhalgh RM: Small abdominal aortic aneurysms, *N Engl J Med* 348:1895-1901, 2003. C
6. La Roy LL et al: Imaging of abdominal aortic aneurysms, *AJR Am J Roentgenol* 152:785, 1989. C
7. Suri S et al: Comparative evaluation of plain films, ultrasound and CT in the diagnosis of intestinal obstruction, *Acta Radiol* 40:422, 1999. B
8. Jalan KN et al: An experience with ulcerative colitis: toxic dilatation in 55 cases, *Gastroenterology* 57:68, 1969. B
9. Balthazar EJ et al: Acute appendicitis: CT and ultrasound correlation in one hundred patients, *Radiology* 190:31, 1994. B
10. Jeffrey RB Jr et al: Acute appendicitis: sonographic criteria based on 250 cases, *Radiology* 167:327, 1988. B
11. Schwartz SI: Appendix. In SI Schwartz, ed: *Principles of surgery,* 6th ed, New York, 1994, McGraw-Hill. C
12. Lee EJ, Kwon HC, Joo HJ, Suh JH, Fleischer AC: Diagnosis of ovarian torsion with color Doppler sonography: depiction of twisted vascular pedicle, *J Ultrasound Med* 17:83-89, 1998. B
13. Taourel PG et al: Acute mesenteric ischemia: diagnosis with contrast-enhanced CT, *Radiology* 199:632, 1996. B
14. Suleiman S, Johnston DE: The abdominal wall: an overlooked source of pain, *Am Fam Physician* 64:431-438, 2001. C
15. Thompson WG et al: Functional bowel disorders. In DA Drossman et al, eds: *Rome II: the functional gastrointestinal disorders,* 2nd ed, McLean, Va, 2000, Degnon Associates. C
16. Olive DL, Pritts EA: Treatment of endometriosis, *N Engl J Med* 345:266-275, 2001. C

30

APPROACH TO ABDOMINAL PAIN

Acute Pancreatitis

Melissa A. Munsell, MD; Geoffrey C. Nguyen, MD; and Mary L. Harris, MD

FAST FACTS

- Acute pancreatitis is a potentially fatal disease with a mortality rate of 5% to 10%.
- Gallstones and alcohol account for 80% of acute pancreatitis.
- Diagnosis is based on clinical findings and confirmed by elevated serum amylase or lipase concentrations three times the upper limit of normal or radiographic findings of pancreatic inflammation or necrosis.
- Assessment of severity by Ranson's score, APACHE-II criteria, or computed tomography (CT) scan is a crucial step in management.
- Prophylactic antibiotics are indicated in acute necrotizing pancreatitis.

I. EPIDEMIOLOGY

1. Acute pancreatitis is inflammation of the pancreas that may involve peripancreatic tissue or remote organs and may also have local complications, such as pancreatic necrosis or pseudocyst formation.[1]
2. Acute pancreatitis is common. The incidence is as high as 38 per 100,000 population per year, with a mortality rate of 5% to 10%.[2,3]
3. Gallstones and alcohol account for more than 80% of cases. Box 31-1 outlines the conditions associated with acute pancreatitis.[4]
4. Most cases of gallstone pancreatitis are associated with transient impaction of a stone in the pancreatic ampulla. Gallstone pancreatitis is more common in women, with peak incidence between 50 and 60 years of age.

II. CLINICAL PRESENTATION

1. The hallmark of acute pancreatitis is continuous, boring, epigastric, right upper quadrant or diffuse abdominal pain. The onset of pain is gradual, peaks in 30 to 60 minutes, and then remains steady. In about half of cases, the abdominal pain may have a bandlike radiation to the back. Nausea and vomiting accompany pain in 90% of cases. Patients may find relief by bending forward.
2. Systemic signs can include fever, tachycardia, tachypnea, and, in severe cases, hypotension.
3. Depending on the severity of the inflammation, the abdominal examination can vary from minimal tenderness to distension with peritoneal signs. Intraabdominal hemorrhage, though uncommon, is manifested by periumbilical (Cullen's sign) or flank (Grey Turner's sign) ecchymoses.[2]

BOX 31-1

COMMON CAUSES OF PANCREATITIS

Gallstones

Alcohol

Idiopathic

Hypertriglyceridemia (usually with serum triglyceride concentrations >1000 mg/dl)

Hypercalcemia

Drugs (thiazides, azathioprine, ethacrynic acid, furosemide, tetracycline, oral contraceptives, 6-mercaptopurine, asparaginase, pentamidine, and didanosine)

Trauma

Previous endoscopic retrograde cholangiopancreatography

Sphincter of Oddi dysfunction

Viral infections (mumps, coxsackievirus, hepatitis A, B, and non-A, non-B, cytomegalovirus)

Anatomical abnormalities (pancreatic divisum)

OTHER CAUSES

Bacterial infection (*Mycoplasma,* legionnaires' disease, *Campylobacter*)

Cardiopulmonary bypass

Crohn's disease

Cystic fibrosis

Toxins (scorpion venom, methyl alcohol)

End-stage renal failure

Familial pancreatitis

Hyperparathyroidism

Hypothermia, idiopathic

Intraductal parasites

Major abdominal surgery

Mesenteric ischemia or embolism

Organ transplantation (cytomegalovirus)

Pancreatic tumors

Penetrating gastric or duodenal ulcer

Pregnancy

Shock

Upper gastrointestinal endoscopy

Vasculitis

4. The clinician should consider other causes of acute abdominal pain. The differential diagnosis of acute pancreatitis is listed in Box 31-2.

III. DIAGNOSIS

Acute pancreatitis is a clinical diagnosis and is confirmed by either serum biological markers or radiologic findings.

A. LABORATORY EVALUATION

1. **Serum amylase** levels rise within 12 hours of the onset of pain. Levels greater than three times the upper limit of normal are characteristic of pancreatitis and usually do not occur in other conditions such as

> **BOX 31-2**
>
> **DIFFERENTIAL DIAGNOSIS OF ACUTE PANCREATITIS**
>
> Acutely perforated ulcer
>
> Acute cholecystitis
>
> Acute intestinal obstruction
>
> Acute mesenteric ischemia
>
> Renal colic
>
> Hyperamylasemia is also seen in mumps, ectopic pregnancy, and renal failure

    salivary injury, viscous perforation, mesenteric ischemia, or renal failure.[5] Serum amylase concentrations usually normalize within 7 days in uncomplicated cases. High triglyceride levels (> 1000 mg/dl) may mask high serum amylase levels.

2. **Serum lipase** concentrations greater than three times the upper limit of normal are characteristic of acute pancreatitis and are associated with a higher sensitivity and specificity than serum amylase concentrations. Lipase remains elevated for 7 to 14 days.

3. **Amylase and lipase levels do not correlate with severity.** For example, in severe necrotizing pancreatitis, serum amylase and lipase may be normal.[6] Daily measurement of serum amylase and lipase has no clinical value.

4. **Alanine aminotransferase level greater than 150 IU/L is highly suggestive of gallstone pancreatitis.**[7] A lipase/amylase ratio greater than 2 suggests alcohol as the cause.[8,9]

B. IMAGING

1. **Abdominal radiograph.** An abdominal radiograph should be obtained to evaluate for other causes of abdominal symptoms (e.g., obstruction). A sentinel loop suggests severe pancreatitis.

2. **Right upper quadrant ultrasound** imaging is the test of choice to detect gallstone pancreatitis and should be performed within 48 hours of presentation to evaluate for cholelithiasis and dilation of common bile duct.

3. **Contrast-enhanced CT** is the test of choice to diagnose and assess the severity of acute pancreatitis. Although findings are normal in 15% to 30% of mild cases, abnormal findings are always present in moderate and severe pancreatitis.

a. Indications for abdominal CT include the following:

    (1) Uncertain clinical diagnosis.

    (2) Hyperamylasemia and severe clinical pancreatitis, abdominal distension, tenderness, high fever (higher than 39° C), and leukocytosis.

    (3) Ranson's score greater than 3 or APACHE-II score greater than 8 (Table 31-1)

    (4) No improvement after 72 hours of initial conservative therapy.

    (5) Acute deterioration after initial clinical improvement.[10]

TABLE 31-1
RANSON'S CRITERIA

At Admission	At 48 Hours
Age > 55 yr	Hematocrit decrease of > 10%
White blood cell count > 16,000/mm³	Blood urea nitrogen level increase of > 5 mg/dl
Glucose level > 200 mg/dl	Calcium level < 8 mg/dl
Lactate dehydrogenase level > 350 IU/L	PaO_2 < 60 mmHg
Aspartate aminotransferase level > 250 IU/L	Base deficit > 4 mEq/L
	Fluid sequestration > 6 L

Risk Factors	Mortality
0-2	< 1%
3-4	15%
5-6	40%
> 6	100%

b. Abdominal CT allows assessment of the degree of pancreatic inflammation and presence of peripancreatic fluid. The use of intravenous (IV) contrast medium can distinguish between pancreatic edema and necrosis because the latter does not enhance.

IV. MANAGEMENT (Fig. 31-1)

A. ASSESSMENT

Assessment of severity is the first step in the management of acute pancreatitis.

1. Most episodes of pancreatitis are mild, and patients typically recover within 7 days with supportive management.
2. Severe pancreatitis is characterized by a Ranson's score > 3 or an APACHE-II score greater than 8; organ failure; or local complications, such as necrosis, abscess, or pseudocyst.
3. Organ failure is the most important indicator of severity and is defined by shock with systolic blood pressure < 90 mmHg, pulmonary insufficiency with $PaO_2 \leq$ 60 mmHg, renal failure with creatinine level > 2 mg/dl, and gastrointestinal bleeding of > 500 ml/24 hr.[6]
4. Severe necrotizing pancreatitis is associated with significantly higher rates of complications and mortality.
5. Scoring systems, CT imaging, and biochemical markers are all used in conjunction with clinical assessment to predict severity.

a. **APACHE-II** provides instantaneous assessment of the severity of pancreatitis and can be implemented on the day of admission. It has superior sensitivity and specificity in distinguishing mild from severe pancreatitis during the initial evaluation and can be monitored on a daily basis. An initial score of 8 or less suggests minimal risk of death, and a score greater than 9 is a strong indicator of severe pancreatitis (see Chapter 17).[6,10-13]

b. **Ranson's criteria** are much simpler than APACHE-II but take 48 hours to complete (see Table 31-1).

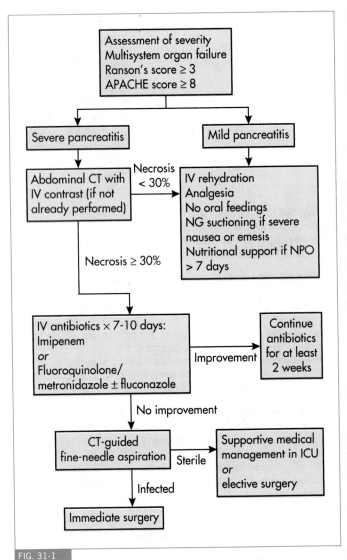

FIG. 31-1
Management of acute pancreatitis. *CT,* computed tomography; *ICU,* intensive care unit; *IV,* intravenous, *NG,* nasogastric; *NPO,* nothing by mouth.

c. **The CT severity index** is based on a combination of prognostic indicators, including extent of pancreatic necrosis and degree of peripancreatic inflammation (Table 31-2). This score has a strong correlation with risk for both local complications and death.[14] A CT scan should be obtained for further risk stratification when severe pancreatitis is suspected on the basis of Ranson's score or APACHE-II criteria.

d. **C-reactive protein** is an acute phase reactant that is a sensitive marker for necrotizing pancreatitis. A peak C-reactive protein level of 210 mg/L on the second, third, or fourth day or a level higher than 120 mg/L on the seventh day predicts severe disease.[15,16]

e. **Hematocrit.** A value of 47% or more at the time of admission is also a risk factor for severe pancreatic necrosis.[17]

B. MANAGEMENT OF MILD PANCREATITIS

1. Mild pancreatitis is characterized by an APACHE-II score of 8 or less and the absence of organ failure, pancreatic necrosis, or high-grade pancreatic inflammation on CT.

2. Treatment is largely supportive and includes IV fluids, analgesia (IV narcotics and patient-controlled analgesia), and nasogastric suctioning for patients with severe nausea or emesis.

3. Patients should take nothing by mouth (NPO) until their need for IV narcotics is minimal or being tapered off. Once abdominal pain has subsided, bowel sounds have returned, and the patient is hungry, a clear liquid diet can be started and advanced as tolerated over several days.[6] Nutritional support should be provided to patients who are NPO for more than 7 days.

ACUTE PANCREATITIS **31**

TABLE 31-2

CTSI

CT Grade	CTSI Points
A: Normal pancreas	0
B: Focal or diffuse enlargement of the pancreas	1
C: Pancreatic abnormalities accompanied by mild peripancreatic inflammation	3
D: Single fluid collection, usually within anterior pararenal space	4
E: Two or more fluid collections near the pancreas or the presence of gas in or adjacent to the pancreas	5

NECROSIS	
None	0
< 33%	2
33-50%	4
> 50%	6

CTSI = CT GRADE(0-5) + NECROSIS (0-6)

Total Points	Complications	Mortality
0-3	8%	< 3%
4-6	35%	6%
7-11	92%	17%

CT, computed tomography; *CTSI,* computed tomography severity index.

C. MANAGEMENT OF SEVERE PANCREATITIS

1. Patients with severe pancreatitis, as defined by organ failure, an APACHE-II score greater than 9, and evidence of necrosis of more than 30% of the pancreas, should be monitored in an intensive care setting.

2. Supportive therapy should include nutritional support, systemic antibiotics, and early surgical consultation if structural complications develop.

3. **Nutrition.** As noted earlier, patients who are NPO for more than 7 days should receive either enteral nutrition through a nasojejunal tube or total parenteral nutrition. Enteral feeding is safe even in severe acute pancreatitis and is preferred because it reduces the risk of catheter-related infections. Furthermore, enteral nutrients are thought to maintain the intestinal barrier.[6,10,18,19]

4. **Prophylactic antibiotics.** Localized infection develops in approximately one third of patients with severe necrotizing pancreatitis and is a leading cause of morbidity and mortality.

   a. Patients with severe pancreatitis should be started on broad-spectrum antibiotics to include gram negatives and anaerobes.[6,10,20-23]

   b. IV antibiotics should be continued for at least 14 days.

   c. Fluconazole should be considered because broad-spectrum antibiotics predispose to fungal infection, which has a higher mortality in necrotizing pancreatitis.[24,25]

5. **Severe pancreatitis without improvement.** Infected necrotic tissue develops in 40% to 70% of cases of necrotizing pancreatitis and is a leading cause of mortality.[26] Patients who do not improve clinically within 14 days on antibiotics should undergo a CT-guided aspiration of the necrotic pancreas to distinguish between sterile and infected necrosis.[22,27,28] Infected pancreatic necrosis evident by Gram stain and confirmed later by culture warrants immediate surgical debridement.[29] Patients with sterile necrosis can be treated with continued medical therapy or elective surgery in several weeks.

6. **Pseudocysts** complicate approximately 1% to 8% of cases of acute pancreatitis[1] and are defined as localized collections of pancreatic secretions that lack an epithelial lining. Most pseudocysts are asymptomatic, are diagnosed by CT scan or ultrasound, and resolve spontaneously. Pseudocysts greater than 5 cm in diameter, those that are symptomatic (e.g., pain or gastric outlet obstruction), and those that are complicated by infection or hemorrhage warrant intervention. Surgical, percutaneous, and endoscopic drainage procedures are options for treatment but have not been adequately compared in controlled trials.[2] The clinical scenario guides the treatment approach.

D. MANAGEMENT OF GALLSTONE PANCREATITIS

1. Most cases of gallstone pancreatitis do not warrant endoscopic retrograde cholangiopancreatography (ERCP) because common bile duct stones usually pass spontaneously into the duodenum. Prompt ERCP should be performed if patients have evidence of obstructive jaundice or cholangitis.[30-32]

2. ERCP may be performed electively for patients with persistent common bile duct stones but without cholangitis or progressive jaundice.
3. Patients with mild gallstone pancreatitis should undergo elective cholecystectomy within 7 days after recovery.
4. Surgery may be delayed for at least 3 weeks in severe gallstone pancreatitis because of an increased risk of infection.[33]

PEARLS AND PITFALLS

- A patient is allowed one episode of pancreatitis of unclear cause without an exhaustive workup for underlying causes.
- ERCP should be performed if a recurrent episode of "idiopathic" pancreatitis occurs.[34]
- After ERCP, only 10% of cases of acute pancreatitis are truly idiopathic.
- Acute pancreatitis is 35 to 800 times more common in patients with the human immunodeficiency virus.[35]
- Drugs such as didanosine and pentamidine are the most common causes of acute pancreatitis in patients with the human immunodeficiency virus.[35]
- Opportunistic infections such as cytomegalovirus should be identified as potential causes of acute pancreatitis and treated aggressively.

REFERENCES

1. Steinberg W, Tenner S: Acute pancreatitis, *N Engl J Med* 330:1198, 1994. C
2. Mergener K, Baillie J: Acute pancreatitis, *BMJ* 316:44, 1998. D
3. Neoptolemos JP et al: Acute pancreatitis: the substantial human and financial costs, *Gut* 42:886, 1998. D
4. Sakorafas GH, Tsiotou AG: Etiology and pathogenesis of acute pancreatitis: current concepts, *J Clin Gastroenterol* 30:343, 2000. C
5. Vissers RJ et al: Amylase and lipase in the emergency department evaluation of acute pancreatitis, *J Emerg Med* 17:1027, 1999. C
6. Banks PA: Practice guidelines in acute pancreatitis, *Am J Gastroenterol* 92:377, 1997. D
7. Tenner S, Dubner H, Steinberg W: Predicting gallstone pancreatitis with laboratory parameters: a meta-analysis, *Am J Gastroenterol* 89:1863, 1994. C
8. Gumaste VV et al: Lipase/amylase ratio: a new index that distinguishes acute episodes of alcoholic from nonalcoholic acute pancreatitis, *Gastroenterology* 101:1361, 1991. B
9. Tenner SM, Steinberg W: The admission serum lipase: amylase ratio differentiates alcoholic from nonalcoholic acute pancreatitis, *Am J Gastroenterol* 87:1755, 1992. B
10. Wyncoll DL: The management of severe acute necrotising pancreatitis: an evidence-based review of the literature, *Intensive Care Med* 25:146, 1999. C
11. Larvin M, McMahon MJ: APACHE-II score for assessment and monitoring of acute pancreatitis, *Lancet* 334:201, 1989. B
12. Dervenis C, Bassi C: Evidence-based assessment of severity and management of acute pancreatitis, *Br J Surg* 87:257, 2000. C
13. Wilson C et al: Prediction of outcome in acute pancreatitis: a comparative study of APACHE-II, clinical assessment and multiple factor scoring systems, *Br J Surg* 77:1260, 1990. B
14. Balthazar EJ et al: Acute pancreatitis: value of CT in establishing prognosis, *Radiology* 174:331, 1990. B

31

ACUTE PANCREATITIS

15. Pezzilli R et al: Serum interleukin-6, interleukin-8, and beta 2-microglobulin in early assessment of severity of acute pancreatitis: comparison with serum C-reactive protein, *Dig Dis Sci* 40:2341, 1995. B

16. Wilson C et al: C-reactive protein, antiproteases and complement factors as objective markers of severity in acute pancreatitis, *Br J Surg* 76:177, 1989. B

17. Baillargeon JD et al: Hemoconcentration as an early risk factor for necrotizing pancreatitis, *Am J Gastroenterol* 93:2130, 1998. B

18. Kalfarentzos F et al: Enteral nutrition is superior to parenteral nutrition in severe acute pancreatitis: results of a randomized prospective trial, *Br J Surg* 84:1665, 1997. A

19. Guillou PJ: Enteral versus parenteral nutrition in acute pancreatitis, *Baillieres Best Pract Res Clin Gastroenterol* 13:345, 1999. D

20. Sainio V et al: Early antibiotic treatment in acute necrotising pancreatitis, *Lancet* 346:663, 1995. A

21. Pederzoli P et al: A randomized multicenter clinical trial of antibiotic prophylaxis of septic complications in acute necrotizing pancreatitis with imipenem, *Surg Gynecol Obstet* 176:480, 1993. A

22. Ratschko M et al: The role of antibiotic prophylaxis in the treatment of acute pancreatitis, *Gastroenterol Clin North Am* 28:641, 1999. C

23. Bassi C et al: Controlled clinical trial of pefloxacin versus imipenem in severe acute pancreatitis, *Gastroenterology* 115:1513, 1998. A

24. Grewe M et al: Fungal infection in acute necrotizing pancreatitis, *J Am Coll Surg* 188:408, 1999. B

25. Gloor B et al: Pancreatic infection in severe pancreatitis: the role of fungus and multiresistant organisms, *Arch Surg* 136:592, 2001. B

26. Isenmann R, Beger HG: Natural history of acute pancreatitis and the role of infection, *Baillieres Best Pract Res Clin Gastroenterol* 13:291, 1999. D

27. Gerzof SG et al: Early diagnosis of pancreatic infection by computed tomography–guided aspiration, *Gastroenterology* 93:1315, 1987. B

28. Widdison AL, Karanjia ND: Pancreatic infection complicating acute pancreatitis, *Br J Surg* 80:148, 1993. C

29. Baron TH, Morgan DE: Acute necrotizing pancreatitis, *N Engl J Med* 340:1412, 1999. C

30. Folsch UR et al: Early ERCP and papillotomy compared with conservative treatment for acute biliary pancreatitis. The German Study Group on Acute Biliary Pancreatitis, *N Engl J Med* 336:237, 1997. A

31. Nitsche R, Folsch UR: Role of ERCP and endoscopic sphincterotomy in acute pancreatitis, *Baillieres Best Pract Res Clin Gastroenterol* 13:331, 1999. C

32. Neoptolemos JP et al: Controlled trial of urgent endoscopic retrograde cholangiopancreatography and endoscopic sphincterotomy versus conservative treatment for acute pancreatitis due to gallstones, *Lancet* 2:979, 1988. A

33. Uhl W et al: Acute gallstone pancreatitis: timing of laparoscopic cholecystectomy in mild and severe disease, *Surg Endosc* 13:1070, 1999. B

34. Somogyi L et al: Recurrent acute pancreatitis: an algorithmic approach to identification and elimination of inciting factors, *Gastroenterology* 120:708, 2001. D

35. Dassopoulos T, Ehrenpreis ED: Acute pancreatitis in human immunodeficiency virus–infected patients: a review, *Am J Med* 107:78, 1999. C

Biliary Tract Disease

Vikesh K. Singh, MD; Jonathan P. Piccini, MD;
and Anthony N. Kalloo, MD

FAST FACTS

- With a sensitivity of 95% for the detection of gallstones, ultrasonography is the diagnostic imaging modality of choice for evaluating right upper quadrant (RUQ) pain and suspected gallstones.
- Cholangitis, or biliary obstruction complicated by infection, is defined by Charcot's triad (RUQ tenderness, fever, and jaundice) and warrants emergent antibiotic therapy and biliary decompression.
- Acalculous cholecystitis accounts for 5% to 10% of acute cholecystitis and often is a cause of occult fevers in the critically ill.

32

Biliary tract diseases comprise a range of disorders affecting the intrahepatic and extrahepatic bile ducts and the gallbladder. These disorders range from molecular disorders of uptake, conjugation, and secretion of bile (e.g., Gilbert's syndrome) to structural disorders of the biliary tree (e.g., choledochal cysts). Ductal obstruction is caused by gallstone impaction in more than 90% of cases and can lead to multiple conditions, including cholecystitis, choledocholithiasis, cholangitis, and pancreatitis. This chapter provides a framework for evaluating and treating diseases related to cholelithiasis.

I. CHOLELITHIASIS

A. EPIDEMIOLOGY AND PATHOPHYSIOLOGY

Cholelithiasis (gallstones) is found in 10% to 15% of all adults. Excess cholesterol saturation of bile, accelerated cholesterol crystal nucleation, and decreased gallbladder motility contribute to gallstone formation.[1]

1. Gallstones are classified as cholesterol, pigment, and mixed gallstones. The prevalence of each varies by geographic locale, with cholesterol and mixed stones accounting for 80% in the United States.
2. **Risk factors for cholesterol gallstone formation** include age older than 40 years, female sex, a high-fat diet, obesity, pregnancy, hyperlipidemia, bile salt loss (ileal disease or resection), diabetes, total parenteral nutrition, cystic fibrosis, and prolonged fasting.
3. Pigmented gallstones include black and brown stones. Black pigment stones are composed of an amorphous bilirubin polymer with calcium salts or bilirubinate. Risk factors include hemolytic anemias, cirrhosis, and advanced age. Brown pigment gallstones can form anywhere in the biliary tree as a consequence of infected bile with either bacteria (e.g.,

Escherichia coli) or helminths (e.g., *Ascaris lumbricoides, Opisthorchis senensis*).

B. PRESENTATION

Gallstones are asymptomatic in 80% of people; however, 1% to 2% of patients with cholelithiasis become symptomatic or develop complications each year.

1. Risk factors for the development of symptomatic cholelithiasis include hemolytic anemia, large gallstones (> 2.5 cm in diameter), and morbid obesity.
2. Symptomatic cholelithiasis or chronic cholecystitis typically presents with constant RUQ or epigastric pain beginning within 1 hour after eating and lasting from 20 minutes to several hours. Patients with symptomatic cholelithiasis may also present with a wide variety of nonspecific abdominal complaints including pain, nausea, and flatulence. Given the high prevalence of asymptomatic gallstones, the challenge is to identify the patients whose symptoms are caused by their gallstones. Testing may be necessary to exclude other gastrointestinal disorders.
3. Other diseases that can present in a similar fashion include peptic ulcer disease, esophageal spasm, acute pancreatitis, and myocardial infarction.
4. There is no role for surgical treatment in asymptomatic cholelithiasis. The risk of prophylactic surgery outweighs the risk of observation.

C. DIAGNOSIS

Ultrasonography is the imaging modality of choice for suspected cholelithiasis because it is 95% sensitive for the detection of gallstones. In contrast, computed tomography has a sensitivity of only 20%.

D. TREATMENT

The treatment of choice for symptomatic gallstones is laparoscopic cholecystectomy. Laparoscopic cholecystectomy has a mortality rate of 0.1% to 0.3%, allows rapid recovery, and prevents recurrence of gallstone disease. The primary disadvantage of the procedure is a slightly higher incidence of common hepatic or bile duct injury when compared with open cholecystectomy. Other treatment options include lithotripsy, bile salt dissolution therapy, and percutaneous cholecystostomy and are reserved for patients unfit for surgery.

II. ACUTE CALCULOUS CHOLECYSTITIS

A. PATHOPHYSIOLOGY

Acute cholecystitis is caused by gallstone impaction in the cystic duct, which leads to gallbladder swelling, an acute inflammatory response, and secondary bacterial infection.

B. PRESENTATION

Acute cholecystitis must be distinguished from uncomplicated biliary colic, which is not associated with obstruction (Table 32-1). Patients may have had attacks of biliary colic in the past or can present with acute cholecystitis as an initial manifestation of gallstone disease.

TABLE 32-1

CLINICAL FEATURES OF BILIARY COLIC AND ACUTE CHOLECYSTITIS

Clinical Findings	Biliary Colic	Acute Cholecystitis
Right upper quadrant pain	Present	Present
Abdominal tenderness	Absent to mild	Moderate to severe, especially over the liver or gallbladder (Murphy's sign)
Fever	Absent	Usually present
Leukocytosis	Absent	Usually > 11,000/μl
Duration of symptoms	< 4 hr	> 6 hr
Ultrasound	Gallstones	Gallstones, thickening of the gallbladder wall
Hydroxyiminodiacetic acid scan	Gallbladder visualized within 4 hr	No filling of the gallbladder

Modified from Goldman L: *Cecil Textbook of Medicine*, 22nd ed, Philadelphia, 2004, Saunders.

C. DIAGNOSIS

Acute calculous cholecystitis is a clinical diagnosis that is confirmed with diagnostic imaging.

1. Ultrasound findings of cholecystitis include a distended gallbladder, pericholecystic fluid, a thickened gallbladder wall, gallstones, and an ultrasonographic Murphy's sign.
2. If the diagnosis remains in doubt after ultrasonography, biliary scintigraphy (hydroxyiminodiacetic acid [HIDA] scan) can be pursued. HIDA scanning is 95% sensitive and is the most specific test for acute cholecystitis. The test involves an intravenous (IV) injection of radiolabeled hydroxyiminodiacetic acid followed by abdominal scanning 1 to 2 hours later. Normally, the isotope is taken up by the liver, excreted in the biliary system, and concentrated in the gallbladder. In acute cholecystitis, the gallbladder does not take up any radiolabeled HIDA and therefore is not seen on abdominal scanning.

D. TREATMENT

The medical management of acute cholecystitis centers on bowel rest, IV hydration, analgesia, and antibiotic therapy.

1. Some patients improve with conservative therapy through spontaneous disimpaction of the gallstone from the cystic duct.
2. When cystic duct obstruction does not subside, complications may arise, including sepsis, gangrenous cholecystitis, gallbladder empyema, or gallbladder perforation. **Patients with fever, patients with elevated total bilirubin levels, and men are more likely to develop complications.**
3. Treatment of acute cholecystitis includes laparoscopic cholecystectomy. When performed within 72 hours of symptoms, cholecystectomy is associated with shorter hospital stays, lower complication rates, and lower conversion rates than open cholecystectomy.

4. The traditional treatment strategy of medical management followed by delayed open cholecystectomy is falling out of favor, although it is still used in patients with high surgical risk. Percutaneous cholecystostomy and endoscopic decompression by endoscopic retrograde cholangiopancreatography (ERCP) are also used in high-risk patients or patients who need a temporizing measure before cholecystectomy.[2]

III. ACUTE ACALCULOUS CHOLECYSTITIS

A. EPIDEMIOLOGY AND PATHOPHYSIOLOGY

1. Acute acalculous cholecystitis (AAC) accounts for 5% to 10% of all cholecystectomies. It usually occurs in older adults and the critically ill.
2. AAC can be caused by ischemia, infection, chemical injury, and nongallstone cystic duct obstruction. Risk factors for AAC are listed in Box 32-1.
3. AAC is more common in patients with human immunodeficiency virus infection. Fifty percent of cases of acute cholecystitis in patients with a CD4 count less than 200 are AAC. *Cytomegalovirus* and *Cryptosporidium* are the two most common causative organisms (see Chapter 51).[3]

B. PRESENTATION

For non–critically ill patients, the presentation may be similar to that of acute cholecystitis. In critically ill patients who are unable to communicate, the initial presentation may be limited to fever, leukocytosis, and abdominal guarding. **Compared with calculous cholecystitis, AAC is associated with a higher risk of complications, including gallbladder perforation and gangrene. Thirty-day mortality is about 20%.**

C. DIAGNOSIS

Ultrasound imaging may be normal early in the clinical course of AAC; however, a distended gallbladder with sludge, a thin wall, and pericholecystic fluid is characteristic of later stages of disease. Bubbles may be visualized in the wall or lumen of the gallbladder, which indicates emphysematous cholecystitis secondary to gas-forming organisms.

D. TREATMENT

Given the high frequency of complications and mortality associated with AAC, the treatment of choice is urgent cholecystostomy or cholecystectomy. Surgical consultation should be pursued immediately once a diagnosis of AAC is made. Percutaneous cholecystostomy and endoscopic decompression by ERCP are also used in high-risk patients or patients who need a temporizing measure before cholecystectomy.

IV. CHOLANGITIS

A. EPIDEMIOLOGY AND PATHOPHYSIOLOGY

1. Cholangitis complicates 1% of cholelithiasis, with a peak incidence in the seventh decade of life.
2. **Cholangitis is caused by obstruction of the common bile duct (CBD), which leads to biliary stasis, bacterial proliferation, and ascending**

BOX 32-1
RISK FACTORS AND PRIMARY ORGANISMS ASSOCIATED WITH ACALCULOUS CHOLECYSTITIS
RISK FACTORS
Fasting
Total parenteral nutrition
Septicemia (biliary infections)
Multiple transfusions
Mechanical ventilation
Opiates
Immunosuppression
Diabetes
Ischemic heart disease
Major trauma
Burns
Major surgery
Childbirth
Malignancy
CAUSATIVE ORGANISMS
Salmonella typhi
Vibrio cholera
Mycobacteria spp.
Cryptosporidium
Clostridium perfringens
Cytomegalovirus
Campylobacter jejuni
Candida spp.

Modified from Table 158-6 in Afdhal NH: Diseases of the gallbladder and bile ducts. In *Cecil textbook of medicine,* 22nd ed, Philadelphia, 2004, Saunders.

32

infection. More than half of cases of cholangitis are caused by gallstone impaction in the CBD; however, biliary stent occlusion, strictures, tumors, and liver flukes (e.g., *Clonorchis sinensis*) can also cause cholangitis.

B. PRESENTATION

1. Clinically, cholangitis is characterized by the presence of Charcot's triad: fever and chills, RUQ pain and tenderness, and jaundice. However, only 50% to 80% of patients present with all three findings. Patients who do present with all three may also have hypotension and change in mental status, a constellation of clinical findings known as Reynolds' pentad. Mortality approaches 70% in patients with Reynolds' pentad.

2. Local and systemic complications of cholangitis include bacteremia, sepsis, pancreatitis, and hepatic abscess formation.

C. DIAGNOSIS

1. In the appropriate clinical context, RUQ ultrasound demonstrating a dilated CBD is diagnostic for cholangitis. The CBD may not be dilated early in presentation or with small choledocholithiasis. Other imaging modalities include ERCP and magnetic resonance cholangiopancreatography.
2. Fifty percent of patients with cholangitis have positive blood cultures, usually with enteric gram-negative organisms (e.g., *E. coli, Klebsiella*).

D. TREATMENT

Treatment involves antibiotic therapy and biliary decompression.

1. Extended-spectrum penicillins with beta-lactamase inhibitors (piperacillin and tazobactam 3.375 g IV every 6 hours) and third- and fourth-generation cephalosporins (ceftriaxone 2 g IV every 12 hours, cefepime 2 g IV every 12 hours) are the antibiotics of choice for acute cholangitis.
2. Decompression of the biliary tree can be accomplished several ways; ERCP with sphincterotomy is the most common method of decompression because it is effective and has a low complication rate.[4] Alternative methods include percutaneous transhepatic external biliary drainage and open surgical decompression.

PEARLS AND PITFALLS

- "Biliary colic" is a misnomer because cystic duct occlusion produces a constant rather than a colicky or cramping pain. It usually occurs between 15 minutes and 1 hour after eating (especially after fatty foods) and may last for several minutes or continue for hours.
- The laboratory abnormalities of cholestasis are characterized by elevation of alkaline phosphatase and gamma-glutamyltransferase; however, acute obstruction of the CBD can present with significantly elevated aspartate aminotransferase and alanine aminotransferase, mimicking acute hepatitis.
- Common causes of drug-induced cholestasis include penicillin antibiotics, erythromycin, nitrofurantoin, oral contraceptives, and phenothiazines.

REFERENCES

1. Johnston DE, Kaplan MM: Pathogenesis and treatment of gallstones, *N Engl J Med* 328(6):412-421, 1993. D
2. Papi C, Catarci M, D'Ambrosio L, et al: Timing of cholecystectomy for acute calculous cholecystitis: a meta-analysis, *Am J Gastroenterol* 99(1):147-155, 2004. C
3. Cacciarelli AG, Naddaf SY, el-Zeftawy HA, et al: Acute cholecystitis in AIDS patients: correlation of Tc-99m hepatobiliary scintigraphy with histopathologic laboratory findings and CD4 counts, *Clin Nucl Med* 23(4):226-228, 1998. B
4. Lai EC, Mok FP, Tan ES, et al: Endoscopic biliary drainage for severe acute cholangitis, *N Engl J Med* 326(24):1582-1586, 1992. A

Acute Liver Failure and Biochemical Liver Testing

Christopher Hoffmann, MD, MPH; David E. Kaplan, MD; and Chloe Thio, MD

> **FAST FACTS**
>
> - Acute liver failure (ALF) is a medical emergency.
> - Fulminant hepatic failure (FHF) is defined as development of encephalopathy within 8 weeks of symptoms or within 2 weeks of jaundice.
> - The most common cause of ALF in industrialized countries is acetaminophen poisoning.
> - Most deaths in FHF are caused by intracranial hypertension, sepsis, and multiorgan failure. Mortality from FHF without transplantation is 80%.[1]
> - N-Acetylcysteine for acetaminophen poisoning is the only proven treatment other than liver transplantation for ALF.
> - Early consultation with a liver transplant team is an important element in management of FHF.

I. INTERPRETATION OF BIOCHEMICAL LIVER TESTS

A. MARKERS OF CHOLESTASIS

1. **Bilirubin.** Unconjugated bilirubin is the product of heme degradation. **Unconjugated bilirubin** (approximated in laboratory testing as indirect bilirubin) is hydrophobic and bound to albumin; it is actively transported across the hepatocyte sinusoidal membrane. In the hepatocyte, it is made water soluble by conjugation to a glucuronide. **Conjugated bilirubin** (approximated in laboratory testing by direct bilirubin) is actively transported from the hepatocyte into the bile canaliculus, from which it is eliminated into the gallbladder and the duodenum via the common bile duct. The kidneys also clear small quantities of conjugated bilirubin; consequently, patients with intact renal function rarely have a bilirubin level higher than 30 mg/dl.
   a. Increased heme turnover or defects in bilirubin processing or elimination lead to hyperbilirubinemia.
   b. Bilirubin levels greater than 2.5 mg/dl can be detected on physical examination as jaundice.
   c. **Unconjugated hyperbilirubinemia usually does not exceed 7 mg/dl and usually is caused by hemolysis and hematoma resorption.** Other causes of elevated unconjugated bilirubin are medications, such as rifampin, which competitively inhibits hepatocyte uptake of bilirubin,

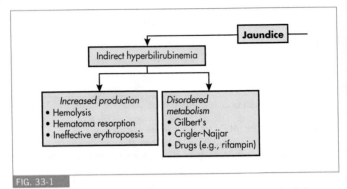

FIG. 33-1

Major causes of hyperbilirubinemia.[2] *ALT,* alanine aminotransferase; *AP,* alkaline phosphate; *CHF,* congestive heart failure.

and Gilbert's and Criglar-Najjar syndromes, disorders of enzymatic defects in the conjugation pathway.

d. **Conjugated hyperbilirubinemia** (more than 50% of total bilirubin) is caused by impaired hepatocyte secretion of bile due to primary hepatocellular causes or impaired secretion due to intrahepatic or extrahepatic bile duct obstruction.

e. **Hyperbilirubinemia** should be evaluated stepwise: First, distinguish between unconjugated and conjugated causes, then differentiate hepatocellular disease from cholestasis, and then differentiate intrahepatic from extrahepatic cholestasis (Fig. 33-1).

2. **Alkaline phosphatase (AP).** AP is an enzyme present in a variety of tissues including liver, bone, kidney, leukocytes, and some tumors; however, the major sources of AP are bone and liver. One can distinguish hepatic AP from other AP sources by either fractionating the AP or measuring gamma glutamyl transpeptidase (GGT). GGT is found in many tissues but not bone. Therefore an elevated AP and gamma glutamyl transpeptidase indicate a hepatobiliary source.

a. Biliary obstruction induces hepatocytes to synthesize AP, with detectable increases occurring 1 to 2 days after obstruction; levels gradually return to baseline over the 1-week half-life of the enzyme.

b. Mild elevations in AP (three times normal) are nonspecific; greater elevations suggest biliary obstruction (intrahepatic or extrahepatic) or infiltrative hepatic disorders such as malignancy, fungal infections, amyloidosis, or sarcoidosis.

B. MARKERS OF HEPATOCELLULAR INJURY: ALANINE AMINOTRANSFERASE AND ASPARTATE AMINOTRANSFERASE

1. Transaminitis is a common laboratory finding among ill inpatients. Alanine aminotransferase (ALT) is specific for hepatocyte necrosis,

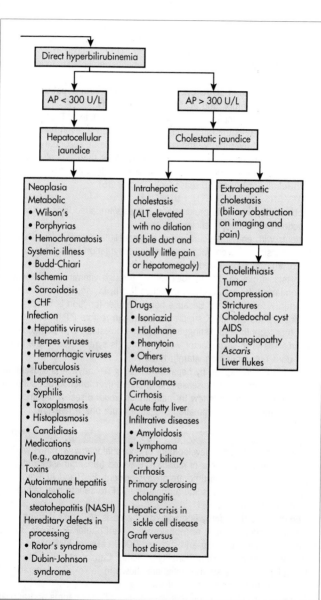

FIG. 33-1—cont'd

whereas aspartate aminotransferase (AST) is found in many tissues, including liver, muscle, kidney, brain, pancreas, and erythrocytes.

2. Modest elevations in AST and ALT (< 500 U/L) are seen in a variety of liver and systemic diseases. Alcoholic hepatitis rarely leads to levels greater than 300 U/L.

3. **Levels greater than 1000 U/L occur with acute viral hepatitis, ischemic liver injury, and acetaminophen toxicity.**

4. In most forms of acute liver injury, the ratio of AST to ALT is < 1. In alcoholic hepatitis the ratio usually is greater than 2, even with superimposed liver injury, and is hypothesized to be secondary to pyridoxine (vitamin B_6) deficiency. A ratio greater than 1 is also often seen with chronic liver disease, and a ratio greater than 3 may be seen with fulminant Wilson's disease (see Chapter 35).

C. MARKERS OF SYNTHETIC FUNCTION

1. **Prothrombin time (PT)** prolongation suggests impaired liver synthetic function or nutritional deficiency.

a. Patients with end-stage cirrhosis or hepatocellular necrosis lose capacity to synthesize sufficient factors (all major coagulation factors except for factor VIII are synthesized by the liver).

b. Cholestasis may lead to a prolonged PT through vitamin K deficiency secondary to fat malabsorption. Factors II, VII, IX, and X depend on vitamin K for synthesis. Because hepatocellular function is intact, subcutaneous vitamin K supplementation can restore PT to normal. Another technique to distinguish between cholestasis and hepatocellular necrosis is to measure factor V level, which is synthesized in the liver but does not depend on vitamin K.

2. **Albumin** is synthesized by hepatocytes (10 g per day). It is a useful in assessing chronic liver disease and impaired liver function but suffers several limitations: It is low in malnutrition, renal disease, chronic illness, and acute inflammation (negative acute phase reactant).

II. FULMINANT HEPATIC FAILURE

1. **FHF** is defined as the development of encephalopathy within 8 weeks of symptoms or 2 weeks of jaundice. Elevated transaminases and prolonged prothrombin time are always present. FHF and ALF are synonymous, although some authors use ALF to denote liver failure without encephalopathy.

2. **Hepatic encephalopathy** is graded on the basis of Conn's grading system of portosystemic encephalopathy (see Chapter 35, Table 35-2).

3. **Epidemiology.** Each year an estimated 2000 cases of FHF occur in the United States, with a mortality of 80%.[3] Causes of FHF with transplantation-free survival rates are shown in Table 33-1; overall survival with transplantation is 84%.

4. **Presentation.** FHF may present with nonspecific symptoms and appear deceptively benign. Jaundice may be the only presenting feature before a catastrophic decline. Further investigation may identify signs of

TABLE 33-1

CAUSES AND SURVIVAL RATES OF FULMINANT HEPATIC FAILURE

Cause	Total Fulminant Hepatic Failure	Transplantation-Free Survival
Acetaminophen	39%	65%
Idiosyncratic drug reaction	13%	25%
Hepatitis B	7%	23%
Ischemic	6%	59%
Hepatitis A	4%	64%
Autoimmune hepatitis	4%	17%
Wilson's disease	3%	0%
Budd-Chiari syndrome	2%	21%
Pregnancy related	2%	50%
Indeterminate or cancer	20%	15%

Reported from a 1998-2001 multicenter U.S. study consisting of 308 patients.[5]

BOX 33-1

KING'S COLLEGE HOSPITAL CRITERIA (MODIFIED LONDON CRITERIA) FOR LIVER TRANSPLANTATION IN FHF[5]

ACETAMINOPHEN-INDUCED FHF

Arterial pH < 7.3

or all 3 of the following: PT > 100 s, serum creatinine > 3.4 mg/dl, grade III-IV hepatic encephalopathy

ALL OTHER CAUSES OF FHF

PT > 100 s

or any 3 of the following: unfavorable cause (non-A, non-B viral hepatitis, drug reaction), jaundice > 7 d before hepatic encephalopathy, age < 10 or > 40 yr, bilirubin > 17.4 mg/dl

FHF, fulminant hepatic failure; PT, prothrombin time.

hepatocellular injury and dysfunction, including ALT and AST elevation, direct hyperbilirubinemia, prolonged PT, increased lactic acid from diminished hepatic metabolism (type B lactic acidosis), hypoglycemia, and elevated ammonia.

5. **Physical examination.** Stigmata of chronic liver disease, spider angiomata, palmar erythema, caput medusae, ascites, and testicular atrophy are absent unless an underlying chronic liver disease preceded the FHF.

6. **Initial evaluation** should include total serum bilirubin, direct bilirubin, sodium, ALT, AST, AP, creatinine, PT, activated partial thromboplastin time, lactate, arterial blood gas determination, ammonia, blood cultures, and diagnosis specific serologies and blood levels. Liver biopsy should be considered early.

7. **King's College criteria are associated with a poor prognosis and help guide transplantation decisions** in acetaminophen-induced and

non–acetaminophen-induced FHF (Box 33-1). Patients who survive FHF usually have no long-term sequelae.

8. **Complications of ALF** include hepatic encephalopathy, cerebral edema, coagulopathy, and bleeding. These complications and their corresponding management are reviewed in Table 33-2. **Cerebral edema is the most common cause of death in FHF.**

III. ETIOLOGY AND TREATMENT OF ALF

1. **Acetaminophen.**
   a. Ingestion of more than 10 g of acetaminophen in a 24-hour period or 4 g in 24 hours in a person who is malnourished, alcoholic, or taking anticonvulsants may cause FHF. Chronic use also decreases the single-day threshold for toxicity. Unintentional overdoses usually occur over several days with an average consumption of 34 g, whereas suicide attempts average 20 g as a single ingestion and often present sooner to medical attention. Unintentional overdoses exceed suicide attempts as a cause of ALF.[6]
   b. **Presentation.** Patients are initially asymptomatic but within the first 24 hours develop malaise, nausea, and vomiting; 24 to 72 hours after ingestion, patients develop jaundice and right upper quadrant tenderness; and 72 to 96 hours after a toxic ingestion, FHF and death occur.
   c. **Diagnosis** rests on the clinical history and serum acetaminophen level (Fig. 33-2).
   d. **Treatment** is with either oral N-acetylcysteine 140 mg/kg as initial dosage then 70 mg/kg every 4 hours for 17 doses (do not give activated charcoal simultaneously) or intravenous N-acetylcysteine 150 mg/kg over 15 minutes followed by 50 mg/kg over 4 hours, then 100 mg/kg over the next 16 hours. Treatment within 15 hours of toxic ingestion markedly improves prognosis. After 15 hours, N-acetyl cysteine reduces the risk of grade IV encephalopathy.

2. **Ethanol.** Although it is usually considered a cause of chronic liver disease, ethanol also causes acute hepatitis and can lead to FHF. Acute alcoholic hepatitis usually occurs in the setting of chronic ethanol ingestion and is thought to be caused by a cytokine-mediated acute inflammatory response rather than direct ethanol toxicity.
   a. Symptoms include low-grade fevers, anorexia, jaundice, and ascites.
   b. **Prognosis can be assessed by the Maddrey discriminant function** (4.6[PT – prothrombin control] + total serum bilirubin; prothrombin control = PT/international normalized ratio). A discriminant factor greater than 32 predicts greater than 50% mortality.[7]
   c. Patients with a discriminant factor greater than 32 should be treated with oral pentoxifylline 400 mg three times a day for 4 weeks (believed to be beneficial because of its anti–tumor necrosis factor-alpha effects)[8] and corticosteroids (may improve outcome if hepatic encephalopathy is also present).[9]

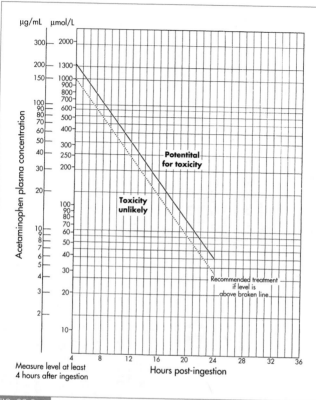

μg/mL   μmol/L

Acetaminophen plasma concentration

Potentital for toxicity

Toxicity unlikely

Recommended treatment
if level is
above broken line

Measure level at least
4 hours after ingestion

Hours post-ingestion

FIG. 33-2

Rumack-Matthew nomogram for acetaminophen poisoning. *(Data from Rumack BH, Matthew H: Pediatrics 55:871, 1975.)*

3. **Mushroom ingestion** (*Amanita phalloides, Lepiota* spp.).
   a. *Amanita* species are found mainly in the Pacific Northwest.
   b. Symptoms develop within 12 hours of ingestion: nausea, vomiting, crampy abdominal pain, and diarrhea. Pancreatic inflammation is a prominent early feature. Symptoms resolve 24 to 48 hours after ingestion. Shortly thereafter the patient abruptly declines.
   c. Treatment includes nasogastric lavage, activated charcoal, forced diuresis, penicillin G 250 mg/kg/day intravenously, and liver transplantation.[10]
4. **MDMA** (3,4-methylenedioxymethamphetamine, Ecstasy).
   a. In some European centers, MDMA is reported to be the second most common cause of liver injury in patients younger than 25 years old.

TABLE 33-2

COMPLICATIONS OF ACUTE LIVER FAILURE

	Pathophysiology	Management
General management	Possible toxin ingestion. Rapid decompensation.	Gastric lavage and activated charcoal if recent toxin exposure. N-acetylcysteine (oral or intravenous) if acetaminophen toxicity is identified by history or acetaminophen level. Risk stratification with laboratory tests: arterial blood gas, prothrombin times, creatinine, and bilirubin and assessment of encephalopathy grade. Activate transplantation workup.
Encephalopathy	Encephalopathy develops in the setting of FHF from elevated intracranial pressure and circulating toxins. (Note: Brain edema rarely occurs in decompensation from chronic liver disease.) Additional causes of encephalopathy in FHF include benzodiazepines, sepsis, and seizures.	Liver transplantation. There is little evidence supporting other interventions. The current empiric interventions are aimed at reducing serum ammonia: a low-protein diet, lactulose 30 g qid, and selective bowel decontamination with metronidazole.
Cerebral edema[13]	35-40% mortality in FHF is attributable to brain herniation thought to be caused by increased osmotic potential from glutamine produced during detoxification of ammonia via a reaction with glutamate. Intracranial hypertension is an ICP > 20 mmHg. Arterial ammonia > 200 µg/dl is associated with cerebral herniation within 24 hr of reaching stage III-IV encephalopathy. Time between onset of jaundice and encephalopathy predicts encephalopathy and survival: with encephalopathy < 1 wk from symptom onset 49% develop intercranial hypertension, acute liver failure (1-4 wk)	Management of grade III-IV encephalopathy with intubation and hyperventilation, intracranial pressure monitoring, mannitol, and hypertonic saline. Maintain the cerebral perfusion pressure (mean arterial pressure − ICP) > 50 mmHg.

Sepsis	Urinary and skin flora are the most common pathogens, with most infections from *Staphylococcus*, *Streptococcus*, and coliforms. Prolonged hospitalization and lengthy courses of antibacterial therapy predispose to fungal infections, predominantly *Candida* spp. 10-80% of patients develop positive blood cultures.	Check frequent surveillance cultures and have a low threshold for administration of antibiotics and antifungals.
Coagulopathy	Decreased coagulation factor synthesis and thrombocytopenia.	Supplement with vitamin K, minimize invasive procedures, and use fresh-frozen plasma and platelets as needed for procedures and bleeding.
Hypoglycemia	Diminished hepatic glyconeogenesis.	Use routine capillary blood glucose monitoring and hypertonic dextrose infusion for hypoglycemia.
Hypotension	Intravascular hypovolemia or sepsis.	Volume repletion with colloid and antibiotics and pressors for sepsis.
Renal failure	Prerenal azotemia from either intravascular hypovolemia or hepatorenal syndrome from splanchnic vasodilation.	Monitor central venous pressures, volume replete with colloid, may need hemofiltration or dialysis. Often requires continuous venovenous hemodialysis because of baseline hypotension.
Gastrointestinal bleeding	Results from stress ulceration and decreased coagulation from coagulopathy and thrombocytopenia.	Stress ulcer prophylaxis with proton pump inhibitor or H_2 receptor antagonist.
		Vitamin K, platelets, and fresh-frozen plasma.

FHF, fulminant hepatic failure; *ICP*, intracranial pressure.

ALF AND BIOCHEMICAL LIVER TESTING

33

b. Clinical suspicion can be confirmed with urine toxicology.

c. Patients present acutely with significantly elevated AST and ALT.

d. MDMA intoxication is associated with a good prognosis. Treatment is largely supportive.

5. **Direct toxins and idiosyncratic drug reactions.** Herbal supplements, phosphorus, carbon tetrachloride, copper salts, arsenicals, valproic acid, carbamazepine, phenytoin, isoniazid, pyrazinamide, ketoconazole, terbinafine, methyldopa, nucleoside reverse transcriptase inhibitors, disulfiram, methotrexate, nefazodone, halothane, propylthiouracil, and tetracycline are all known causes of ALF. Toxicity may develop after brief or long-term exposure and may lead to fulminant or subacute hepatic failure.

6. **Viral hepatitis** is discussed in Chapter 34; however, several points regarding FHF and viral hepatitis merit emphasis here.

a. Less than 1% of patients with hepatitis A develop FHF. Hepatitis A is more likely to cause FHF in the setting of chronic hepatitis B or C.

b. Hepatitis B–related FHF often progresses rapidly, leading to death within 10 days of the onset of jaundice.[11] Rash, arthralgias or arthritis, and loss of taste for smoking are nonspecific symptoms that may precede hepatic symptoms in acute hepatitis B by several weeks.

c. Reactivation hepatitis B may occur during immune reconstitution in patients with the human immunodeficiency virus who are on antiretroviral therapy. Symptoms and disease progression may parallel de novo acute hepatitis B infection.

d. Antiviral medications (lamivudine 300 mg daily or tenofovir 300 mg daily) may improve outcome in reactivation hepatitis B and severe acute hepatitis B.[12]

e. Hepatitis C rarely presents as acute hepatitis and is not a reported cause of ALF in the United States, although there are case reports of hepatitis C–associated FHF in Japan.

7. **Herpes viruses (cytomegalovirus, Epstein-Barr virus, herpes simplex virus, varicella-zoster virus)** can lead to ALF, especially among immunocompromised patients. Patients usually present with nonspecific signs and symptoms, including anorexia, nausea, lethargy, fever, and abdominal pain. Patients with herpes simplex virus hepatitis often are anicteric. Those with varicella may have a rash. Diagnosis is based on serologic testing, quantitative polymerase chain reaction, and liver biopsy demonstrating viral inclusion bodies. Antiviral therapy is the mainstay of treatment: ganciclovir for cytomegalovirus and acyclovir for herpes simplex virus and varicella-zoster virus.

8. **The Budd-Chiari syndrome** is hepatic venous outflow obstruction of any origin. Common predisposing conditions include polycythemia vera (10% to 40% of cases), myeloproliferative disorders, other hypercoagulable states, and tumor invasion.[13]

a. Symptoms usually are nonspecific and include nausea, vomiting, and mild jaundice. Disease onset may range from fulminant to chronic. The degree of liver failure depends on acuity of onset (and subsequent development of venous collaterals).

b. Doppler ultrasound of the liver is 85% sensitive and specific. Magnetic resonance imaging and computed tomography have better sensitivity, but venography is the diagnostic gold standard.

c. Treatment depends on the extent of hepatic necrosis and impairment and includes anticoagulation, thrombolytics, angioplasty, transjugular intrahepatic portosystemic shunt, and liver transplantation.

9. **Venoocclusive disease (VOD)** is a common complication of stem cell transplantation (> 50%) and is thought to be caused by chemotherapy- and radiation-associated endothelial dysfunction in the terminal hepatic venules.

a. VOD is a clinical diagnosis characterized by the triad of painful hepatomegaly, fluid retention (> 5% weight gain), and jaundice (bilirubin greater than 15 mg/dl).

b. Doppler ultrasonography of the hepatic vein may demonstrate flow reversal but is not diagnostic; imaging is most useful to exclude other diagnoses (e.g., hepatic vein thrombosis).

c. Risk of VOD can be reduced by the use of ursodeoxycholic acid and heparin.

d. VOD complicated by FHF carries a grave prognosis. Options for treatment include tissue plasminogen activator and liver transplantation.

10. **Autoimmune hepatitis** usually is not a fulminant process but can progress to fulminant decompensation (see Chapter 35).

11. **Wilson's disease** can present with ALF. Twenty-four–hour urine copper and examination for Kayser-Fleischer rings around the iris should be included early in evaluation of acute liver disease. Ceruloplasmin has limited sensitivity and specificity in acute hepatitis. For more details, see Chapter 35.

12. **Ischemia (shock liver)** occurs with severe systemic hypotension, usually accompanied by multiorgan failure. A known episode of hypotension followed by rapid rise (often > 1000 U/L) and fall in transaminases is diagnostic. Treatment is supportive, and the outcome usually is good if the underlying precipitant resolves.

13. **Neoplastic infiltration of the liver** can present with ALF, most commonly the lymphoproliferative disorders (especially lymphomas) and melanoma. Patients often present with abdominal pain or jaundice. Treatment is directed at the underlying malignancy.

14. **Reye's syndrome** is a syndrome of acute encephalopathy and ALF, usually with a history of antecedent viral illness and salicylate therapy. It is most commonly seen in children 6 to 9 years old; however, it is rare in adults.

PEARLS AND PITFALLS

- Apparently mild and resolving hepatitis can suddenly and precipitously decompensate. Always complete a thorough history and evaluation

at the earliest time and be prepared to refer the patient for liver transplantation.
- Isolated hyperbilirubinemia is a common finding among hospitalized patients. It can be caused by immune phenomenon and is seen with some medications and infections such as leptospirosis.
- Pay close attention to signs of intracranial hypertension and sepsis because these are the leading causes of mortality in FHF.
- Hemochromatosis is an important cause of cirrhosis but does not cause acute hepatitis or acute liver failure. Iron studies drawn in patients with FHF awaiting transplantation in the setting of acute hepatitis often are abnormal, with high transferrin saturation, ferritin, and plasma iron; these values should not be misinterpreted to represent hemochromatosis.
- A prodrome of myalgias, arthralgias, rash, or constitutional symptoms weeks to months before rising transaminases suggests an infectious cause such as hepatitis B virus.
- Transaminase elevations occurring during an inpatient admission usually are related to medications.

REFERENCES

1. Trey C: The fulminant hepatic failure surveillance study. Brief review of the effects of presumed etiology and age of survival, Can Med Assoc J 106(Suppl):525-527, 1972. B
2. Feldman M, Friedman LS, Sleisenger MH: Sleisenger & Fordtran's gastrointestinal and liver disease, 7th ed, Philadelphia, 2002, WB Saunders. C
3. Lee W: Acute liver failure, N Engl J Med 329:1862-1872, 1993. B
4. Ostapowitcz G et al: Results of a prospective study of acute liver failure at 17 tertiary care centers in the United States, Ann Intern Med 137:947-954, 2002. B
5. Dhiman RK et al: Prognostic evaluation of early indicators in fulminant hepatic failure by multivariate analysis, Dig Dis Sci 43:1311, 1998. B
6. Lee W: Acetaminophen and the US Acute Liver Failure Study Group, Hepatology 40:6-9, 2004. B
7. Maddrey WC et al: Corticosteroid therapy of alcoholic hepatitis, Gastroenterology 75:193-199, 1978. B
8. Akriviadis et al: Pentoxifylline improves short-term survival in severe acute alcoholic hepatitis, Gastroenterology 119:1637-1648, 2000. A
9. Mathurin et al: Survival and prognostic factors in patients with severe alcoholic hepatitis treated with prednisolone, Gastroenterology 110:685-690, 1996. B
10. Broussard C et al: Mushroom poisoning, Am J Gastroenterol 96: 3195-3198, 2001. C
11. Mandell: Principles and practice of infectious diseases, 5th ed, London, 2000, Churchill Livingstone. C
12. Torii N et al: Effectiveness and long-term outcome of lamivudine therapy for acute hepatitis B, Hepatol Res 24:34-41, 2002. B
13. Menon KVN et al: The Budd-Chiari syndrome, N Engl J Med 350:578-585, 2004. B

Viral Hepatitis

Brady Stein, MD; Kelly Brungardt, MD; John Clarke, MD; and Rudra Rai, MD

FAST FACTS

- Acute hepatitis A typically is diagnosed by detection of hepatitis A virus (HAV) immunoglobulin M (IgM) antibody. It is transmitted by a fecal-oral route and remains the most common form of acute viral hepatitis in many parts of the world.
- Between 3% and 5% of adults infected with hepatitis B (HBV) become chronic carriers, defined by hepatitis B surface antigen (HBsAg) positivity for more than 6 months. IgM HBV core antibody may be the only marker of the window period between the disappearance of HBsAg and appearance of anti-HBsAg. Presence of hepatitis B e antigen (HBeAg), HBV DNA, and HBsAg are important markers used to assess disease activity.
- Between 55% and 85% of patients with acute exposure to hepatitis C become chronically infected. Hepatitis C antibody (HCV Ab) is used to screen for hepatitis C infection, and HCV RNA quantifies viremia. HCV Ab may be falsely negative (e.g., acute infections, immunosuppressed patients) or falsely positive (e.g., passive transfer of maternal antibodies in infants, autoimmune conditions) and may be confirmed by the recombinant immunoblot assay.
- HCV genotype studies help determine those more likely to achieve a sustained virologic response. Patients with genotype 1 are least likely to respond to treatment.

34

I. HEPATITIS A

A. VIROLOGY AND EPIDEMIOLOGY

1. HAV is a small nonenveloped RNA hepatovirus (picornavirus family) that is transmitted by the fecal-oral route. After absorption in the small intestine and replication in the liver, HAV is secreted into bile and shed in feces for 1 to 2 weeks before clinical illness and approximately 1 week after the onset of jaundice. The incubation period is 15 to 50 days.[1] There is no chronic carrier state.

2. Hepatitis A is particularly prevalent in the economically developing regions of Africa, Asia, and Latin America, where seroprevalence rates approach 100% and most infections occur by 5 years of age. In contrast, seroprevalence rates are approximately 33% in the United States.[2]

3. The rates of hepatitis A have been steadily decreasing over the past 2 decades. This decline correlates with the use of HAV vaccine in high-risk areas but also reflects improvements in hygiene, sewage disposal, crowding, and food safety.[3]

B. CLINICAL PRESENTATION

1. Hepatitis A may begin with a nonspecific prodrome of fever, malaise, weakness, anorexia, nausea, vomiting, arthralgias, myalgias, and upper respiratory symptoms; this is often followed in 1 to 2 weeks by dark urine, jaundice, mild pruritus, and slight liver enlargement and tenderness.

2. Laboratory studies reflect hepatocellular injury, and serum aminotransferase levels may be elevated between 500 and 5000 U/L. Serum bilirubin usually peaks later than transaminase levels but often remains less than 10 mg/dl.

3. Hepatitis A usually has a benign course in young, healthy people and is associated with a low mortality.[4,5] Illness usually is more severe in adults than in children, in whom HAV infection often is asymptomatic. Older adults, immunosuppressed patients, or those with chronic liver disease usually have greater morbidity.

4. Most patients have complete clinical recovery and normalization of liver function tests within 6 months after onset of symptoms. Atypical disease courses such as fulminant liver failure, cholestatic hepatitis, and relapsing hepatitis are rare.

C. DIAGNOSIS

Diagnosis of HAV requires presence of serum HAV IgM antibody during the acute phase of the illness. IgM antibody persists for 3 to 6 months after onset of symptoms. Detection of HAV IgG antibody without the presence of IgM antibody indicates past infection; it persists for decades after acute HAV infection and indicates recovery and resistance to subsequent HAV infections.[4] A typical serologic course for HAV infection is shown in Fig. 34-1.

D. MANAGEMENT

1. Given the generally benign nature of hepatitis A, most patients can be treated at home with supportive therapies. Some patients must be hospitalized (largely those older than 45) because of persistent anorexia, nausea, or vomiting.

2. No specific antiviral treatment is available for hepatitis A. Intake of hepatotoxic substances, such as acetaminophen, should be avoided.

E. PROPHYLAXIS

1. Two forms of prophylaxis are available for hepatitis A: immune globulin and an inactivated HAV vaccine.

2. Immune globulin should be given within 14 days of exposure and will prevent disease in more than 85% of patients. It is also recommended for preexposure prophylaxis for people traveling to endemic areas in the following 2 weeks.

3. Inactivated hepatitis A vaccine (Box 34-1) is highly immunogenic. More than 94% of patients have antibodies 1 month after vaccination, and clinical efficacy is maintained for 7 to 9 years. Models suggest that immunity is likely to exist for 20 years without the need for boosters.[2] Responses may be lower in people with chronic liver disease, older

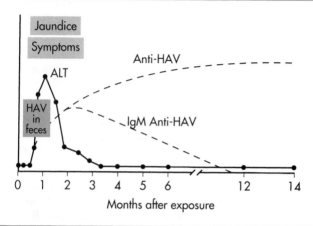

FIG. 34-1

Hepatitis A serology. *ALT*, alanine aminotransferase; *anti-HAV*, total antibody against hepatitis A infection; *IgM anti-HAV*, acute immunoglobulin M reaction to hepatitis A infection. (*Accessed June 6, 2004, at www.cdc.gov/ncidod/diseases/hepatitis/slideset/hep_a.*)

BOX 34-1

INDICATIONS FOR HEPATITIS A VACCINATION[2]

People planning to travel to endemic areas
Men who have sex with men
Illicit drug users
Recipients of clotting factor concentrates
People with chronic liver disease

adults, and immunocompromised people. The only contraindication to vaccination is previous allergic reaction. A two-dose schedule is recommended with 6 months between doses.

II. HEPATITIS B

A. VIROLOGY AND EPIDEMIOLOGY

1. HBV is a DNA hepadnavirus that consists of double-stranded DNA surrounded by an outer lipoprotein envelope and an inner core composed of nucleocapsid proteins.
2. In the United States, 1.25 million people have chronic hepatitis B.[6] The prevalence of HBV varies markedly worldwide, with 45% of the world's population living in areas of high prevalence, defined as more than 8% of population HBsAg positive and most transmissions occurring

perinatally or in early childhood. In areas of low prevalence (United States, northern Europe, Australia) less than 2% of the population is HBsAg positive, and transmission primarily occurs in adolescents and young adults.

3. HBV is present in large quantities in blood and serous fluids, and lower concentrations are found in semen, saliva, and vaginal secretions. In developed countries, most infections occur via sexual transmission or injection drug use.

B. CLINICAL PRESENTATION

1. The incubation period ranges from 45 days to 180 days. Acute infection usually is asymptomatic in infants and children; the clinical presentation in adults ranges from asymptomatic infection to cholestatic hepatitis, and rarely acute liver failure. Jaundice occurs in approximately 30% to 50% of adults.

2. Fulminant liver failure occurs in 1% of acute infections in adults and is characterized by coagulopathy, encephalopathy, and cerebral edema.[7] Fulminant infection occasionally complicates chronic hepatitis B infection after the withdrawal of immunosuppressive agents.

3. The rate of viral clearance varies significantly based on age and immune response. Fortunately, **less than 5% of adults infected with HBV remain chronically infected.**[8]

4. HBV is not directly cytotoxic to hepatocytes; instead, it is the host immune response to viral antigens displayed on infected hepatocytes that is the principal determinant of hepatocellular injury.

5. Cirrhosis develops in approximately 20% of people with chronic hepatitis B. Compared with those without hepatitis B, **chronic carriers have a 100-fold higher risk of developing hepatocellular carcinoma.**[8]

C. DIAGNOSIS

1. In primary HBV infection, HBsAg typically appears 4 to 10 weeks after acute exposure to HBV, before the development of symptoms. Shortly thereafter, patients become symptomatic, and HBV core antibody (initially IgM) appears in the serum. Biochemical abnormalities develop, including elevated aminotransferases (often > 500 U/L) and modest bilirubin elevations (5 to 10 mg/dl). With resolving infection, patients develop antibodies to HBsAg, and the HBsAg disappears. Rarely, there is a window period in which neither HBsAg nor anti-HBsAg is detectable, and IgM HBV core antibody is the only marker of infection. A history of hepatitis B infection is diagnosed by the presence of anti-HBsAg antibody plus IgG anti–hepatitis B core antibody (Fig. 34-2).

2. **Chronic HBV infection is defined by HBsAg positivity for more than 6 months.**

3. Active inflammation and fibrosis in the liver are reflected by fluctuating transaminitis, HBeAg positivity, and a high HBV viral load (HBV DNA). Approximately 5% to 10% of those infected will develop anti-HBeAg

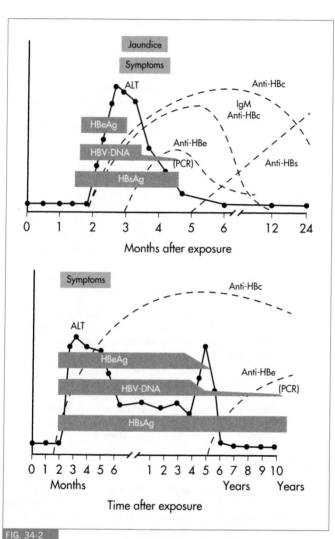

FIG. 34-2

Hepatitis B serology in acute and chronic infection. *ALT,* alanine aminotransferase; *anti-HBc,* total antibody to hepatitis B core antigen; *anti-HBe,* antibody to hepatitis B e antigen; *anti-HBs,* antibody to hepatitis B antigen; *HBeAg,* hepatitis B e antigen; *HBsAg,* hepatitis B surface antigen; *HBV,* hepatitis B virus; *IgM anti-HBc,* acute IgM antibody to hepatitis B core antigen; *PCR,* polymerase chain reaction. (*Accessed June 6, 2004, at www.cdc.gov/ncidod/diseases/hepatitis/b/ aasld_update_chronichep_b.*)

antibodies each year, which is often associated with a transient rise in alanine aminotransferase (ALT). Anti-HBe antibodies herald the development of low levels of HBV viremia and normal aminotransferases. However, a small percentage of patients continue to have high titers of HBV DNA despite anti-HBe antibodies because a precore mutation creates a truncated version of HBeAg.

4. Up to 20% of carriers in the inactive phase can have exacerbations of hepatitis, evidenced by elevated aminotransferases, active inflammation and fibrosis of the liver, and rarely reversions from anti-HBe antibody to HBeAg positivity.[9]

D. MANAGEMENT

1. Acute hepatitis B infection has no specific treatment. Therapy is largely supportive.

2. The goals of treatment of chronic hepatitis B are sustained suppression of HBV DNA replication and remission of liver disease. The endpoints used to assess treatment response are normalization of serum aminotransferases, undetectable HBV DNA (by an unamplified assay), serum conversion from HBeAg to anti-HBe antibody, and improvement in liver histology.

a. Patients with elevated liver transaminases, HBV DNA, and HBeAg positivity with or without cirrhosis may be evaluated by liver biopsy in preparation for treatment.

b. Chronic hepatitis B with HBeAg positivity and normal ALT levels (< twice the upper limits of normal) should have ALT measured every 3 to 6 months, but treatment is not currently recommended.

c. Inactive carriers should have serum transaminase determinations every 6 to 12 months to detect disease reactivation.[9]

3. The U.S. Food and Drug Administration (FDA) has approved three treatments for chronic hepatitis B: interferon alfa, lamivudine, and adefovir. Entecavir received preliminary FDA approval in March 2005. Other treatments include emtricitabine and tenofovir, which are available for off-label use, and telbivudine, which is currently in phase III trials.

a. **Interferon alfa** is a recombinant cytokine with immunomodulatory, antiviral, and antiproliferative effects. Its advantages include finite duration of treatment, more durable response, and lack of resistant mutants. Approximately 30% of patients who tolerate the regiment have a successful, sustained response (decline in ALT, loss of HBeAg). It is most effective in those with chronic hepatitis B infection who have elevated ALT and lower levels of HBV DNA.[9]

b. **Lamivudine** is an oral nucleoside analog that rapidly suppresses HBV DNA by 3 to 4 log and leads to HBeAg seroconversion in 65% of cases in which the pretreatment ALT was more than five times the upper limit of normal and 26% in patients with ALT two to five times the upper limit of normal. Three years of lamivudine treatment reduces necroinflammatory activity and reverses fibrosis in most patients.[10]

Lamivudine is conveniently given as a daily pill with few side effects. Treatment can be stopped 6 to 9 months after HBeAg seroconversion. Lamivudine therapy leads to the emergence of resistant variants (YMDD mutants) in 15% to 20% of patients after 1 year of therapy and approximately 67% of patients by 4 years of lamivudine treatment.[8]

c. **Adefovir** is a nucleotide analog that inhibits the HBV DNA polymerase. It is associated with a 3- to 4-log decrease in HBV DNA, HBeAg seroconversion in 12%, and normalization of ALT in 48% of patients after 48 weeks of treatment. Resistance to adefovir is rare (2.5% after 2 years of treatment). Adefovir may be used in lamivudine-resistant patients.[11] It is dosed daily and has minimal side effects at low dosages (only the 10-mg dosage is approved by the FDA). Rarely, it is associated with nephrotoxicity.[12]

d. **Entecavir** is a cyclopentyl guanine analog with activity against both wild type and lamivudine-resistant HBV. Entecavir is associated with effective HBV inhibition even with low ALT, and phase III data showed little or no reported resistance after 48 weeks of treatment.[13]

e. **Tenofovir,** an adenine nucleoside analog that is approved for treatment of the human immunodeficiency virus (HIV), also has activity against the HBV polymerase. It has not received FDA approval for the treatment of hepatitis B.[14]

4. **HBV reinfection occurs in 80% of patients after liver transplantation** if no measures are taken to prevent reinfection. Current post-transplantation prophylaxis consists of hepatitis B immune globulin and lamivudine. This regimen reduces the rate of reinfection to 10% and the HBV-free survival to 80%.[8]

E. PROPHYLAXIS

1. The plasma hepatitis B vaccine (Box 34-2) was introduced in 1982 and results in antibody formation to HBsAg. It has largely been replaced in the United States by recombinant formulations.

2. Protective serum titers of anti-HBsAg antibody develop in 95% of healthy adults who receive a series of three intramuscular doses.[15] Immunocompromised patients and those undergoing hemodialysis

34

VIRAL HEPATITIS

BOX 34-2

CENTERS FOR DISEASE CONTROL GUIDELINES FOR HEPATITIS B VACCINATION

Universal infant immunization

All children who have not been previously vaccinated

Health care workers

Inmates of correctional facilities

Intravenous drug users

Persons at risk for sexually transmitted diseases

Household members of a person with chronic hepatitis B infection

International travelers traveling for > 6 mo to endemic hepatitis B areas

Accessed June 6, 2004 at http://www.cdc.gov/idu/hepatitis/vaccines.pdf

have a lower seroconversion, and postvaccination testing may be necessary.

3. In addition to vaccination, postexposure prophylaxis can be provided with HBV-specific immunoglobin administration and the first HBV vaccine dose given simultaneously in separate sites.

III. HEPATITIS C

A. VIROLOGY AND EPIDEMIOLOGY

1. In the United States approximately 1.8% of the population is HCV seropositive (4 million people), and 2.7 million people are estimated to have ongoing HCV infection, with a peak prevalence in those aged 40 to 59 years[16] (Box 34-3).

2. The incidence of HCV in the United States has been declining, largely because of improvements in blood donor screening programs; however, a fourfold increase in the number of people diagnosed with hepatitis C is projected over the next decade.[17] **HCV is the leading indication for liver transplantation.**[18]

3. The hepatitis C virus is a single-stranded RNA flavivirus with six genotypes and more than 50 subtypes. Genotypes 1a and 1b are the most common in the United States.[19]

B. CLINICAL PRESENTATION

1. HCV infection is infrequently diagnosed during the acute phase of illness because the majority of patients have few or no symptoms. When they do occur, clinical manifestations typically begin 7 to 8 weeks (range 2 to 26 weeks) after exposure to HCV and generally consist of jaundice, malaise, and nausea. Acute fulminant hepatitis C infection is documented but rare.[20]

2. Spontaneous clearance of viremia, once infection has been established, is rare. Between 55% and 85% of those infected become chronic carriers. Among this group, 5% to 20% develop cirrhosis over the next 20 to 25 years. Once cirrhosis develops, the risk of hepatocellular carcinoma is 1% to 4% per year (see Chapter 35).[21]

BOX 34-3
RISK FACTORS FOR HEPATITIS C INFECTION[17]
Intravenous drug use
Blood transfusions before 1992
Exposure to an infected sexual partner*
Perinatal exposure*
Frequent exposure to infected blood among health care workers*
Tattooing*
Body piercing*
Folk medicine practices including acupuncture*

*Less efficient mode of transmission.

3. In addition to duration of infection, risk factors associated with progression of fibrosis include older age, male sex, alcohol use, HIV, low CD4 count, high body mass index, and diabetes.[19,22]

C. DIAGNOSIS

1. Diagnosis of HCV is based on both serologic testing and viral RNA amplification. HCV antibody testing is extremely sensitive and specific, and it is the initial screening test of choice. Anti-HCV antibodies are present approximately 8 weeks after exposure. False negative results can occur in acute infection, immunosuppressed patients with HIV, and those on chronic hemodialysis.[23] Typical serologic patterns of acute and chronic hepatitis C infection are shown in Fig. 34-3.

2. HCV RNA testing is used to confirm diagnosis by documenting viremia, which is detectable 1 to 2 weeks after exposure.

3. Biopsy is recommended during the initial assessment of those with chronic hepatitis C and helps stage the severity of disease, grade the degree of necrosis and inflammation, and identify those who may or may not benefit from treatment.

34

VIRAL HEPATITIS

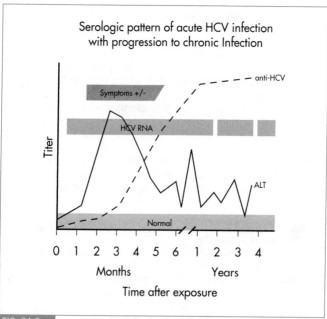

Serologic pattern of acute HCV infection with progression to chronic Infection

FIG. 34-3

Hepatitis C acute and chronic serology. *anti-HCV,* total antibody to hepatitis C infection; *HCV,* hepatitis C virus. (*Accessed June 6, 2004, at www.cdc.gov/ncidod/diseases/hepatitis/slideset/hep_c.*)

D. MANAGEMENT

1. **Treatment of hepatitis C is generally considered for all patients without specific contraindications** but may be prioritized and recommended for patients with a higher likelihood of developing cirrhosis, including those with persistently elevated transaminase levels, detectable HCV RNA greater than 50 U/L, and histologic evidence of fibrosis or inflammation.[17] Treatment is also recommended for patients with significant extrahepatic manifestations of HCV infection.[22]

2. **Baseline HCV RNA should be measured before treatment, after 12 weeks of treatment, and at the end of treatment.** HCV genotyping should be completed before treatment because viral genotype is the strongest predictor of response.

3. **The current standard of care for the treatment of chronic hepatitis C infection is weekly subcutaneous peginterferon alfa paired with daily ribavirin therapy.** When compared with patients treated with interferon alfa in combination with ribavirin or peginterferon alone, patients treated with peginterferon with ribavirin demonstrated significantly better end-of-treatment response and sustained virologic response (SVR)[24] (Box 34-4).

4. **Patients with genotype 1 HCV infection** should be treated for 48 weeks. Patients who do not show early virologic response after 12 weeks of treatment may discontinue therapy because 97% of these patients will also fail to achieve SVR.[24] In patients with genotype 1 infection and low levels of viremia (< 2 million copies/ml), 64% achieve SVR compared with 46% among those with high levels of viremia.[25]

5. **Patients with genotype 2 and 3 HCV infections** achieve higher SVR rates (74% to 81% depending on low or high levels of viremia) and should be treated with peginterferon plus ribavirin for 24 weeks.[25]

6. Other than genotype, several factors predict higher response rates to HCV treatment: lower pretreatment HCV RNA, younger age, lower body weight, and absence of bridging fibrosis and cirrhosis.[22]

BOX 34-4

HCV TREATMENT DEFINITIONS[22]

Sustained virologic response: absence of HCV RNA in serum at the end of treatment and 6 mo later.

Early virologic response: 2-log drop or loss of viral HCV RNA 12 wk into therapy.

End-of-treatment response: absence of detectable virus as the termination of treatment.

Nonresponder has stable HCV RNA levels despite treatment.

Partial responder has a declining HCV RNA level, but levels never become undetectable.

HCV, hepatitis C virus.

African American patients with genotype 1 were recently shown to have significantly lower rates of SVR than non-Hispanic white patients.[26]

E. PROPHYLAXIS

1. No clinical benefit has been shown with immune globulin prophylaxis, and it is not recommended after exposure. There is no available vaccine for hepatitis C.

2. Needlestick transmission of HCV is an important concern for health care workers. It is not possible to prevent infection after exposure to HCV, and HCV infection will develop in an estimated 2% to 10% of exposed individuals.

3. Because clinical symptoms may be minimal, HCV antibody, HCV RNA, and ALT levels should be measured within several days of exposure and 6 months thereafter.[27]

4. There are no clear recommendations about the timing or duration of treatment for acute hepatitis C infection. Excellent results have been achieved in uncontrolled trials with interferon alone. These results are confounded because most patients present with symptomatic acute infection, which has been associated with higher rates of spontaneous clearance (52%).[28]

PEARLS AND PITFALLS

- All patients with chronic viral hepatitis should be vaccinated against hepatitis A and B.
- Extrahepatic disease is associated with both hepatitis B and hepatitis C infections.
- In acute hepatitis B infection, arthralgias and rashes occur in 25% of cases. Polyarteritis nodosa can occur with either acute or chronic infection. Chronic hepatitis B is associated with immune complex–mediated diseases such as membranoproliferative glomerulonephritis; leukocytoclastic vasculitis; and, rarely, type II mixed cryoglobinemia.[6]
- Hepatitis C is the primary cause of essential mixed cryoglobinemia, and cryoglobulins can be found in up to half of people with HCV infection (although few people have symptomatic disease).[29,30] Hepatitis C has also been associated with membranoproliferative glomerulonephritis, lichen planus, sicca syndrome, porphyria cutanea tarda, and non-Hodgkin's lymphoma.[31]
- Interferon alfa has significant side effects, including flulike symptoms, fatigue, leukopenia, thrombocytopenia, and depression. It is given as a subcutaneous injection either daily or three times per week. Pegylated interferon is created by the addition of a polyethylene glycol moiety to the interferon molecule. This addition extends the half-life and duration of therapeutic levels, resulting in a sustained serum concentration and allowing once-a-week dosing. Ribavirin side effects include hemolysis, nausea, anemia, nasal congestion, and pruritus.
- Hepatitis D is a defective single-stranded RNA virus that needs hepatitis B surface antigen for replication.

- Hepatitis D is acquired via percutaneous and sexual exposure. It is uncommon in the United States except among intravenous drug users.
- Hepatitis B and D coinfection occurs when the viruses are acquired together and leads to a more severe acute hepatitis and higher risk of fulminant hepatic failure. However, the risk of chronic liver disease is lower.
- Hepatitis D superinfection occurs in hepatitis B surface antigen–positive patients who acquire hepatitis D. Superinfection is associated with a higher risk of chronic liver disease.
- HDV is detected by measurement of anti-HDV antibodies or HDV RNA amplification.
- Hepatitis E is an RNA virus that is transmitted by the fecal-oral route and causes acute hepatitis outbreaks in developing countries through contaminated drinking water.
- The incubation period of hepatitis E is approximately 40 days, and the severity of illness increases with age. There is no chronic disease associated with hepatitis E.
- Fatal fulminant hepatitis occurs in 15% to 25% of women infected during the third trimester of pregnancy.

REFERENCES

1. Koff RS: Hepatitis A, *Lancet* 351:1643, 1998. C
2. Craig AS et al: Prevention of hepatitis A with hepatitis vaccine, *N Engl J Med* 350:476-481, 2004. C
3. Berenguer M et al: Viral hepatitis. In Feldman M, Friedman LS, Sleisenger MH: *Sleisenger & Fordtran's gastrointestinal and liver disease,* 7th ed, Philadelphia, 2002, WB Saunders. C
4. Lednar WM et al: Frequency of illness associated with epidemic hepatitis A virus infections in adults, *Am J Epidemiol* 122:226, 1985. B
5. Tong MJ et al: Clinical manifestations of hepatitis A: recent experience in a community teaching hospital, *J Infect Dis* 171S1:S15, 1995. B
6. Lee WM: Hepatitis B virus infection, *N Engl J Med* 337:1733, 1997. C
7. Lee WM: Acute liver failure, *N Engl J Med* 329:1862, 1993. C
8. Ganem D et al: Hepatitis B virus infection: natural history and clinical consequences, *N Engl J Med* 350:1118-1129, 2004. C
9. Lok AS, McMahon BJ: Chronic hepatitis B. AASLD practice guidelines, *Hepatology* 34:1225-1241, 2001. D
10. Dienstag JL et al: Durability of serologic response after lamivudine treatment of chronic hepatitis B, *Hepatology* 37:748-755, 2003. A
11. Marcellin P et al: Adefovir dipivoxil for the treatment of hepatitis e antigen-positive chronic hepatitis, *N Engl J Med* 348:808-816, 2003. A
12. Lok AS, McMahon BJ: Chronic hepatitis B: Update of recommendations, *Hepatology* 39:857-861, 2004. D
13. Baraclude (TM) (entecavir) Prescribing Information, 2005, Bristol Myers Squib Company, New York. B
14. Dore GJ et al: Efficacy of tenofovir disoproxil fumarate in antiretroviral therapy-naive and -experienced patients coinfected with HIV-1 and hepatitis B virus, *J Infect Dis* 189:1185-1192, 2004. A

15. Lemon SM, Thomas DL: Vaccines to prevent viral hepatitis, *N Engl J Med* 336:196, 1997. C
16. Alter MJ et al: The prevalence of hepatitis C virus infection in the United States, 1988 through 1994, *N Engl J Med* 341:556, 1999. B
17. National Institutes of Health: *NIH consensus statement on the management of hepatitis C: 2002,* Volume 19, Number 3, Bethesda, Md, 2002, Author. D
18. Poynard T et al: Viral hepatitis C, *Lancet* 362:2095-2100, 2003. C
19. Lauer GM, Walker BD: Hepatitis C virus infection, *N Engl J Med* 345:41-52, 2001. C
20. Farci P et al: Hepatitis C virus–associated fulminant hepatic failure, *N Engl J Med* 335:631, 1996. B
21. Di Besceglie AM: Hepatitis C and hepatocellular carcinoma, *Hepatology* 26:S34-S38, 1997. C
22. Strader DB et al: Diagnosis, management, and treatment of hepatitis C, *Hepatology* 39:1147-1171, 2004. D
23. Pawlotsky JM: Use and interpretation of virological tests for hepatitis C, *Hepatology* 36:S65-S73, 2002. C
24. Fried MW et al: Peginterferon alfa-2a plus ribavirin for chronic hepatitis C virus infection, *N Engl J Med* 347:975-981, 2002. A
25. Hadziyannis SJ et al: Peginterferon alfa-2a and ribavirin combination therapy in chronic hepatitis C: randomized study of the effect of treatment duration and ribavirin dose, *Ann Intern Med* 140:346-355, 2004. A
26. Muir AJ et al: Peginterferon alpha-2b and ribavirin for the treatment of chronic hepatitis C in blacks and non-Hispanic whites, *N Engl J Med* 350:2265-2271, 2004. A
27. Sulkowski MS et al: Needlestick transmission of hepatitis C, *JAMA* 287:2406, 2002. B
28. Gerlach JT et al: Acute hepatitis C: high rate of both spontaneous and treatment-induced viral clearance, *Gastroenterology* 125:80-88, 2003. B
29. Agnello V et al: A role for hepatitis C virus infection in type II cryoglobulinemia, *N Engl J Med* 327:1490, 1992. B
30. Cacoub P et al: Mixed cryoglobulinemia and hepatitis C virus, *Am J Med* 96:124-132, 1994. B
31. Mehta S et al: Extrahepatic manifestations of infection with hepatitis C virus, *Clin Liver Dis* 5:1-19, 2001. C

34

VIRAL HEPATITIS

End-Stage Liver Disease

Carlos Alves, MD; Kelly Brungardt, MD; Brady Stein, MD;
Jonathan P. Piccini, MD; and Rudra Rai, MD

35

> ### FAST FACTS
>
> - Chronic liver disease includes a broad differential diagnosis of infectious, autoimmune, inherited, metabolic, toxic, and acquired origins (Box 35-1).
> - The most common causes of cirrhosis in the United States are alcoholic liver disease and chronic hepatitis C infection.
> - Nonalcoholic fatty liver disease (NAFLD) is the most common explanation for persistently elevated alanine aminotransferase (ALT) after excluding hepatitis C.
> - The clinical sequelae of cirrhosis are caused by impaired hepatic synthetic function (jaundice and coagulopathy) and portal hypertension (ascites and variceal bleeding).
> - Hepatic encephalopathy can be precipitated by infection, dehydration, hypokalemia, alkalosis, and sedating medications.
> - Among patients with cirrhosis, the cumulative incidence of hepatocellular carcinoma is 4% to 7% per year.
> - Patients with autoimmune hepatitis are commonly female; diagnosis is suggested by the detection of characteristic laboratory abnormalities, including predominant aminotransferase elevation, hypergammaglobulinemia, and antinuclear antibodies, smooth muscle autoantibodies, or autoantibodies against liver and kidney microsomal antigens.
> - A workup for metabolic and inherited causes of chronic liver disease involves iron studies and *HFE* mutation analysis if hemochromatosis is suspected, ceruloplasmin and 24-hour urinary copper if Wilson's disease is suspected, and alpha-1 antitrypsin phenotype studies if alpha-1 antitrypsin deficiency is suspected.
> - The Model for End-Stage Liver Disease (MELD) score, which uses serum creatinine, bilirubin, and international normalized ratio, is an independent predictor of mortality in patients with cirrhosis and those who are awaiting liver transplantation.[1]
> - Patients who have cirrhosis and are admitted to an intensive care unit have a median survival of 1 month.[2]

I. EVALUATION OF THE CIRRHOTIC PATIENT

1. **Epidemiology.** Cirrhosis is a pathologically defined disorder and represents a late stage of progressive hepatic fibrosis characterized by distortion of the normal hepatic architecture and the formation of regenerative nodules. Cirrhosis generally is irreversible in its advanced

> **BOX 35-1**
>
> **COMMON CAUSES OF CIRRHOSIS**
>
> **INFECTIOUS**
>
> | | |
> |---|---|
> | Viral hepatitis | Toxoplasmosis |
> | Schistosomiasis | Echinococcosis |
>
> **INHERITED**
>
> | | |
> |---|---|
> | Hereditary hemochromatosis | Fanconi's syndrome |
> | Alpha-1 antitrypsin deficiency | Gaucher's disease |
> | Wilson's disease | Hereditary tyrosinemia |
> | Galactosemia and other glycogen storage diseases | |
>
> **DRUGS AND TOXINS**
>
> | | |
> |---|---|
> | Alcohol | Isoniazid |
> | Amiodarone | Arsenicals |
>
> **CARDIAC AND VASCULAR CAUSES**
>
> | | |
> |---|---|
> | Chronic right heart failure | Chronic portal vein thrombosis |
> | Budd-Chiari syndrome | Veno-occlusive disease |
>
> **OTHER CAUSES**
>
> | | |
> |---|---|
> | Sarcoidosis | Nonalcoholic steatohepatitis |
> | Primary biliary cirrhosis | Cystic fibrosis |
> | Secondary biliary cirrhosis | Graft versus host disease |
> | Primary sclerosing cholangitis | |

35

END-STAGE LIVER DISEASE

stages, at which point the only option may be liver transplantation. Patients with cirrhosis are susceptible to a variety of complications, and their life expectancy is markedly reduced. Cirrhosis is the twelfth leading cause of death in the United States, accounting for approximately 27,000 deaths in 2003.[3]

2. **Clinical presentation.** Cirrhosis may be asymptomatic for a long period of time before the insidious or, less often, abrupt onset of symptoms. Weakness, fatigability, disturbed sleep, muscle cramps, and weight loss are common. In advanced cirrhosis, anorexia usually is present and may be extreme, with associated nausea and occasional vomiting. Abdominal pain may be present and is related to hepatic enlargement and stretching of Glisson's capsule or to the presence of ascites. Menstrual abnormalities (usually amenorrhea), impotence, loss of libido, sterility, and gynecomastia in men may occur.

3. **Physical examination** usually reveals an enlarged, palpable, and firm liver with a sharp or nodular edge.

a. **Common skin manifestations** include spider angiomata (invariably on the upper half of the body), palmar erythema (mottled redness of the thenar and hypothenar eminences), and Dupuytren's contractures. Evidence of vitamin deficiency (glossitis and cheilosis) is common.

b. **Jaundice** is mild at first (usually not detectable until serum bilirubin is > 2 mg/dl) but increases in severity during the later stages of the disease and may lead to elevated urobilinogen levels and "cola urine."

c. **Findings of portal hypertension.** Splenomegaly, dilated superficial veins of the abdomen and thorax, and rectal varices reflect the intrahepatic obstruction to portal blood flow. The Cryrveilhier-Baum murmur is a venous hum that may be heard in patients with portal hypertension and results from collateral connections between the portal system and the remnant of the umbilical vein. It is best appreciated when the stethoscope is placed over the epigastrium and is augmented by maneuvers that increase intraabdominal pressure.

d. **Late findings** include ascites, pleural effusions, peripheral edema, ecchymotic lesions. Encephalopathy is also a late finding, except when precipitated by an acute hepatocellular insult or an episode of gastrointestinal bleeding.

4. **Diagnostic imaging.**

a. **Abdominal ultrasound** is routinely used during evaluation of the cirrhotic patient. In advanced cirrhosis, the liver may appear small and nodular. Surface nodularity and increased echogenicity with irregular-appearing areas are consistent with cirrhosis but can also be seen in hepatic steatosis. Findings of portal hypertension include an enlargement of the portal vein and the presence of collateral veins. Ultrasonography is also useful for detecting splenomegaly, ascites, and portal vein thrombosis.

b. **Computed tomography** often is used to evaluate the liver parenchyma and mass lesions.

c. **Magnetic resonance imaging** may reveal iron overload and provide an estimate of the hepatic iron concentration. **Magnetic resonance angiography is more sensitive than ultrasonography in diagnosing vascular complications of cirrhosis such as portal vein thrombosis.**

5. **Laboratory evaluation.** Patients with cirrhosis often have several laboratory abnormalities. Transaminitis reflects underlying hepatocellular inflammation and injury. Hyperbilirubinemia, hypoalbuminemia, and coagulopathy reflect the impaired synthetic function in end-stage liver disease (see Chapter 33). Excessive renal vasoconstriction and levels of antidiuretic hormone can lead to renal failure and hyponatremia. Finally, cirrhotic patients often have several hematologic abnormalities, including anemia and thrombocytopenia (see Chapters 41 and 43).

6. **Liver biopsy** is the gold standard for diagnosis of cirrhosis, during which a sample of the liver is obtained by either a percutaneous, transjugular, laparoscopic, or radiographically guided fine needle approach depending on the clinical setting. The sensitivity of liver biopsy is 80% to 100% depending on the method used and the size and number of specimens obtained. Liver biopsy may not be necessary if the clinical, laboratory, and radiologic data strongly suggest the presence of cirrhosis. Liver biopsy may also suggest the cause of

liver failure, as is often the case in hereditary hemochromatosis, nonalcoholic steatohepatitis (NASH), Wilson's disease, and alpha-1 antitrypsin deficiency.

II. ACQUIRED FORMS OF CHRONIC LIVER DISEASE

A. ALCOHOLIC LIVER DISEASE

1. **Epidemiology.**

a. Alcoholic liver disease is the second most common indication for liver transplantation in the United States.[4] The relative risk of clinical alcoholic liver disease begins to increase in those who consume more than 30 g of ethanol each day and is substantially higher in those drinking more than 80 g per day (8 beers, 1 L wine, or a half pint of distilled spirit) over 10 years.[5]

b. Estimates suggest that 90% to 100% of heavy drinkers display fatty liver, whereas 10% to 35% develop alcoholic hepatitis and 8% to 20% develop cirrhosis.[6] Female sex and coinfection with viral hepatitis C are important risk factors for the development of more severe disease.

2. **Evaluation.** A history of alcohol abuse or dependence aids diagnosis but may be denied by the patient. Questioning family members and the primary care provider and using questionnaires such as CAGE may be helpful (see Chapter 79).

a. **Laboratory abnormalities** that may suggest excessive alcohol consumption lack sensitivity but have reasonable specificity and include an elevated gamma glutamyl transpeptidase (GGT) and mean corpuscular volume (MCV). Associated metabolic abnormalities include hypertriglyceridemia, hyperuricemia, and elevated high-density lipoproteins. The most common pattern of aminotransferase elevation is aspartate aminotransferase (AST) greater than alanine aminotransferase (ALT) by a ratio of at least 2:1.

b. **Liver biopsy** is useful to confirm diagnosis, evaluate for concomitant liver disease, and determine the extent of liver injury. Typical histologic findings include polymorphonuclear infiltrates, centrilobular hepatocyte swelling, steatosis, Mallory bodies, and fibrosis.

3. **Management.** Abstinence is the only effective therapy, and in some cases it leads to spontaneous recovery. Patients must complete a 6-month period of confirmed abstinence before becoming eligible for transplantation. Patients undergoing liver transplantation for alcoholic liver disease experience outcomes similar to those who undergo transplantation for nonalcoholic liver disease.

B. NASH AND NAFLD

1. **Epidemiology**

a. Ludwig et al. introduced the term *NASH* (nonalcoholic steatohepatitis) in 1980 to describe a histology that was indistinguishable from that of alcoholic hepatitis in patients who did not abuse alcohol.[7] NASH is an intermediate stage in the spectrum of NAFLD, which includes a range of liver damage including simple steatosis, steatohepatitis, fibrosis, and cirrhosis. It has been suggested that NAFLD may account for 70% of cases of cryptogenic cirrhosis.[8]

b. NASH has been reported in all age groups, although the highest prevalence probably is between 40 and 60 years of age. NASH occurs with equal frequency in men and women.

c. Features of the metabolic syndrome are highly associated (obesity, type 2 diabetes mellitus, hyperglycemia, glucose intolerance, and hyperlipidemia).[9,10]

d. In a large cross-sectional study, age older than 45 years, high body mass index, the presence of diabetes, and an AST/ALT ratio greater than 1 were found to be independent predictors of advanced liver fibrosis.[11]

2. **Evaluation.** Most patients are asymptomatic and often are diagnosed based on abnormal findings on routine laboratory evaluation. NAFLD is the most common explanation for persistently elevated ALT after hepatitis C.

a. Most patients present with mild elevations in aminotransferases (1:4 normal values). Serum and hepatic iron stores often are elevated. For unclear reasons, a small percentage of patients are antinuclear antibody positive.[12]

b. **Other causes of chronic liver disease should be excluded.** NASH must be distinguished from alcoholic hepatitis as well, and significant alcohol use must be ruled out by interviews with the patient, family members, and primary provider.

c. The **role of liver biopsy** in the diagnostic workup is debated, but it remains the only diagnostic test that can detect NASH accurately and determine long-term prognosis.[8]

3. **Management.**

a. **Lifestyle modification including weight loss of 10% or more and control of blood glucose and lipids is the cornerstone of management.** Small studies have shown that gradual weight loss may lead to a decrease in aminotransferase levels and possible improvement in liver histology. On the other hand, rapid weight loss (> 1 kg/week) and starvation may lead to increased fibrosis and focal necrosis.[10,13]

b. Most studies involving pharmacologic intervention are small and uncontrolled, with a short duration of follow-up and inconsistent data on postintervention liver histology. To date, agents such as ursodeoxycholic acid, vitamin E, gemfibrozil, metformin, and troglitazone have been evaluated.[14]

C. **CHRONIC VIRAL HEPATITIS (See Chapter 34)**

D. **AUTOIMMUNE HEPATITIS**

1. **Epidemiology.** Autoimmune hepatitis (AIH) is an unresolving inflammation of the liver of unknown cause, predominantly affecting women (4:1). AIH accounts for 20% of chronic hepatitis and 6% of transplants in the United States.[15]

2. **The spectrum of clinical presentation is broad,** ranging from asymptomatic disease to acute hepatitis in 25% or, rarely, fulminant hepatic failure. Approximately one third of patients have cirrhosis at presentation. Approximately 10% to 50% of patients with AIH display associated extrahepatic autoimmune disorders including thyroid disease, rheumatoid arthritis, and ulcerative colitis.[15]

3. Evaluation.

a. **Serologic findings** include the presence of antinuclear antibody or anti–smooth muscle antibody in type I disease (70% to 80% of patients), anti liver-kidney microsomal antibody (3% to 4%) in type II disease, and anti–soluble liver antigen/liver-pancreas antigen in type III disease. Perinuclear antineutrophil cytoplasmic antibody, commonly associated with primary sclerosing cholangitis (PSC), is also found in 60% to 90% of patients with AIH.[16]

b. **Other laboratory findings** should be present, including predominant aminotransferase elevation, hypergammaglobulinemia or elevated immunoglobulin G to 1.5 times normal, and the absence of antimitochondrial antibody.

c. **Definitive diagnosis requires the exclusion of other forms of chronic liver disease.**

d. **Liver biopsy** should be performed, which may reveal interface hepatitis and may help in ruling out other autoimmune liver diseases.[17,18]

4. Management.

a. **Corticosteroid monotherapy (starting dosage: prednisone 20 to 30 mg) and low-dose prednisone (5 to 10 mg) in combination with azathioprine (50 to 150 mg) are effective treatments for AIH.** The latter regimen is preferred to reduce the complications of steroid use. Treatment leads to clinical and histologic improvement and a 20-year life expectancy greater than 80%.[19]

b. According to professional guidelines, **absolute indications for treatment** include aminotransferase levels greater than 10 times normal, aminotransferase levels 5 times normal in conjunction with a serum gamma globulin level at least twice the upper limit of normal, and histologic features of bridging necrosis or multiacinar necrosis.[20]

c. **Therapy is continued until remission, treatment failure, incomplete response, or drug toxicity occurs. Eighty percent of patients achieve remission after 3 years.**

d. **Liver transplantation** is effective in decompensated disease unresponsive to conventional therapy and has an associated 5-year survival of patient and graft from 83% to 92%.[21]

E. **PRIMARY BILIARY CIRRHOSIS**

1. **Epidemiology and presentation.** PBC is a progressive cholestatic disorder characterized by inflammatory destruction of the interlobular bile ducts, which progresses to end-stage liver disease. It occurs

predominantly in middle-aged women. Clinical illness is insidious and is heralded by fatigue and pruritus, which is often worse at night.

2. **Laboratory evaluation** reveals cholestasis with elevation of alkaline phosphatase, cholesterol (especially low-density lipoprotein), and later bilirubin. ALT and AST may be mildly elevated. Antimitochondrial antibodies (directed against pyruvate dehydrogenase) are present in 95% of patients, and serum immunoglobulin M levels are elevated.

3. **Diagnosis** is suggested by the presence of cholestasis, elevated serum immunoglobulin M, and antimitochondrial antibodies and is confirmed by characteristic histology on liver biopsy. Abdominal ultrasound should be performed to exclude other causes of cholestasis. PBC must be differentiated from chronic biliary tract obstruction secondary to stone or stricture; carcinoma of the bile ducts; primary sclerosing cholangitis; sarcoidosis; cholestatic drug toxicity; and, in some cases, chronic hepatitis.

4. **Management** is initially directed at symptom relief and, later, management of end-stage liver disease and its complications.[22]

a. **Cholestyramine or colestipol can be used to treat pruritus.** Opioid antagonists (e.g., naloxone or naltrexone), rifampicin, and the 5-HT_3 serotonin receptor antagonist ondansetron may be beneficial in cases of refractory pruritus.[23]

b. **Deficiencies of vitamins A, K, and D** may occur if steatorrhea is present and is aggravated when cholestyramine or colestipol is administered.

c. Patients are at **high risk of developing osteoporosis** and may benefit from bisphosphonate therapy.[24]

d. Because of its lack of toxicity, **ursodeoxycholic acid** (13 to 15 mg/kg/day) is the preferred medical treatment and has been shown to slow the progression of disease, improve long-term survival, and delay the need for liver transplantation.[25,26] Ursodeoxycholic acid should not be administered within 4 hours of cholestyramine.

5. **Liver transplantation** is the treatment of choice for patients with advanced disease and is associated with a 1-year survival rate of 85% to 90%. Unfortunately, disease recurs in the graft in 20% of patients by 3 years.[27] Without liver transplantation, survival averages 7 to 10 years once symptoms develop.

F. **PRIMARY SCLEROSING CHOLANGITIS**

1. **Epidemiology and clinical presentation.**

a. PSC is an inflammatory cholestatic disease that leads to fibrosis and stricturing of the intrahepatic and extrahepatic biliary ducts. Although PSC is an uncommon disease, it is among the leading indications for liver transplantation in the United States.

b. PSC affects predominantly men aged 20 to 40 and is closely associated with ulcerative colitis (and occasionally Crohn's disease), which is present in approximately two thirds of patients with PSC.

c. Patients present with progressive obstructive jaundice, often associated with malaise, pruritus, anorexia, and indigestion. Patients may be diagnosed before symptoms develop because of an elevated alkaline phosphatase level.

2. **Diagnosis.**

a. **Antineutrophil cytoplasmic antibodies** are found in 70% of patients, and serum antinuclear, anticardiolipin, antithyroperoxidase antibodies, and rheumatoid factor may also be positive but lack specificity.

b. The diagnosis of primary sclerosing cholangitis is generally made by **endoscopic retrograde cholangiopancreatography (ERCP).** Magnetic resonance **cholangiopancreatography** may be used as a noninvasive alternative, but it is less sensitive than ERCP for visualizing the intrahepatic ducts. PSC may be confined to small intrahepatic bile ducts, in which case ERCP is normal and the diagnosis is suggested by liver biopsy.

c. **Liver biopsy** is required for staging, which is based on the degree of inflammation and fibrosis.

3. **Management.**

a. Corticosteroids have been used with inconsistent and unpredictable results. **High-dose ursodeoxycholic acid** may reduce cholangiographic progression and liver fibrosis.[28] If there is a major stricture, stent placement may relieve symptoms and improve biochemical abnormalities.

b. In patients with ulcerative colitis, PSC is an independent risk factor for the development of **colorectal dysplasia and cancer,** and strict adherence to a colonoscopic surveillance program is advisable.

c. **Cholangiocarcinoma** may complicate the course of primary sclerosing cholangitis in at least 10% of cases and may be difficult to diagnose by cytologic examination because of false-negative results. A serum CA 19-9 level more than 100 U/ml is suggestive but not diagnostic of cholangiocarcinoma.

d. **Complications of chronic cholestasis,** such as osteoporosis and malabsorption of fat-soluble vitamins, may occur.

4. **Liver transplantation** is the preferred treatment for those with end-stage liver disease. Actuarial survival rates with liver transplantation are as high as 85% at 5 years,[29] but rates are much lower once cholangiocarcinoma has developed. After transplantation, patients have a higher risk of nonanastomotic biliary strictures.

III. GENETIC AND METABOLIC FORMS OF CHRONIC LIVER DISEASE

A. HEREDITARY HEMOCHROMATOSIS

1. Hereditary hemochromatosis is an autosomal recessive inherited form of iron overload characterized by inappropriately high intestinal iron absorption. The disorder is associated with a defect in the *HFE* gene

on chromosome 6; the C282Y mutation is the most common, and homozygosity for this mutation can be found in 5 in 1000 people of northern European descent.[30]

2. Previously undiagnosed patients often present in the fourth or fifth decade with fatigue, malaise, and arthralgia. Hypothyroidism, hypogonadism, and restrictive cardiomyopathy often develop. The classic triad consists of diabetes, bronze skin pigmentation, and cirrhosis but is rare because of earlier diagnosis.

3. Mild transaminitis is present in nearly half of patients; many patients come to a physician's attention because of an elevated transferrin saturation (more than 45%) found on routine iron studies. Transferrin saturation is more sensitive and specific than serum ferritin, which can be elevated in many forms of chronic liver disease. The combination of an elevated ferritin and transferrin saturation is 93% sensitive in otherwise healthy patients. Genetic testing involving *HFE* mutation analysis (C282Y and H63D) helps confirm the diagnosis.[17] Liver biopsy is necessary for definitive diagnosis.

4. **Treatment** involves weekly phlebotomy of 500 ml of blood until the hematocrit is less than 37%; when the ferritin is less than 50 and the transferrin saturation is less than 50%, maintenance phlebotomy can occur every 2 to 3 months. Once a proband is identified, family screening becomes necessary.[17]

5. **Liver transplantation** is the only effective treatment for patients with decompensated cirrhosis. Posttransplant survival is worse than with other forms of end-stage liver disease because of the higher rates of postoperative infection and hereditary hemochromatosis–associated cardiomyopathy.[31]

B. ALPHA-1 ANTITRYPSIN DEFICIENCY

1. Alpha-1 antitrypsin deficiency is an autosomal recessive metabolic disorder that can affect the lungs, liver, kidneys, and pancreas. Approximately 1 in 1600 people is affected. Alpha-1 antitrypsin functions as a protease inhibitor, degrading serine proteases including neutrophil elastase. The normal allelic representation is PiMM; the most common pathologic form is the PiZZ variant, which causes both lung and liver disease.

2. Liver disease in these patients is related to accumulation of abnormal alpha-1 antitrypsin within hepatocytes as opposed to pulmonary manifestations, which depend largely on the amount of functional glycoprotein.

3. Patients with alpha-1 antitrypsin deficiency can develop symptomatic disease or cirrhosis at any age. PiZZ homozygotes who do not display liver disease in childhood have an approximate 10% chance of developing cirrhosis as adults, with men at higher risk.[17]

4. If the cause of cirrhosis is unclear, diagnosis can be secured by measuring alpha-1 antitrypsin in the serum and characterizing the protease inhibitor phenotype. The absence of emphysema does not rule out the disease.

5. The only treatment for alpha-1 antitrypsin deficiency–associated cirrhosis is liver transplantation.

C. WILSON'S DISEASE

1. Wilson's disease is an autosomal recessive disorder of copper overload with a prevalence in most populations of 1 in 30,000. There are more than 200 distinct mutations of the Wilson's disease gene *ATP7b*, which makes genetic testing complicated.

2. Wilson's disease may present with liver disease (35%), progressive neurologic disease (35%), or psychiatric illness (20%). Patients with liver disease may present with asymptomatic transaminase elevation, chronic active hepatitis, or fulminant liver failure with severe coagulopathy and encephalopathy. Patients with neurologic manifestations usually present in their 20s, although patients with Wilson's disease can present after age 30.[32]

3. The Kayser-Fleischer ring is caused by copper deposition at the Descemet membrane on the cornea; it is present in approximately 50% of patients presenting with liver disease and almost all patients with neurologic or psychiatric involvement.

4. Diagnosis is based on the clinical presentation and laboratory evaluation, but liver biopsy remains the gold standard (Box 35-2).

5. Chelation is the first-line treatment for Wilson's disease and allows patients to live healthy, symptom-free lives. The three most commonly used chelation agents are penicillamine, trientine, and tetrathiomolybdate.[16] Zinc supplementation may be used as maintenance therapy to inhibit copper absorption in the gastrointestinal tract. Patients must also adopt dietary modifications to limit copper intake.

6. Patients who present with fulminant hepatic failure or advanced liver disease and those who fail chelation therapy should be referred for liver transplantation.

IV. RISK STRATIFICATION AND PROGNOSIS

1. Risk stratification and prognosis are vitally important in end-stage liver disease for both patient management and transplant organ allocation.

2. Traditionally, prognosis in end-stage liver disease has been determined using the Child-Pugh classification system.[33] Although widely used, the Child-Pugh classification suffers from the use of tiered rather than

35
END-STAGE LIVER DISEASE

BOX 35-2

DIAGNOSIS OF WILSON'S DISEASE

Serum ceruloplasmin: low in 85% of patients with Wilson's disease

24-hour urine copper

Kayser-Fleischer rings: 99% with neuropsychiatric findings; 30% to 50% with hepatic presentation

Liver biopsy with quantitative copper assay; copper stains unreliable

MODIFIED CHILD-PUGH CLASSIFICATION AND THE MELD SURVIVAL MODEL

Parameter	Numerical Score		
	1	2	3
Ascites	None	Slight	Moderate or severe
Encephalopathy	None	Grade 1-2	Grade 3-4
Bilirubin (mg/dl)	< 2	2-3	> 3
Albumin (mg/L)	> 3.5	2.8-3.5	< 2.8
Prothrombin time (seconds increased)	1-3	4-6	> 6

Total Numerical Score	Child-Pugh Class
5-6	A
7-9	B
10-15	C

MELD = [0.957 × log(creatinine) + 0.378 × log(bilirubin) + 1.12 × log(international normalized ratio) + 0.643] × 10*

Modified from Goldman L: *Cecil textbook of medicine,* 22nd ed, Philadelphia, 2004, Saunders.
MELD, Model for End-Stage Liver Disease.
*See www.mayo.edu/int-med/gi/model/mayomodl-5-unos.htm to calculate MELD score directly.

continuous variables and subjective bias in the estimation of the degree of ascites and encephalopathy (Table 35-1).
3. The Model for End-Stage Liver Disease (MELD) score has replaced the Child-Pugh classification as the predominant prognostic model in end-stage liver disease.[21,34] The MELD score, initially validated in patients undergoing elective transjugular intrahepatic portosystemic shunting, uses serum creatinine, bilirubin, and international normalized ratio. It is an independent predictor of mortality in patients with cirrhosis or those who are awaiting liver transplantation.[1]
4. The MELD formula is shown in Table 35-1. The MELD score ranges from 6 to 40. Patients who have had dialysis twice within the last week are assigned a serum creatinine of 4 mg/dl. Generally, patients with a MELD greater than 24 are considered for transplantation, and those with a MELD greater than 30 are critically ill.

V. COMPLICATIONS OF CIRRHOSIS
1. **Portal hypertensive gastropathy** is a complication of portal hypertension diagnosed on endoscopic examination. The mucosal layer appears engorged and friable, and bleeding occurs indolently rather than briskly as in variceal hemorrhage. Treatment includes the prevention of bleeding complications through beta-adrenergic blockade with propranolol, which reduces splanchnic arterial and venous pressure.
2. **Gastroesophageal varices** (see Chapter 37).
3. **Ascites, spontaneous bacterial peritonitis, and the hepatorenal syndrome** (see Chapter 36).
4. **Hepatic encephalopathy** is a complex state of disordered central nervous system function resulting from failure of the liver to detoxify

noxious agents because of hepatocellular dysfunction and portosystemic shunting.

a. **Early signs of encephalopathy** include disturbances of sleep with reversal of sleep-wake cycles (Table 35-2). Alterations in personality, mood disturbances, confusion, deterioration in self-care and handwriting, and daytime somnolence are additional clinical features of hepatic encephalopathy. Later findings include fluctuating level of consciousness, fetor hepaticus (a musty odor of the breath and urine believed to be caused by mercaptans), and neurologic signs such as flapping tremor (asterixis). The diagnosis usually is one of exclusion but should be considered in patients with acute or chronic liver disease and altered mental status.

b. **Treatment** is aimed at eliminating or treating precipitating factors (Box 35-3) and lowering blood toxin levels by decreasing the absorption of protein and nitrogenous products from the gastrointestinal tract.

   (1) **Lactulose,** a nonabsorbable disaccharide that acts as an osmotic laxative, can be administered in a dosage of 30 to 60 ml every hour until diarrhea occurs; thereafter the dosage is adjusted so that the patient has two to four soft stools daily.[35]

35

END-STAGE LIVER DISEASE

TABLE 35-2

STAGES OF HEPATIC ENCEPHALOPATHY

Stage	Mental Status	Asterixis	Electroencephalogram
I	Mild confusion, slurred or disordered speech	+/−	Triphasic waves
II	Lethargy	+	Triphasic waves
III	Marked confusion, incoherent speech, stupor	+	Triphasic waves
IV	Coma	−	Delta waves

BOX 35-3

PRECIPITANTS OF HEPATIC ENCEPHALOPATHY

ELEVATED NITROGENOUS COMPOUNDS

Gastrointestinal bleeding	Renal failure
Excessive protein intake	

ELECTROLYTE ABNORMALITIES

Hypokalemia	Alkalosis
Hyponatremia	

MEDICATIONS

Sedatives	Opioids
Hypnotics	

OTHER PRECIPITANTS

Infection (especially spontaneous bacterial peritonitis)	Superimposed acute liver disease
	Surgery
Progressive liver disease	Worsening portosystemic shunts

(2) Intestinal ammonia production by bacteria can also be decreased by oral administration of a "nonabsorbable" antibiotic such as **neomycin** (0.5 to 1 g every 6 hours), but neomycin may reach sufficient concentrations in the bloodstream to cause renal toxicity and ototoxicity. Similar benefits may be achieved with broad-spectrum antibiotics such as **metronidazole and off-label use of other novel nonabsorbable antibiotics (e.g., rifaximin).**

(3) **Chronic encephalopathy may be controlled by lactulose administration and dietary protein restriction (usually to 60 g/d).**

5. **Hepatopulmonary syndrome** is characterized by hypoxemia, platypnea (worsening dyspnea with standing), and orthodeoxia (decreased oxygen saturation with standing), resulting from right-to-left intrapulmonary shunts, which are usually located in the dependent portions of the lung. These dilations in intrapulmonary vessels can be detected by contrast-enhanced echocardiography or a macroaggregated albumin lung perfusion scan.[18] Large arteriovenous shunts may be embolized. Liver transplantation addresses the underlying metabolic disturbances responsible for causing the shunts and may eventually lead to amelioration of the hepatopulmonary syndrome in cases that have not yet been complicated by advanced pulmonary hypertension.

6. **Hepatocellular carcinoma.**

a. **Epidemiology.** Hepatocellular carcinoma (HCC) is one of the most common tumors in the world. In the United States, the annual incidence of HCC is 2.4 in 100,000, and 60% to 90% of HCC tumors occur in cirrhotic patients. The incidence is four times higher in men than in women.

b. **Diagnosis.** Patients may present with abdominal pain or an asymptomatic right upper quadrant mass. Alpha-fetoprotein levels greater than 500 ng/ml are found in about 70% of patients with HCC. In patients at high risk for HCC, screening programs have been initiated to identify small tumors when they are still resectable. Because 20% of patients with early hepatocellular carcinoma do not have elevated alpha-fetoprotein levels, ultrasonographic screening should be used, as well as alpha-fetoprotein determination. No randomized study has yet shown survival benefit for screening patients at high risk of developing hepatocellular carcinoma.

c. **Treatment.** Surgical resection offers the only chance for cure; however, few patients have a resectable tumor at the time of presentation because of underlying cirrhosis, involvement of both hepatic lobes, or distant metastases (common sites are lung, brain, bone, and adrenal), and so the 5-year survival is low.

(1) **Liver transplantation** is a therapeutic option, but tumor recurrence and metastases are the major problems. Patients who have a single lesion no larger than 5 cm or three or fewer lesions no

larger than 3 cm have survival after liver transplantation that is the same as survival after transplantation for nonmalignant liver disease.

(2) **Other approaches** include transarterial chemoembolization, radiofrequency ablation, ultrasound-guided percutaneous ethanol injection, and cryoablation. Treatment options for unresectable disease are limited, with systemic chemotherapy and radiation demonstrating poor efficacy.

PEARLS AND PITFALLS

- Patients with cirrhosis should undergo routine screening for HCC, including alpha-fetoprotein determination every 6 to 12 months and annual hepatic imaging via ultrasound or computed tomography.
- The risk of osteoporosis is elevated in patients with chronic liver disease.
- Patients with hemochromatosis and end-stage liver disease are at higher risk of infection with siderophilic organisms such as *Vibrio vulnificus, Listeria monocytogenes,* and *Yersinia enterocolitica.*
- Patients who present with right upper quadrant pain, rapid-onset ascites, or decompensated liver failure should be evaluated for hepatic vein thrombosis (Budd-Chiari syndrome).
- The diagnosis of Wilson's disease can be difficult in acute liver failure because patients without Wilson's disease may have low serum ceruloplasmin and elevated urinary copper.

REFERENCES

1. Wiesner R, Edwards E, Freeman R, et al: United Network for Organ Sharing Liver Disease Severity Score Committee: Model for end-stage liver disease (MELD) and allocation of donor livers, *Gastroenterology* 124(1):91-96, 2003. B
2. Gildea TR, Cook WC, Nelson DR, et al: Predictors of long-term mortality in patients with cirrhosis of the liver admitted to a medical ICU, *Chest* 126(5): 1598-1603, 2004. B
3. Hoyert DL, Kung HC, Smith BL: Deaths: preliminary data for 2003, *National Vital Statistics Report* 53(15), Hyattsville, Md, 2005, National Center for Health Statistics. B
4. Narayanan MK: Pathogenesis, diagnosis, and treatment of alcoholic liver disease, *Mayo Clin Proc* 76:1021-1029, 2001. C
5. Moseley RH: Evaluation of abnormal liver function tests, *Med Clin North Am* 80(5):887-906, 1996. C
6. McCullough AJ: Alcoholic liver disease: proposed recommendations for the American College of Gastroenterology, *Am J Gastroenterol* 93:2022-2035, 2040, 1998. D
7. Neuschwander-Tetri BA et al: Nonalcoholic steatohepatitis: summary of an AASLD single topic conference, *Hepatology* 37:1202-1217, 2003. D
8. Clark J et al: Nonalcoholic fatty liver disease, *Gastroenterology* 122:1649-1657, 2002. C
9. te Sligte K et al: Non-alcoholic steatohepatitis: review of a growing medical problem, *Eur J Intern Med* 15:10-21, 2004. C
10. Angulo P, Lindor KD: Treatment of non-alcoholic steatohepatitis, *Best Pract Res Clin Gastroenterol* 16:797-810, 2002. C

11. Angulo P et al: Independent predictors of liver fibrosis in patients with nonalcoholic steatohepatitis, *Hepatology* 30:1356-1362, 1999. B
12. Reid AE: Nonalcoholic steatohepatitis, *Gastroenterology* 121:710-723, 2001. C
13. American Gastroenterological Association technical review on nonalcoholic fatty liver disease, *Gastroenterology* 123:1705-1725, 2002. D
14. Angulo P, Lindor KD: Treatment of non-alcoholic steatohepatitis, *Best Pract Res Clin Gastroenterol* 16:797-810, 2002. C
15. Czaja AJ: Autoimmune hepatitis. In Feldman M et al: *Sleisenger & Fordtran's gastrointestinal and liver disease,* 7th ed, Philadelphia, 2002, Elsevier. C
16. Schilsky ML: Treatment of Wilson's disease: what are the relative roles of penicillamine, trientine, and zinc supplementation? *Curr Gastroenterol Rep* 3:54-59, 2001. C
17. Maher JJ: Inherited, infiltrative, and metabolic disorders involving the liver. In Goldman L ed: *Cecil textbook of medicine,* 21st ed, Philadelphia, 2000, Elsevier. C
18. Abrams GA et al: Use of macroaggregated albumin lung scan to diagnose hepatopulmonary syndrome: a new approach, *Gastroenterology* 114:305, 1998. C
19. Sanchez-Urdazpal LS et al: Prognostic features and role of liver transplantation in severe corticosteroid-treated autoimmune chronic active hepatitis, *Hepatology* 15:215-221, 1992. B
20. Czaja AJ, Freese DK: Diagnosis and treatment of autoimmune hepatitis, *Hepatology* 36:479-497, 2002. D
21. Kamath P et al: A model to predict survival in patients with end-stage liver disease, *Hepatology* 33:464-470, 2001. B
22. Heathcote EJ, American Association for the Study of Liver Diseases Practice Guideline: Management of primary biliary cirrhosis, *Hepatology* 31:1005-1013, 2003. D
23. Terg R et al: Efficacy and safety of oral naltrexone treatment for pruritus of cholestasis, a crossover, double blind, placebo-controlled study, *J Hepatol* 37:717-722, 2002. A
24. Wolfhagen FH et al: Cyclical etidronate in the prevention of bone loss in corticosteroid-treated primary biliary cirrhosis. A prospective, controlled pilot study, *J Hepatol* 26: 325-330, 1997. A
25. Poupon RE, Poupon R, Balkau B: Ursodiol for the long-term treatment of primary biliary cirrhosis. The UDCA-PBC Study Group, *N Engl J Med* 330:1342-1347, 1994. A
26. Combes B et al: A randomized, double-blind, placebo-controlled trial of ursodeoxycholic acid in primary biliary cirrhosis, *Hepatology* 22:759, 1995. A
27. Neuberger J: Transplantation for primary biliary cirrhosis, *Semin Liver Dis* 17:137-146, 1997. C
28. Mitchell SA et al: A preliminary trial of high-dose ursodeoxycholic acid in primary sclerosing cholangitis, *Gastroenterology* 121:900-907, 2001. A
29. Graziadei IW et al: Long-term results of patients undergoing liver transplantation for primary sclerosing cholangitis, *Hepatology* 30:1121-1127, 1999. B
30. Leonis MA: Inherited and metabolic disorders of the liver. In Feldman M et al: ed: *Sleisenger & Fordtran's gastrointestinal and liver disease,* 7th ed, Philadelphia, 2000, Elsevier. C
31. Carithers RL: AASLD practice guidelines: liver transplantation. *Liver Transpl* 6:122-135, 2000. D

32. Gow PJ et al: Diagnosis of Wilson's disease: an experience over three decades, *Gut* 46:415-419, 2000. B
33. Pugh RNH et al: Transection of the oesophagus for bleeding oesophageal varices, *Br J Surg* 60:646-649, 1973. B
34. Christensen E: Prognostic models including the Child-Pugh, MELD, and Mayo risk scores: where are we and where should we go? *J Hepatol* 41:344-350, 2004. C
35. Morgan MY, Hawley KE: Lactitol vs. lactulose in the treatment of acute hepatic encephalopathy in cirrhotic patients: a double-blind randomized study, *Hepatology* 7:1278, 1987. A

35

END-STAGE LIVER DISEASE

Ascites

Daniel J. Mollura, MD; Raquel Charles, MD;
Michal L. Melamed, MD; and Rudra Rai, MD

FAST FACTS

- Cirrhosis is the most common cause of ascites, yet up to 15% of patients with ascites do not have liver disease.
- Ascites is the most common complication of cirrhosis and is associated with significant morbidity, including spontaneous bacterial peritonitis (SBP), hepatorenal syndrome, and hepatic hydrothorax.
- SBP is present when there are more than 250 polymorphonuclear cells per cubic milliliter of ascites or when organisms are present on Gram stain of the peritoneal fluid.
- Paracentesis is the gold standard for the diagnosis of SBP and provides data that are helpful in determining the cause of the patient's ascites.

I. EPIDEMIOLOGY

1. Cirrhosis is the most common cause of ascites: 85% of patients with ascites have cirrhosis. Among the major complications of liver cirrhosis, ascites is more common than variceal hemorrhage or hepatic encephalopathy.[1]
2. Five percent of patients with ascites have more than one contributing factor. These patients are said to have mixed ascites.[2]
3. Effective management of ascites entails consideration of a broad differential diagnosis and accurate identification of the underlying cause (Table 36-1).

II. CLINICAL PRESENTATION

A. HISTORY

1. Ascites is a pathological accumulation of fluid in the peritoneal space.
2. Patients should be asked about risk factors for ascites, which may help determine the cause.
   a. Alcohol abuse suggests a diagnosis of alcoholic cirrhosis, although, alcohol consumption can exacerbate underlying liver disease with an alternative origin (e.g., alcohol abuse in a patient with hemochromatosis). Intravenous (IV) drug use, sexual exposure, tattoos, and blood transfusions increase the risk of hepatitis C infection.
   b. Foreign travel (endemic exposures).
   c. Obesity, diabetes, and dyslipidemia suggest a diagnosis of nonalcoholic steatohepatitis, which is becoming more prevalent in Western countries.
   d. History of malignancy. Breast, lung, pancreatic, gastric, and colonic malignancies can cause ascites via peritoneal metastases and

TABLE 36-1

CAUSES OF ASCITES

Cause of Ascites	Comments
Portal hypertension	
Cirrhosis	Accounts for 80% of ascites in the United States.
Fulminant hepatic failure	Rarely causes ascites.
Hepatic outflow obstruction	Ascites is a characteristic clinical feature of hepatic outflow obstruction.
Congestive heart failure	
Constrictive or restrictive cardiomyopathy	
Budd-Chiari syndrome (hepatic vein or inferior vena cava occlusion)	Most commonly associated with an underlying thrombotic disorder.
Veno-occlusive disease	Important cause of ascites in bone marrow transplant recipients.
Portal vein occlusion	Rarely causes ascites.
Malignancy	Accounts for 10% of ascites in the United States; peritoneal carcinomatosis causes 50% of malignant ascites.
Infection	
Peritoneal tuberculosis	See Tables 36-2 and 36-3.
Fitz-Hugh-Curtis syndrome	Perihepatitis associated with fibrous perihepatic exudate usually is caused by *Neisseria gonorrhoeae* or *Chlamydia trachomatis*.
Infectious peritonitis in patients infected with human immunodeficiency virus	
Renal	
Nephrotic syndrome	Covert cirrhosis should be excluded.
Nephrogenous in hemodialysis recipients	Covert cirrhosis should be excluded.
Endocrine	
Myxedema	
Meigs's syndrome	
Struma ovarii	
Ovarian stimulation syndrome	
Pancreatic ascites	Associated with pancreatitis, raised ascitic amylase concentration.
Biliary leak	Previous surgery, including laparoscopic cholecystectomy, gangrenous gallbladder, trauma, percutaneous liver biopsy.
Urine ascites	Urinary leak into the peritoneum.
Systemic lupus erythematosus	
Miscellaneous	Idiopathic chronic nonspecific peritonitis in patients infected with human immunodeficiency virus.
Mixed causes	See text.

Modified from Goldman L, Bennett JC: *Cecil textbook of medicine,* 21st ed, Philadelphia, 2000, WB Saunders.

carcinomatosis. Malignant ascites often is painful, whereas cirrhotic ascites is not (unless a superimposed infection, such as SBP, is present).

e. Sudden-onset ascites in a patient with stable cirrhosis suggests primary hepatic malignancy.

f. A history of biventricular or right-sided heart failure caused by coronary ischemia, myocarditis (autoimmune or infectious), cardiotoxic medications, restrictive cardiomyopathy, or constrictive pericarditis (radiation, infection, malignancy) can lead to the development of ascites.

g. History of renal failure, proteinuria, or hematuria.

h. Clotting disorders leading to vascular thrombosis of the inferior vena cava, hepatic veins, or portal veins also cause ascites.

i. Prior mycobacterial infection, tuberculosis exposure, or immunocompromise should raise suspicion for intraperitoneal tuberculosis (Tables 36-2 and 36-3).

j. Hemophagocytic syndrome can masquerade as cirrhosis with ascites, fever, jaundice, and hepatosplenomegaly with lymphoma or leukemia.[3]

B. PHYSICAL EXAMINATION

1. The physical examination often is unreliable in diagnosing ascites. The accuracy of the physical examination in detecting ascites is less than 60%. The examination of the patient with suspected ascites begins with inspection for a full, bulging abdomen. The most informative examination finding is dullness to percussion. If there is no dullness on percussion of the flanks, the probability of ascites is less than 10%.[4] Dullness requires 1500 ml of fluid. Testing for a fluid wave is not useful.[5]

TABLE 36-2

CLINICAL CHARACTERISTICS OF PERITONEAL TUBERCULOSIS

Clinical Characteristic	Frequency (%)*
Ascites	80-100
Abdominal swelling	65-100
Abdominal pain	36-93
Weight loss	37-87
Fever	56-100
Diarrhea	9-27
Abdominal tenderness	65-87
Anemia	46-68
Positive purified protein derivative test	55-100

Modified from Goldman L, Bennett JC: *Cecil textbook of medicine,* 21st ed, Philadelphia, 2000, WB Saunders.

*These percentages represent the frequency with which these features have been observed in peritoneal tuberculosis. These data antedate studies of tuberculosis in patients infected with human immunodeficiency virus.

TABLE 36-3

DIAGNOSTIC TESTS OF PERITONEAL TUBERCULOSIS

Diagnostic Test	Comments
Paracentesis	
With smear	< 3% positive
With culture	20%-80% positive
With measurement of ascitic adenosine deaminase	≤ 32.3 U/L; low ascitic protein levels (i.e., cirrhosis) may cause false negative results; not validated in U.S. patients
With lactate dehydrogenase level ≤ 90 U/L	
Laparoscopy with biopsy	Best test; up to 100% positive
Needle biopsy of the peritoneum	Largely replaced by laparoscopy
Diagnostic laparotomy	Should be considered if laparoscopy not available

Modified from Goldman L, Bennett JC: *Cecil textbook of medicine*, 21st ed, Philadelphia, 2000, WB Saunders.

36

ASCITES

2. Gaseous distension and ovarian masses can mimic ascites. On percussion the presence of gas is apparent as diffuse tympani, and the presence of ovarian masses causes central dullness and tympanitic flanks. Detecting ascites in obese patients can be challenging and may entail abdominal ultrasound.

3. It is important to look for the stigmata of advanced liver disease (see Chapter 35). Visible veins on the patient's back suggest blockage of the inferior vena cava. An immobile mass at the umbilicus (Sister Mary Joseph nodule) is highly suggestive of peritoneal carcinomatosis. Elevated jugular venous pressures point to concomitant heart failure or constrictive pericarditis. Patients with nephritic syndrome as the cause of their ascites may have anasarca.

4. SBP, which often has a subtle presentation, is an important consideration. The clinician should maintain a high index of suspicion for SBP because it can develop in any patient with ascites. Symptoms of SBP include abdominal pain, fever, and gastrointestinal complaints such as nausea, vomiting, and diarrhea. Signs of impaired liver function, such as hepatic encephalopathy or renal failure, may be the sole presenting feature.

III. DIAGNOSIS

A. ULTRASOUND

1. Ultrasound can detect as little as 100 ml of abdominal fluid. Ultrasound marking of the abdomen can assist paracentesis by identifying optimal location and loculation of the peritoneal fluid.

B. PARACENTESIS

1. Paracentesis is the gold standard for the proper diagnosis of ascites and is often important in treating discomfort from elevated intraabdominal pressure. Paracentesis is indicated for the following conditions:

a. New-onset ascites.
b. Fever in a patient with known ascites in order to evaluate for SBP.
c. Symptomatic relief.
d. Decompensated liver failure, including new renal failure or encephalopathy, to evaluate for SBP.

2. Bowel perforation and hemoperitoneum are rare complications of paracentesis (< 1 in 1000 patients). Prophylactic transfusion of fresh frozen plasma or platelets in coagulopathic-cirrhotic patients is not indicated and is not recommended because of the low risk of bleeding. Coagulopathy precludes paracentesis only when fibrinolysis or DIC is present.[1,6]

3. Information on how to perform paracentesis can be found in Chapter 2. Ascitic fluid should be sent for a complete blood cell count with differential, albumin levels, and cultures. Studies show that inoculation of 10 to 20 ml of ascitic fluid into two blood culture bottles at the bedside optimizes results.[7]

4. If a concurrent serum albumin level is ordered, the serum-ascites gradient (SAAG) can be calculated as serum albumin minus ascitic albumin and is useful in determining the cause of ascites.[6] A SAAG greater than 1.1 g/dl is 97% accurate in the diagnosis of portal hypertension (Box 36-1).

5. Total protein, glucose, lactate dehydrogenase, carcinoembryonic antigen, and ascitic alkaline phosphatase can help distinguish primary from secondary SBP.

6. Cytologic analysis is 96.7% sensitive for detecting peritoneal carcinomatosis if three samples are sent.

7. Ascitic mycobacterial cultures are 50% sensitive. High clinical suspicion for mycobacterial infection may warrant laparoscopy with biopsy.

8. An ascitic amylase level greater than 20,000 U/L suggests pancreatic ascites from a ruptured pancreatic duct or leaking pseudocyst. Lower but elevated amylase concentrations are seen in acute pancreatitis. Similarly, markedly elevated bilirubin in ascitic fluid may indicate a bile leak from fistulas or anastomotic leaks after liver transplantation.

9. Elevated ascitic triglyceride levels or chylous ascites are consistent with intraabdominal lymphatic obstruction secondary to trauma, tumor, tuberculosis, congenital malformation, or filariasis but may also be seen in nephrotic ascites.

IV. MANAGEMENT

The management of ascites depends on the underlying cause.

1. **Portal hypertension (high-SAAG or cirrhotic ascites).** The conceptual physiologic goal is to achieve negative sodium balance because ascites is caused primarily by sodium retention.

a. **Abstinence from alcohol** reverses ascites and improves mortality in alcohol-induced liver injury.[8]

BOX 36-1

CAUSES OF ASCITES BASED ON SERUM-ASCITES ALBUMIN GRADIENT

HIGH GRADIENT ($\geq$ 1.1 g/dl)

Cirrhosis	Portal vein thrombosis
Alcoholic hepatitis	Veno-occlusive disease
Cardiac failure	Fatty liver of pregnancy
Massive liver metastases	Myxedema
Fulminant hepatic failure	Mixed ascites
Budd-Chiari syndrome	

LOW GRADIENT (< 1.1 g/dl)

Peritoneal carcinomatosis	Nephrotic syndrome
Peritoneal tuberculosis	Serositis
Pancreatic ascites	Bowel obstruction or infarction
Biliary ascites	

Data from Runyon BA et al: *Ann Intern Med* 117(3):215, 1992.

b. **A sodium-restricted diet** (88 mmol/day or 2000 mg/day). A 24-hour urine sodium level greater than 78 mmol/day (88 mmol/day intake, 10 mmol/day nonurinary excretion in afebrile and nondiarrheic patient) suggests dietary noncompliance with sodium restriction. More simply, spot urine sodium concentrations greater than simultaneous spot urine potassium indicate sodium excretion greater than 78 mmol/day with 90% accuracy.[1,9]

c. **Diuretic** therapy of ascites is best achieved with oral spironolactone and furosemide in a 100:40 ratio, with maximum dosages of 400 mg and 160 mg, respectively, to sustain normokalemia. Titrate at 3- to 5-day intervals. Amiloride (10 to 40 mg daily), triamterene (50 to 100 mg twice daily), and eplerenone (selective aldosterone blockade) can be substituted for spironolactone if tender gynecomastia develops.[10] Recommended fluid weight loss is 300 to 500 g/d with peripheral edema and 800 to 1000 g/d without peripheral edema.[11]

d. **Free water restriction is not recommended** unless the serum sodium level is less than 125 mmol/L. **Large-volume therapeutic paracentesis** is appropriate for patients with tense ascites. If more than 4 L is to be removed, give 8 to 10 g albumin per liter of ascites removed.[12] Because diuretics and sodium restriction are the first-line treatment, serial paracentesis (every 2 weeks) is warranted mainly for diuretic-resistant patients.[13] **Referral for liver transplantation** is appropriate, especially when ascites is refractory to medical treatment.[11] (See Chapter 35).

e. Treatment alternatives for patients who develop diuretic-resistant ascites or recurrent hepatohydrothorax include transjugular intrahepatic portosystemic shunting and peritoneovenous shunting. Several large-scale, multicenter randomized controlled trials comparing transjugular intrahepatic portosystemic shunting with sequential large-volume paracentesis have demonstrated better control of ascites with shunting.[14,15] Patients should be monitored in an intensive care setting after the shunt is placed because of the risk of hemoperitoneum. Patients should also be monitored for more common complications including encephalopathy, which is related to the portosystemic shunt. It occurs in approximately 30% of patients and usually presents 2 to 3 weeks after the procedure.[16] Other complications include hemolytic anemia; severe hyperbilirubinemia; vegetative infections; and stenosis leading to recurrent portal hypertension or variceal bleeding. The role of peritoneovenous shunts has diminished in recent years because of the high rate of complications, including fungal infections and disseminated intravascular coagulation.

2. **Low-SAAG ascites.** In low-SAAG ascites, the underlying disorder (usually extrahepatic) must be identified and treated (Box 36-1).

3. **Spontaneous bacterial peritonitis.**

a. Patients with an ascitic fluid polymorphonuclear cell count greater than 250/mm^3 are considered to have SBP and should receive empirical treatment with a third-generation cephalosporin (e.g., cefotaxime 2 g IV every 8 hours or ceftriaxone 1 g every 12 hours).[17] When culture and sensitivity results return, the antibiotic coverage can be narrowed. The three most common isolates from ascitic fluid are *Escherichia coli*, *Klebsiella pneumoniae*, and *Streptococcus pneumoniae.* **Inability to identify an organism from ascitic fluid cultures does not rule out SBP.**

b. After 48 hours of appropriate antimicrobial treatment the ascites neutrophil count should decrease. Patients with a neutrophil count less than 250/mm^3 but with signs and symptoms of systemic illness also need empiric antibiotic treatment until ascites culture results are reported.[1]

c. In patients with cirrhosis and SBP, treatment with IV albumin (1.5 g/kg within 6 hours of the diagnostic paracentesis, followed by 1 g/kg on day 3) in addition to an antibiotic results in a lower incidence of renal impairment and death than does treatment with an antibiotic alone.[18] Secondary peritonitis differs from SBP in that it is a surgically treatable form of peritonitis usually arising from perforation or abscess. Secondary peritonitis often has ascites neutrophil counts in the thousands, polymicrobial infection, and two or three of the following: total protein level greater than 1 g/dl, lactate dehydrogenase level greater than the upper limit of normal for serum, or glucose level less than 70 mg/dl. These criteria offer 100% sensitivity but only 45% specificity for secondary peritonitis.[19] **Polymicrobial SBP is presumed to be caused by bowel perforation until proven otherwise.**

d. **SBP prophylaxis.** For patients at high risk for SBP (ascitic total protein measurements less than 1 g/dl, a prior history of SBP, or acute variceal hemorrhage), oral norfloxacin 400 mg daily is recommended.[20] In the setting of short-term prophylaxis for a high-risk procedure, an alternative is oral ciprofloxacin 500 mg twice a day for 7 days[21] or an IV quinolone (ofloxacin 400 mg daily).[22]

4. **Hepatorenal syndrome** (HRS) is characterized by worsening azotemia with avid sodium retention and oliguria in a patient with advanced liver disease in the absence of primary causes of renal dysfunction. The exact cause remains to be identified; however, altered renal hemodynamics and renal cortical vasoconstriction, caused by imbalances in the production of vasoactive metabolites, play a pathogenic role. The diagnostic criteria for HRS include the following:[11]

a. Liver failure (acute or chronic).

b. Serum creatinine greater than 1.5 or creatinine clearance less than 40 ml/min.

c. Low urine sodium (< 10 mEq/L).

d. No evidence of septic or hypovolemic shock, or use of nephrotoxic medications.

e. No improvement in renal function with volume expansion (IV fluid administration or diuretic cessation).

f. Less than 500 mg/day proteinuria and no ultrasound evidence of obstructive renal failure or parenchymal renal disease.

5. Type 1 HRS is a rapidly progressive renal failure. Creatinine doubles to more than 2.5 mg/dl or creatinine clearance decreases to less than 20 ml/min in less than 2 weeks. Type 2 HRS is slowly progressive and chronic.

6. **Management of HRS.**[11] Patients with type 1 HRS should be referred for liver transplantation. Experimental medical regiments for HRS include combinations of the following:

a. Oral midodrine 7.5 to 12.5 mg three times a day with subcutaneous octreotide 100 to 200 μg three times a day.

b. Norepinephrine 0.5 to 3 mg/hr IV infusion was used in patients in the intensive care unit in one small pilot study with some initial success. However, this intervention remains controversial.

c. In combination with the aforementioned medications, albumin 1 g/kg IV on day 1, followed by 20 to 40 g daily.

d. Duration of therapy is 5 to 15 days, with a goal creatinine of 1.5 mg/dl or less.

e. Hemodialysis may be used as a bridge to liver transplantation if hepatorenal failure is refractory to medical therapy, but dialysis does not improve outcome without transplantation.

PEARLS AND PITFALLS

- The history and physical examination may suggest the cause of ascites, but the gold standard for diagnosis is paracentesis.
- SBP is a common complication of ascites and is associated with myriad presentations. All patients with newly diagnosed ascites, ascites and fever, or decompensation in the setting of known ascites should undergo urgent diagnostic paracentesis.

- Patients with end-stage liver disease often have low blood pressures; however, patients with ascites who have hypotension that does not respond to fluid bolus should be admitted to the intensive care unit.
- Aminoglycosides should not be used to treat SBP because they can exacerbate underlying renal dysfunction.
- Patients receiving appropriate antibiotic treatment for SBP should show clinical improvement within 48 hours. If a patient does not improve, a repeat diagnostic paracentesis is indicated to determine whether the neutrophil count has decreased and to culture the fluid for the possibility of another microbiological cause.

REFERENCES

1. Runyon BA: Management of adult patients with ascites due to cirrhosis, *Hepatology* 39:1-16, 2004. D
2. Runyon BA, Montano AA, Akriviadis EA, Antillon MR, Irving MA, McHutchison JG: The serum-ascites albumin gradient is superior to the exudates-transudate concept in the differential diagnosis of ascites, *Ann Intern Med* 117:215-220, 1992. B
3. de Kerguenec C, Hillaire S, Molinie V, et al: Hepatic manifestations of hemophagocytic syndrome: a study of 30 cases, *Am J Gastroenterology* 96:852-857, 2001. B
4. Williams JW, Simel DL: Does this patient have ascites? How to divine fluid in the abdomen, *JAMA* 267:2645, 1992. C
5. Cattau EL Jr et al: The accuracy of the physical examination in the diagnosis of suspected ascites, *JAMA* 247(8):1164, 1982. A
6. Runyon BA: Paracentesis of ascitic fluid: a safe procedure, *Arch Intern Med* 146:2259-2261, 1986. B
7. Runyon BA, Canawati HN, Akriviadis EA: Optimization of ascitic fluid culture technique, *Gastroenterology* 95(5):1351, 1988. A
8. Veldt BJ, Laine F, Guillogomarc'h A, et al: Indication of liver transplantation in severe alcoholic liver cirrhosis: quantitative evaluation and optimal timing, *J Hepatol* 36:93-98, 2002. B
9. Stiehm AJ, Mendler MH, Runyon BA: Detection of diuretic-resistance or diuretic-sensitivity by the spot urine Na/K ratio in 729 cirrhotics with ascites: approximately 90% accuracy as compared to 24 hour urine Na excretion [abstract], *Hepatology* 36:222A, 2002. B
10. Angeli P, Pria MD, De Bei E, et al: Randomized clinical study of the efficacy of amiloride and potassium anrenoate in nonazotemic cirrhotic patients with ascites, *Hepatology* 19:72-79, 1994. A
11. Gines P, Cardenas A, Arroyo V, Rodes J: Management of cirrhosis and ascites, *N Engl J Med* 350:1646-1654, 2004. C
12. Gines P, Tito L, Arroyo V, et al: Randomized comparative study of therapeutic paracentesis with and without intravenous albumin in cirrhosis, *Gastroenterology* 94:1493-1502, 1988. A
13. Gines P, Arroyo V, Quintero E, et al: Comparison of paracentesis and diuretics in the treatment of cirrhotics with tense ascites: results of a randomized study, *Gastroenterology* 93:234-241, 1987. A
14. Sanyal A, Genning C, Reddy K, et al: The North American study for the treatment of refractory ascites, *Gastroenterology* 124:634-641, 2003. A

15. Rossle M, Ochs A, Gulberg V, et al: A comparison of paracentesis and transjugular intrahepatic portosystemic shunting in patients with ascites, *N Engl J Med* 342:1701-1707, 2000. A

16. Russo M, Sood A, Jacobson I, Brown R: Transjugular intrahepatic portosystemic shunt for refractory ascites: an analysis of the literature on efficacy, morbidity, and mortality, *Am J Gastroenterol* 98:2521-2527, 2003. C

17. Felisart J et al: Cefotaxime is more effective than is ampicillin-tobramycin in cirrhotics with severe infections, *Hepatology* 5(3):457, 1985. A

18. Sort P et al: Effect of intravenous albumin on renal impairment and mortality in patients with cirrhosis and spontaneous bacterial peritonitis, *N Engl J Med* 341:403, 1999. A

19. Akriviadis EA, Runyon BA: The value of an algorithm in differentiating spontaneous from secondary bacterial peritonitis, *Gastroenterology* 98:127-133, 1990. B

20. Gines P, Rimola A, Planas R, et al: Norfloxacin prevents spontaneous bacterial peritonitis recurrence in cirrhosis: results of a double-blind, placebo-controlled trial, *Hepatology* 12:716-724, 1990. A

21. Hsieh W, Lin H, Hwang S, et al: The effect of ciprofloxacin in the prevention of bacterial infection in patients with cirrhosis after upper gastrointestinal bleeding, *Am J Gastroenterol* 93:962-966, 1998. A

22. Blasise M, Paterson D, Trinchet JC, Levacheher S, Ceaugrand M, Pourriat JL: Systemic antibiotic therapy prevents bacterial infection in cirrhotic patients with gastrointestinal hemorrhage, *Hepatology* 20:34-38, 1994. A

36

ASCITES

Gastrointestinal Bleeding

Elizabeth Griffiths, MD, and Sergey Kantsevoy, MD

FAST FACTS

- The first step in managing gastrointestinal (GI) hemorrhage is to assess the hemodynamic stability of the patient and resuscitate if needed.
- Upper GI hemorrhage is defined by bleeding proximal to the ligament of Treitz.
- Eighty percent of patients with GI hemorrhage stop bleeding spontaneously.
- The most common causes of upper GI bleeding (UGIB) are peptic ulcer disease and esophageal varices.
- Mortality from nonvariceal GI bleeding is between 6% and 10%.[1-4]
- Variceal bleeding is associated with > 30% mortality.[5-7]
- Patients with orthostasis, hemodynamic instability, or active bleeding should be evaluated by the intensive care unit.
- The most common causes of lower GI bleeding (LGIB) are diverticulosis and angiodysplasia.
- After a first episode of LGIB all patients should undergo elective outpatient colonoscopy to evaluate for neoplasia.

I. UPPER GI BLEEDING

A. EPIDEMIOLOGY

1. UGIB results in approximately 300,000 hospital admissions annually in the United States.[1,7] Table 37-1 lists the most common causes of acute UGIB.[3,4,8,9]
2. Eighty percent of patients stop bleeding spontaneously; most of the morbidity and mortality with UGIB occurs in the remaining 20%.[7]
3. Ninety percent of patients with liver disease and cirrhosis have gastric varices, and 29% of these patients bleed.[10,11]

B. CLINICAL PRESENTATION

1. The presence of acute UGIB is suggested by hematemesis (bloody or coffee-ground vomit), which is seen in 56% of patients.[3]
2. Distinguishing between UGIB and LGIB on the basis of stool color can be difficult. Seventy percent of patients with UGIB have melena, which can result from as little as 50 ml of blood.[9,12] Hematochezia usually is associated with a lower GI source of bleeding but can also be seen with large-volume (> 1000 ml), brisk UGIB.[12,13] As many as 11% of patients suspected initially to have LGIB ultimately are found to have an upper GI source.[2]
3. The first priority in patients who present with GI bleeding is hemodynamic stability, which should be achieved with appropriate

TABLE 37-1

CAUSES OF ACUTE UPPER GASTROINTESTINAL HEMORRHAGE

Most Common Causes

Diagnosis	Incidence (%)
Peptic ulcer disease (stomach or duodenum)	47-79
Gastric erosions	6-30
Esophageal varices	8-16
No diagnosis determined	8-22

Less Common Causes

Esophagitis
Erosive duodenitis
Mallory-Weiss tear
Neoplasm
Esophageal ulcer
Osler-Weber-Rendu telangiectasia

volume resuscitation and blood pressure stabilization. Resting tachycardia suggests 10% volume loss, and postural hypotension occurs after 20% to 30% loss of circulating volume. Shock (suggested by a supine blood pressure < 100 mmHg and pulse > 100 beats/min) indicates a 40% loss of intravascular volume and is associated with mortality rates up to 30%. This evaluation should be followed by clinical risk stratification and, for those at high risk, early endoscopy[7] (Box 37-1).

4. Although UGIB can be dramatic, it may also be asymptomatic. The most common presentation is iron deficiency anemia or repeatedly positive stool occult blood tests.[14] These findings should prompt a reasonably quick but not emergent evaluation beginning with elective outpatient upper and lower endoscopy.

C. DIAGNOSIS

1. Nasogastric (NG) aspirate and lavage.

a. **When UGIB is strongly suspected, a NG tube should be placed and lavage performed with 500 ml water.**[13] The suspicion of varices should not preclude placement of an NG tube except in the event of a recent banding procedure. NG lavage that reveals bright red blood confirms the diagnosis of active UGIB and in many studies has been shown to predict poor outcome.[7,13] If lavage produces only coffee-ground material, this probably represents recent but not ongoing UGIB.

b. If initial lavage reveals a large amount of fresh blood, gastric lavage with tap water should be continued in an attempt to clear the stomach contents before esophagogastroduodenoscopy (EGD).

c. **Negative lavage does not rule out UGIB** because the bleeding may have stopped or may be occurring at a site beyond the gastric pylorus; bilious return is more reassuring.[3]

d. Positive findings can also be misleading: only 30% of those with coffee grounds and 50% with red blood on aspiration had active bleeding at endoscopy.[15]

BOX 37-1	
RISK STRATIFICATION IN GASTROINTESTINAL BLEEDING	
CLINICAL PREDICTORS OF MORBIDITY	CLINICAL PREDICTORS OF MORTALITY
Age > 65	Age > 60
Shock	Shock
Poor overall health	Poor health
Comorbid illness	Comorbid illness
Low initial hemoglobin	Continued bleeding or rebleeding
Melena	Fresh blood from above or below
Need for transfusion	Bleeding while in hospital for another
Fresh red blood on rectal examination,	reason
in emesis, or in the nasogastric	Elevated urea, creatinine, or
aspirate	aminotransferases

2. Admission laboratory studies (Table 37-2).

3. **Diagnostic studies.**

a. **Endoscopy.** EGD should be performed to localize the site of bleeding and allow possible therapeutic intervention. EGD within the first 24 hours of hospitalization can allow safe discharge of patients at low risk of rebleeding.[7]

b. **Tagged red blood cell scan.** A tagged red blood cell scan may be helpful in finding the site of bleeding in patients with brisk bleeding (> 0.1 ml/min) if EGD is not available or cannot find the source, although its utility and accuracy are controversial.[16]

c. **Selective mesenteric arteriography** is another alternative to EGD. Angiography has a sensitivity of 75% but is helpful only in the setting of brisk bleeding (arterial blood loss of 0.5 to 0.6 ml/min).[11]

d. **Chest radiograph.** This should be performed in those with significant hematemesis or altered mental status to evaluate for sequelae of aspiration.

e. **Barium contrast studies** should be avoided because they may interfere with subsequent EGD, angiography, or surgery.

D. **MANAGEMENT**

1. **Hemodynamic stabilization.**

a. All patients with GI bleeding should have two large-bore (≥ 18-gauge) peripheral intravenous lines or a large central venous line at all times to facilitate rapid, large-volume infusions in the case of sudden GI hemorrhage.

b. Hemodynamic status should be assessed immediately. If indicated, resuscitation should begin with normal saline and subsequently with blood products.

c. Elective endotracheal intubation for airway protection during EGD in cases of copious UGIB is controversial. It should be considered in those with massive bleeding, altered mental status, or severe agitation.

2. **Supportive transfusions.**

TABLE 37-2

RECOMMENDED LABORATORY EVALUATION OF GI BLEEDING

Laboratory Study	Recommendations
Hemoglobin and hematocrit	May take 48-72 hr to reflect blood loss because this entails equilibration between the intravascular and extravascular space. Hematocrits should be checked every 4-6 hr while patient is bleeding.[17]
Prothrombin time and partial thromboplastin time	These should be checked on admission and, if abnormal, should be corrected to within 1.5 times normal with infusion of fresh frozen plasma and subcutaneous vitamin K.
Platelet count	Patients with platelets < 50,000 should receive platelet transfusions to keep platelets above this value.
Blood urea nitrogen/creatinine	A ratio > 35 suggests absorption of blood from the GI tract in patients with normal renal function and suggests upper GI or proximal lower GI bleeding.[18,19]
ABO and Rh antibody type and crossmatch	Patients with the diagnosis of GI bleeding should always have an active type and screen. If there is ongoing bleeding, 2-4 units of crossmatched blood should be kept on reserve.

GI, gastrointestinal.

a. Transfuse with packed red blood cells to a goal hematocrit > 25%. **Transfusion should increase the hematocrit approximately 2% to 3% per unit transfused; failure to increase appropriately suggests ongoing blood loss.**

b. Calcium levels should be monitored after multiple transfusions (i.e., > 5) because calcium chelation with EDTA may cause hypocalcemia. Fresh frozen plasma should be given if dilutional coagulopathy becomes a concern.

3. **Empiric therapy with acid suppression** before EGD is based largely on biological plausibility. Proton pump inhibitors (PPI) or histamine receptor antagonists should be initiated early (i.e., before EGD results).[7]

4. **Specific causes.**

a. **Erosive esophagitis** causes up to 6% of UGIB and is caused by gastroesophageal reflux disease, fungal (*Candida* sp.) or viral (herpes simplex virus, cytomegalovirus) infections, and pills in the esophagus (bisphosphonates, tetracycline, potassium, and nonsteroidal antiinflammatory drugs [NSAIDs]). Treatment is based on the underlying cause.[2]

b. A **Mallory Weiss tear** is a linear mucosal tear near the esophagogastric junction, usually caused by retching; 23% of such tears bleed, accounting for 3% to 15% of all UGIB. These lesions usually stop bleeding spontaneously, but they can occasionally be more serious, and in these cases therapy is largely endoscopic.[11]

c. Peptic ulcers.
   (1) The endoscopic appearance of ulcers has been correlated with the risk of rebleeding and mortality (Table 37-3).
   (2) Low-risk patients are those with clean-based ulcers or nonprotuberant clot on an ulcer bed. High-risk lesions include those with visible vessels or actively bleeding ulcers.
   (3) **Recurrent bleeding is the most important predictor of adverse outcome and is associated with a five- to sixteenfold increase in mortality.**[20]
   (4) Patients who experience recurrent bleeding should undergo a second attempt at endoscopic management.[21] If bleeding continues despite repeat EGD or if the patient remains hemodynamically unstable despite aggressive resuscitation, the patient should be referred for surgery.[21] Arterial embolization can be considered in poor surgical candidates.[22]
   (5) Control of gastric acidity can promote healing and prevent recurrent bleeding in high-risk patients. Those with severe bleeding and high-risk findings on EGD should receive a bolus followed by continuous intravenous infusion of a PPI.[7,23]
   (6) Follow-up elective EGD should be performed in those with a gastric ulcer to ensure healing and exclude an underlying malignancy.
   (7) The two primary risk factors for ulcers are *Helicobacter pylori* infection and use of NSAIDs. Therefore when endoscopic biopsy reveals *H. pylori*, the patient should be treated for eradication of the organism. All NSAIDs (including aspirin) should be avoided.[25]
d. Varices.
   (1) **In a patient with known cirrhosis and portal hypertension, the most likely source of bleeding is an esophagogastric varix.**
   (2) Intravenous octreotide (a long-acting analog of somatostatin) should be started once the patient is hemodynamically stable (administered as an initial 50-µg bolus followed by 50 µg/hr continuous infusion for 3 to 5 days). A combination of octreotide and endoscopic therapy appears to be more effective than either modality alone.[26]

TABLE 37-3

ASSOCIATION BETWEEN ENDOSCOPIC APPEARANCE OF ULCERS AND RISK OF REBLEEDING AND MORTALITY[24]

Endoscopic Characteristic	Prevalence (%)	Rebleeding (%)	Surgery (%)	Mortality (%)
Clean base	42	5	0.5	2
Flat spot	20	10	6	3
Adherent clot	17	22	10	7
Nonbleeding visible vessel	17	43	34	11
Active bleeding	18	55	35	11

(3) EGD can allow therapeutic interventions such as sclerotherapy and band ligation. If these techniques do not stop bleeding, balloon tamponade (e.g., with a Sengstaken-Blakemore or Minnesota tube) should be attempted.

(4) Once the patient has stopped actively bleeding, combination medical treatment with a nonselective beta-blocker (e.g., nadolol or propranolol) and isosorbide mononitrate has been found to be more effective than either agent alone.[27] Beta-blockers should be started first and titrated to a goal heart rate of 55 to 60 beats/min. Isosorbide mononitrate can be added and titrated to a goal systolic blood pressure of 95 to 105 mmHg. Endoscopic therapy with band ligation has recently been shown to be as effective as beta-blockers in decreasing the incidence of first bleeding episodes and rebleeding.[28]

(5) Patients with recurrent variceal bleeding should be considered for transjugular intrahepatic portosystemic shunt placement.[29,30]

(6) Bleeding from varices stops spontaneously in about 50% of patients, but without intervention, the rebleeding rate is 60% to 70%. If variceal bleeding is continuous, the mortality approaches 80%.

e. **Obscure GI bleeding** accounts for 3% to 5% of all UGIB and includes angiodysplasia, Dieulafoy lesions (submucosal arteriolar bleeding through a small vessel protruding through otherwise normal mucosa), Cameron erosions (erosions within a large hiatal hernia), malignancy, and hemobilia.[11,14]

II. LOWER GI BLEEDING
A. EPIDEMIOLOGY
1. LGIB is distal to the ligament of Treitz and accounts for approximately 24% to 33% of all hospital admissions for GI bleeding.[31]
2. The relative risk of LGIB increases 200-fold with an increase in age from 20 to 80.[32] This increase is explained primarily by the development of diverticular disease and angiodysplasia with aging.

B. CLINICAL PRESENTATION
1. Acute LGIB usually presents as hematochezia, melena, or dark blood with clots. Hematochezia most commonly results from LGIB, although 1 in 10 patients with hematochezia are found to have a brisk UGIB.
2. Melena suggests a bleeding source proximal to the cecum, and dark red blood with clots usually is from a source in the ascending colon. Acute LGIB usually warrants hospital admission and further evaluation.
3. A significant number of patients presenting with acute LGIB experience severe, persistent bleeding, and these patients account for most of the morbidity and mortality. It is essential to identify these patients for early, aggressive resuscitation and intervention. Table 37-4 reviews the findings most predictive of severe bleeding.
4. LGIB may also present with progressive iron deficiency anemia or Hemoccult-positive stool on routine screening. These findings suggest a

INDEPENDENT RISK FACTORS FOR SEVERE* LOWER GASTROINTESTINAL BLEEDING

Predictor	Odds Ratio (95% Confidence Interval)	P Value
Heart rate > 100	3.67 (1.78-7.57)	< 0.001
Systolic blood pressure < 115	3.45 (1.54-7.72)	0.003
Syncope	2.82 (1.06-7.46)	0.04
Nontender abdominal examination	2.43 (1.22-4.85)	0.01
Persistent bleeding (gross blood on rectal examination, bleeding during the first 4 hr of presentation)	2.32 (1.28-4.2)	0.005
Aspirin use (any daily aspirin)	2.07 (1.12-3.82)	0.02
> 2 Comorbid illnesses	1.93 (1.08-3.44)	0.02

Modified from Strate LL, Orav EJ, Syngal SS: *Arch Intern Med* 163:838-843, 2003.
*> 2 units of packed red blood cells, > 20% decrease in hematocrit, or recurrent bleeding after 24 hr causing hematocrit drop of > 20%, necessitating additional transfusions or readmission to the hospital within 1 week.

MORTALITY AND CAUSES OF LOWER GASTROINTESTINAL BLEEDING

Source of Bleeding	Percentage of Cases
Diverticulosis	15-48
Angiodysplasia	3-37
Cancer or polyps	9-30
Colitis or ulcerations	6-22
Anorectal pathology	0-9
Other	4-14
Overall mortality	2-5

slightly different differential diagnosis and usually can be evaluated with colonoscopy and managed on an outpatient basis.

C. INITIAL EVALUATION AND MANAGEMENT

All patients presenting with acute LGIB should be assessed for hemodynamic instability, and initial resuscitation should proceed with volume repletion, vascular access, and correction of coagulopathy, as with UGIB. Table 37-2 details the appropriate admission laboratory studies. A complete history and physical examination help to formulate a differential diagnosis for the cause of bleeding.

D. DIFFERENTIAL DIAGNOSIS OF LGIB

Table 37-5 lists the causes and mortality associated with LGIB. This section reviews the specific features of diagnosis and management for the most common causes of bleeding.

1. **Diverticular disease.**
a. In most cases, colonic diverticula are acquired lesions, associated with increasing age.[33] Most diverticula occur in the sigmoid colon between

the tenia coli, are paired, and are distributed regularly along the length of the colon, paralleling the location of penetrating vessels.[33] The incidence of diverticulosis ranges from 2% to 10%; however, most patients are asymptomatic.[34]

b. **Diverticulosis is the most common cause of LGIB.** Diverticular bleeding usually is painless; however, it can also present with mild abdominal cramping followed by passage of large-volume red or maroon blood and clots.

c. Bleeding resolves spontaneously in 70% to 80% of cases, but 22% to 38% of patients rebleed.[35,36] NSAID and aspirin use, particularly in combination, is considered one of the greatest risk factors for severe diverticular bleeding.

2. **Angiodysplasia.**

a. Arteriovenous malformations (AVMs), or angiodysplasia, are small, dilated submucosal veins responsible for 20% to 30% of acute LGIB. These lesions increase in frequency with age and are distributed throughout the small and large intestine. In the colon, AVMs usually are found in the cecum and proximal ascending colon.[37]

b. AVMs can cause a range of bleeding from Hemoccult-positive stools to life-threatening acute LGIB.[38]

c. Although angiography remains the standard for diagnosis, colonoscopy with intervention on these lesions is a well-studied and effective form of management with a sensitivity better than 80% with good bowel preparation.[38] Treatment of these patients with estrogen is controversial and may not be effective.[39] Surgery should be considered in patients with a well-localized source of bleeding who do not respond to conservative therapy.

d. Angiodysplasia in the setting of aortic stenosis is called Heyde's syndrome and is thought to be caused by acquired von Willebrand deficiency (see Chapter 45). The clinician should keep this association in mind because the presence of aortic stenosis may alter hemodynamic management.

3. **Neoplastic disease.** Rectal bleeding is concerning for colorectal cancer, especially in older adults. Among patients presenting with LGIB, polyps or cancers are present in 2% to 35% of patients.[40]

4. **Colitis.**

a. **Ischemic colitis.**

(1) Colonic ischemia is most commonly encountered in older patients with multiple comorbidities; however, this entity has been described in a broad range of age groups in the context of shock, vasculitis, coagulopathy, long-distance running, cocaine abuse, and as a side effect of medications (5-hydroxytryptamine antagonists).

(2) Clinically, patients present with an unexplained GI illness with Hemoccult-positive diarrhea or frank LGIB with or without an acute abdomen.[41] Risk factors for a poor prognosis include end-stage

renal disease and atherosclerotic disease.[41] Overall mortality approaches 30% in patients on hemodialysis.[41]

   (3) Colonoscopic examination demonstrates ulceration, and histology reveals necrosis. Persistent chronic ischemia can lead to stricturing and may necessitate colonic resection.

b. **Inflammatory colitis.** Acute LGIB is an uncommon complication of inflammatory bowel disease. The incidence is < 5%, with major bleeding occurring more commonly in patients with Crohn's disease than ulcerative colitis (see Chapter 38).[42]

c. **Infectious colitis.** Bacteria, viruses, and parasites can all cause bloody diarrhea (see Chapter 39).

d. **Radiation colitis.** Rectal bleeding is the most common complication of radiation therapy for cancers of the prostate and cervix. The incidence ranges from 5% to 30% and correlates with the total dosage of radiation delivered. Because of radiation-induced scarring, surgery should be considered a last resort.

5. **Hemorrhoids.** Many people who present with LGIB have hemorrhoids, but the degree to which they represent a true source of bleeding is less well established. Two percent to nine percent of patients with significant hematochezia have a hemorrhoidal source.

E. DIAGNOSTIC AND THERAPEUTIC EVALUATION

Evaluation for the source of LGIB bleeding can be difficult. Various diagnostic and therapeutic options exist. Initial evaluation usually includes colonoscopy, angiography, or tagged red cell scan.

1. **Tagged red blood cell scan** can detect rates of bleeding as low as 0.1 ml/min, but higher rates of bleeding usually are necessary for accurate detection and localization. This test is most accurate when positive results are obtained within 2 hours of injection. Positive results localize the bleeding to a particular area in the abdomen, and the utility of these scans is primarily to demonstrate that the rate of bleeding is adequate to be visualized with angiography.

2. **Angiography** can allow identification of the site of bleeding if the rate is greater than 0.5 ml/min and can also provide therapeutic options such as local vasopressin infusion and selective embolization.

3. **Colonoscopy** has shown promise for management of LGIB. Although the data for colonoscopic intervention in patients with acute LGIB are limited, early studies have demonstrated good bleeding control, with fewer complications than angiography.[43] An algorithm for the timely management of lower GI bleeding is shown in Figs. 37-1 and 37-2.

4. **Surgery** should be considered in patients with brisk, ongoing bleeding necessitating transfusion of > 4 units of blood, those who rebleed despite angiographic or endoscopic management, and those with hemorrhagic shock despite resuscitation.

F. OUTCOMES

The mortality rate for LGIB is < 5%. Patients who develop LGIB while in the hospital have a significantly higher mortality than those who present and are admitted with symptoms of LGIB.

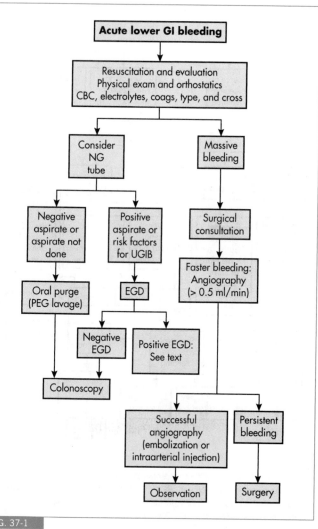

FIG. 37-1

Algorithm for the timely management of acute lower GI bleeding. *GI*, gastrointestinal; *CBC*, complete blood cell count; *NG*, nasogastric; *UGIB*, upper gastrointestinal bleeding; *EGD*, esophagogastroduodenoscopy. *(From Eisen GM et al: Gastrointest Endosc 53(7):859-863, 2001.)*

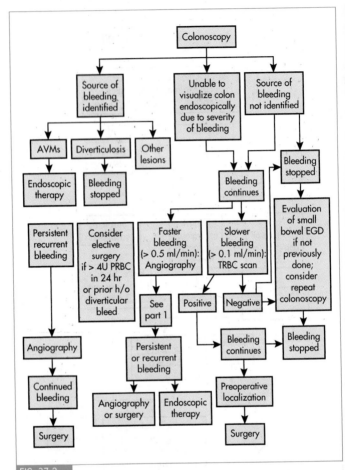

FIG. 37-2

Algorithm for colonoscopy in the setting of acute lower GI bleeding. *AVM*, arteriovenous malformation; *U*, unit; *PRBC*, packed red blood cells; *TRBC*, tagged red blood cell; *EGD*, esophagogastroduodenoscopy. *(From Eisen GM et al: Gastrointest Endosc 53(7):859-863, 2001.)*

PEARLS AND PITFALLS
- In patients with a history of coronary artery disease, special care should be taken to assess for myocardial ischemia in the setting of UGIB. Recent history of myocardial infarction does not preclude EGD unless the patient is hypotensive or very ill.[44]

- Indications for intensive care unit evaluation include hemodynamic instability, orthostasis, shock, active bleeding, ongoing hematemesis or hematochezia, and nasogastric lavage with bright red blood that does not clear after 500-ml lavage.
- Predictors of adverse outcome (defined as death, need for any operation, recurrent hematemesis, recurrent melena after initial clearing, or a falling hematocrit value despite transfusion) at initial evaluation include initial hematocrit < 30%, initial systolic blood pressure < 100 mmHg, red blood in the nasogastric lavage, evidence of portal hypertension (e.g., history of cirrhosis or ascites on examination), and hematemesis.[45]
- Predictors of mortality include age older than 60 years and the presence of serious comorbid disease. The mortality rate is 12% to 25% in patients older than 60 years and 10% in patients younger than 60 years. In patients with GI bleeding, as the number of comorbidities (cardiac, central nervous system, GI, hepatic, neoplastic, pulmonary, and renal) increases from none to six, mortality rates increase from 3% to 7%, 10%, 15%, 27%, 44%, and 67%, respectively.

REFERENCES

1. Cutler JA, Mendeloff AI: Upper gastrointestinal bleeding: nature and magnitude of the problem in the U.S., *Dig Dis Sci* 26(suppl):90S, 1981. B
2. Silverstein FE et al: The national ASGE survey on upper gastrointestinal bleeding. II. Clinical prognostic factors, *Gastrointest Endosc* 27:80, 1981. B
3. Gilbert DA et al: The national ASGE survey on upper gastrointestinal bleeding. III. Endoscopy in upper gastrointestinal bleeding, *Gastrointest Endosc* 27:94, 1981. B
4. Yavorski RT et al: Analysis of 3294 cases of upper gastrointestinal bleeding in military medical facilities, *Am J Gastroenterol* 90:568, 1995. B
5. Graham DY, Smith JL: The course of patients after variceal hemorrhage, *Gastroenterology* 80:800, 1981. B
6. Thomsen BL, Moller S, Sorensen TIA: Copenhagen Esophageal Varices Sclerotherapy Project: optimized analysis of recurrent bleeding and death in patients with cirrhosis and esophageal varices, *J Hepatol* 21:367, 1994. B
7. Barkun A, Bardou M, Marshall JK: Consensus recommendations for managing patients with nonvariceal upper gastrointestinal bleeding, *Ann Intern Med* 139:843-857, 2003. B
8. Longstreth GF, Feitelberg SP: Hospital care of acute nonvariceal upper gastrointestinal bleeding: 1991 & 1981, *J Clin Gastroenterol* 19:189, 1994. B
9. Daniel WA Jr, Egan S: The quantity of blood required to produce a tarry stool, *JAMA* 113:2232, 1939. B
10. Kleber G et al: Prediction of variceal hemorrhage in cirrhosis: a prospective follow up study, *Gastroenterology* 100(5 pt 1):1332-1337, 1991. A
11. Exon DJ, Sydney Chung SC: Endoscopic therapy for upper gastrointestinal bleeding, *Best Pract Res Clin Gastroenterol* 18(1):77-98, 2004. C
12. Schiff L et al: Observations on the oral administration of citrated blood in man. II. The effect on the stools, *Am J Med Sci* 203:409, 1942. B
13. Luk GD, Bynum TE, Hendrix TR: Gastric aspiration in localization of gastrointestinal hemorrhage, *JAMA* 241:576, 1979. B

37

GASTROINTESTINAL BLEEDING

14. Leighton JA et al: Obscure gastrointestinal bleeding, *Gastrointest Endosc* 58(5):650-655, 2003. D
15. Peter DJ, Dougherty JM: Evaluation of the patient with gastrointestinal bleeding: an evidence based approach, *Emerg Med Clin North Am* 17:239, 1999. C
16. Garofalo TE, Abdu RA: Accuracy and efficacy of nuclear scintigraphy for the detection of gastrointestinal bleeding, *Arch Surg* 132:196, 1997. B
17. Ebert RV, Stead EA, Gibson JG: Response of normal subjects to acute blood loss, *Arch Intern Med* 68:687, 1941. B
18. Richards RJ, Donica MB, Grayer D: Can the blood urea nitrogen/creatinine ratio distinguish upper from lower gastrointestinal bleeding? *J Clin Gastroenterol* 12:500, 1990. B
19. Chalasani N, et al: Blood urea nitrogen-to-creatinine concentration in gastrointestinal bleeding: a reappraisal, *Am J Gastroenterol* 92:1796, 1997. B
20. Rockall TA, Logan RF, Devlin HB, Northfield TC: Risk assessment after acute upper gastrointestinal haemorrhage, *Gut* 38(3):316-321, 1996. B
21. Lau JYW et al: Endoscopic retreatment compared with surgery in patients with recurrent bleeding after initial endoscopic control of bleeding ulcers, *N Engl J Med* 340:751, 1999. A
22. Lieberman DA et al: Arterial embolization for massive upper gastrointestinal tract bleeding in poor surgical candidates, *Gastroenterology* 86:876, 1984. B
23. Lau JY et al: Effect of intravenous omeprazole on recurrent bleeding after endoscopic treatment of bleeding peptic ulcers, *N Engl J Med* 343:310, 2000. A
24. Laine L, Peterson WL: Bleeding peptic ulcer, *N Engl J Med* 331:717, 1994. C
25. Somerville K, Faulkner G, Langman M: Non-steroidal anti-inflammatory drugs and bleeding peptic ulcer, *Lancet* 1:462, 1986. B
26. Avgerinos A et al: Early administration of somatostatin and efficacy of sclerotherapy in active oesophageal variceal bleeds: the European Acute Bleeding Oesophageal Variceal Episodes (ABOVE) randomised trial, *Lancet* 350:1495, 1997. A
27. Villanueva C et al: Nadolol plus isosorbide mononitrate compared with sclerotherapy for the prevention of variceal rebleeding, *N Engl J Med* 334:1624, 1996. A
28. Zaman A: Current management of esophageal varices, *Curr Treat Options Gastroenterol* 6(6):499-507, 2003. C
29. Cabrera J et al: Transjugular intrahepatic portosystemic shunt versus sclerotherapy in the elective treatment of variceal hemorrhage, *Gastroenterology* 110:832, 1996. A
30. Rossle M et al: Randomised trial of transjugular-intrahepatic-portosystemic shunt versus endoscopy plus propranolol for prevention of variceal rebleeding, *Lancet* 349:1043, 1997. A
31. Peura DA et al: The American College of Gastroenterology Bleeding Registry: preliminary findings, *Am J Gastroenterol* 92(6):924, 1997. D
32. Longstreth GF: Epidemiology and outcome of patients hospitalized with acute lower gastrointestinal hemorrhage: a population-based study, *Am J Gastroenterol* 92(3):206, 1997. B
33. West AM, Losada M: The pathology of diverticular disease, *J Clin Gastroenterol* 38:S11-S16, 2004. C
34. Stollman N, Raskin JB: Diverticular disease of the colon, *Lancet* 363:631-639, 2004. C
35. McGuire HH Jr, Haynes BW Jr: Massive hemorrhage from diverticulitis of the colon: guidelines for therapy based on bleeding patterns in fifty cases, *Ann Surg* 175:847-855, 1972. B

36. Zuckerman GR, Prakash C: Acute lower intestinal bleeding. II. Etiology, therapy, and outcomes, *Gastrointest Endosc* 49(2):228, 1999. C

37. Bounds BC, Friedman LS: Lower gastrointestinal bleeding, *Gastroenterol Clin North Am* 32(4):1107-1125, 2003. C

38. Richter JM et al: Angiodysplasia. Clinical presentation and colonoscopic diagnosis, *Dig Dis Sci* 29(6):481-485, 1984. B

39. Hodgson H: Hormonal therapy for gastrointestinal angiodysplasia, *Lancet* 359(9318):1630-1631, 2002. C

40. Ferraris R et al: Predictive value of rectal bleeding for distal colonic neoplastic lesions in a screened population, *Eur J Cancer* 40:245-252, 2004. B

41. Scharff JR et al: Ischemic colitis: spectrum of disease and outcome, *Surgery* 134(4):624-629, 2003. B

42. Pardi DS et al: Acute major gastrointestinal hemorrhage in inflammatory bowel disease, *Gastrointest Endosc* 49(2):153-157, 1999. B

43. Jensen DM et al: Urgent colonoscopy for the diagnosis and treatment of severe diverticular hemorrhage, *N Engl J Med* 342:78-82, 2000. B

44. Cappell MS, Iacovone FM Jr: Safety and efficacy of esophagogastroduodenoscopy after myocardial infarction, *Am J Med* 106:29, 1999. B

45. Corley DA et al: Early indicators of prognosis in upper gastrointestinal hemorrhage, *Am J Gastroenterol* 93:336, 1998. B

37

Inflammatory Bowel Disease

Lynn B. Eckert, MD; Geoffrey C. Nguyen, MD; and Mary L. Harris, MD

FAST FACTS

- *Inflammatory bowel disease (IBD)* refers to ulcerative colitis (UC) and Crohn's disease, idiopathic diseases affecting the gastrointestinal tract that are distinguished from each other by clinical, histologic, and endoscopic characteristics (Table 38-1).
- Although the clinical course of IBD is chronic and often relapsing and remitting, mortality is generally not greater than in the general population.
- UC is confined to the mucosa and submucosa of the colon and invariably involves the rectum.
- Crohn's disease may affect any component of the gastrointestinal tract in a discontinuous pattern of "skip lesions."
- UC and Crohn's disease have clinical and therapeutic similarities, and approximately 10% of patients have indeterminate IBD in which the clinical picture does not allow distinction between the two entities.

I. EPIDEMIOLOGY

1. The incidence and prevalence of UC in the United States are 7.3 and 116 per 100,000, respectively. The incidence of Crohn's disease is 7 in 100,000, and the prevalence is 104 in 100,000.[1]
2. The peak age at onset for both diseases is between 15 and 25 years, with a smaller second peak between the ages of 40 and 60. Men and women are affected equally.
3. The incidence of UC and Crohn's disease is higher among people of Ashkenazi Jewish and Scandinavian descent and lower among Hispanics and African Americans.
4. Interestingly, there is a strong association between Crohn's disease and cigarette smoking but a weaker association between ulcerative colitis and tobacco use.

II. CLINICAL PRESENTATION

A. ULCERATIVE COLITIS

1. The typical presentation of UC is bloody diarrhea characterized by frequent small, loose stools and often associated with tenesmus. However, symptoms depend on severity and location of disease. Severity of disease is assessed by clinical, physical, and laboratory criteria as shown in Table 38-2.

TABLE 38-1

COMPARISON OF ULCERATIVE COLITIS AND CROHN'S DISEASE

	Ulcerative Colitis	Crohn's Disease
CLINICAL FEATURES		
Diarrhea	Often bloody	Usually occult blood
Constitutional symptoms	In severe disease	Common
Abdominal pain	In severe disease	Often prominent
Perianal disease	None	Common
Fistulas	None	Common
Small bowel involvement	Never with exception of backwash ileitis	Common
Surgery	Curative	Recurs after surgery
Increased cancer risk	Yes	Yes
ENDOSCOPIC FEATURES		
Rectal involvement	Always	Rectal sparing common
Lesions	Continuous and circumferential	Skip lesions
Aphthous ulcers	Uncommon	Common
Cobblestoning	No	Yes
PATHOLOGIC FEATURES		
Inflammation	Mucosal and submucosal	Transmural
Granuloma	No	Diagnostic when present

TABLE 38-2

CRITERIA FOR EVALUATING THE SEVERITY OF ULCERATIVE COLITIS

Criterion	Mild Disease	Severe Disease	Fulminant Disease
Stool frequency (per day)	≤ 4	5-10	> 10
Hematochezia	Intermittent	Frequent	Continuous
Temperature (°C)	Normal	> 37.5	> 37.5
Heart rate (beats/min)	Normal	> 90	> 90
Hematocrit value	Normal	< 75% of normal	Transfusion needed
Erythrocyte sedimentation rate	Normal	Elevated	Elevated
Colonic features on radiography	—	Air, edematous wall	Dilation, thumbprinting
Clinical signs	—	Abdominal tenderness	Abdominal distension and tenderness

Modified from Hanauer SB: *N Engl J Med* 334:841, 1996.

2. UC invariably involves the rectum and is called ulcerative proctitis when it is limited to this area. Proctosigmoiditis extends into the mid–sigmoid colon, and left-sided UC involves the regions up to the splenic flexure. Pancolitis is inflammation that affects colonic mucosa beyond the splenic flexure.

3. More than half of patients initially have a mild and indolent disease that involves the rectum and sigmoid, characterized by self-limited episodes of rectal bleeding and tenesmus, although nonbloody diarrhea is not uncommon. At presentation, approximately one third have moderately severe disease (see Table 38-2). Severe or fulminant UC is characterized by more than 10 bloody stools per day, severe abdominal cramping, severe anemia, high-grade fever, hypoalbuminemia, and weight loss.

4. The rectal examination may reveal bright red blood, but the physical examination usually is normal in mild UC. Patients with moderate disease may have low-grade fever and abdominal tenderness. In severe cases, however, presenting features of UC may include fever, tachycardia, orthostatic hypotension, severe abdominal tenderness with rebound over the colon, and decreased bowel sounds.

5. A deadly complication of UC is toxic megacolon resulting from transmural inflammation. The inflammation paralyzes smooth muscle layers, resulting in colonic dilation associated with systemic symptoms. Bloody diarrhea with abdominal distension and tenderness is typical, and patients appear acutely toxic. Diagnosis is based on radiographic evidence of colonic dilation and the clinical criteria outlined in Box 38-1. Management of toxic megacolon is detailed in Chapter 30.

6. The differential diagnosis of UC depends on the presentation. If the patient has proctitis, the physician should consider other causes of rectal blood, including internal hemorrhoids, diverticulosis, arteriovenous malformations, colorectal cancer, infectious proctitis, and radiation proctitis in those with history of exposure. For patients with bloody diarrhea, infectious colitis (e.g., *Shigella, Campylobacter, Yersinia*) and ischemic colitis should be included in the differential diagnosis.

B. CROHN'S DISEASE

1. The clinical presentation of Crohn's disease is more variable than that of UC. The predominant symptoms are diarrhea, abdominal pain, and weight loss, often associated with low-grade fever and malaise.

2. Crohn's disease most often affects the ileum and colon (40%) but may be confined to the distal ileum (30%) or limited to the colon (25%).[2]

BOX 38-1

CRITERIA FOR TOXIC MEGACOLON

1. Chronic dilation plus	3. One of the following:
2. Three of the following:	Dehydration
Fever > 38°C	Altered mental status
Tachycardia >120 beats/min	Hypotension
Leukocytosis >10,500/mm³	Electrolyte disturbances
Anemia	
plus	

The clinical course can follow three patterns: inflammatory, perforating and fistulizing, and stenosing or stricturing. The inflammatory type involves diarrhea caused by multiple factors, including increased secretion and impaired fluid reabsorption resulting from inflammation of the ileum or colon. Bile malabsorption and steatorrhea may also result from ileal disease or resection. Patients with inflammatory Crohn's disease often have colicky abdominal pain, often in the right lower quadrant. Perforating disease may occur when transmural inflammation leads to serosal penetration and subsequent localized peritonitis with fever and abdominal pain with rebound or guarding. Penetration of the bowel wall may also result in fistulization.

3. Although enteroenteric fistulas may be asymptomatic, enterovesicular fistulas may lead to recurrent polymicrobial urinary tract infections and pneumaturia. Psoas and retroperitoneal abscesses may arise from fistulas in the retroperitoneum. Perianal disease (perianal abscesses, fissures, ulcers, strictures, and stenoses) may occur in one third of patients and is characterized by pain and drainage.

4. **The differential diagnosis of Crohn's disease** includes infections, caused by such organisms as *Yersinia, Shigella, Campylobacter,* and *Giardia,* and ileocecal tuberculosis. Other diseases that may mimic Crohn's disease include intestinal lymphoma, amyloidosis, lymphocytic and collagenous colitis, and diverticulitis. Behçet's disease, in particular, can be manifested as inflammation of the terminal ileum and aphthous ulcers and can have such extraintestinal manifestations as uveitis, arthritis, erythema nodosum, and iridocyclitis.

C. EXTRAINTESTINAL MANIFESTATIONS

1. **IBD is commonly associated with extraintestinal manifestations.**[3] The sacroiliac joints often are affected, resulting in a seronegative spondyloarthropathy. Patients may also have peripheral oligoarthritis in larger joints such as the knees, hips, elbows, and wrists.

2. **Common skin manifestations** include erythema nodosum and pyoderma gangrenosum. Inflammation may also involve the eyes, resulting in anterior uveitis or episcleritis.

3. Sclerosing cholangitis is a serious hepatic complication more commonly seen in UC than in Crohn's disease (see Chapter 35). Patients initially have an elevated alkaline phosphatase level. Nephrolithiasis is commonly seen in Crohn's disease and results from calcium malabsorption and increased absorption of oxalate, resulting in calcium oxalate nephrolithiasis. The incidence of thromboembolism also is higher in IBD.[4]

III. DIAGNOSIS

A. LABORATORY TESTS

1. Stool studies, including fecal leukocytes, culture, ova, and parasites, and a *Clostridium difficile* toxin screen should be obtained for patients with suspected IBD to rule out an infectious cause. Nonspecific markers

of inflammation, such as the erythrocyte sedimentation rate (ESR) and the C-reactive protein level (CRP), may be elevated during acute flareups. In addition, patients with suspected IBD should have a complete blood cell count to evaluate for leukocytosis and severe anemia. Hypoalbuminemia may reflect poor nutritional status, and electrolyte abnormalities may indicate severe diarrhea.

2. The serologic markers perinuclear antineutrophilic cytoplasmic antibody (P-ANCA) and anti–*Sacchromyces cerevisiae* antibody (ASCA) may help distinguish between UC and Crohn's disease, especially in indeterminate cases. In several studies patients with positive tests for P-ANCA and negative tests for ASCA were more likely to have UC, whereas those who were P-ANCA negative and ASCA positive were more likely to have Crohn's disease.[5] Although these tests have a specificity greater than 90%, they have a low sensitivity (40% to 60%) and should be used only as an adjunct to endoscopy and radiography in diagnosis.

B. ENDOSCOPY

1. **Colonoscopy with ileoscopy and biopsy is the primary tool for diagnosing IBD and determining the extent of disease.** In most cases endoscopy can be used to differentiate between UC and Crohn's disease (see Table 38-1). Endoscopic features that may be observed in both diseases include pseudopolyps, fibrotic strictures, loss of haustral folds, and linear superficial scars.

2. **Findings that may be more specific to Crohn's disease** include aphthous ulcers, which may involve the entire wall of the colon; cobblestoning; and the presence of discontinuous lesions. Sparing of the rectum is also more suggestive of Crohn's disease because UC invariably involves the rectum. However, patients with UC who have been treated with 5-aminosalicylic acid (5-ASA) and steroid suppositories may also demonstrate rectal sparing. Isolated involvement of the terminal ileum also suggests Crohn's disease.

3. **Typical endoscopic findings in UC** include erythema, mucosal edema, friability, loss of fine vascular pattern, and mucosal granularity. These features typically begin at the anal verge and extend proximally in a continuous and circumferential manner. In addition to its utility in the diagnosis, colonoscopy during a UC flare may predict clinical severity and need for surgery.[6] Biopsy may also detect superimposed cytomegalovirus colitis. In severe cases of suspected UC, sigmoidoscopy is preferable to colonoscopy because of the lower risk of perforation. Colonoscopy is contraindicated in suspected cases of toxic megacolon.

C. IMAGING

1. **Fluoroscopic studies play an important role in the diagnosis of Crohn's disease.** The dedicated small bowel series and upper gastrointestinal series are particularly important in detecting Crohn's disease proximal to the terminal ileum and not accessible by ileoscopy. Findings may

include multiple aphthous ulcers, a cobblestone appearance, fistulas, and a "string sign" caused by luminal narrowing.

2. Radiographic imaging is a powerful adjunct in diagnosing many of the complications of IBD. Plain films are helpful in assessing suspected toxic megacolon or small bowel obstruction. Single contrast studies are particularly valuable in defining strictures, fistulas, and tumors. Abdominal computed tomography with contrast medium may be used to identify abscesses, microperforations, fluid collections, or colonic thickening. Findings consistent with UC on double-contrast radiographic studies include pseudopolyps, mucosal granularity, fibrosis, and loss of haustral folds.

IV. MANAGEMENT

1. **IBD is managed predominantly in the outpatient setting.** Hospitalized patients with IBD tend to have more severe manifestations of the disease. Some patients are admitted for severe exacerbations of known disease, whereas in other hospitalized patients the disease is diagnosed for the first time.

2. **The goal of treatment is to achieve remission and then to maintain this state with a variety of agents.** In general, the first line of treatment for both Crohn's disease and UC is the use of 5-ASA derivatives. Steroids often are used for acute flareups, and immunomodulators are used to maintain remission of severe refractory disease.

A. MANAGEMENT OF ULCERATIVE COLITIS[7] (Fig. 38-1)

1. **Mild to moderate cases of UC** may be encountered in the inpatient setting when patients are initially admitted for lower gastrointestinal bleeding. The 5-ASA (mesalamine) drugs are the first-line agents in both induction and remission therapy for mild to moderate UC. The parent compound, sulfasalazine, is a less expensive alternative but has more frequent side effects. In patients with ulcerative proctitis, topical 5-ASA drugs such as 5-ASA suppositories or topical corticosteroids (Cortifoam) applied twice daily are effective in achieving remission. Rowasa enemas (5-ASA) may be implemented at 4 g daily for disease extending to the proctosigmoid and distal colon. In patients with moderate to severe UC, oral prednisone may be initiated at a dosage of 40 to 60 mg daily and then slowly tapered after remission is achieved.

2. **Patients with fulminant UC** necessitating hospitalization are at greater risk for severe gastrointestinal (GI) bleeding, toxic megacolon, and perforation. The mainstays of treatment for these patients are parenteral steroids, strict bowel rest, and nutritional support. Those with severe GI bleeding need immediate assessment of their hemodynamic status and management of the bleeding. Parenteral steroids (methylprednisolone 20 mg intravenously every 8 hours or prednisolone 30 mg intravenously every 12 hours) can be

Condition	Treatment			
Proctitis	5-ASA enemas, 5-ASA suppositories, oral 5-ASA drugs, or corticosteroid enemas	*Continued activity* → Prednisone or immunomodulators	*Continued activity* → Proctectomy	
Mild to moderate pancolitis	Oral 5-ASA drugs	*Continued activity* → Prednisone	*Continued activity or steroid dependence* → Immunomodulators or colectomy	
Severe or fulminant pancolitis	Parenteral steroids	*Continued activity* → Cyclosporine or colectomy		
Disease in remission	Maintenance with oral 5-ASA drugs			

FIG. 38-1

Treatment of ulcerative colitis. *ASA*, aminosalicylic acid. *(Modified from Goldman L, Bennett JC: Cecil textbook of medicine, 21st ed, Philadelphia, 2000, WB Saunders.)*

administered. For patients who do not improve within 7 to 10 days, cyclosporine 4 mg/kg given as a continuous intravenous infusion over 24 hours may be used in conjunction with steroids. This therapy may yield an initial response in 50% to 80% of patients.[8] The serum total cholesterol level should be checked before initiation of therapy because levels less than 120 mg/dl may predispose to seizures.

3. Once hospitalized, **patients with fulminant UC should be monitored for signs and symptoms of toxic megacolon and perforation.** Vital signs should be measured as often as every 4 hours, and abdominal examinations should be performed frequently (see Chapter 30).

4. **Once remission is achieved, patients should be started on a maintenance regimen.** Because steroids are ineffective as maintenance agents, orally administered prednisone should be initiated and gradually tapered, and a 5-ASA agent should be started. Patients who initially respond to intravenous cyclosporine should be switched to orally administered cyclosporine for several months and simultaneously be started on a regimen of 6-mercaptopurine (6-MP) or its prodrug azathioprine for maintenance.

5. **Surgical intervention** should be considered for patients whose fulminant UC is refractory to medical therapy. Other indications for surgery include toxic megacolon, severe bleeding, impending perforation, strictures, high-grade dysplasia, and severe extraintestinal manifestations. It should be noted that the progressive course of primary sclerosing cholangitis is unchanged by surgery. Surgery is curative for UC.

B. MANAGEMENT OF CROHN'S DISEASE (Fig. 38-2)

1. **The management of Crohn's disease depends on the clinical presentation.** In patients with mild inflammatory symptoms of abdominal pain and diarrhea, the 5-ASA agents are the first line of therapy, and the choice of formulation depends on the target region.[9] Pentasa is a sustained-released granular formulation that targets the upper gastrointestinal tract and the ileum and colon. Asacol is pH sensitive and targets the ileum and colon, whereas sulfasalazine is active only in the colon.

2. **Patients who do not respond to mesalamine** at maximum dosages of 4.8 g/day after 3 to 4 weeks should be started on metronidazole at 10 mg/kg in divided doses alone or in combination with ciprofloxacin 500 mg twice daily.[10] For patients who do not respond to antibiotics or who have moderately severe symptoms, oral prednisone 40 mg/day should be started. A slow-release form of budesonide (Entocort EC), at a dosage of 9 mg/day, is also effective in achieving remission in patients with disease affecting the ileum to the ascending colon. This corticosteroid is associated with fewer systemic side effects because > 90% is metabolized by the liver via first-pass effect.[11]

3. **Patients whose disease is refractory to the preceding measures or who are chronically dependent on steroids should be started on immunomodulators,** including azathioprine or its metabolite 6-MP at

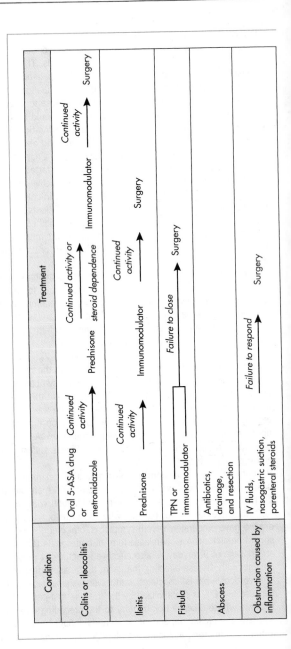

Condition	Treatment			
Colitis or ileocolitis	Oral 5-ASA drug or metronidazole	*Continued activity* → Prednisone	*Continued activity or steroid dependence* → Immunomodulator	*Continued activity* → Surgery
Ileitis	Prednisone	*Continued activity* → Immunomodulator	*Continued activity* → Surgery	
Fistula	TPN or immunomodulator	*Failure to close* → Surgery		
Abscess	Antibiotics, drainage, and resection			
Obstruction caused by inflammation	IV fluids, nasogastric suction, parenteral steroids	*Failure to respond* → Surgery		

		Failure to respond	
Obstruction caused by scarring	IV fluids, nasogastric suction	→ Surgery	
Perianal disease	Antibiotics and surgical drainage		
Disease in remission	Maintenance with oral 5-ASA drugs or immunomodulators		

FIG. 38-2

Treatment of Crohn's disease. *ASA,* aminosalicylic acid; *IV,* intravenous; *TPN,* total parenteral nutrition. (*Modified from Goldman L, Bennett JC: Cecil textbook of medicine, 21st ed, Philadelphia, 2000, WB Saunders.*)

38

INFLAMMATORY BOWEL DISEASE

50 mg/day. Myelosuppression is a common adverse effect, and patients need monthly monitoring of blood cell counts. Methotrexate, at an initial weekly dosage of 25 mg intramuscularly, is an alternative for patients who cannot tolerate azathioprine.[12]

4. **The tumor necrosis factor–alpha (TNF-α) antagonist infliximab** is the next line of therapy for moderate to severe Crohn's disease that is refractory to the aforementioned measures. Infliximab is administered as 5 mg/kg at 0, 2, and 6 weeks and then subsequently given every 8 weeks. Infliximab is generally well tolerated, but clinicians must be aware of the occurrence of infrequent complications including opportunistic infections, sepsis, autoimmune disorders, and a serum sickness–like reaction.[13] For those who continue to have active disease despite immunomodulator therapy, long-term low-dose steroid therapy or complete bowel rest with total parenteral nutrition may be necessary. Purified protein derivative (PPD) testing should be performed in patients before initiation of TNF-α antagonist therapy, due to high incidence of Tb reactivation on these medications.

5. **Once remission has been achieved, maintenance therapy should be initiated** with mesalamine. Patients who achieve remission with azathioprine or 6-MP should be maintained on these regimens.[14] Similarly, patients with refractory disease who needed infliximab to achieve remission should continue to receive infusions at 6- to 8-week intervals.[15]

6. **Perineal abscesses and draining fistulas** that are not amenable to surgery are initially managed with metronidazole, ciprofloxacin, or both. Relapse after discontinuation of antibiotics is common, however, and long-term therapy may be necessary. If perineal disease remains refractory, 6-MP, infliximab, or surgery may be indicated. Other fistulization in Crohn's disease should be treated with azathioprine or 6-MP because fistulas generally are not successfully closed with steroids or sulfasalazine. If this therapy is unsuccessful, infliximab therapy should be initiated.[16] Patients with enterovesical fistulas and resultant urinary tract infections need antibiotics and often surgery.

7. Patients with Crohn's disease commonly need hospitalization for microperforation, obstructive symptoms, or severe bleeding. Those with evidence of localized abscesses or microperforation should be treated with bowel rest and broad-spectrum antibiotics and may need surgery. Whether steroids should be used in this situation is controversial. Initially, pelvic and abdominal abscesses should be managed conservatively. Although surgical resection of affected bowel segments yields a lower rate of recurrence, medical therapy and percutaneous drainage have been found to avert subsequent surgery in the majority of patients and may be an alternative to surgery.[17] Unless small bowel obstruction (SBO) occurs in the setting of previous adhesions, it is usually partial and is managed initially with intravenous fluids,

parenteral nutrition, and nasogastric suction. Failure to improve or development of complete obstruction is an indication for surgery. Ulceration in Crohn's disease may also lead to severe bleeding and warrants supportive management, parenterally administered steroids, and possibly surgery.

8. The most common **indications for surgery in Crohn's disease** are high-grade SBO, perforation, massive hemorrhage, and refractoriness to medical therapy. High-grade dysplasia on surveillance biopsy also warrants surgical intervention. Surgical options depend on the regions involved. Perforation or stricture of the small bowel may be managed by segmental resection and anastomosis. Stricturoplasty may relieve intestinal obstruction while averting short gut syndrome. Treatment of colorectal involvement ranges from segmental colectomy to total proctocolectomy, depending on extent of the disease. Unlike UC, Crohn's disease commonly recurs after surgery; endoscopically discovered relapse occurs at a rate of 70% per year and clinically apparent recurrence at 15% per year. Postoperative prophylaxis with mesalamine or metronidazole may reduce this recurrence rate.[18,19]

C. SURVEILLANCE FOR COLORECTAL CANCER

Both UC and Crohn's colitis predispose patients to colorectal cancer. The cancer risk for UC is 0.5% to 1% per year after 10 years.[20] Patients who have had UC and Crohn's disease involving the colon for more than 8 years should undergo annual examination with colonoscopy. Multiple contiguous surveillance biopsy specimens should be obtained.

D. IBD AND PREGNANCY

Fertility is a common concern of patients with IBD. Fertility is most often normal in UC and inactive Crohn's disease; however, active Crohn's disease impairs fertility. Advise patients to take folic acid before conception. Maintenance treatment should be continued because it has been shown that disease activity is more harmful than most medications, including 6-MP.[21] Surgery (ileal pouch–anal anastomosis) for UC has been shown to reduce female fecundity.[22]

PEARLS AND PITFALLS

- Colonoscopy with ileoscopy is the primary diagnostic tool in IBD.
- Patients taking steroids on a long-term basis should also take calcium and vitamin D supplements and undergo dual-energy x-ray absorptiometry during the first 3 to 6 months of steroid therapy because maximal bone loss occurs in this period.
- Patients with Crohn's disease of the small bowel have a predisposition to iron, folate, and vitamin B_{12} malabsorption and should be screened for these deficiencies.
- Bile salt malabsorption is a common cause of diarrhea in patients who have undergone ileal resections of less than 100 cm. This diarrhea may respond to cholestyramine.
- Steroids, sulfasalazine, or mesalamine is the therapy of choice for IBD during pregnancy.

38

INFLAMMATORY BOWEL DISEASE

- Surgery is curative for UC but not for Crohn's disease, which has a clinical recurrence as high as 20% 1 year after surgery.
- Prophylaxis against deep venous thrombosis is an important aspect of management because patients with IBD have an elevated risk of thromboembolic events.
- The risk of colorectal cancer is elevated in both UC and Crohn's colitis, and patients who have had disease longer than 8 years should have annual colonoscopies.
- Irritable bowel syndrome occurs in 15% to 20% of the general population and is a common comorbid condition in IBD.[23]
- If patients have symptoms of irritable bowel syndrome, this does not rule out IBD or vice versa.
- Irritable bowel syndrome occurring concomitantly with IBD may not respond to antiinflammatory agents, but supportive care with antidiarrheal or antispasmodic medications may alleviate symptoms.
- Endoscopy may be useful in distinguishing irritable bowel symptoms from active IBD.

REFERENCES

1. Farrokhyar R, Swarbrick ET, Irvine EJ: A critical review of epidemiological studies in inflammatory bowel disease, *Scand J Gastroenterol* 36:2, 2001. C
2. Farmer RG, Hawk WA, Turnbull RBJ: Clinical patterns in Crohn's disease: a statistical study of 615 cases, *Gastroenterology* 68:627, 1975. B
3. Bernstein CN et al: The prevalence of extraintestinal diseases in inflammatory bowel disease: a population-based study, *Am J Gastroenterol* 96:1116, 2001. B
4. Koutroubakis IE: Role of thrombotic vascular risk factors in inflammatory bowel disease, *Dig Dis* 18:161, 2000. C
5. Peeters M et al: Diagnostic value of anti–*Saccharomyces cerevisiae* and antineutrophil cytoplasmic autoantibodies in inflammatory bowel disease, *Am J Gastroenterol* 96:730, 2001. B
6. Carbonnel F et al: Colonoscopy of acute colitis: a safe and reliable tool for assessment of severity, *Dig Dis Sci* 39:1550, 1994. B
7. Hanauer SB, Dassopoulos T: Evolving treatment strategies for inflammatory bowel disease, *Annu Rev Med* 52:299, 2001. C
8. Lichtiger S et al: Cyclosporine in severe ulcerative colitis refractory to steroid therapy, *N Engl J Med* 330:1841, 1994. A
9. Prantera C et al: Mesalamine in the treatment of mild to moderate active Crohn's ileitis: results of a randomized, multicenter trial, *Gastroenterology* 116:521, 1999. A
10. Sutherland L et al: Double blind, placebo controlled trial of metronidazole in Crohn's disease, *Gut* 32:1071, 1991. A
11. Thomsen OO et al: A comparison of budesonide and mesalamine for active Crohn's disease, *N Engl J Med* 339:370, 1998. A
12. Feagan BG et al: Methotrexate for the treatment of Crohn's disease. North American Crohn's Study Group Investigators, *N Engl J Med* 332:292, 1995. A
13. Colombel JF et al: The safety profile of infliximab in patients with Crohn's disease: the Mayo clinic experience in 500 patients, *Gastroenterology* 126:19, 2004. B

14. Candy S et al: A controlled double blind study of azathioprine in the management of Crohn's disease, *Gut* 37:674, 1995. A
15. Rutgeerts P et al: Efficacy and safety of retreatment with anti-tumor necrosis factor antibody (infliximab) to maintain remission in Crohn's disease, *Gastroenterology* 117:761, 1999. A
16. Present DH et al: Infliximab for the treatment of fistulas in patients with Crohn's disease, *N Engl J Med* 340:1398, 1999. A
17. Garcia JC et al: Abscesses in Crohn's disease: outcome of medical versus surgical treatment, *J Clin Gastroenterol* 32:409, 2001. B
18. McLeod RS et al: Prophylactic mesalamine treatment decreases postoperative recurrence of Crohn's disease, *Gastroenterology* 109:404, 1995. A
19. Rutgeerts P et al: Controlled trial of metronidazole treatment for prevention of Crohn's recurrence after ileal resection, *Gastroenterology* 108:1617, 1995. A
20. Kornbluth A, Sachar DB: Ulcerative colitis practice guidelines in adults. American College of Gastroenterology, Practice Parameters Committee, *Am J Gastroenterol* 92:204, 1997. D
21. Francella A et al: The safety of 6-mercaptopurine for childbearing patients with inflammatory bowel disease: a retrospective cohort study, *Gastroenterology* 124:9, 2003. B
22. Ording Olsen K et al: Ulcerative colitis: female fecundity before diagnosis, during disease, and after surgery compared with a population sample, *Gastroenterology* 122:15, 2002. B
23. Bayless TM, Harris ML: Inflammatory bowel disease and irritable bowel syndrome, *Med Clin North Am* 74:21, 1990. C

38

INFLAMMATORY BOWEL DISEASE

Diarrhea

Melissa A. Munsell, MD; Gregory B. Ang, MD; Mark Donowitz, MD; and Cynthia L. Sears, MD

39

FAST FACTS

- Diarrhea is a change in bowel habits with abnormally loose stools, usually associated with excessive frequency of defecation and more than 200 g stool per day.[1]
- Diarrhea develops through the following mechanisms: decreased rate of intestinal nutrient and salt absorption, net electrolyte secretion, rapid intestinal transit, and the ingestion of poorly absorbable substances, increasing intraluminal osmotic activity.[2]
- Diarrhea is classified as acute (lasting < 14 days), persistent (14 to 28 days), or chronic (> 4 weeks).
- Acute diarrhea usually is caused by infection and is self-limited. It usually does not warrant antibiotics[3] but does necessitate oral rehydration therapy.
- Chronic diarrhea is less likely to be caused by infection, is more often a symptom of other disorders, and is generally classified as watery, inflammatory, or fatty.[4]
- Watery diarrhea can be further classified as secretory versus osmotic, which can be distinguished by the response to fasting. Osmotic diarrhea resolves by 48 hours of fasting, whereas secretory diarrhea persists after 48 hours of fasting.[5]

I. EPIDEMIOLOGY

Globally, diarrheal diseases account for more than 2 million deaths each year.[6] In the United States, the incidence of diarrheal illness is estimated to be 1.4 episodes per person per year, or 211,000,000 cases per year.[6] Chronic diarrhea is estimated to affect 3,080,000 people per year in the United States.[7] Infectious diarrhea is the most common cause of diarrhea worldwide.[2]

II. ACUTE DIARRHEA: CLINICAL PRESENTATION AND DIAGNOSIS

1. **Presentation.** Acute diarrhea can be classified as noninflammatory or inflammatory diarrhea.
a. **Noninflammatory infectious diarrhea** presents with watery diarrhea that may be more than 1 L per day. It is usually self-limited and is not associated with severe abdominal pain or stool containing blood or pus. Fever can be variable.[1]
b. **Inflammatory diarrhea** may present with watery diarrhea or dysentery. Dysentery is frequent, small-volume stools that are mucoid or bloody and may be accompanied by fever, severe abdominal pain, and tenesmus.[1]

2. **The history** should focus on relevant clinical and epidemiologic features.
   a. **Relevant clinical features** include when and how the illness began, stool characteristics, frequency of bowel movements, stool quantity, presence of dysenteric symptoms, and symptoms of volume depletion.
   b. **Relevant epidemiologic features** include travel history, day care center contact, consumption of uncooked foods (e.g., raw or uncooked meat or seafood, unpasteurized milk products or apple cider, and foods sitting at room temperature more than 2 hours), swimming or drinking from a lake or stream, animal contact, sick contacts, medications, human immunodeficiency virus infection, or immunosuppression.[8]
3. **The physical examination** generally is not helpful in making a specific diagnosis but **is used to assess the patient's volume status:** orthostatic vital signs, dry mucus membranes, resting tachycardia, and skin turgor. The abdominal examination should assess bowel sounds, tenderness, and distension. Examination should also include visual inspection of the stool and occult blood determination.
4. **Laboratory findings.**
   a. Leukocytosis with a left shift suggests an inflammatory cause because noninflammatory diarrhea generally is associated with a normal white blood cell count.
   b. Serum electrolytes, urea nitrogen, and creatinine should be analyzed for evidence of volume contraction, renal failure, and electrolyte depletion.
5. **Etiology** (Table 39-1[8,9] and Box 39-1).
6. **Evaluation.** Most cases of acute diarrhea last less than 24 hours and do not warrant investigation. Thorough evaluation should be undertaken in patients with more severe illness, as indicated by any of the following features:
   - Profuse, watery diarrhea with volume depletion, as evidenced by orthostatic hypotension.
   - Dysentery (frequent stools with blood and mucus).
   - Fever.
   - Diarrhea with severe abdominal pain.
   - Diarrhea in older adults.
   - Immunocompromised patients (e.g., acquired immunodeficiency syndrome, posttransplant state, chemotherapy, diabetes).
   a. A careful history and laboratory evaluation will aid in the diagnosis and management of acute diarrhea. Laboratory evaluation should be undertaken in patients who are severely ill, those meeting the criteria outlined earlier, or those with a prior history of antibiotic therapy.
   b. **Stool examination.**
      (1) **Stool cultures** should be obtained in patients meeting the criteria outlined earlier, those appearing clinically ill, or those with stools positive for fecal leukocytes, lactoferrin, or occult blood.[10]
      (2) Evaluation of stools for **ova and parasites (O & P)** is indicated in the setting of persistent or chronic diarrhea, travel to developing

39

DIARRHEA

TABLE 39-1

DIFFERENTIAL DIAGNOSIS OF ACUTE INFECTIOUS DIARRHEA

Agent	Clinical Features	Pathogen-Specific Treatment*
VIRUSES		
Norwalk agent	Schools, hospitals, nursing homes, cruise ships; waterborne, foodborne	None.
Rotavirus	Day care centers, contact with young children	None.
Adenovirus		None.
BACTERIA		
Salmonella (non-typhi)	Foodborne (many vehicles, e.g., eggs, meat, dairy)	No therapy for healthy host with mild to moderate symptoms; TMP/SMX 1 DS bid (if susceptible) or FQ × 5-7 d (e.g., ciprofloxacin 500 mg PO bid) or ceftriaxone 100 mg/kg/d in 1 or 2 divided doses if severe illness.
Shigella	20% foodborne; primarily person-to-person (e.g., day care centers)	TMP/SMX 1 DS bid × 3 d (if acquired in U.S. and if susceptible); FQ (e.g., ciprofloxacin 500 mg PO bid × 1-3 d).
Campylobacter jejuni	Foodborne (e.g., undercooked poultry); 0.1% associated with Guillain-Barré syndrome	No therapy for healthy host with mild to moderate symptoms; if severe, erythromycin 500 mg bid,† FQ, or azithromycin × 5 d.
Staphylococcus aureus	Food poisoning; emesis more prominent than diarrhea within 6 hr of exposure to ingested toxin	None
Bacillus cereus	Two syndromes: similar to S. aureus, onset of emesis within 6 hr, often caused by fried rice; or similar to C. perfringens, watery diarrhea, longer incubation	None.
Clostridium perfringens	Food poisoning; watery diarrhea, incubation period 8-24 hr	None.
Vibrio cholerae O1 or O139	Contaminated shellfish, raw seafood (e.g., sushi)	Doxycycline 300 mg × 1 dose or tetracycline 500 mg qid × 3 d.

Escherichia coli O157:H7 (EHEC or STEC) ETEC, EAEC	Foodborne (e.g., undercooked hamburger, contaminated water or other foods); nonbloody or bloody diarrhea, associated with HUS Travelers	Avoid use of antibiotics because of potential increased risk of HUS.[9] FQ × 1-3 d or TMP/SMX 1 DS bid × 1-3 d (if susceptible).
Clostridium difficile	Recent antimicrobial therapy (within the past 2 mo)	Metronidazole 250 mg qid to 500 mg tid × 10 d or vancomycin 125 mg qid.
Yersinia enterocolitica	Pseudoappendicitis; pork products, unpasteurized dairy	Usually none.
PROTOZOA		
Cryptosporidium spp.	HIV or immunocompetent hosts; foodborne, waterborne; day care	Nitazoxanide‡ 500 mg q12hr × 3 d[11] or paromomycin 500 mg tid × 7 d with azithromycin. Treatment not needed in immunocompetent hosts.
Microsporidia	HIV (importance in immunocompetent host is unclear)	Albendazole 400 mg bid × 3 wk or fumagillin 60 mg qd × 2 wk if immunocompromised.
Isospora belli	HIV, travel	TMP/SMX 1 DS bid × 7-10 d.
Cyclospora	Foodborne; travel; duration >2 wk	TMP/SMX 1 DS bid × 7 d.
Giardia lamblia	Ingestion of stream water, travel	Metronidazole 250 mg tid × 5-7 d or tinidazole 2 g dose × 1.
Entamoeba histolytica	Travel to endemic areas, anal intercourse	Metronidazole 750 mg tid × 5-10 d and paromomycin 500 mg tid × 7 d.

39

DIARRHEA

Modified from Guerrant RL et al: *Clin Infect Dis* 32:331, 2001; and Thielman NM et al: *N Engl J Med* 350:38, 2004.

DS, double strength; *EAEC,* enteroadherent *Escherichia coli; EHEC,* enterohemorrhagic *E. coli; ETEC,* enterotoxigenic *E. coli; FQ,* fluoroquinolone, such as ciprofloxacin 500 mg PO bid; *HIV,* human immunodeficiency virus; *HUS,* hemolytic-uremic syndrome; *STEC,* Shiga toxin-producing *E. coli; TMP/SMX,* trimethoprim-sulfamethoxazole.

*Treatment in immunocompetent patients. Hydration, preferably oral, is essential in all cases. A lactose-free diet trial may help decrease stool volume.

†Erythromycin can cause gastrointestinal upset, so an alternative drug may be considered to treat *C. jejuni.*

‡From *Med Lett Drugs Ther* 45:29, 2003.

BOX 39-1

DIFFERENTIAL DIAGNOSIS OF ACUTE NONINFECTIOUS DIARRHEA

Drugs and toxins (e.g., magnesium, caffeine, theophylline, laxatives, opiates, lactulose, colchicine, metformin, digitalis, iron, methyldopa, hydralazine, sorbitol, quinidine, fructose, mannitol, arsenic, cadmium, mercury, mushrooms)

Irritable bowel syndrome

Inflammatory bowel disease

Ischemic bowel disease

Food allergies

Lactase deficiency

Onset of chronic diarrhea of any cause (e.g., vasoactive intestinal peptide–secreting tumor)

countries or mountainous areas, exposure to children attending day care centers, receptive anal intercourse, acquired immunodeficiency syndrome, other immune-compromised states, community waterborne outbreaks, and bloody diarrhea with few or no fecal leukocytes. There is no utility of evaluation for O & P in patients with onset of diarrhea > 72 hours after hospitalization.

(3) Evaluation for *Clostridium difficile* toxin is indicated in patients who have received antimicrobial therapy within the past 2 months and patients hospitalized for more than 72 hours. Generally, two consecutive stool examinations have a sensitivity of 90% in detecting *C. difficile*.[12]

c. **Flexible sigmoidoscopy** with or without upper gastrointestinal endoscopy should be considered for recipients of anal intercourse, immunocompromised hosts, and patients with persistent diarrhea (> 14 days) not responding to antimicrobial therapy or without a diagnosis after laboratory evaluation, including at least two complete stool examinations for culture, ova and parasites, and *C. difficile*.

d. In patients who appear to have been exposed to toxins, abdominal radiographs or abdominal computed tomograms should be obtained to evaluate for the presence and extent of colitis and to evaluate for megacolon or ileus.[13]

III. ACUTE INFECTIOUS DIARRHEA: MANAGEMENT

1. The management of patients with diarrhea who need medical evaluation and are volume depleted begins with rehydration.

2. According to the Infectious Diseases Society of America, the preferred form of fluid replacement is an oral glucose- or starch-containing electrolyte solution (oral rehydration solution) such as Ceralyte or Pedialyte.[8]

3. **Empiric antibiotics may be considered in the following patients.**

a. Traveler's diarrhea can be treated with fluoroquinolone therapy (e.g., oral ciprofloxacin 500 mg twice a day) because it can reduce the duration of illness from 3 to 5 days to less than 2 days according to Infectious Diseases Society of America guidelines.[8] Alternatively, travelers can prophylactically take bismuth subsalicylate (one to two 262-mg tablets four times a day), which has been shown to decrease the incidence of traveler's diarrhea by 35% to 65% and appears to be safe for up to 3 weeks.[6]

b. Patients with diarrhea lasting longer than 10 days, in whom giardiasis is suspected and other evaluations are negative, may be treated empirically with metronidazole 250 to 750 mg orally three times a day for 7 days.[8]

c. Patients with severe febrile diarrheal illnesses may be treated empirically with a fluoroquinolone if they appear toxic or unstable. If possible, antibiotic therapy should be delayed until Shiga toxin–producing *Escherichia coli* is ruled out by fecal testing because of concern for increased risk of hemolytic-uremic syndrome (HUS).[9] If intravenous therapy is deemed necessary because of systemic toxicity (e.g., salmonellosis), a fluoroquinolone or intravenous third-generation cephalosporin is reasonable empiric treatment.

4. **Use of antimotility agents.**

a. Adults with nondysenteric diarrhea can be given antimotility agents such as loperamide (4 mg initially, then 2 mg after each unformed stool, not to exceed 16 mg daily) or diphenoxylate with atropine (4 mg four times a day) without ill effect.

b. **Antimotility agents should be avoided in patients with bloody diarrhea or proven infection with Shiga toxin–producing *E. coli* or *Clostridium difficile*.**[8]

c. In children and older adults with enterohemorrhagic *E. coli* infection, antimotility agents may trigger HUS[14] and lead to worsening neurologic symptoms.[15]

5. Culture-directed antimicrobial therapy is used when specific pathogens are identified in stool samples and illness has not resolved (see Table 39-1). Of the four leading bacterial pathogens (*Salmonella, Shigella, Campylobacter jejuni,* and Shiga toxin–producing *E. coli*), only *Shigella* spp. infection is routinely treated. Treating *Salmonella* with antibiotic therapy increases the frequency and duration of intestinal carriage of the organisms.

6. A systematic approach to the evaluation and management of acute diarrhea is outlined in Fig. 39-1.[16-18]

IV. CHRONIC DIARRHEA: DIAGNOSIS

1. **Diarrhea of more than 4 weeks' duration warrants an evaluation for chronic diarrheal illnesses.**[5] The evaluation of patients with chronic diarrhea is more complex than that of patients with acute diarrhea because of the broad range of possible causes (Box 39-2).

2. Any acute infectious diarrhea can lead to chronic diarrhea; therefore the first step in evaluating chronic diarrhea is to rule out infectious causes.

3. Stool samples should be taken at two separate times for cultures, three times for O & P, acid-fast staining (to evaluate for *Cryptosporidium, Cyclospora,* and *Isospora belli*), and *Giardia* antigen testing (enzyme-

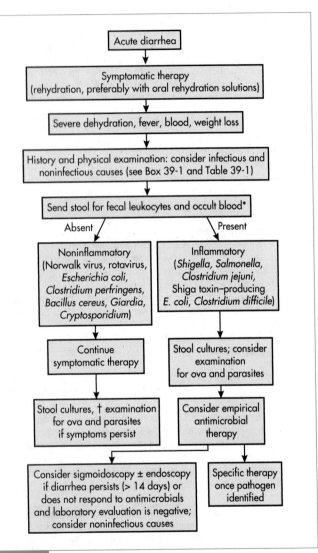

FIG. 39-1

Approach to acute diarrhea. *Send stool for *Clostridium difficile* toxin test if the patient has a history of antibiotic use within the past 2 months. Twenty-five percent of *C. difficile* disease occurs in the outpatient setting. †Of patients with *Shigella*, *Salmonella*, and *C. difficile* infections, 30% or more do not have fecal leukocytes or occult blood.[17,18] *(Modified from Guerrant RL, Bobak DA: N Engl J Med 325:327, 1991.)*

BOX 39-2

CAUSES OF CHRONIC DIARRHEA

OSMOTIC WATERY DIARRHEA

Osmotic laxatives (magnesium, phosphate, sulfate)

Carbohydrate malabsorption

SECRETORY WATERY DIARRHEA

Congenital syndromes

Bacterial toxins

Inflammatory bowel disease

Vasculitis

Drugs and poisons (see Box 39-1)

Laxative abuse

Disordered motility or regulation

Endocrine diarrhea (hyperthyroidism, hypothyroidism, Addison's disease,
   gastrinoma, vasoactive intestinal peptide–secreting tumor, somatostatinoma,
   carcinoid syndrome, medullary thyroid carcinoma, mastocytosis)

Other tumors (colon carcinoma, lymphoma, villous adenoma)

IDIOPATHIC SECRETORY DIARRHEA

Epidemic secretory (Brainerd's) diarrhea

INFLAMMATORY DIARRHEA

Inflammatory bowel disease

Infectious diseases

Ischemic colitis

Radiation colitis

FATTY DIARRHEA (50% WATERY)

Malabsorption syndromes (celiac disease, Whipple's disease, short bowel
   syndrome, small bowel bacterial overgrowth)

Maldigestion (pancreatic exocrine insufficiency, inadequate luminal bile acids)

Modified from Schiller LR: *Med Clin North Am* 84:1259, 2000.

linked immunosorbent assay). *C. difficile* testing should be performed if
there has been any antibiotic use within the past 2 months.

4. A lactose-free diet should be followed for several days because acute
   diarrhea may lead to secondary lactase deficiency.[5]

5. Along with excluding infectious causes and lactase deficiency, previous
   gastric surgery, ileal resection, medications, and systemic disease
   should be excluded as causes of chronic diarrhea.[5]

6. In addition to the history, physical examination, and routine laboratory
   blood work, a quantitative stool collection and analysis often are
   necessary to classify the diarrhea and to assist in making a specific
   diagnosis once infectious causes have been excluded (Table 39-2).[19]

7. Additional blood, urine, radiologic, endoscopic, or other studies may be
   considered for further evaluation of chronic diarrhea (Table 39-3).

8. The response to fasting often is used to distinguish secretory from
   nonsecretory diarrhea. Secretory diarrhea persists after 48 hours of
   fasting, whereas nonsecretory diarrhea ceases by 48 hours of fasting.[5]

TABLE 39-2

STOOL STUDIES IN NONINFECTIOUS CHRONIC DIARRHEA

Study	Comments
Stool Na^+, K^+	Osmotic gap < 50 mOsm/kg suggests secretory diarrhea; > 50 mOsm/kg suggests osmotic diarrhea; fecal osmotic gap = 290 − 2(stool Na^+ + K^+).*
Stool pH	pH < 5.6 suggests carbohydrate malabsorption.*
Fecal occult blood	Positive test suggests the presence of inflammatory bowel disease, neoplastic diseases, ischemia, radiation.
Fecal leukocytes	Presence suggests inflammatory or infectious diarrhea.
Sudan stain; 72-hr fecal fat (on 75- to 100-g fat/d diet)	Steatorrhea (> 14 g fat/d) indicates malabsorption (normally < 7 g fat/d); 7-14 g fat/day may result from large stool volume.
Stool alkalinization or thin-layer chromatography	Evaluation for laxative abuse (bisacodyl, phenolphthalein, anthraquinones).
Stool weight	Diarrhea defined by stool weight > 200 g/d.
Stool osmolality	Osmolality < 250 mOsm/kg implies dilution of stool with water or urine.
Stool Mg^+, sulfate, phosphate	Stool Mg^+ > 45 mM suggests inadvertent Mg^+ ingestion in mineral supplements or antacids or surreptitious laxative abuse.

*Data from Eherer AJ, Fordtran JS: Gastroenterology 103:545, 1992.

V. CHRONIC DIARRHEA: MANAGEMENT

1. As with acute diarrhea, patients with chronic diarrhea must receive adequate hydration, preferably with an oral rehydration solution.
2. **Empiric therapy is advocated for patients with chronic diarrhea in the following situations**[4]:
   a. As initial or temporizing therapy before diagnostic testing.
   b. After exhaustive investigation fails to reveal a specific cause.
   c. When a diagnosis has been made but no specific treatment is available or specific treatment fails.[10]
3. **Empiric treatment may include the following:**
   a. Antibiotics (e.g., metronidazole, fluoroquinolones, or TMP-SMX) if bacterial or protozoal infection is suspected based on the patient's history.
   b. Opiates (e.g., loperamide) for symptomatic control.
   c. Bile acid–binding resins (e.g., cholestyramine).
   d. Octreotide is used as a secondary agent, usually in secretory diarrhea, dumping syndrome, and chemotherapy-induced diarrhea.

PEARLS AND PITFALLS

- Antibiotic prophylaxis is not recommended for healthy people traveling to high-risk areas unless the traveler has significant predisposing illness such as acquired immunodeficiency syndrome, inflammatory bowel

TABLE 39-3

ADDITIONAL STUDIES IN EVALUATING CHRONIC DIARRHEA

Radiologic	Urine	Blood	Endoscopic	Other
Abdominal radiographic findings (for pancreatic calcification)	5-HIAA (for carcinoid syndrome)	Gastrin,* calcitonin,* VIP,* somatostatin*	Sigmoidoscopy with biopsy	Test of bile acid or other breath test for bacterial overgrowth
Barium studies of the upper gastrointestinal tract, small bowel, and colon	Thin-layer chromatography (for laxatives)	Thyroid function tests	Colonoscopy and ileoscopy with biopsy (for right-sided colitis, amebiasis, Crohn's disease, and microscopic and collagenous colitis)	Nutritionist-supervised lactose-free diet for 3-5 d
Abdominal computed tomography			Upper endoscopy, including small bowel biopsy	

5-HIAA, 5-hydroxyindoleacetic acid; *VIP,* vasoactive intestinal peptide.
*Should not be performed unless stool volume is >1 L/day or severe hypokalemia is present.

disease, hypochlorhydria secondary to prior gastric surgery or use of a proton pump inhibitor, insulin-dependent diabetes mellitus, or severe vascular, cardiac, or renal disease or malignancy.[20] Fluoroquinolones are the agent of choice for traveler's diarrhea unless the patient is traveling to southeast Asia, where more than 90% of *Campylobacter* strains are quinolone resistant.[21,22]

- Symptomatic food handlers and health care workers with acute, presumed infectious diarrhea should be barred from directly handling food and from caring for patients. Asymptomatic food handlers and health care workers with diagnosed *Salmonella* should have two consecutive negative stool samples taken 24 hours apart and at least 48 hours after resolution of symptoms before returning to their jobs.[8]

- Patients with diarrhea who have been the recipients of anal intercourse are at risk for proctitis and colitis resulting from direct rectal inoculation of pathogens. In addition to the more common bacterial enteropathogens, *Neisseria gonorrhoeae, Chlamydia trachomatis,* herpes simplex virus, and *Treponema pallidum* should be considered as causative agents.

- Immunocompromised patients, such as transplant recipients, patients undergoing chemotherapy, patients with human immunodeficiency virus infection, and patients with primary immunodeficiencies, are susceptible to an additional range of pathogens, which are beyond the scope of this chapter (see Chapter 51 and Chapter 62).

REFERENCES

1. Aranda-Michel J, Giannella RA: Acute diarrhea: a practical review, *Am J Med* 106:670, 1999. C
2. Casburn-Jones AC, Farthing MJ: Management of infectious diarrhoea, *Gut* 53:296, 2004. C
3. Schiller LR: Diarrhea, *Med Clin North Am* 84:1259, 2000. C
4. American Gastroenterological Association Medical Position Statement: Guidelines for the evaluation and management of chronic diarrhea, *Gastroenterology* 116:1461, 1999. D
5. Donowitz M et al: Evaluation of patients with chronic diarrhea, *N Engl J Med* 332:725, 1995. C
6. Thielman NM, Guerrant RL: Acute infectious diarrhea, *N Engl J Med* 350:38, 2004. C
7. *The burden of gastrointestinal diseases,* Bethesda, Md, 2001, American Gastroenterological Association. D
8. Guerrant RL et al: Practice guidelines for the management of infectious diarrhea, *Clin Infect Dis* 32:331, 2001. D
9. Wong CS et al: The risk of the hemolytic-uremic syndrome after antibiotic treatment of *Escherichia coli* O157:H7 infections, *N Engl J Med* 342:1930, 2000. B
10. DuPont HL: Guidelines on acute infectious diarrhea in adults, *Am J Gastroenterol* 92:1962, 1997. D
11. Rossignol JF et al: Treatment of diarrhea caused by *Cryptoporidium parvum*: a prospective randomized, double-blind, placebo-controlled study of nitazoxanide, *J Infect Dis* 184:103-106, 2001. A
12. Manabe YC et al: *Clostridium difficile* colitis: an efficient clinical approach to diagnosis, *Ann Intern Med* 123:835, 1995. B
13. Schiller LR: Diarrheal diseases, *ACP Medicine,* WebMD, April 2003. C
14. Cimolai N et al: Risk factors for the progression of *Escherichia coli* O157:H7 enteritis to hemolytic-uremic syndrome, *J Pediatr* 116:589, 1990. B
15. Cimolai N et al: Risk factors for the central nervous system manifestations of gastroenteritis-associated hemolytic-uremic syndrome, *Pediatrics* 90:616, 1992. B
16. Guerrant RL, Bobak DA: Bacterial and protozoal gastroenteritis, *N Engl J Med* 325:327, 1991. C
17. Slutsker L et al: *Escherichia coli* O157:H7 diarrhea in the United States: clinical and epidemiologic features, *Ann Intern Med* 126:505, 1997. B
18. Talan DA et al: Etiology of bloody diarrhea among patients presenting to United States emergency departments: prevalence of *Escherichia coli* O157:H7 and other enteropathogens, *Clin Infect Dis* 32:573, 2001. B
19. Eherer AJ, Fordtran JS: Fecal osmotic gap and pH in experimental diarrhea of various causes, *Gastroenterology* 103:545, 1992. A
20. DuPont H, Ericsson C: Prevention and treatment of traveler's diarrhea, *N Engl J Med* 328:1821, 1993. C
21. Hoge CW et al: Trends in antibiotic resistance among diarrheal pathogens isolated in Thailand over 15 years, *Clin Infect Dis* 26:341, 1998. B
22. Sanders JW et al: An observational clinic-based study of diarrheal illness in deployed United States military personnel in Thailand: presentation and outcome of *Campylobacter* infection, *Am J Trop Med Hyg* 67:533-538, 2002. B

Transfusion Medicine

Kent R. Nilsson Jr., MD, MA; Johan Bakken, MS; and Jerry Spivak, MD

FAST FACTS

- In hemodynamically stable patients, packed red blood cells (PRBCs) may be transfused at a rate of 2 to 4 ml/kg/hr. In patients at risk for volume overload, the rate of infusion should be slowed to 1 ml/kg/hr. Because 1 unit of PRBCs is about 300 ml, a healthy 70-kg person can be transfused 1 unit of PRBCs over 1 to 2 hours.
- As a rule, 1 unit of PRBCs increases hematocrit by 3 points, 1 unit of FFP provides 7% of the coagulation factor activity of a 70-kg patient, and 1 unit of platelets increases platelet count by 5000 to 10,000.
- When a transfusion reaction is suspected, the transfusion should be stopped immediately, and the nature of the transfusion reaction should be determined.
- Aggressive volume resuscitation with blood products can cause dilutional coagulopathy, hypothermia, thrombocytopenia, electrolyte imbalances (i.e., potassium, calcium), and acid-base disturbances.

Although transfusion of blood products offers life-saving benefits, an increasing body of literature suggests that routine transfusion for laboratory abnormalities puts the patient at risk for untoward outcomes. In addition to traditional risks such as transmission of bloodborne pathogens, transfusions have been associated with immunosuppression, microcirculatory dysfunction, and venous thromboembolism. As a result, efforts have been made to more strictly define which patient populations benefit from transfusion.

I. COMPONENTS AND INDICATIONS
A. RED BLOOD CELL COMPONENTS

1. **Whole blood.** Though rarely used, whole blood contains all coagulation factors except factors V and VIII and can be used in coagulopathic, hypovolemic patients in need of greater oxygen-carrying capacity.
2. **PRBCs.** Prepared from whole blood, PRBCs are the most frequently used blood product component (see Fig. 40-1 for indications).[1] Recent research favors a conservative strategy in most patients. In Hebert and colleagues' study of 838 critically ill euvolemic patients randomized to receive transfusions when hemoglobin concentration fell below either 7 or 10 g/dl, there was no difference in 30-day mortality. However, subgroup analysis demonstrated lower mortality in younger, less acutely ill patients using the restrictive approach.[2] Additional research has demonstrated that patients with congestive heart failure and patients

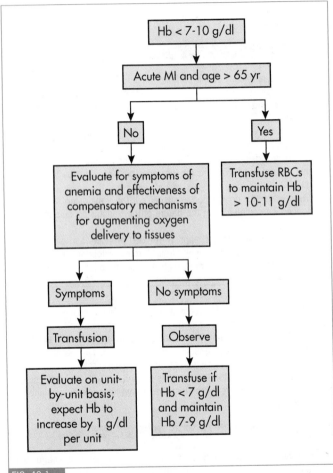

FIG. 40-1
An approach to transfusion. Note: The role of transfusion in anemic patients with acute coronary syndromes remains controversial.[5,6] *Hb,* hemoglobin; *MI,* myocardial infarction; *RBCs,* red blood cells. *(Adapted from Goldman L, Ausiello D: Cecil textbook of medicine, 22nd ed, Philadelphia, 2004, WB Saunders.)*

with sickle cell anemia undergoing surgery benefit from more aggressive transfusion strategies.[3,4] The role of transfusion in patients with coronary artery disease is unclear.[5,6]

3. **Leukoreduced red blood cells.** Leukocytes present in blood products are responsible for a number of complications associated with transfusion,

including human leukocyte antigen (HLA) alloimmunization, immunomodulation, and febrile nonhemolytic transfusion reactions. In addition, nucleated cells serve as reservoirs for several pathogens including human T-cell lymphotropic virus (HTLV) and cytomegalovirus. Leukocyte depletion at the time of collection or at the bedside reduces the risk of these complications and is indicated in patients who need multiple transfusions, who have suffered febrile transfusion reactions, or who are immunosuppressed and need cytomegalovirus-negative blood when none is available.

4. **Washed red blood cells.** Washing red blood cells with saline removes proteins, including immunoglobulins, and is indicated in patients who have allergic reactions, such as immunoglobulin A–deficient patients.

5. **Irradiated red blood cells.** Radiation eliminates the proliferative potential of T-lymphocytes contained in blood products and thereby reduces the risk of graft versus host disease. Indications include bone marrow transplantation, blood products from relatives or HLA-matched donors, and certain immunodeficient states.

B. PLATELETS

1. Unlike those of PRBC transfusion, indications for platelet transfusion are much more dependent on the particular clinical situation (see Fig. 40-2 for accepted transfusion thresholds).[1] In general, platelet transfusion should be considered for patients without fever or infection when platelet levels drop below 10,000/μl and in unstable inpatients with levels below 20,000/μl.

2. Platelet counts should be measured after transfusion, generally after 10 minutes or more, and counts should increase by about 5000 to 10,000 per unit transfused. Inappropriately low increases may result from alloimmunization, splenomegaly, sepsis, or disseminated intravascular coagulation (DIC). The half-life of transfused platelets is shorter than that of native platelets, and elimination may be further accelerated in systemic inflammatory states.

C. FRESH FROZEN PLASMA

1. Fresh frozen plasma (FFP) provides coagulation factors, including plasma proteins such as fibrinogen, protein C, and protein S.

2. Indications for transfusion of FFP include hemorrhage in a coagulopathic patient, correction of a coagulopathy before an invasive procedure, and replacement fluid for patients with thrombotic thrombocytopenic purpura (see Chapter 43) undergoing plasmapheresis. FFP is also indicated for correction of vitamin K deficiency and warfarin overdose.

3. One unit of FFP (about 300 ml) provides 7% of the necessary coagulation factors for a 70-kg person. Because coagulation factor concentrations of 20% to 30% normal levels provide effective hemostasis, transfusion of 10 to 15 ml/kg of FFP (2 to 6 units of FFP) usually corrects most underlying coagulopathies.

40

TRANSFUSION MEDICINE

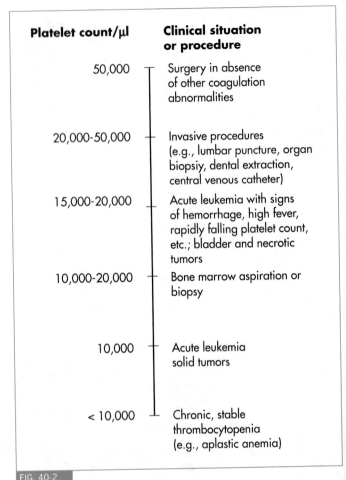

Platelet count/μl	Clinical situation or procedure
50,000	Surgery in absence of other coagulation abnormalities
20,000-50,000	Invasive procedures (e.g., lumbar puncture, organ biopsiy, dental extraction, central venous catheter)
15,000-20,000	Acute leukemia with signs of hemorrhage, high fever, rapidly falling platelet count, etc.; bladder and necrotic tumors
10,000-20,000	Bone marrow aspiration or biopsy
10,000	Acute leukemia solid tumors
< 10,000	Chronic, stable thrombocytopenia (e.g., aplastic anemia)

FIG. 40-2

Threshold for platelet transfusions. *(Adapted from Goldman L, Ausiello D: Cecil textbook of medicine, 22nd ed, Philadelphia, 2004, WB Saunders.)*

4. In the absence of active consumption of coagulation factors, correction of a coagulopathy with FFP lasts about 6 hours.

D. CRYOPRECIPITATE

1. Cryoprecipitate is composed of proteins that precipitate out of plasma at cold temperatures, including fibrinogen, factor VIII, and von Willebrand factor.

2. Indications for cryoprecipitate include fibrinogen deficiency, factor XIII deficiency; tissue plasminogen activator-related life-threatening hemorrhage; massive transfusion; and, rarely, factor VIII or von Willebrand factor deficiency. Cryoprecipitate may also be used when renal disease causes a functional platelet deficit.
3. Because the concentration of cryoprecipitate varies, dosing should be done in consultation with the hospital's blood bank.

II. RISKS OF TRANSFUSION AND ADVERSE REACTIONS
A. INFECTIOUS
Despite improvements in donor screening and laboratory testing, transfusion-associated disease transmission can still occur. See Table 40-1 for risks of common pathogens.[1]
B. ACUTE ADVERSE REACTIONS
1. **Hemolytic transfusion reactions.** Accounting for the majority of transfusion-related deaths, acute hemolytic transfusion reactions occur as a result of preformed antibodies directed against donor erythrocytes and present with fever, chills, dyspnea, nausea, vomiting, or flank pain. Disseminated intravascular coogulation (DIC), acute renal failure, and shock may develop quickly.
a. Laboratory tests show evidence of hemolysis (hemoglobinuria, elevated lactate dehydrogenase, decreased haptoglobin, and indirect hyperbilirubinemia). A direct Coombs test will be positive (unless all infused cells have been destroyed) and is considered diagnostic. Patients should be monitored for DIC and acute renal failure.
b. If a transfusion reaction is suspected, the transfusion should be stopped immediately and sent for repeat crossmatch with a new sample of the patient's blood. The patient should receive aggressive volume resuscitation. Alkalinization of the urine to a pH greater than 7 and the use of diuretics may reduce the risk of acute renal failure.
2. **Febrile nonhemolytic transfusion reaction.** A febrile response to transfusion is the most common transfusion reaction and results from donor lymphocyte production of cytokines. Symptoms include fever, chills, and headache, which occur within 1 to 6 hours of transfusion.
a. Diagnosis is made after hemolysis and anaphylaxis are ruled out.
b. Treatment is with acetaminophen (650 mg), diphenhydramine (25 mg), and glucocorticoids, if necessary.

TABLE 40-1

COMMON PATHOGENS AND ASSOCIATED RISK OF TRANSMISSION PER UNIT	
Human immunodeficiency virus	1:2,135,000
Hepatitis B virus	1:205,000-488,000
Hepatitis C virus	1:1,935,000
HTLV	1:2,993,000
Malaria	1:4,000,000
Cytomegalovirus	Varies according to the clinical situation

Modified from *Cecil textbook of medicine,* 22nd ed, Philadelphia, 2004, WB Saunders.

40

TRANSFUSION MEDICINE

c. Leukodepleted blood is useful for patients who have suffered repeated febrile episodes.

3. **Transfusion-related acute lung injury (TRALI).** TRALI is a rare complication of transfusion but accounts for about 13% of deaths. Occurring 1 to 6 hours after transfusion, TRALI is most often associated with FFP. Although the pathophysiology is unclear, HLA and granulocyte sensitization in multiparous female donors appears to play a role.[7] Clinically, TRALI is characterized by severe dyspnea and hypoxia caused by noncardiogenic pulmonary edema. Fever, hypotension, and hemoptysis are not uncommon.

a. Chest radiographs demonstrate diffuse, bilateral interstitial infiltrates.

b. Treatment is supportive and may include full ventilatory support. Symptoms usually resolve within 72 hours.

4. **Allergic reaction.** Allergic reactions to transfused blood result from recipient immunoglobulin E antibodies directed against proteins in the transfused blood. Reactions range from urticaria to anaphylaxis.

a. Whereas urticarial eruptions can be treated symptomatically with antihistamines and temporary cessation of transfusion, anaphylaxis may necessitate ventilatory and circulatory support.

b. Future transfusions should be with washed blood products.

5. **Bacterial contamination.** Though uncommon, bacterial contamination of blood products by transient donor bacteremia or ineffective antisepsis at the time of phlebotomy is the second leading cause of transfusion-associated death. Patients develop dyspnea, tachycardia, back pain, fever, and rigors about 45 minutes after the start of infusion. Treatment includes discontinuation of the transfusion, broad-spectrum antibiotics, and supportive care. *Yersinia enterocolitica* is the most common bacterial contaminant in PRBCs.[8]

6. **Volume overload.** Patients with heart failure or noncompliant vasculature are at risk for developing volume overload. Patients at risk for volume overload should be transfused at a slower rate (1 ml/kg/min). Diuretics may be necessary in symptomatic patients.

C. **DELAYED ADVERSE REACTIONS**

1. **Delayed hemolytic transfusion reaction.** A delayed hemolytic reaction can occur days to weeks after transfusion as a result of newly formed or anamnestically stimulated alloantibodies. The resulting extravascular hemolysis can cause a hemolytic anemia less severe than that seen with the intravascular hemolysis associated with acute hemolytic transfusion anemia, although renal failure can occur. Laboratory tests show evidence of hemolysis (hemoglobinuria, elevated lactate dehydrogenase, decreased haptoglobin, and indirect hyperbilirubinemia). A direct Coombs test will be positive. In general, treatment is supportive.

2. **Graft versus host disease (GVHD).** GVHD occurs when viable donor lymphocytes engraft and react against the recipient's cells. Patients at

high risk for GVHD include those with impaired CD8+ and natural killer cell function. Clinical manifestations of GVHD occur days to weeks after transfusion and include fever, erythroderma, and epidermolysis. Although GVHD is rare, mortality approaches 90%. Patients at high risk for developing GVHD should receive irradiated blood products.

3. **Posttransfusion purpura.** Posttransfusion purpura is an uncommon reaction that typically occurs 7 to 10 days after transfusion in parous women. It is characterized by severe thrombocytopenia as a result of an anamnestic antibody response to the PLA-1 (HPA1-a) antigen. Treatment consists of intravenous immunoglobulin or plasmapheresis. Immediate platelet transfusion should be avoided because it may worsen the thrombocytopenia.

D. LONG-TERM TRANSFUSION CONSEQUENCES

Patients with more than 100 units of transfused red blood cells are at risk for secondary hemochromatosis if they have not received iron chelation therapy.

III. MASSIVE TRANSFUSION

Massive transfusion is variably defined but involves the administration of large numbers of blood products in a short period of time. As a result, patients may develop hypothermia and coagulation, acid-base, and electrolyte disturbances.

A. COAGULOPATHY

The administration of plasma-poor PRBCs often leads to a dilutional coagulopathy that is exacerbated by the coexistent acidosis, hypothermia, and DIC seen in exsanguinating patients. Although replacement of coagulation factors and platelets ideally would be guided by laboratory values, an unstable patient may need empiric administration of blood products. FFP is indicated for prothrombin time and activated partial thromboplastin time ratios more than 1.5 times control, and platelet transfusions are indicated for platelet values less than 50,000.[9] Dilutional coagulopathy typically occurs after 10 units and dilutional thrombocytopenia after 20 units of PRBCs.

B. METABOLIC DISTURBANCES

To prevent the coagulation of stored blood, citrate is added in order to chelate calcium and inhibit the coagulation cascade. In the setting of massive transfusion, the infusion of large quantities of citrate can lead to hypocalcemia. In addition, the metabolism of citrate into bicarbonate can cause a metabolic alkalosis, which is the most common acid-base disturbance associated with transfusion. Patients with renal and liver impairment are at particularly high risk. In addition, patients may develop hypokalemia or hyperkalemia.[9]

C. HYPOTHERMIA

PRBCs are stored at 1° C to 6° C, so massive transfusion can quickly lower the core temperature and in severe cases may cause arrhythmias. In-line blood warmers should be used for infusion of blood components.[9]

PEARLS AND PITFALLS

- Patients on angiotensin-converting enzyme inhibitors who undergo bedside leukocyte reduction of blood may develop profound hypotension as a result of bradykinin production.
- Maintaining body temperature during massive transfusion is crucial to correcting coagulopathy.
- Platelets should never be given to patients with thrombotic thrombocytopenic purpura because it worsens neurologic deficits.
- Care must be given when giving platelets or FFP to patients with pulmonary hypertension because the presence of vasoactive substances such as serotonin can cause abrupt hemodynamic decompensation.
- Patients with uremic bleeding may benefit from the administration of desmopressin acetate (0.3 mg/kg intravenously), which increases platelet adhesiveness through unknown mechanisms. Cryoprecipitate may also be beneficial.

REFERENCES

1. *Cecil textbook of medicine,* 22nd ed, Philadelphia, 2004, WB Saunders. D
2. Hebert PC, Wells G, Blajchman MA, et al: A multicenter, randomized, controlled clinical trial of transfusion requirements in critical care, *N Engl J Med* 340(6):409-417, 1999. A
3. Vichinsky EP, Haberkern CM, Neumayr L, et al: A comparison of conservative and aggressive transfusion regimens in the perioperative management of sickle cell disease. The Preoperative Transfusion in Sickle Cell Disease Study Group, *N Engl J Med* 333(4):206-213, 1995. A
4. Silverberg DS, Wexler D, Sheps D: The effect of correction of mild anemia in severe, resistant congestive heart failure using subcutaneous erythropoietin and intravenous iron: a randomized controlled study, *J Am Coll Cardiol* 37(7):1775-1780, 2001. A
5. Wu WC, Rathore SS, Wang Y, et al: Blood transfusion in elderly patients with acute myocardial infarction, *N Engl J Med* 345(17):1230-1236, 2001. B
6. Rao SV, Jollis JG, Harrington RA: Relationship of blood transfusion and clinical outcomes in patients with acute coronary syndromes, *JAMA* 292(13):1555-1562, 2004. B
7. Palfi M, Berg S, Ernerudh J, Berlin G: A randomized controlled trial of transfusion-related acute lung injury: is plasma from multiparous blood donors dangerous? *Transfusion* 41(3):317-322, 2001. A
8. Goodnough LT, Brecher ME, Kanter MH, AuBuchon JP: Transfusion medicine (2 parts), *N Engl J Med* 340(6):438-447, 1999. C
9. Crosson JT: Massive transfusion, *Clin Lab Med* 16(4):873-882, 1996. C

Anemia and Erythrocytosis

Sigrid Berg, MD, MPH; Julie-Aurore Losman, MD, PhD; Hetty Carraway,
MD; and Michael Streiff, MD

FAST FACTS

- The most common cause of anemia is iron deficiency.
- Anemia is defined as a hematocrit less than 37% in women and 40% in men or a hemoglobin less than 12 g/dl in women and 14 g/dl in men.
- Analysis of the peripheral blood smear is essential to the diagnosis of any patient with anemia.
- Classic patterns of anemia are shown in Table 41-1.
- The most common cause of erythrocytosis is hypoxia caused by chronic pulmonary disease.
- Erythrocytosis is defined by a hematocrit greater than 48% in women and 51% in men or a hemoglobin greater than 16.5 g/dl in women and 18.5 g/dl in men.

Anemia

I. EPIDEMIOLOGY

1. Iron deficiency is the most common cause of anemia in the United States. Iron deficiency anemia affects 10% of premenopausal women, 25% of pregnant women, 5% of children, and 2.5% to 5% of men and postmenopausal women. Children, pregnant women, and older adults are the most commonly affected by anemia.

2. All patients with anemia should undergo an evaluation. Data show that after evaluation, 40% of older adults with anemia have a change in therapy.

II. CLINICAL PRESENTATION

1. **Patients often present with fatigue or low energy.** An adequate history is vital and should include an evaluation for energy level, cold intolerance, substance abuse (including alcohol ingestion, type of diet, medications, and vitamins), pica, neurologic complaints (which may occur with vitamin B_{12} or iron deficiency), family history of anemia or hemoglobinopathies, gastrointestinal bleeding, menorrhagia, or kidney problems. Allergies or medications can precipitate hemolysis, especially in patients with glucose-6-phosphate dehydrogenase deficiency or hemolytic anemia.

2. **Physical examination** should assess for pallor, skin creases, nails (spoon nails are associated with iron deficiency), angular stomatitis (iron deficiency), glossitis (iron deficiency and megaloblastic anemia),

TABLE 41-1

CLASSIC ANEMIA PATTERNS

Type	Serum Iron	Total Iron-Binding Capacity	Transferrin Percentage Saturation	Ferritin	Reticulocyte Count
Iron deficiency	Low	High	Low	Low	Low
Anemia of chronic disease	Low-normal	Low-normal	Low-normal	Normal-high	Low
Sideroblastic anemia	High	High	High	High	Low

orthostatic hypotension (acute bleeding), jaundice (hemolytic anemia, liver disease), bruising (suggests thrombocytopenia that can be associated with underlying bone marrow disease), telangiectasias, and splenomegaly.

III. DIAGNOSIS (Fig. 41-1)

1. The American Task Force Guidelines recommend that all infants and pregnant women be screened for anemia. Routine screening of other patients is not recommended unless they are symptomatic.
2. All patients with anemia should have a complete blood cell count with differential, basic metabolic panel (to evaluate renal function), reticulocyte count, peripheral blood smear, and screening stool for occult blood.
3. A **peripheral blood smear** is most helpful if a patient has not received a blood transfusion recently. The peripheral blood smear, a thin smear processed with Wright-Giemsa stain, is helpful in distinguishing the type of anemia based on the size, shape, and color of the red blood cells (RBCs). For example, patients with iron deficiency have abnormally shaped RBCs (poikilocytosis), small RBCs (microcytosis), high RBC distribution width (anisocytosis), and lack of pigmentation (hypochromia). In megaloblastic anemia, macro-ovalocytes, hypersegmented neutrophils, and Howell-Jolly bodies are seen. A peripheral blood smear from a patient with anemia of chronic disease would be expected to have normal or microcytic RBCs. In patients with liver disease, thin macrocytes, target cells, and acanthocytes (spur cells) may be present.
4. The **RBC shape** often is the most helpful clue in the differential diagnosis of hemolytic disorders. Diagnostic findings include fragmentation of RBCs from traumatic hemolysis on artificial heart valves, spherocytosis as a marker of hereditary spherocytosis, sickle cells and oakleaf cells in sickle cell disease, target cells in thalassemia, and blister forms in glucose-6-phosphate dehydrogenase deficiency.
5. The **mean corpuscular volume** (MCV) is a direct measure of the average size of the RBC. Normal MCV ranges from 80 to 100 fl. The

characterization of anemia according to the size of the erythrocytes is an efficient and organized approach to diagnosing causative factors in anemia. Microcytic anemia (MCV < 80 fl), macrocytic anemia (MCV > 100 fl), and normocytic anemia (MCV 80 to 100 fl) are discussed in detail later in this chapter.

6. A low **mean corpuscular hemoglobin concentration** often points to a diagnosis of iron deficiency, thalassemia, or sideroblastic anemia.

7. The **RBC distribution width** reveals the variation of red cell volumes. A high RBC distribution width suggests possible iron, vitamin B_{12}, or folate deficiency but may also be the result of any process that increases the reticulocyte count (including chronic bleeding or hemolysis).

8. The **reticulocyte count** is determined after a blood film is stained for reticulin (the remains of the cellular RNA). Early reticulocytes are bigger than mature red cells, so a high reticulocyte count elevates the MCV. The reticulocyte count usually is expressed as a percentage of cells examined in an individual patient. This number must be corrected for the presence of anemia because the initial count, expressed as a percentage of RBCs present, is spuriously elevated when it is related to a reduced anemic RBC pool. The corrected reticulocyte count, or reticulocyte index, is equal to the patient's hematocrit divided by 45 and multiplied by the percentage of reticulocytes. See Table 41-2 for the significance of reticulocyte indices.

$$\text{Reticulocyte index} = \% \text{ Reticulocytes} \times \text{Hematocrit}/45$$

9. **Ferritin** is the major iron storage protein. The ferritin assay is the most sensitive and specific laboratory test for assessing iron stores. A low ferritin level (< 12 ng/ml in women and < 30 ng/ml in men) is evidence of iron deficiency. Ferritin is also an acute phase reactant. Elevated levels of ferritin can be seen in acute illness, inflammation, and infection, even in the presence of iron deficiency. However, high ferritin levels make iron deficiency unlikely.

10. The measurement of **serum iron** is affected by many variables, including free hemoglobin, inflammation, infection, and iron ingestion. Often a low serum iron level is helpful in the diagnosis of anemia of chronic disease in addition to the diagnosis of iron deficiency anemia.

11. **Total iron-binding capacity (TIBC)** is a laboratory measurement of the ability of serum to bind iron. TIBC is determined largely by transferrin,

TABLE 41-2

RETICULOCYTE INDICES

Reticulocyte Index	Significance
< 1	Inadequate RBC production
1-2	Indeterminate
> 2	Adequate RBC production or ongoing RBC loss

RBC, red blood cell.

41

ANEMIA AND ERYTHROCYTOSIS

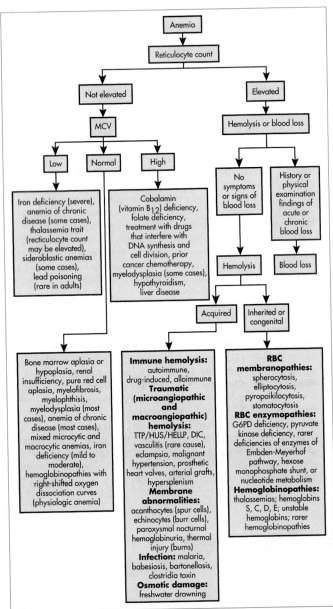

FIG. 41-1

See legend on the opposite page

a beta-globulin that regulates absorption and transport of iron. TIBC typically is low in anemia of chronic disease and elevated in iron deficiency anemia.

12. **Transferrin saturation** is equal to the serum iron divided by the TIBC. A transferrin saturation less than 10% suggests iron deficiency. This is not specific, however, because up to 30% of patients with a low saturation are not iron deficient. Like ferritin, transferrin is also an acute phase reactant, so TIBC can be affected by acute illness. Therefore, the transferrin saturation can be misleading: A falsely elevated TIBC can result in a low transferrin saturation, just as a low TIBC and low serum iron level (as seen in anemia of chronic disease) can result in a normal transferrin saturation.

13. A **bone marrow aspirate** stained for hemosiderin is the gold standard test for diagnosis of iron deficiency anemia, but this test is not always performed because it is painful, expensive, and associated with sampling errors.

IV. MANAGEMENT[2]

1. The **role of transfusion** in anemia is not well defined (see Chapter 40).

2. In the United States, **erythropoietin therapy** has been approved by the Food and Drug Administration for patients with selected medical conditions,[3] including those with chronic renal failure, those with human immunodeficiency virus infection receiving zidovudine therapy, patients with cancer, and patients undergoing surgery. In one study, erythropoietin was most beneficial for surgical patients whose initial hematocrit value was 33% to 39% and whose anticipated blood losses were 1 to 3 L.

3. **Iron deficiency anemia.**[4-6]

a. **Diagnosis** of iron deficiency anemia is made when a patient has a low hematocrit value along with microcytic anemia (MCV < 80 fl) and a low ferritin level (< 12 ng/ml in women and < 30 ng/ml in men). Iron saturation is less than 15%. A bone marrow examination is almost never indicated because a trial of iron therapy usually establishes the diagnosis with less discomfort and expense.

b. The average adult has 2 to 5 g of iron (1 g in storage form). Blood loss is the only way to excrete iron. The total iron loss in pregnancy is

Diagnosis of anemias. *DIC,* disseminated intravascular coagulation; *G6PD,* glucose-6-phosphate dehydrogenase; *HELLP,* hepatomegaly, elevated liver function tests, low platelets; *HUS,* hemolytic-uremic syndrome; *MCV,* mean corpuscular volume; *RBC,* red blood cell; *TTP,* thrombotic thrombocytopenic purpura. *(Modified from Goldman L, Bennett JC: Cecil textbook of medicine, 21st ed, Philadelphia, 2000, WB Saunders.)*

41

ANEMIA AND ERYTHROCYTOSIS

1 g, including the estimated blood loss at delivery. Pregnant women are placed on a folate and iron regimen. The average loss of blood with each menstrual cycle in women is 22 mg. Menstruating young women with microcytic anemia can be treated presumptively with iron if they will be available for follow-up to determine their response. A careful family history should be obtained to identify cases of thalassemia. However, most patients with iron deficiency anemia should be assumed to have a gastrointestinal blood loss. Testing these patients for fecal occult blood is essential.

c. Iron is absorbed in the duodenum. **Treatment for iron deficiency anemia** is ferrous sulfate 325 mg (60 mg elemental iron) taken orally three times a day with meals for 6 to 12 months. Scratching the tablet or having patients take it with an acidic beverage is thought to increase gastrointestinal absorption. Leading causes of treatment failure are poor compliance (because of nausea and constipation from iron) and poor absorption (caused by concomitant antacid use).

d. **Treatment response.** The reticulocyte count increases in 1 week and peaks 10 days after iron therapy has begun. Hemoglobin levels should normalize in about 2 months. If iron therapy fails, gastrointestinal malabsorption (e.g., sprue) should be considered as a possible cause of anemia. If oral iron therapy is unsuccessful, intravenous iron replacement can be considered.

4. **Anemia of chronic disease.**[7,8]

a. **Diagnosis** of anemia of chronic disease is made when a patient has a low hematocrit value along with microcytic or normocytic anemia and a normal or high ferritin level. Transferrin and iron saturation are normal with a low TIBC. Bone marrow biopsy usually is not indicated, but if one is performed, the results are normal. Anemia of chronic disease is a diagnosis of exclusion; drug toxicity and chronic blood loss should be excluded before a final diagnosis of anemia of chronic disease is established.

b. Anemia of chronic disease has a slow onset with few symptoms. The **pathophysiology** is not well understood, but this condition probably evolved as a cytokine-mediated defense against microbial pathogens. The result is that iron is withheld from microbes, as well as from erythroid precursors. Ultimately, RBC survival is shortened, and the marrow compensatory response is impaired because of disturbed iron metabolism and impaired erythropoietin production.

c. Anemia of chronic disease improves only when the underlying disorder has been identified and treated.

5. **Megaloblastic anemia.**[9,10]

a. Macrocytic anemia (MCV < 100 fl) can be divided into two major groups: the megaloblastic anemias and nonmegaloblastic anemias. The presence of hypersegmented neutrophils and large platelets on peripheral blood smear leads to the diagnosis of megaloblastic anemia. Megaloblastic anemia affects all three cell lines, and pancytopenia may be found at presentation. Normal neutrophils and platelets in the presence of an elevated MCV signify that the patient has a nonmegaloblastic anemia.

b. **Nonmegaloblastic anemias** usually reflect membrane cholesterol defects related to systemic abnormalities such as liver disease or hypothyroidism.

c. **Further evaluation of megaloblastic anemia includes assays for serum vitamin B_{12}, methylmalonic acid (if low or low-normal vitamin B_{12} levels), and RBC folate levels.** Deficiency of vitamin B_{12} (usually because of impaired absorption) or folate (because of poor nutrition or increased demand) is the most common cause of this anemia. Vitamin B_{12} deficiency often is present even with a low normal serum B_{12} concentration and can be confirmed by an elevated serum methylmalonic acid level and elevated homocysteine level.

d. **Intestinal malabsorption or defective secretion of intrinsic factor** may cause vitamin B_{12} deficiency. Defective secretion of intrinsic factor can be caused by autoimmune destruction of stomach parietal cells (pernicious anemia) or by surgical removal of the parietal cells when part of the stomach is removed (gastrectomy). Patients who have small bowel disease, blind loop syndrome, or intestinal parasites may have vitamin B_{12} deficiency because of lack of absorption in the ileum.

e. In vitamin B_{12} deficiency, patients may have symptoms of neurologic compromise that predates the onset of anemia or macrocytosis. The daily vitamin B_{12} requirement is 2 to 5 µg. Liver stores equal 2 to 5 mg, so clinical manifestations of vitamin B_{12} deficiency may take years to develop.

f. **Folate deficiency** may be caused by poor nutrition (alcoholism), malabsorption (jejunal disease), or increased needs (pregnancy, dialysis, hemolytic anemia). Anticonvulsant drugs and oral contraceptives have been associated with megaloblastic anemia caused by folate deficiency. Homocysteine levels may be elevated in this condition, but the methylmalonic acid level should be normal.

g. Within 48 hours of parenteral **vitamin B_{12} or folate administration,** marrow abnormalities begin to normalize. Complete normalization occurs within 2 to 3 days. Reticulocyte count peaks in 4 to 10 days. If response is blunted, an underlying iron deficiency anemia should be suspected. Folate treatment of vitamin B_{12}-deficient patients may partially correct the anemia and marrow abnormalities but may accelerate the development of neurologic abnormalities. The vitamin B_{12} dosage is 1000 µg/day for 1 to 2 weeks, then 1000 µg/week for 4 weeks, then a maintenance dosage of 100 or 1000 µg intramuscularly for life. Folate replacement is 1 mg/day orally.

6. **Sickle cell anemia** (see Chapter 42).

7. **Hemolytic anemias.** See Fig. 41-1 for a list of some of the more common hemolytic anemias. An elevated bilirubin, elevated reticulocyte count, elevated lactate dehydrogenase, or undetectable haptoglobin may

be seen in such conditions. A detailed assessment of the varied hemolytic anemias is beyond the scope of this chapter.

Erythrocytosis

I. EPIDEMIOLOGY

1. Erythrocytosis is defined by a hematocrit above 48% in women and 51% in men or a hemoglobin greater than 16.5 g/dl in women and 18.5 g/dl in men.
2. **The most common cause of erythrocytosis is hypoxia secondary to pulmonary disease.** Other important causes include polycythemia vera, paraneoplastic phenomena, renal transplantation, and familial disorders.
3. Polycythemia vera[11,12] is a clonal disorder of a multipotent hematopoietic stem cell, characterized by leukocytosis, thrombocytosis, and erythrocytosis.
   a. The annual incidence is 2.3 cases per 100,000, the mean age at diagnosis is 51 years, and the disorder presents earlier in women.
   b. The male-to-female ratio is 1.3:1. Polycythemia vera is rare in blacks, and the incidence is higher in people of European Jewish ancestry.
   c. There is no recognized association with radiation exposure, no genetic marker, and no familial predisposition.

II. CLINICAL PRESENTATION

1. A thorough **history** and review of systems are critical. Patients with pulmonary symptoms (i.e., dyspnea, chronic cough, daytime somnolence, cyanosis) or patients who spend a great deal of time at high altitude could develop erythrocytosis secondary to hypoxia. Pulmonary disease, intracardiac shunt, renal transplant, and tobacco abuse are associated with secondary erythrocytosis. Hypervolemia, a hypermetabolic state, episodic pruritus (classically after having bathed), and a history of hemorrhagic or thrombotic events suggest polycythemia vera. Erythrocytosis may be familial, so a family history of erythrocytosis would be important to obtain. Home and occupational exposures (e.g., carbon monoxide or cobalt) must be assessed as well.
2. Important findings on **physical examination** include the presence or absence of findings consistent with cardiopulmonary abnormalities (dyspnea, abnormal breath sounds, cyanosis, clubbing, abnormal heart sounds), arteriovenous shunting (murmurs, bruits), Cushing's syndrome (e.g., striae, buffalo hump, central obesity), pheochromocytoma (labile blood pressure, diaphoresis), polycythemia vera (hypertension, painful areas of erythema, engorged retinal and lingual veins, flushed facies, dusky cyanosis, hepatosplenomegaly), or erythropoietin-secreting malignancies (hepatosplenomegaly).

III. DIAGNOSIS (Table 41-3)[11]

1. **Initial evaluation** for erythrocytosis should include measurement of a complete blood cell count, including RBC mass and plasma volume.

TABLE 41-3

DIFFERENTIAL DIAGNOSES FOR ERYTHROCYTOSIS

Type	Category	Causes
Primary	Polycythemia vera	Abnormal proliferation of myeloid stem cells
	Congenital	Activating erythropoietin receptor mutations
Secondary (in presence of hypoxia)	Carboxyhemoglobinemia	Carbon monoxide poisoning, chronic smoking
	Alveolar hypoventilation	Sleep apnea, Pickwickian syndrome
	Chronic lung disease	Chronic obstructive pulmonary disease
	High-altitude environment	
	Arteriovenous shunting	Arteriovenous malformations, right-to-left cardiopulmonary shunting, pulmonary arteriovenous malformations (hereditary hemorrhagic telangiectasia)
	Renal	Renal artery stenosis
	Congenital	2,3-Diphosphoglycerate mutase deficiency, high–oxygen affinity hemoglobinopathy, congenital methemoglobinemia
	Drugs	Cobalt (cytotoxic hypoxia)
Secondary (in absence of hypoxia)	Paraneoplastic	Ovarian cancer, renal cell carcinoma, hepatocellular carcinoma, parathyroid carcinoma, cerebellar hemangioblastoma, uterine leiomyomata, meningioma
	Renal	Polycystic kidney disease, chronic dialysis, Bartter's syndrome, post–renal transplant erythrocytosis
	Adrenal	Pheochromocytoma, Cushing's syndrome, stress
	Congenital	Chuvash polycythemia (abnormal oxygen homeostasis), high set point for erythropoietin production, idiopathic familial erythropoiesis
	Drugs	Androgen doping, erythropoietin doping, transfusion
Relative	Reduced plasma volume	Diuretics, dehydration, diarrhea, vomiting, severe burns, capillary leak syndrome, smoking
	Gaisböck syndrome (stress polycythemia)	Associated with nephropathy, hypertension, and anxiety in obese patients
	High-normal value	> 95th percentile

41

ANEMIA AND ERYTHROCYTOSIS

Concomitant elevations of white cell count or platelet count raise suspicion for polycythemia vera. An elevated RBC count in the setting of a normal or low hematocrit is consistent with thalassemia trait. Red cell mass and plasma volume may help differentiate between a relative and a true erythrocytosis.

2. A **serum erythropoietin level** can help differentiate between polycythemia vera and secondary causes of erythrocytosis. Generally, a low erythropoietin level can be seen with polycythemia vera (unless a congenital erythropoietin receptor mutation is suspected). Normal erythropoietin levels are indeterminate. Elevated erythropoietin levels are associated with both hypoxia-dependent and hypoxia-independent secondary polycythemias, although erythropoietin levels may be normal in cases of secondary erythrocytosis in which feedback inhibition occurs, erythropoiesis is directly stimulated, or erythropoietin sensitivity is high.

3. **Arterial blood gas** sampling can be helpful in cases of chronic hypoxia or carbon monoxide poisoning. Postambulatory or nocturnal desaturations may reveal underlying cardiopulmonary disease.

4. **Congenital polycythemias** tend to appear early in life, and such patients often present with a positive family history. Hemoglobin electrophoresis can detect the presence of abnormal hemoglobin with high oxygen affinity. Measurement of the oxygen pressure at 50% oxygen saturation (P-50) may also be helpful.

5. Basic chemistries and liver function tests are useful in seeking secondary causes of erythrocytosis, such as hepatocellular carcinoma and secretory endocrine tumors. Urinalysis may reveal hematuria consistent with renal cell carcinoma.

6. Radiographic studies may be warranted to search for cardiopulmonary, renal, or malignant sources of abnormal erythrocytosis.

7. **Diagnostic criteria for polycythemia vera** are listed in Table 41-4.[11,12]

IV. MANAGEMENT

1. **Polycythemia vera.**[11,12]

a. Median survival is 15 to 25 years. The major causes of death are arterial and venous thrombosis and bleeding.

b. Other complications include bone marrow failure, iron deficiency anemia, and transformation into acute myeloblastic leukemia (AML) (risk of transformation is significantly higher after treatment with radiophosphorus or chlorambucil).

c. Definitive treatment consists of phlebotomy to hematocrit less than 45% in men, less than 42% in women, and less than 36% during pregnancy.

d. Symptomatic treatment consists of antihistamines, selective serotonin reuptake inhibitors, phototherapy, or interferon-alpha for pruritus; low-dose aspirin or anagrelide for erythromelalgia; and interferon-alpha, imatinib, or hydroxyurea for extramedullary hematopoiesis.

TABLE 41-4	
DIAGNOSTIC CRITERIA FOR POLYCYTHEMIA VERA	
A1	Red blood cell mass > 25% above mean normal predicted value
A2	Arterial O_2 saturation ≥ 92%
A3	Splenomegaly
B1	Thrombocytosis (> 400,000 cells/μl)
B2	Leukocytosis (> 12,000 cells/μl)
B3	Erythroid and megakaryocytic hyperplasia on bone marrow biopsy
B4	Low serum erythropoietin levels

Diagnosis of polycythemia vera: A1 + A2, A1 + A3, or A1 + two B criteria.

41

ANEMIA AND ERYTHROCYTOSIS

2. Management of other sources of erythrocytosis is best accomplished through successful diagnosis and treatment of the underlying disorder, when possible.

PEARLS AND PITFALLS

- In patients with chronic kidney disease, perform an anemia workup before initiating erythropoietin therapy to exclude any component of anemia not caused by renal insufficiency. Patients on erythropoietin therapy can also benefit from iron supplementation if their baseline iron stores are low.
- The incidence of anemia is as high as 70% in patients with acquired immunodeficiency syndrome. Anemia in human immunodeficiency virus–infected patients usually is a multifactorial process. See Chapter 48.
- The findings of four prospective, randomized, double-blind, placebo-controlled clinical trials support the use of erythropoietin in patients infected with HIV when symptomatically anemic patients have baseline serum erythropoietin levels less than 500 IU/L. In these studies, 70% of patients had significant increases over baseline hematocrit and a reduction in transfusion needs as a result of erythropoietin therapy. Erythropoietin should be given as 100 IU/kg subcutaneously three times a week.[13]
- An elevated RBC count in the setting of a normal or low hematocrit suggests the presence of thalassemia trait and should be evaluated further via peripheral smear, hemoglobinopathy screen, and detailed family history.
- The five most common tumors associated with erythrocytosis are renal cell carcinoma, hepatocellular carcinoma, cerebellar hemangioblastoma, pheochromocytoma, and uterine myoma.

REFERENCES

1. Wu WC et al: Blood transfusion in elderly patients with acute myocardial infarction, *N Engl J Med* 345:1230, 2001. B
2. Beutler E: The common anemias, *JAMA* 259:2433, 1988. C
3. Goodnough L et al: Erythropoietin therapy, *N Engl J Med* 336:933, 1997. B

4. Guyatt GH: Diagnosis of iron-deficiency anemia in the elderly, *Am J Med* 88:205, 1990. B

5. Lipshitz DA et al: A clinical evaluation of serum ferritin as an index of iron stores, *N Engl J Med* 290:1213, 1974. B

6. Brown RG: Determining the cause of anemia: general approach, with emphasis on microcytic hypochromic anemias, *Postgrad Med* 89:161, 1991. C

7. Cash JM et al: The anemia of chronic disease: spectrum of associated diseases in a series of unselected hospitalized patients, *Am J Med* 87:638, 1989. B

8. Andrews N: Disorders of iron metabolism, *N Engl J Med* 341:1986, 1999. C

9. Carmel R: Pernicious anemia: the expected findings of very low serum cobalamin levels, anemia, and macrocytosis are often lacking, *Arch Intern Med* 148:1712, 1988. B

10. Ledrele FA: Oral cobalamin for pernicious anemia: medicine's best kept secret? *JAMA* 265:94, 1991. B

11. Tefferi A: Polycythemia vera: a comprehensive review and clinical recommendations, *Mayo Clin Proc* 78:174, 2003. C

12. Spivak JL: Polycythemia vera: myths, mechanisms, and management, *Blood* 100:4272, 2002. C

13. Henry DH: Experience with epoetin alfa and acquired immunodeficiency syndrome anemia, *Semin Oncol* 25:64, 1998. B

Sickle Cell Anemia

Elizabeth Griffiths, MD; Rosalyn Juergens, MD;
and Sophie Lanzkron, MD

FAST FACTS

- Vaso-occlusion is the most common reason for hospital admission and is treated with aggressive hydration, parenteral pain control, oxygen if the patient is hypoxic, and treatment of the precipitating cause.
- Hospitalized patients should be provided with an incentive spirometer and encouraged to use it every 2 hours while awake.
- Indications for transfusion and exchange transfusion include chest crisis, strokes and transient ischemic attacks, priapism, splenic and hepatic sequestration crisis, and multisystem organ failure.
- The incidence of sudden death in sickle cell disease is high and probably is related to the high incidence of pulmonary hypertension (about 30%).
- Chronic sickling can affect every organ system.

42

I. EPIDEMIOLOGY[1]

1. One in every 400 African Americans in the United States has sickle cell disease (SCD). The mean survival for people with sickle cell anemia is 48 years for women and 42 years for men.
2. SCD is defined as hemoglobin SS disease (sickle cell anemia), hemoglobin SC disease, or sickle cell β thalassemia. Eight percent of African Americans are heterozygous carriers of the sickle cell trait. Hemoglobin S results from a substitution of a valine for glutamic acid as the sixth amino acid of the β-globin chain. Two of these abnormal β-globin chains form when part of a tetramer with two α-globin chains form a polymer that is poorly soluble when deoxygenated and distorts the erythrocyte into a sickled form.

II. CLINICAL PRESENTATION, DIAGNOSIS, AND MANAGEMENT OF ACUTE CRISES

A. VASO-OCCLUSIVE CRISIS

1. **Vaso-occlusive crisis is the most common reason for patients with SCD to seek medical care.**
2. The frequency of attacks varies from patient to patient, but in one large study 33% of patients with SCD rarely had pain, 33% had two to six pain crises necessitating hospitalization per year, and 33% had more than six pain-related crises per year.[2]
3. More frequent pain crises are associated with higher mortality.[3]

4. Acute pain is the result of tissue ischemia caused by occlusion of capillaries by sickled erythrocytes.[1] Chronic pain is the residua of destroyed bones, joints, and visceral organs from previous pain crises.

5. An acute pain crisis typically lasts 5 to 7 days and often is precipitated by dehydration, infection, low oxygen tension, acidosis, pregnancy, alcohol, stress, or cold weather.

6. **Treatment of acute crises**[4] is mainly supportive and includes aggressive hydration and adequate pain management (Table 42-1). Patient-controlled analgesia is a way to meet the dual goals of prompt delivery of pain medication and prevention of oversedation.

7. **Supplemental oxygen** has been shown to have benefit only when hypoxia is present. Withdrawal of oxygen can cause rebound sickling if the Po_2 decreases precipitously.[5]

8. **Transfusion** has not been shown to shorten the duration of acute pain crises.

9. **Incentive spirometry** has been demonstrated in a randomized controlled trial to prevent the development of atelectasis and infiltrates, particularly in patients with chest wall pain.[6]

10. **Hydroxyurea** increases the production of hemoglobin F and can be used as a means of decreasing the number and severity of acute pain crises in the chronic setting (Table 42-2). The dosage is started at 15 mg/kg by mouth daily and can be increased to the maximum tolerated dosage (white blood cell count 2500 to 3000/mm³) or a maximum of 2 g per day.[7] A hematology consultation should be considered when this medication is used.

B. ACUTE CHEST SYNDROME

1. Acute chest syndrome has been defined in clinical studies as the presence of **pulmonary infiltrates on chest radiograph, chest pain, and fever**.

2. Chest crises can be precipitated by pulmonary fat embolism (from infarctions of long bone), bacterial and viral infection, pulmonary edema, asthma and microvascular or macrovascular lung infarction.[6]

3. **Initial management** includes analgesia (with care taken to avoid respiratory depression), cautious administration of intravenous (IV) fluids, oxygen supplementation, and empirical antibiotics while culture results are awaited.

4. **Transfusion.** If the patient has multilobar involvement in the setting of anemia or thrombocytopenia, rapidly progressive disease, underlying cardiac disease, or respiratory failure, transfusion is indicated.

a. Standard transfusions can be used for patients who are more anemic than their baseline hemoglobin; however, increasing the hemoglobin concentration to more than 11 g/dl may lead to complications caused by increased viscosity.[8]

b. Exchange transfusions can be used for patients who are not significantly more anemic than baseline but who have a high concentration of hemoglobin SS (usual goal is < 30%).

TABLE 42-1

RECOMMENDED DOSAGE AND INTERVAL OF ANALGESICS NECESSARY TO OBTAIN ADEQUATE PAIN CONTROL IN SICKLE CELL DISEASE

Analgesic	Dosage or Rate	Comments
SEVERE OR MODERATE PAIN		
Morphine	Parenteral: 0.1-0.15 mg/kg q3-4h; recommended maximum single dose 10 mg PO: 0.3-0.6 mg/kg q4h	Drug of choice for pain; lower dosages are used in older adults and in patients with liver failure or impaired ventilation.
Meperidine	Parenteral: 0.75-1.5 mg/kg q2-4h; recommended maximum dosage 100 mg PO: 1.5 mg/kg q4h	Higher incidence of seizures; avoid use in patients with renal or neurologic disease or those who receive monoamine oxidase inhibitors.
Hydromorphone	Parenteral: 0.01-0.02 mg/kg q3-4h PO: 0.04-0.06 mg/kg q4h	
Oxycodone	PO: 0.15 mg/kg/dose q4h	
Ketorolac	Intramuscular, adults: 30 or 60 mg initial dose, followed by 15-30 mg	Equal efficacy to 6 mg morphine sulfate; helps narcotic-sparing effect; not to exceed 5 days; maximum 150 mg first day, 120 mg subsequent days; may cause gastric irritation.
Butorphanol	Parenteral: 2 mg q3-4h	Agonist-antagonist; can precipitate withdrawal if given to patients who are being treated with agonists.
MILD PAIN		
Codeine	PO: 0.5-1 mg/kg q4h; maximum dosage 60 mg	Mild to moderate pain not relieved by aspirin or acetaminophen; can cause nausea and vomiting.
Aspirin	PO: 0.3-6 mg q4-6h	Often given with a narcotic to enhance analgesia; can cause gastric irritation.
Acetaminophen	PO: 0.3-0.6 mg q4h	Often given with a narcotic to enhance analgesia.
Ibuprofen	PO: 300-400 mg q4h	Can cause gastric irritation.
Naproxen	PO: 500 mg/dose initially, then 250 mg q8-12h	Long duration of action; can cause gastric irritation.
Indomethacin	PO: 25 mg q8h	Contraindicated in psychiatric, neurologic, and renal diseases; high incidence of gastric irritation; useful in gout.

Data from Charache S et al: *Medicine (Baltimore)* 75:300, 1996. In Hoffman R et al: *Hematology: basic principles and practice*, 3rd ed, New York, 2000, Churchill Livingstone.

SICKLE CELL ANEMIA

42

TABLE 42-2

TABLE 42-2

CLINICAL EFFECTS OF HYDROXYUREA THERAPY

Variable	Hydroxyurea	Placebo	p Value
Acute pain crisis rate	2.5/yr	4.5/yr	< 0.0001
Hospitalization rate for acute pain crisis	1/yr	2.4/yr	< 0.0001
Interval to first pain crisis	3 mo	1.5 mo	< 0.0001
Interval to second pain crisis	8.8 mo	4.6 mo	< 0.0001
Acute chest syndrome	25	51	< 0.0001
Patients receiving transfusions	48	73	0.0001
Blood units transfused	336	586	0.0004

Data from Charache S et al: *Medicine (Baltimore)* 75:300, 1996. In Hoffman R et al: *Hematology: basic principles and practice,* 3rd ed, New York, 2000, Churchill Livingstone.

5. Unless there is a proven diagnosis of venous thromboembolism, anticoagulation is not indicated.
6. Aggressive chronic transfusion therapy decreases the incidence of acute chest syndrome in patients with SCD; however, **hydroxyurea is the first-line treatment for prevention of recurrent episodes of acute chest syndrome.**[9]

C. APLASTIC CRISIS

1. Aplastic crisis is caused by a transient arrest in erythropoiesis accompanied by an abrupt fall in hemoglobin concentration. Most cases are associated with parvovirus B19, but aplastic crises have also been reported with *Streptococcus pneumoniae, Salmonella,* and Epstein-Barr virus.
2. The treatment for aplastic crisis is transfusion therapy, which may be necessary for several weeks. If the patient has a refractory parvovirus B19 infection, IV immune globulin can be administered.

D. SPLENIC SEQUESTRATION CRISIS[1,2,10]

1. Vaso-occlusion in the spleen causes a marked decrease in hemoglobin concentration. This occurs primarily in those who have not undergone splenic autoinfarction (more common in hemoglobin SC or sickle thalassemia).
2. It is treated with exchange transfusion and often recurs. Splenectomy usually is recommended after an acute episode.

III. ORGAN SYSTEM INVOLVEMENT (Table 42-3)

A. CENTRAL NERVOUS SYSTEM

1. **There is a higher incidence of both ischemic and hemorrhagic stroke in patients with SCD.** It is important to have a high index of suspicion for stroke in patients with SCD and altered mental status. These patients may present with a global decrease in consciousness rather than focal neurologic deficits.
2. **Ischemic stroke** affects 6% to 12% of patients with SCD and is one of the leading causes of death in both children and adults with SCD.[11]

TABLE 42-3

SEQUELAE AND COMORBIDITIES IN SICKLE CELL DISEASE WITH ASSOCIATED PREVALENCE DATA

Stroke	25%[24]
Pulmonary hypertension	20%-40%
Chronic renal insufficiency	5%[10]
Priapism	89% by adulthood[10]
Cholelithiasis	40%[24]

a. Use of exchange transfusion to keep the hemoglobin S concentration below 30% during an acute stroke is beneficial.[12]

b. Major risk factors for ischemic stroke as identified in the Cooperative Study of Sickle Cell Disease[13] include previous transient ischemic attack (relative risk [RR] 56), low steady state hemoglobin (RR 1.9 per 1-g/dl decrease), frequent history of acute chest syndrome (RR 2.4 per event per year), an episode of acute chest syndrome within the previous 2 weeks (RR 7), and an elevated systolic blood pressure (RR 1.3 per 10-mmHg increase).

c. The efficacy of aspirin or warfarin therapy in preventing recurrent stroke has not been established.

3. **Intracranial hemorrhage** accounts for one third of strokes in patients with SCD and has a very high immediate mortality.[14] The peak incidence of intracranial hemorrhage is between the ages of 20 and 29 years, whereas ischemic infarction is much more common in children.

a. The two leading risk factors for hemorrhagic stroke are low steady state hemoglobin (RR 1.6 per 1-g/dl decrease) and elevated steady state leukocyte count (RR 1.9 per 5000/µl increase).[1]

b. Patients present with headache, elevated intracranial pressure, altered level of consciousness, and focal neurologic deficits.

c. Immediate exchange transfusion is recommended for patients with intracranial hemorrhage.

B. EYES

1. Proliferative sickle retinopathy is the most common ocular sequela of SCD (greater frequency in hemoglobin SC disease).[15] Neovascularization generally is asymptomatic; however, vitreous hemorrhage and retinal detachment may result. Proliferation is treated with laser photocoagulation, which can prevent further complications.

2. Central retinal artery occlusion can occur, presenting as sudden loss of vision. This is an emergency that should prompt immediate transfusion and ophthalmology consultation.

C. LUNGS

1. **Acute chest syndrome.**

2. **Pulmonary hypertension** affects 20% to 40% of patients with SCD.[16]

a. Risk factors include a history of renal or cardiovascular problems, elevated systolic blood pressure, frequent transfusions (more than 10 lifetime), and (in men) a history of priapism. Serum markers of elevated hemolysis also are associated with higher rates of pulmonary hypertension; these include low hemoglobin, elevated serum lactate dehydrogenase, alkaline phosphatase, direct bilirubin, aspartate aminotransferase, and low serum transferrin.

b. Patients can be assessed accurately with two-dimensional echocardiography, and those with pulmonary hypertension may be candidates for therapy.

c. Two-year mortality (about 50%) in these patients approaches that of patients with primary pulmonary hypertension. Mortality in patients with SCD and pulmonary hypertension is significantly higher than in those with SCD alone and may account for the higher incidence of sudden death in patients with sickle cell anemia.

D. CARDIOVASCULAR SYSTEM

1. **Hypertension** reflects underlying renal disease.[1,2,10] First-line therapy should include beta-blockers and calcium channel blockers. Diuretics should be used with caution because they can cause dehydration and sickling. In small studies, angiotensin-converting enzyme inhibitors have been shown to be useful in those with proteinuria.

2. **Atherosclerotic coronary disease** is less common in this population; however, myocardial infarctions in the absence of significant atherosclerotic disease do occur. If risk stratification is indicated, radionuclide or echocardiographic studies are more helpful than electrocardiography-based tests because of a high rate of false-positive results.

E. HEPATOBILIARY SYSTEM[4,15]

1. Elevated bilirubin production from chronic hemolysis puts patients with SCD at higher risk of gallstones, affecting 75% of patients with SCD by age 30.[17]

2. **Hepatic crisis.** Vaso-occlusion in the liver causes right upper quadrant pain, hepatomegaly, and fever associated with acute transaminitis, hyperbilirubinemia, and an elevated alkaline phosphatase. Vaso-occlusive liver disease is a diagnosis of exclusion, so other causes of acute liver disease (e.g., cholecystitis, viral hepatitis) must be evaluated and ruled out. Hepatic crisis usually is self-limited but on rare occasion can progress to fulminant liver failure and necessitate exchange transfusion. Treatment is otherwise the same as in any vaso-occlusive crisis.

3. **Hepatic sequestration.** Sequestration of red cells in the liver can cause hepatomegaly associated with a falling hemoglobin and increasing reticulocyte count. Exchange transfusion may be necessary in these cases.

F. RENAL SYSTEM

1. **Hyposthenuria** (inability to maximally concentrate urine) generally is present by age 3 and is characterized by obligatory urine output of more than 2 L per day. It may predispose patients to dehydration and more frequent sickling.

2. **Renal tubular acidosis** is the most common cause of metabolic acidosis in SCD. Usually a type IV tubular acidosis, which results from damage to the distal renal tubule, it should be corrected by sodium bicarbonate therapy if acidemia is present.

3. **Gross hematuria** (painless) is commonly seen in SCD and may also develop in sickle cell trait carriers.[18] Evaluation includes renal ultrasound, cystoscopy, and culture. Treatment includes aggressive hydration to maintain a high urinary flow rate, alkalinization of the urine, and bed rest. If the bleeding is refractory, aminocaproic acid can be used but is associated with an elevated risk of clot formation in the urinary tract.

4. **Proteinuria** is present in 25% of adults with SCD.[19] It can progress to nephrotic syndrome in cases caused by membranoproliferative glomerulonephritis. Patients should be screened yearly for proteinuria, and angiotensin-converting enzyme inhibitors are recommended in those who develop it.

5. **Renal papillary necrosis** is a common and usually asymptomatic cause of hematuria and proteinuria in SCD.[18] It is associated with interstitial nephritis from nonsteroidal antiinflammatory drug use.

6. **Chronic kidney disease** occurs in up to 5% of patients with SCD and usually is heralded by worsening proteinuria.[20] SCD is not a contraindication to hemodialysis or renal transplantation.

G. MUSCULOSKELETAL SYSTEM

1. **Lower extremity ulcers** are found in 10% to 20% of patients with SCD and are more prevalent in men.[21] The mainstay of treatment is aggressive wound care. Transfusions may be used when ulcers are refractory to treatment (> 6 months), but their effectiveness remains unclear.

2. **Avascular necrosis** of the femoral and humeral heads is common in SCD and should be evaluated with magnetic resonance imaging. Peak incidence is between 25 and 35 years. Total joint replacement may be necessary to treat pain and to improve function.

3. **Joint effusions** may be caused by synovial infarction, but gout, septic arthritis, osteoarthritis, or rheumatic causes should be considered. Treatment includes nonsteroidal antiinflammatory drugs and local heat.

H. GENITOURINARY SYSTEM

Between 30% and 50% of men with SCD report at least one episode of acute priapism in their lifetime. Failure of an erection to subside after several hours is a urologic emergency. Management includes aggressive IV hydration; IV narcotic analgesia; and, if necessary, exchange transfusion. If these measures do not work, penile aspiration may be necessary.

I. HEMATOPOIETIC SYSTEM[7]

1. The anemia of SCD is a chronic hemolytic anemia with an appropriate reticulocytosis.

2. Mean hemoglobin concentrations are approximately 8 g/dl in patients with SS disease, although they are usually higher in patients with SC disease or S/β-thalassemia.

42

SICKLE CELL ANEMIA

3. Folate deficiency is common, and 20% of patients with SCD are iron deficient, so supplementation is necessary.

4. Patients who undergo chronic transfusion are at risk for iron overload, which can lead to cardiomyopathy, endocrine failure, and cirrhosis. Ferritin is not an accurate measure of total body iron stores; rather, total body iron should be evaluated through liver biopsy and iron quantitation (> 7 mg/g dry weight warrants chelation therapy).

5. White blood cell counts are higher than normal (12,000 to 15,000/mm^3) even in the absence of infection. Thrombocytosis may also be present.

6. Bone marrow transplantation is potentially curative for SCD, but the short- and long-term complications prevent widespread use.

J. INFECTIOUS DISEASE

1. Fevers can occur as a result of vaso-occlusion, but a persistent fever higher than 38.3° C should prompt an evaluation for infection.

2. Infections tend to occur in areas damaged by chronic sickling such as the lungs, kidneys, and bones.

3. These patients should be considered functionally asplenic because splenic autoinfarction usually occurs by early childhood.

4. Common infections.[2,10]

a. **Pneumonia.** Common organisms include atypical bacteria such as *Mycoplasma*, *Chlamydia*, and *Legionella*. Because of immunizations, *Streptococcus pneumoniae* and *Haemophilus influenzae* are becoming less common pathogens.

b. **Urinary tract infections** can recur and can lead to urosepsis. A follow-up urine culture 2 weeks after treatment is recommended.

c. **Osteomyelitis and septic arthritis** must be differentiated from vaso-occlusive bony pain. The epidemiology of osteomyelitis in SCD is unique because *Salmonella* species are the most common causative organisms, whereas *Staphylococcus aureus* is the infectious agent in approximately 25% of cases. Chronic *Salmonella* osteomyelitis necessitates prolonged antibiotic therapy with 1 month of recommended IV treatment followed by months of oral therapy.[22]

PEARLS AND PITFALLS

- Chronic pain can be present in SCD and must be treated adequately, often with long-acting narcotics such as sustained-release morphine or methadone on a two- or three-times-daily schedule. Breakthrough pain should be managed with short-acting analgesics including narcotics and nonsteroidal antiinflammatory drugs (see Table 42-1).

- Patients with SCD have been shown to have a higher rate of surgical complications than the general population (30% rate of serious complications).[23] Preoperative transfusion is recommended. Studies comparing transfusion to a hemoglobin level greater than 10 g/dl and exchange transfusion (goal hemoglobin SS < 30%) have found no significant difference in operative morbidity and mortality.

- Postoperative acute chest syndrome develops in 10% of patients who undergo surgery.
- The main complication of transfusion is the higher incidence of new alloantibody formation.
- Routine health maintenance is paramount in the care of patients with sickle cell disease. All adults should be immunized against *S. pneumoniae,* hepatitis B virus, and influenza. Patients should undergo yearly urinalysis to evaluate for proteinuria, yearly echocardiography to screen for pulmonary hypertension, and annual retinal examinations to detect early proliferative retinopathy.
- Folic acid should be given daily (1 mg orally each day).
- No additional risk of oral contraceptive use is associated with SCD.
- Genetic counseling should be offered to all patients with SCD.

REFERENCES

1. Bunn HF: Pathogenesis and treatment of sickle cell disease, *N Engl J Med* 337:762, 1997. C
2. Powars DR: Natural history of sickle cell disease: the first ten years, *Semin Hematol* 12:267, 1975. C
3. Platt OS et al: Pain in sickle cell disease: rates and risk factors, *N Engl J Med* 325:11, 1991. C
4. Steinberg M: Management of sickle cell disease, *N Engl J Med* 340:1021, 1999. C
5. Embury SH et al: Effects of oxygen inhalation on endogenous erythropoiesis, and properties of blood cells in sickle-cell anemia, *N Engl J Med* 311:291, 1984. C
6. Bellet PS et al: Incentive spirometry to prevent acute pulmonary complications in sickle cell disease, *N Engl J Med* 333:699, 1995. A
7. Charache S et al: Effect of hydroxyurea on the frequency of painful crises in sickle cell anemia, *N Engl J Med* 332:1317, 1995. A
8. Schmalzer EA et al: Viscosity of mixtures of sickle cells and normal red cells at varying hematocrit levels: implications for transfusion, *Transfusion* 1987:228, 1987. A
9. Miller ST et al: Impact of chronic transfusion therapy on incidence of pain and acute chest syndrome during the stroke prevention trial in sickle cell anemia, *J Pediatr* 139:785, 2001. B
10. Claster S, Vinchinski EP: Managing sickle cell disease, *BMJ* 327:1151, 2003. C
11. Powars DR et al: The natural history of stroke in sickle cell disease, *Am J Med* 65:461, 1978. C
12. Cohen AR et al: A modified transfusion program for prevention of stroke in sickle cell disease, *Blood* 79:1657, 1992. C
13. Ohene-Frempong F et al: Cerebrovascular accidents in sickle cell disease: rates and risk factors, *Blood* 91:288, 1998. C
14. Adams RJ: Stroke prevention in sickle cell disease, *Curr Opin Hematol* 7:101, 2000. C
15. Hayes RJ et al: Haematological factors associated with proliferative retinopathy in homozygous sickle cell disease, *Br J Ophthalmol* 65:712, 1981. C

42

SICKLE CELL ANEMIA

16. Gladwin MT et al: Pulmonary hypertension as a risk factor for death in patients with sickle cell disease, *N Engl J Med* 350:886, 2004. B
17. Sheehy TW et al: Exchange transfusion for sickle cell intrahepatic cholestasis, *Arch Intern Med* 140:1364, 1980. C
18. Pham PT et al: Renal abnormalities in sickle cell disease, *Kidney Int* 57:1, 2000. C
19. Falk RH et al: Sickle cell nephropathy, *Adv Nephrol* 23:133, 1994. C
20. Abbott KC et al: Sickle cell nephropathy at end-stage renal disease in the United States: patient characteristics and survival, *Clin Nephrol* 58:9, 2002. C
21. Koshy M et al: Leg ulcers in patients with sickle cell disease, *Blood* 74:1403, 1989. C
22. Anand AJ, Glatt AE: Salmonella osteomyelitis and arthritis in sickle cell disease, *Semin Arthritis Rheum* 24:211, 1994. C
23. Vichinsky EP et al: A comparison of conservative and aggressive transfusion regimens in the perioperative management of sickle cell disease, *N Engl J Med* 333:206, 1995. B
24. Childs JW: Sickle cell disease: the clinical manifestations, *J Am Osteopath Assoc* 95:593, 1995. D

Thrombocytopenia

Ann Mullally, MD; Susan Lee Limb, MD; and Alison Moliterno, MD

FAST FACTS

- Spontaneous bleeding usually does not occur until platelet counts are less than 10,000/µl.
- Platelet counts should be kept above 20,000/µl in patients with systemic illness (i.e., infection) and above 50,000/µl patients undergoing any procedure.
- The most common medications causing thrombocytopenia are heparin, sulfa drugs, piperacillin, linezolid, rifampin, quinine and quinidine, cimetidine, and valproic acid.
- Emergency treatment of idiopathic thrombocytopenic purpura (ITP) includes intravenous immunoglobulin (IVIG) 1 g/kg/day for 2 days, intravenous methylprednisolone 1 g/day for 3 days, and platelet transfusion.
- In heparin-naive patients, the thrombocytopenia caused by heparin-induced thrombocytopenia (HIT) develops within 7 days of heparin exposure.
- Cessation of heparin alone is not sufficient in patients with suspected HIT. Alternative anticoagulation should be initiated, even in the absence of clinically apparent thrombosis.
- Plasmapheresis should be initiated as early as possible in the course of thrombotic thrombocytopenic purpura (TTP). In the absence of life-threatening bleeding, platelet transfusions should be avoided because they may worsen thrombosis.

43

1. Thrombocytopenia is defined as a platelet count less than 150,000/µl of whole blood (normal values range from 150,000 to 350,000/µl).
2. Generally, bleeding caused by minor trauma is not observed until platelet counts fall below 50,000/µl.[1] Spontaneous bleeding usually occurs when counts are less than 10,000/µl. Although exceedingly rare, intracranial bleeding is the main cause of death from thrombocytopenia.
3. Thrombocytopenia usually presents with self-limited small vessel bleeding in the gastrointestinal and genitourinary tracts, including gingival bleeding, epistaxis, and menorrhagia. In the absence of trauma, gross hematuria and gastrointestinal bleeding are uncommon. Petechiae and ecchymoses may also be present.
4. Patients with a consumptive process (e.g., ITP, hypersplenism) have a lower risk of bleeding than patients with impaired production.

I. APPROACH TO THE PATIENT WITH THROMBOCYTOPENIA

1. When evaluating a patient with newly identified thrombocytopenia, it is useful to first distinguish the otherwise healthy patient from the patient with systemic illness. The algorithm in Fig. 43-1 illustrates the investigation of isolated thrombocytopenia in otherwise healthy patients.

2. When evaluating the acutely ill or hospitalized patient with thrombocytopenia, it is useful to distinguish thrombocytopenia caused by increased platelet destruction from thrombocytopenia caused by impaired platelet production. The algorithms in Fig. 43-2 and Fig. 43-3 illustrate this approach.

II. THROMBOCYTOPENIA IN THE OTHERWISE HEALTHY PATIENT

A. PSEUDOTHROMBOCYTOPENIA

1. Before embarking on an extensive workup, consider pseudothrombocytopenia as a potential explanation for reduced platelet count.

2. Pseudothrombocytopenia usually is caused by platelet clumping in the blood sample, arising from inadequate anticoagulation of the sample or immunoglobulin-mediated agglutination, leading to an underestimation of platelets by automated cell counters.

3. Pseudothrombocytopenia is confirmed by collection of a blood sample in a tube containing heparin or sodium citrate as the anticoagulant (rather than edetic acid, which exposes the IIb/IIIa epitope and mediates autoantibody agglutination) or by manual inspection of a peripheral blood smear taken directly from a fingerstick.[2]

B. IDIOPATHIC THROMBOCYTOPENIC PURPURA

1. **Epidemiology.**

a. ITP, also called primary immune thrombocytopenia, is an organ-specific autoimmune disorder in which platelets coated with immunoglobulin G autoantibodies undergo accelerated clearance through Fcγ receptors expressed by tissue macrophages, predominantly in the spleen and liver.

b. The true incidence is difficult to estimate because many cases are asymptomatic, and no gold standard for diagnosis exists. Adult ITP is more common in women (female-to-male ratio 1.7:1). Despite the usual impression that ITP is a disease of younger and middle-aged adults, the mean age at diagnosis is 56 years.[3]

2. **Presentation.** In adults, ITP typically has an insidious onset and a chronic course. A history of preceding viral or other illness is uncommon. Symptoms and signs at presentation are highly variable, ranging from no symptoms to mild bruising and mucosal bleeding to frank hemorrhage from any site.

3. **Diagnosis.**

a. **The diagnosis of ITP remains one of exclusion.** Secondary forms of the disease can occur in association with systemic lupus erythematosus,

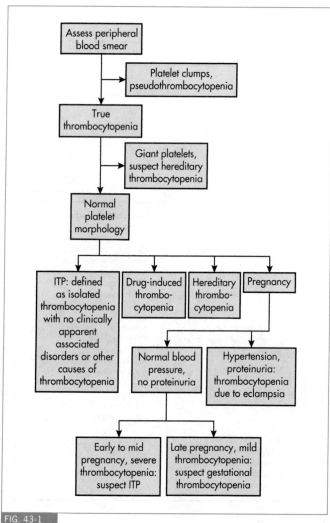

FIG. 43-1

Algorithm for investigating isolated thrombocytopenia in an otherwise healthy person.
ITP, idiopathic thrombocytopenic purpura. *(From George JN:* Lancet
355(9214):1531-1539, 2000, Fig. 3.)

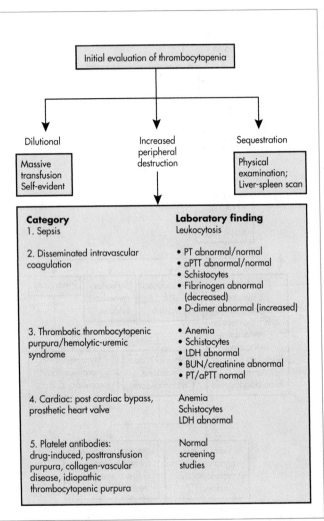

FIG. 43-2

Initial evaluation for thrombocytopenia in the patient with systemic illness.
aPTT, activated partial thromboplastin time; *BUN,* blood urea nitrogen; *LDH,* lactate dehydrogenase; *PT,* prothrombin time. *(From Goldman L, Bennett JC: Cecil textbook of medicine, 21st ed, Philadelphia, 1999, WB Saunders.)*

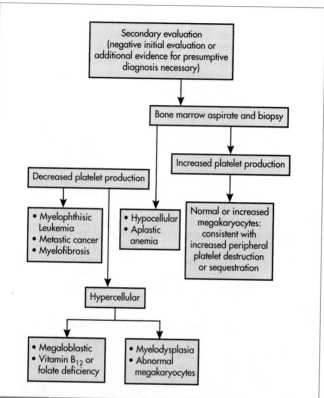

43

THROMBOCYTOPENIA

FIG. 43-3

Secondary evaluation for thrombocytopenia. (*From Goldman L, Bennett JC: Cecil textbook of medicine, 21st ed, Philadelphia, 1999, WB Saunders.*)

the antiphospholipid syndrome, infection with the human immunodeficiency virus or hepatitis C, and lymphoproliferative disorders (chronic lymphocytic leukemia, large granular lymphocytic leukemia, and lymphoma).

b. **Laboratory investigation should begin with a complete blood cell count and peripheral blood smear.**

c. **Antiplatelet antibody assays** have an estimated sensitivity of 50% to 65%, an estimated specificity of 80% to 90%, and an estimated positive predictive value of 80%.[4] A negative test does not exclude the diagnosis, and measurement is not recommended by the American Society of Hematology.[5]

d. Equally controversial is the need for **bone marrow aspiration.** Guidelines from the American Society of Hematology state that bone marrow aspiration is not necessary in adults younger than 60 years if the presentation is typical, but it should be performed before splenectomy.[5] In practice, bone marrow aspiration is generally reserved for patients older than 40 years of age (to exclude lymphoproliferative disorders or bone marrow failure),[6] for those with atypical features (e.g., unexplained symptoms, additional cytopenias, unexplained macrocytosis, abnormalities on peripheral blood smear), or for those who do not improve quickly.

4. **Management.** ITP is a heterogeneous disease and is unpredictable in its response to therapy. Deciding which patients need treatment can be complicated. Important factors that should be considered before treatment include the presence of active bleeding, absolute platelet count, patient age (higher age increases risk), patient lifestyle (sedentary vs. active), additional risk factors for bleeding (uremia, liver disease), treatment side effects, and patient preference. Therapeutic guidelines are based on expert opinion rather than on evidence because few clinical trials have been completed.

a. **Acute management.** Patients with active bleeding need emergent treatment. The standard management in such cases begins with IVIG 1 g/kg/day for 2 days, intravenous methylprednisolone 1 g/day for 3 days, and platelet transfusions. Bleeding patients may also benefit from the antifibrinolytic agent aminocaproic acid (5-g loading dose followed by 1 g every 6 hours intravenously or orally).

b. **Long-term management.**

   (1) **Corticosteroids.** For patients without evidence of bleeding, corticosteroids remain the standard initial therapy for ITP. A 4- to 6-week course of prednisone (1 mg/kg daily) with a slow taper is the usual starting regimen. Approximately two thirds of patients respond to steroids and achieve full or partial remission, usually within the first week of therapy. Unfortunately, the majority of patients relapse after withdrawal of treatment.

   (2) **IVIG and anti-Rh(D).** Patients with corticosteroid-refractory disease can be treated with IVIG or anti-Rh(D) immunoglobulin (RhoGAM). The dosage of IVIG is the same dosage given for emergency treatment (1 g/kg/day for 2 days). Rh-positive nonsplenectomized patients can be given 50 to 75 μg/kg anti-Rh(D). Approximately 70% of patients respond transiently to IVIG or anti-D, but neither agent achieves a long-term remission.

   (3) **Splenectomy** should be reserved for patients with refractory thrombocytopenia 4 to 6 weeks after diagnosis or patients who are steroid-dependent, needing a daily dosage of prednisone greater than 10 mg.[5] However, there has never been a randomized trial comparing splenectomy with drug therapy. Roughly three quarters of patients who undergo splenectomy achieve a complete remission, with approximately 60% still in remission at 10 years.[7] Immunization against *Streptococcus pneumoniae, Haemophilus*

influenzae B, and *Neisseria meningitidis* is generally advised at least 2 weeks before splenectomy.[5]

(4) **Refractory ITP.** Approximately one third of all adult patients with ITP fail second-line therapy (splenectomy) and can be defined as having chronic refractory ITP. Multiple therapies have been attempted in these patients, including chronic low-dose steroids (5 to 10 mg/day), high-dose dexamethasone (40 mg/day),[8] and various immunosuppressive agents. Rituximab (anti-CD20 monoclonal antibody), Campath-1H (anti-CD52 monoclonal antibody), and the androgen analog danazol have also been used with some success. More recently, eradication of *Helicobacter pylori* infection has been reported to be associated with clinical response in ITP.[9]

C. DRUG-INDUCED THROMBOCYTOPENIA

1. **Drug-induced thrombocytopenia is common and usually is immune mediated.** Antibody-drug complexes on the surface of platelets trigger complement activation and subsequent removal from the circulation.
2. Drug-induced thrombocytopenia typically develops 2 to 3 weeks after initial exposure to the drug.[5] The antithrombotic glycoprotein IIb/IIIa receptor inhibitors are a notable exception. Because of preformed antibodies to the glycoprotein IIb/IIIa receptor, platelet counts can fall within 30 minutes to 24 hours of drug exposure.[10]
3. Almost every drug has been associated with some degree of thrombocytopenia. The most common causes include heparin, quinine and quinidine, cimetidine, rifampin, piperacillin, linezolid, sulfa drugs, and anticonvulsants such as valproic acid.[5]
4. Generally, thrombocytopenia caused by drug antibodies resolves within 10 days after discontinuation of the medication but can persist longer.

D. THROMBOCYTOPENIA ASSOCIATED WITH PREGNANCY

Gestational thrombocytopenia is mild, asymptomatic, and present in 5% of pregnant women at term.[11] More severe thrombocytopenia (platelets < 70,000 cells/μl) occurring earlier in pregnancy should raise suspicion for ITP.

E. HEREDITARY THROMBOCYTOPENIA

Hereditary thrombocytopenia is rare, although many different subtypes, including May-Hegglin syndrome (giant platelets), have been described.

III. THROMBOCYTOPENIA IN THE PATIENT WITH SYSTEMIC ILLNESS

A. INFECTION

1. Viral (e.g., human immunodeficiency virus, Epstein-Barr virus, cytomegalovirus, hantavirus), rickettsial (e.g., *Ehrlichia,* Rocky Mountain spotted fever, Lyme), and parasitic (e.g., malaria) infections can result in thrombocytopenia by interfering with platelet production.
2. **Sepsis is a common and often overlooked cause of thrombocytopenia in the critically ill.** Sepsis is associated with elevated concentrations of

43

THROMBOCYTOPENIA

macrophage colony-stimulating factor, which leads to histiocyte engulfment of megakaryocytes (hemophagocytic syndrome).[12]

B. THROMBOTIC MICROANGIOPATHIES

1. **Epidemiology.** The thrombotic microangiopathies are characterized by excessive platelet aggregation, which leads to microvascular occlusion, thrombocytopenia, and mechanical injury to erythrocytes (microangiopathic hemolytic anemia).[13]

a. Platelet aggregation primarily within the systemic microvasculature causes TTP, whereas that affecting predominantly the renal circulation is known as hemolytic-uremic syndrome (HUS). Clinical distinction between the two entities is not always straightforward, and they are often described as a single disorder. However, studies demonstrate distinct histopathologic findings in the two disease states, suggesting different underlying pathophysiologies.[14]

b. Thrombotic microangiopathy has also been described in association with certain drugs (e.g., ticlopidine, mitomycin), after allogenic bone marrow transplantation, during pregnancy, and postpartum.

2. **Pathophysiology.**

a. The microvascular thrombi that characterize TTP and HUS consist of platelet aggregates with abundant von Willebrand factor (vWF). Endothelial cells and megakaryocytes produce multimers of vWF that bind to platelet glycoprotein Ib receptors. ADAMTS 13 is a vWF-cleaving metalloprotease present in plasma. In TTP plasma, ADAMTS 13 activity is less than 5% of normal. As a result, the large multimers of vWF are not cleaved; instead, they remain anchored to the endothelium, allowing passing platelets to adhere and form potentially occlusive platelet thrombi.

b. In contrast, plasma ADAMTS 13 activity is largely normal in HUS. Shiga toxin–producing *Escherichia coli* (*E. coli* O157) is believed to be the predominant etiological agent of HUS in children and occasionally causes HUS in adults. Shiga toxin enters the circulation and attaches to the glomerular capillary endothelial cells, where it induces the endothelial cells to secrete large multimers of vWF, causing platelet activation and microthrombus formation.

3. **Presentation.**

a. More than 90% of patients exhibit the classic pentad of signs and symptoms characteristic of TTP: thrombocytopenia, microangiopathic hemolytic anemia, neurologic abnormalities, renal abnormalities, and fever.[15]

b. In practice, however, **the triad of thrombocytopenia, schistocytosis, and elevated lactate dehydrogenase should raise the physician's suspicion of TTP,** particularly in the absence of an alternative explanation for these abnormalities.

c. The extent of microvascular aggregation is reflected in the degree of thrombocytopenia, erythrocyte fragmentation (schistocytes, helmet cells), and elevation of lactate dehydrogenase.

4. **Diagnosis.** The availability of effective treatment for TTP makes early diagnosis essential. This urgency has led to decreased stringency in the five diagnostic criteria as they were originally described in 1966.

5. **Management.**

a. A single randomized clinical trial demonstrating the superiority of plasma exchange over plasma infusion[16] provides the only firm evidence on which to base recommendations for treatment in TTP.

b. Plasma exchange is the combination of plasmapheresis (which may remove unusually large multimers of vWF and autoantibodies against ADAMTS 13) and infusion of fresh frozen plasma or cryosupernatant (containing additional metalloprotease). It is the primary treatment of adults with acquired acute idiopathic TTP and should be initiated as early as possible in the course of the disease. Its increased availability over the past 20 years has dramatically improved survival rates in this disease from 10% to approximately 90%. Initially, plasma exchange should be performed once daily. The value of additional treatment modalities (including glucocorticoids) is unknown.

c. In the absence of life-threatening hemorrhage or intracranial bleeding, **platelet transfusions should be avoided** because they can exacerbate microvascular thrombosis.

d. The role of plasma exchange in adults with HUS is much less clear, and it is generally felt to be ineffective in this patient group.

C. HEPARIN-INDUCED THROMBOCYTOPENIA

1. **Epidemiology and pathophysiology.**

a. HIT type 2 is a complication of heparin therapy characterized by a decreased platelet count after treatment with heparin, platelet activation, and thrombosis. **HIT type 2 is an immune-mediated process that produces an acquired, transient hypercoagulable state.** Immunoglobulin G antibodies form against a complex of heparin and platelet factor 4.[17] These antibodies then bind to the Fc receptors on platelets, resulting in platelet activation, increased thrombin generation, and an increased risk of thromboembolism.

b. HIT type 1 is a benign nonimmune disorder resulting in mild thrombocytopenia that typically occurs in the first 3 days of heparin administration.

c. The incidence of true HIT type 2 ranges from 0.3% to 3% depending on the clinical scenario in which it is studied. It is more common in surgical patients (in particular after cardiac surgery) than in medical patients.

2. **Presentation.**

a. In heparin-naive patients with type 2 HIT, the platelet count does not fall before day 5 of heparin administration, although thrombosis can occur before the onset of true (platelet count $< 150,000/\mu l$) thrombocytopenia.[18]

b. A more rapid decline (10.5 hours) in platelet count may be seen in patients with heparin exposure in the previous 100 days.[19]

c. Type 2 HIT can be severe, and even small dosages of heparin, such as the amount used in intravenous line flushes, can cause significant thrombocytopenia and thrombosis.

d. Typically platelet counts drop to less than 100,000/μl or decrease by more than 50% of the pretreatment level.

3. **Diagnosis.** The diagnosis of HIT type 2 can be difficult. Most laboratories use an enzyme-linked immunosorbent assay to detect HIT immunoglobulin G antibodies. The test is approximately 75% sensitive and not very specific, making false positive results common.

4. **Management.**

a. The first step in management of type 2 HIT is the avoidance of all heparin products (including intravenous line flushes). However, heparin cessation alone is not sufficient. **Alternative anticoagulation should be initiated in patients with suspected type 2 HIT** even in the absence of clinically apparent thrombosis because there is 25% to 50% risk of developing symptomatic thrombosis, including 5% risk of sudden thrombotic death.[20,21]

b. Alternative anticoagulation with direct thrombin inhibitors is necessary until the platelet count increases and plateaus. Two direct thrombin inhibitors (lepirudin and argatroban) are approved for treating HIT.

c. Warfarin should be started only after the patient has achieved therapeutic anticoagulation and the thrombocytopenia has resolved because of the risk of warfarin-induced skin necrosis (including venous limb gangrene).[22] There should be at least a 5-day overlap of direct thrombin inhibitor and warfarin.

d. Although unfractionated heparin is at least 10 times more likely to cause HIT than low molecular weight heparin,[18] up to 90% of patients with HIT display cross-reactivity with low molecular weight heparins, and so their use should be avoided.

D. DISSEMINATED INTRAVASCULAR COAGULATION

1. Disseminated intravascular coagulation (DIC) is characterized by systemic activation of coagulation cascade, which leads to the intravascular formation of fibrin, thrombotic occlusion of small and medium-sized vessels, and subsequent organ ischemia. This process consumes and depletes platelets and coagulation factors, which can result in hemorrhage. DIC is an acquired disorder associated with multiple disease states and conditions, most commonly infection, cancer, and pregnancy (Box 43-1).

2. Microangiopathic hemolysis is invariably present in TTP and HUS, whereas it is seen only sometimes in patients with severe DIC, as a result of the thrombotic occlusion of the microvasculature by intravascular fibrin (Table 43-1).

3. See Chapter 45 for further discussion of DIC, including diagnosis and management.

E. CHRONIC LIVER DISEASE

Thrombocytopenia is a common complication of chronic liver disease, especially in patients with cirrhosis. The thrombocytopenia of chronic liver

---

BOX 43-1

CLINICAL CONDITIONS THAT MAY BE ASSOCIATED WITH DISSEMINATED INTRAVASCULAR COAGULATION

Sepsis or severe infection (any microorganism)

Trauma (e.g., polytrauma, neurotrauma, fat embolism)

Organ destruction (e.g., severe pancreatitis)

Malignancy (e.g., solid tumors, myeloprolific and lymphoproliferative malignancies)

Obstetric calamities (e.g., amniotic fluid embolism, abrupto placentae)

Vascular abnormalities (e.g., Kasabach-Merritt syndrome, large vascular aneurysms)

Severe hepatic failure

Severe toxic or immunologic reactions (e.g., snake bites, recreational drugs, transfusion reactions, transplant rejection)

Modified from Levi M, de Jonge E: *Blood Rev* 16(4):217-223, 2002, Table 1.

TABLE 43-1

DISTINGUISHING FEATURES BETWEEN THROMBOTIC MICROANGIOPATHY AND DISSEMINATED INTRAVASCULAR COAGULATION

	Thrombotic Microangiopathy	Disseminated Intravascular Coagulation
Clinical setting	Previously healthy subjects	Patients with a severe underlying disorder
Partial thromboplastin time	Normal or short	Usually long
Prothrombin time	Usually normal	Long
Thrombin time	Normal	Always long
Fibrinogen	Normal or elevated	Usually low
D-dimer	Slightly elevated	Markedly elevated

From Sagripanti A, Sarteschi LM: *Biomed Pharmacother* 54(8-9):423-430, 2000, Table IV.

---

disease is multifactorial, although the most commonly stated reason is portal hypertension, with congestive splenomegaly leading to platelet sequestration. Thrombopoietin, the main regulator of thrombopoiesis, is produced predominantly by the hepatic parenchyma. **In patients with cirrhosis, there is an inappropriate thrombopoietin response to decreased platelet levels.**[23] Thrombocytopenia resolves and **thrombopoietin** levels return to normal after liver transplantation.[24]

F. POSTTRANSFUSION PURPURA

Posttransfusion purpura is an uncommon transfusion reaction that results in severe thrombocytopenia (see Chapter 40).

G. OTHER CAUSES OF THROMBOCYTOPENIA

1. Autoimmune disorders (e.g., systemic lupus erythematosus, rheumatoid arthritis, and antiphospholipid syndrome) are associated with immune-mediated thrombocytopenia.

2. Myelodysplastic syndrome, vitamin B_{12} deficiency, and folate deficiency may present initially with isolated thrombocytopenia.

3. Physical destruction of platelets from shear stress may occur during cardiopulmonary bypass or be caused by prosthetic heart valves.
4. An uncommon cause of increased platelet destruction is type IIB von Willebrand disease.

PEARLS AND PITFALLS

- Before low platelet counts are evaluated, pseudothrombocytopenia should be excluded.
- A negative antiplatelet antibody assay does not rule out TTP.
- HIT can develop despite very low dosages of heparin, such as the amount used in intravenous line flushes.
- In type 2 HIT a rapid decline (10.5 hours) in platelet count may be seen in patients previously exposed to heparin within 100 days of presentation.
- Laboratory tests for HIT are approximately 75% sensitive but lack specificity.
- Although unfractionated heparin is 10 times more likely to cause HIT than low molecular weight heparin, almost all patients with HIT display cross-reactivity, and so low molecular weight heparin should be avoided.
- The triad of thrombocytopenia, schistocytosis, and elevated lactate dehydrogenase should raise suspicion of TTP.

REFERENCES

1. Lacey JV, Penner JA: Management of idiopathic thrombocytopenic purpura in the adult, *Semin Thromb Haemost* 3(3):160, 1977. C
2. Payne BA, Pierre RV: Pseudothrombocytopenia: a laboratory artifact with potentially serious consequences, *Mayo Clinic Proc* 59(2):123, 1984. E
3. Frederiksen H, Schmidt K: The incidence of idiopathic thrombocytopenia purpura increases with age, *Blood* 94:909-913, 1999. B
4. Warner MN, Moore JC: A prospective study of protein-specific assays used to investigate idiopathic thrombocytopenic purpura, *Br J Haematol* 104:442, 1999. B
5. George JN et al: Idiopathic thrombocytopenic purpura: a practice guideline developed by explicit methods for the American Society of Hematology, *Blood* 88(1):3, 1996. D
6. Najean Y, Lecompte T: Chronic pure thrombocytopenia in elderly patients: an aspect of myelodysplastic syndrome, *Cancer* 64(12):2506, 1989. B
7. Stasi R et al: Long-term observation of 208 adults with chronic idiopathic thrombocytopenic purpura, *Am J Med* 98(5):436, 1995. B
8. Andersen JC: Response of resistant idiopathic thrombocytopenic purpura to pulsed high-dose dexamethasone therapy, *N Engl J Med* 330:1560-1564, 1994. (Published correction appears in *N Engl J Med* 331:283, 1994.) B
9. Michel M, Cooper N: Does *Helicobacter pylori* initiate or perpetuate immune thrombocytopenic purpura? *Blood* 103:890-896, 2004. B
10. Curtis BR et al: Thrombocytopenia after second exposure to abciximab is caused by antibodies that recognize abciximab-coated platelets, *Blood* 99(6):2054, 2002. B
11. Burrows RF, Kelton JG: Fetal thrombocytopenia and its relation to maternal thrombocytopenia, *N Engl J Med* 329:1463-1466, 1993. B

12. Francois B et al: Thrombocytopenia in the sepsis syndrome: role of hemophagocytosis and macrophage colony-stimulating factor, *Am J Med* 103(2):114, 1997. B

13. Moake JL: Thrombotic microangiopathies, *N Engl J Med* 347:589-600, 2002. C

14. Hosler GA, Cusumano AM: Thrombotic thrombocytopenic purpura and hemolytic uremic syndrome are distinct pathologic entities. A review of 56 autopsy cases, *Arch Pathol Lab Med* 127(7):834-839, 2003. B

15. Amorosi EL, Ultmann JE: Thrombotic thrombocytopenic purpura: report of 16 cases and review of the literature, *Medicine (Baltimore)* 45:139-159, 1966. B

16. Rock GA, Shumak KH, Buskard NA, et al: Comparison of plasma exchange with plasma infusion in the treatment of thrombotic thrombocytopenic purpura, *N Engl J Med* 325:93-397, 1991. A

17. Amiral J et al: Platelet factor 4 complexed to heparin is the target for antibodies generated in heparin-induced thrombocytopenia, *Thromb Haemost* 68:95, 1992. B

18. Warkentin TE et al: Heparin-induced thrombocytopenia in patients treated with low-molecular-weight heparin or unfractionated heparin, *N Engl J Med* 332(20):1330, 1995. A

19. Warkentin TE, Kelton JG: Temporal aspects of heparin-induced thrombocytopenia, *N Engl J Med* 344:1286, 2001. B

20. Warkentin TE: Heparin-induced thrombocytopenia: pathogenesis and management, *Br J Haematol* 121:535-555, 2003. C

21. Warkentin TE, Kelton JG: A 14-year study of heparin-induced thrombocytopenia, *Am J Med* 101:502-507, 1996. B

22. Warkentin TE et al: The pathogenesis of venous limb gangrene associated with heparin-induced thrombocytopenia, *Ann Intern Med* 127(9):804, 1997. B

23. Espanol I, Gallego A: Thrombocytopenia associated with liver cirrhosis and hepatitis C viral infection: role of thrombopoietin, *Hepatogastroenterology* 47:1404-1406, 2000. B

24. Peck-Radosavljevic M, Zacherl J: Is inadequate thrombopoietin production a major cause of thrombocytopenia in cirrhosis of the liver? *J Hepatol* 27:127-131, 1997. B

43

THROMBOCYTOPENIA

Bone Marrow Failure

Catherine S. Magid, MD; and Robert Brodsky, MD

FAST FACTS

- Aplastic anemia is a disorder of bone marrow failure characterized by peripheral pancytopenia and a hypocellular bone marrow.
- Pancytopenia is a deficiency of all cellular blood elements (anemia, neutropenia, and thrombocytopenia).
- Aplastic anemia may be congenital or acquired. More than 90% of aplastic anemia is acquired, and in most cases pancytopenia results from autoimmune-mediated bone marrow failure.
- Aplastic anemia predominantly affects children and young adults but may occur at any age.
- The presenting symptoms of pancytopenia are nonspecific: fatigue, dyspnea on exertion, fever, easy bruising, and increased susceptibility to infections.
- Bone marrow examination in patients with aplastic anemia demonstrates hypocellularity (< 25%) without malignant cells.

I. EPIDEMIOLOGY

1. More than 80% of diagnosed cases of aplastic anemia are classified as idiopathic.[1]
2. The best estimate of the incidence of aplastic anemia in western Europe is two cases per million, but in Southeast Asia the incidence may be two to three times higher.[2,3]
3. Acquired aplastic anemia has been associated with drug use, benzene exposure, insecticides, viruses, and other agents. Although drugs are often cited as a cause of aplastic anemia, a population-based control study in Thailand found that drugs were the cause of only 5% of newly diagnosed cases of aplastic anemia.[4,5]

II. CLINICAL PRESENTATION

1. The most common presenting symptoms in the patient with pancytopenia often are nonspecific and reflective of the low blood counts: fatigue, dyspnea on exertion, menorrhagia, easy bruising, epistaxis, gingival bleeding, fever, and headache. Symptoms may develop abruptly or may present insidiously over weeks to months.
2. Increased susceptibility to bacterial and fungal infections is a common consequence of neutropenia and increases with decreasing neutrophil count (absolute neutrophil count < 200).
3. Physical examination generally is nonfocal but may demonstrate pallor and petechiae. The liver and spleen generally are not enlarged.

4. The complete blood cell count demonstrates pancytopenia with reticulocytopenia. The peripheral blood smear confirms thrombocytopenia and a decrease in granulocytes and monocytes. Erythrocytes may be macrocytic, but the morphology of the remaining elements is normal.

III. ETIOLOGY

1. In most cases of acquired aplastic anemia, the autoimmune destruction of hematopoietic stem cells is mediated by cytotoxic T lymphocytes and involves inhibitory Th1 cytokines and the Fas-dependent cell death pathway.

2. There is an association with seronegative hepatitis, affecting approximately 1% of newly diagnosed cases, predominating in young males, and occurring within 2 to 3 months after the onset of hepatitis. The origin of aplastic anemia in this population is thought to be autoimmune because most cases respond to immunosuppressive therapy.[6]

3. When diagnosing aplastic anemia it is important to exclude other (potentially reversible) causes of pancytopenia. Common causes and associations of pancytopenia are listed in Box 44-1.

4. **It is important to differentiate between aplastic anemia and PNH.**

   a. Almost 70% of patients with aplastic anemia have detectable PNH cells at diagnosis by certain assays, and many patients who receive immunosuppressive treatment with antithymocyte globulin recover with evidence of PNH.

   b. PNH is caused by somatic mutations in the PIG-A gene, which results in a failure to synthesize glycosylphosphatidyl-inositol anchors, a moiety that is necessary to anchor certain proteins to the cell membrane.

   c. This leads to partial or complete absence of glycosylphosphatidyl-inositol–anchored proteins, particularly CD55 and CD59.

   d. CD55 and CD59 are complement regulatory proteins; their absence explains the complement-mediated hemolysis that is often seen in PNH.

   e. Patients with PNH also have a higher risk of thrombosis, although the mechanism is unclear.

IV. DIAGNOSIS

1. The diagnostic approach to the patient with newly diagnosed pancytopenia should include a thorough history, including family history, duration and type of symptoms, occupational exposures, history of infections, and medications.

2. Physical examination should focus on eliciting findings that point to a specific diagnosis, such as splenomegaly (Epstein-Barr virus, hairy cell leukemia), congenital abnormalities such as short stature, radial abnormalities, and café-au-lait spots (Fanconi's anemia).

3. Initial laboratory testing should include complete blood cell count with differential, reticulocyte count, peripheral blood smear, liver function

44

BONE MARROW FAILURE

BOX 44-1

CAUSES OF PANCYTOPENIA

CONGENITAL

Fanconi's anemia

Schwachman-Diamond syndrome

Amegakaryoctyic thrombocytopenia

Reticular dysgenesis

Dyskeratosis congenita

ACQUIRED

Toxins

Benzene (sources of exposure include gasoline, other petroleum products, and
rubber manufacturing)

Arsenicals

Ionizing radiation

Medication (i.e., chemotherapeutic agents, antiepileptics, ticlopidine)

Hematologic

Paroxysmal nocturnal hemoglobinuria

Myelodysplastic syndrome

Large granular lymphocyte leukemia

Acute leukemia

Hairy cell leukemia

Myelofibrosis

Bone marrow replacement by metastatic cancer

Polycythemia vera (fibrotic phase)

Infections

Hepatitis (non-A, non-B, non-C)

Human immunodeficiency virus infection

Cytomegalovirus

Epstein-Barr virus

Others

Graft versus host disease

Anorexia nervosa

Pregnancy

Thymoma, thyroid carcinoma

---

tests with hepatitis serologies, vitamin B_{12} and folate levels, and lactate
dehydrogenase.

4. Peripheral blood flow cytometry should be performed to exclude PNH.
   Anti-CD59 is the most commonly used antibody for the diagnosis of
   PNH. A newer, more sensitive and specific assay (flourescent labeled
   inactive variant of aerolysin [FLAER]) is increasingly being used to
   detect an absence of glycosylphosphatidyl-inositol–anchored proteins on
   the cells surface. Chromosome fragility studies with diepoxybutane
   should be performed on patients younger than 40 years old to rule out
   Fanconi's anemia.

5. **Bone marrow aspirate, biopsy, and cytogenetics confirm the diagnosis.**
It is sometimes necessary to perform more than one biopsy to clearly
establish the diagnosis. The core biopsy should be at least 1 cm long.

V. RISK STRATIFICATION AND PROGNOSIS

1. The clinical course of an untreated patient with aplastic anemia can be
predicted on the basis of the peripheral blood counts. Without successful
treatment, more than 70% of patients with severe aplastic anemia and
very severe aplastic anemia will die within 1 year[7] (Box 44-2).
2. At any degree of severity, outcomes are worse for older patients. The
greater mortality among older patients results primarily from infection
and bleeding.

VI. TREATMENT

1. Supportive care is vital. Identify and discontinue any potentially toxic
medications or exposures. Diagnose and treat any potentially reversible
causes of bone marrow failure.
2. Definitive therapies for aplastic anemia include allogeneic bone
marrow transplantation, immunosuppression, and high-dose
cyclophosphamide.
3. Transfusions may be used to support blood counts while awaiting
definitive therapy. Note that they should be limited to prevent
sensitization in patients who are candidates for bone marrow
transplantation. Transfusion should be with cytomegalovirus-negative,
irradiated, or filtered products.
4. Allogeneic bone marrow transplantation is the treatment of choice for
young patients with a human leukocyte antigen–matched sibling (in
general, patients younger than 30 years old). The incidence of graft
versus host disease and infection is higher in patients older than 20
years and limits the success of bone marrow transplantation in this
population.[8]

BOX 44-2

NOMENCLATURE AND STAGING

SEVERE APLASTIC ANEMIA

Hypocellular bone marrow and the presence of at least two of the following:

Neutrophils < 500/ml

Platelets < 20,000/ml

Corrected reticulocytes < 1% (< 60,000 absolute reticulocyte count)

VERY SEVERE APLASTIC ANEMIA

Meets criteria for severe aplastic anemia, but additionally neutrophils are
< 200/ml

NONSEVERE APLASTIC ANEMIA

Hypocellular marrow and pancytopenia but does not meet criteria for severe
aplastic anemia

5. For patients who are older than 40 (some institutions use 50) and those who do not have a matched sibling donor, the likelihood of severe graft versus host disease is too high for transplantation to be a viable option. For these patients, immunosuppression is the treatment of choice, either with antithymocyte globulin (ATG) and cyclosporine or with high-dose cyclophosphamide.

6. ATG and cyclosporine are well tolerated but often not curative. Additionally, there is a high incidence of late clonal disorders (PNH, myelodysplastic syndrome, AML) in patients treated with ATG and cyclosporine. Of patients with aplastic anemia who are treated with ATG, 15% to 33% recover with evidence of PNH.[9]

7. High-dose cyclophosphamide has higher immediate toxicity than ATG and cyclosporine but is potentially curative, both as an up-front regimen and as salvage therapy.[10] In a study by Brodsky et al., 19 patients received high-dose cyclophosphamide, with a median neutropenic duration of 49 days. There were three deaths in patients older than 50 years old. The remainder of patients remained alive, without disease and without evidence of clonal disorder.[11]

PEARLS AND PITFALLS

- Age at presentation may provide a clue to the underlying cause.
- In a young adult presenting with pancytopenia and congenital physical abnormalities, consider Fanconi's anemia.
- Less than 5% of aplastic anemia is drug induced.
- Residual bone marrow cellularity may be patchy; a cellular bone marrow aspirate in a patient with clinical findings otherwise suggestive of aplastic anemia suggests the need for repeat biopsies from additional sites.
- Patients who are treated with antithymocyte globulin should undergo regular screening for development of secondary clonal disorders.
- Nonsevere aplastic anemia does not warrant treatment, but patients should be followed for possible disease progression.

REFERENCES

1. Issararagrisil S et al: Low drug attributability of aplastic anemia in Thailand. The Aplastic Anemia Study Group, *Blood* 89:4034-4039, 1997. B
2. Issararagrisil S et al: Incidence of aplastic anemia in Bangkok. The Aplastic Anemia Study Group, *Blood* 77:2166-2168, 1991. B
3. Issararagrisil S: Epidemiology of aplastic anemia in Thailand. The Aplastic Anemia Study Group, *Int J Hematol* 70:137-140, 1999. C
4. Shapiro S et al: Agranulocytosis in Bangkok, Thailand: a predominantly drug-induced disease with an unusually low incidence. Aplastic Anemia Study Group, *Am J Trop Med Hyg* 60:573-577, 1999. B
5. Issararagrisil S et al: Incidence and non-drug etiologies of aplastic anemia in Thailand. The Thai Aplastic Anemia Study Group, *Eur J Haematol Suppl* 60:31-34, 1996. B
6. Brown KE et al: Hepatitis associated aplastic anemia, *N Engl J Med* 336:1059-1064, 1997. B

7. Young NS: Aplastic anemia, *Lancet* 346:228, 1995. C
8. Kernan NA et al: Analysis of 462 transplantations from unrelated donors facilitated by the National Marrow Donor Program, *N Engl J Med* 328:593, 1993. B
9. Socie G et al: Malignant tumors occurring after immunosuppressive treatment. A report from the European Bone Marrow Transplantation Group: Severe Aplastic Anemia Working Party, *N Engl J Med* 329:1152, 1993. B
10. Brodsky RA et al: Durable treatment-free remission after high dose cyclophosphamide therapy for previously untreated severe aplastic anemia, *Ann Intern Med* 135:477, 2001. B
11. Brodsky RA et al: Complete remission in severe aplastic anemia after high dose cyclophosphamide without bone marrow transplantation, *Blood* 87:491, 1996. B

44

BONE MARROW FAILURE

Bleeding Disorders

Susan Cheng, MD; and Michael Streiff, MD

> ## FAST FACTS
>
> - Bleeding disorders are inherited or acquired. The most important inherited disorders are von Willebrand disease (vWD) and hemophilia. The most common acquired disorders are caused by liver disease, vitamin K deficiency, and antiplatelet or anticoagulation therapy.
> - Clinically significant vWD tends to present with mucosal bleeding and easy bruising, whereas hemophilias are more likely to present with deep, soft tissue bleeds (e.g., hemarthroses or hematomas).
> - A family history of bleeding diathesis or a need for chronic transfusions or iron replacement increases the likelihood of a bleeding disorder.
> - The leading cause of hemorrhagic death in hemophilia is cerebral bleeding.

I. EPIDEMIOLOGY

1. **Inherited bleeding disorders** are caused by dysfunction or deficiency of coagulation factors (Fig. 45-1 and Fig. 45-2).
   a. The prevalence of vWD is 1% worldwide, affecting all sexes, races, and ethnicities equally. Although vWD is the most common inherited bleeding disorder, less than 10% of those affected are symptomatic.
   b. Hemophilia A and B are X-linked recessive (1 in 5000 and 1 in 25,000 males, respectively). Hemophilia C is autosomal recessive (1 in 100,000), with a higher prevalence among Ashkenazi Jews, up to 10% of whom are heterozygotes.[1,2]
   c. Much less common are disorders involving a deficiency of fibrinogen, prothrombin, or factors V, VII, or X.
2. **Acquired bleeding disorders** are caused by liver disease, vitamin K deficiency, antiplatelet or anticoagulation therapy, disseminated intravascular coagulation (DIC), and factor inhibitors.

II. CLINICAL PRESENTATION

1. In **vWD**, as in platelet disorders, the history often reveals easy bruisability or mucosal bleeding (e.g., epistaxis, gum bleeding, menorrhagia).
2. **Hemophilia** is characterized by deep, soft tissue bleeds (e.g., hemarthrosis, intramuscular bleeding) and may present with palpable ecchymoses. Postoperative bleeds tend to be delayed and severe.
   a. Common sites of bleeding include weight-bearing joints, extremity muscles, and the gastrointestinal and genitourinary tracts (up to 90% of patients have hematuria).

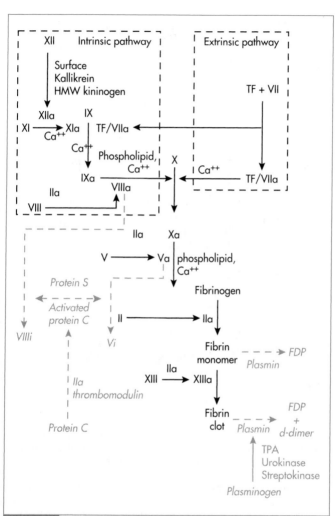

FIG. 45-1

Classic coagulation cascade. *FDP,* fibrin degradation product; *HMW,* high molecular weight; *TF,* tissue factor; *TPA,* tissue plasminogen activator.

TABLE 45-1

CHARACTERISTICS OF COAGULATION FACTORS

Location of Synthesis	Factors (approximate half-life, hr)
Liver, dependent on vitamin K	VII (6), IX (24), X (36), II (60), protein C (7), protein S (42)
Liver	V (12-36), I (120)
Probably liver	XI (40-84), XII (50), XIII (96-180)
Endothelial cells and elsewhere	VIII (12)

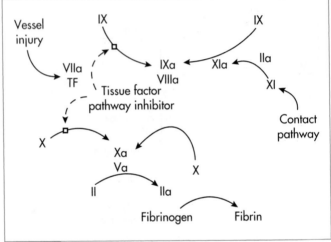

FIG. 45-2

Revised coagulation cascade.[3] *TF*, tissue factor.

b. Maintain a high index of suspicion for cerebral hemorrhage (high mortality) or iliopsoas bleeding (high morbidity). In all extremity bleeds, maintain a high index of suspicion for compartment syndrome, a surgical emergency.

3. The presentation of patients with **factor inhibitors** is similar to that of hemophilia.

4. Because only severe disease results in significant spontaneous bleeding, the physical examination in most patients with a bleeding diathesis often is normal.

III. ETIOLOGY

1. Bleeding disorders can be divided into those that are inherited or acquired. Other than platelet disorders (discussed in Chapter 43), bleeding diatheses are caused by deficiency or dysfunction of coagulation factors or the presence of an inhibitor to a coagulation factor.

2. **Inherited.**

a. **vWD** is caused by a deficiency or defect in von Willebrand factor (vWF), a large multimeric glycoprotein, synthesized in endothelial cells and megakaryocytes, that functions in platelet adherence and as a plasma carrier of factor VIII.

   (1) **Type 1** (autosomal dominant with variable penetrance, 60% to 80% of cases) is a partial quantitative factor deficiency.

   (2) **Type 2** (autosomal dominant or recessive, 15% to 20% of cases) consists primarily of qualitative factor defects. There are four known subtypes, the most common of which is **type 2A** (10% to 15% of vWD cases), which involves the loss of large and intermediate-sized multimers.

   (3) **Type 3** (autosomal recessive, rare) involves a severe deficiency of vWF and factor VIII and lacks response to transfusion or desmopressin acetate (DDAVP).

b. **Hemophilias** include inherited deficiencies of individual factors. Disease severity is classified by the percentage of normal factor activity: mild (5% to 25%), moderate (1% to 5%), or severe (< 1%). The types of hemophilia include the following:

   (1) Hemophilia A (classic hemophilia, X-linked): factor VIII deficiency.

   (2) Hemophilia B (Christmas disease, X-linked): factor IX deficiency.

   (3) Hemophilia C (autosomal recessive): factor XI deficiency.

3. **Acquired.**

a. **Vitamin K deficiency** is caused by malnutrition, decreased absorption (antibiotic suppression of intestinal flora or malabsorption), or warfarin.

b. **Liver disease** impairs the production of coagulation factors (Table 45-1) to a degree proportional to the extent of liver damage, whether acute or chronic.

c. **Supratherapeutic effects of anticoagulation therapy** (warfarin or heparin) usually occur just after therapy initiation and during dosage adjustment.

d. **DIC** can cause bleeding problems under conditions described later in this chapter.

e. **Factor inhibitors** are antibodies that accelerate the clearance of or impair the activity of coagulation factors. Inhibitors include anti–factor VIII alloantibodies acquired after multiple treatments of hemophilia A with factor VIII concentrate.

IV. DIAGNOSIS

1. The history and examination should review any bleeding manifestations in childhood; with menstruation and pregnancies, if applicable; and following surgeries and dental work. Screen for a family history of bleeding disorders. Review all medications, especially anticoagulation therapy and medications that commonly interact with warfarin (Box 45-1).

45

BLEEDING DISORDERS

BOX 45-1

COMMONLY USED MEDICATIONS THAT INTERACT WITH WARFARIN

MAJOR EFFECT

Antifungal agents, barbiturates, danazol, phenytoin, trimethoprim-sulfamethoxazole

MODERATE EFFECT

Allopurinol, amiodarone, antithyroid drugs, binding resins, carbamazepine, cephalosporins, corticosteroids, diflunisal, disulfiram, ethanol, fluvoxamine, isoniazid, metronidazole, nalidixic acid, paroxetine, penicillins, propafenone, quinolones, rifampin, statins, sulfinpyrazone, thyroid hormones, vitamin K

BOX 45-2

MIXING STUDIES EXPLAINED

Mixing studies help determine whether an isolated aPTT elevation is caused by a factor deficiency or factor inhibitor. The patient's plasma is mixed in a 1:1 ratio with normal pooled plasma, and the aPTT test is repeated.

If the repeat aPTT is normal (i.e., "corrects"), there is a factor deficiency. Only a 50% presence of clotting factors is necessary to achieve normal clotting if no inhibitors are present. If the presence of a factor deficiency is found, individual factor assays can reveal which factors are deficient.

If the repeat aPTT is still elevated (i.e., "does not correct"), a factor inhibitor is present. Most inhibitors have a clinical effect after 1:1 dilution, but to see the effect of some, the 1:1 diluted sample must be incubated for up to 2 hr at average body temperature. The most common inhibitors are the following:

Presence of heparin in the sample

Antiphospholipid antibodies

Inhibitors against factors VIII, IX, or X

Inhibitors against thrombin (e.g., fibrin or fibrin degradation product)

aPTT, activated partial thromboplastin time.

---

2. **Laboratory evaluation** should begin with a platelet count, prothrombin time (PT), and activated partial thromboplastin time (aPTT). If these are normal, consider measuring a thrombin time or fibrinogen level.
a. An **isolated elevation in the aPTT** suggests heparin therapy, antiphospholipid antibody syndrome, hemophilia, factor inhibitor, or possibly DIC.
b. An **elevated PT,** with or without elevated aPTT, is found in warfarin therapy, vitamin K deficiency, liver disease, and possibly DIC.
c. An **isolated thrombin elevation** suggests heparin therapy, fibrinogen abnormality, or thrombin inhibitor.
d. A DIC screen should be done if the clinical picture is suggestive.
e. Consider mixing studies for an elevated PT or aPTT (Box 45-2).

f. Consider measuring individual factor levels if mixing studies suggest a factor deficiency. Begin with the factors most likely to be deficient (e.g., factors VIII and IX). In DIC, all factors are consumed. In liver disease, factors synthesized in the liver are low (all except VIII). In vitamin K deficiency, only selected factors are low (see Table 45-1).

g. See Chapter 43 if thrombocytopenia is suspected.

3. **Narrowing the diagnosis.**

a. **In vWD, the bleeding time and aPTT have limited utility.** The most useful assays are the vWF antigen and ristocetin cofactor assays. The vWF antigen reflects the amount of vWF protein in the sample; the ristocetin cofactor assay measures vWF function.

   (1) vWF levels may be increased by age, pregnancy, adrenergic stimulation, estrogen therapy, and inflammation. vWF levels also can be 25% lower in patients with blood type O than in patients of other blood groups.

   (2) Patients suspected of having vWD but having only slightly low laboratory results may need to be retested on several occasions, separated by weeks, to make the diagnosis.

b. In **vitamin K deficiency,** the PT is elevated, with or without an elevation in aPTT. A deficiency of vitamin K–dependent factors can be found.

c. In **hemophilias,** the PT and vWF levels usually are normal. The aPTT typically is elevated and normalizes with mixing studies. Factor level testing reveals a low VIII, IX, or XI level.

4. If a congenital bleeding disorder is found, family members should be tested.

V. PROGNOSIS

1. In vWD, morbidity depends on the type and severity of disease. Many patients are asymptomatic or have mild cutaneous or mucous membrane bleeding. Patients with type 3 vWD can have severe bleeding symptoms similar to those of hemophilia.

2. Life expectancy for patients with hemophilia is 50 to 60 years. Excluding the sequelae of hepatitis, human immunodeficiency virus, and cirrhosis, overall mortality with severe hemophilia is still 20% higher than in age-matched controls.

3. For acquired bleeding disorders, outcomes are determined by the underlying disease.

VI. MANAGEMENT

1. In **vWD,** the goal of therapy is to achieve hemostasis. The mainstays of treatment are DDAVP (which releases vWF from endothelial storage sites) and plasma-derived factor VIII concentrates (containing factor VIII and vWF).[4]

a. In patients known to respond to **DDAVP,** it can be used preoperatively or to treat bleeding complications. Type 1 vWD is more likely than type 2 to respond to DDAVP because the endogenous vWF moiety in type 1 is deficient but functionally normal. Type 3 vWD will not respond because vWD stores are absent. Effects of intravenous DDAVP are seen in 30 to 60 minutes. A repeat dose can be given in 12 to 24 hours for continued bleeding or postoperative use.

b. For patients receiving **plasma-derived factor VIII concentrates** (e.g., Humate-P), factor VIII levels should be followed daily to ensure hemostasis and avoid supranormal levels, which can cause thromboembolism. Cryoprecipitate (enriched for vWF) should be used only if factor VIII concentrates are not available.

c. Adjunctive therapies include fibrinolysis inhibitors (e.g., aminocaproic acid), platelet concentrates, and oral estrogen-progesterone preparations.

2. In **hemophilia,** the goals of treatment are to achieve hemostasis, relieve symptoms, and provide prophylaxis against future bleeds and their sequelae.

a. For mild to moderate factor deficiency, therapies include factor VIII or IX concentrate and DDAVP (for factor VIII deficiency). For severe factor deficiency, factor concentrates are the mainstay of treatment.

   (1) **Factor VIII.** 1 U/kg increases plasma levels by 2%, and the half-life is 8 to 12 hours.

   (2) **Factor IX.** 1 U/kg increases plasma levels by 1%, and the half-life is 16 hours.

b. Adjunctive therapies include DDAVP and antifibrinolytics (aminocaproic acid). Advise caution during physical activity, which can trigger soft tissue bleeds. Consider prophylactic factor replacement to help prevent bleeding and subsequent chronic articular and muscular damage.

3. **Vitamin K deficiency** is treated with vitamin K supplementation as needed. Guidelines for treating vitamin K deficiency in the setting of warfarin therapy are listed in Part III, Table 8. Intravenous vitamin K decreases PT more effectively than when given subcutaneously or orally but tends to overshoot therapeutic goals and risks anaphylaxis. The next most effective and preferred route is oral, although the subcutaneous route may be easier in certain situations.[5]

4. **Coagulopathy caused by liver disease** is best managed by treating the underlying liver disorder. Vitamin K can be given but will achieve only a partial response because the loss of vitamin K–dependent clotting factors results primarily from hepatocellular damage in addition to any concurrent vitamin K deficiency. Fresh frozen plasma administration is effective for achieving hemostasis in the setting of active bleeding or around procedures.

5. Most cases of **supratherapeutic anticoagulation** (e.g., warfarin, heparin) are not life threatening and are treated by holding or decreasing dosages of the agent in use. Fresh frozen plasma and vitamin K may be given for active bleeding. Protamine sulfate may be given for heparin overdose.

BOX 45-3

DISEASE STATES COMMONLY ASSOCIATED WITH DIC

ACUTE DIC

Sepsis or severe infection (especially gram-negative), obstetric complications, collagen vascular disease (e.g., systemic lupus erythematosus with antiphospholipid syndrome [APS]), acute tissue injuries (e.g., trauma, fat embolism), organ destruction (e.g., severe pancreatitis)

SUBACUTE DIC

Solid or hematologic malignancies (e.g., leukemias, neuroblastomas, rhabdomyosarcomas, and mucin-producing adenocarcinomas associated with Trousseau's syndrome), certain connective tissue disorders, thrombophilias, marantic endocarditis

DIC, disseminated intravascular coagulation.

45

BLEEDING DISORDERS

VII. SPECIAL CONSIDERATION: DIC

1. **Epidemiology.** DIC often occurs in severe systemic illness (Box 45-3) and increases mortality risk above that associated with the primary disease.[6]
2. **Presentation.** Symptoms depend on disease severity and chronicity, ranging from asymptomatic compensated DIC to shock and death.
   a. Acute DIC usually is hemorrhagic, presenting with petechiae and ecchymoses at sites of trauma. Thromboses and bleeding may also be present. Purpura fulminans, cutaneous purpuric or hemorrhagic lesions, can develop, spread rapidly, and progress to frank gangrene.
   b. Chronic or subacute DIC typically manifests as thrombosis in a variety of sites.
3. **Etiology.** DIC is a consumption coagulopathy in which proinflammatory cytokines lead to excess thrombin formation and massive activation of the coagulation system. An acute hemorrhagic state can result from the depletion of platelets and clotting factors and excessive plasmin formation. A subacute, chronic state occurs when there is partial compensation for the consumption coagulopathy but excessive thrombin formation persists.
4. **Diagnosis.** Both clinical evaluation and laboratory tests are necessary to diagnose DIC. Suggestive screening tests include elevated PT and aPTT, low platelet count, elevated D-dimer or fibrin (split) degradation products, and low fibrinogen, protein C, and antithrombin levels.
   a. Serial tests may reveal abnormal trends and are more helpful than single results.
   b. D-dimer and fibrin degradation products are nonspecific and often elevated in trauma or recent surgery.
   c. Because fibrinogen is an acute phase reactant, serum levels may be normal despite an ongoing consumption coagulopathy.
   d. Schistocytes may be seen in the peripheral smear but are a nonspecific finding.

e. The presence of a disorder known to be associated with DIC, combined with abnormal test results, increases the likelihood of DIC. Scoring systems to aid the diagnosis have been developed but await validation.[7]

5. **Prognosis.** DIC usually is associated with a high mortality rate caused by the underlying disorder. Sequelae of DIC, including thrombosis, acral cyanosis, and limb ischemia, can lead to significant morbidity, which can be reduced by early recognition and treatment.

6. **Management.** Treat the underlying disease and, if necessary, replace deficient blood products using platelets, fresh frozen plasma, or cryoprecipitate if the fibrinogen level is less than 100 mg/dl (with a maintained goal of 100 to 150 mg/dl).

a. The notion that giving blood products, particularly fresh frozen plasma, may worsen DIC by adding more coagulation factors for consumption ("adding fuel to the fire") has never been proven by clinical or experimental studies.[7]

b. Consider treating sepsis-related DIC with activated protein C (see Chapter 21).[8]

c. Heparin therapy may help inhibit coagulation activation, but its benefit has not been shown in trials,[7] so heparin is best reserved for patients with digital ischemia, acral cyanosis, or purpura fulminans, where the treatment goal is based on a parameter such as fall in fibrin degradation products or D-dimer or a rise in fibrinogen level.

PEARLS AND PITFALLS

- Always screen for a history of bleeding with surgical or dental procedures.
- Patients presenting with a severe bleeding diathesis should be evaluated for intramuscular iliopsoas hemorrhage given the risk of large-volume blood loss and femoral nerve compression.
- If the patient has an intramuscular bleed, maintain a high suspicion for compartment syndrome. If the clinical picture is suggestive, compartment pressures must be measured after factor replacement is given.
- Mild vWD or hemophilia A may be masked by the factors that elevate factor VIII levels.
- Heyde's syndrome occurs in patients with aortic stenosis who develop an acquired form of vWD. Blood flow across a severely stenotic aortic valve results in shearing of von Willebrand multimers and bleeding of preexisting vascular malformations such as angiodysplasias in the gastrointestinal tract. The bleeding manifestation of this syndrome resolves with aortic valve replacement.[9]
- Given the exposure to blood products in patients with hemophilia, the risk of transfusion-related infections is high.

REFERENCES

1. Bolton-Maggs PH: Factor XI deficiency and its management, *Haemophilia* 6(Suppl 1):100-109, 2000. C

2. Rick ME, Walsh CE, Key NS: Congenital bleeding disorders, *Hematology (Am Soc Hematol Educ Program)* 559-574, 2003. C
3. Streiff MB, Bray PF, Kickler TS: *Johns Hopkins coagulation laboratory guide,* 2nd ed, Baltimore, 2002. C
4. Mannucci PM: Treatment of von Willebrand's disease, *N Engl J Med* 351(7):683-694, 2004. C
5. Whitling AM, Bussey HI, Lyons RM: Comparing different routes and doses of phytonadione for reversing excessive anticoagulation, *Arch Intern Med* 158(19):2136-2140, 1998. B
6. Toh CH, Dennis M: Disseminated intravascular coagulation: old disease, new hope, *BMJ* 327(7421):974-977, 2003. C
7. Hambleton J, Leung LL, Levi M: Coagulation: consultative hemostasis, *Hematology (Am Soc Hematol Educ Program)* 335-352, 2002. C
8. Bernard GR, Vincent JL, Laterre PF, et al: Efficacy and safety of recombinant human activated protein C for severe sepsis, *N Engl J Med* 344(10):699-709, 2001. A
9. Vincentelli A, Susen S, Le Tourneau T, et al: Acquired von Willebrand syndrome in aortic stenosis, *N Engl J Med* 349(4):343-349, 2003. B

45

BLEEDING DISORDERS

Hypercoagulable States

Susan Cheng, MD; and Michael Streiff, MD

I. EPIDEMIOLOGY

1. Venous thromboembolism is increasingly being viewed as a chronic disease, with recurrence rates of 17.5% at 2 years and 30.3% at 8 years.[1]
2. Of all inherited thrombophilias, factor V Leiden mutation and the prothrombin gene mutation account for 50% to 60%; most of the remaining are protein S deficiency, protein C deficiency, and antithrombin deficiency (Table 46-1).
3. There are few data about thrombophilias in non-Caucasian populations, but studies suggest that factor V Leiden and the prothrombin mutation are rare in non-Caucasians.

II. CLINICAL PRESENTATION

1. **Thromboses can present in many forms,** including superficial venous thrombosis (SVT), deep vein thrombosis (DVT) with or without pulmonary embolus, myocardial infarction, and stroke.

BOX 46-1

CAUSES OF HYPERCOAGULABLE STATES

PRIMARY

Decreased Antithrombotic Activity

Protein S deficiency

Protein C deficiency

Antithrombin III deficiency

Less common causes, including fibrinolytic system abnormalities (e.g., plasminogen abnormality or deficiency) or heparin cofactor II deficiency

Increased Prothrombotic Activity

Factor V Leiden mutation (most common cause of activated protein C resistance)

Activated protein C resistance exclusive of factor V Leiden mutation

Prothrombin G20210A mutation

Elevated levels or activity of factors XI, IX, or VIII

Less common causes, such as dysfibrinogenemia

SECONDARY

Situational risk factors

Postoperative states

Trauma

Pregnancy

Hormone therapy

Immobility

Certain chemotherapeutic agents

Vascular abnormalities (e.g., congenital IVC malformations, May-Thurner syndrome, Paget–von Schrötter syndrome, chronic extrinsic vascular compression)

Associated with systemic disease

Malignancy

Congestive heart failure

Hyperhomocysteinemia

Antiphospholipid syndrome

Myeloproliferative disorders: polycythemia vera, essential thrombocythemia

Hyperviscosity: Waldenström's macroglobulinemia, multiple myeloma

Other disease states: nephrotic syndrome, heparin-induced thrombocytopenia and thrombotic syndrome, paroxysmal nocturnal hemoglobinuria, Behçet's disease, inflammatory bowel disease

IVC, inferior vena cava.

a. Classic findings of SVT include a firm, tender, erythematous fibrous cord, usually in the area of previous varicose or normal-appearing vein.

b. Classic findings of DVT include mild to moderate edema; erythema; tenderness; and, rarely, a discrete palpable cord. Recurrence of lower extremity DVT is in the contralateral leg 50% of the time.

c. **Unusual sites of thrombosis may suggest an underlying cause.** Visceral clots are most common in paroxysmal nocturnal hematuria, Behçet's

TABLE 46-1

ESTIMATED PREVALENCE OF THROMBOPHILIAS IN PATIENTS WITH VENOUS THROMBOEMBOLISM[2,3]

Thrombophilia	Prevalence (%)
Factor V Leiden	20-40
Hyperhomocystinemia	10-20
Prothrombin G20210A mutation	14
Antiphospholipid syndrome	14
Elevated factor VIII levels	10-15
Antithrombin III deficiency	3-4
Protein C deficiency	3-4
Protein S deficiency	3-4

syndrome, and myeloproliferative disorders; cerebral venous sinus thromboses have been described in inflammatory bowel disease and oral contraceptive use; portal vein thrombosis is most common in liver disease.

3. Clinical histories highly suggestive of a primary thrombotic disorder include the following:
a. Thrombosis at a young age (usually younger than 50).
b. Family history of thrombosis, especially in at least one first-degree relative.
c. Thrombosis without precipitating factor.
d. Recurrent thrombosis, even with precipitating factors.
e. Recurrent pregnancy loss and thrombosis at unusual sites (e.g., cerebral, mesenteric, portal, or hepatic veins).

4. Female patients should be screened for hormone therapy use (including oral contraceptives, hormone replacement, tamoxifen). A history of recurrent fetal loss suggests an inherited thrombophilia or antiphospholipid antibodies.

5. Past medical history should screen for collagen-vascular diseases, myeloproliferative diseases, atherosclerotic disease, and nephrotic syndrome.

6. Medications that can induce antiphospholipid syndrome include hydralazine, procainamide, and phenothiazines.

7. It is always important to evaluate for malignancy.

III. ETIOLOGY

1. A venous thromboembolism typically has multiple causes, usually a primary or genetic basis in addition to secondary or acquired factors.[1] A predisposing genetic cause is found in up to 50% of patients with venous thromboembolism, and a secondary factor is found in more than 80% of patients.[4]

2. The primary hypercoagulable states are caused by either a defect or deficiency of antithrombotic protein activity or an increase in prothrombic protein activity.[1] See Figs. 45-1 and 45-2 and Table 45-1

in Chapter 45 to recall the coagulation cascade and characteristics of coagulation factors.

IV. DIAGNOSIS

1. The physical examination is neither sensitive nor specific for the diagnosis of SVT or DVT; pain or tenderness along course of major veins in the thighs, calf tenderness, and Homan's sign are discussed in Chapter 86. Special attention should be paid to the signs of Budd-Chiari syndrome (ascites, hepatomegaly, edema) or nephrotic syndrome (edema).

2. **Initial laboratory tests** should include complete blood cell count, prothrombin time, activated partial thromboplastin time, chemistries including liver and renal function tests, and urinalysis. New or recurrent thrombosis in the setting of heparin therapy and a drop in platelet count by 50% or more from baseline suggest the possibility of HIT-TS (see Chapter 43 for diagnosis of HIT).

3. If the history and physical examination are suggestive, consider a workup for malignancy, which can initially present as an unprecipitated venous thromboembolism.[5,6]

4. Red cell fragments seen on a peripheral blood smear may be helpful if disseminated intravascular coagulation is suspected. Although disseminated intravascular coagulation usually presents with bleeding, it can present as a low-grade consumptive coagulopathy with venous or arterial thrombosis, especially in the setting of malignancy.

5. **Special tests** are not likely to change management in most cases of first-time, explainable thromboembolism.[7] However, the presence of an easily identifiable predisposing factor should not prevent special testing if the history is otherwise suggestive of a primary hypercoagulable state (Box 46-2).

a. In addition to strongly thrombophilic factors listed in Box 46-2, consider a full screen for presentations of thrombosis in connection with oral contraceptive or hormone use, pregnancy, or a history of warfarin-induced skin necrosis.

b. The presence of a primary hypercoagulable state alters management regarding the duration of anticoagulation, prophylaxis for future procedures or events (e.g., surgery and pregnancy), and potential family screening.

c. Timing is important for special tests, as outlined in Box 46-3.

6. Confirmed arterial thrombosis necessitates an evaluation for antiphospholipid syndrome (APS), hyperhomocysteinemia, malignancy, and possibly dysfibrinogenemia. Also consider clonal disorders such as polycythemia vera and essential thrombocythemia.

V. PROGNOSIS

1. There are few data on the outcomes of patients with primary hypercoagulable states.

46

HYPERCOAGULABLE STATES

BOX 46-2

WHEN TO ORDER SPECIAL TESTS[8]

Determine whether the patient has any of the following 3 characteristics:

First thrombosis at younger than 50 years of age.

More than 1 thrombotic event or multiple thrombotic defects at first presentation.

First-degree relative with thrombotic event at younger than 50 years of age.

If patient has none of the aforementioned characteristics, he or she is weakly thrombophilic, so consider testing for APC deficiency, prothrombin mutation, antiphospholipid syndrome, and hyperhomocysteinemia.

If the patient has any of the aforementioned characteristics, he or she is strongly thrombophilic, so consider testing for APC deficiency, prothrombin mutation, antiphospholipid syndrome, hyperhomocysteinemia, antithrombin deficiency, protein C deficiency, and protein S deficiency.

BOX 46-3

WHICH TESTS TO ORDER WHEN[6]

INITIAL SCREENING TESTS

APC resistance: clotting-based assay, molecular-based assay for factor V Leiden

Antiphospholipid antibodies: lupus anticoagulant assay (Russell's viper venom time), enzyme-linked immunosorbent assay for anticardiolipin antibody

Prothrombin G20210A mutation

Fasting homocysteine level

Factor VIII level

TESTS TO PERFORM REMOTE FROM ACUTE EVENT*

Antithrombin activity

Protein C activity

Protein S activity, free and total levels

---

*Antithrombin, protein C, and protein S levels are ideally measured 2 weeks after a 3- to 6-month course of anticoagulant therapy after a thrombotic event. For protein C or protein S level measurements, the patient may continue to be on heparin or enoxaparin as long as he or she has been off warfarin for 2 weeks.[8] If antithrombin, protein C, or protein S levels are normal at presentation, they are unlikely to be deficient.

2. Studies show that heterozygotes of the factor V Leiden mutation or the prothrombin mutation do not have a higher risk of a repeat thrombosis than noncarriers after the same initial thrombosis. However, carriers of both the factor V Leiden mutation and the prothrombin mutation have a higher overall risk of thrombosis.[10]

3. For patients with secondary hypercoagulable states, morbidity and mortality are related to the underlying condition.

VI. MANAGEMENT AND PREVENTION

1. Acute therapy.

a. **Uncomplicated venous thromboembolism** can be treated with unfractionated heparin or low molecular weight heparin.[1,11]

(1) Low molecular weight heparin therapy does not usually necessitate monitoring. Antifactor Xa levels can be measured in obese patients (> 150 kg) or in renal insufficiency (creatinine clearance < 30), given limited data on appropriate dosing in these patients.

(2) Heparins do not cross the placenta and so are safe in pregnancy.

b. If the patient has a history of or is suspected to have **heparin-induced thrombocytopenia** (HIT), with or without thrombotic complications (HIT-TS), the patient should be anticoagulated with a direct thrombin inhibitor (DTI) such as argatroban or lepirudin.[12]

(1) Remember to stop all exposure to heparin.

(2) Argatroban is preferred in renal failure because it is eliminated by the liver and excreted in bile. Lepirudin is preferred in liver dysfunction because it is eliminated primarily via the kidneys (Table 46-2).

(3) Before discontinuing a DTI, ensure that the platelet count has reached at least 100,000 and that warfarin is at a therapeutic dosage such that the international normalized ratio has been more than 2.0 for at least 2 days.

(4) In HIT, warfarin should never be initiated on its own because of the risk of venous gangrene and warfarin-induced skin necrosis.

2. **Long-term anticoagulation** guidelines are listed in Table 46-3. There is not yet consensus on which thrombophilias necessitate lifelong therapy after a first thrombosis.[10] However, consider indefinite therapy for factor V Leiden homozygotes, heterozygotes of both factor V Leiden and the prothrombin mutation, and deficiencies of protein C, S, or antithrombin.[8]

3. New anticoagulants being studied include bivalirudin, a low molecular weight synthetic DTI with a short half-life; ximelagatran, an orally absorbed DTI; and fondaparinux, a factor Xa inhibitor.[12,13]

4. If an inherited thrombotic state is found, consider testing family members.

VII. SPECIAL CONSIDERATION: ANTIPHOSPHOLIPID SYNDROME (APS)

1. **Epidemiology.** Of patients with systemic lupus erythematosus, 12% to 30% have anticardiolipin antibodies and 15% to 34% have a lupus anticoagulant; 50% of patients with systemic lupus erythematosus and antiphospholipid antibodies have a history of venous or arterial thrombosis.[15]

2. **Presentation.** Recurrent episodes tend to mimic the original event, with venous thromboses following venous events, and arterial thromboses following arterial events.

a. Overall, **venous thromboses are more common than arterial thromboses,** occurring in up to 55% of patients, half of whom will also have pulmonary embolus.[15] Among arterial events, up to 50% are cerebrovascular.

46

HYPERCOAGULABLE STATES

TABLE 46-2

ANTICOAGULATION THERAPY

Drug	Half-Life	Metabolism	Dosing	Therapeutic Goal
Unfractionated heparin	1-2 hr	Hepatic	12 U/kg/hr IV for ACS or 16-18 U/kg/hr IV for deep vein thrombosis or pulmonary embolus with titrations q4-6h prn	aPTT ratio = 1.5-2.5
Enoxaparin	2-8 hr	Renal	1 mg/kg SC q12h or 1.5 mg/kg SC q24h	Antifactor Xa = 0.6-1
Warfarin	20-60 hr	Hepatic	5-10 mg qd for 2 d, then 2-10 mg qd	International normalized ratio = 2-3
Argatroban	45 min	Hepatic	2 μg/kg/min IV with titrations prn	aPTT ratio = 1.5-3
Lepirudin	60-90 min	Renal	0.4 mg/kg bolus, then 0.15 mg/kg/hr IV with titrations prn	aPTT ratio = 2-3

aPTT, activated partial thromboplastin time; *ACS,* acute coronary syndrome.

b. In **pregnancy,** there is a higher risk of fetal loss and premature delivery caused by pregnancy-associated hypertension and placental insufficiency.

c. **Catastrophic APS** is very rare (0.8% in one series[16]), involving multiple thromboses in at least three different organ systems, which include the kidneys, lungs, central nervous system, heart, and skin in 50% of patients. Distinguishing catastrophic APS from thrombotic thrombocytopenic purpura is critical for deciding appropriate management.

3. **Etiology.** APS involves the production of antibodies against phospholipids or phospholipid-binding proteins (e.g., β_2 glycoprotein). In vitro, they inhibit phospholipid-dependent coagulation activity to varying degrees. In vivo, however, APS produces a prothrombic state, the cause of which remains a subject of active research.

4. **Diagnosis.** Diagnosis can be made using the Sapporo criteria (Boxes 46-4 and 46-5), which have a 71% sensitivity and 98% specificity. Patients not meeting these criteria may still warrant diagnosis on the basis of other findings (e.g., livedo reticularis, valvular disease, cerebrovascular events, hemolytic anemia, and thrombocytopenia). To aid the diagnosis, it is also possible to measure antibodies to β_2-glycoprotein-I, prothrombin, and the antibodies resulting in a false positive syphilis serology (low sensitivity and specificity).

TABLE 46-3

RECOMMENDED DURATION OF TREATMENT IN VENOUS THROMBOEMBOLIC DISEASE[17]

Patient Characteristics	Length of Treatment
Most patients	≥ 3 mo (international normalized ratio 2-3 if warfarin, or can use low molecular weight heparin or unfractionated heparin).
1st event with reversible or time-limited factor	≥ 3 mo.
1st episode of idiopathic venous thromboembolism	≥ 6 mo.
Recurrent idiopathic venous thromboembolism, or a continuing risk factor (e.g., cancer, antithrombin deficiency, antiphospholipid syndrome)	≥ 12 mo.
Symptomatic isolated calf thrombosis	6 to 12 wk; if anticoagulation cannot be given, perform serial noninvasive studies of lower extremity over next 10-14 d to assess for proximal extension of the thrombus.

BOX 46-4

SAPPORO CRITERIA FOR DIAGNOSING ANTIPHOSPHOLIPID SYNDROME[14]

At least one clinical criterion and one laboratory criterion must be present.

CLINICAL CRITERIA

Confirmed vascular thrombosis.

Pregnancy morbidity: ≥ 1 unexplained deaths of normal fetus at ≥ 10 wk gestation; ≥ 1 premature births at ≤ 34 wk due to severe preeclampsia, eclampsia, or severe placental insufficiency; or ≥ 3 unexplained consecutive spontaneous abortions at < 10 wk, excluding chromosomal abnormalities.

LABORATORY CRITERIA

Anticardiolipin antibodies (immunoglobulin G or M) in medium or high titer on ≥ 2 occasions, measured ≥ 6 wk apart.

Lupus anticoagulant found on 2 occasions, measured ≥ 6 wk apart, detected according to international guidelines in the following steps:

1. Phospholipid-dependent coagulation test is prolonged (e.g., activated partial thromboplastin sign, kaolin clotting time, dilute Russell's viper venom time, dilute prothrombin time, Textarin time).
2. Prolonged coagulation time does not correct in mixing studies.
3. Coagulation time shortens with addition of excess phospholipid.
4. Other coagulopathies have been excluded (e.g., factor VIII inhibitor, heparin).

5. **Prognosis.** Morbidity and mortality are related to the risks of thrombosis
   from the APS itself, the risks of bleeding during anticoagulation and a
   higher incidence of malignancy and risk factors for cardiovascular
   disease.[18]
6. **Management.** The mainstay of treatment is anticoagulation rather than
   immunosuppression, which has been shown to be ineffective.
a. **Prevention.** For patients without clinical manifestations of APS, aspirin
   325 mg daily and hydroxychloroquine may provide protection from
   thrombosis. All procoagulant factors, including oral contraceptives,
   should be avoided, and all cardiovascular risk factors should be
   modified aggressively.
b. **Treatment.** Even a single thrombotic event warrants lifelong
   anticoagulation because the risk of recurrence is 20% to 70%.[15]
   In most patients, unfractionated heparin or low molecular weight
   heparin can be followed by warfarin therapy with a goal international
   normalized ratio of 2.0 to 3.0.[19] Patients in whom this treatment fails
   may need a higher goal international normalized ratio of 3.0 to 4.0.[20]

PEARLS AND PITFALLS
- The types of malignancies most likely to be associated with recurrent
  thromboses are lung, brain, gastrointestinal (particularly pancreas), and
  genitourinary.[21]
- A spontaneous upper extremity thrombosis without a history of an
  indwelling catheter may be caused by a thoracic outlet abnormality
  (Paget–von Schrötter syndrome) or other hypercoagulable state.[22,23]
- Venous thrombi may manifest as cerebrovascular events from emboli
  traveling across a patent foramen ovale to cause cryptogenic strokes.[1]
- Anemia, leukopenia, and thrombocytopenia often are found in
  paroxysmal nocturnal hemoglobinuria, and clots are almost exclusively
  in the visceral venous network or central nervous system.

- Patients with coagulopathy secondary to liver cirrhosis still need deep vein thrombosis prophylaxis. Severe liver disease can predispose to thrombosis through impaired synthesis of natural plasma anticoagulants and has been associated with portal vein thrombosis.[24]
- Atherosclerosis-associated thrombosis[25] probably occurs through activation of the coagulation system. Statins may reduce the risk of venous thromboembolism.[26]
- Hyperhomocysteinemia, a significant risk factor for cardiovascular disease and venous thromboembolism, can be treated safely and inexpensively, making the diagnosis worthwhile. If the serum homocysteine is elevated, measure vitamin B_{12} and methylmalonic acid levels to rule out a primary vitamin B_{12} deficiency.
- If anticardiolipin antibodies are found, syphilis and the human immunodeficiency virus must be excluded as potential causes.

REFERENCES

1. Schafer AI, Levine MN, Konkle BA, Kearon C: Thrombotic disorders: diagnosis and treatment, *Hematology (Am Soc Hematol Educ Program)* 520-539, 2003. C
2. Barger AP, Hurley R: Evaluation of the hypercoagulable state. Whom to screen, how to test and treat, *Postgrad Med* 108(4):59-66, 2000. C
3. Seligsohn U, Lubetsky A: Genetic susceptibility to venous thrombosis, *N Engl J Med* 344(16):1222-1231, 2001. C
4. Makris M, Rosendaal FR, Preston FE: Familial thrombophilia: genetic risk factors and management, *J Intern Med Suppl* 740:9-15, 1997. C
5. Piccioli A, Prandoni P: Idiopathic venous thromboembolism as a first manifestation of cancer, *Haemostasis* 31(Suppl 1):37-39, 2001. B
6. Prandoni P: Cancer and thromboembolic disease: how important is the risk of thrombosis? *Cancer Treat Rev* 28(3):133-136, 2002. C
7. Baglin T, Luddington R, Brown K, Baglin C: Incidence of recurrent venous thromboembolism in relation to clinical and thrombophilic risk factors: prospective cohort study, *Lancet* 362(9383):523-526, 2003. B
8. Bauer KA: The thrombophilias: well-defined risk factors with uncertain therapeutic implications, *Ann Intern Med* 135(5):367-373, 2001. C
9. Streiff MB, Bray PF, Kickler TS: *Johns Hopkins coagulation laboratory guide,* 2nd ed, Baltimore, Md, 2002. C
10. De Stefano V, Martinelli I, Mannucci PM, et al: The risk of recurrent deep venous thrombosis among heterozygous carriers of both factor V Leiden and the G20210A prothrombin mutation, *N Engl J Med* 341(11):801-806, 1999. B
11. Dolovich LR, Ginsberg JS, Douketis JD, Holbrook AM, Cheah G: A meta-analysis comparing low-molecular-weight heparins with unfractionated heparin in the treatment of venous thromboembolism: examining some unanswered questions regarding location of treatment, product type, and dosing frequency, *Arch Intern Med* 160(2):181-188, 2000. C
12. Hirsh J, Heddle N, Kelton JG: Treatment of heparin-induced thrombocytopenia: a critical review, *Arch Intern Med* 164(4):361-369, 2004. C
13. Shapiro SS: Treating thrombosis in the 21st century, *N Engl J Med* 349(18):1762-1764, 2003. C

14. Buller HR, Davidson BL, Decousus H, et al: Fondaparinux or enoxaparin for the initial treatment of symptomatic deep venous thrombosis: a randomized trial, *Ann Intern Med* 140(11):867-873, 2004. A

15. Hanly JG: Antiphospholipid syndrome: an overview, *CMAJ* 168(13):1675-1682, 2003. C

16. Cervera R, Piette JC, Font J, et al: Antiphospholipid syndrome: clinical and immunologic manifestations and patterns of disease expression in a cohort of 1,000 patients, *Arthritis Rheum* 46(4):1019-1027, 2002. B

17. Ansell J, Hirsh J, Dalen J, et al: Managing oral anticoagulant therapy, *Chest* 119(1 Suppl):22S-38S, 2001. D

18. Tanne D, D'Olhaberriague L, Trivedi AM, Salowich-Palm L, Schultz LR, Levine SR: Anticardiolipin antibodies and mortality in patients with ischemic stroke: a prospective follow-up study, *Neuroepidemiology* 21(2):93-99, 2002. B

19. Crowther MA, Ginsberg JS, Julian J, et al: A comparison of two intensities of warfarin for the prevention of recurrent thrombosis in patients with the antiphospholipid antibody syndrome, *N Engl J Med* 349(12):1133-1138, 2003. A

20. Ruiz-Irastorza G, Khamashta MA, Hunt BJ, Escudero A, Cuadrado MJ, Hughes GR: Bleeding and recurrent thrombosis in definite antiphospholipid syndrome: analysis of a series of 66 patients treated with oral anticoagulation to a target international normalized ratio of 3.5, *Arch Intern Med* 162(10):1164-1169, 2002. B

21. Prandoni P, Piccioli A, Pagnan A: Recurrent thromboembolism in cancer patients: incidence and risk factors, *Semin Thromb Hemost* 29(Suppl 1):3-8, 2003. B

22. Martinelli I, Cattaneo M, Panzeri D, Taioli E, Mannucci PM: Risk factors for deep venous thrombosis of the upper extremities, *Ann Intern Med* 126(9):707-711, 1997. B

23. Heron E, Lozinguez O, Alhenc-Gelas M, Emmerich J, Fiessinger JN: Hypercoagulable states in primary upper-extremity deep vein thrombosis, *Arch Intern Med* 160(3):382-386, 2000. B

24. Harper PL, Edgar PF, Luddington RJ, et al: Protein C deficiency and portal thrombosis in liver transplantation in children, *Lancet* 2(8617):924-927, 1988. B

25. Prandoni P, Bilora F, Marchiori A, et al: An association between atherosclerosis and venous thrombosis, *N Engl J Med* 348(15):1435-1441, 2003. B

26. Ray JG, Mamdani M, Tsuyuki RT, Anderson DR, Yeo EL, Laupacis A: Use of statins and the subsequent development of deep vein thrombosis, *Arch Intern Med* 161(11):1405-1410, 2001. B

Oncologic Emergencies

*Justin Bekelman, MD; Nadine Jackson, MD, MPH;
and Ross C. Donehower, MD*

FAST FACTS

- Magnetic resonance imaging (MRI) with gadolinium is the test of choice for detecting intracranial metastases. Patients found to have intracranial metastases and evidence of mass effect should be started on corticosteroid therapy emergently.
- The clinical hallmark of neoplastic meningitis is multifocal central nervous system symptoms. Patients with suspected neoplastic meningitis should undergo MRI of the brain and spine followed by lumbar puncture.
- Any new or worsening back pain in a patient with cancer warrants urgent radiographic evaluation with a screening MRI to evaluate for epidural spinal cord compression. Awaiting MRI confirmation of the diagnosis before instituting steroids is almost never warranted.
- Neutropenic fever is defined as a single temperature of 38.3° C (101° F) or higher or 1 hour of temperatures 38° C (100.4° F) or higher in the setting of an absolute neutrophil count (ANC) less than 500 cells/mm³ or less than 1000 cells/mm³ with predicted decline to less than 500 cells/mm³.
- Neutropenic fever is a medical emergency and warrants immediate blood cultures and antibiotic therapy.
- Hypercalcemia is the most common metabolic complication of malignancy. Patients often present with lethargy, dehydration, constipation, and altered mental status. Acute renal failure is common.
- Tumor lysis syndrome usually occurs in patients with hematologic malignancies, when rapid tumor cell turnover leads to metabolic derangements including hyperuricemia, hyperphosphatemia, hyperkalemia, hypocalcemia, and subsequent renal failure.
- Patients at risk for tumor lysis syndrome should be treated with aggressive hydration and allopurinol.

I. INTRACRANIAL METASTASES

A. CLINICAL PRESENTATION AND DIAGNOSIS

1. Headache (especially early morning) or other signs of elevated intracranial pressure, focal weakness, sensory loss, gait instability, seizures, and intractable nausea and vomiting are all common signs and symptoms of intracranial metastases.
2. The diagnostic test of choice is MRI with gadolinium and (to a lesser extent) contrast-enhanced computed tomography (CT).

3. There are no pathognomonic features on MRI or CT that distinguish brain metastases from other mass lesions; however, a peripheral location, spherical shape, ring enhancement with prominent edema, and multiple lesions all suggest metastatic disease in the proper clinical context.

B. MANAGEMENT

1. The optimal therapy for brain metastases (whether single or multiple) remains controversial. Corticosteroids, radiotherapy, surgical management, and radiosurgery all have an established place in management.

2. **Corticosteroids.** Patients with symptoms or evidence of cerebral edema should be started on corticosteroid therapy. Steroids are thought to stabilize the endothelial cells lining the blood-brain barrier, minimizing permeability and edema. Dexamethasone (10 mg intravenously [IV] every 6 hours) is the corticosteroid of choice, largely because of its minimal mineralocorticoid effect. Proton pump inhibitors should be prescribed with high-dose steroids.

3. **Anticonvulsants** should be given only to patients who have had a seizure because prophylactic anticonvulsants do not prevent first seizures in patients with newly diagnosed brain metastases.[1]

4. Surgery is reserved for patients who otherwise have a good performance status and life expectancy with a **single brain metastasis**, or as many as three metastases if there is significant mass effect. Patients with single metastases appear to survive longer when treated with surgery and whole brain radiotherapy (WBRT) than when treated with WBRT alone (median survival 9 to 10 vs. 3 to 6 months).[2,3]

5. More than 70% of patients have **multiple brain metastases** at diagnosis and are best treated with WBRT alone.

6. **Stereotactic radiosurgery** delivers intense focal irradiation and may serve as a substitute for surgical treatment in patients with lesions less than 3 cm in diameter. Stereotactic radiosurgery does not relieve mass effect or the need for steroids. For single brain metastases, local control and overall survival with radiosurgery and WBRT are comparable to those in patients treated with conventional surgery and WBRT.[4]

II. NEOPLASTIC MENINGITIS

A. EPIDEMIOLOGY AND CLINICAL PRESENTATION

1. Meningeal involvement is the first manifestation of systemic carcinoma in 5% to 10% of patients who develop neoplastic meningitis. Leptomeningeal involvement occurs more often with non-Hodgkin's lymphomas and leukemias and less often with solid tumors.

2. **The clinical hallmark of neoplastic meningitis is the presence of multifocal cranial nerve and spinal root lesions or hydrocephalus.**

3. Most patients present with nonspecific, nonlocalizing symptoms related to elevated intracranial pressure, including pain (80%), diffuse

headache (25%), or pain in a spinal, radicular, or meningeal pattern (> 50%).

B. DIAGNOSIS

1. Once neoplastic meningitis is suspected clinically, the diagnosis rests on a combination of cerebrospinal fluid (CSF) studies and neuroimaging. Fig. 47-1 outlines the evaluation and treatment of patients with suspected neoplastic meningitis.[5]
2. All patients should have an MRI of the brain and spine with gadolinium to exclude large parenchymal masses and obstructive hydrocephalus before lumbar puncture because of the potential for brain herniation.
3. If hydrocephalus is present, a shunt may be placed. CSF can be obtained at that time, but if no malignant cells are found, a lumbar puncture should be performed.
4. In the absence of hydrocephalus, a lumbar puncture (LP) should be performed and a large volume of CSF (10 to 20 ml) should be sent for cytologic examination. Initial cytology reveals evidence of malignancy in more than half of CSF samples, and the yield increases to approximately 90% after three lumbar punctures.

C. MANAGEMENT

1. Prognosis is generally poor. Without treatment, irreversible neurologic dysfunction and death occur within 6 weeks. Standard therapy extends survival to 3 to 6 months and is considered palliative.
2. Once the diagnosis is established, patients should be stratified into "poor risk" and "good risk" categories on the basis of performance status, degree of neurologic deficits, extent of systemic disease, and available treatment options (see Fig. 47-1).
3. Patients in the "good risk" group may be candidates for aggressive chemoradiation therapy. Intrathecal administration of chemotherapy through a subcutaneous (Ommaya) reservoir and intraventricular catheter has become standard. Methotrexate, cytosine arabinoside, and thiotepa are the agents commonly used. Cytosine arabinoside is effective mainly against leukemias and lymphomas. Methotrexate and thiotepa appear to be equivalent in efficacy and toxicity.[6,7]
4. CSF is analyzed monthly until cytologic studies become normal and every 2 months thereafter.

III. EPIDURAL SPINAL CORD COMPRESSION

A. EPIDEMIOLOGY

1. Epidural spinal cord compression (ESCC) is defined as compression of the thecal sac by tumor in the epidural space at the level of the spinal cord or cauda equina.
2. It is estimated that 5% of patients dying of cancer develop ESCC. Cord compression may be the initial presentation of malignancy in 20% of cases of ESCC.
3. Metastatic prostate cancer, breast cancer, and lung cancer each account for approximately 15% to 20% of cases, whereas renal cell cancer,

47

ONCOLOGIC EMERGENCIES

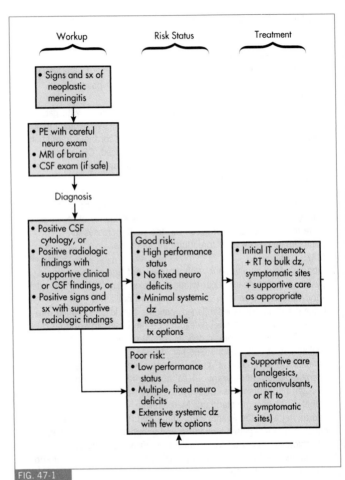

FIG. 47-1

The evaluation and treatment of neoplastic meningitis. *chemotx,* chemotherapy; *CSF,* cerebrospinal fluid; *dz,* disease; *IT,* intrathecal; *MRI,* magnetic resonance imaging; *PE,* physical examination; *RT,* radiation therapy; *sx,* symptoms; *tx,* treatment.

non-Hodgkin's lymphoma, and multiple myeloma account for approximately 5% to 10% of cases.

B. CLINICAL PRESENTATION

1. Pain occurs in 95% of patients with ESCC, is present for a median of 7 weeks before diagnosis, and usually worsens with recumbency (as opposed to lumbar herniation of degenerative disk disease).

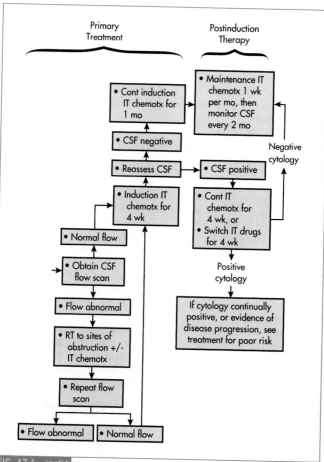

FIG. 47-1—cont'd

2. Weakness usually is symmetric. Radicular symptoms are more common with ESCC of the lumbosacral spine than ESCC of the thoracic spine. Bladder and bowel dysfunction are late symptoms.

3. Pretreatment neurologic status is the most important predictor of posttreatment function, hence the need for early and rapid diagnosis.[8,9]

C. DIAGNOSIS

1. **Any new or worsening back pain in a patient with cancer mandates urgent radiographic evaluation.** Malignant epidural cord compression should progress to paralysis only when the patient delays seeking medical attention.

2. MRI with gadolinium is the most rapid and cost-effective means of diagnosis and should be the first procedure performed (Fig. 47-2).[9] Plain radiographs, CT, and bone scans are not sensitive in the detection of ESCC; however, CT myelography is useful when MRI is contraindicated.

3. If weakness or other signs of myelopathy are found, institute high-dose steroids and obtain an MRI of the entire spine. Awaiting MRI confirmation of the diagnosis before instituting steroids is almost never warranted.

D. MANAGEMENT

1. Corticosteroids can relieve cord compression caused by edema. Patients who receive steroids are more likely to remain ambulatory 6 months after ESCC (59% versus 33%).[10] The recommended regimen includes a 10-mg bolus of dexamethasone, followed by 4 mg every 6 hours, with a one-third taper in the dosage every 3 to 4 days. Higher dosages may be used in patients with deteriorating neurologic function.

2. Corticosteroid treatment followed by radiotherapy is the standard of care. To minimize the harmful effects of radiation on normal tissues, radiation usually is fractionated into small doses administered over a few days to weeks.

3. Patients with neurologic symptoms treated with radical decompressive surgery followed by postoperative radiation therapy regain the ability to walk more often and maintain ambulation longer than patients treated with radiation alone.[11]

4. Management should also include aggressive analgesia (usually opiates), scheduled bowel regimens, and deep venous thrombosis prophylaxis.

5. The median survival in patients undergoing radiotherapy for ESCC ranges from 3 to 6 months. Survival rates are higher in patients who are ambulatory either before or after radiation.[12]

IV. NEUTROPENIC FEVER

A. EPIDEMIOLOGY

1. Chemotherapy-associated neutropenic fever is the most common indication for nonelective admission of patients with cancer.

2. Historically, gram-negative organisms were the most commonly identified pathogens in patients with neutropenic fever. More recently, *Streptococcus* and *Staphylococcus* have become the most common isolates, probably because of the increased use of indwelling catheters and antimicrobial prophylaxis.

3. Among patients with leukemia, a threefold to eightfold increase in the incidence of fungal infections has occurred in recent decades. Approximately 80% of these fungal infections are caused by *Candida* species.

B. CLINICAL PRESENTATION

1. Neutropenic fever is defined as a single temperature of 38.3° C (101° F) or higher or 1 hour of temperatures 38° C (100.4° F) or

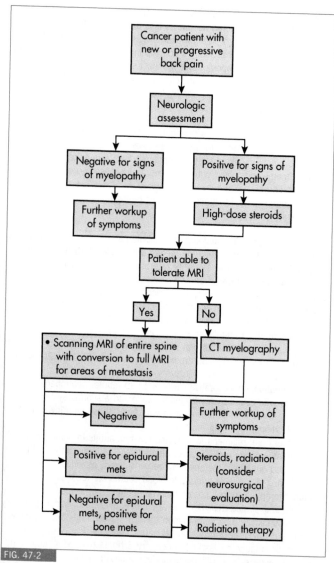

FIG. 47-2

Approach to a patient with cancer and back pain. *CT,* computed tomography; *mets,* metastases; *MRI,* magnetic resonance imaging. *(Modified from Ruckdeschel JC: Spinal cord compression. In Clinical oncology, 2nd ed, New York, 2000, Churchill Livingstone.)*

higher in the setting of an ANC less than 500/mm^3 or less than 1000 cells/mm^3 with predicted decline to less than 500 cells/mm^3.[13]

2. Signs and symptoms of inflammation may be minimal or absent in the neutropenic patient, especially if accompanied by anemia. The majority of infections in neutropenic fever manifest solely as bacteremia.

3. Commonly identified sites of infection in a neutropenic host are the oropharynx, sinuses, lungs, urinary tract, perirectal area, and skin, especially around the site of an indwelling catheter.

C. DIAGNOSIS

1. Initial evaluation includes a thorough physical examination, complete blood cell count, chemistries (to assess electrolytes and renal and hepatic function), blood cultures (obtained from a peripheral vein and catheter ports), and cultures of any lesion observed on physical examination.

2. Urine cultures, stool cultures, and chest radiographs should be obtained if clinically indicated.

D. MANAGEMENT

1. Withholding empiric antibiotics from febrile patients with neutropenia is associated with a mortality rate greater than 80%. **With the use of empiric antibiotics, the mortality rate associated with neutropenic fever has fallen to less than 10%.**

2. The Infectious Disease Society of America has proposed guidelines for the use of antimicrobial agents in febrile neutropenic patients. A management algorithm is shown in Fig. 47-3.[13]

3. Low-risk adults. Carefully screened adults who are low risk for complications may use an oral treatment regimen (ciprofloxacin 500 mg per os [PO] twice daily and amoxicillin-clavulanate 500 mg PO every 8 hours).[14,15]

a. An international collaborative study of 1139 febrile, neutropenic patients with established malignancy validated a scoring system to identify, at the time of presentation with fever, those with low risk for complications, including mortality (Table 47-1).[16]

b. Outpatient oral regimens for selected low-risk adults in stable social situations are safe and effective. Alternatively, early discharge with continued outpatient therapy may be considered, provided close monitoring is available and white blood counts are recovering.

4. **Monotherapy.** In uncomplicated febrile neutropenia, several studies have demonstrated that monotherapy has equivalent or superior efficacy with less toxicity than combination therapy.[17] Recommended regimens include ceftazidime 2 g IV every 8 hours, cefepime 2 g IV every 8 hours, or imipenem-cilastin 1 g IV every 6 hours (use with caution in patients with renal insufficiency in view of seizure potential).

5. **Combination therapy.** For complicated febrile neutropenia, an aminoglycoside in combination with the antimicrobials listed as monotherapy has the potential advantages of synergistic effects against gram-negative rods and a lower risk of drug resistance. These

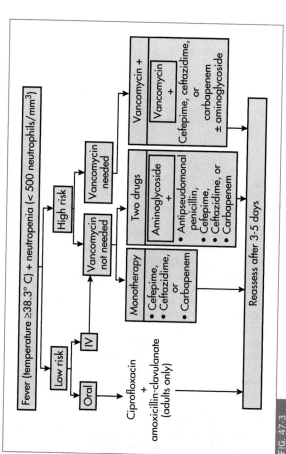

FIG. 47-3

Algorithm for antibiotic selection in neutropenic fever. *IV,* intravenous.

47

ONCOLOGIC EMERGENCIES

TABLE 47-1

SCORING INDEX FOR IDENTIFICATION OF FEBRILE NEUTROPENIC PATIENTS
AT LOW RISK FOR COMPLICATIONS

Characteristic	Score
Extent of illness (choose 1 item only)	
No or mild symptoms	5
Moderate symptoms	3
No hypotension	5
No chronic obstructive pulmonary disease	4
Solid tumor or no fungal infection	4
No dehydration	3
Outpatient at onset of fever	3
Age < 60 yr	2

Note: The highest possible score is 26. A risk index score of ≥ 21 indicates that the patient is likely to be at low risk for complications and morbidity (positive predictive value 91%, sensitivity 71%, specificity 68%) in identifying patients without serious complications at 5 days.[13,16]

    advantages are tempered by aminoglycoside-associated nephrotoxicity and ototoxicity. Recommended regimens include gentamicin 2 mg/kg every 8 hours or 5 mg/kg IV every 24 hours or amikacin 15 mg/kg/day or divided every 8 to 12 hours (once-daily dosing is preferred for less toxicity; check peak and trough levels). See Fig. 47-3.

6. **Vancomycin.** If a patient presents with an obvious catheter-associated infection, severe mucositis, or hypotension, the patient is receiving fluoroquinolone prophylaxis, or there is a high prevalence of methicillin-resistant *Staphylococcus* or cephalosporin-resistant *Streptococcus,* vancomycin therapy should be considered. There is no evidence to support routine use of vancomycin as part of the initial empiric regimen for neutropenic fever.[18]

7. **Afebrile patients.** Patients who become afebrile over a 3- to 5-day period should be maintained on antibiotics for at least 7 days or until the ANC is greater than 500 cells/mm^3 (Fig. 47-4).

8. **Febrile patients.** The median time to defervescence in adequately treated patients is 5 days (range 2 to 7 days). Therefore, initial antibiotic choices should not be modified unless there is clinical deterioration or new culture data[13,14] (Fig. 47-5).

9. **Patients with persistent fever despite 3 to 5 days of broad-spectrum antibiotics should be reassessed. If warranted, vancomycin or empiric antifungal coverage can be added.**

a. Before the addition of antifungal therapy, evaluation should include biopsy of skin lesions, CT of chest, abdomen, and sinuses, nasal endoscopy (if indicated), and repeat cultures.

b. Recommended regimens include amphotericin B 1 mg/kg/day (increase to 1.5 mg/kg/day for persistent fever after 24 hours at a given dosage) or liposomal amphotericin B 3 to 5 mg/kg/day (as effective as

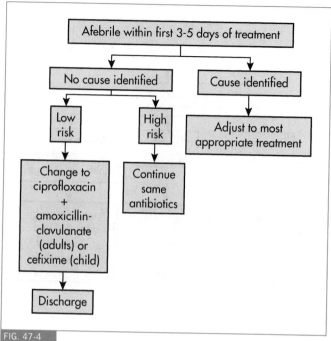

FIG. 47-4

Antibiotic management in patients who defervesce.

conventional amphotericin B with less nephrotoxicity and other side effects).[19]

c. Caspofungin (70 mg on day 1 and 50 mg once daily thereafter) was recently shown to be as effective and generally better tolerated than liposomal amphotericin B when given as empiric antifungal therapy.[20]

d. Voriconazole, available in an oral form, has been found to be more effective than amphotericin in treating suspected invasive aspergillosis.[21] Recommended therapy is voriconazole 6 mg/kg IV every 12 hours for two doses, then 4 mg/kg IV every 12 hours for at least 7 days, followed by 200 mg PO twice daily. Patients with severe mucositis or other cause of malabsorption should not receive oral voriconazole.

10. **Duration of antibiotic therapy.** The single most important determinant of successful discontinuation of antibiotics is the neutrophil count.[13]

a. Regardless of febrile status, patients with ANC less than 100 cells/mm^3, mucositis, or unstable vital signs should be maintained on antibiotics.

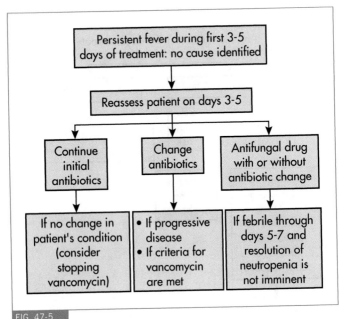

FIG. 47-5
Management of persistent neutropenic fever.

b. Patients with persistent fever but recovering marrow may discontinue antibiotics 4 to 5 days after ANC exceeds 500 cells/mm³. If ANC remains less than 500 cells/mm³, antibiotics should be continued, with reassessment after 14 days.

11. **Antivirals.** Empiric use of antiviral drugs is not recommended. However, if skin or mucus membrane lesions test positive for herpes simplex virus or varicella-zoster virus, oral acyclovir can prevent herpes simplex virus outbreaks and promote mucositis healing. Newer agents such as valacyclovir may be better absorbed.

12. **Colony-stimulating factors.** Trials evaluating the routine use of hematopoietic growth factors such as granulocyte colony-stimulating factor or granulocyte-macrophage colony-stimulating factor in febrile neutropenic patients have failed to show a significant improvement in clinical outcomes or survival.[22] The American Society of Clinical Oncology guidelines recommend against the use of growth factors in uncomplicated cases of febrile neutropenia. However, use of growth factors in high-risk patients (pneumonia, hypotension, sepsis, systemic fungal infections, or severe cellulitis) with prolonged neutropenia appears to have some value.[23]

13. **Antibiotic prophylaxis.** Routine pharmacologic prophylaxis, although of variable efficacy in preventing bacteremia, has not been shown to decrease infection-related mortality and selects for antimicrobial resistance both in the community and in the individual patient.[13,24]

a. We recommend trimethoprim-sulfamethoxazole therapy for patients at risk for Pneumocystis *jirovecii* pneumonitis (those with leukemias, certain solid tumors, histiocytosis, or acquired immunodeficiency syndrome), regardless of the presence or absence of neutropenia.

b. To date, consensus guidelines recommend fluconazole only for preventing candidiasis in patients undergoing hematopoietic stem cell transplantation (400 mg/day from the day of transplantation until engraftment).[25] Most centers continue fluconazole through day + 100 given evidence for short- and long-term benefit.[26]

V. HYPERCALCEMIA

A. EPIDEMIOLOGY AND ETIOLOGY

1. Hypercalcemia develops in 10% to 20% of patients with cancer. It occurs most often in squamous lung cancer, breast cancer, and multiple myeloma. For a discussion of hypercalcemia not associated with malignancy please see Chapter 29.

2. Malignant tumors can increase serum calcium through several mechanisms, including local osteolysis via bone metastases and tumor secretion of osteoclast-activating factors, parathyroid hormone–related protein, and calcitriol.

B. MANAGEMENT

1. **Initial treatment involves restoration of intravascular volume with 0.9% saline.** This lowers the calcium concentration by dilution and increases renal calcium excretion by restoring the glomerular filtration rate. Administration of 3 to 4 L/day should lead to euvolemia and maintain a brisk diuresis.

2. **Glucocorticoids.** For hypercalcemia associated with multiple myeloma and lymphoma, prednisone 20 to 40 mg/day reduces calcium concentration within 2 to 5 days.

3. **Loop diuretics** promote calcium excretion but should be used cautiously because they may lead to persistent hypovolemia.

4. **Bisphosphonates** inhibit bone resorption, thereby acting directly on the source of hypercalcemia. Several agents have been shown to reduce serum calcium levels in the setting of malignancy. Although pamidronate was the most commonly used bisphosphonate, zoledronate has been shown to be more effective.[27] Zoledronic acid also has a shorter infusion time of 15 minutes (maximum dosage of 4 mg). Normal calcium levels are achieved by day 10 in 90% of patients using zoledronate, compared with 70% of patients using pamidronate.

5. **Calcitonin.** Salmon calcitonin works more rapidly than pamidronate and should be used for severe hypercalcemia. It inhibits bone resorption and increases urinary calcium excretion. Dosages of 4 to 8 IU/kg

intramuscularly or subcutaneously every 6 to 12 hours lower the calcium concentration by 1 to 2 mg/dl within 6 hours. Calcitonin's usefulness is limited by tachyphylaxis, which develops in most patients. Calcitonin has a prolonged effect when a bisphosphonate is administered concomitantly.[28] Calcitonin also has potent analgesic effects on bone pain caused by skeletal metastases. Side effects include flushing, nausea, and abdominal cramping. Allergic reactions have been reported.

VI. HYPERVISCOSITY SYNDROME

A. EPIDEMIOLOGY

1. Paraproteinemia is the most common cause of hyperviscosity syndrome (HVS). Protein-protein interaction of large molecules results in the formation of multimolecular aggregates and thereby increases viscosity.
2. Of the paraproteinemias, Waldenström's macroglobulinemia with lymphoplasmacytic lymphoma (immunoglobulin M gammopathy associated with low-grade B-cell lymphoma) accounts for the majority of cases. Ten to thirty percent of patients with Waldenström's macroglobulinemia develop HVS.[29]
3. The second most common paraproteinemia associated with HVS is multiple myeloma. The incidence of HVS is 4.2% in patients with immunoglobulin G myeloma and up to 25% in those with immunoglobulin A myeloma.[30]
4. Elevated whole blood viscosity is more common and is clinically more important than elevated serum viscosity.

B. CLINICAL PRESENTATION

1. **The classic triad of symptoms includes visual disturbances, bleeding, and neurologic manifestations.**
2. Visual disturbances with occasional visual loss can be caused by retinopathy characterized by "sausage link" or "boxcar" venous engorgement of the retinal veins that leads to bleeding, exudates, microaneurysms, and rarely papilledema.
3. Bleeding from mucosal surfaces, including the gastrointestinal tract, is thought to be related to impaired platelet function.
4. Neurologic manifestations include headache, dizziness, vertigo, hearing impairment, somnolence, seizures, stroke, and coma. Cardiopulmonary findings may include pulmonary edema, myocardial infarction, and valvular abnormalities.

C. DIAGNOSIS

1. Laboratory evaluation should include a complete blood cell count, serum chemistries, plasma viscosity, whole blood viscosity, and coagulation profiles. Serum and urine protein electrophoresis should be requested if the patient is being evaluated for paraproteinemia.
2. **Normal relative plasma viscosity is between 1.4 and 1.8. Values from 2 to 4 are abnormal but rarely symptomatic. Values above 4 often are**

symptomatic and are an indication for emergency treatment. A value above 4 corresponds roughly to a serum immunoglobulin M (IgM) level greater than 3 g/dl, an immunoglobulin G (IgG) level greater than 4 g/dl, and an immunoglobulin A (IgA) level greater than 6 g/dl.[31]

3. **Measurement of whole blood viscosity is a better measure of hyperviscosity than measure of serum viscosity or plasma viscosity alone.** Whole blood viscosity is reported as being comparable to a sample with a certain hematocrit (e.g., a patient's whole blood has a viscosity comparable to that of a patient with a hematocrit of 65%).

4. Relative whole blood viscosity of 55% or greater increases the risk of HVS.

D. MANAGEMENT

1. Plasma exchange via plasmapheresis is the gold standard of treatment. Plasmapheresis uses centrifugation to separate patient's plasma containing excess proteins from cellular blood elements and replacing it with albumin or fresh frozen plasma.

2. Large-bore access is necessary for exchange. A dialysis catheter is adequate in the emergency setting. More permanent catheters (e.g., Quinton) often are placed by surgeons or interventional radiologists.

3. A larger percentage of IgG and IgA is extravascular (smaller molecules than IgM), and so paraproteinemia from IgG or IgA may necessitate larger plasmapheresis volumes and repeated procedures to adequately reduce viscosity.[32] IgM is predominantly intravascular and often can be cleared in one or two treatments.

4. Complications of plasmapheresis include paresthesias, muscle cramps, and tetany caused by depletion of ionized calcium as it binds to citrate used in automated plasmapheresis.

5. Packed red blood cell transfusions increase blood viscosity and exacerbate symptoms. They should be withheld until the viscosity is measured and appropriately lowered.

6. Diuretics and volume depletion also increase viscosity, and their use should be avoided.

VII. SUPERIOR VENA CAVA SYNDROME

A. EPIDEMIOLOGY

1. Superior vena cava (SVC) syndrome results from invasion or external compression of the SVC or thrombosis of blood within the SVC; 85% of cases are caused by malignancy. The remainder of cases are caused by infection or its complications, such as fibrosing mediastinitis.

2. Among malignancies, lung cancer and lymphoma cause 94% of cases.[33]

3. Small cell lung cancer is more likely than non–small cell lung cancer to cause SVC syndrome because the former tends to develop centrally and the latter peripherally. SVC syndrome develops in 20% of patients with small cell lung cancer.

47

ONCOLOGIC EMERGENCIES

B. CLINICAL PRESENTATION

1. Dyspnea is the most common presenting symptom, followed by edema of the face, trunk, or extremities. Patients may also have jugular venous distension, distension of thoracic veins, and facial plethora.
2. Most patients with SVC syndrome have an abnormal chest radiograph at presentation.

C. DIAGNOSIS

1. Accurate diagnosis should be established before treatment unless the patient is in extremis with stridor, indicating central airway obstruction or laryngeal edema. Radiation therapy may prevent the determination of tissue diagnosis in up to 40% of cases.[34]
2. **Radiographic studies** are necessary to demonstrate SVC compression or obstruction, to assess collateral blood flow, and to determine the location of the tumor or lymph nodes causing the obstruction.
   a. **Chest radiographs** are abnormal in approximately 80% of cases. The most common findings on chest film include mediastinal widening and pleural effusion. Superior mediastinal and right hilar masses may also be seen.
   b. **Contrast-enhanced chest CT** defines extent of venous blockage and potential cause of venous obstruction. MRI is an alternative to CT scanning for patients with a contrast dye allergy.
3. **Tissue diagnosis** can be obtained in two thirds of cases by sputum cytology, pleural fluid cytology, or biopsy of enlarged peripheral lymph nodes. Bone marrow biopsy may be used to diagnose non-Hodgkin's lymphoma or small cell lung cancer and to provide staging information.

D. MANAGEMENT

1. If stridor is present, prompt otolaryngology consultation should be obtained for possible tracheostomy. Administration of steroids to decrease laryngeal edema should be considered. Positive-pressure ventilation, with 20% oxygen and 80% helium, and frequent suctioning to control secretions may also be helpful in the interim.
2. Supportive measures, such as diuretics and elevation of the head of the bed, may provide symptomatic relief.
3. The nonemergent management of SVC syndrome includes radiation therapy with or without chemotherapy. Tumors that most commonly cause SVC syndrome are sensitive to chemotherapy, and in those instances chemotherapy alone may be appropriate. Combination therapy decreases local recurrence rates of non-Hodgkin's lymphomas and improves survival in limited-stage small cell lung cancer. Radiation relieves symptoms in 70% of patients within 2 weeks.
4. Non–small cell lung cancers respond poorly to therapy, and the development of SVC syndrome is a poor prognostic factor with a median survival of 5 months.

5. Endovascular stent placement may be considered for patients who cannot tolerate radiation or chemotherapy or for whom such treatments are unlikely to be successful.

VIII. TUMOR LYSIS SYNDROME

A. EPIDEMIOLOGY

1. Tumor lysis syndrome occurs in patients with acute leukemia and high-grade lymphoma (i.e., Burkitt's) because of the heavy tumor burden and rapid cell turnover. It has also been reported to occur rarely in patients with small cell lung carcinoma, breast carcinoma, sarcoma, ovarian malignancies, germ cell tumors, and medulloblastoma.

2. Risk factors include large tumor burden, lactate dehydrogenase (LDH) level greater than 1500 IU, extensive bone marrow involvement, and high tumor sensitivity to chemotherapeutic agents. Other risk factors include younger than 25 years, male sex, advanced disease with abdominal involvement, prior volume depletion, and concentrated acidic urine.[35]

3. Tumor lysis can occur either spontaneously or after therapy (including preparative regimens for bone marrow transplantation). Spontaneous tumor lysis syndrome may complicate one third of high-grade lymphomas (e.g., lymphoblastic lymphoma and Burkitt's lymphoma).[36]

4. Metabolic derangements arise from rapid tumor cell death and release of intracellular potassium, phosphate, and purines. Severity of the metabolic derangements depends on the timing and intensity of chemotherapy, intracellular electrolyte and solute levels, prophylactic measures, acid-base status, and glomerular filtration rate.[37]

B. CLINICAL PRESENTATION AND DIAGNOSIS

1. **Hyperkalemia** typically occurs 6 to 72 hours after the initiation of chemotherapy and is exacerbated by chronic kidney disease, acute renal failure, and metabolic acidosis.

2. **Hyperphosphatemia or hypocalcemia** usually occurs 24 to 48 hours after initiation of chemotherapy. Cell lysis liberates intracellular stores of phosphorus, which exceeds the renal clearance threshold. When the calcium-phosphate solubility product exceeds 70 there is a risk of calcium-phosphate precipitation, which can lead to hypocalcemia.

3. **Hyperuricemia** occurs 48 to 72 hours after initiation of chemotherapy. Uric acid is the end product of purine metabolism. Hyperuricosuria leads to crystallization of uric acid in renal tubules and collecting ducts, which is promoted by the acidic environment of the renal medulla. Crystallization leads to intraluminal tubular obstruction and damage to the renal tubular epithelial cells. Urine uric acid concentrations are more accurate than plasma uric acid levels in predicting the risk of developing uric acid nephropathy. Patients with uric acid nephropathy may have a urine uric acid/creatinine ratio greater than 1, whereas patients with acute renal failure from other causes have ratios less than 1.[38]

47

ONCOLOGIC EMERGENCIES

BOX 47-1

CAUSES OF RENAL FAILURE IN PATIENTS WITH CANCER

Urinary obstruction	Calcium and phosphate nephropathy
Severe volume depletion	Myeloma kidney (cast nephropathy)
Parenchymal disease	Drug nephrotoxicity
Glomerulonephritis (e.g., cryoglobulinemia)	Methotrexate
Vasculitis	Cis-platinum
Hypercalcemic nephropathy	Mitomycin C
Tumor replacement	Interferon-alfa
Tumor lysis syndrome	Interleukin-2
Acute uric acid nephropathy	Antibiotics

Modified from Arrambide K, Toto RD: *Semin Nephrol* 13(3):273, 1993.

4. Tumor lysis syndrome should be anticipated in a patient who has a tumor known to cause the syndrome and at presentation a high LDH, hyperuricemia (usually > 15 mg/dl), hyperphosphatemia (usually > 8 mg/dl), hyperkalemia, hypocalcemia, and renal failure. Other causes of renal failure in patients with cancer must be excluded (Box 47-1).

C. MANAGEMENT

1. The goals of management include prevention and the preservation of renal function or management of renal failure and its complications.

2. **Prevention includes the administration of allopurinol (initial dosage of 600 to 900 mg PO, then 300 to 600 mg PO daily) and aggressive hydration with intravenous fluids containing bicarbonate (50 to 100 mEq/L) administered at a rate of 200 to 300 ml/hr. The goal urine pH should be 7 to 7.5. Daily urine output should exceed 2500 ml.** If possible, allopurinol should be started at least 48 hours before initiation of cytoreductive therapy.[39] Often, however, chemotherapy cannot be delayed. Overzealous alkalinization should be avoided because this can precipitate further calcium phosphate deposition and worsen hypocalcemia by shifting calcium to its nonionized form.

3. **Rasburicase** is a genetically engineered urate oxidase used to treat hyperuricemia and tumor lysis.[40] Uric oxidase converts less soluble uric acid to highly soluble allantoin. Rasburicase reduces plasma uric acid levels within 4 hours of first dose, and dosage adjustment for renal failure is unnecessary. Exercise caution when using rasburicase in patient with glucose-6-phosphate dehydrogenase deficiency because it can cause hemolytic anemia.[41]

4. **Acetazolamide** 5 mg/kg/day can be given to maintain the solubility of uric acid. Because acetazolamide alkalinizes urine, it can also paradoxically cause calcium phosphate deposition and shift calcium to its nonionized form.

5. **Hyperkalemia** should be treated aggressively with potassium restriction, sodium polystyrene sulfonate, and loop diuretics. Maneuvers to shift potassium intracellularly should be used only as a temporizing measure.

6. **Hyperphosphatemia** should be treated with phosphate binders such as Amphojel.

7. **Only symptomatic hypocalcemia should be treated** because exogenous calcium administration in the setting of hyperphosphatemia may produce metastatic calcification.

8. **Hemodialysis is indicated in acute renal failure accompanied by uremia, metabolic acidosis, electrolyte disorders, or volume overload.** At present, hemodialysis is preferred over peritoneal dialysis because of the higher uric acid and phosphorus clearance rates. Peritoneal dialysis may also be contraindicated in patients with abdominal disease.

9. Fluid intake and output should be strictly monitored, and electrolyte levels (potassium, phosphate, uric acid, and calcium) should be checked twice daily.

IX. HEMORRHAGIC CYSTITIS

A. EPIDEMIOLOGY

1. Hemorrhagic cystitis can occur secondary to complications of chemotherapy, radiation therapy, or opportunistic infections in the immunocompromised host.

2. Up to 20% of patients receiving cyclophosphamide or busulfan (and less commonly ifosfamide) develop hemorrhage cystitis.

3. Approximately 20% of patients who receive pelvic irradiation will develop a urologic complication. Hematuria develops in 5%, increasing in frequency with increasing duration since therapy.[42]

4. Viruses that may be associated with hemorrhagic cystitis include adenovirus type 11, influenza, cytomegalovirus, herpes simplex virus, and BK virus. This should be considered in bone marrow transplant recipients.

B. DIAGNOSIS

1. Patients present with urgency, frequency, dysuria, suprapubic pain, and hematuria. Men may have referred pain from bladder spasms at the glans of the penis.

2. Workup includes urinalysis, urine culture, coagulation parameters, plain radiographs, ultrasonography, and cystoscopy and intravenous pyelography to assess for structural changes and identify the source of bleeding.

C. MANAGEMENT

1. **Prophylaxis of cyclophosphamide-induced hemorrhagic cystitis includes intravenous hydration** with forced diuresis or bladder irrigation. Intravenous hydration should begin 12 to 24 hours before administration of cyclophosphamide and continue for 24 to 48 hours

47

ONCOLOGIC EMERGENCIES

after completion. Loop diuretics should be used to maintain a urine output greater than 100 ml/m²/hr.

2. In addition to intravenous hydration, diuresis, and bladder irrigation, **2-mercaptoethane sulfonate (MESNA)** should be administered. MESNA binds the metabolized product of cyclophosphamide, acrolein, which is toxic to the bladder. A MESNA dose that is 20% of the total cyclophosphamide dosage (i.e., 200 mg MESNA for 1000 mg cyclophosphamide) is given at the time of cyclophosphamide administration, and then two or three additional 20% doses are given 4 hours apart. Side effects include mild nausea and occasional vomiting. **MESNA has decreased the incidence of hematuria and hemorrhagic cystitis after cyclophosphamide therapy.**

3. In general, when drug-induced hemorrhagic cystitis is suspected, management includes discontinuation of the offending agent, optimization of coagulation parameters, repletion of platelets, and symptomatic treatment (use of antispasmodics or narcotic analgesics). Packed red blood cells should be transfused as needed.

4. Hematuria may be classified as mild, moderate, or severe depending on response to therapeutic maneuvers and transfusion needs. Treatment of hemorrhagic cystitis is summarized in Table 47-2.

5. **Aminocaproic acid** (Amicar) inhibits fibrinolysis by inhibiting plasminogen activator substances. The loading dose is 5 g PO, followed by 1 to 1.5 g hourly to a maximum of 30 g in a 24-hour period. Upper urinary tract bleeding must be ruled out because aminocaproic acid can cause clots to become more dense and difficult to pass.

TABLE 47-2		
GRADING AND TREATMENT OF HEMORRHAGIC CYSTITIS		
Grade of Hematuria	**Grade Definition**	**Treatment**
Mild	Stable hematocrit	Bladder irrigation with water, saline, silver nitrate, or alum.
Moderate	Decrease in hematocrit necessitating < 6 U PRBCs	Evacuate clots. Prevent clot formation by using continuous bladder irrigation with water or saline. Consider aminocaproic acid or bladder instillation with alum or silver nitrate.
Severe	Hemorrhage refractory to simple irrigations, instillations, or aminocaproic acid and necessitating > 6 U PRBCs	Formalin instillation with the patient under general anesthesia. Selective embolization of the anterior branches of the hypogastric artery, cystotomy with bladder packing or urinary diversion and partial cystectomy if formalin fails.

PRBCs, packed red blood cells.

PEARLS AND PITFALLS

- For patients who present with calcium concentrations of 18 to 20 mg/dl, hemodialysis or peritoneal dialysis with a calcium-free dialysate bath can be effective.
- Most patients with SVC syndrome die as a result of progression of their underlying disease rather than from complications of SVC syndrome.
- SVC syndrome develops in some patients with malignancy because of clot extension from central venous catheters. Such patients can be treated with thrombolytic therapy (if there are no contraindications) with or without percutaneous transluminal angioplasty, followed by anticoagulant therapy.
- Cerebellar metastases may cause more severe symptoms than supratentorial metastases and be more difficult to identify because there are fewer localizing symptoms. Symptoms may include nausea, vomiting, headache, and gait disturbance.
- Emergency treatment of elevated intracranial pressure includes hyperventilation to a Pco_2 between 25 and 30 mmHg, osmotic diuresis with mannitol (20% to 25% solution given as 0.5 to 2 g/kg IV over 20 to 30 minutes), and dexamethasone.
- MRI with gadolinium and limited sagittal views is the most rapid and cost-effective means of diagnosing epidural spinal cord compression. However, awaiting MRI confirmation of the diagnosis before instituting steroids is almost never warranted.
- Carefully screened adults who are low risk for complications may use an oral treatment regimen for neutropenic fever.
- For uncomplicated neutropenic fever, monotherapy has equivalent or superior efficacy with less toxicity than combination therapy.
- There is no evidence to support routine use of vancomycin as part of the initial empirical regimen for neutropenic fever.
- Avoid diuretics in patients with hyperviscosity syndrome because they can increase blood viscosity.
- The classic triad of symptoms of hyperviscosity syndrome includes visual disturbances, bleeding, and neurologic manifestations.
- Prophylaxis of cyclophosphamide-induced hemorrhagic cystitis includes intravenous hydration with forced diuresis or bladder irrigation. Intravenous hydration should begin 12 to 24 hours before administration of cyclophosphamide and continue for 24 to 48 hours after completion of the dose. Loop diuretics should be used to maintain a urine output greater than 100 ml/m^2/hr.
- In tumor lysis syndrome, allopurinol may cause rash (including Stevens-Johnson syndrome) or interstitial nephritis, lead to xanthine stone formation, or cause pneumopathy. An intravenous formulation is available in patients unable to tolerate oral medications.

47

ONCOLOGIC EMERGENCIES

REFERENCES

1. Glantz M: Practice parameter: anticonvulsant prophylaxis in patients with newly diagnosed brain tumors. Report of the Quality Standards Subcommittee of the American Academy of Neurology, *Neurology* 54:1886-1893, 2000. D
2. Patchell R et al: A randomized trial of surgery in the treatment of single metastases to the brain, *N Engl J Med* 322:494, 1990. A
3. Vecht C et al: Treatment of single brain metastasis: radiotherapy alone or combined with neurosurgery? *Ann Neurol* 33:583, 1993. B
4. Sperduto P et al: A phase III trial comparing whole brain irradiation alone versus whole brain irradiation plus stereotactic radiosurgery for patients with one to three brain metastases, *Int J Radiat Oncol Phys* 51:3, 2002. A
5. *Practice guidelines in oncology: carcinomatous/lymphomatous meningitis,* Version 1.2003, 2/27/04. National Comprehensive Cancer Network. Accessed at www.nccn.org on May 23, 2004. D
6. Grossman S et al: Randomized prospective comparison of intraventricular methotrexate and thiotepa in patents with previously untreated neoplastic meningitis, *J Clin Oncol* 11:561, 1993. A
7. Glantz M et al: High dose intravenous methotrexate for patients with nonleukemic leptomeningeal cancer: is intrathecal chemotherapy necessary? *J Clin Oncol* 16:1561-1567, 1998. C
8. Maranzano E, Latini P, Beneventi S, et al: Comparison of two different radiotherapy schedules for spinal cord compression in prostate cancer, *Tumori* 84:472-477, 1998. B
9. Ruckdeschel J: Spinal cord compression. In *Clinical oncology,* 2nd ed, New York, 2000, Churchill Livingstone. D
10. Sorensen S et al: Effect of high-dose dexamethasone in carcinomatous metastatic spinal cord compression treated with radiotherapy: a randomized trial, *Eur J Cancer* 30A:22, 1994. A
11. Patchell R et al: A randomized trial of direct decompressive surgical resection in the treatment of spinal cord compression caused by metastasis, *Proc Am Soc Clin Oncol* 22:21 (abstr 22), 2003. A
12. Helweg-Larsen S, Sorensen P, Kreiner S: Prognostic factors in metastatic spinal cord compression: a prospective study using multivariate analysis of variables influencing survival and gait function in 153 patients, *Int J Radiat Oncol Biol Phys* 46:1163-1169, 2000. B
13. Hughes W et al: 2002 guidelines for the use of antimicrobial agents in neutropenic patients with cancer, *Clin Infect Dis* 34(6):730-751, 2002. D
14. Khalil G, Ghanem K, Auwaerter P: Fever and neutropenia. In *Johns Hopkins Division of Infectious Disease antibiotic guide, 2003.* Accessed at www.hopkins-abxguide.org on March 25, 2004. C
15. Freifeld A et al: A double-blind comparison of empirical oral and intravenous antibiotic therapy for low-risk febrile patients with neutropenia during cancer chemotherapy, *N Engl J Med* 341:305, 1999. A
16. Klatersky J et al, Multinational Association of Supportive Care in Cancer: The Multinational Association of Supportive Care in Cancer risk index: a multinational scoring system for identifying low-risk febrile neutropenic cancer patients, *J Clin Oncol* 18:3038, 2000. B
17. Sanders J et al: Ceftazidime monotherapy for empiric treatment of febrile, neutropenic patients: a meta-analysis, *J Infect Dis* 164:907, 1992. C
18. EROTC. International Antimicrobial Therapy Cooperative Group and the National Cancer Institute of Canada: Vancomycin added to empirical combination

antibiotic therapy for fever in granulocytopenic cancer patients, *J Infect Dis* 163:951, 1991. C

19. Wingard J, White M, Anaissie E, et al: A randomized, double-blind comparative trial evaluating the safety of liposomal amphotericin B versus amphotericin lipid complex in the empirical treatment of febrile neutropenia, *Clin Infect Dis* 31:1155-1163, 2000. A

20. Walsh T et al: Caspofungin versus liposomal amphotericin B for empirical antifungal therapy in patients with persistent fever and neutropenia, *N Engl J Med* 351(14):1391-1402, 2004. A

21. Herbrecht R et al: Voriconazole versus amphotericin B for primary therapy of invasive aspergillosis, *N Engl J Med* 347:408, 2002. B

22. Annaissie E et al: Randomized comparison between antibiotics alone and antibiotics plus granulocyte-macrophage colony-stimulating factor in cancer patients with fever and neutropenia, *Am J Med* 100:17, 1996. A

23. Ozer H et al: 2000 update of recommendations for the use of hematopoietic colony-stimulating factors: evidence-based clinical practice guidelines, *J Clin Oncol* 18:3558-3585, 2000. D

24. Cruciani M et al: Prophylaxis with fluoroquinolones for bacterial infections in neutropenic patients: a meta-analysis, *Clin Infect Dis* 23:795, 1996. C

25. Centers for Disease Control and Prevention: Guidelines for preventing opportunistic infections among hematopoietic stem cell transplant recipients: recommendations of CDC, the Infectious Diseases Society of America, and the American Society of Blood and Transplantation, *MMWR Morb Mortal Wkly Rep* 1-125 49:RR-10, 2000. D

26. Marr KA et al: Prolonged fluconazole prophylaxis is associated with persistent protection against candidiasis-related death in allogenic marrow transplant recipients: long-term follow-up of a randomized, placebo-controlled trial, *Blood* 96:2055-2061, 2001.

27. Smith MR et al: Randomized controlled trial of zoledronic acid to prevent bone loss in men receiving androgen deprivation therapy for nonmetastatic prostate cancer, *J Urol* 169(6):2008-2012, 2003. A

28. Bilezikian JP: Management of hypercalcemia, *J Clin Endocrinol Metab* 77:1445, 1993. C

29. Mehta J, Singhal S: Hyperviscosity syndrome in plasma cell dyscrasias, *Semin Thromb Hemost* 29:467-471, 2003. C

30. Whittaker JA, Tuddenham EG, Bradley J: Hyperviscosity syndrome in IgA multiple myeloma, *Lancet* 2:572, 1973. C

31. Bloch KJ, Maki DG: Hyperviscosity syndromes associated with immunoglobulin abnormalities, *Semin Hematol* 10:113, 1973. C

32. Zarkovic M, Kwaan HC: Correction of hyperviscosity by apheresis, *Semin Thromb Hemost* 29(5):535-542, 2003. C

33. Abner A: Approach to the patient who presents with superior vena cava obstruction, *Chest* 103:394S, 1993. C

34. Loeffler JS et al: Emergency prebiopsy radiation for mediastinal masses: impact on subsequent pathologic diagnosis and outcome, *J Clin Oncol* 4:716, 1986. C

35. Arrambide K, Toto RD: Tumor lysis syndrome, *Semin Nephrol* 13:273, 1993. C

36. Cohen LF et al: Acute tumor lysis syndrome: a review of 37 patients with Burkitt's lymphoma, *Am J Med* 68:486, 1980. B

37. Jones DP, Mahmoud H, Chesney RW: Tumor lysis syndrome: pathogenesis and management, *Pediatr Nephrol* 9:206, 1995. C

47

ONCOLOGIC EMERGENCIES

38. Kelton J, Kelley WN, Holmes EW: A rapid method for the detection of acute uric acid nephropathy, *Arch Intern Med* 138:612, 1978. B
39. Razis E et al: Incidence and treatment of tumor lysis syndrome in patients with acute leukemia, *Acta Haematol* 91:171, 1994. B
40. Pui CH et al: Recombinant urate oxidase for the prophylaxis or treatment of hyperuricemia in patients with leukemia or lymphoma, *J Clin Oncol* 19:697-704, 2001. B
41. Davidson MB et al: Pathophysiology, clinical consequences, and treatment of tumor lysis syndrome, *Am J Med* 116:546-564, 2004. C
42. Crew JP, Jephcott CR, Reynard JM: Radiation-induced haemorrhagic cystitis, *Eur Urol* 40:111-123, 2001. C

Acute Retroviral Syndrome and General Management of the Human Immunodeficiency Virus

Christopher Hoffmann, MD, MPH; and John Bartlett, MD

FAST FACTS

- Acute retroviral syndrome occurs in 40% to 90% of patients newly infected with the human immunodeficiency virus (HIV) and in some patients with chronic HIV who discontinue antiretroviral therapy. Common presenting symptoms are fever, malaise, myalgia, and rash.
- Acute HIV infection can be diagnosed by a negative or equivocal HIV antibody test plus a high HIV RNA viral load (> 100,000) by quantitative reverse transcription polymerase chain reaction (PCR).
- Acquired immunodeficiency syndrome (AIDS) is defined as HIV with either a CD4 lymphocyte count < 200 or an AIDS indicator condition (candidiasis other than oropharyngeal, cervical cancer, cryptococcosis, cryptosporidiosis or isosporosis with chronic diarrhea, cytomegalovirus, herpes with chronic ulcer, disseminated histoplasmosis, HIV-associated dementia, HIV-associated wasting, Kaposi's sarcoma, lymphoma, disseminated mycobacterium avium intracellulare (MAI), tuberculosis, recurrent bacterial pneumonia [2 or more infections in 12 months], progressive multifocal leukoencephalopathy (PML), or toxoplasmosis of internal organ).
- During care for HIV-infected patients, CD4 T-lymphocyte levels should be monitored routinely for risk of opportunistic infections; in contrast, HIV viral load is monitored to evaluate response to therapy.
- Antiretroviral (ARV) therapy usually is started in the outpatient setting in patients with a CD4 count of ≤ 350 or AIDS.
- Immune reconstitution syndrome occurs when effective antiretroviral therapy suppresses viral replication, allowing immune recovery. It is an important cause of fever in patients on antiretroviral therapy.

48

AIDS was first reported in the United States in 1981 and has since become a major disease worldwide. This chapter reviews diagnosis and management of primary HIV infection and important general issues that arise among hospitalized patients with HIV. Subsequent chapters address specific systemic, neurologic, pulmonary, gastrointestinal, and dermatologic diseases encountered in HIV-infected patients.

I. ACUTE RETROVIRAL SYNDROME

A. EPIDEMIOLOGY

1. In the United States the prevalence of AIDS is increasing as people with AIDS live longer. Since the introduction of highly active antiretroviral therapy in 1996, HIV has gone from a universally fatal disease to a potentially chronic infection. In 2003, 405,926 people in the United States had AIDS.[1]
2. Ninety percent of people with AIDS live in developing countries.
3. Sexual intercourse is the most common mode of HIV transmission. Risk of transmission varies with the nature of sexual exposure (e.g., insertive anal sex is the highest risk), presence of other sexually transmitted diseases or mucosal injury, and HIV viral load. Other important modes of transmission include intravenous drug use, oral-genital contact, maternal-fetal transmission, and transfusion of contaminated blood products.
4. Risk of transmission is highest during primary infection because of high viral load.

B. PRESENTATION

1. **Pathophysiology.**
a. Infection in sexually transmitted HIV begins with viral fusion of the HIV surface protein gp120 to the cellular CD4 receptor and chemokine coreceptor on mucosal dendritic cells. After fusion, HIV RNA is transcribed by the enzyme reverse transcriptase into DNA, which is subsequently integrated into the host genome. Within 48 hours of infection, the infected dendritic cells have migrated into lymph nodes. From there, the virus infects CD4 T-lymphocytes, leading to systemic dissemination and viremia, usually within 7 days.[2]
b. Serum levels of HIV RNA (viral load) rise rapidly (to > 100,000/ml) and peak 3 to 7 weeks after infection before rapidly declining to a steady state known as the set point. CD4 T-lymphocyte counts acutely decline (may be < 500/mm³) in mirror image of the viral load rise and transiently rebound as the viral load falls. Without treatment, the CD4 count slowly trends down at a rate dependent on viral load and host characteristics. Untreated HIV results in death in an average of 10 years (Fig. 48-1).
2. **Symptoms of acute HIV infection** (Table 48-1). Symptoms develop 5 to 29 days after exposure in 40% to 90% of patients and typically last 1 to 2 weeks.[3] Similar symptoms may also occur among patients with chronic HIV after discontinuation of effective ARV therapy.

C. DIAGNOSIS

1. Evaluation for primary HIV infection includes HIV antibody (enzyme-linked immunosorbent assay [ELISA]) and Western blot of specific HIV antigens (note that antibodies do not appear until 2 to 12 weeks after HIV infection), quantitative viral load of RNA by reverse transcription PCR, and CD4 count. In addition, other tests based on clinical history and epidemiology (Box 48-1) should be sent.

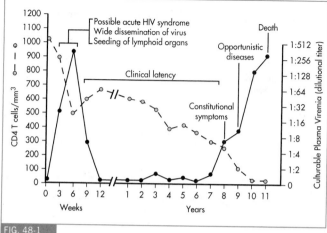

FIG. 48-1
Natural history of HIV. *(From Abbas A: Diseases of immunity. In Kumar V et al: Robbins and Cotran's pathologic basis of disease, 7th ed, Philadelphia, 2005, Elsevier, originally redrawn from Fauci AS, Lane HC: Human immunodeficiency virus disease: AIDS and related conditions. In Fauci AS et al, eds: Harrison's principles of internal medicine, 14th ed, New York, 1997, McGraw-Hill.)*

2. Primary HIV infection is diagnosed if there is either a negative or equivocal HIV ELISA or Western blot with a high viral load (> 100,000) or a positive HIV ELISA with a recent negative ELISA.

D. MANAGEMENT

1. Patients with acute retroviral illness are at higher risk for other sexually transmitted diseases. Tests for syphilis, chlamydia and gonorrhea (e.g., urethral or cervical DNA probe), and cervical cancer should be sent.
2. Viral genotyping for viral resistance patterns has been shown to improve ARV selection and should be obtained at the time of diagnosis.[5]
3. Antiretroviral therapy for primary HIV infection is not supported by randomized clinical trials; current U.S. Department of Health and Human Services guidelines list therapy as optional.
4. All patients should receive counseling on the risk of sexual transmission and safe sex.

II. GENERAL MANAGEMENT OF HIV AND AIDS

The following section describes hematologic and endocrine complications of HIV, immune reconstitution syndrome, and complications of ARVs.

A. HEMATOLOGIC ABNORMALITIES

1. Anemia (Box 48-2) is the most common hematologic abnormality among patients with HIV. Laboratory data are consistent with anemia of

48

ACUTE RETROVIRAL SYNDROME AND MANAGEMENT OF HIV

TABLE 48-1

COMMON PRESENTING SYMPTOMS AND SIGNS OF ACUTE RETROVIRAL SYNDROME[4]

Sign or Symptom	Frequency
Fever	90%
Malaise	70%
Myalgia or arthralgia	60%
Rash (usually maculopapular)	60%
Night sweats	50%
Headache	50%

Pharyngitis, lymphadenopathy, oral ulcers, mild transaminitis, aseptic meningitis, thrombocytopenia and neutropenia, and weight loss (average 10 lb) occur less often.

BOX 48-1

DIFFERENTIAL DIAGNOSIS OF ACUTE RETROVIRAL ILLNESS

Infectious mononucleosis
Cytomegalovirus
Primary herpes simplex virus
Influenza
Early viral hepatitis
Lymphoma
Systemic lupus erythematosus
Streptococcal pharyngitis
Lyme disease
Rickettsial disease
Secondary syphilis
Adult Still disease

BOX 48-2

COMMON CAUSES OF ANEMIA WITH HIV

Medications: zidovudine, dapsone, ganciclovir, primaquine, trimethoprim-sulfamethoxazole
Bacteremia and sepsis
Viruses: parvovirus B19, cytomegalovirus, Epstein-Barr virus
Lymphoma
Disseminated mycobacterial and fungal infections
Autoimmune hemolytic anemia, thrombotic thrombocytopenic purpura
Drug-induced hemolytic anemia
Nutritional deficiencies

chronic disease (i.e., normocytic anemia and normal iron studies). Zidovudine may cause mild anemia to severe red cell aplasia.[6]

2. Thrombocytopenia (Box 48-3) occurs in about 40% of patients with HIV and can occur at any stage of illness, including primary HIV infection. The most common cause is idiopathic thrombocytopenic purpura.

B. ENDOCRINE ABNORMALITIES

Adrenal insufficiency is common among patients with AIDS, occurring in up to 50% of critically ill patients with HIV.[7] Common causes include

---

BOX 48-3

CAUSES OF THROMBOCYTOPENIA WITH HIV

Human immunodeficiency virus–related idiopathic thrombocytopenic purpura

Thrombotic thrombocytopenic purpura

Sepsis

Disseminated mycobacterial and fungal diseases

Lymphoma

Cytomegalovirus, rubella

Toxoplasmosis

Medications: acyclovir, flucytosine, ganciclovir, interferon, pentamidine, rifampin

---

cytomegalovirus, mycobacterial infection, *Cryptococcus neoformans, Toxoplasma gondii,* and *Histoplasma capsulatum.* See Chapter 26 for a discussion of symptoms, diagnosis, and management of adrenal insufficiency.

C. ARV THERAPY AND COMPLICATIONS (Table 48-2)

ARV therapy works by suppressing viral replication and allowing recovery of CD4 counts. Current initial therapy always includes three drugs, usually two nucleoside reverse transcription inhibitors and either a nonnucleoside reverse transcription inhibitor or a protease inhibitor. If a patient is on a stable regimen as an outpatient, it should be continued during hospitalization unless it is responsible for significant adverse effects.

D. IMMUNE RECONSTITUTION SYNDROME

1. Immune reconstitution syndrome is a paradoxical worsening in clinical status after initiation of ARV therapy. It occurs as a consequence of improved immune surveillance of antigens from resolved or ongoing chronic infections. Affected patients usually have low initial CD4 counts ($< 50/mm^3$) and develop symptoms 1 week to several months after initiation of ARV therapy.

2. The most common cause is mycobacterial infection; others are listed in Table 48-3. The differential diagnosis also includes medication side effects, acute infections, and tumors. Management should focus on treating the underlying infection (if active). Steroids may provide benefit, especially for central nervous system symptoms and lymphadenitis. ARV therapy usually is continued.[8]

E. PROPHYLAXIS FOR OPPORTUNISTIC INFECTIONS (Table 48-4)

All patients who meet criteria should receive prophylaxis because it significantly decreases rehospitalization and mortality. Initiation during hospitalization usually is appropriate.

III. OCCUPATIONAL POSTEXPOSURE PROPHYLAXIS

Rapid initiation (within 2 hours) of ARV therapy after a potential exposure reduces the risk of HIV infection. If a health care provider is exposed, the hospital postexposure office or on-call physician should be contacted immediately. In addition to risk assessment, postexposure testing is

TABLE 48-2		
ANTIRETROVIRALS AND COMMON SIDE EFFECTS		
Sign or Symptom	Medication	Comments
NEUROLOGIC		
Peripheral neuropathy	ddI, d4T	
Central nervous system effects	Efavirenz	Abnormal dreams, agitation, hallucinations.
GASTROINTESTINAL		
Abdominal pain	All PIs, AZT, ddI	
Nausea, emesis, diarrhea	Lopinavir, saquinavir, nelfinavir, ritonavir	
Pancreatitis	ddI, d4T, ddC	
Lactic acidosis and hepatic steatosis	AZT, ddI, d4T	Lactic acidosis often accompanied by nausea and emesis, with frequent weight loss or wasting. Discontinue antiretroviral therapy immediately.
↑ Indirect bilirubin	Atazanavir, indinavir	Benign
Transaminitis or hepatitis	Nevirapine, efavirenz, all PIs	Initiation of nevirapine is contraindicated in women with CD4 counts >250 and men with CD4 counts >400 because of risk of fulminant liver failure.
HEMATOLOGIC		
Anemia and macrocytosis	AZT	Mean corpuscular volume >100.
Neutropenia	AZT	
ENDOCRINE		
Hyperlipidemia	Protease inhibitors (except atazanavir), d4T	
Hyperglycemia	Most protease inhibitors	
DERMATOLOGIC		
Abacavir hypersensitivity	Abacavir	Fever, skin rash, malaise, nausea, emesis, dyspnea, and cough. Usually occurs during first 4-6 wk of therapy; consult with expert before discontinuing therapy.
Rash	Nevirapine, efavirenz, abacavir, amprenavir	Benign and self-limited unless Stevens-Johnson or TEN.
MISCELLANEOUS		
Nephrolithiasis	Indinavir	
Fanconi's syndrome	Tenofovir	
Cannabinoid-positive urine drug screen	Efavirenz	With some assays.

AZT, zidovudine; d4T, didehydrodideoxythymidine; ddC, dideoxycytidine; ddI, dideoxyinosine; PI, protease inhibitor; SJS, Stevens-Johnson syndrome; TEN, toxic epidermolysis.

TABLE 48-3

IMMUNE RECONSTITUTION SYNDROME

Manifestation	Pathogens
Pulmonary infiltrates, pneumonitis	TB, MAI, *Pneumocystis jirovecii*
Lymphadenitis (peripheral or central)	TB, MAI
Cerebritis, meningitis, encephalitis	TB, *Cryptococcus,* herpes simplex virus, parvovirus B19
Hepatitis	Hepatitis B, hepatitis C, *Cryptococcus,* MAI
Guillain-Barré	Unknown
Uveitis, vitreitis	Cytomegalovirus
Zoster flares	Varicella-zoster virus
Gut perforation	TB

MAI, Mycobacterium avium; *TB,* Mycobacterium tuberculosis.

48

TABLE 48-4

PROPHYLAXIS FOR OPPORTUNISTIC INFECTIONS

Organism	CD4 Threshold	First-Line Prophylaxis
Pneumocystis jirovecii	<200/µl	TMP-SMX single-strength PO qd
Toxoplasma gondii	<100/µl and IgG positive	TMP-SMX double-strength PO qd
Mycobacterium avium	<50/µl	Azithromycin 1200 mg PO weekly
Cytomegalovirus	<200/µl and history of active cytomegalovirus	Valganciclovir 900 mg PO qd
Cryptococcus	History of cryptococcal meningitis	Fluconazole 200 mg PO qd

See www.aidsinfo.nih.gov/guidelines for more information.

IgG, immunoglobin G; *PO,* per os; *TMP-SMX,* trimethoprim-sulfamethoxazole.

standard and involves testing the source (for HIV and hepatitis B and C if the status is unknown) and the exposed person for baseline HIV and hepatitis B and C. See www.aidsinfo.nih.gov/guidelines/ for further details and risk stratification.

PEARLS AND PITFALLS

- Acute retroviral illness has nonspecific symptoms and is often missed. It should be considered even in patients who may not seem to be at high risk. One of the fastest-growing demographics of HIV is African-American and Latin women who are in monogamous relationships with men who engage in high-risk behavior.
- CD4 T-lymphocyte levels are suppressed in many acute infections, which may lead to low counts in patients without HIV or other immunodeficiency states.
- Drug interactions must be considered whenever a new medication (e.g., statins, opioids) is prescribed for a patient on ARV therapy.

- Many antiretrovirals must be dose-adjusted for renal insufficiency.
- ARV resistance mutations are archived. Prior genotyping of the HIV virus provides useful information in prescribing ARVs. For this reason, among others, one should not stop or change a patient's ARV regimen without contacting the patient's primary care provider.

REFERENCES

1. *HIV/AIDS surveillance report (2003)* 15(2), Atlanta, 2003, CDC, Department of Health and Human Services. B
2. Pilcher CD et al: Acute HIV revisited, *J Clin Invest* 113:937-945, 2004. C
3. Schacker T, Collier AC, Hughes J, et al: Clinical and epidemiological features of primary HIV infection, *Ann Intern Med* 125:257-264, 1996. B
4. Daar E, Little S, Pitt J, et al: Diagnosis of primary HIV-1 infection, *Ann Intern Med* 134:25-29, 2001. B
5. Weinstock HS et al: The epidemiology of antiretroviral drug resistance among drug-naïve HIV-1-infected persons in 10 US cities, *J Infect Dis* 189:2174-2180, 2004. B
6. Evans RH, Scadden DT: Haematological aspects of HIV infection, *Bailliere Clin Haematol* 13:215-230, 2000. C
7. Marik PE et al: Adrenal insufficiency in critically ill patients with human immunodeficiency virus, *Crit Care Med* 30:1267-1273, 2002. A
8. Hirsch HH, Kaufmann G, Sendi P, Battegay M: Immune reconstitution in HIV-infected patients, *Clin Infect Dis* 38:1159-1166, 2004. C

Central Nervous System Involvement in Human Immunodeficiency Virus Infection

David Riedel, MD; Nimalie Stone, MD; and Avindra Nath, MD

FAST FACTS

- Most neurologic manifestations of human immunodeficiency virus (HIV) infection occur with advanced immunodeficiency; the prevalence of neurologic disorders approaches two thirds of patients with symptomatic HIV infection.[1]
- The most common central nervous system (CNS) mass lesions are toxoplasmosis, primary CNS lymphoma (PCNSL), and progressive multifocal leukoencephalopathy (PML), but these are difficult to differentiate on the basis of history and physical examination alone; nearly 50% of clinical diagnoses are incorrect.
- The prevalence of HIV dementia (HIVD) is increasing as patients with HIV infection are living longer in the era of highly active antiretroviral therapy (HAART).[2]
- A headache in a patient with acquired immunodeficiency syndrome (AIDS) should never be overlooked. It should be investigated with a serum cryptococcal antigen, head computed tomography (CT), or lumbar puncture (LP) as clinically indicated.
- Given the higher prevalence of mass lesions in immunocompromised patients, a noncontrast head CT should be obtained before LP.
- Cerebrospinal fluid (CSF) analysis often is abnormal in HIV-infected patients, even in the asymptomatic stage.[3]
- With cryptococcal meningitis (CM), management of elevated intracranial pressure (ICP) is the most important step for reducing morbidity and mortality.[4]

HIV affects the CNS in myriad ways. It acts both in direct and indirect ways to damage the CNS; there are direct toxic effects, and in the latter case, HIV facilitates opportunistic infection by destroying host immunity. The neurologic manifestations of HIV infection occur most often with advanced disease: up to two thirds of patients with AIDS have clinically relevant neurologic disease.[1] Even in asymptomatic patients, CSF often is abnormal, with 50% having an elevated protein or pleocytosis.[3] It is important to remember that HIV-infected patients may have more than one CNS process occurring simultaneously. This chapter addresses the most common neurologic infections and conditions in patients with HIV; the incidence of each process has been declining since the introduction of HAART in 1996.[5]

I. CRYPTOCOCCAL MENINGITIS

A. EPIDEMIOLOGY AND ETIOLOGY

1. *Cryptococcus neoformans* is an encapsulated yeast that is acquired from the environment via inhalation. Cryptococcal infection represents dissemination of active pulmonary infection rather than reactivation of latent infection.[6]

2. The organism causes a basilar meningitis, which is exacerbated by the blockage of arachnoid granulations by its polysaccharide capsule, leading to a communicating hydrocephalus; occasionally it also causes intraparenchymal CNS cryptococcomas.

3. Up to 10% of HIV-infected patients develop CM as an AIDS-defining illness.[6] Risk is related to the level of immunosuppression; patients are most susceptible when the CD4 count has fallen below 100 (Table 49-1).

B. PRESENTATION

Presentation usually is subacute, with symptoms worsening over days to weeks. Findings include headache (75%), fever (> 65%), altered mental status, and rarely meningismus; up to 10% have a typical, umbilicated papular rash.

C. DIAGNOSIS

1. Serum cryptococcal antigen is positive in > 99% of cases of CM.[4] Blood cultures often reveal fungemia.

2. Brain imaging should be obtained before LP, although both CT and magnetic resonance imaging (MRI) usually are normal.

3. Diagnosis ultimately depends on demonstration of the organism in the CSF. CSF may be normal; other findings include elevated protein, hypoglycorrhachia, and a mononuclear pleocytosis.

TABLE 49-1	
THE ASSOCIATION BETWEEN CD4 COUNT AND CNS PROCESSES	
CNS Process	CD4 Count at Presentation (cells/μl)
Cryptococcal meningitis	<100
Cytomegalovirus encephalitis	<50
CNS toxoplasmosis	<100
Primary CNS lymphoma	<50
Progressive multifocal leukoencephalopathy	<100*
Human immunodeficiency virus dementia	<200†

Modified from Bartlett JG, Gallant JE: *2003 medical management of HIV infection*, Baltimore, 2003, Johns Hopkins University, Division of Infectious Diseases and AIDS Service.
CNS, central nervous system.
*Up to 25% of cases can be found with CD4 > 200.
†Cases are now more common with CD4 > 200.

4. CSF cryptococcal antigen and microscopic evaluation of smears can give a presumptive diagnosis.[6] Opening pressure should be measured carefully because it is often markedly elevated.

D. MANAGEMENT AND TREATMENT

1. Treatment is divided into induction, consolidation, and maintenance phases.[3] Recommended treatment consists of induction (2 weeks) with amphotericin B 0.7 to 1 mg/kg/day intravenously (IV) plus flucytosine 100 mg/kg/day per os (PO) divided into four doses; this is followed by 10 weeks of fluconazole 400 mg/day PO.[4] Long-term suppression with fluconazole 200 mg PO is necessary to prevent relapse unless immune reconstitution is achieved.[3]

2. Management of elevated ICP is a crucial component of treating CM because this complication is the major cause of morbidity and mortality.[4] Options include serial LPs with CSF drainage or placement of either a lumbar drain or ventriculoperitoneal shunt. Symptoms of recurrent headache or change in mental status are indications to repeat the LP with repeat opening pressure measurement. Drain placement usually is deferred unless ICP remains elevated after 2 weeks of serial LP drainage.

E. PROGNOSIS

1. Several factors have been found to predict poor prognosis, the most important of which is altered mental status at presentation.[7] Other factors include high initial opening pressure, low CSF white count, and fungemia.[7]

2. Without treatment, CM is fatal. Mortality with treatment is approximately 5%.[8]

II. CYTOMEGALOVIRUS ENCEPHALITIS

A. EPIDEMIOLOGY AND ETIOLOGY

Reactivation of cytomegalovirus (CMV) within the CNS usually occurs when the CD4 count is < 50 and may cause retinitis, encephalitis, polyradiculitis, polyradiculomyelitis, and peripheral neuropathies.

B. PRESENTATION

CMV infection of the brain may have several unique presentations, and it may also resemble encephalitis caused by other viruses. CMV encephalitis has three distinct forms: subacute dementia, ventriculoencephalitis, and focal infection.

C. DIAGNOSIS

1. At diagnosis, most patients have other organ systems affected by CMV besides the CNS, so establishing the presence of CMV elsewhere may aid in the diagnostic evaluation.

2. Serologic testing usually reveals immunoglobulin G (IgG) positivity.

3. CSF often is abnormal but nonspecific; findings include pleocytosis, elevated protein, and hypoglycorrhachia.

4. CMV polymerase chain reaction of the CSF has a specificity greater than 90%, but sensitivity is lower (around 80%).[1] However, detection of

49

CNS INVOLVEMENT IN HIV INFECTION

CMV DNA by polymerase chain reaction in the CSF does not always indicate active disease because latent infection can also be detected by this method.[9]

5. MRI is better than CT for detecting abnormalities; findings may include periventricular enhancement with enlarged ventricles.

6. Definitive diagnosis entails brain biopsy.

D. TREATMENT

Ganciclovir 5 mg/kg IV twice daily and foscarnet 90 mg/kg IV twice daily for 3 to 6 weeks has become standard therapy; one study showed better survival with this combination than in historical controls receiving only monotherapy (median survival 94 vs. 42 days).[10] Each of these drugs has significant side effects.

E. PROGNOSIS

Prognosis is poor; median survival in one study was < 5 weeks.[11]

III. CNS MASS LESIONS

A. EPIDEMIOLOGY AND ETIOLOGY

1. CNS mass lesions prevalent in HIV-infected patients include CNS toxoplasmosis, PCNSL, PML, tuberculomas, cryptococcomas, and CMV encephalitis. It is important to consider all other brain lesions (e.g., primary brain tumor, metastatic tumors).

2. With the exception of tuberculosis and PML (up to 25% of patients),[1] each of these disorders occurs with advanced immunosuppression (i.e., CD4 less than 100).

3. Cerebral toxoplasmosis is caused by reactivation of the latent parasitic infection *Toxoplasma gondii*. PCNSL is driven by Epstein-Barr virus reactivation in the CNS. Reactivation of the JC virus leads to PML.

B. PRESENTATION

In general, the common CNS diseases that occur in an HIV-infected patient are difficult to differentiate by history and physical examination alone (Table 49-2). However, nearly all patients with HIV infection who present with hemiballism or hemichorea have cerebral toxoplasmosis.[12]

C. DIAGNOSIS

See Table 49-3.

D. MANAGEMENT (Table 49-4)

1. If *Toxoplasma* IgG is positive and the lesion is typical for toxoplasmosis, empiric toxoplasmosis treatment is recommended for a 2-week course with a repeat MRI to assess for improvement at the end of this trial period.[3] Of patients who respond to treatment, 95% show radiographic improvement by the end of 2 weeks.[1]

2. If the clinical workup is inconclusive or if empiric treatment for toxoplasmosis is unsuccessful, proceed to brain biopsy. Most studies show a yield greater than 90% for biopsy.[1] In a recent study, 6% had more than one diagnosis from the single biopsy site, and 3% had tumors not typical of AIDS.[13] Studies have shown that nearly half of diagnoses made before brain biopsy were inaccurate.[1]

TABLE 49-2

COMPARISON OF SYMPTOMS, SIGNS, AND CLINICAL COURSE OF HUMAN IMMUNODEFICIENCY VIRUS CNS MASS LESIONS

CNS Process	Common Clinical Signs and Symptoms	Disease Progression
Toxoplasmosis[1]	Focal neurologic deficits (69%), headache (55%), confusion (52%), fever (47%), seizures (29%)	Subacute (days to weeks)
Primary CNS lymphoma	Altered mental status (60%), focal neurologic deficits, headache, seizures (15%), afebrile	Insidious (2 to 8 wk)
Progressive multifocal leukoencephalopathy	Progressive focal neurologic deficits (affecting speech, vision, or motor function), afebrile, no headache	Gradual (weeks to months)

Modified from Bartlett JG, Gallant JE: 2003 medical management of HIV infection, Baltimore, 2003, Johns Hopkins University, Division of Infectious Diseases and AIDS Service.
CNS, central nervous system.

3. CNS mass lesions often are complicated by cerebral edema. Steroids to control edema should be used only with severe swelling or signs of impending herniation because they may confound a subsequent brain biopsy result by partially treating PCNSL.

E. PROGNOSIS

Median survival for patients with PCNSL is 3 to 4 months with treatment,[6] although several newer studies have shown prolonged survival with the addition of HAART.[14,15] Survival for patients with PML without treatment usually is < 6 months.[1]

IV. HIV DEMENTIA

A. EPIDEMIOLOGY

HIVD has gone by various names, including HIV-associated dementia, HIV-associated encephalitis, and AIDS dementia complex. Before the advent of HAART, the cumulative lifetime risk of HIVD was 15% to 20% in adults.[16] Since the widespread use of HAART, the incidence of HIVD has fallen significantly,[5] but the prevalence has actually increased because of longer survival with AIDS.[2] However, more cases of HIVD are presenting with higher CD4 counts (i.e., > 200).[5]

B. PRESENTATION

1. HIVD usually is described as a subcortical dementia that includes dysfunction of cognitive, behavioral, and motor systems. Symptoms often are of insidious onset and are often overlooked. Early signs include apathy, mental slowing, memory loss, and reading and comprehension difficulties.

2. Progression occurs at variable rates.[18] HIVD can be a significant cause of morbidity as activities of daily living become impaired.

TABLE 49-3

COMPARISON OF LABORATORY AND RADIOGRAPHIC FINDINGS IN HUMAN IMMUNODEFICIENCY VIRUS CNS MASS LESIONS

CNS Process	CSF Findings	Radiologic Findings	Other Studies
Toxoplasmosis	Normal in 20-30%; variable protein; white blood cells (mono), 0 to 40.	Often multiple; 1- to 2-cm simple ring lesions; located in basal ganglia and gray-white junction; moderate edema or mass effect; prominent enhancement.	Serum Toxoplasma immunoglobulin G false negative in <5%. PCR can be done on CSF but is only 50% sensitive.
PCNSL	Normal in up to 50%; Epstein-Barr virus PCR 80% sensitive and >94% specific.	One or multiple; 2-6 cm; solid but irregular; more are periventricular; prominent edema or mass effect; prominent enhancement.	Thallium-201 single-photon emission computed tomography scan is 90% specific and sensitive (positive for PCNSL; negative for toxoplasmosis). Brain biopsy usually is needed and shows a B cell lymphoma.
Progressive multifocal leukoencephalopathy	Normal; JC virus PCR 80% sensitive and >95% specific.	Multiple lesions often involving posterior fossa; variable location; no mass effect; no enhancement.	Brain biopsy shows JC virus by immunostaining or by in situ hybridization in nuclei of oligodendrocytes and astroglia.

Modified from Bartlett JG, Gallant JE: 2003 medical management of HIV infection, Baltimore, 2003, Johns Hopkins University, Division of Infectious Diseases and AIDS Service. CNS, central nervous system; CSF, cerebrospinal fluid; PCNSL, primary CNS lymphoma; PCR, polymerase chain reaction.

TABLE 49-4		
RECOMMENDED TREATMENT REGIMENS		
CNS Process	Recommended Therapy	Alternative Therapy
Toxoplasmosis	Pyrimethamine 200 mg loading dose, then 50-75 mg/d PO and leucovorin 10-20 mg/d PO and sulfadiazine 1000-1500 mg q6h PO for 3-6 wk. If CD4 cell count remains < 200/mm³, indefinite maintenance therapy is necessary.	For sulfa-allergic patients, may substitute clindamycin 600 mg q6h intravenously (for sulfadiazine).
PCNSL	Radiation and steroids.	Two recent trials have shown marked improvement in survival in patients receiving HAART in addition to radiation.
Progressive multifocal leukoencephalopathy	None proven. Response to HAART suggested by some studies.	Conflicting evidence for cidofovir.

Modified from Bartlett JG, Gallant JE: *2003 medical management of HIV infection*, Baltimore, 2003, Johns Hopkins University, Division of Infectious Diseases and AIDS Services.
CNS, central nervous system; *HAART*, highly active antiretroviral therapy; *PO*, per os.

C. DIAGNOSIS
1. HIVD is a diagnosis of exclusion. There must be no evidence of CNS opportunistic infection or other neurologic processes. A battery of neuropsychological testing often is used to aid diagnosis in the research setting.
2. CSF analysis may show a nonspecific pleocytosis or a mildly elevated protein level. The value of measuring CSF HIV RNA levels or immune markers is unclear. MRI shows cortical and central atrophy.

D. PROGNOSIS
Before HAART, HIVD progressed to death, usually in < a year.

E. MANAGEMENT
Because HIVD is an AIDS-defining illness, its diagnosis is an indication to initiate HAART.

PEARLS AND PITFALLS
- Cryptococcal meningitis can have very mild symptoms initially, and subtle changes in mental status should not be overlooked.
- If a serum cryptococcal antigen is positive, further investigation with LP, chest radiograph, and blood cultures is mandatory; even if all studies are negative, treatment with fluconazole is still necessary to prevent disease progression.
- CMV encephalitis often is accompanied by CMV involvement of another organ system (e.g., retina, gastrointestinal tract, adrenals, or blood).

- Serum *Toxoplasma* IgG has greater than 95% sensitivity; other diseases should be considered more likely even when lesions resemble toxoplasmosis but serology is negative.
- PML can occur at any CD4 count (up to 25% of patients have CD4 counts > 100).
- HIVD is an important diagnosis to make because it may have significant effects on a patient's ability to perform activities of daily living and comply with HAART medication regimens.[1]

REFERENCES

1. Skiest DJ: Focal neurological disease in patients with acquired immunodeficiency syndrome, *Clin Infect Dis* 34:103, 2002. C
2. McArthur JC et al: Human immunodeficiency virus-associated dementia: an evolving disease, *J Neurovirol* 9:205, 2003. C
3. Bartlett JG, Gallant JE: *2003 medical management of HIV infection,* Baltimore, 2003, Johns Hopkins University, Division of Infectious Diseases and AIDS Service. C
4. Saag MS et al: Practice guidelines for the management of cryptococcal disease, *Clin Infect Dis* 30:710, 2000. D
5. Sacktor N: The epidemiology of human immunodeficiency virus–associated neurological disease in the era of highly active antiretroviral therapy, *J Neurovirol* 8(s.2):115, 2002. C
6. Mamidi A, DeSimone JA, Pomerantz RJ: Central nervous system infections in individuals with HIV-1 infection, *J Neurovirol* 8:158, 2002. C
7. Powderly WG: Current approach to the acute management of cryptococcal infections, *J Infect* 41:18, 2000. C
8. Van der Horst CM et al: Treatment of cryptococcal meningitis associated with the acquired immunodeficiency syndrome, *N Engl J Med* 337:15, 1997. A
9. Maschke M, Kastrup O, Diener HC: CNS manifestations of cytomegalovirus infections: diagnosis and treatment, *CNS Drugs* 16:303, 2002. C
10. Anduze-Faris BM et al: Induction and maintenance therapy of cytomegalovirus central nervous system infection in HIV-infected patients, *AIDS* 14:517, 2000. B
11. Holland NR et al: Cytomegalovirus encephalitis in acquired immunodeficiency syndrome (AIDS), *Neurology* 44:507, 1994. B
12. Nath A, Hobson DE, Russell A: Movement disorders with cerebral toxoplasmosis and AIDS, *Mov Disord* 8:107, 1993. B
13. Gildenberg PL, Gathe JC, Kim JH: Stereotactic biopsy of cerebral lesions in AIDS, *Clin Infect Dis* 30:491, 2000. B
14. Hoffmann C et al: Survival of AIDS patients with primary central nervous system lymphoma is dramatically improved by HAART-induced immune recovery, *AIDS* 15:2119, 2001. B
15. Skiest DJ, Crosby C: Survival is prolonged by highly active antiretroviral therapy in AIDS patients with primary central nervous system lymphoma, *AIDS* 17:1787, 2003. B
16. McArthur JC et al: Dementia in AIDS patients: incidence and risk factors. Multicenter AIDS Cohort Study, *Neurology* 43:2245, 1993. B
17. Bouwman FH et al: Variable progression of HIV-associated dementia, *Neurology* 50:1814, 1998. B

Pulmonary Involvement in Human Immunodeficiency Virus

Catherine Passaretti, MD; Josh Lauring, MD, PhD; and Stuart Ray, MD

FAST FACTS

- Recurrent bacterial pneumonia and *Pneumocystis jiroveci* pneumonia (PCP) are common pulmonary infections in patients with the human immunodeficiency virus (HIV), and both occur at higher rates in patients with lower CD4 counts. Acute onset of symptoms (i.e., < 7 days) suggests a bacterial process, whereas subacute onset of symptoms (i.e., weeks to months) suggests PCP, other fungal pneumonias, or a mycobacterial process.
- *Streptococcus pneumoniae* and *Haemophilus influenzae* are the most common causes of bacterial pneumonia in patients with HIV.
- Patients with acquired immunodeficiency syndrome (AIDS) are at a higher risk for developing severe pulmonary or disseminated disease from endemic mycoses. Histoplasmosis is the most common endemic fungal infection in patients with HIV.
- Ninety-five percent of cases of PCP occur in patients with CD4 counts less than 200/mm^3.
- Adjunctive corticosteroids reduce mortality and respiratory failure in patients with PCP and a PaO_2 < 70 or a PAO_2-PaO_2 gradient > 35 on room air.
- After initiation of therapy for PCP, patients may have rapid deterioration in clinical status before improvement.
- If PCP is suspected and an induced sputum is negative, bronchoalveolar lavage (BAL) should be pursued.

50

Pulmonary manifestations of HIV are very common. Recurrent bacterial pneumonia, PCP, and fungal pneumonias are major causes of morbidity and mortality in patients with HIV. This chapter focuses on pulmonary disease processes and management unique to patients with HIV.

I. BACTERIAL PNEUMONIA

A. EPIDEMIOLOGY

1. Patients with HIV at any stage of immunosuppression are at a higher risk for developing bacterial pneumonia. One study showed 5.5 cases of bacterial pneumonia per 100 person-years in patients with HIV compared with only 0.9 cases per 100 person-years in the control group. In addition, the risk of developing bacterial pneumonia if the patient has HIV increases substantially as the CD4 count declines.[1]

2. HIV-positive patients are at a higher risk of recurrence of bacterial pneumonia; as many as 13% of cases of pneumococcal pneumonia recur within 6 months.[2] Case mortality is 5% to 11%.[1]

B. CLINICAL PRESENTATION

The clinical presentation in patients with HIV is similar to that in those who are immunocompetent (see Chapter 55).

C. ETIOLOGY

1. The most common identifiable agent is *S. pneumoniae,* whose incidence is about 200 times higher than in the general population. Atypical agents including *Chlamydia pneumoniae, Mycoplasma pneumoniae,* and *Legionella* spp. have an incidence similar to that in the HIV-negative population.
2. Causative agents in cavitary pneumonia include *Staphylococcus aureus, Pseudomonas aeruginosa, Klebsiella* spp., *Rhodococcus equi, Mycobacterium tuberculosis,* and *Mycobacterium kansasii.* Polymicrobial infection is quite common.
  a. Patients with cavitary pneumonia from a bacterial agent tend to have higher CD4 counts than those with cavitation caused by nonbacterial agents.
  b. Nonbacterial culprits for cavitation include *Pneumocystis jiroveci,* Kaposi's sarcoma, and non-Hodgkin's lymphoma.

D. DIAGNOSIS

Evaluation of bacterial pneumonia includes chest radiograph, Gram stain and culture of expectorated sputum (obtained prior to antibiotics), complete blood cell count and differential, and blood cultures (see Fig. 50-1).

E. TREATMENT

1. Treatment is the same as in the immunocompetent host (see Chapter 55).
2. Pneumococcal vaccination should be offered with revaccination at 5-year intervals. Some studies indicate that vaccination is more effective if the patient has a CD4 count > 500/mm³.

II. *PNEUMOCYSTIS CARINII (JIROVECI)* PNEUMONIA

A. EPIDEMIOLOGY

1. PCP is the most common AIDS-defining illness, occurring in 15% to 28% of patients infected with HIV.
2. *Pneumocystis carinii,* a fungus, was renamed *Pneumocystis jiroveci* in 1999 because of differences between rat and human pathogen DNA sequences.[3]
3. The incidence of PCP increases as the CD4 count declines. Ninety-five percent of cases occur at CD4 counts < 200/mm³. The risk of developing PCP in a patient with a CD4 count less than 100/mm³ is 60% to 70% per year if no prophylaxis is used and 40% to 50% per year if on prophylaxis.[4]

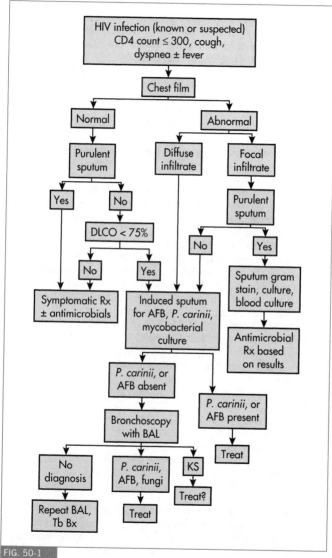

50

FIG. 50-1

Evaluation of a patient with the human immunodeficiency virus (HIV) and pulmonary symptoms. *AFB,* acid-fast bacillus; *BAL,* bronchoalveolar lavage; *DLCO,* diffusing capacity of the lung for carbon dioxide; *KS,* Kaposi's sarcoma; *Rx,* medication; *Tb Bx,* transbronchial biopsy. *(From L Goldman, ed: Cecil textbook of medicine, 21st ed, Philadelphia, 2000, WB Saunders.)*

4. Caucasian race, prior PCP, recurrent undiagnosed fevers, thrush, and weight loss, despite a CD4 count > 200/mm^3, carry a higher risk for PCP.

5. Short-term mortality for PCP ranges from 10% to 20%. If respiratory failure is present, mortality increases to 60%.[5]

B. CLINICAL PRESENTATION

1. Classic symptoms include fever (79% to 100%), progressive dyspnea on exertion (95%), and cough (present in 95%, nonproductive in 70%).

2. Symptoms often are mild initially and progress slowly over the course of weeks.

3. Physical examination usually reveals fever and tachypnea. The lung examination sometimes reveals rales or rhonchi but can be normal in up to 50% of cases.

4. Extrapulmonary manifestations of PCP are more common if aerosolized pentamidine is used for prophylaxis. The most common nonpulmonary sites include lymph nodes, bone marrow, spleen, and liver.

C. DIAGNOSIS

1. See Fig. 50-1 for a diagnostic algorithm.

2. The chest radiograph (CXR) is abnormal in more than 80% of cases. CXR usually shows diffuse bilateral interstitial or alveolar infiltrates, but this presentation is only 84% to 97% specific for PCP. Similar findings on CXR can be seen with bacterial pneumonia, tuberculosis, and pulmonary Kaposi's sarcoma.[6] The presence of pneumothorax in a patient with HIV represents PCP in 77% of cases.[7]

3. In about 10% of patients with PCP the CXR is completely normal. If the CXR is normal, high-resolution chest computed tomography (CT) usually shows typical patchy or nodular ground glass changes. When these changes were present, one study showed that CT carried a sensitivity of 100% and specificity of 89% in identifying PCP.[8]

4. Serum lactate dehydrogenase (LDH) levels are elevated in > 90% of patients with PCP and have been shown to increase with the onset of symptoms and decrease during recovery.[9] LDH often is elevated in other pulmonary conditions LDH such as bacterial pneumonia, tuberculosis, and lymphoma. Therefore a normal LDH level makes the diagnosis of PCP unlikely, but an elevated level is not diagnostic.

5. Several studies have shown that exercise-associated arterial O_2 desaturation is sensitive but not specific for a diagnosis of PCP if performed under standardized conditions.[10] No studies have looked at O_2 saturation before and after ambulation in a hospital ward; therefore lack of desaturation should not be used to rule out PCP.

6. Definitive diagnosis of PCP entails identification of the organism in a respiratory specimen, usually obtained via sputum induction (sensitivity

55% to 95%) or BAL, both of which are 99% specific for the diagnosis of PCP.

7. If sputum induction is nondiagnostic, bronchoscopy with BAL should be pursued. In HIV-positive patients, BAL has a sensitivity of 89% to 98% for PCP.[11]

D. TREATMENT

1. **Prevention of PCP** (Table 50-1). Prophylaxis against PCP is highly effective in reducing the risk of developing PCP and decreasing mortality. Prophylaxis is recommended for HIV-infected patients with CD4 counts < 200/mm³, unexplained fever for > 2 weeks, oropharyngeal candidiasis, or a history of PCP. Discontinuation of prophylaxis is safe when the patient has documented CD4 counts > 200/mm³ for 3 months.[12]

2. **Treatment regimens for PCP.** See Table 50-2.

3. **Adjunctive steroids for moderate to severe PCP.** Multiple studies have shown the beneficial effects of corticosteroids on reducing mortality, reducing the risk of respiratory failure, and preventing early

50

PULMONARY INVOLVEMENT IN HIV

TABLE 50-1

PROPHYLACTIC REGIMENS FOR PCP

Drug	Dosage
Trimethoprim-sulfamethoxazole	1 single-strength PO daily or 1 double-strength PO 3 times/wk
Dapsone	100 mg PO daily
Atovaquone	1500 mg PO daily
Aerosolized pentamidine*	300 mg inhaled per month via Respirgard II nebulizer

PCP, Pneumocystis jiroveci pneumonia, PO, per os.
*PCP infections that occur despite treatment with aerosolized pentamidine usually are localized to upper lobes, involve pneumothoraces or extrapulmonary manifestations, and result in lower yield on bronchoalveolar lavage.

TABLE 50-2

DRUG THERAPY FOR *PNEUMOCYSTIS JIROVECI* PNEUMONIA

Drug	Dosage
Trimethoprim-sulfamethoxazole (therapy of choice)	Trimethoprim 15 mg/kg/d and sulfamethoxazole 75 mg/kg/day IV, divided tid or qid for 21 d; usual oral dosage is 2 double-strength tid
Clindamycin-primaquine	Clindamycin 600 mg IV q8h or 300-450 mg PO qid and primaquine 15-30 mg/d for a total of 21 d
Atovaquone	750 mg PO tid for 21 d

IV, intravenously; PO, per os.

deterioration in patients with moderate to severe PCP (arterial O_2 tension $\leq$ 70 mmHg or an A-a gradient of $\geq$ 35 mmHg on room air). Although no studies have been completed on the optimal corticosteroid regimen, current recommendations are to use prednisone 40 mg orally twice daily for 5 days, followed by 40 mg daily for 5 days, followed by 20 mg daily for 11 days.[13]

III. MYCOBACTERIAL DISEASE
See Chapter 52.

IV. OTHER FUNGAL PULMONARY INFECTIONS
See Table 50-3.

PEARLS AND PITFALLS

- Cytomegalovirus (CMV) is commonly isolated from BAL in patients with HIV; however, the significance of this agent as a pulmonary pathogen remains unclear. Studies have shown that anti-CMV treatment does not affect survival in patients with pneumonia and positive BAL cultures, especially if other pulmonary pathogens are present. Currently, for a diagnosis of CMV, four criteria must be met: pulmonary infiltrates must be present; CMV must be detected by culture, antigen, or nucleic studies of pulmonary secretions; characteristic intracellular inclusions must be present in lung tissue or BAL macrophages; and no other pulmonary pathogen can be present.[19] Only if all of these criteria are met should therapy with ganciclovir, foscarnet, or valganciclovir be initiated.
- **Empiric therapy for PCP should not be initiated without plans to complete a full evaluation.** Even with typical symptoms and infiltrates on CXR, < 50% of patients in one large series had PCP on BAL. Because *P. jiroveci* can be detected in BAL specimens for many days after initiation of therapy, therapy should not be withheld while a diagnosis is being pursued.
- Noninfectious causes of pulmonary symptoms such as pulmonary Kaposi's sarcoma, non-Hodgkin's lymphoma, lymphocytic interstitial pneumonitis, and nonspecific pneumonitis can all present with subacute to chronic cough, dyspnea, fevers, fatigue, and weight loss.
- The incidence of PCP in non-HIV immunosuppressed patients (e.g., organ transplant recipients) has increased in the past two decades. Compared with HIV-infected patients, non-HIV immunosuppressed patients tend to have a more fulminant presentation with a higher incidence of respiratory failure (43%) and death (35% to 40%). Patients at elevated risk for developing PCP (e.g., those on prolonged high-dose steroids) should receive PCP prophylaxis.
- PCP is one of the few causes of bilateral pneumothoraces.

TABLE 50-3

PULMONARY FUNGAL INFECTIONS IN HIV

Fungus*	Epidemiology	Clinical Presentation	Chest Radiograph	Diagnosis and Treatment
Histoplasma capsulatum[14]	Most common endemic mycose in HIV, occurring in 5% to 27% of patients with AIDS in endemic areas. Location: Mississippi River valley, Caribbean, and Latin America.	Isolated pulmonary involvement in < 5% of patients with HIV; disseminated disease is much more common (95%). Usual presentation is subacute (~1-3 mo), with development of fever, fatigue, weight loss. 50% have cough and dyspnea. Oral ulcers are common.	Diffuse interstitial or reticulonodular infiltrates. Focal infiltrates or nodules (~10% of cases). Mediastinal lymphadenopathy is rare.	Histoplasma polysaccharide antigen (sensitivity: urine 93%, blood 89%, BAL 89%). Blood cultures with a fungal isolator may take weeks to grow. In 40% of cases, the organism is visible on Wright's stained smears of peripheral blood or buffy coat. Serology is of limited value. Bronchoscopy with BAL and transbronchial biopsy usually is necessary if pulmonary symptoms are present. Inpatient treatment: amphotericin B or itraconazole (12-wk induction). Chronic suppressive treatment: fluconazole or itraconazole.
Coccidioides immitis[15,16]	Occurs in < 2% of patients with AIDS in most endemic areas. Most common if CD4 count is < 250/mm³.	80% present with diffuse or focal pulmonary involvement. Common symptoms include fever, cough, dyspnea, fatigue, chest pain, weight loss.	Diffuse reticulonodular infiltrates (~45%). Focal infiltrates (~35%).	Sputum cultures low yield (<16%). Bronchoscopy and BAL usually necessary with cytologic exam (positive in 40%) and culture

cont'd

50

PULMONARY INVOLVEMENT IN HIV

TABLE 50-3

PULMONARY FUNGAL INFECTIONS IN HIV—cont'd

Fungus*	Epidemiology	Clinical Presentation	Chest Radiograph	Diagnosis and Treatment
	Poor prognosis, with mortality of 70% if diffuse lung involvement. Location: southwestern US and Latin America.	Skin findings in 5%. Subacute onset of symptoms over weeks to months. Extrapulmonary sites of infections also include central nervous system, bone, and eye.		(takes 3-5 d to grow). Blood cultures infrequently positive. Treatment with fluconazole, itraconazole, or amphotericin B.
Blastomyces dermatitidis[17]	Uncommon but fulminant in patients with HIV. Most common in patients with CD4 <200/mm³. ~40% mortality. Location: midwestern and south central US.	Fever, cough, dyspnea, weight loss, fatigue. Localized pulmonary involvement occurs in about 50% of patients; the rest have disseminated disease. Cutaneous lesions less common in patients with AIDS.	Focal lobar infiltrates (~40%). Diffuse interstitial infiltrates (~40%). Nodules, cavities, and pleural effusions may also be seen.	Demonstration of organisms from culture of exam of BAL and lung biopsy needed. Culture may take weeks but is positive in more than 90% of patients. Treatment: amphotericin B or itraconazole if less ill. Chronic suppressive treatment: itraconazole.
Aspergillus fumigatus[18]	1% to 4% of patients with HIV. Risk factors: neutropenia and corticosteroid use. Location: worldwide.	Fever, cough, dyspnea, chest pain, and hemoptysis.	Upper lobe cavities (36%). Focal infiltrate (22%) or bilateral interstitial or reticulonodular infiltrates.	Definitive diagnosis requires tissue biopsy because aspergillus is a common airway colonizer. Treatment: amphotericin B or itraconazole.

AIDS, acquired immunodeficiency syndrome; *BAL*, bronchoalveolar lavage; *HIV*, human immunodeficiency virus.
*For *Cryptococcus neoformans*, see Chapter 49.

REFERENCES

1. Hirschtick RE, Glassroth J, Jordan MC, et al: Bacterial pneumonia in persons infected with the human immunodeficiency virus, *N Engl J Med* 333(13):845-851, 1995. B
2. Bartlett JG: Pneumonia in the patient with HIV infection, *Infect Dis Clin North Am* 12:807-820, 1998. C
3. Stringer JR, Beard CB, Miller RF, Wakefield AE: A new name (*Pneumocystis jiroveci*) for *Pneumocystis* from humans, *Emerg Infect Dis* 8(9):891-896, 2002. C
4. Phair J, Munoz A, Detels R, et al: The risk of *Pneumocystis carinii* pneumonia among men infected with human immunodeficiency virus type I, *N Engl J Med* 322:161-165, 1990. B
5. Mansharamani NG, Garland R, Delaney D, Kosiel H: Management and outcome patterns for adult *Pneumocystis carinii* pneumonia, 1985-1995: comparison of HIV-associated cases to other immunocompromised states, *Chest* 118(3):704-711, 2000. B
6. Baughman RP, Dohn MN, Frame PT: The continuing utility of bronchoalveolar lavage to diagnose opportunistic infection in AIDS patients, *Am J Med* 97(6):515-522, 1994. B
7. Metersky ML, Colt HG, Olson LK, Shanks TG: AIDS-related spontaneous pneumothorax. Risk factors and treatment, *Chest* 108(4):946-951, 1995. B
8. Gruden JF, Huang L, Turner J, et al: High resolution CT in the evaluation of clinically suspected *Pneumocystis carinii* pneumonia in AIDS patients with normal, equivocal or nonspecific radiographic findings, *AJR Am J Roentgenol* 169:967-975, 1997. B
9. Zaman MK, White DA: Serum lactate dehydrogenase levels and *Pneumocystis carinii* pneumonia, *Am Rev Respir Dis* 137:796-800, 1988. B
10. Smith DE, Wyatt J, McLuckie A, et al: Severe exercise hypoxaemia with normal or near normal x-rays: a feature of *Pneumocystis carinii* infection, *Lancet* 2(8619):1049-1051, 1988. B
11. Huang L, Hecht FM, Stansell JD, et al: Suspected *Pneumocystis carinii* pneumonia with a negative induced sputum examination: is early bronchoscopy useful? *Am J Respir Crit Care Med* 151:1866-1871, 1995. B
12. Lopez Bernaldo de Quiros JC, Miro JM, Pena JM, et al: A randomized trial of the discontinuation of primary and secondary prophylaxis against *Pneumocystis carinii* pneumonia after highly active antiretroviral therapy in patients with HIV infection. Grupo de Estudio del SIDA, *N Engl J Med* 344(3):159-167, 2001. A
13. Gagnon S, Boota AM, Fischl MA, et al: Corticosteroids as adjunctive therapy for severe *Pneumocystis carinii* pneumonia in the acquired immunodeficiency syndrome. A double-blind, placebo controlled trial, *N Engl J Med* 323(21):1444-1450, 1990. A
14. McKinsey DS, Spiegel RA, Hutwagner L, et al: Prospective study of histoplasmosis in patients infected with human immunodeficiency virus: incidence, risk factors and pathophysiology, *Clin Infect Dis* 24(6):1195-1203, 1997. B
15. Bronniman DA, Adam RD, Galgiani JN, et al: Coccidioidomycosis in the acquired immunodeficiency syndrome, *Ann Intern Med* 106:372, 1987. C
16. DiTomasso JO, Ampel NM, Sobonya RE, Bloom JW: Bronchoscopic diagnosis of pulmonary coccidioidomycosis: comparison of cytology, culture and transbronchial biopsy, *Diagn Microbiol Infect Dis* 18:83, 1994. B

17. Pappas PG, Pottage JC, Powderly WG, et al: Blastomycosis in patients with the acquired immunodeficiency syndrome, *Ann Intern Med* 116: 847, 1992. C
18. Denning DW, Follansbee SE, Scolaro M, et al: Pulmonary aspergillosis in the acquired immunodeficiency syndrome, *N Engl J Med* 324:654-662, 1991. B
19. Rodriguez-Barradas MC, Stool E, Musher DM, et al: Diagnosing and treating cytomegalovirus pneumonia in patients with AIDS, *Clin Infect Dis* 23(1):76-81, 1996. B

Gastrointestinal Disorders in Patients with the Human Immunodeficiency Virus

Pennan Barry, MD, MPH; and Peter Belitsos, MD

FAST FACTS

- One third of patients with acquired immunodeficiency syndrome (AIDS) develop esophageal symptoms, with candidal esophagitis being the most common cause.
- Empiric fluconazole completely resolves esophageal symptoms in 82% of patients.
- Cholestasis associated with the human immunodeficiency virus (HIV) is seen in up to 55% of HIV-infected patients.
- Acute diarrhea lasting more than 5 days warrants further investigation.
- Stool analysis of chronic diarrhea should include stool culture and stain for ova and parasites including special stains for *Cryptosporidium, Isospora,* microsporidia, and acid-fast bacillus. Medication side effects should also be considered as a cause of diarrhea.

HIV-infected patients often present with a variety of gastrointestinal (GI) complaints. Although the HIV-infected patient is susceptible to a variety of illnesses that an immunocompetent person is not, it is important to consider common GI illnesses when generating a differential diagnosis. This chapter focuses on HIV-associated GI illness.

I. THRUSH (OROPHARYNGEAL CANDIDIASIS)

A. EPIDEMIOLOGY

More than 90% of patients with AIDS develop oropharyngeal candidiasis at some time during their illness.[1]

B. PRESENTATION AND DIAGNOSIS

Thrush appears as adherent white plaques in the mouth with or without erythema, often with angular cheilitis. Risk factors include CD4 < 250/mm^3, steroids, or antibiotics.

C. MANAGEMENT (Table 51-1)

1. Thrush should be treated for 10 to 14 days, preferably with nystatin or clotrimazole. Symptoms should respond within 5 days but may not completely resolve for 10 to 14 days. Relapse is common.[2]
2. Antifungal prophylaxis may be indicated in patients with several recurrences of symptomatic oropharyngeal candidiasis. Patients with

TABLE 51-1

TREATMENT OPTIONS FOR OROPHARYNGEAL CANDIDIASIS

Medication	Dosage	Comments
Clotrimazole troches	10 mg 5×/d	Preferred initial therapy. Tastes bad.
Nystatin	500,000 units gargled 4-5×/d	Less effective than clotrimazole or fluconazole.
Fluconazole	100 mg PO qd	Dosage may be increased for resistant infections.
Itraconazole	100 mg PO qd liquid	Many drug interactions.
Caspofungin	70 mg IV × 1, then 50 mg IV qd	Effective in fluconazole- and amphotericin-resistant infections.
Amphotericin B	0.3-0.5 mg/kg IV qd	Toxicity and side effects may limit use.

IV, intravenously; *PO,* per os.

CD4 counts < 50/mm^3 benefit most from prophylaxis.[1] The optimal prophylactic regimen is not known, but fluconazole dosages from 200 mg orally once weekly to 200 mg once daily have been found to be effective.[3,4]

Note: See Table 51-2 and Fig. 51-1 for the presentation and treatment of esophagitis.

II. HIV CHOLANGIOPATHY

A. EPIDEMIOLOGY

Elevated alkaline phosphatase and gamma-glutamyl transpeptidase can be seen in up to 55% of HIV-infected patients.[5]

B. PRESENTATION

1. HIV cholangiopathy is seen in patients with advanced HIV disease and CD4 counts < 200/mm.[3,6] Regardless of etiologic pathogen, patients usually are symptomatic and present with sharp right upper quadrant pain or epigastric pain that may radiate to the back. In 50%, nausea, vomiting, and low-grade fever are also present.[6] High spiking fevers suggest cholangitis.[6] Pruritus and jaundice are uncommon.
2. Typical laboratory values include elevated alkaline phosphatase (to more than five times the upper limit of normal), normal to mildly elevated bilirubin, and moderate transaminitis.

C. DIFFERENTIAL DIAGNOSIS (Box 51-1)

1. *Cryptosporidium* is the single most common identifiable pathogen in the biliary tract in patients with HIV cholangiopathy and often can be isolated from the stool.[7]
2. Cytomegalovirus is the second most isolated pathogen; microsporidia may be the underlying cause in many cases with an unknown pathogen.[8]

TABLE 51-2				
ESOPHAGEAL DISEASE IN PATIENTS WITH THE HUMAN IMMUNODEFICIENCY VIRUS				
	Candida	*CMV*	*HSV*	*Aphthous Ulcers*
Frequency as cause of symptoms	50-70%	10-20%	2-5%	10-20%
CLINICAL FEATURES				
Dysphagia	+++	+	+	
Odynophagia	++	+++	+++	+++
Thrush	50%-70%	<25%	<25%	<25%
Oral ulcers	Rare	Uncommon	Common	Uncommon
Pain	Diffuse	Focal	Focal	Focal
Fever	Uncommon	Common	Uncommon	Uncommon
DIAGNOSIS				
Endoscopy	Usually treated empirically. Pseudomembranous plaques; may involve entire esophagus.	Biopsy needed for treatment. Erythema and erosions or ulcers, single or multiple discrete lesions, often distal.	Biopsy needed for treatment. Erythema and erosions or ulcers, usually small, coalescing, shallow.	Similar in appearance and location to CMV ulcers.
Microbiology	Brush: yeast and pseudomycelium on potassium hydroxide prep or periodic acid–Schiff stain. Culture with sensitivities may be useful with suspected resistance.	Biopsy: Intracellular inclusions or positive culture. Highest yield with histopathology of biopsy and culture. Culture often is not recommended because of false positives.	Brush and biopsy: intracytoplasmic inclusions and multinucleate giant cells, fluorescent antibody (FA) stain, or positive culture.	Negative studies for *Candida*, HSV, CMV, and other diagnoses.

cont'd

51

GASTROINTESTINAL DISORDERS IN PATIENTS WITH HIV

TABLE 51-2
ESOPHAGEAL DISEASE IN PATIENTS WITH THE HUMAN IMMUNODEFICIENCY VIRUS—cont'd

	Candida	CMV	HSV	Aphthous Ulcers
TREATMENT				
Acute	Fluconazole 200 mg/d PO, up to 800 mg/d. Efficacy of fluconazole is 82%.[19] Refractory cases: itraconazole 200 mg/d or voriconazole 200-300 mg PO or IV bid. Amphotericin 0.5-0.7 mg/kg/d IV. Caspofungin 70 mg/d IV × 1, then 50 mg/d.	Ganciclovir 5 mg/kg IV bid × 2-3 wk or valganciclovir 900 mg bid × 3 wk, then 900 mg/d (when able to swallow). Foscarnet 40-60 mg/kg q8h × 2-3 wk. Efficacy of antiviral treatment is 75%.	Acyclovir 200-800 mg PO 5x/d or 5 mg/kg IV q8h × 2-3 wk or valacyclovir 1 g PO tid (when able to swallow).	Prednisone 40 mg/day PO × 7-14 d, then taper < 10 mg/wk. Consider fluconazole prophylaxis with prednisone course. Thalidomide 200 mg PO daily. Corticosteroids by intralesional injection.
Maintenance	Fluconazole 100 mg/d PO (indicated with frequent or severe occurrences). Lower dosage or less frequent dosing may reduce resistance.	Maintenance treatment is arbitrary. May await relapse, then ganciclovir 5 mg/kg/d IV. Possible role for oral ganciclovir.	Maintenance treatment is arbitrary. Acyclovir 200-400 mg PO 3-5x daily.	None.

Modified from Bartlett JG, Gallant JE: *Medical management of HIV infection*, Baltimore, 2003, Johns Hopkins University, Division of Infectious Diseases and AIDS Service.
CMV, cytomegalovirus; *HSV*, herpes simplex virus; *IV*, intravenously; *PO*, per os.

BOX 51-1

CAUSES OF CHOLESTASIS IN PATIENTS WITH HIV

Medications
  Antiretrovirals
  Antimicrobials including macrolides, trimethoprim-sulfamethoxazole,
    pentamidine, azole antifungals, isoniazid, rifampin, and pyrazinamide
Infections
  Bacteria: *Bartonella henselae*
  Mycobacteria: *Mycobacterium tuberculosis, Mycobacterium avium-intracellulare*
    complex
  Viral: CMV
  Fungal: *Cryptococcus neoformans*
  Parasitic: *Cryptosporidium,* microsporidia
Neoplasms
  Kaposi's sarcoma
  Lymphoma
Causes of cholestasis in non-HIV-infected patients (e.g., alcohol, gallstones)

Modified from Te HS: *Clin Liver Dis* 8(1), 213-228, 2004.

D. DIAGNOSIS
1. Studies have found ultrasound to be up to 98% accurate in predicting normal or abnormal endoscopic retrograde cholangiopancreatogram (ERCP) examinations in patients suspected of having AIDS cholangiopathy.[9] Although other studies have challenged this figure, the low cost and low morbidity make ultrasound the preferred initial imaging test.[10]
2. Magnetic resonance cholangiopancreatography often is used as an intermediate step between ultrasound and ERCP.
3. ERCP remains the gold standard and allows both therapeutic intervention and biopsy. A pathogen is identified up to 75% of the time.[6]
4. Computed tomography (CT) is more sensitive for intrahepatic biliary disease and is the best method for imaging neoplastic disease.[6]

E. MANAGEMENT
1. Sphincterotomy has been shown in several studies to achieve pain relief but has not been reliably shown to decrease cholestatic liver enzymes or improve mortality.[7,11]
2. Antimicrobial management alone is ineffective.[6]

III. DIARRHEA

Diarrhea occurs in a majority of patients with AIDS. Acute diarrhea can occur at any CD4 count, whereas chronic persistent diarrhea, defined as > 3 loose or watery stools a day for > 30 days, is more common at CD4 counts < 200/mm^3. The differential diagnosis for both acute and

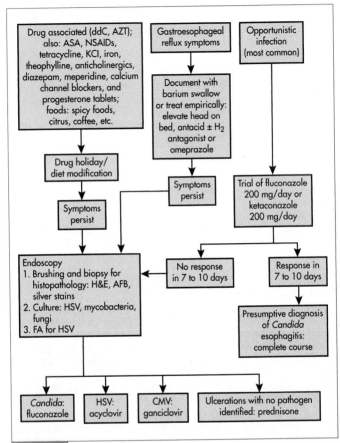

FIG. 51-1
Approach to odynophagia in patients with acquired immunodeficiency syndrome. *AFB*, acid-fast bacillus; *ASA*, aspirin; *AZT*, zidovudine; *CMV*, cytomegalovirus; *ddC*, dideoxycytidine; *FA*, fluorescent antibody stain; *H&E*, hematoxylin and eosin; *HSV*, herpes simplex virus; *NSAIDs*, nonsteroidal antiinflammatory drugs. *(Modified from Bartlett JG, Gallant JE: Medical management of HIV infection, Baltimore, 2003, Johns Hopkins University, Division of Infectious Diseases and AIDS Service.)*

chronic diarrhea includes disorders seen in immunocompetent hosts
(see Chapter 39).

A. ACUTE DIARRHEA

Acute causes of diarrhea unique to patients with HIV include diarrhea
secondary to antiretroviral therapy (especially nelfinavir and amprenavir),
Kaposi's sarcoma, and lymphoma.

B. CHRONIC DIARRHEA

1. **Presentation and differential diagnosis.** Medications, particularly
   protease inhibitors and antibiotics, are important causes of idiopathic
   chronic diarrhea (Table 51-3).
2. **Diagnosis.**
a. See stepwise approach in Box 51-2.[12]
b. Three sets of stool studies yields a diagnosis in 47% of patients,[12,13]
   and endoscopy can yield a diagnosis in almost 50% of the remaining
   cases. Yield is higher and more cost effective if CD4 count is
   < 100/mm.[3,14]
c. Stains for *Cryptosporidium*, microsporidia, and *Isospora* should be
   specified when stool samples are sent to the laboratory because these
   stains are not routinely performed by most laboratories.
d. CT may be helpful in patients who also have fever or abdominal
   pain to diagnose CMV colitis, *Clostridium difficile* colitis, and
   lymphoma.[2]
e. Colonoscopy is best used to investigate CMV, Kaposi's sarcoma, or
   lymphoma.[2]
3. **Management.**
a. Mild to moderate diarrhea may be controlled with frequent small meals;
   caffeine avoidance; and a low-lactose, low-fat, high-fiber diet.[2]

BOX 51-2

DIAGNOSTIC APPROACH TO DIARRHEA ASSOCIATED WITH AIDS

Step 1:
  Review medications.
  3 stool samples for culture, ova, and parasites with stains for *Isospora*,
    microsporidia, and *Cryptosporidium*.
  Stool for *Clostridium difficile* toxin assay, fecal leukocytes and lactoferrin assay,
    and hemoccult.
  Routine blood work for electrolyte disturbances.
  Blood culture if febrile.
  Blood culture for mycobacteria if CD4 count is <100/mm³.
Step 2 (if no pathogen is identified by Step 1):
  Sigmoidoscopy or colonoscopy with mucosal biopsies.
Step 3 (if no pathogen is identified by Step 2):
  Upper endoscopy with duodenal biopsies.

Modified from Cohen J, West AB, Bini EJ: *Gastroenterol Clin North Am* 30(3):637-664, 2001.

TABLE 51-3

CAUSES OF HIV-ASSOCIATED CHRONIC DIARRHEA: PRESENTATION, DIAGNOSIS, AND THERAPY

Pathogen and Incidence in Patients with AIDS	Clinical Presentation	Diagnostic Test*	Stool White Blood Cells	Standard Therapy	Comments
Cryptosporidium 10-30%	Watery diarrhea, cramps, nausea, vomiting, dehydration, wasting	Acid-fast stain	−	ARVs. No regimen works well. Paromomycin 500-1000 mg PO bid. Symptom control.	Best results with ARVs, sometimes with only small CD4 increase.[2]
Cytomegalovirus 15-40%	Diarrhea, cramps, tenesmus, fever, abdominal pain, weight loss, hematochezia	Polymerase chain reaction Hematoxylin and eosin stain of biopsy specimen	+	ARVs. Valganciclovir 900 mg PO bid × 3 wk, then 900 mg PO qd. Ganciclovir 5 mg/kg IV bid × 2 wk, then valganciclovir 900 PO qd. Foscarnet 40-60 mg/kg IV q8h × 2 wk, then 90 mg/kg/d.	Response to treatment is variable.[20]
Idiopathic 20-30%	Usually small volume, controlled with antidiarrheals; weight loss uncommon; can resolve spontaneously	All tests negative	−	Symptom control.	Must rule out Kaposi's sarcoma and lymphoma with large-volume idiopathic diarrhea.[2] Medications, particularly protease inhibitors and antibiotics, are important causes.

Microsporidia: *Enterocytozoon bieneusi* or *Enterocytozoon (septata) intestinalis* 15-30%	Diarrhea, cramps, weight loss, wasting, malabsorption; fever uncommon	Modified trichrome stain (Calcofluor stain)	ARVs. *E. intestinalis* (10-20%): albendazole 400 mg PO bid × > 3 wk. *E. bieneusi* (80-90%): fumagillin 60 mg/d × 14 d (high rate of neutropenia and thrombocytopenia). Symptom control.	ARVs are best therapy. Non-ARV treatment often ineffective.
Mycobacterium avium-intracellulare complex 10-20%	Diarrhea, abdominal pain, weight loss, anemia, night sweats, fever, hepatosplenomegaly	Acid-fast stain Culture Duodenum biopsy	Clarithromycin 500 mg PO bid and ethambutol 15 mg/kg/d. Azithromycin 600 mg/d and ethambutol 15 mg/kg/d +/- rifabutin 300 mg/d. Aspirin or nonsteroidal antiinflammatory drugs for symptoms.	Use 3 drugs for severe disease. Slow response to treatment over weeks.
Mycobacterium tuberculosis	Diarrhea, abdominal pain, fever, weight loss, night sweats, hematochezia	Acid-fast stain Culture	Isoniazid. Rifampin. Pyrazinamide. Ethambutol.	
Cyclospora <1%	Chronic intermittent diarrhea, weight loss	Acid-fast stain	TMP-SMX 1 DS PO bid × 3 d.	
Isospora belli 1-3%	Profuse watery diarrhea, cramps, eosinophilia, malabsorption	Acid-fast stain	TMP-SMX 3-4 DS PO per day. Pyrimethamine 50-75 mg/day PO × 7-10 d.	Most respond quickly to therapy. Most common in Haiti.

cont'd

51

GASTROINTESTINAL DISORDERS IN PATIENTS WITH HIV

TABLE 51-3

CAUSES OF HIV-ASSOCIATED CHRONIC DIARRHEA: PRESENTATION, DIAGNOSIS, AND THERAPY—cont'd

Pathogen and Incidence in Patients with AIDS	Clinical Presentation	Diagnostic Test*	Stool White Blood Cells	Standard Therapy	Comments
Histoplasmosis	Diarrhea, hematochezia, weight loss, fever, abdominal pain	GMS stain Fungal culture of biopsy Urine antigen	–	Amphotericin B 0.7-1 mg/kg IV, then itraconazole 200 mg PO bid. Itraconazole 200 mg PO tid × 3 d, then bid.	
Herpes simplex virus	Proctitis, distal colitis, diarrhea, tenesmus, rectal pain, hematochezia	Viral culture	+ or –	Acyclovir 200 mg PO 5×/d. Acyclovir 400 mg PO tid. Famciclovir 500 mg PO bid or valacyclovir 1 g PO bid.	
Giardia lamblia 1-3%	Enteritis, watery diarrhea, malabsorption, bloating, flatulence	Wet mount Enzyme-linked immunosorbent assay	–	Metronidazole 250 mg PO tid × 10 d.	Travelers, recent immigrants, or those with ingestion of untreated surface water.
Entamoeba histolytica 1-3%	Invasive colitis, cramps, hematochezia, self-limited diarrhea; most asymptomatic carriers	Wet mount	+ or –	Metronidazole 500-750 mg PO or IV tid × 5-10 d (then iodoquinol 650 mg PO tid × 21 d or paromomycin 500 mg PO qid × 7 d).	Travelers or recent immigrants.

Modified from Cohen J, West AB, Bini EJ: *Gastroenterol Clin North Am* 30(3):637-664, 2001, with additional data from Bartlett JG, Gallant JE: *Medical management of HIV infection*, Baltimore, 2003, Johns Hopkins University, Division of Infectious Diseases and AIDS Service.

AIDS, acquired immunodeficiency syndrome; *ARV*, antiretroviral; *DS*, double strength; *GMS*, gomori methamine silver; *HIV*, human immunodeficiency virus; *IV*, intravenously; *PO*, per os; *TMP-SMX*, trimethoprim-sulfamethoxazole.

*Parentheses indicate secondary means of detection or therapy.

b. Symptomatic control with antimotility agents (e.g., diphenoxylate and atropine, loperamide, tincture of opium) can be used when inflammatory and invasive causes of diarrhea have been ruled out. These agents can be used at maximal dosages with safety.

c. Bulking agents such as fiber supplements may also be useful.

d. A trial of pancreatic enzyme supplementation is worthwhile in refractory cases because AIDS-associated diarrhea can be associated with fat malabsorption.[15]

IV. PANCREATITIS

A. EPIDEMIOLOGY

1. Acute pancreatitis is 35 to 800 times more common in patients with AIDS than in the general population and has an annual incidence between 0.7% and 14%.[16]

2. Risk of pancreatitis increases with advancing HIV disease.[16]

B. PRESENTATION

Presentation is similar to that of pancreatitis in non-HIV infected patients, with symptoms of epigastric pain, nausea, vomiting, and low-grade fever.

C. DIFFERENTIAL DIAGNOSIS (Box 51-3)

1. Several medications used in HIV-infected patients can cause pancreatitis, of which dideoxyinosine (ddI) and pentamidine have been the most studied.

2. The rate of pancreatitis with ddI is 4.4% to 7%, with a fatality rate of 6%.[17] ddI-associated pancreatitis typically occurs in the first 6 months of therapy but does not occur immediately after drug initiation.

BOX 51-3

CAUSES OF PANCREATITIS IN HIV-INFECTED PATIENTS[2,16]

Medications
  NRTIs, especially ddI
    ddI, dideoxycytidine, didehydrodideoxythymidine
    May be a result of NRTI-associated lactic acidosis
  Protease inhibitor–induced hypertriglyceridemia
  Pentamidine (directly toxic to pancreatic islet cells, leading to glucose abnormalities)
  Others: sulfonamides, corticosteroids, octreotide, isoniazid, rifampin, paromomycin
Infections: cytomegalovirus, toxoplasmosis, *Mycobacterium avium-intracellulare* complex, tuberculosis, cryptosporidiosis, HIV
Causes of pancreatitis in non–HIV-infected patients (see Chapter 31)

ddI, dideoxyinosine; *HIV*, human immunodeficiency virus; *NRTI*, nucleoside reverse transcriptase inhibitor.

51

GASTROINTESTINAL DISORDERS IN PATIENTS WITH HIV

3. Pancreatic involvement of opportunistic infections usually is associated with disseminated infection.[16]

D. DIAGNOSIS

1. Pancreatitis is a clinical diagnosis with associated elevations in amylase and lipase.

2. Note that 60% of HIV-positive patients have mildly elevated amylase or lipase (14% have elevations more than twice the upper limit of normal), without clinical pancreatitis.[18]

3. Lactic acid levels should be checked, especially in patients taking nucleoside reverse transcriptase inhibitors.

4. Abdominal CT or ultrasound can provide additional information in patients with suspected pseudocyst, hemorrhage, necrosis, or biliary obstruction.

E. MANAGEMENT

1. Supportive management with fluids and pain control is the mainstay of treatment (see Chapter 31).

2. All pancreatotoxic medications should be stopped immediately.

PEARLS AND PITFALLS

- Dysphagia caused by *Candida* esophagitis usually is described as a feeling of food getting stuck in the chest, not in the throat.

- Herpes is a rare cause of esophageal ulcers (5%) that is exquisitely painful.

- Chronic large-volume diarrhea without a known cause must be investigated to rule out lymphoma or Kaposi's sarcoma.

- Disseminated *Mycobacterium avium-intracellulare* complex may present as diffuse abdominal pain.

- Nucleoside reverse transcriptase inhibitors (particularly ddI, dideoxycytidine, and didehydrodideoxythymidine) can all cause pancreatitis.

- A high degree of suspicion of medication-induced pancreatitis is essential in patients presenting with abdominal pain, and lactic acid levels should be checked, especially in patients on nucleoside reverse transcriptase inhibitors.

REFERENCES

1. Vazquez JA: Therapeutic options for the management of oropharyngeal and esophageal candidiasis in HIV/AIDS patients, *HIV Clin Trials* 1(1):47-59, 2000. C

2. Bartlett JG, Gallant JE: *Medical management of HIV infection,* Baltimore, Md, 2003, Johns Hopkins University Division of Infectious Diseases and AIDS Service. C

3. Powderly WG, Finkelstein D, Feinberg J, et al: A randomized trial comparing fluconazole with clotrimazole troches for the prevention of fungal infections in patients with advanced human immunodeficiency virus infection. NIAID AIDS Clinical Trials Group, *N Engl J Med* 332(11):700-705, 1995. A

4. Schuman P, Capps L, Peng G, et al: Weekly fluconazole for the prevention of mucosal candidiasis in women with HIV infection. A randomized, double-blind,

placebo-controlled trial. Terry Beirn Community Programs for Clinical Research on AIDS, *Ann Intern Med* 126(9):689-696, 1997. A

5. Te HS: Cholestasis in HIV-infected patients, *Clin Liver Dis* 8(1), 2004. C
6. Mahajani RV, Uzer MF: Cholangiopathy in HIV-infected patients, *Clin Liver Dis* 3(3):669-684, 1999. C
7. Bouche H, Housset C, Dumont JL, et al: AIDS-related cholangitis: diagnostic features and course in 15 patients, *J Hepatol* 17(1):34-39, 1993. B
8. Pol S, Romana CA, Richard S, et al: Microsporidia infection in patients with the human immunodeficiency virus and unexplained cholangitis, *N Engl J Med* 328(2):95-99, 1993. B
9. Daly CA, Padley SP: Sonographic prediction of a normal or abnormal ERCP in suspected AIDS related sclerosing cholangitis, *Clin Radiol* 51(9):618-621, 1996. B
10. Urbain D, Jeanmart J, Lemone M, et al: Cholestasis in patients with the acquired immune deficiency syndrome: comparison between ultrasonographic and cholangiographic findings, *Am J Gastroenterol* 86(5):574-576, 1991. B
11. Cello JP, Chan MF: Long-term follow-up of endoscopic retrograde cholangiopancreatography sphincterotomy for patients with acquired immune deficiency syndrome papillary stenosis, *Am J Med* 99(6):600-603, 1995. B
12. Cohen J, West AB, Bini EJ: Infectious diarrhea in human immunodeficiency virus, *Gastroenterol Clin North Am* 30(3):637-664, 2001. C
13. Blanshard C, Francis N, Gazzard BG: Investigation of chronic diarrhoea in acquired immunodeficiency syndrome. A prospective study of 155 patients, *Gut* 39(96):824-832, 1996. B
14. Bini EJ, Cohen J: Diagnostic yield and cost-effectiveness of endoscopy in chronic human immunodeficiency virus-related diarrhea, *Gastrointest Endosc* 48(4):354-361, 1998. B
15. Poles MA, Fuerst M, McGowan I, et al: HIV-related diarrhea is multifactorial and fat malabsorption is commonly present, independent of HAART, *Am J Gastroenterol* 96(6):1831-1837, 2001. B
16. Dassopoulos T, Ehrenpreis ED: Acute pancreatitis in human immunodeficiency virus-infected patients: a review. *Am J Med* 107(1):78-84, 1999. C
17. Schindzielorz A, Pike I, Daniels M, Pacelli L, Smaldone L: Rates and risk factors for adverse events associated with didanosine in the expanded access program, *Clin Infect Dis* 19(6):1076-1083, 1994. B
18. Argiris A, Mathur-Wagh U, Wilets I, Mildvan D: Abnormalities of serum amylase and lipase in HIV-positive patients, *Am J Gastroenterol* 94(5):1248-1252, 1999. B
19. Wilcox CM, Alexander LN, Clark WS, Thompson SE III: Fluconazole compared with endoscopy for human immunodeficiency virus-infected patients with esophageal symptoms, *Gastroenterology* 110(6):1803-1809, 1996. A
20. Reed EC, Wolford JL, Kopecky KJ, et al: Ganciclovir for the treatment of cytomegalovirus gastroenteritis in bone marrow transplant patients. A randomized, placebo-controlled trial, *Ann Intern Med* 112(7):505-510, 1990. A

51

Systemic Manifestations of the Human Immunodeficiency Virus

David Riedel, MD; and Cynthia L. Sears, MD

> **FAST FACTS**
>
> - Opportunistic infections (OIs) are the major cause of morbidity and mortality in patients infected with the human immunodeficiency virus (HIV); incidence is inversely correlated with CD4 count.
> - Cytomegalovirus (CMV) retinitis affects 30% of HIV-infected patients with CD4 counts < 50/mm³ and is associated with significant visual morbidity; more than one third of eyes at 1 year progress to legal blindness (20/200 vision).[1,2]
> - *Mycobacterium avium-intracellulare* complex (MAC) is one of the three most common OIs afflicting HIV-infected patients (*Pneumocystis carinii* pneumonia and esophageal candidiasis are the other 2).[3]
> - The clinical definition of HIV-associated fever of unknown origin (FUO) is similar to that of classic FUO; however, unlike classic FUO, the causes of FUO in HIV-infected patients usually are infectious diseases.[4,5]

HIV affects the body in myriad ways, having both direct and indirect effects via destruction of the immune system. In the latter case, the resultant immunosuppression permits the development of OIs, the defining feature of the acquired immunodeficiency syndrome (AIDS). The majority of OIs are encountered when HIV is most advanced and immune suppression is greatest. Table 52-1 presents HIV-associated conditions and the approximate CD4 count at which each usually occurs. This chapter addresses two common OIs (CMV retinitis and MAC disease) not covered elsewhere, and a common diagnostic problem: FUO in the HIV-infected patient.

I. CMV RETINITIS

A. EPIDEMIOLOGY

CMV retinitis occurs primarily with advanced immunosuppression (i.e., CD4 < 50/mm³).

B. PRESENTATION

Symptoms of CMV retinitis are nonspecific, and patients may be asymptomatic initially.[6] Complaints include photopsia (flashing lights), scotomata (blind spots), floaters, and blurring or loss of central vision.[6,7] Patients do not have conjunctivitis, photophobia, or pain.[6]

TABLE 52-1

CD4 COUNT AND HIV-ASSOCIATED COMPLICATIONS

CD4 Cell Count	Infectious Complications	Noninfectious Complications
> 500/mm³	Acute retroviral syndrome Candidal vaginitis	Persistent generalized lymphadenopathy Guillain-Barré syndrome Myopathy Aseptic meningitis

200-500/mm³	Bacterial pneumonia
	Pulmonary TB
	Herpes zoster
	Oropharyngeal candidiasis
	Cryptosporidiosis (self-limited)
	Kaposi's sarcoma
	Oral hairy leukoplakia
	Cervical intraepithelial neoplasia
	Cervical cancer
	B-cell lymphoma
		Anemia
		Mononeuritis multiplex
		Idiopathic thrombocytopenic
		  purpura
		Hodgkin's lymphoma
		Lymphocytic interstitial
		  pneumonitis

< 200/mm³	*Pneumocystis carinii* pneumonia Disseminated histoplasmosis and coccidioidomycosis Miliary or extrapulmonary TB	Wasting Peripheral neuropathy HIV-associated dementia Cardiomyopathy Vacuolar myelopathy Progressive polyradiculopathy Non-Hodgkin's lymphoma
< 100/mm³	Disseminated herpes simplex CNS toxoplasmosis Cryptococcosis Cryptosporidiosis (chronic) Candidal esophagitis	

< 50/mm³	Progressive multifocal
	  leukoencephalopathy
	Primary CNS lymphoma
	Disseminated cytomegalovirus
	Disseminated *Mycobacterium*
	  avium-intracellulare complex	

Modified from Bartlett JG, Gallant JE: *2004 medical management of HIV infection,* Baltimore, 2004, Johns Hopkins University, Division of Infectious Diseases and AIDS Service.
CNS, central nervous system; *HIV,* human immunodeficiency virus; *TB,* tuberculosis.

C. CAUSES

CMV retinitis results from reactivation of latent CMV disease and subsequent viremic spread to the eye.[1]

D. DIAGNOSIS

1. Diagnosis is clinical, via dilated funduscopic examination by an ophthalmologist. CMV lesions sometimes are described as cotton-wool spots and consist of yellow-white areas of retinal necrosis and edema (sometimes hemorrhagic) that follow a vascular distribution.

2. The diagnosis of CMV retinitis should prompt thorough evaluation for extraocular CMV disease; likewise, detection of extraocular CMV disease necessitates an ophthalmologic examination.

E. TREATMENT

1. Treatment generally is divided into induction and maintenance regimens.

a. Induction therapy consists of intraocular ganciclovir implant and valganciclovir 900 mg orally (PO) twice a day (to prevent spread to the other eye). Highly active antiretroviral therapy (HAART) should be initiated as well.[1]

b. The maintenance regimen includes both valganciclovir 900 mg PO daily and intraocular ganciclovir implants, which are replaced every 6 months. Induction therapy is for 14 to 21 days, whereas maintenance therapy is either lifelong or continued until immune reconstitution is achieved with HAART.[1]

2. Relapse or presentation in the contralateral eye, especially after 6 months of therapy, is a sign of ganciclovir resistance.[1]

F. PROGNOSIS AND MORTALITY

CMV retinitis is associated with a significant amount of visual morbidity, with more than one third of eyes progressing to 20/200 vision (i.e., legal blindness) at 1 year.[2] Complications of CMV retinitis include blindness, retinal detachment, relapse, and immune recovery uveitis (associated with HAART).[1] Any visual loss occurring before treatment usually is irreversible.

II. MAC DISEASE

A. EPIDEMIOLOGY

The major risk factor for development of MAC disease is the level of immunosuppression, with the majority of cases occurring with CD4 < 50/mm^3.

B. PRESENTATION

1. Symptoms of MAC disease are varied and nonspecific. Nearly all organ systems may be involved, but those most often affected include blood, bone marrow, liver, spleen, intestinal tract, and lymph nodes. Patients most often have a protracted illness with persistent, high, spiking fevers (often in the evening) and weight loss in association with night sweats. Intractable diarrhea with significant malabsorption is common, as is abdominal pain.

2. Laboratory data may demonstrate evidence of either hepatic (e.g., elevated alkaline phosphatase) or bone marrow (e.g., pancytopenia) involvement. The pancytopenia often is associated with intractable anemia that necessitates frequent transfusions.

C. CAUSES

MAC disease is caused by two related species: *M. avium* and *M. intracellulare*. Disseminated MAC infection results from primary acquisition (not reactivation) from the environment via colonization of the gastrointestinal or respiratory tract. In an early study in patients with CD4 < 50/mm³, if MAC was found colonizing either the gastrointestinal or respiratory tract, the risk of subsequent bacteremia within 1 year was about 60%.[8]

D. DIAGNOSIS

Diagnosis is verified by blood culture. The sensitivity of blood cultures is 90% to 95%, although positive results may take from several days up to a month.[1] Ninety-eight percent of autopsy-confirmed cases of MAC have positive blood cultures.[9] With MAC dissemination, organ involvement is common; biopsies of liver, lymph nodes, small bowel, or bone marrow usually are positive.

E. TREATMENT

1. Treatment is initiated with ethambutol 15 mg/kg/day PO plus either clarithromycin 500 mg PO twice a day or azithromycin 600 mg PO once a day.[1] One study showed clearance of bacteremia after 16 weeks of treatment to be significantly greater with clarithromycin than azithromycin (85.7% vs. 37.5%)[10]; however, a second study found no significant difference in clearance of bacteremia at 24 weeks and similar mortality.[11] With more severe disease or symptoms, a third drug (ciprofloxacin, levofloxacin, rifabutin, or amikacin) often is added,[1] although these regimens are not well studied.

2. Blood cultures often remain positive for many weeks (median time to clearance is 16 weeks) after initiation of therapy, but follow-up blood cultures usually are not performed.

3. Treatment duration is at least 1 year in patients who have immune reconstitution with HAART; without immune recovery, therapy is lifelong.

F. PROGNOSIS AND MORTALITY

In the pre-HAART era, 23% of patients with untreated bacteremia died within 28 days of diagnosis, whereas treatment with antimycobacterials nearly doubled survival time (from 139 to 263 days).[12]

III. HIV-ASSOCIATED FUO

A. EPIDEMIOLOGY

FUO in HIV-infected patients is common; one series reported 3.5% of HIV admissions satisfying FUO criteria.[13] The patient's ethnicity and travel history must be considered in the differential diagnosis for FUO; for instance, visceral leishmaniasis is a cause of FUO in Western Europe but uncommon in the United States.

B. PRESENTATION

The general criteria for HIV-associated FUO are similar to those of classic FUO and are derived from Durack and Street[14] (Box 52-1).

C. CAUSES

HIV infection itself is **rarely** the cause of FUO. Common causes of FUO in HIV-infected patients (based on studies from the United States and

---

BOX 52-1

CRITERIA FOR FEVER OF UNKNOWN ORIGIN IN PATIENTS WITH HIV

Temperature >101° F on multiple occasions.
Fever of > 4 wk duration for outpatients, > 3 d duration for inpatients.
Diagnosis remains uncertain after 3 d despite appropriate investigation.

Modified from Durack DT, Street AC: Fever of unknown origin: reexamined and redefined, *Curr Clin Top Infect Dis* 11:35, 1991.

BOX 52-2

COMMON CAUSES OF FEVER OF UNKNOWN ORIGIN IN PATIENTS WITH HIV

Disseminated *Mycobacterium avium-intracellulare* complex
Tuberculosis (pulmonary and extrapulmonary)
Pneumocystis jiroveci pneumonia (PCP)
Histoplasmosis
Disseminated cytomegalovirus infection
Visceral leishmaniasis*
Lymphoma
Esophageal candidiasis
Drug fever
Sinusitis
Cryptococcosis
Bartonella infection

Modified from Armstrong WS, Katz JT, Kazanjian PH: *Clin Infect Dis* 28:341, 1999; Lozano F et al: *Eur J Clin Microbiol Infect Dis* 15:705, 1996; and Mayo J, Collazos J, Martinez E: *Scand J Infect Dis* 29:327, 1997.
*Reported from endemic regions in Europe.

Europe) are listed in Box 52-2. Multiple causes for FUO are found in 15.8% to 19% of patients, and no cause is found in 6.3% to 19%.[5,13]

D. DIAGNOSIS (Fig. 52-1)

1. Knowledge of both the patient's most recent CD4 count and infectious diseases endemic to the region is crucial in developing a differential diagnosis.

2. Imaging.

   a. It is important to note that fever can precede the development of radiographic findings in both *Pneumocystis jiroveci* pneumonia and tuberculosis; chest radiographs can be normal in 20% of the former and 40% of the latter.[16]

   b. The yield of head, thoracic, and abdominal computed tomography scans in obtaining a diagnosis is 17%, 50%, and 19%, respectively.[15] Occasionally, magnetic resonance imaging of the brain with contrast may yield a diagnosis (e.g., cerebral toxoplasmosis).

   c. An echocardiogram should be obtained in patients at risk for endocarditis, such as intravenous drug abusers.[15]

52

SYSTEMIC MANIFESTATIONS OF HIV

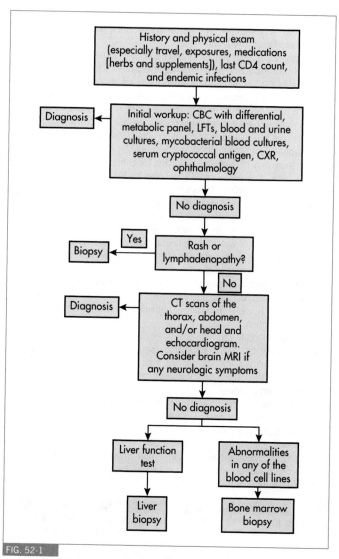

FIG. 52-1

Diagnostic algorithm for fever of unknown origin in a patient with HIV. *CBC*, complete blood cell count; *CT*, computed tomography; *CXR*, chest radiograph; *LFTs*, liver function tests; *MRI*, magnetic resonance imaging.

3. Histopathology.

a. Localizing abnormalities on physical examination, such as a rash or lymphadenopathy, warrant biopsy.

b. Should the diagnosis remain uncertain, liver or bone marrow biopsy should be considered. As in HIV-negative patients, liver biopsy in HIV-associated FUO is most useful when there are abnormal liver function tests (especially elevated alkaline phosphatase); it has been reported to have a 45% diagnostic yield (higher in cases of disseminated MAC). Bone marrow biopsy is most helpful if there are peripheral cytopenias; a diagnosis is obtained in this way in about 25% of cases.[15]

4. Occasionally, an empiric treatment trial may be attempted, particularly when there is a high clinical suspicion for either MAC or tuberculosis; in this case, a response should be noted for MAC within 10 days and for tuberculosis within 14 days.[17]

5. An empiric trial of drug discontinuation may also be attempted because some medicines used for prophylaxis (e.g., sulfa drugs) or treatment in HIV-infected patients can produce fever.

6. Finally, a period of watchful waiting and careful observation may be prudent because certain diseases declare themselves over time.

E. PROGNOSIS AND MORTALITY
A diagnosis is reached in about 80% of cases of HIV-associated FUO.[17] Of those in whom no cause for fever is found, nearly one third resolve spontaneously; however, survival for patients with undiagnosed FUO is low (58% at 6 months).[15]

PEARLS AND PITFALLS
- Blood cultures for MAC are the best diagnostic tests and should be obtained on all HIV-infected patients with low CD4 counts who are admitted with fever or systemic symptoms, but they can take up to a month to turn positive.
- Fever can precede the development of radiographic findings in both *Pneumocystis jiroveci* pneumonia and tuberculosis; chest radiographs can be normal in 20% of the former and 40% of the latter.[16]
- In the evaluation of HIV-associated FUO, noninvasive diagnostic methods should be exhausted before more invasive means are attempted because the former often secure the diagnosis, and the latter may cause morbidity.[5]

REFERENCES
1. Bartlett JG, Gallant JE: *2004 medical management of HIV infection,* Baltimore, 2004, Johns Hopkins University, Division of Infectious Diseases and AIDS Service. C
2. Kempen JH et al: Risk of vision loss in patients with cytomegalovirus retinitis and the acquired immunodeficiency syndrome, *Arch Ophthalmol* 121:466, 2003. B
3. Kaplan JE et al: Epidemiology of human immunodeficiency virus–associated opportunistic infections in the United States in the era of highly active anti-retroviral therapy, *Clin Infect Dis* 30:S5, 2000. C

4. Mayo J, Collazos J, Martinez E: Fever of unknown origin in the setting of HIV infection: guidelines for a rational approach, *AIDS Patient Care STDs* 12:373, 1998. D

5. Armstrong WS, Katz JT, Kazanjian PH: Human immunodeficiency virus–associated fever of unknown origin: a study of 70 patients in the United States and review, *Clin Infect Dis* 28:341, 1999. B

6. Whitley RJ et al: Guidelines for the treatment of cytomegalovirus diseases in patients with AIDS in the era of potent antiretroviral therapy, *Arch Intern Med* 158:957, 1998. D

7. Jacobson MA: Treatment of cytomegalovirus retinitis in patients with the acquired immunodeficiency syndrome, *N Engl J Med* 337:105, 1997. C

8. Chin DP et al: Mycobacterium avium complex in the respiratory or gastrointestinal tract and the risk of M. avium complex bacteremia in patients with human immunodeficiency virus infection, *J Infect Dis* 169:289, 1994. B

9. Hawkins CC et al: Mycobacterium avium complex infections in patients with the acquired immunodeficiency syndrome, *Ann Intern Med* 105:184, 1986. B

10. Ward TT et al: Randomized, open-label trial of azithromycin plus ethambutol vs. clarithromycin plus ethambutol as therapy for Mycobacterium avium complex bacteremia in patients with human immunodeficiency virus infection, *Clin Infect Dis* 27:1278, 1998. B

11. Dunne M: A randomized, double-blind trial comparing azithromycin and clarithromycin in the treatment of disseminated Mycobacterium avium infection in patients with human immunodeficiency virus, *Clin Infect Dis* 31:1245, 2000. B

12. Chin DP et al: The impact of Mycobacterium avium complex bacteremia and its treatment on survival of AIDS patients: a prospective study, *J Infect Dis* 170:578, 1994. B

13. Lozano F et al: Prospective evaluation of fever of unknown origin in patients infected with the human immunodeficiency virus, *Eur J Clin Microbiol Infect Dis* 15:705, 1996. B

14. Durack DT, Street AC: Fever of unknown origin: reexamined and redefined, *Curr Clin Top Infect Dis* 11:35, 1991. C

15. Mayo J, Collazos J, Martinez E: Fever of unknown origin in the HIV-infected patient: new scenario for an old problem, *Scand J Infect Dis* 29:327, 1997. C

16. Sullivan M, Feinberg J, Bartlett JG: Fever in patients with HIV infection, *Infect Dis Clin North Am* 10:149, 1996. C

17. Sepkowitz KA: FUO and AIDS, *Curr Clin Top Infect Dis* 19:1, 1999. C

52

SYSTEMIC MANIFESTATIONS OF HIV

Fever of Unknown Origin

Scott Kim, MD; Rachel Damico, MD, PhD; and Paul Auwaerter, MD

I. EPIDEMIOLOGY

1. The majority of identifiable causes of FUO can be grouped into four specific disease categories: infections, neoplasms, noninfectious inflammatory diseases, and miscellaneous causes.[3]
2. The prevalence of different causes has changed over the past five decades including an increase in the relative proportion of patients who remain undiagnosed because of improvements in laboratory and radiologic diagnostic techniques (Fig. 53-1).[4]
3. FUO often is subdivided into four subcategories: classic FUO, FUO associated with the human immunodeficiency virus (HIV; see Chapter 52), neutropenic FUO, and nosocomial FUO (Table 53-1).[5]
4. Tuberculosis, endocarditis, and intraabdominal abscesses are the most commonly reported infectious causes of FUO, although more extensive use of computed tomography (CT) scanning is leading to earlier diagnosis of intraabdominal abscesses. The most common malignancies implicated in FUO are Hodgkin's lymphoma and non-Hodgkin's lymphoma. Temporal arteritis accounts for 15% to 16% of FUO diagnoses in older adults.[5]

II. CLINICAL PRESENTATION

1. Because FUO is caused by a wide range of entities, the clinical manifestations may be protean. Associated clinical signs such as cardiac murmurs, skin lesions, lymphadenopathy, temporal artery

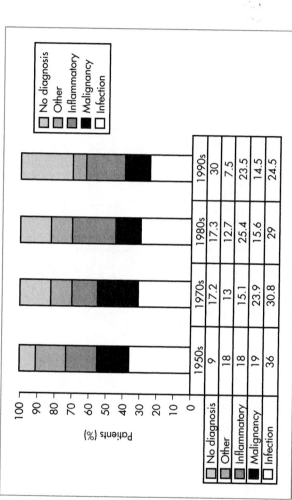

	1950s	1970s	1980s	1990s
No diagnosis	9	17.2	17.3	30
Other	18	13	12.7	7.5
Inflammatory	18	15.1	25.4	23.5
Malignancy	19	23.9	15.6	14.5
Infection	36	30.8	29	24.5

FIG. 53-1

Trends in the causes of fever of unknown origin. *(Modified from Mourad O et al: Arch Intern Med 163:545-551, 2003.)*

53

FEVER OF UNKNOWN ORIGIN

TABLE 53-1

CLASSIFICATION OF FEVER OF UNKNOWN ORIGIN

Category	Patient Population	Minimal Duration of Investigation	Typical Causes
HIV associated	Confirmed HIV positive	3 d of inpatient investigation or 4 wk of outpatient studies	Mycobacterial infection (*Mycobacterium avium-intracellulare* and *Mycobacterium tuberculosis*), non-Hodgkin's disease, drug fever
Neutropenic	Absolute neutrophil count ≤ 500/mm^3 or in decline	3 d	Bacterial infections, aspergillosis, candidemia
Nosocomial	Hospitalized in an acute care setting (not admitted with infection)	3 d	Pulmonary embolus, sinusitis, *Clostridium difficile* colitis, drug fever
Classic	All others with fever ≥ 3 wk	3 d of inpatient investigation or 3 outpatient visits	Infection, neoplasm, noninfectious inflammatory diseases

Modified from Durack DT, Street AC: Fever of unknown origin: reexamined and redefined. In Remington JS, Swartz MN, eds: *Current topics in infectious diseases*, Cambridge, Mass, 1991, Blackwell.
HIV, human immunodeficiency virus.

thickening or tenderness, organomegaly, or constitutional signs of decline including weight loss should be sought aggressively.

2. Temporal and physiologic patterns of the fever occasionally are useful in suggesting a diagnosis.[5]

a. Persistently elevated body temperature with minimal variation ($< 1°$ F per day) can be seen with rickettsial infections or lobar pneumonia.

b. Intermittent or hectic fever, an exaggeration of normal circadian rhythms, can be seen with endocarditis, abscesses, malignancies, and drug fever.

c. Double-quotidian fevers (i.e., two extreme variations per day) are associated with Still's disease and, less commonly, right-sided gonococcal endocarditis and visceral leishmaniasis (kala-azar).[6]

d. Relapsing fevers, recurring over intervals of days or weeks, can be characteristic of a wide variety of causes (Box 53-1).

e. Tertian fevers, fever paroxysms on cycles of days 1 and 3, are typically seen with synchronization of *Plasmodium vivax* red blood cell lysis.[6] These are generally not seen in travelers but rather in residents of endemic regions with semi-immunity to malaria.

f. Quartan fevers, paroxysms occurring on cycles of days 1 and 4, are seen with *Plasmodium malariae*. Like tertian fevers, these are generally seen in residents of endemic regions with semi-immunity to malaria.

g. Pel-Ebstein fevers are episodic fevers lasting 3 to 10 days with intervening afebrile periods of similar duration. Classically these fevers are associated with Hodgkin's and other types of lymphomas.[6]

h. Relative bradycardia, defined as a lower heart rate than expected for the temperature, is also known as temperature-pulse dissociation. The fever must be greater than $102°$ F, with an observed pulse less than the expected pulse, as defined by the following algorithm: Normal pulse = ([Last digit of $°F - 1$] × 10) + 100; for example, for $104°$ F, $([4 - 1] × 10) + 100 = 130$ bpm. The patients should not be on beta-blockers. Causes include atypical pneumonia, Q fever (*Coxiella* infection), psittacosis, leptospirosis, brucellosis, and drug fever.

3. Some common causes.

a. Infections.

(1) *Mycobacterium tuberculosis* (see Chapter 56).

(2) Abscesses.

(a) Liver abscesses cause symptoms of right upper quadrant tenderness, jaundice, and hepatomegaly in 50% of patients; an equal number present only with fever. The liver is involved either through hematogenous spread or by contiguous involvement from another intraabdominal source. Amebic abscesses (*Entamoeba histolytica*) commonly involve the liver, whereas hepatosplenic candidiasis is seen in patients recovering from chemotherapy-induced neutropenia.

BOX 53-1
RELAPSING FEVER
INFECTIOUS CAUSES
Babesiosis
Blastomycosis
Borrelia recurrentis
Brucellosis
Histoplasmosis
Rat bite fever
Syphilis
Coccidioidomycosis
Colorado tick fever
Cytomegalovirus
Dengue fever
Epstein-Barr virus
Trench fever
Visceral leishmaniasis
Lymphocytic choriomeningitis
Leptospirosis
Lyme disease
Malaria
Q fever (*Coxiella burnetii*)
Tuberculosis
Typhus
NONINFECTIOUS CAUSES
Drug fever
Behçet's disease
Still's disease
Crohn's disease
Familial Mediterranean fever
Systemic lupus erythematosus
Hyperimmunoglobulin D syndrome

Modified from Cunha B: *Infect Dis Clin North Am* 10:33, 1996.

   (b) Splenic abscesses are far less common than liver abscesses, but
       if untreated they have a high mortality. Only half of patients
       with splenic abscesses have left-sided pain and splenomegaly.
   (c) Perinephric abscesses usually develop as a consequence of
       ascending urinary tract infections. Persistent fever and sterile
       pyuria may suggest a perinephric abscess.
(3) Bacterial endocarditis (see Chapter 57). If infectious endocarditis
    is suspected but blood cultures remain negative after 72 hours,
    fastidious and culture-negative organisms should be considered and
    sought by prolonging incubation of blood cultures and obtaining
    serologic studies for *Coxiella burnetii*, *Bartonella*, and *Brucella*.

TABLE 53-2
LABORATORY STUDIES FOR ORGANISMS CAUSING ENDOCARDITIS

Organism	Approach
Abiotrophia species	Growth on supplemented media
Bartonella	Serologic assays
Coxiella burnetii (Q fever)	Serologic assays
HACEK organisms (*Haemophilus, Actinobacillus, Cardiobacterium, Eikenella, Kingella*)	Prolonged incubation of blood cultures
Chlamydia (*Chlamydia psittaci*)	Serologic assays
Tropheryma whippelii	
Legionella	Subculture and serologic assays
Fungi	
Candida	Bacterial or fungal blood cultures
Histoplasma	Urine or serum *Histoplasma* antigen
Aspergillus	Serologic tests not approved; rare

Modified from Mylonakis E, Calderwood SB: *N Engl J Med* 345:1318, 2001.

Rarely, fungal and mycobacterial organisms can cause endocarditis (Table 53-2).

b. Malignancies.

(1) **Lymphoma.** Malignancies of reticuloendothelial origin (lymphomas and leukemias) are the cancers most commonly identified as causes of FUO. The diagnosis of lymphoma is based on histologic evaluation of tissue, typically an excisional biopsy of an abnormal lymph node. Fine-needle aspiration is suboptimal because tissue architecture is lost.

(2) **Renal cell carcinoma** (hypernephroma). The classic triad of flank pain, gross hematuria, and a palpable abdominal mass is present in only 10% of cases, whereas microscopic hematuria is seen in more than half.

c. Noninfectious inflammatory diseases.

(1) **Temporal arteritis and giant cell arteritis.** Classic manifestations of giant cell arteritis include headache, fever, anemia, and an elevated erythrocyte sedimentation rate. Abrupt loss of vision, known as amaurosis fugax, and scalp tenderness along the temporal arteries are seen in some. Patients may have the systemic symptoms of polymyalgia rheumatica, including proximal muscle stiffness and pain. In some series, giant cell arteritis is responsible for FUO in 15% to 16% of patients 65 years and older.[3]

(2) **Still's disease** (adult-onset juvenile rheumatoid arthritis). Still's disease is a clinical diagnosis of exclusion suggested by the triad of arthritis or arthralgia, high fevers (double-quotidian pattern), and evanescent rash, particularly on the trunk. Fevers may antedate manifestations of arthritis by a year. Additional symptoms or findings may include sore throat, lymphadenopathy, splenomegaly,

and pleurisy. There are no definitive serologic markers, but serum ferritin levels are markedly elevated during flareups.
   (3) **Thyroiditis.** Patients may present with isolated fevers. Consider checking thyroid-stimulating hormone levels in all patients with FUO.
 d. Drug fevers.
   (1) Fever as the only sign of an adverse drug reaction is uncommon, reported as the sole manifestation in only 3% to 4% of adverse drug reactions.[7]
   (2) Drug fevers typically occur 7 to 10 days after initiation and resolve within 48 hours after the offending agent is discontinued.
   (3) Although they are classically described as low-grade, sustained fevers, observational data suggest that drug fevers are more often spiking, reflecting exaggerated normal diurnal variation of body temperature.
   (4) Penicillins, cephalosporins, antituberculous medications, quinidine, procainamide, methyldopa, and phenytoin are among the most common agents causing drug fever.[7]
   (5) The best practical approach for diagnosing drug fever is to discontinue the suspected medication. Rechallenge, though confirmatory, is rarely performed.

III. DIAGNOSIS

A. NONINVASIVE LABORATORY TESTING

1. There is no consensus in the literature on what laboratory evaluations make up a sufficient initial evaluation of FUO. Box 53-2 represents a suggested preliminary evaluation. Early HIV testing may help direct the differential diagnosis.
2. Testing should be guided by clues from the history and physical examination. A focused approach based on one or two findings is more likely to yield results than a scattered evaluation.
3. A prospective, multicenter study of FUO in an immunocompetent population found that blood chemistry studies are useful to guide further studies.[7] The erythrocyte sedimentation rate and C-reactive protein are nonspecific measures of inflammation often done to evaluate FUO because they may point to inflammatory conditions or chronic infection if elevated.
4. In the absence of historical, physical, and laboratory clues pointing to infection, blindly performed microbiological serologic tests have a low yield.

B. IMAGING TECHNIQUES

1. Chest radiography can be informative even in the absence of symptoms or abnormal examination findings[8]; imaging of the chest and abdomen should be part of the initial evaluation for FUO.
2. In a retrospective study, abdominal CT had a diagnostic yield of 19%, with falsely normal findings in only 1 of 47 cases.[7]

```
BOX 53-2
PRELIMINARY LABORATORY TESTS AND IMAGING IN FEVER OF
UNKNOWN ORIGIN

Complete blood cell count with differential
Blood chemistries
Liver enzymes with bilirubin
Lactate dehydrogenase
Creatine phosphokinase
Erythrocyte sedimentation rate
Antinuclear antibodies
Rheumatoid factor
Human immunodeficiency virus antibody and polymerase chain reaction
Serologic tests for cytomegalovirus and Epstein-Barr virus
Blood cultures from samples taken on 3 occasions while patient is not receiving
    antibiotics
Urinalysis
Purified protein derivative test
Ferritin
Chest radiography
Abdominal and pelvic imaging (computed tomography or ultrasound)
```

53

FEVER OF UNKNOWN ORIGIN

3. Abdominal ultrasound is less sensitive than abdominal CT,[9] but it may be helpful for the specific assessment of the hepatobiliary system and gallbladder.

4. Brain and sinus CT imaging may assist in diagnosing brain abscess, sinusitis, mastoiditis, and oral abscesses. Data on the use of CT in diagnosing febrile neutropenic pediatric oncology patients suggests that brain CT rarely has diagnostic utility in febrile patients without localizing symptoms.[10]

5. Nuclear medicine studies generally demonstrate poor sensitivity in FUO evaluation, with reported sensitivities for various modalities ranging from 40% to 54%.[3] Fluorine-18 2-fluoro-2-deoxy-D-glucose positron emission tomography (FDG-PET) may have specific utility in determining metabolic activity of CT-diagnosed lesions, and it has also been noted to detect vasculitic causes of FUO, including giant cell arteritis.[11] Tagged leukocyte and immunoglobulin scans using indium-111 and technetium-99 tracers are theoretically more specific than gallium and FDG-PET in identifying infectious causes such as osteomyelitis.

6. Venous Doppler imaging can detect deep vein thromboses, which may cause FUO in 2% to 6% of cases.[7]

7. Color duplex ultrasound of the temporal arteries may be a noninvasive alternative to temporal artery biopsy in the diagnosis of temporal

arteritis, with a reported sensitivity and specificity of 93% when a halo, stenosis, or occlusion is identified.[12]

8. The primary role of imaging modalities is to direct further invasive testing, including possible aspiration, biopsy, or laparotomy. One fourth to one half of diagnoses are derived by noninvasive means.[2,3,11]

C. HISTOLOGIC TECHNIQUES

1. In immunocompetent patients, blind tissue sampling rarely is fruitful as a screening study, but yields increase when sampling is directed by diagnostic clues and noninvasive studies. An exception may be temporal artery biopsy as a screen for giant cell arteritis in older adults, even in those without headache but with an elevated erythrocyte sedimentation rate or C-reactive protein.[3]

2. Biopsy of the lymph nodes, liver, and bone marrow appears to have a higher diagnostic yield in HIV-associated FUO than in classic FUO.[11,13,14]

3. Suspicious skin lesions should be sampled and evaluated by histology and by culture. Biopsies of anterior cervical and inguinal lymph nodes appear to have low diagnostic yield in immunocompetent patients with FUO, especially if they are less than a centimeter in size.[15] Supraclavicular lymph nodes should always be considered pathologic until proven otherwise. Visceral biopsy of enlarged lymph nodes can be pursued if peripheral nodes are unrevealing and bone marrow biopsy is nondiagnostic.

4. Bone marrow biopsy is most useful in evaluating miliary tuberculosis, fungal infections, and malignancies. In immunocompetent patients, bone marrow biopsy and culture have a low yield without significant anemia.[16] If analysis of blood cultures and more easily obtainable tissues is not diagnostic, bone marrow biopsy for pathology and culture is an appropriate next step for many patients. Bone marrow biopsy has a higher diagnostic yield when performed at this later stage of the workup of classic FUO.[9]

5. Even in the absence of localizing symptoms, temporal arteritis has been found to be the most common cause of fever in older adults with FUO, identified in 16% to 17% of patients in some series.[3,17] Some advocate temporal artery biopsy as a primary screen for patients 65 years and older.[6] Biopsy should be considered in all older patients, and certainly before the empirical use of corticosteroids.

6. Nonspecific liver chemical abnormalities often are identified in patients with FUO (50%), although specific liver diseases are responsible for fevers in only a small minority (4%).[9] Liver biopsy can help in the diagnosis of granulomatous diseases such as granulomatous hepatitis, sarcoidosis, and miliary tuberculosis. Given the often nonspecific findings of liver biopsies in FUO, this procedure should be considered only after exhaustive study, but yields may be higher in patients with significant hepatomegaly.[18]

IV. MANAGEMENT

1. There is no agreed-upon diagnostic or therapeutic approach to the FUO because of the many causes. Any pretest probability for an individual cause is generally low. Therapy hinges on elucidating the specific cause of fever.

2. Overall, there are three approaches to FUO that remain elusive after significant evaluation:

a. The wait-and-see approach is most sensible for patients in good clinical condition. Undiagnosed FUO carries a favorable long-term prognosis.

b. A staged diagnostic approach usually means that considered tests have increasing rates of complications (e.g., liver biopsy, exploratory laparotomy) and therefore are pursued only after careful contemplation.

c. Therapeutic trials with antibiotics or steroids are indicated only in patients with clinical deterioration. One group of investigators favors the use of tetracyclines over beta-lactams, on the basis of their efficacy in unusual infectious causes of FUO.[17] Empiric antitubercular drugs should always be considered before a patient is ill enough to need care in the ICU.

V. OUTCOMES

Patients with FUO whose cause remains undiagnosed after extensive study tend to have favorable outcomes. For example, in a cohort of 61 patients with FUO who were discharged without a specific diagnosis, the mortality rate at 5 years was only 3.2%.[4]

PEARLS AND PITFALLS

- Although it may be tempting to treat FUO empirically with antibiotics, they should not be given to stable patients. The empiric use of antibiotics may contribute to difficulty in identifying the cause of FUO. For example, the fever of miliary tuberculosis may be suppressed by aminoglycosides or fluoroquinolones.

- Eliminate as many medications as possible; drug-related reactions are common and may be unpredictable.

- Empiric use of corticosteroids should be avoided unless there is reasonable suspicion of temporal arteritis and biopsy is planned, or all measures have been exhausted in the investigation of the inflammatory disorder.

REFERENCES

1. Bryan C: Fever of unknown origin: the evolving definition, *Arch Intern Med* 163:1003-1004, 2003. D

2. Knockaert DC, Dujardin KS, Bobbaers HJ: Long-term follow-up of patients with undiagnosed fever of unknown origin, *Arch Intern Med* 156:618, 1996. B

3. Mourad O, Palda V, Detsky AS: Comprehensive evidence-based approach to fever of unknown origin, *Arch Intern Med* 163:546-550, 2003. C

4. Cunha B: The clinical significance of fever patterns, *Infect Dis Clin North Am* 10:33, 1996. C

5. Durack DT, Street AC: Fever of unknown origin-reexamined and redefined. In Remington JS and Swartz MN, eds: *Current clinical topics in infectious diseases,* Cambridge, Mass, 1991, Blackwell. C

6. Quinn MJ, Sheedy PF, Stephens DH, Haltery RR: Computed tomography of the abdomen in evaluation of patients with fever of unknown origin, *Radiology* 136:407-411, 1980. B

7. Tabor P: Drug-induced fever, *Drug Intell Clin Pharm* 20:414-416, 1986. C

8. de Kleijn EM, Vandenbroucke JP, van der Meer JW: Fever of unknown origin. II. Diagnostic procedures in a prospective multicenter study of 167 patients, *Medicine* 76:410, 1997. B

9. Dooley KE, Golub J, Goes FS, Merz WG, Sterling TR: Empiric treatment of community-acquired pneumonia with fluoroquinolones, and delays in the treatment of tuberculosis, *Clin Infect Dis* 34:1607-1612, 2002. B

10. Archibald S et al: Computed tomography in the evaluation of febrile neutropenic pediatric oncology patients, *Pediatr Infect Dis J* 20:5-10, 2001. B

11. Knockaert DC, Vanderschueren S, Blockmans D: Fever of unknown origin in adults: 40 years on, *J Intern Med* 253:269, 2003. C

12. Schmidt WA, Kraft HE, Vorpahl K, Volker L, Gromnica-Ihle EJ: Color duplex ultrasonography in the diagnosis of temporal arteritis, *N Engl J Med* 337:1336-1342, 1997. B

13. Fernandez-Aviles F et al: The usefulness of the bone marrow examination in the etiological diagnosis of prolonged fever in patients with HIV infection, *Med Clin* 112:641, 1999. B

14. Volk EE et al: The diagnostic usefulness of bone marrow cultures in patients with fever of unknown origin, *Am J Clin Pathol* 110:150, 1998. B

15. de Kleijn EM, van der Meer JW: Inquiry into the diagnostic workup of patients with fever of unknown origin, *Neth J Med* 50:69, 1997. B

16. Volk E, Miller ML, Kirskley BA, Washington JA: The diagnostic usefulness of bone marrow cultures in patients with fever of unknown origin, *Am J Clin Pathol* 110:150-153, 1998. B

17. Esposito AL, Gleckman RA: Fever of unknown origin in the elderly, *J Am Geriatr Soc* 27:498-505, 1978. C

Central Nervous System Infection

Adam Spivak, MD; Alan Cheng, MD; Aimee Zaas, MD; and Paul Auwaerter, MD

FAST FACTS

- Acute bacterial meningitis (ABM) is a medical emergency. Instituting appropriate empiric antibiotic treatment as soon as possible is essential.
- Bacterial meningitis often presents with nonspecific constitutional or upper respiratory symptoms followed by confusion, delirium, or obtundation. Consider meningitis in any patient with altered sensorium, meningismus, headache, or fever.
- A lumbar puncture should be performed as soon as possible if meningitis is suspected. Computed tomography of the head before a lumbar puncture should be obtained in older adults; immunosuppressed patients; and those with a history of central nervous system (CNS) disease, seizure within the past week, evidence of papilledema, focal neurologic deficits, coma, or a suspected mass lesion. Imaging and subsequent lumbar puncture should not delay antibiotic treatment.
- The case fatality rate for ABM is 21% for *Streptococcus pneumoniae*, 6% for *Haemophilus influenzae,* and 3% for *Neisseria meningitidis.*

54

I. MENINGITIS

A. EPIDEMIOLOGY

1. The typical pathogens of ABM depend on the age of the host and the presence of comorbidities (Table 54-1).
2. Although acute aseptic meningitis typically has a viral cause (especially enteroviruses), medications such as nonsteroidal antiinflammatory drugs may also cause aseptic meningitis (Table 54-2). Partially treated bacterial meningitis may have a sterile cerebrospinal fluid (CSF) with cell counts typical of viral meningitis.
3. Infectious risk factors for community-acquired ABM are numerous and include a recent history of respiratory tract infection (otitis media, sinusitis, pneumonia), diabetes mellitus, and intravenous drug use. Comorbid conditions impairing cellular immunity (human immunodeficiency virus [HIV], steroid use, organ transplantation, cytotoxic chemotherapy) increase the risk of acquiring *Listeria monocytogenes,* whereas conditions that alter immunoglobulin

TABLE 54-1

EMPIRIC THERAPY FOR BACTERIAL MENINGITIS IN ADULTS

Patient Group	Likely Pathogen	Antibiotic
18-50 yr old	*Streptococcus pneumoniae, Neisseria meningitidis*	3rd-generation cephalosporin and vancomycin
>50 yr old	*S. pneumoniae, Listeria monocytogenes,* or gram-negative bacilli	Ampicillin, vancomycin, and 3rd-generation cephalosporin
Impaired cellular immunity	*L. monocytogenes* or gram-negative bacilli	Ampicillin, vancomycin, and ceftazidime
Head trauma, neurosurgery, cerebrospinal fluid shunt, or nosocomial infection	Staphylococci, gram-negative bacilli, or *S. pneumoniae*	Vancomycin and ceftazidime

Modified from Tunkel AR et al: *Clin Infect Dis* 39(1), 2004.

production (splenectomy, hypogammaglobulinemia, multiple myeloma) increase the risk of acquiring *S. pneumoniae* meningitis.[1]

4. Risk factors for nosocomially acquired meningitis include recent surgical instrumentation, immunocompromised states, CSF leak, and history of head trauma.[2]

B. CLINICAL PRESENTATION

1. Signs and symptoms of ABM include headache (> 90% of patients), fever (> 90%), meningismus (> 85%), and altered sensorium (> 80%). Seizures, nausea, vomiting, and focal neurologic signs are present in a minority of patients. Clinical history is notoriously nonspecific.

2. Fever, neck stiffness, and change in mental status are highly sensitive findings for acute meningitis; ABM can be excluded in a patient with none of these symptoms.[3]

3. Kernig's sign (pain elicited when the patient's knee is extended while the hip is flexed at 90 degrees) and Brudzinski's sign (patient flexes hips, knees, or both with passive flexion of the neck) are classically described signs of meningeal inflammation, but they have poor diagnostic sensitivity.[4]

4. Certain microbial agents are associated with distinct clinical presentations.

a. *N. meningitidis* is present in 73% of patients with ABM who have a rash (often petechial).[2] The differential diagnosis includes Rocky Mountain spotted fever, echovirus type 9, *S. pneumoniae, H. influenzae, Acinetobacter,* and *Staphylococcus aureus* meningitis with sepsis.

b. Patients with aseptic meningitis caused by enteroviruses may present with chest or abdominal pain, upper respiratory symptoms, or a rash. In addition, constitutional symptoms are prominent, and a biphasic fever curve may be present.

TABLE 54-2

DIFFERENTIAL DIAGNOSIS OF ACUTE MENINGITIS

Infectious Etiologies	Noninfectious Etiologies
Bacteria	*Medications*
Streptococcus pneumoniae	Antimicrobials (trimethoprim-
Neisseria meningitidis	sulfamethoxazole, ciprofloxacin, penicillin,
Haemophilus influenzae	isoniazid)
Listeria monocytogenes	Nonsteroidal antiinflammatory drugs
Salmonella spp.	Chemotherapies
Nocardia spp.	Azathioprine
Mycobacterium tuberculosis	Carbamazepine
Pseudomonas aeruginosa	Immune globulin
	Ranitidine
	Phenazopyridine
Viruses	*Intracranial Tumors and Cysts*
Nonpolio enteroviruses	Craniopharyngioma
Mumps virus	Dermoid and epidermoid cysts
Arboviruses	Teratoma
Herpes viruses	
Lymphocytic choriomeningitis virus	
Human immunodeficiency virus	
Adenovirus	
Influenza virus	
Measles virus	
Other	*Other*
Rickettsia rickettsii (Rocky Mountain	Neurosurgery
spotted fever)	Spinal anesthesia
Ehrlichia spp.	Intrathecal injections
Treponema pallidum	Systemic lupus erythematosus
Viral postinfectious syndromes	Seizures
Leptospira spp.	Migraine
Borrelia burgdorferi	

Modified from Mandell GL, Bennett JE, Dolin R, eds: *Mandell, Douglas, and Bennett's principles and practice of infectious diseases*, 5th ed, New York, 2000, Churchill Livingstone.

5. Subacute meningitis develops over a period of weeks, with mental status changes, headache, neck pain, and fever. Tuberculous meningitis should be suspected in alcoholic patients, HIV-positive patients, and immigrants from countries in which the infection is endemic. The differential diagnosis also includes sarcoidosis, fungal infections, syphilis, brucellosis, listeriosis, acanthamoebiasis, strongyloidiasis, Sjögren's disease, and Behçet's disease.

C. DIAGNOSIS

1. Lumbar puncture (LP) should be performed immediately in a patient who does not have a bleeding diathesis. See Table 54-3 for CSF characteristics in meningitis. Routine head computed tomography (CT) before LP is controversial. Head CT is more likely to influence management decisions in patients older than 60 years,

TABLE 54.3

CHARACTERISTICS OF CEREBROSPINAL FLUID ANALYSIS IN MENINGITIS

	Normal Cerebrospinal Fluid	Bloody Tap	Viral Meningitis	Bacterial Meningitis
Opening pressure (cm H$_2$O)	5-20	Normal	Normal to mildly elevated	> 18
WBC count (cells/mm^3)	< 10 monocytes < 1 polymorphonuclear cell	WBC to RBC ratio 1:700	10-1000, lymphocyte predominance	1000-5000, neutrophil predominance
RBC count (cells/mm^3)	< 2	WBC to RBC ratio 1:700	Normal	Normal
Protein (mg/dl)	< 45	15-45	Normal	100-500
Glucose (mg/dl)	> 50% serum levels	Normal	Normal	< 40

Modified from Bartlett JG: *Pocket book of infectious disease therapy*, 10th ed, Baltimore, 1999, Williams & Wilkins.
RBC, red blood cell; *WBC*, white blood cell.

immunocompromised patients and those with CNS disease including seizures within 1 week of presentation, obtundation, or a focal neurologic deficit.[5] Head CT should not delay the initiation of antibiotic therapy.

2. The sensitivity of Gram staining correlates with the bacterial load in the CSF: 25% of patients with fewer than 10^3 colony-forming units (CFUs) per milliliter have positive Gram stains, whereas 97% of those with more than 10^5 CFUs/ml have positive Gram stains. Gram staining is also pathogen dependent and ranges from about 90% for *S. pneumoniae* and *H. influenzae* to less than 50% for *L. monocytogenes*.[6,7]

D. MANAGEMENT

1. Prompt initiation of antibiotics is imperative. When the results of rapid diagnostic tests, such as Gram staining, are positive, pathogen-specific therapy should be initiated. If Gram staining is nondiagnostic, initial therapy should target the most likely organisms (see Table 54-1).

2. Antibiotics should be initiated after LP is performed and blood cultures are obtained. If head CT is indicated to ensure the safety of LP, blood cultures should be obtained and antibiotics started before imaging.

3. Administering corticosteroids *before* antimicrobials in adults with pneumococcal meningitis reduces serious sequelae.[8] Dexamethasone 10 mg intravenously every 6 hours should be given when pneumococcal meningitis is suspected. Steroids should be discontinued if the CSF Gram stain shows gram-negative organisms, if other types of meningitis are diagnosed, or if no organism is isolated after 4 days of therapy.[9,10] If the *S. pneumoniae* isolate is penicillin resistant or the physician has a high suspicion of penicillin resistance, dexamethasone should not be used because steroids may decrease CSF levels of vancomycin.

4. Meningitis prophylaxis is recommended for close contacts of patients with *N. meningitidis* ABM in order to eradicate pharyngeal carriage (oral ciprofloxacin 500 mg once or rifampin 600 mg every 12 hours for four doses). A meningococcal vaccine is available for those at risk of epidemic meningitis and often is recommended for dormitory-housed college students.

II. ENCEPHALITIS

A. EPIDEMIOLOGY

1. Encephalitis, an infection of the brain parenchyma, occurs worldwide, and often is of viral origin (Box 54-1).

2. Epidemics caused by arboviruses, such as West Nile virus, typically occur in the summer and fall. These viruses are transmitted to humans by insect vectors, with other mammals often serving as reservoirs.

3. Sporadic cases of encephalitis are most commonly caused by herpes simplex virus (HSV type 1), varicella-zoster virus, or enteroviruses.

54

CENTRAL NERVOUS SYSTEM INFECTION

BOX 54-1
VIRUSES COMMONLY CAUSING ENCEPHALITIS
EPIDEMIC AND SEASONAL VIRUSES (SUMMER AND FALL)
Arboviruses (summer and fall): West Nile virus, western equine encephalitis virus, eastern encephalitis virus, St. Louis encephalitis, Powassan virus, LaCrosse virus, California encephalitis virus
Enteroviruses (late summer and fall): Coxsackie viruses, echovirus, poliovirus, enterovirus
SPORADIC VIRUSES (OCCURRING YEAR-ROUND)
Herpes simplex virus 1 and 2
Varicella-zoster virus
Epstein-Barr virus
Mumps
Measles
Rabies
Cytomegalovirus
Adenovirus
Human immunodeficiency virus

Modified from Mandell GL, Bennett JE, Dolin R, eds: *Mandell, Douglas, and Bennett's principles and practice of infectious diseases,* 5th ed, New York, 2000, Churchill Livingstone.

B. CLINICAL PRESENTATION

1. Patients with encephalitis often have a prodrome consistent with a nonspecific viral illness. Typically this progresses to headache, fever, and nuchal rigidity. Often a rapid, global decline in mental status occurs, but focal neurologic involvement is not uncommon. Ataxia, hemiparesis, aphasia, cranial nerve involvement, and psychosis can be present depending on the affected area of the CNS. Seizures occur in 50% of patients.
2. Clues in the history or physical examination may narrow the differential diagnosis.
a. A history of recent travel, outdoor exposure, and tick bites suggest an arbovirus.
b. Parotitis, orchitis, and pancreatitis suggest mumps encephalitis.
c. Aphasia, hallucinations, and acute personality changes suggest HSV encephalitis.[11] Note that both varicella-zoster virus and HSV encephalitis can occur with a concomitant cutaneous vesicular outbreak, although this is uncommon.

C. DIAGNOSIS

1. If not contraindicated, LP should be performed as soon as possible after presentation. CSF results in viral encephalitis typically do not differ from those of viral meningitis. See Box 54-2 for the differential diagnosis of encephalitis.
a. Elevated red blood cell counts in the absence of a traumatic tap suggest HSV encephalitis; other causes of elevated red blood cell counts in the

BOX 54-2

DIFFERENTIAL DIAGNOSIS OF ENCEPHALITIS

Subdural hematoma

Fungal, parasitic, rickettsial, or tuberculous infection

Brain abscess

Vasculitis

Reye's syndrome

Toxic encephalopathy

Neoplasm

Systemic lupus erythematosus

Sarcoid

Behçet's disease

Modified from Mandell GL, Bennett JE, Dolin R, eds: *Mandell, Douglas, and Bennett's principles and practice of infectious diseases,* 5th ed, New York, 2000, Churchill Livingstone.

54

CENTRAL NERVOUS SYSTEM INFECTION

CSF include hemorrhagic encephalitis caused by Colorado tick fever virus or California encephalitis virus.

b. CSF polymerase chain reaction (PCR) is available for HSV 1 and 2, CMV, Epstein-Barr virus, varicella-zoster virus, West Nile Virus, and the enteroviruses. Results are available quickly and have excellent predictive value.

c. In addition, coxsackie viruses, echovirus, lymphocytic choriomeningitis virus, mumps virus, and some arboviruses can be grown in culture.

2. HIV antibodies and PCR should be obtained if risk factors are present.

3. Acute and convalescent sera antibody titers can be used to diagnose arboviruses.

4. Brain biopsy is reserved for patients with nondiagnostic CSF evaluation who demonstrate clinical decline despite empiric therapy.

5. Electroencephalography and imaging studies such as magnetic resonance imaging often are obtained in patients with encephalitis and can help to identify a region of involvement and exclude other processes. These studies can suggest a specific viral entity.

a. HSV has a predilection for temporal and inferofrontal lobe involvement.

b. Eastern equine encephalitis may involve the basal ganglia and thalami.

D. MANAGEMENT

1. Acyclovir (10 mg/kg intravenously every 8 hours) should be started empirically for any patient suspected of having HSV encephalitis. In patients with PCR-positive HSV encephalitis, a repeat CSF PCR at 2 weeks can help determine duration of treatment. If the second PCR is negative, some experts believe that acyclovir can be stopped. Oral agents do not currently have a role in treating encephalitis and should not be used. Early treatment reduces mortality from 70% to 19%.[11]

2. Treatment for arbovirus-related encephalitis, including West Nile virus, is supportive. Patients often need an intensive care setting. Despite the lack of specific treatments, diagnosis is important in shaping understanding of outbreak patterns.
3. The incidence and degree of residual neurologic deficits after recovery depend on the viral cause. Eastern equine encephalitis causes severe neurologic sequelae in about 80% of patients,[12] whereas other viruses, such as Epstein-Barr virus and California encephalitis virus, have a more benign postinfection course.

III. BRAIN AND EPIDURAL ABSCESS

A. EPIDEMIOLOGY

1. Once a rare infection, CNS abscesses have become more common with the advent of HIV infection and the increasing population of patients receiving immunosuppressive therapy.
2. CNS abscesses often are polymicrobial infections (Table 54-4). Streptococci are the most commonly isolated bacterial pathogen and are thought to spread from the oral cavity, gastrointestinal tract, and female genital tract.
3. Neurocysticercosis, caused by the helminth *Taenia solium,* is a common cause of brain abscess in developing countries and often presents with seizures.

TABLE 54-4
MICROBIOLOGY OF CENTRAL NERVOUS SYSTEM ABSCESS

Predisposing Condition	Usual Microbial Isolates
Otitis media or mastoiditis	Streptococci (anaerobic or aerobic), *Bacteroides* and *Prevotella* spp., Enterobacteriaceae
Sinusitis	Streptococci, *Bacteroides* spp., Enterobacteriaceae, *Staphylococcus aureus, Haemophilus* spp.
Dental sepsis	Mixed *Fusobacterium, Prevotella,* and *Bacteroides* spp., streptococci
Penetrating trauma or neurosurgery	*S. aureus,* streptococci, Enterobacteriaceae, *Clostridium* spp.
Lung abscess, empyema, bronchiectasis	*Fusobacterium, Actinomyces, Bacteroides,* and *Prevotella* spp., streptococci, *Nocardia* spp.
Bacterial endocarditis	*S. aureus,* streptococci
Congenital heart disease	Streptococci, *Haemophilus* spp.
Neutropenia	Aerobic gram-negative bacilli, *Aspergillus* spp., *Zygomycetes, Candida* spp.
Transplantation	*Aspergillus* spp., *Candida* spp., *Zygomycetes,* Enterobacteriaceae, *Nocardia* spp., *Toxoplasma gondii*
Human immunodeficiency virus infection	*Toxoplasma gondii, Nocardia* spp., *Mycobacterium* spp., *Listeria monocytogenes, Cryptococcus neoformans*

Modified from Mandell GL, Bennett JE, Dolin R, eds: *Mandell, Douglas, and Bennett's principles and practice of infectious diseases,* 5th ed, New York, 2000, Churchill Livingstone.

B. CLINICAL PRESENTATION

1. CNS abscesses can arise from a contiguous focus of infection (e.g., otitis media) or hematogenous spread of a primary source (e.g., endocarditis). Penetrating head trauma is another mechanism for local abscess formation. Brain abscesses usually present with unilateral headache. Fever occurs in about 50% of patients. Focal neurologic complaints related to the location of the abscess can guide the clinician toward the diagnosis but are not always present.

2. Epidural abscesses can also be caused by a contiguous focus of infection (e.g., osteomyelitis of the spine, pressure ulcers, or instrumentation) or hematogenous spread. *S. aureus* is the most common organism recovered in these infections. Local tenderness, pain with progression to a radiculitis, and nuchal rigidity are clinical signs suggesting epidural abscess. Loss of motor, bowel, or bladder function is a neurosurgical emergency. The thoracic spine is most commonly involved, followed by the lumbar region.

C. DIAGNOSIS

1. CT scan, though not as sensitive as magnetic resonance imaging, is an acceptable test and should be performed with intravenous contrast if an abscess is suspected. Findings depend on the temporal course of the lesion. Cerebritis is seen early on without a rim of inflammation; this progresses to a ring-enhancing lesion.

2. Magnetic resonance imaging is superior to CT scanning for identifying spinal epidural abscesses. Plain films of the spine are insensitive and not recommended.

3. LP is contraindicated in patients with parenchymal or epidural abscess because of the risk of herniation. This underscores the importance of rapid imaging in patients suspected of having mass lesions.

D. MANAGEMENT

1. When a CNS abscess is suspected on the basis of presentation and imaging studies, aspiration to guide antibiotic management should be considered.[13] Empiric, broad-spectrum antibiotics should be initiated (Table 54-5) and narrowed based on culture results.

2. Steroids are recommended only when there is both mass effect and decreased mental status. In such circumstances, dexamethasone (10 mg intravenous loading dose followed by 4 mg intravenously every 6 hours) should be given. Steroids should be discontinued as soon as possible because they can impair antibiotic penetration into the abscess.

3. Criteria regarding need for surgical intervention do not exist. However, masses larger than 2.5 cm generally do not resolve without surgical management. Consultation with a neurosurgeon is imperative at the time of diagnosis.

4. Duration of antibiotic treatment in CNS abscess has not been studied extensively. Six to 8 weeks of intravenous antibiotics is a common recommendation.

54

CENTRAL NERVOUS SYSTEM INFECTION

TABLE 54-5
ANTIMICROBIAL TREATMENT OF CENTRAL NERVOUS SYSTEM ABSCESS

Predisposing Condition	Antimicrobial Regimen
Otitis media or mastoiditis	Metronidazole and 3rd-generation cephalosporin*
Sinusitis (frontoethmoid or sphenoid)	Metronidazole and 3rd-generation cephalosporin; add vancomycin if methicillin-resistant *Staphylococcus Aureus* is suspected
Dental sepsis	Penicillin and metronidazole
Penetrating trauma or neurosurgery	Vancomycin and 3rd-generation cephalosporin
Lung abscess, empyema, bronchiectasis	Penicillin, metronidazole, and sulfonamide (if *Nocardia* suspected)
Bacterial endocarditis	Vancomycin, ampicillin, and gentamicin or nafcillin
Congenital heart disease	3rd-generation cephalosporin
Unknown	Vancomycin, metronidazole, 3rd-generation cephalosporin

Modified from Mandell GL, Bennett JE, Dolin R, eds: *Mandell, Douglas, and Bennett's principles and practice of infectious diseases*, 5th ed, New York, 2000, Churchill Livingstone.
*3rd-generation cephalosporins include cefotaxime and ceftriaxone. Ceftazidime or the 4th-generation (cephalosporin cefepime) can be used if *Pseudomonas aeruginosa* is suspected.

PEARLS AND PITFALLS

- Patients with meningitis should respond to the antibiotics indicated by clinical improvement within 36 hours.
- Opening pressure is accurate only if the patient's legs are straight and the patient is lying down when this parameter is measured.
- Ten to 20 percent of HIV-infected patients with cryptococcal meningitis have elevated intracranial pressure that warrants serial large-volume LPs or ventriculoperitoneal shunting. If hydrocephalus or focal abscesses are not present, large-volume CSF removal by LP is effective in most patients. It is recommended that CSF pressure be decreased by 50% and maintained at less than 30 cm H_2O.
- College students, splenectomized patients, travelers to endemic areas, patients deficient in terminal complement components, and those with Hodgkin's disease should receive meningococcal vaccination.
- In patients diagnosed with encephalitis, intravenous acyclovir should be initiated and maintained until HSV has been ruled out as the etiologic agent. The negative predictive value of PCR for HSV in the CSF is adequate to rule out this diagnosis.

REFERENCES
1. Aronin SI, Quagliarello VJ: New perspectives on pneumococcal meningitis, *Hosp Pract* 36:43, 2001. C
2. Durand ML et al: Acute bacterial meningitis in adults: a review of 493 episodes, *N Engl J Med* 328:21, 1993. C

3. Attia J, Hatala R, Cook DJ, Wong JG: The rational clinical examination. Does this adult patient have acute meningitis? *JAMA* 282(2):175-181, 1999. C

4. Thomas KE, Hasbun R, Jekel J, Quagliarello VJ: The diagnostic accuracy of Kernig's sign, Brudzinski's sign, and nuchal rigidity in adults with suspected meningitis, *Clin Infect Dis* 35(1):46-52, 2002. B

5. Tunkel AR et al: Practice guidelines for the management of bacterial meningitis, *Clin Infect Dis* 39(1), 2004. D

6. Gray LD, Fedorko DP: Laboratory diagnosis of bacterial meningitis, *Clin Microbiol Rev* 5:130, 1992. C

7. Greenlee JE: Approach to the diagnosis of meningitis: cerebrospinal fluid evaluation, *Infect Dis Clin North Am* 4:483, 1990. C

8. de Gans J, van de Beek D: Dexamethasone in adults with bacterial meningitis. European Dexamethasone in Adulthood Bacterial Meningitis Study Investigators, *N Engl J Med* 347:1549, 2002. A

9. van de Beek D, de Gans J, McIntyre P, Prasad K: Steroids in adults with acute bacterial meningitis: a systematic review, *Lancet Infect Dis* 4(3):139-143, 2004. C

10. Chaudhuri A: Adjunctive dexamethasone treatment in acute bacterial meningitis, *Lancet Neurol* 3(1):54-62, 2004. C

11. Whitley RJ, Lakeman F: Herpes simplex virus infections of the central nervous system: therapeutic and diagnostic considerations, *Clin Infect Dis* 20(2):414-420, 1995. C

12. Deresiewicz RL, Thaler SJ, Hsu L, Zamani AA: Clinical and neuroradiographic manifestations of eastern equine encephalitis, *N Engl J Med* 336(26):1867-1874, 1997. C

13. Shahzadi S, Lozano AM, Bernstein M, et al: Stereotactic management of bacterial brain abscesses, *Can J Neurol Sci* 23(1):34-39, 1996. B

54

CENTRAL NERVOUS SYSTEM INFECTION

Pneumonia

Nicola Zetola, MD; Aimee Zaas, MD; and John Bartlett, MD

55

FAST FACTS

- Antibiotic treatment for community-acquired pneumonia (CAP) should begin within 4 hours of presentation.
- The most common etiologic agents in CAP are *Streptococcus pneumoniae, Haemophilus influenzae,* and possibly *Chlamydia pneumoniae.* Although not routinely recognized, viruses (e.g., influenza, parainfluenza, and respiratory syncytial virus) account for 10% to 23% of all CAP.
- The most common etiologic agents in lethal pneumonia are *S. pneumoniae* and *Legionella.*
- Factors that portend a poor prognosis of CAP include advanced age, multilobar involvement, bacteremia, and severe medical comorbidities.
- Failure of CAP to respond to antibiotics usually is caused by delay in initiation of treatment or host factors.
- Nosocomial pneumonia (NP) should be suspected in any hospitalized patient with purulent respiratory secretions, fever, or worsening hypoxia plus an abnormal chest radiograph (CXR).
- Mechanical ventilation is the most important risk factor for the development of NP.
- Antibiotics can be safely stopped in patients with low likelihood of NP after a short course of treatment.

Pneumonia is both a common reason for inpatient admission and a common nosocomial infection. This chapter provides a framework for treating and evaluating both CAP and NP.

I. COMMUNITY-ACQUIRED PNEUMONIA

A. EPIDEMIOLOGY

1. CAP is an acute infection of the pulmonary parenchyma that is accompanied by either an acute infiltrate on CXR or auscultatory findings consistent with pneumonia. CAP can be diagnosed only in patients who have not been hospitalized or lived in a long-term care facility for the 14 days before presentation.[1]
2. Given the emergence of antibiotic resistance and the potential hazards of antibiotic treatment failures, a definitive microbiological diagnosis is desirable. However, 40% to 60% of CAP cases have no identified etiologic agent (Table 55-1).[2]
3. The average mortality for hospitalized patients with CAP is 14%.[3]

TABLE 55-1

MICROBIOLOGICAL PATHOGENS IN CAP AND VAP

Microbiological Agent or Cause	CAP*	VAP†
Streptococcus pneumoniae	20-60%	4%
Haemophilus influenzae	3-10%	10%
Staphylococcus aureus	3-5%	20%
Enterobacteriaceae	3-10%	14%
Pseudomonas aeruginosa	—	25%
Acinetobacter spp.	—	8%
Miscellaneous (*Moraxella catarrhalis*, group A		
Streptococcus, Neisseria meningitidis)	3-5%	2%
Streptococcus spp.	—	8%
Atypical agents	10-20%	—
Legionella	2-8%	—
Mycoplasma pneumoniae	1-6%	—
Chlamydia pneumoniae	4-6%	—
Viruses (influenza, parainfluenza,		
respiratory syncytial virus)	2-15%	—
Aspiration	6-10%	—

CAP, community-acquired pneumonia; VAP, ventilator-associated pneumonia.
*Data from Bartlett JG, Mundy L: *N Engl J Med* 333:1618, 1995. Based on 15 published reports from North America. None of these studies used techniques adequate to detect anaerobes in respiratory secretions; these organisms account for 20-30% of cases in some reports. *Pneumocystis jiroveci* is also excluded but may account for up to 15% in recent reports from urban centers.
†Data from Chastre J et al: *Am J Respir Crit Care Med* 165:867-903, 2002. Based on bronchoscopic techniques in 24 studies, for a total of 1689 episodes and 2490 pathogens.

55

PNEUMONIA

B. CLINICAL PRESENTATION

1. CAP is a clinical diagnosis based on the patient's history, physical examination, and CXR. There is no gold standard method of diagnosis.
2. A specific etiologic agent cannot be definitely identified by presentation or radiologic findings; however, the patient's presentation can suggest a possible organism.

a. Pneumococcal pneumonia classically presents with sudden onset of chills and fever with rigors, productive cough, pleuritic chest pain, and focal infiltrates on CXR.

b. *Legionella* pneumonia often is preceded by gastrointestinal complaints and accompanied by hyponatremia, elevated lactate dehydrogenase, and delirium.

c. *Haemophilus* is commonly found in smokers with chronic obstructive pulmonary disease and often causes patchy lobar infiltrates and productive cough.

d. Staphylococcal pneumonia may be rapidly progressive and often is associated with bilateral lobar involvement and cavity formation. It often follows influenza infection.

e. *Klebsiella* pneumonia presents classically, albeit rarely, with red "currant jelly" sputum.

f. Atypical organisms (*Mycoplasma pneumoniae*, *Chlamydia pneumoniae*) often have an insidious presentation, with dry cough and scattered infiltrates on CXR. *Legionella* and *Mycoplasma* often present with extrapulmonary symptoms (e.g., headaches, myalgias, arthralgias).

g. *Mycobacterium tuberculosis* pneumonia causes chronic cough, weight loss, fevers, and night sweats.

C. **DIAGNOSIS**

1. Conceptually, the diagnosis of CAP can be divided into etiologic agents that must be diagnosed, etiologic agents that can be diagnosed, and etiologic agents that cannot be diagnosed (Box 55-1).

2. Basic labs, including a complete blood cell count with differential and a chemistry panel (including glucose, serum sodium, liver function tests, and renal function tests), should be obtained in every patient.

3. A CXR with demonstrable infiltrate is necessary to diagnose CAP.[1] The only important exception is *Pneumocystis jiroveci* pneumonia (formerly known as *Pneumocystis carinii*), in which a normal CXR does not rule out the diagnosis.

4. Microbiology and immunology.

a. A sputum sample by a deep cough expectoration should be obtained before antibiotic therapy. Adequate sputum for culture has fewer than 10 epithelial cells and more than 25 polymorphonuclear cells per low-power field. For maximum yield, a sputum sample should reach the laboratory less than 2 hours after collection.[4]

b. Blood cultures should be obtained in every patient admitted for CAP. About 11% of patients hospitalized with CAP have positive blood cultures, with *S. pneumoniae* accounting for 67%.[2]

c. When available, urine antigen testing is a quick, noninvasive way to identify the pathogen. The pneumococcal assay has a sensitivity of

BOX 55-1
ETIOLOGIC AGENTS OF COMMUNITY-ACQUIRED PNEUMONIA ACCORDING TO THE IMPORTANCE OF ESTABLISHING THE DIAGNOSIS
ORGANISMS WE NEED TO KNOW
Agents of bioterrorism
Legionella
Community-acquired methicillin-resistant *Staphylococcus aureus*
Severe acute respiratory syndrome
Influenza (particularly avian influenza, including H5, 7, and 9 strains)
ORGANISMS WE WOULD LIKE TO KNOW
Streptococcus pneumoniae
Haemophilus influenzae
ORGANISMS WE CANNOT KNOW
Chlamydia pneumoniae
Anaerobes
Mycoplasma pneumoniae

50% to 80% and a specificity of 90%,[4] and the *Legionella* assay has a sensitivity of 60% to 90% and specificity of 95%. The latter should be ordered in all cases of severe CAP, immunosuppression, or failure to respond to beta-lactam treatment.

    d. Nasopharyngeal aspirates should be checked for influenza during the influenza season.[1]

5. Bronchoscopy should be performed only in highly unusual situations or in severe nosocomial pneumonia.

6. Other considerations.

    a. Patients with cough for more than 1 month, chronic fevers, night sweats, weight loss, or a suggestive CXR should be evaluated for *M. tuberculosis* (see Chapter 56).

    b. Human immunodeficiency virus (HIV) testing should be done for people 15 to 54 years of age in hospitals with more than 1 newly diagnosed case per 1000 discharges.

    c. A high level of suspicion is necessary to diagnose infections caused by acts of bioterrorism. To diagnose inhaled anthrax, blood cultures and computed tomography scan are necessary. For plague and tularemia, blood cultures, sputum cultures, and Gram stains should be ordered.

D. MANAGEMENT

1. Guidelines for antibiotic selection in CAP are provided by the Infectious Disease Society of America.[1] If the etiologic agent is known, antibiotic selection is based on in vitro susceptibility testing or data from clinical trials (Tables 55-2 and 55-3).

2. Antibiotic treatment for CAP should begin within 4 hours of presentation.[5]

3. Duration of treatment has not been standardized through randomized controlled trials. The generally accepted treatment duration is 5 to 10 days for common bacterial pneumonia, 10 to 14 days for *Mycoplasma* or *Chlamydia*, and 10 to 14 days for *Legionella*. Patients with infections involving *Staphylococcus aureus* and *Pseudomonas* often need longer treatment. Therapy can change from intravenous to oral once the patient begins to improve.

4. Lack of response necessitates a reassessment of the diagnosis and a determination of whether the problem is related to the host (e.g., empyema), the medications (e.g., inappropriate dosage regimen), or the pathogen (e.g., microbiological resistance or misdiagnosis).[1] It is important to remember that many patients do not respond despite appropriate antibiotic therapy, as evidenced by the 17% mortality rate associated with properly treated pneumococcal pneumonia with bacteremia.

E. PROGNOSIS

1. Several systems have been developed for risk stratifying patients with pneumonia, with the goal of appropriate triage to outpatient care, general hospital ward, or more closely monitored settings.

TABLE 55-2
RECOMMENDED EMPIRIC ANTIMICROBIAL THERAPY FOR PNEUMONIA

	Clinical Setting		Recommended Therapy*
Community-acquired pneumonia	General medical ward (preferred agents)		Extended-spectrum cephalosporin or β-lactam and β-lactamase inhibitor with a macrolide
			Fluoroquinolone
	Intensive care unit (preferred agents)		Extended-spectrum cephalosporin or β-lactam and β-lactamase inhibitor with either a macrolide or a fluoroquinolone
	Modifying factors and special situations		Structural disease of the lung (bronchiectasis): antipseudomonal agents plus a fluoroquinolone
			β-Lactam allergy: fluoroquinolone with or without clindamycin
			Suspected aspiration: fluoroquinolone plus clindamycin, metronidazole, or a β-lactam and β-lactamase inhibitor
Nosocomial pneumonia	Early onset (without specific risk factors)	Enteric gram-negative† Haemophilus influenzae Methicillin-susceptible Staphylococcus aureus Streptococcus pneumoniae	2nd- or 3rd-generation cephalosporins or β-lactam and β-lactamase inhibitor
			If allergic to penicillin: fluoroquinolone or clindamycin with aztreonam
	Late onset	Include early-onset core organisms plus: Pseudomonas aeruginosa Acinetobacter Methicillin-resistant Staphylococcus aureus	Aminoglycoside or ciprofloxacin with one of the following: β-lactam and β-lactamase inhibitor, ceftazidime, cefepime, imipenem, or aztreonam
			Vancomycin linezolid⁶

Modified from Chastre J et al: *Am J Respir Crit Care Med* 165:867-903, 2002.

*Extended-spectrum cephalosporin, cefotaxime or ceftriaxone; macrolide, azithromycin, clarithromycin, or erythromycin; fluoroquinolone, levofloxacin, gatifloxacin, moxifloxacin, or another fluoroquinolone with enhanced activity against S. pneumoniae; β-lactam and β-lactamase inhibitor, piperacillin-tazobactam; β-lactam and β-lactamase inhibitor for structural diseases of the lung, piperacillin-tazobactam; antipseudomonal agents, piperacillin, piperacillin-tazobactam, carbapenem, or cefepime.

†Include Enterobacter spp., Escherichia coli, Klebsiella spp., Proteus spp., and Serratia spp.

TABLE 55-3

PATHOGEN-DIRECTED ANTIMICROBIAL THERAPY FOR PNEUMONIA

Organism	Preferred	Alternative
Streptococcus pneumoniae		
Penicillin susceptible (MIC <2 μg/ml)	Penicillin G, amoxicillin	Cephalosporins, imipenem, macrolide, clindamycin, doxycycline, or fluoroquinolone
Penicillin resistant (MIC ≥2 μg/ml)	Agents based on in vitro susceptibility tests, including cefotaxime, ceftriaxone, and fluoroquinolone	Vancomycin, telithromycin, and linezolid
Haemophilus influenzae	Cephalosporin (2nd or 3rd generation), TMP/SMX, doxycycline, β-lactam and β-lactamase inhibitor, macrolide	Fluoroquinolone, clarithromycin
Moraxella catarrhalis	Cephalosporin (2nd or 3rd generation), TMP/SMX, β-lactam and β-lactamase inhibitor, macrolide	Fluoroquinolone
Anaerobe	β-Lactam and β-lactamase inhibitor, clindamycin	Imipenem
Staphylococcus aureus		
Methicillin susceptible	Nafcillin and oxacillin rifampin or gentamicin	Cefazolin, cefuroxime, vancomycin, clindamycin, TMP/SMX
Methicillin resistant	Linezolid or vancomycin	Rifampin or gentamicin
Escherichia coli, Klebsiella, Proteus, or Enterobacter	3rd-generation cephalosporin aminoglycoside, carbapenem	Aztreonam, β-lactam and β-lactamase inhibitor, fluoroquinolone
Pseudomonas aeruginosa	Aminoglycoside antipseudomonal β-lactam: ticarcillin, piperacillin, mezlocillin, ceftazidime, cefepime, aztreonam, or carbapenem	Aminoglycoside ciprofloxacin; ciprofloxacin antipseudomonal β-lactam
Acinetobacter baumannii	Same as for Pseudomonas aeruginosa	
Legionella	Azithromycin, rifampin; fluoroquinolone (including ciprofloxacin)	Doxycycline, rifampin

Modified from Mandell LA et al: *Clin Infect Dis* 37:1405-1433, 2003.
MIC, minimum inhibitory concentration; *TMP/SMX*, trimethoprim-sulfamethoxazole.

55

PNEUMONIA

2. Investigators from the Pneumonia Outcomes Research Trial (PORT) study created a model predicting mortality that can help to guide hospital admission.[7] Although it is well validated, this system is complex and cumbersome.[1,7]

3. A faster tool for risk stratifying patients with CAP is the CURB-65 system (the *C* stands for impaired consciousness, *U* for urea nitrogen more than 7 mmol/L [about 42 mg/dl], *R* for respiratory rate > 30/minute, *B* for blood pressure < 90 systolic, and 65 for older than 65). Each component has a value of 1 point. When summed, a score of 0 to 1 predicts a mortality of 1.5%, probably suitable for outpatient treatment. A score of 2 has intermediate mortality of 9%, and the patient probably would benefit from inpatient treatment. A score of 3 or more predicts a mortality of 22%; the patient should be hospitalized, possibly in an intensive care unit.[8]

II. NOSOCOMIAL PNEUMONIA

NP is the second most common hospital-acquired infection (after urinary tract infections). This section discusses important clues, diagnostic criteria, and antibiotic selection.

A. EPIDEMIOLOGY

1. NP is defined clinically as the presence of a new lung infiltrate in the setting of a systemic inflammatory response in a hospitalized patient. It is the most common infection acquired in the intensive care unit.

2. Intubation is the most important risk factor for NP and is associated with a twenty-one-fold higher risk.[9] In ventilated patients with NP, the condition often is called ventilator-associated pneumonia.

3. Because of differences in etiologic pathogens and resistance patterns, NP has been traditionally divided in early- and late-onset NP.

a. Early-onset NP occurs before the fifth day of hospitalization, and it is usually secondary to aspiration of community-acquired pathogens during endotracheal intubation or secondary to impaired consciousness. The most common pathogens are *S. pneumoniae, Haemophilus influenzae, S. aureus*, or *Moraxella catarrhalis*.[10,11] Anaerobes should also be considered.

b. Late-onset NP occurs after the fifth day and is caused by the aspiration of potentially multidrug-resistant organisms acquired from the nosocomial flora.[10] Prolonged mechanical intubation and previous use of broad-spectrum antibiotics are strongly associated with resistant pathogens.[12,13]

B. CLINICAL PRESENTATION

1. NP develops as a result of the patient's continuous aspiration of small quantities of bacteria. This progresses into a bronchopneumonia that is manifested by purulent respiratory secretions. The absence of purulent secretions makes the diagnosis of NP less likely.[13]

2. NP should be considered in any intubated patient who develops evidence of infection or sepsis.

C. DIAGNOSIS

1. Qualitative tracheobronchial aspiration has a high negative predictive value and can be used to rule out NP when the clinical picture is not clear.
2. Given the high prevalence of multidrug-resistant pathogens causing NP, great efforts should be done to establish a microbiological diagnosis to guide the therapy.
a. Quantitative cultures provide more reliable detection of infection and can be obtained via tracheobronchial aspiration or with more invasive methods such as protected specimen brush washings or bronchoalveolar lavage. Using the threshold of 10,000 colony-forming units per milliliter, quantitative tracheobronchial aspiration showed higher sensitivities (82% vs. 64%) and lower specificity (83% vs. 96%) than invasive methods.[14]
b. Protected specimen brush washings and bronchoalveolar lavage have comparable diagnostic yields. Most studies show sensitivities ranging from 70% to 90% and specificities from 70% to 95%.
c. Four randomized studies have evaluated noninvasive and invasive approaches to diagnosing NP.[15-18] Only one of them showed that invasive approaches were superior to noninvasive methods in terms of morbidity and mortality.[15]
3. It is important to note that no method can confidently confirm the diagnosis of NP or its etiologic agents.

D. MANAGEMENT

1. Risk factor modification may help to prevent the development of NP[13] (Table 55-4).
2. Because delays in therapy have been associated with increased mortality, empiric antibiotic therapy directed against the most likely etiologic agents should be administered while further evaluation proceeds (see Table 55-2).
3. Because of the high mortality attributable to NP, it is appropriate to use antibiotics even in patients with low likelihood of infection. Antibiotics can be safely stopped in these patients after a short course of treatment.

55

PNEUMONIA

TABLE 55-4	
RISK FACTORS FOR NOSOCOMIAL PNEUMONIA AND PREVENTIVE STRATEGIES	
Risk Factors	**Preventive Measures**
Intubation	Noninvasive ventilation
Nasotracheal intubation	Oral intubation
Supine body position	Semirecumbent body position
Pharmacologic paralysis	Avoidance of muscle relaxants
Daily change of ventilator circuits	Change ventilator circuits not more than once per week

Modified from Ewig S et al: *Thorax* 57:366-371, 2002.

4. A comparative trial showed linezolid to be a safe and effective alternative antibiotic for MRSA NP.[19]

PEARLS AND PITFALLS

- Beta-lactams (amoxicillin, cefotaxime, cefprozil, and cefpodoxime) are the preferred drugs for penicillin-sensitive strains of *S. pneumoniae*. Many consider cefotaxime and ceftriaxone the best drugs for pneumococcal pneumonia (because of efficacy and ease of administration). Empiric treatment for penicillin-resistant strains should be with a fluoroquinolone, vancomycin, telithromycin, or an agent selected on the basis of in vitro tests.
- Older adults with CAP may present with nonspecific symptoms such as delirium.
- The urinary antigen test for *Legionella* detects only the serogroup 1, which accounts for 70% to 80% of community-acquired cases but a smaller percentage of nosocomial cases.[20]
- Aspiration pneumonia should be suspected in patients with depressed levels of consciousness or dysphagia and radiographic evidence of an infiltrate in a dependent pulmonary segment (posterior segment of an upper lobe or superior segment of a lower lobe). The drug of choice for community-acquired aspiration pneumonia is clindamycin or a beta-lactam and beta-lactamase inhibitor. Nosocomial aspiration pneumonia usually is caused by gram-negative bacilli or *S. aureus*.
- Patients hospitalized more than 3 days have hospital-acquired oral flora (including resistant gram-negative rods and *S. aureus*).
- Soluble triggering receptor expressed on myeloid cells (TREM-1) in bronchoalveolar lavage fluid was more accurate than clinical values in diagnosing ventilator-associated pneumonia.[21]

REFERENCES

1. Mandell LA et al: Update of practice guidelines for the management of community-acquired pneumonia in immunocompetent adults, *Clin Infect Dis* 37:1405-1433, 2003. D
2. Bartlett JG, Mundy L: Community-acquired pneumonia, *N Engl J Med* 333:1618, 1995. C
3. Fine MJ et al: Prognosis and outcomes of patients with community-acquired pneumonia: a meta-analysis, *JAMA* 275:134, 1996. A
4. Jefferson H et al: Transportation delay and the microbiological quality of clinical specimens, *Am J Clin Pathol* 64:689, 1975. B
5. Houck PM et al: Timing of antibiotic administration and outcomes for Medicare patients hospitalized with community-acquired pneumonia, *Arch Intern Med* 164(6):637-644, 2004. B
6. Guidlines for the management of adults with hospital-acquired, ventilator-associated, and healthcare-associated pneumonia, *Am J Respir Crit Care Med* 171:388-416, 2005.
7. Fine MJ et al: A prediction rule to identify low-risk patients with community-acquired pneumonia, *N Engl J Med* 336:243, 1997. A

8. Lim WS, van der Eerden MM, Laing R, et al: Defining community acquired pneumonia severity on presentation to hospital: an international derivation and validation study, *Thorax* 58(5):377-382, 2003. A

9. Haley RW, Hooton TM, Culver DH, et al: Nosocomial infections in US hospitals, 1975-76: estimated frequency by selected characteristics of patients, *Am J Med* 70:947-959, 1981. B

10. American Thoracic Society: Hospital-acquired pneumonia in adults: diagnosis, assessment, initial severity, and prevention. A consensus statement, *Am J Respir Crit Care Med* 153:1711-1725, 1996. D

11. Akca O, Koltka K, Uzel S, et al: Risk factors for early-onset, ventilator-associated pneumonia in critical care patients: selected multiresistant versus nonresistant bacteria, *Anesthesiology* 93:638-645, 2000. B

12. Chastre J, Fagon JY: Ventilator-associated pneumonia, *Am J Respir Crit Care Med* 165:867-903, 2002. D

13. Ewig S, Bauer T, Torres A: The pulmonary physician in critical care * 4: nosocomial pneumonia, *Thorax* 57(4):366-371, 2002.

14. Marquette CH et al: Diagnostic efficiency of endotracheal aspirates with quantitative bacterial cultures in intubated patients with suspected pneumonia. Comparison with the protected specimen brush, *Am Rev Respir Dis* 148:138-144, 1993. A

15. Sanchez-Nieto JM, Torres A, Garcia-Cordoba F, et al: Impact of invasive and noninvasive quantitative culture sampling on outcome of ventilator-associated pneumonia: a pilot study, *Am J Respir Crit Care Med* 157:371-376, 1998. A

16. Ruiz M, Torres A, Ewig S, et al: Noninvasive versus invasive microbial investigation in ventilator-associated pneumonia: evaluation of outcome, *Am J Respir Crit Care Med* 162:119-125, 2000. A

17. Sole Violan J, Fernandez JA, Benitez AB, et al: Impact of quantitative invasive diagnostic techniques in the management and outcome of mechanically ventilated patients with suspected pneumonia, *Crit Care Med* 28:2737-2741, 2000. A

18. Fagon JY, Chastre J, Wolff M, et al: Invasive and noninvasive strategies for management of suspected ventilator-associated pneumonia. A randomized trial, *Ann Intern Med* 132:621-630, 2000. A

19. Wunderink RG, Rello J, Cammarata SK, et al: Linezolid vs vancomycin: analysis of two double-blind studies of patients with methicillin-resistant *Staphylococcus aureus* nosocomial pneumonia, *Chest* 124(5):1789-1797, 2003. A

20. Helbig JH, Uldum SA, Bernander S, et al: Clinical utility of urinary antigen detection for diagnosis of community-acquired, travel-associated, and nosocomial Legionnaires' disease, *J Clin Microbiol* 41(2):838-840, 2003. B

21. Gibot S et al: Soluble triggering receptor expressed on myeloid cells and the diagnosis of pneumonia, *N Engl J Med* 350:451-458, 2004.

55

PNEUMONIA

Tuberculosis

Joshua Schiffer, MD; and Eric Nuermberger, MD

TB is any disease state that results from infection with *Mycobacterium tuberculosis*. The lungs are the most common portal of entry and site of disease for *M. tuberculosis,* but almost any body site may be involved. Latent TB infection (LTBI) represents asymptomatic infection with *M. tuberculosis* and, unless treated, confers a lifelong risk of reactivation TB. Coinfection with human immunodeficiency virus (HIV) dramatically increases the likelihood of progression from latent to active TB and accounts for the large burden of TB morbidity and mortality in many developing countries.

Identification and appropriate treatment of people with active pulmonary TB prevents the ongoing transmission of disease. In the setting of appropriate directly observed therapy, treatment response rates in active disease are high for both HIV-negative and HIV-positive patients. Treatment of latent TB prevents progression to active disease and is therefore another important means of TB control.

I. EPIDEMIOLOGY

1. Roughly 30% of the world's population (about 1.8 billion people) is latently infected with *M. tuberculosis*. There were 8 million new cases of active TB and 2 million TB-related deaths in 2000.
2. In the United States, there are roughly 16,000 cases per year, of which 26% are attributable to HIV infection.[1] TB remains most common among the urban poor, alcoholics, intravenous drug users, the homeless, migrant farm workers, and prison inmates.
3. The lifetime risk of progression from LTBI to active disease is 10% to 20%, with most of the risk occurring within 5 years of primary

infection.[2] With HIV coinfection, the yearly risk of reactivation is about 10%.[3]

4. HIV is the strongest risk factor for progression to active TB. Malnutrition, alcoholism, homelessness, incarceration, renal failure, and immunosuppressive medicines (e.g., tumor necrosis factor-alpha inhibitors) also increase the likelihood of progression from LTBI to disease.

5. Multidrug-resistant TB (MDR-TB) accounted for only 1.2% of new cases in the United States in 1997.[4] Risk factors for MDR-TB include exposure to a person with MDR-TB or recent TB treatment failure, or recent travel to an area with high rates of drug resistance such as Eastern Europe.

II. PRESENTATION

A. PATHOGENESIS

1. Infection with *M. tuberculosis* is acquired through inhalation of aerosolized droplet nuclei containing tubercle bacilli, generated by a contact with pulmonary TB. The odds of transmission increase with duration and closeness of exposure and with contact with a highly contagious host with active cough and cavitary lung disease.[5]

2. After local proliferation in nonimmune alveolar macrophages, bacilli are transported to hilar lymph nodes and spread hematogenously, lodging preferentially in tissues with high oxygen tension. These latent foci account for the diverse array of clinical syndromes possible during reactivation.

3. Evolution of cell-mediated immunity in the host leads to macrophage activation and tissue-damaging immune response that contains or kills the tubercle bacilli, resulting in involution of the primary lung lesion and other pulmonary and extrapulmonary foci.

4. Although usually subclinical, primary TB may result in overt disease, including miliary disease or progressive pneumonia in those who fail to contain the initial infection (often older adults or people with HIV or another immunodeficiency).

5. Reactivation TB may occur months, years, or decades after primary infection when latent foci reactivate and proliferating bacilli trigger a granulomatous host response. In the lung, this response leads to caseous foci that undergo liquefaction to form cavities. Enlarging cavities erode into airways, and the resultant high oxygen content leads to exponential bacillary growth. The infectious cycle is completed when these bacilli are expectorated in a cough-generated aerosol and inhaled by a new host.

B. ACTIVE TB

1. **Primary TB** typically is subclinical in adults but may result in a pneumonic illness with cough, fever, and pleurisy. In children, the chest radiograph classically reveals characteristic middle or lower lobe infiltrates with ipsilateral hilar adenopathy (Gohn focus). Adults often

56

TUBERCULOSIS

develop an apical metastatic focus of fibrosis or calcification during primary infection either with or without evidence of infiltrates in the area around the Gohn focus.

2. Older adults and HIV-positive patients can develop a more aggressive primary cavitating pneumonia and occasionally develop miliary TB without achieving latency.

3. Symptoms of **reactivation TB** typically are organ specific, but prominent systemic symptoms are common and include a protracted fever, night sweats, anorexia, weight loss, and malaise.

4. Symptoms of **pulmonary TB** relate directly to the presence of pulmonary infiltrates and apical cavities and include productive cough, dyspnea, and fever. Although uncommon, hemoptysis implies advanced disease.

5. Chest radiography is a key component in the diagnostic evaluation for TB, and characteristic findings on chest radiograph may predate the onset of pulmonary symptoms or findings on physical examination. In the immunocompetent host, the most typical location for reactivation in the lungs is the posterior aspect of an upper lobe or the posterior, superior aspect of a lower lobe.

6. Although the differential diagnosis for cavitary lung lesions is large, apical cavities seen in a patient with a known TB contact or risk factor should be regarded as TB until proven otherwise. In patients with the acquired immunodeficiency syndrome, the predictive value of apical cavities for TB is much lower, and diffuse infiltrates are more commonly seen.[6]

7. **Extrapulmonary TB** (Table 56-1) results from reactivation of foci established during the lymphohematogenous phase of primary infection but may occur during primary infection in an immunocompromised patient.

8. **Miliary TB** is characterized by disseminated disease with systemic symptoms. Diffuse 0.5- to 1-mm lesions are seen on chest radiograph. Pleuritis, mediastinal lymphadenitis, adrenalitis, meningitis, and abdominal lymphadenitis leading to peritonitis are common late features. Hyponatremia is also common and may be caused by meningitis-related syndrome of inappropriate antidiuretic hormone secretion (SIADH) or adrenal insufficiency. Anemia of chronic disease is typical, but neutropenia or thrombocytopenia may indicate marrow involvement. Granulomatous hepatitis may mimic cholangitis, with elevated bilirubin and alkaline phosphatase but only mildly elevated transaminases.

9. Other very rare forms of extrapulmonary disease include interstitial nephritis, monoarthritis, otitis, uveitis, laryngitis, and gastrointestinal tract disease.

10. Active TB has several atypical features in HIV-positive patients with CD4 lymphocyte count less than 200/mm^3 (Table 56-2).

TABLE 56-1
COMMON SITES OF EXTRAPULMONARY TB

Syndrome	Presentation	Body Fluid	Notes
Meningitis	Headache, fever, and malaise, progressing to mental status changes and focal neurologic deficits, particularly in the cranial nerves.	Cerebrospinal fluid: 5-2000 WBCs with mononuclear predominance, although neutrophils may predominate early in infection. Protein moderately elevated and glucose usually low.	Rarely presents acutely with obtundation, high fever, and meningismus. Masslike tuberculoma may cause seizure or focal deficit.[7] Focal vasculitis may cause stroke.[7]
Pleural effusion	Mild to moderate in size. Unilateral except in miliary disease.	Pleural: 500-2500 WBCs, mostly lymphocytes; initial phase of neutrophil predominance. pH usually < 7.3, and cell count is < 5% mesothelial cells.	In a young host the usual cause is rupture of a subpleural focus during primary infection. An increasing proportion of cases are related to reactivation TB in older patients.[8] Usually in presence of pleural effusion. Typically affects middle-aged adults.
Pericardial effusion			
Genitourinary tract	May involve any genitourinary site. Significant destruction may occur before dysuria, renal colic, and diagnosis. Often no systemic symptoms.	As above. Sterile pyuria. Ureteral strictures and hydronephrosis on intravenous pyelogram.	Renal failure, testicular mass, infertility, and menstrual disorders are rare presentations.[9]
Osteomyelitis (Pott's disease)	Tender spine. Often no systemic symptoms. Can progress to cord compression.	Magnetic resonance imaging: anterior wedging of two adjacent vertebral bodies and destruction of intervening disk.	Lower thoracic > lumbar > cervical > sacral spine involvement.[10]

TB, tuberculosis; *WBC*, white blood cell.

56

TUBERCULOSIS

TABLE 56-2

CLINICAL MANIFESTATIONS OF ACTIVE TUBERCULOSIS IN EARLY AND LATE
HUMAN IMMUNODEFICIENCY VIRUS INFECTION

	CD4 < 200/mm³	CD4 > 300/mm³
Tuberculin test	Usually negative	Usually positive
Adenopathy	Common	Unusual
Pulmonary distribution	Lower and middle lobe	Upper lobe
Cavitation	Typically absent	Often present
Extrapulmonary disease	> 50%	10-15%

Reproduced from Haas D: Mycobacterial diseases (Chapter 240: *Mycobacterium* tuberculosis).
In Mandell GL, Bennett JE, Dolin R, eds: *Mandell, Douglas, and Bennett's principles and practice of infectious diseases*, 5th ed, New York, 2000, Churchill Livingstone.

C. LATENT TB

LTBI is defined as the presence of a positive tuberculin skin test in an asymptomatic patient with no sign of active disease. Residual apical fibrosis or calcification (Simon's focus) or a Ghon lesion plus a calcified hilar node (together known as a Ranke complex) may be observed.

III. DIAGNOSIS

A. ACTIVE TB

1. *M. tuberculosis* is an aerobic, slowly dividing bacillus. Therefore, rapid diagnosis can be made only by demonstrating acid-fast bacilli in a specimen from a patient with compatible disease or by nucleic acid amplification technology, if available. Confirmation requires prolonged culture.

2. When pulmonary TB is suspected, three expectorated morning sputum samples should be sent for acid-fast smear and culture. Because **nontuberculous mycobacteria** are also acid-fast, positive smears may be tested for *M. tuberculosis* DNA by polymerase chain reaction in order to confirm the diagnosis.

3. The BACTEC liquid culture system generally detects *M. tuberculosis* within 16 days and is used to increase sensitivity and determine drug sensitivities. Biopsy with both culture and microscopic examination for caseating granulomas is necessary in certain culture-negative cases.

4. Cerebrospinal fluid culture lacks absolute sensitivity, but yield is substantially higher with multiple large-volume lumbar punctures.[8] Polymerase chain reaction may also be helpful for cases in which cerebrospinal fluid cultures are negative but suspicion of TB remains high. Because 75% of cases involve other organs, other features suggestive of systemic TB increase the likelihood of TB meningitis in the setting of a sterile pleocytosis.

5. The sensitivity of pleural fluid smear and culture is only 15% to 20% for effusions related to primary TB. Pleural biopsy (sensitivity of 75%) with culture often is necessary for a definitive diagnosis. For patients with reactivation pulmonary TB and an effusion, both smear (50%) and

culture (60%) are slightly more sensitive than pleural biopsy and should be repeated before biopsy is attempted.[11] Pleural fluid with more than 5% mesothelial cells makes the diagnosis of TB very unlikely.

6. Urine culture identifies approximately 90% of cases of genitourinary TB.[12]

B. LATENT TB

1. Placement of 5000 units or 0.1 ml purified protein derivative of tuberculin intradermally is the standard method for detecting LTBI in an immunocompetent patient.

2. A tuberculin skin test is interpreted as positive when the indurated area (not the erythematous area) exceeds a predetermined diameter 48 to 72 hours after being placed (Table 56-3).

3. Only those who would be at high risk of reactivation or those with a high pretest probability of having latent TB infection should receive a tuberculin skin test.

4. Because bacille Calmette-Guérin vaccination has highly variable effects on delayed type hypersensitivity, history of bacille Calmette-Guérin vaccination should be ignored when deciding whether to place a tuberculin skin test and when interpreting the result.

5. All people with a positive tuberculin skin test should be ruled out for active disease by history, physical examination, and chest radiography.

IV. MANAGEMENT

A. ACTIVE TB

1. Patients with smear-positive pulmonary TB are contagious and should be isolated in a negative pressure room to protect other patients and hospital staff. Patients with drug-susceptible TB generally become noncontagious with elimination of cough and decrease in bacillary load within 2 weeks of the initiation of therapy.

TABLE 56-3

CUTOFF VALUES FOR A POSITIVE TUBERCULIN SKIN TEST

Size	Populations
> 5 mm	HIV positive, recent TB exposure, chest radiograph consistent with old TB, organ transplant, ≥ 15 mg qd prednisone
> 10 mm	Skin test conversion within 2 yr; intravenous drug abuse; diabetes; medical immunosuppression; head, neck, or hematologic malignancy; weight loss; gastrectomy; jejunoileal bypass; member of high-incidence immigrant group; underserved population or long-term care facility
> 15 mm	Low-incidence group

Modified from Sterling TR: Mycobacterial infections. In Miller RG, Sisson SD, Ashar BM, eds: *The Johns Hopkins internal medicine board review*, St Louis, 2004, Mosby.
TB, tuberculosis.

2. Empiric treatment should be started before culture confirmation for seriously ill patients suspected of having TB.

3. Stable patients with clinical features of TB whose initial cultures and smears are negative should also be strongly considered for empiric treatment once an appropriate negative workup for alternative causes of disease is completed.

4. Recent treatment guidelines recommend 2 months of isoniazid (INH), rifampin, pyrazinamide, and ethambutol followed by 4 months of INH and rifampin or INH and rifapentine.[13] Various dosing intervals may be considered, but for HIV-positive people with CD4 counts less than 100/mm^3 treatment should be administered daily or thrice weekly.

5. The duration of therapy should be extended to 9 months if sputum culture remains positive after 2 months of therapy and initial chest radiograph reveals cavitation. Treatment for central nervous system TB should be given for 9 to 12 months. TB osteomyelitis or arthritis may also warrant extended therapy depending on clinical response.

6. Adjunctive corticosteroids (prednisone 60 mg/day for the first 4 weeks, tapered over the next 7 weeks) are recommended for TB pericarditis. Dexamethasone (12 mg/day for the first 3 weeks, tapered over the next 3 weeks) is recommended for patients with central nervous system TB, especially with depressed consciousness.

7. Treatment of TB in HIV-infected patients is associated with several unique problems including paradoxical worsening, highly active retroviral therapy (HAART) and anti-TB drug interactions, and acquired rifamycin resistance. Paradoxical worsening or immune reconstitution inflammatory syndrome is defined as clinical or radiographic worsening of the original TB symptoms after initiation of HAART or anti-TB treatment despite successful bacillary clearance. A thorough evaluation for other opportunistic infection or TB treatment failure should be undertaken before this diagnosis is made. Biopsy often shows sterile granulomas. Severe cases generally respond well to steroids.[14] For patients newly diagnosed with HIV and TB coinfection, delay of initiation of HAART until 4 to 8 weeks after starting therapy for TB should be considered.

8. Treatment with anti-TB drugs in the context of HAART warrants consultation with an expert. Rifabutin generally is substituted for rifampin because it has fewer adverse interactions with antiretroviral agents.

9. Baseline evaluation of all patients treated for TB should include testing for HIV (if status is unknown); measurements of liver enzymes, serum creatinine, and platelet count; and testing of visual acuity and color vision (when ethambutol is to be used). It is not necessary to monitor these blood tests unless baseline abnormalities are present or new symptoms develop. Patients should be questioned monthly about symptoms of hepatitis and visual disturbances (the latter only while receiving ethambutol).

10. MDR-TB, defined as resistance to at least INH and rifampin, usually is identified by drug susceptibility testing. Therapy is complex and entails 18 to 24 months of specialized treatment with a combination of toxic- first and second-line agents. An expert should supervise treatment of MDR-TB.

B. LATENT TB

1. Standard treatment for LTBI is 6 to 9 months of daily INH.[15] An alternative regimen is rifampin for 4 months.
2. Treatment for 2 months with rifampin and pyrazinamide has been associated with inordinate risk of fulminant hepatic failure and generally should not be used.[16]
3. For treatment of people exposed to a contagious contact with MDR-TB, treatment with pyrazinamide plus either ethambutol or a fluoroquinolone for 6 to 12 months is recommended.

V. PROGNOSIS

1. Patients with cavitary disease and positive cultures after 2 months of therapy have a relapse and failure rate of 21%, compared with 5% to 6% in people with one of these risk factors and 2% for patients with neither risk factor.[17]
2. HIV-positive and HIV-negative patients have nearly equivalent response rates to TB treatment.[18]

PEARLS AND PITFALLS

- Because of impaired cellular immunity, TB can present in a subtle fashion in older adults and should be considered in the differential diagnosis for failure to thrive, particularly in the setting of a nonresolving pneumonitis.
- Erythema nodosum and a severe unilateral conjunctivitis are allergic complications that occasionally present with the onset of hypersensitivity to *M. tuberculosis* after primary infection.
- In patients with CD4 counts less than $50/mm^3$, pulmonary *Mycobacterium kansasii* infection is clinically indistinguishable from TB.[19]
- Apical cavities are common sites of superinfection with *Aspergillus* and nontuberculous mycobacterium.
- An adenosine deaminase level is a highly specific test for TB in pleural or peritoneal fluid and can be interpreted in a shorter period of time than mycobacterial culture.
- The tuberculin skin test may be falsely negative in approximately one in four patients with active TB.
- In 5% to 10% of miliary TB, patients decompensate before evolution of chest radiograph findings. This syndrome is called cryptic miliary TB and is a protean and often fatal cause of fever of unknown origin.
- TB monoarthritis is one of the few instances in which synovial biopsy may be necessary for diagnosis.

- All patients who are started on an anti–tumor necrosis factor-alpha inhibitor should have a tuberculin skin test placed and evaluated before treatment because of the high risk of progression to active disease in patients with LTBI treated with these medications.
- The empiric use of fluoroquinolones for community-acquired respiratory infections may result in transient clinical improvement and a diminished yield of culture in patients with TB, delaying diagnosis and the initiation of appropriate therapy.[20]

REFERENCES

1. Corbett EL, Watt CJ, Walker N, et al: The growing burden of TB: global trends and interactions with the HIV epidemic, *Arch Intern Med* 163(9):1009-1021, 2003. C
2. Sutherland I: Recent studies in the epidemiology of tuberculosis, based on the risk of being infected with tubercle bacilli, *Adv Tuberc Res* 19:1-63, 1976. B
3. Selwyn PA, Hartel D, Lewis VA, et al: A prospective study of the risk of tuberculosis among intravenous drug users with human immunodeficiency virus infection, *N Engl J Med* 320:545-550, 1989. B
4. Espinal MA, Laszlo A, Simonsen L, et al: Global trends in resistance to antituberculosis drugs. World Health Organization–International Union Against Tuberculosis and Lung Disease Working Group on Anti-Tuberculosis Drug Resistance Surveillance, *N Engl J Med* 344(17):1294-1303, 2001. C
5. Houk VH, Kent DC, Baker JH, et al: The Byrd study. In-depth analysis of a micro-outbreak of tuberculosis in a closed environment, *Arch Environ Health* 16(1):4-6, 1968. B
6. Chaisson RE, Schecter GF, Theuer CP, et al: Tuberculosis in patients with the acquired immunodeficiency syndrome. Clinical features, response to therapy, and survival, *Am Rev Respir Dis* 136(3):570-574, 1987. B
7. Kennedy DH, Fallon RJ: Tuberculous meningitis, *JAMA* 241:264-268, 1979. C
8. Epstein DM, Kline LR, Albelda SM, et al: Tuberculous pleural effusions, *Chest* 91:106-109, 1987. B
9. Simon HB, Weinstein AJ, Pasternak MS, et al: Genitourinary tuberculosis: clinical features in a general hospital population, *Am J Med* 63:410, 1977. B
10. Pertuiset E, Beaudreuil J, et al: Spinal tuberculosis in adults. A study of 103 cases in a developed country, 1980-94, *Medicine (Baltimore)* 78:309, 1999. B
11. Antoniskis D, Amin K, Barnes PF: Pleuritis as a manifestation of reactivation tuberculosis, *Am J Med* 89(4):447-450, 1990. C
12. Christensen WI: Genitourinary tuberculosis: review of 102 cases, *Medicine* 53:377-390, 1974. B
13. American Thoracic Society/Centers for Disease Control and Prevention/Infectious Diseases Society of America: Treatment of tuberculosis, *Am J Respir Crit Care Med* 167:603-662, 2003. A
14. Narita M, Ashkin D, Hollender ES, Pitchenik AE: Paradoxical worsening of tuberculosis following antiretroviral therapy in patients with AIDS, *Am J Respir Crit Care Med* 158(1):157-161, 1998. B
15. Comstock GW: How much isoniazid is needed for prevention of tuberculosis among immunocompetent adults? *Int J Tuberc Lung Dis* 3:847-850, 1999. B
16. Jasmer RM, Saukkonen JJ, Blumberg H, et al: Short-course rifampin and pyrazinamide compared with isoniazid for latent tuberculosis infection: a multicenter clinical trial, *Ann Intern Med* 137:640-647, 2002. A

17. Benator D, Bhattacharya M, et al, Tuberculosis Trials Consortium: Rifapentine and isoniazid once a week versus rifampicin and isoniazid twice a week for treatment of drug-susceptible pulmonary tuberculosis in HIV-negative patients: a randomised clinical trial, *Lancet* 360(9332):528-534, 2002. A
18. Dean GL, Edwards SG, et al: Starting HAART early in severely immunosuppressed HIV positive patients presenting with TB is associated with decreased mortality and lower rates of progression, *AIDS* 1:75-84, 2002. B
19. Benator DA, Gordin FM: Nontuberculous mycobacteria in patients with human immunodeficiency virus infection, *Semin Respir Infect* 11:285, 1996. C
20. Dooley KE, Golub J, Goes FS, et al: Empiric treatment of community-acquired pneumonia with fluoroquinolones, and delays in the treatment of tuberculosis, *Clin Infect Dis* 34(12):1607-1612, 2002. B

Infective Endocarditis

Nicola Zetola, MD; David A. Zidar, MD; and Stuart Ray, MD

FAST FACTS

- Infective endocarditis (IE) has a wide variety of clinical presentations characterized by nonspecific or constitutional symptoms associated with cardiac, embolic, and immunologic manifestations.
- The clinical presentations of right- and left-sided IE differ. The absence of cardiac murmurs but the presence of complications from the involvement of the pulmonary vasculature (e.g., septic pulmonary emboli) is notorious in the presentation of right-sided IE. In contrast, left-sided IE may present with systemic embolization or symptoms of valvular insufficiency.
- The current gold standard for the diagnosis of IE is the pathological study of valvular vegetation. However, in its absence the combination of clinical, microbiological, and echocardiographic data specified in the Duke criteria is considered appropriate.
- In cases of suspected endocarditis, rapid initiation of empiric therapy before microbiology results are available is appropriate.

IE is an infection of the endothelial surface of the heart associated with an adherent vegetation composed of platelets, fibrin, and microorganisms. IE is classified as native valve IE (NVE), prosthetic valve IE (PVE), IE associated with intravenous drug use (IDU), and nosocomial IE. Hemodialysis-associated IE and IE in older adults also have differing epidemiology and can be classified separately.[1] NVE typically involves valves of the left side of the heart, as opposed to IDU-associated IE, in which the right side is more commonly involved.

I. EPIDEMIOLOGY AND ETIOLOGY

1. The epidemiology of IE has changed markedly over the past century with changes in the incidence of risk factors. Risk factors include rheumatic heart disease, congenital heart disease, mitral valve prolapse, degenerative heart disease, IDU, and indwelling catheters.
2. The annual incidence of NVE is 3.6 per 100,000 patients, with a median in-hospital mortality of 16%.[1] In contrast, IE associated with IDU occurs at a rate of 2% to 5% per year.[2] The incidence of health care–associated IE is rapidly increasing with the extended use of indwelling catheters and invasive procedures. The risk of PVE is greatest within the first 6 weeks after surgery.[3] The cumulative incidence is 1.4% to 3.1% at 12 months and 3.2% to 5.7% after 5 years.[4,5]

3. Important variability exists regarding which valves are affected. NVE usually is left-sided, whereas IDU and indwelling catheters increase the likelihood of right-sided involvement.

4. See Table 57-1 for causative organisms by IE classification.

a. Transient bacteremia is common and is probably the source of most NVE.

b. The HACEK organisms (*Haemophilus* species, *Actinobacillus actinomycetemcomitans*, *Cardiobacterium hominis*, *Eikenella* species, and *Kingella kingae*) are an uncommon cause of NVE, but they are important to note both because they are difficult to grow and because they are oxacillin resistant. The microbiology laboratory must be alerted if one of them is suspected.

c. IDU-associated IE typically is secondary to skin flora, with *Staphylococcus aureus* being the most common pathogen.[6,7] Polymicrobial, fungal, or pseudomonal IE also are more common.

d. PVE is classified as having early (< 2 months) or late (> 6 months) onset because endothelialization of the prosthetic valve within the first 6 months reduces the risk of infection. Early-onset PVE is most commonly caused by coagulase-negative staphylococci or *S. aureus* (often methicillin-resistant *S. aureus*), whereas organisms involved in late-onset PVE are similar to those in native valves.

TABLE 57-1

MICROBIOLOGY OF IE

	Native Valve IE (%)	IE in Intravenous Drug Users (%)	Prosthetic Valve IE (%)	
			Early (< 2 mo)	*Late (> 6 mo)*
Staphylococci	44	69	67	46
S. aureus	38	69	20	21
Coagulase negative	6	0	47	25
Streptococci	31	8	0	35
Oral streptococci	21	3	0	26
Others*	10	5	0	8
Enterococcus spp.[†]	8	2	7	7
HACEK[‡]	4	0	0	1
Polymicrobial	2	9	0	1
Other[§]	4	5	0	3
Fungi	1	2	0	0
Culture negative	6	5	27	7

Data from Moreillon P et al: *Lancet* 363(9403):139-149, 2004.

IE, infective endocarditis.

*Including *S. agalactiae, S. bovis, S. pneumoniae, S. pyogenes,* group G *Streptococcus,* and *Abiotrophia* spp.

[†]> 80% *Enterococcus faecalis.*

[‡]Includes *Haemophilus* spp., *Actinobacillus actinomycetemcomitans, Cardiobacterium hominis, Eikenella corrodens,* and *Kingella kingae.*

[§]Includes *Escherichia coli, Corynebacterium* spp., *Proteus mirabilis, Mycobacterium tuberculosis,* and *Bacteroides fragilis.*

e. Antibiotic use before presentation is the most common cause of "culture-negative" endocarditis.

II. CLINICAL PRESENTATION

A. SYMPTOMS

1. IE can resemble a number of both infectious and noninfectious processes. Most patients have only nonspecific or constitutional symptoms; however, patients may appear toxic.
2. The most common symptoms are fever, chills, and sweats. Fever may be absent in older adults or chronically ill patients. Anorexia, weight loss, and malaise are common. Headaches, confusion, stroke, myalgias, arthralgias, back pain, abdominal pain, nausea, and vomiting are also common.
3. Chest pain, dyspnea, cough, and hemoptysis suggest septic pulmonary embolism.

B. PHYSICAL EXAMINATION

1. The most important physical finding is the presence of a new murmur suggestive of regurgitation. However, the absence of a murmur should not preclude consideration of the diagnosis.
2. Right-sided endocarditis often presents without murmurs because the low pressure gradient makes auscultation of murmurs difficult.[8,9] In addition, because the blood is filtered in the lungs, peripheral embolic manifestations typically are absent; rather, symptoms arise from septic pulmonary emboli, causing chest pain, dyspnea, cough, and hemoptysis.
3. Manifestations of embolic or inflammatory phenomena, which are more common with left-sided endocarditis, include splenomegaly (15% to 50%), petechiae (10% to 40%), splinter hemorrhages (5% to 15%), Osler nodes (7% to 10%), Janeway lesions, and Roth spots (4% to 10%). Focal neurologic deficits, ischemic digits, and abdominal tenderness resulting from systemic embolism may also be present.
4. Septic pulmonary emboli, renal emboli, and renal insufficiency from acute glomerulonephritis are seldom appreciated on physical examination but are important components of the clinical picture (Box 57-1).

III. DIAGNOSIS

1. The workup should start with a thorough history, physical examination, and serial blood cultures.
2. If the suspicion for endocarditis is high, echocardiography should be performed. Transthoracic echocardiography is noninvasive and highly specific if a vegetation is detected, so it is often the initial test of choice. However, transthoracic echocardiography is up to 65% sensitive in NVE and 16% to 36% sensitive in PVE. In contrast, transesophageal echocardiography is 90% to 100% sensitive in NVE and 82% to 96%

BOX 57-1

COMPLICATIONS OF INFECTIVE ENDOCARDITIS

CARDIAC

Valvular destruction with or without congestive heart failure

Conduction system disruption from myocardial abscess

Purulent pericarditis from extension of myocardial abscess

EMBOLIC

Septic pulmonary emboli resulting from tricuspid or pulmonic valve ("right-sided") endocarditis

Cerebral, renal, splenic, hepatic, soft tissue emboli with concomitant abscess resulting from mitral or aortic valve ("left-sided") endocarditis

IMMUNOLOGIC

Glomerulonephritis

Arthritis

Constitutional symptoms

---

sensitive in PVE.[10,11] Transesophageal echocardiography is also the modality of choice for detecting abscess formation (28% vs. 87% sensitivity).

3. The Duke criteria (Box 57-2)[12] incorporate echocardiographic, microbiological, and clinical findings and have been validated in the diagnosis of both PVE and NVE.[13]

IV. MANAGEMENT

A. MEDICAL THERAPY

1. Treatment of IE should be directed at the causative agent, if known. However, patients with acute IE often need empiric antibiotics, which should cover common risk factor–associated pathogens (e.g., *S. aureus* in IDU-associated IE). Empiric antibiotics should be given only after adequate culture specimens are obtained (Table 57-2).

2. Patients in whom IE is strongly suspected and who have recent (within the preceding year) prosthetic valve implantation or an indwelling vascular catheter are at high risk for coagulase-negative staphylococcal endocarditis, and empiric therapy with vancomycin should be considered.

3. The synergistic effect of aminoglycosides with a penicillin is important for the optimal treatment of enterococcal IE[14] and reduces the time until blood culture negativity in cases involving other gram-positive organisms.[15] The value of aminoglycosides in other forms of endocarditis is less clear, so their use should be avoided for patients at highest risk of nephrotoxicity and ototoxicity, including those 65 years or older, those with renal dysfunction, and those with preexisting eighth nerve dysfunction.

BOX 57-2

DUKE CRITERIA

MAJOR CRITERIA

1. Positive blood culture for IE:
   a. Typical microorganism for IE from 2 separate blood cultures: *Streptococcus viridans*, *Streptococcus bovis*, HACEK group, *Staphylococcus aureus*, or enterococci in the absence of a primary focus
   b. Persistently positive blood culture, defined as recovery of a microorganism consistent with IE from cultures drawn ≥ 12 hr apart, or all of 3 or a majority of 4 or more separate cultures, with the first and last being drawn ≥ 1 hr apart
   c. Culture positive for *Coxiella burnetii* (Q fever) or antiphase I immunoglobulin G titer > 1:800.
2. Evidence of endocardial involvement:
   a. Positive echocardiogram for IE:
      i. Oscillating intracardiac mass on valve or supporting structures, in the path of regurgitant jets, or on implanted material, in the absence of an alternative anatomic explanation, or
      ii. Abscess, or
      iii. New partial dehiscence of prosthetic valve
   OR
   b. New valvular regurgitation (↑ or change in preexisting murmur not sufficient)

MINOR CRITERIA

1. Predisposition: predisposing heart condition or intravenous drug use
2. Fever: > 38° C
3. Vascular phenomena: major arterial emboli, septic pulmonary infarcts, mycotic aneurysms, intracranial hemorrhage, conjunctival hemorrhages, Janeway lesions
4. Immunologic phenomena: glomerulonephritis, Osler nodes, Roth spots, rheumatoid factor
5. Microbiological evidence: positive blood cultures but not meeting major criteria (excluding single positive culture for coagulase-negative staphylococci and organisms not known to cause IE) as noted previously or serologic evidence of active infection with organism consistent with IE

DIAGNOSIS

A definitive diagnosis is made with 2 major criteria, 1 major and 3 minor criteria, or 5 minor criteria.

Modified from Durak DT, Lukes AS, Bright DK: *Am J Med* 96:200, 1994; and Li J et al: *Clin Infect Dis* 30:633, 2000.
HACEK, *Haemophilus* spp., *Actinobacillus actinomycetemcomitans, Cardiobacterium hominis, Eikenella corrodens,* and *Kingella kingae*; IE, infective endocarditis.

TABLE 57-2
SUGGESTED TREATMENT FOR ENDOCARDITIS

Pathogen	Native Valve		Prosthetic Valve	
	Treatment	Time (wk)	Treatment	Time (wk)
PCN-susceptible S. viridans, S. bovis, or other Streptococcus	PCN or ceftriaxone	4		
	PCN or ceftriaxone with gentamicin*		PCN or ceftriaxone with gentamicin*	6
Intermediate–PCN-resistant S. viridans, S. bovis, or other Streptococcus	PCN or ceftriaxone with gentamicin*	4	PCN or ceftriaxone with gentamicin†	6
	Vancomycin	4		
Enterococcus spp. (susceptible)	PCN, ampicillin, or vancomycin with gentamicin	4-6	PCN, ampicillin, or vancomycin with gentamicin	6
HACEK group	Ceftriaxone	4	Ceftriaxone	6
Methicillin-sensitive Staphylococcus aureus	Oxacillin or nafcillin ± gentamicin‡	4-6	Oxacillin or nafcillin with RFP and gentamicin§	≥ 6
Methicillin-resistant Staphylococcus aureus	Vancomycin ± gentamicin‡	4-6	Vancomycin with RFP and gentamicin§	≥ 6
Culture-negative endocarditis¶	Vancomycin with gentamicin* ± ceftriaxone	4	Vancomycin with gentamicin* ± ceftriaxone	≥ 6

Modified from Moreillon P et al: Lancet 363:139-149, 2004; Wilson WR et al.: JAMA 274:1706-1713, 1995; Mylonakis et al: N Engl J Med 345:1318-1330, 2001.
HACEK, Haemophilus spp., Actinobacillus actinomycetemcomitans, Cardiobacterium hominis, Eikenella corrodens, and Kingella kingae; PCN, penicillin; RFP, rifampin.
*Low-dose gentamicin for 2 wk. Once-daily doses might be adequate.
†Low-dose gentamicin could be extended to 4 wk. Once-daily doses might be adequate.
‡Low-dose gentamicin could be added for the first 3-5 d.
§Low-dose gentamicin for 2 wk.
¶Individualize for each patient.

57

INFECTIVE ENDOCARDITIS

BOX 57-3

SURGICAL INDICATIONS IN INFECTIVE ENDOCARDITIS

Moderate to severe congestive heart failure caused by valve dysfunction

Unstable prosthesis

Perivalvular extension of infection or intracardiac fistula

Large (>10 mm diameter), hypermobile vegetation (with or without prior arterial embolus)

Uncontrolled infection despite optimal antimicrobial therapy

Unavailability of effective antimicrobial therapy: endocarditis caused by fungi, *Brucella*, *Pseudomonas aeruginosa* (aortic or mitral valves), highly resistant enterococci, or poorly responsive *Staphylococcus aureus* (aortic or mitral valves)

PVE caused by *S. aureus* with an intracardiac complication

Relapse of NVE or PVE after optimal therapy

Culture-negative NVE or PVE with persistent fever (> 10 d)

Modified from Karchmer AW: Infective endocarditis. In Braunwald E, ed: *Heart disease: a textbook of cardiovascular medicine,* 6th ed, Philadelphia, 2001, WB Saunders.
NVE, native valve endocarditis; *PVE,* prosthetic valve endocarditis.

4. Surveillance electrocardiograms should be performed daily while the patient is febrile, then periodically during treatment. Particular attention should be given to the identification of PR segment prolongation that may signify the development of a valve ring abscess.

B. SURGICAL THERAPY

See Box 57-3 for indications for valve replacement.

C. PROGNOSIS

1. Patients who are receiving appropriate antibiotics for IE may continue to have fever and appear toxic for several days; this does not portend a poor outcome.

2. Five features are independently associated with 6-month mortality in IE: presence of associated illness, abnormal mental status, moderate to severe congestive heart failure, bacterial cause other than *Streptococcus viridans,* and medical therapy without valve surgery.[16]

PEARLS AND PITFALLS

- Obtaining blood cultures before starting antibiotics is critical because antibiotic use before presentation is the most common cause of "culture-negative" endocarditis.

- The association between *Streptococcus bovis* endocarditis and colonic disorders has long been recognized. Therefore, identification of *S. bovis* endocarditis should prompt an evaluation for gastrointestinal disorders, particularly malignancies.

- The diagnosis of IE should also be considered when one encounters bacteremia without an obvious source of infection, bacteremia typical for IE (*S. aureus,* HACEK), or persistent bacteremia while on antibiotics. IE can also mimic rheumatologic illness.

- Community-acquired methicillin-resistant *S. aureus* is an increasingly common cause of IDU-associated IE.
- Endocarditis prophylaxis before invasive procedures should be considered in all patients with murmurs.

REFERENCES

1. Moreillon P, Que YA: Infective endocarditis, *Lancet* 363(9403):139-149, 2004. C
2. Graves MK, Soto L: Left-sided endocarditis in parental drug abusers: recent experience at a large community hospital, *South Med J* 85:378, 1992. B
3. Hogevik H et al: Epidemiologic aspects of infective endocarditis in an urban population: a 5-year prospective study, *Medicine* 74:324, 1995. B
4. Rutledge R, Kim J, Applebaum RE: Actuarial analysis of the risk of prosthetic valve endocarditis in 1,598 patients with mechanical and bioprosthetic valves, *Arch Surg* 120:469, 1985. B
5. Calderwood SB et al: Risk factors for the development of prosthetic valve endocarditis, *Circulation* 72:31, 1985. B
6. Mathew J et al: Clinical features, site of involvement, bacteriologic findings, and outcome of infective endocarditis in intravenous drug users, *Arch Intern Med* 155:1641, 1995. B
7. Hecht SR, Berger M: Right-sided endocarditis in intravenous drug users: prognostic features in 102 episodes, *Ann Intern Med* 17:560, 1992. B
8. Roder BL et al: Clinical features of *Staphylococcus aureus* endocarditis: a 10-year experience in Denmark, *Arch Intern Med* 159:462, 1999. B
9. Fowler VG Jr et al: Infective endocarditis due to *Staphylococcus aureus:* 59 prospectively identified cases with follow-up, *Clin Infect Dis* 28:106, 1999. B
10. Daniel WG, Mugge A: Transesophageal echocardiography, *N Engl J Med* 332:1268, 1995. C
11. Daniel WG et al: Comparison of transthoracic and transesophageal echocardiography for detection of abnormalities of prosthetic and bioprosthetic valves in the mitral and aortic positions, *Am J Cardiol* 71:210, 1993. A
12. Durak DT, Lukes AS, Bright DK: New criteria for diagnosis of infective endocarditis: utilization of specific echocardiographic findings, *Am J Med* 96:200, 1994. B
13. Nettles RE et al: An evaluation of the Duke criteria in 25 pathologically confirmed cases of prosthetic valve endocarditis, *Clin Infect Dis* 25:1401, 1997. B
14. Eliopoulos GM: Enterococcal endocarditis. In Kaye D, ed: *Infective endocarditis,* 2nd ed, New York, 1992, Raven Press. C
15. Fantin B, Carbon C: In vivo antibiotic synergism: contribution of animal models, *Antimicrob Agents Chemother* 36:907, 1992. B
16. Hasbun R, Vikram HR, Barakat LA, et al: Complicated left-sided native valve endocarditis in adults: risk classification for mortality, *JAMA* 289(15):1933-1940, 2003. B

57

INFECTIVE ENDOCARDITIS

Central Venous Catheter Infections

Nicola Zetola, MD; Aimee Zaas, MD; and Stuart Ray, MD

> **FAST FACTS**
>
> - *Staphylococcus* spp. (gram-positive cocci in clusters) are the most common cause of catheter-related bloodstream infections (CR-BSIs). The presence of the coagulase enzyme differentiates *S. aureus* (coagulase positive) from the less virulent coagulase-negative staphylococci (e.g., *S. epidermidis*, *S. saprophyticus*).
> - Among *Staphylococcus* spp., coagulase-negative staphylococci predominate in CR-BSIs. Coagulase-negative staphylococci are the leading pathogens of indwelling catheters because of their ubiquity as human commensals and propensity to adhere to polymers and form biofilm (bacteria and extracellular glycoprotein matrix). Biofilm enhances bacterial adherence and provides protection from antibiotic and immune destruction.
> - The mortality rate of *S. aureus* CR-BSI is significantly higher than that of any other organism.[1]
> - Blood cultures from specimens drawn through central venous catheters have a 90% sensitivity and a 92% specificity for diagnosing CR-BSI.[2]
> - Unstable patients with CR-BSI need immediate removal of the catheter and intravenous antibiotics.
> - Only stable patients with coagulase-negative staphylococcal CR-BSI can be treated safely without removal of the catheter. High rates of recurrence are associated with this practice.

Central venous catheters are a major source of nosocomial infections that increase hospital length of stay, morbidity, and mortality. This chapter outlines the diagnosis and prevention of CR-BSIs.

I. EPIDEMIOLOGY

1. Intravascular catheters are the source of most primary bloodstream infections.[3] The skin at the insertion site is the most common source of infection during the first 10 days after insertion, whereas hub contamination becomes a predominant factor when catheters are left in place more than 10 days.
2. Microbial epidemiology of CR-BSI is outlined in Table 58-1.

TABLE 58-1

MICROBIAL EPIDEMIOLOGY OF CATHETER-RELATED BLOODSTREAM INFECTIONS

Pathogen	Percentage (%)
Gram-positive cocci	**54**
Coagulase-negative *Staphylococcus*	35
Staphylococcus aureus	6
Enterococci	10
Streptococcus spp.	3
Gram-positive bacilli	**5**
Bacillus spp.	2
Corynebacterium spp.	3
Gram-negative bacilli	**24**
Pseudomonas aeruginosa	14
Acinetobacter spp.	1
Enterobacteria*	9

Modified from Pearson ML: *Am J Infect Control* 24:262, 1996.
*Escherichia coli (4%), Proteus spp. (1%), Serratia spp. (2%), Klebsiella spp. (2%).

II. CLINICAL PRESENTATION

1. Central venous catheter infections should be suspected when a patient with a central venous catheter has unexplained fever, leukocytosis, or hypotension.
2. Catheter exit site infections generally manifest clinically as purulence, erythema, or induration at the site.

III. DIAGNOSIS

1. Because surveillance cultures in asymptomatic patients have not been shown to have clinical benefit, the Centers for Disease Control advises culturing of catheters only when clinically indicated (e.g., fever, hypotension).
2. A semiquantitative culture of the catheter tip can be used to diagnose CR-BSI by rolling the tip (distal 4 cm) of the catheter across an agar plate and counting the colonies that form after an overnight incubation. A positive culture is more than 15 colony-forming units. Semiquantitative culture has a sensitivity of 85%, specificity of 83%, and negative predictive value of 99.7%.[4]
3. An alternative approach to diagnosing CR-BSI is with paired blood cultures (two sets of blood cultures: one from the catheter and one from a peripheral vein). Wormser and colleagues evaluated this approach to the diagnosis of CR-BSI in 200 patients in the intensive care unit with indwelling central venous catheters and found a 96% sensitivity and 98% specificity when the peripheral blood culture result was used as the gold standard.[2]
4. Differential time to positivity is also useful in the diagnosis of CR-BSI.[5] In a large prospective study, Raad and colleagues found that differential

time to positivity (central venous catheter blood culture turning positive before a paired peripheral culture) had a sensitivity of 89% and specificity of 83%.[6]

5. Coagulase-negative staphylococci often contaminate blood cultures; the clinical picture should correlate with the microbiological criteria.

IV. TREATMENT

1. For treatment of CR-BSI, see Table 58-2.
2. Coagulase-negative staphylococcal CR-BSIs are the only CR-BSIs that can be treated safely without removal of the catheter (only if the patient is clinically stable); this recommendation is based on a case-controlled

TABLE 58-2

TREATMENT OF CATHETER-RELATED BLOODSTREAM INFECTION BASED ON PATHOGEN

Organism	Antimicrobial	Rapid Response	Slow Response
Staphylococcus aureus* (methicillin susceptible)	Oxacillin, nafcillin, cefazolin	10-14 d	4 wk
S. aureus* (methicillin resistant)	Vancomycin	10-14 d	4 wk
Staphylococcus epidermidis	Vancomycin (most isolates are methicillin resistant)	7 d (if catheter is removed)	10-14 d (if catheter remains)
Gram-negative bacilli	According to sensitivity of isolate	10-14 d	Prolonged
Escherichia coli and Klebsiella	3rd-generation cephalosporin or quinolone		
Enterobacter and Serratia	Carbapenem, cefepime, or 3rd-generation quinolone		
Acinetobacter	Ampicillin-sulbactam or carbapenem		
Stenotrophomonas maltophilia	Trimethoprim-sulfamethoxazole		
Pseudomonas aeruginosa	3rd or 4th-generation cephalosporin or antipseudomonal penicillin with aminoglycoside		
Candida spp.	Fluconazole, amphotericin B, or caspofungin[7]	14 d after last positive culture	Prolonged

Data from *Clin Infect Dis* 32:1249, 2001.

*Infections complicated by endocarditis or septic emboli or in patients with underlying cardiac valvular abnormalities are treated for 4-6 wk. Synergistic gentamicin 1 mg/kg q8h for 5 d can be used for complicated *S. aureus* bacteremia.

study of 70 oncology patients in which equal mortality (11%) was observed in the group whose catheters remained in place and in the group whose catheters were removed.[8]

3. *S. aureus* is never considered a contaminant, and metastatic foci are of particular concern (endocarditis, osteomyelitis, septic emboli, abscesses). Evaluation for endocarditis (by echocardiogram) is warranted.

4. *Candida* spp.: Removal of the intravascular catheter and treatment with parenteral antifungal therapy are recommended, starting with amphotericin or caspofungin in severely ill patients.[8,10] See Chapter 61 for additional details.

PEARLS AND PITFALLS

- The practice of routinely changing central catheters to prevent infection is not useful.[3]
- In a stable patient with suspected CR-BSI, the offending catheter can be removed over a guidewire and a new catheter inserted at the same site. If a CR-BSI is diagnosed, the new catheter should be removed and a catheter inserted at a new site.[3]
- When sending the catheter tip for culture, always send the distal 4 to 6 cm. (Culture the tip only when infection is suspected.)
- If blood culture results are negative and the catheter tip has more than 15 colony-forming units, monitor closely and repeat blood cultures.
- Subclavian central venous catheters are less likely than femoral or internal jugular catheters to become infected. In one study, colonization rates in patients in the intensive care unit were 47% for femoral, 22% for internal jugular, and 10% for subclavian catheters.[11]
- Chlorhexidine is superior to povidone-iodine for skin cleansing at the time of insertion, yielding an 84% decrease in catheter colonization.[12]
- Prophylactic antimicrobial use during catheter insertion does not reduce the risk of infection.[13]
- The best method for preventing CR-BSI is use of maximal sterile barriers during catheter insertion. Such barriers include covering the patient with a sterile drape and wearing a mask, cap, sterile gown, and gloves. A landmark randomized, prospective study by Raad and associates compared maximal sterile barrier precautions against standard precautions during the insertion of nontunneled, noncuffed central venous catheters in oncology patients.[14] The incidence of catheter-related sepsis was six times greater in the control group than in the maximal sterile barrier group.

58

CENTRAL VENOUS CATHETER INFECTIONS

REFERENCES

1. Byers K et al: Case fatality rate for catheter-related bloodstream infections (CRBSI): a meta-analysis [Abstract 43]. In *Proceedings of the fifth annual meeting of the Society for Hospital Epidemiology of America, 1995.* A
2. Wormser GP et al: Sensitivity and specificity of blood cultures obtained through intravascular catheters, *Crit Care Med* 18:152, 1990. A

3. Pearson ML and the Hospital Infection Control Practices Advisory Committee: Guideline for prevention of intravascular device-related infections, *Am J Infect Control* 24:262, 1996. D

4. Collignon PJ et al: Is semiquantitative culture of central vein catheter tips useful in the diagnosis of catheter associated bacteremia? *J Clin Microbiol* 24:532, 1996. D

5. Blot F et al: Earlier positivity of central-venous- versus peripheral-blood cultures is highly predictive of catheter-related sepsis, *J Clin Microbiol* 36:105, 1998. A

6. Raad I, Hanna HA, Alakech B, et al: Differential time to positivity: a useful method for diagnosing catheter-related bloodstream infections, *Ann Intern Med* 140:18-25, 2004. B

7. Mora-Duarte J et al: Comparison of caspofungin and amphotericin B for invasive candidiasis, *N Engl J Med* 347(25):2020, 2002. A

8. Raad II et al: Catheter removal affects recurrence of coagulase negative staphylococcal bacteremia, *Infect Control Hosp Epidemiol* 13:215, 1992. B

9. Nguyen MH et al: Therapeutic approaches in patients with candidemia: evaluation in a multicenter, prospective, observational study, *Arch Intern Med* 155:2429, 1995. B

10. Rex JH et al: A randomized trial comparing fluconazole with amphotericin B for the treatment of candidemia in patients without neutropenia. Candidemia Study Group and the National Institute, *N Engl J Med* 331:1325, 1994. A

11. Gil RT et al: Triple vs single lumen central venous catheters: a prospective study in a critically ill population, *Arch Intern Med* 149:1139, 1989. A

12. Maki DG, Ringer M, Alvarado CJ: Prospective randomized trial of povidone-iodine, alcohol, and chlorhexidine for prevention of infection associated with central venous and arterial catheters, *Lancet* 338:339, 1991. A

13. Ranson MR et al: Double-blind placebo controlled study of vancomycin prophylaxis for central venous catheter insertion in cancer patients, *J Hosp Infect* 15:95, 1990. A

14. Raad II et al: Prevention of central venous catheter-related infections by using maximal sterile barrier precautions during insertion, *Infect Control Hosp Epidemiol* 15:231, 1994. A

Urinary Tract Infections

Catherine Passaretti, MD; Hossein Ardehali, MD, PhD;
and Eric Nuermberger, MD

FAST FACTS

- Urinary tract infections (UTIs) may involve the lower or upper urinary tract. Acute cystitis is an infection of the bladder epithelium. Presenting symptoms include dysuria, frequency, urgency, suprapubic pain, and hematuria. Acute pyelonephritis is an infection of the renal parenchyma and collecting system. Presenting symptoms include symptoms of acute cystitis and fever, chills, flank pain, nausea, and vomiting.

- In women, the gold standard for diagnosis of a UTI is a urine culture from a midstream voided sample containing more than 10^5 colony-forming units (CFUs) per milliliter or a specimen containing more than 10^2 CFUs/ml obtained from a symptomatic woman with pyuria (> 8000 leukocytes/ml of uncentrifuged urine or > 5 leukocytes per high-power field in a centrifuged sediment). In men, a diagnosis of UTI is achieved with more than 10^3 CFUs/ml.

- Causative pathogens for uncomplicated UTIs include *Escherichia coli* (80%), *Staphylococcus saprophyticus*, *Klebsiella* spp., and *Enterococcus faecalis*.

- Empiric treatment of acute uncomplicated cystitis in women without a urine culture is an accepted practice. In most areas, empiric treatment consists of a 3-day course of trimethoprim-sulfamethoxazole (TMP-SMX). In geographic locations with rates of resistant *E. coli* greater than 20%, either a 3-day course of a fluoroquinolone or a 7-day course of nitrofurantoin is recommended.[1]

- Acute uncomplicated pyelonephritis can be treated in outpatients with an oral fluoroquinolone unless persistent high fever, inability to tolerate oral intake, nausea and vomiting, or high white blood cell count is present. In these cases, the patient should be admitted and treated with intravenous antibiotics, then switched to oral therapy once stable. Treatment duration is 10 to 14 days.

UTIs are a common problem that leads to substantial morbidity and expense. Acute cystitis alone results in up to 3.6 million visits to physicians' offices[2] and more than 1 million hospital admissions per year. This chapter provides an approach to the management of common urinary tract infections.

I. EPIDEMIOLOGY

1. Acute cystitis, the clinical syndrome resulting from infection of the bladder epithelium, is a common malady that disproportionately affects

women. Forty to fifty percent of women report having at least one UTI in their lifetime. The incidence of acute cystitis is particularly high in young, sexually active women, who experience 0.5 to 0.7 episodes per person year.[3] Cystitis is much less common in men, with an annual incidence of 5 episodes per 10,000.[4]

2. Complicated UTIs are infections associated with an underlying condition that increases the risk of therapeutic failure, such as old age, instrumentation, catheter use, spinal cord injury, diabetes, pregnancy, obstruction, immunosuppression, and renal failure.

3. Asymptomatic bacteriuria is defined as the presence of a positive urine culture in the absence of symptoms. The prevalence of asymptomatic bacteriuria in the general population is about 3.5% and increases with age, pregnancy, diabetes, and history of UTI.

4. Acute pyelonephritis is the clinical syndrome caused by infection of the renal parenchyma and collecting system. Approximately 250,000 cases of pyelonephritis occur annually in the United States.[5]

5. Chronic pyelonephritis is inflammation, scarring, and atrophy of the renal parenchyma caused by persistent or recurrent infection and is most commonly seen in patients with long-term vesicoureteral reflux.

6. Recurrent UTIs may be caused by **reinfection** with a different isolate or **relapse** of infection with the original isolate within 2 weeks after completion of therapy. Approximately one third of women with a UTI have a recurrent infection, often less than 6 months after diagnosis.[6]

7. Acute prostatitis is infection of the prostate, often caused by ascending colonization of the urinary tract. Symptoms include acute onset of fever, dysuria, pelvic or perineal pain, dribbling, and hesitancy.

8. Chronic prostatitis is a more subacute process characterized by recurrent prostatic infection and typically manifests as recurrent UTI, dysuria, or pelvic pain.[7]

II. CLINICAL PRESENTATION

1. Symptoms of acute cystitis include dysuria, frequency, urgency, and suprapubic pain. Hematuria is present in approximately 30% of cases. Patients may also complain of cloudy, malodorous urine. Urethritis may cause similar symptoms of dysuria and frequency, but the symptoms often are milder and more gradual in onset. Causative agents for acute urethritis include *Chlamydia trachomatis*; *Neisseria gonorrhoeae*; *Ureaplasma urealyticum*; herpes simplex virus; and, less commonly, *E. coli* or other uropathogens.

2. Acute pyelonephritis, in contrast to cystitis, usually presents with a fever higher than 38.4° C, chills, and flank pain or costovertebral angle tenderness. Systemic symptoms such as general malaise, myalgias, nausea, vomiting, and anorexia may also be present.

3. Older adults may have a paucity of symptoms with either cystitis or pyelonephritis.

III. CAUSES

1. Most UTIs are caused by Enterobacteriaceae originating from the digestive tract, with *E. coli* being the most common causative agent (Table 59-1). In women the most common route of infection is migration of the organism from the rectum to the vaginal introitus, colonization of the distal urethra, and ascension to the bladder. Women are more prone to UTIs than men because of the proximity of the urethra[6] to the anus and the short length of the urethra (about 4 cm). Sexual intercourse and the use of spermicidal agents and diaphragms also increase the risk of UTIs in women.
2. Normal host defenses against UTI include urinary flow, increased urea concentrations, increased osmolarity, and the antiadherent and antibacterial properties of the bladder mucosa.
3. Risk factors for UTI are listed in Box 59-1.
4. Pyelonephritis usually occurs as a result of ascending infection, but bacteremic spread can also occur (most commonly with *Staphylococcus aureus*).

IV. DIAGNOSIS

1. In young to middle-aged women, the diagnosis of acute uncomplicated UTI can be made on the basis of typical clinical presentation in the absence of vaginal discharge or irritation. Ninety percent of women who

TABLE 59-1
BACTERIAL ETIOLOGY OF URINARY TRACT INFECTIONS[8]

	% Uncomplicated	% Complicated*
GRAM NEGATIVE		
Escherichia coli	70-95	21-54
Proteus mirabilis	1-2	1-10
Klebsiella spp.	1-2	2-17
Citrobacter spp.	<1	5
Enterobacter spp.	<1	2-10
Pseudomonas aeruginosa	<1	2-19
Other	<1	6-20
GRAM POSITIVE		
Coagulase-negative staphylococci	5-10[†]	1-4
Enterococci	1-2	1-23
Group B streptococci	<1	1-4
Staphylococcus aureus	<1	1-2
Other	<1	2

Modified from Hooton TM: The current management strategies for community acquired urinary tract infection, *Infect Dis Clin North Am* 17(2):303-332, 2003.
*Data from Nicolle LE: A practical guide to the management of complicated urinary tract infection, *Drugs* 53:583-592, 1997.
[†]*Staphylococcus saprophyticus*.

BOX 59-1
FACTORS THAT INCREASE SUSCEPTIBILITY TO URINARY TRACT INFECTION[5]

BIOLOGIC
Prior history of urinary tract infection
Urinary obstruction
Congenital abnormalities of the urinary tract
Diabetes

BEHAVIORAL
Sexual intercourse
Diaphragm use
Condom use
Spermicide use

OTHER
Urogenital surgery
Estrogen deficiency

fit these criteria have a UTI. A good history should help differentiate between symptoms of cystitis, urethritis, and vaginitis.[9,10]

2. Pretreatment cultures do not improve outcomes in acute uncomplicated cystitis and are not necessary before initiation of treatment.

3. Urinalysis and culture are recommended for patients with an unclear diagnosis, recurrent or relapsing cystitis, pyelonephritis, or complicated UTIs.[10]

4. Pyuria (defined as 8000 leukocytes per milliliter of uncentrifuged urine or > 5 leukocytes per high-power field in a centrifuged sediment) on urinalysis is present in almost all women with a UTI (95% sensitivity, 71% specificity).[2] White blood cell casts on urinalysis are diagnostic of a UTI.

5. Urine culture obtained from a midstream voided specimen traditionally has been considered positive if more than 10^5 CFUs/ml are present. In women with acute symptoms and pyuria, a culture can be considered positive if more than 10^2 CFUs/ml are present.[11]

6. Urine dipstick testing may also suggest UTI. A positive leukocyte esterase test has been shown to be 75% to 96% sensitive and 94% to 98% specific in detecting pyuria. A positive nitrite test is a fairly sensitive test for the presence of Enterobacteriaceae (which convert urinary nitrate to nitrite), but it lacks specificity.[11]

7. In cases of suspected pyelonephritis, evaluation includes complete blood cell count with differential, serum creatinine, urinalysis, urine culture, and blood cultures (obtained before antibiotic therapy).

8. Imaging studies are not routinely indicated in a patient with acute pyelonephritis or cystitis unless the patient has recurrent pyelonephritis; has symptoms suggestive of stone, obstruction, or abscess; or does not respond to antibiotic therapy within 72 hours. Computed tomography

with contrast is more sensitive than ultrasound for detecting stones, abscesses, or other abnormalities.

V. MANAGEMENT

1. Forty to seventy percent of lower UTIs clear spontaneously if untreated, although symptoms may persist for weeks to months. In one study comparing a 3-day course of nitrofurantoin with placebo in the treatment of uncomplicated UTI, 41% of patients receiving placebo and 74% of patients receiving nitrofurantoin achieved bacteriological cure at 7 days. More importantly, 1 out of 38 women receiving placebo went on to develop pyelonephritis.[12]

2. Trimethoprim-sulfamethoxazole (TMP-SMX) remains highly effective in treating cystitis and acute pyelonephritis and is the treatment of choice unless the patient lives in an area where resistance rates among *E. coli* isolates are greater than 20%. Risk factors for infection with TMP-SMX-resistant bacteria include diabetes, recent treatment with antimicrobials (especially TMP-SMX), recent UTI, and recent hospitalization. Clinical and microbiologic response rates are clearly lower in patients with TMP-SMX-resistant isolates.[13]

3. Fluoroquinolones are at least as effective in treating cystitis and pyelonephritis as TMP-SMX. A recent study comparing a 7-day course of ciprofloxacin with a 14-day course of TMP-SMX for acute pyelonephritis showed significantly higher clinical and bacteriologic cure rates in patients treated with ciprofloxacin.[14] However, use of fluoroquinolones for acute uncomplicated cystitis should be limited by their greater cost and concerns about selecting for drug-resistant bacteria. Currently, in the United States 10% of TMP-SMX-resistant *E. coli* is also fluoroquinolone resistant.[15]

4. Nitrofurantoin is associated with lower cure rates (85% vs. 90% to 95%) than TMP-SMX or the fluoroquinolones, but it is a favorable alternative to the latter drugs for acute uncomplicated cystitis because resistance remains low among common uropathogens. Nitrofurantoin does not achieve acceptable serum concentrations and should not be used in patients with pyelonephritis or renal failure.

5. Use of amoxicillin or oral cephalosporins is currently out of favor because of the prevalence of drug resistance and the need for a 7-day regimen.

6. Single-dose oral fosfomycin is less effective in treating acute cystitis than TMP/SMX and fluoroquinolones, especially for treating infections caused by *Staphylococcus saprophyticus*.[2] Advantages of fosfomycin therapy include ease of administration, low rates of resistance, and reduced fluoroquinolone usage. One disadvantage is its higher cost.

7. Table 59-2 and Box 59-2 provide guidelines for the duration of treatment and dosage for each antibiotic regimen. For most antibiotics, longer treatment durations are associated with greater cost, lower compliance, and a higher rate of adverse effects with no increase in efficacy.[8,16]

59

URINARY TRACT INFECTIONS

TABLE 59-2	
INFECTIOUS DISEASES SOCIETY OF AMERICA GUIDELINES: ACUTE UNCOMPLICATED URINARY TRACT INFECTIONS[16]	
Resistance	Recommended Drug Dosage
TMP-SMX resistance < 20%	TMP/SMX 1 double-strength tablet (160/800 mg) bid × 3 d
TMP-SMX resistance > 20%	Fluoroquinolone × 3 d (e.g., ciprofloxacin 250 mg bid)
	Nitrofurantoin (macrocrystals 50-100 mg qid × 7 d or monohydrate and macrocrystals (Macrobid) 100 mg bid × 7 d)
	Fosfomycin trometamol 3 g single-dose treatment

TMP-SMX, trimethoprim-sulfamethoxazole.

BOX 59-2
INFECTIOUS DISEASES SOCIETY OF AMERICA GUIDELINES: ACUTE UNCOMPLICATED PYELONEPHRITIS[16]
MILD OR MODERATE SYMPTOMS IN A COMPLIANT PATIENT: OUTPATIENT TREATMENT (TOTAL OF 7-14 D)
May need 12-24 hr initial observation in emergency department (parenteral or oral treatment)
Oral treatment:
Fluoroquinolone
Trimethoprim-sulfamethoxazole, if uropathogen known to be susceptible
Amoxicillin or amoxicillin-clavulanate, if gram-positive pathogen
SEVERE SYMPTOMS OR NONCOMPLIANT PATIENT: INPATIENT TREATMENT
Parenteral therapy until afebrile:
Aminoglycoside + ampicillin or
Fluoroquinolone or
Extended-spectrum cephalosporin + aminoglycoside
Change to oral agent (based on pretherapy urine culture and sensitivities) to finish course once patient is stable and signs and symptoms are improving

8. In women with acute **complicated** cystitis, fluoroquinolones are the therapy of choice. Treatment duration in these patients should be extended to 7 to 14 days.

PEARLS AND PITFALLS

- For women who have more than two episodes of acute cystitis in 6 months or three episodes in 1 year, consider long-term (6-12 months) prophylactic antibiotics or postcoital prophylaxis.[17] Antimicrobial options for prophylaxis include daily TMP-SMX, trimethoprim alone, nitrofurantoin, or thrice-weekly TMP-SMX or norfloxacin.[2] Avoiding the use of diaphragms or spermicides, voiding after intercourse, using topical estrogen (for postmenopausal women), and drinking liberal amounts of fluids may also help decrease the risk of recurrent UTIs.

Several studies have shown that 200 to 750 ml of cranberry juice per day may help decrease the risk of symptomatic, recurrent infection.[2]

- Pregnant women should be screened and treated for asymptomatic bacteriuria (ASB) because 20% to 40% of women with ASB progress to pyelonephritis, and ASB is associated with low birth weight and higher likelihood of preterm delivery.[18] Treatment options include nitrofurantoin, amoxicillin-clavulanate, amoxicillin, or cephalosporins.[19]

- ASB should also be treated when it occurs in renal transplant recipients, patients who have recently undergone a urologic procedure, and patients with neutropenia. ASB in older adults, in patients with indwelling bladder catheters, or in those with diabetes generally should not be treated.

- Risk factors for acute cystitis in men include increased age, lack of circumcision, HIV infection (especially with lower CD4 counts), anatomic abnormalities such as benign prostatic hypertrophy or urethral strictures, and sexual activity (especially insertive anal intercourse). Thirty percent of young men with bacteriuria have an anatomic abnormality. For this reason, all young men without the aforementioned risk factors for UTI should be evaluated for an anatomic or functional abnormality. Given the higher likelihood of developing a complicated infection, all men with UTIs should be treated for 7 to 10 days with TMP-SMX or fluoroquinolones.[20]

- Recurrent UTIs in men should prompt an investigation for nephrolithiasis or prostatitis.

- Twenty-five percent of male genitourinary complaints are attributable to prostatitis. Traditionally, the diagnosis of prostatitis is based on clinical findings and the "four-cup test." The four-cup test involves collecting four specimens: #1 is the first 10 ml of voided urine, #2 is a midstream specimen, #3 is collection of prostatic secretions after prostatic massage, and #4 is the first 10 ml of urine collected after prostatic massage. In prostatitis, cultures of #1 and #2 should be negative, whereas cultures of #3 and #4 should be positive.[21] Empiric treatment of acute prostatitis consists of ciprofloxacin or TMP-SMX for 4 weeks. Chronic bacterial prostatitis should be treated with a fluoroquinolone, TMP-SMX, or doxycycline for 6 to 12 weeks.

- In patients with indwelling catheters, pyuria is less strongly correlated with UTI than in patients without catheters.[22] Treatment with antibiotics should be given only when symptoms occur with evidence of infected urine. Obtaining routine urine cultures in the absence of symptoms is discouraged. An essential component of the treatment of UTI in a patient with an indwelling catheter is removal of the old catheter. Given that up to 17% of nosocomial bacteremia is the result of UTIs caused by indwelling catheters, preventive measures such as avoiding or discontinuing the use of catheters whenever possible, changing catheters every 2 to 4 weeks, and using closed drainage systems should be emphasized.

59

URINARY TRACT INFECTIONS

- Sterile pyuria (i.e., pyuria in the absence of bacteriuria) may indicate infection with bacteria such as *Ureaplasma urealyticum, Chlamydia trachomatis, Mycobacterium tuberculosis,* or fungi. It may also indicate noninfectious causes such as calculi, interstitial nephritis, and polycystic kidney disease.
- Treatment of asymptomatic candiduria is not recommended in nonneutropenic catheterized patients because recurrence is likely as long as the Foley catheter remains in place. Treatment of candiduria with fluconazole or amphotericin B for 7 to 14 days is recommended in patients who are either symptomatic or neutropenic or have undergone renal transplantation or recent urologic manipulation.[23]

REFERENCES

1. Warren JW, Abrutyn E, Hebel JR, et al: Guidelines for antimicrobial treatment of uncomplicated urinary tract infection, *Infect Dis Clin North Am* 11:551-581, 1997. D
2. Fihn SD: Acute uncomplicated urinary tract infection in women, *N Engl J Med* 349(3):259-266, 2003. C
3. Hooton TM, Scholes D, Hughes JP, et al: Prospective study of risk factors for symptomatic UTIs in young women, *N Engl J Med* 335(7):468-474, 1996. B
4. Krieger JN, Ross SO, Simonsen JMJ: Urinary tract infections in healthy university men, *J Urol* 149(5):1046-1048, 1993. B
5. Foxman B: Epidemiology of urinary tract infections: incidence, morbidity and economic costs, *Am J Med* 113(suppl 1A):5S-13S, 2002. C
6. McLaughlin SP, Carson CC: Urinary tract infections in women, *Med Clin North Am* 88(2):417-429, 2004. C
7. Hua VN, Schaeffer AJ: Acute and chronic prostatitis, *Med Clin North Am* 88(2):483-494, 2004. C
8. Hooton TM: The current management strategies for community-acquired urinary tract infection, *Infect Dis Clin North Am* 17(2):303-332, 2003. D
9. Bent S, Nallamothu BK, Simel DL, et al: Does this woman have an acute uncomplicated urinary tract infection? *JAMA* 287(20):2701-2710, 2002. C
10. Bent S: The optimal use of diagnostic testing in women with acute uncomplicated cystitis, *Am J Med* 113(Suppl 1A):20S-28S, 2002. C
11. Pappas PG: Laboratory in the diagnosis and management of urinary tract infections, *Med Clin North Am* 75(2):313-325, 1991. C
12. Christiaens TC, DeMeyere M, Verschraegen G, et al: Randomized controlled trial of nitrofurantoin versus placebo in the treatment of uncomplicated urinary tract infection in adult women, *Br J Gen Pract* 52(482):708-710, 2002. A
13. Raz R, Chazan B, Kennes Y, et al: Empiric use of trimethoprim-sulfamethoxazole (TMP-SMX) in the treatment of women with uncomplicated urinary tract infections, in a geographical area with a high prevalence of TMP-SMX–resistant uropathogens, *Clin Infect Dis* 34(9):1165-1169, 2002. B
14. Talan DA, Stamm WE, Hooton TM, et al: Comparison of ciprofloxacin (7 days) and trimethoprim-sulfamethoxazole (14 days) for acute uncomplicated pyelonephritis in women: a randomized trial, *JAMA* 283:1583-1590, 2000. A
15. Karlowsky JA, Thornsberry C, Jones ME, et al: Susceptibility of antimicrobial-resistant urinary *Escherichia coli* isolates to fluoroquinolones and nitrofurantoin, *Clin Infect Dis* 36(2):183-187, 2003. B

16. Nicolle LE: Urinary tract infection: traditional pharmacologic therapies, *Dis Mon* 49(2):111-128, 2003. C
17. Hooton TM: Recurrent urinary tract infection in women, *Int J Antimicrob Agents* 17:259-268, 2001. C
18. Mittendorf R, Williams MA, Kass EH: Prevention of preterm delivery and low birth weight associated with asymptomatic bacteriuria, *Clin Infect Dis* 14(4):927-932, 1992. C
19. Millar LK, Cox SM: Urinary tract infections complicating pregnancy, *Infect Dis Clin North Am* 11(1):13-26, 1997. C
20. Lipsky BA: Urinary tract infections in men. Epidemiology, pathophysiology, diagnosis, and treatment, *Ann Intern Med* 110(2):138-150, 1989. C
21. Lipsky BA: Prostatitis and urinary tract infection in men: what's new; what's true? *Am J Med* 106(3):327-334, 1999. C
22. Tambyah PA, Maki DG: The relationship between pyuria and infection in patients with indwelling urinary catheters: a prospective study of 761 patients, *Arch Intern Med* 160(5):673-677, 2000. B
23. Lundstrom T, Sobel J: Nosocomial candiduria: a review, *Clin Infect Dis* 32(11):1602-1607, 2001. C

Soft Tissue and Bone Infection

Adam Spivak, MD; Patrick Sosnay, MD; and Sara Cosgrove, MD

> ### FAST FACTS
>
> - The most common causes of cellulitis are *Streptococcus* species and *Staphylococcus aureus*. Osteomyelitis is most commonly caused by *S. aureus*.
> - Cellulitis often is treated empirically. In contrast, antimicrobial therapy for osteomyelitis should be guided by microbiologic data. Culture of infected bone is the gold standard.
> - Patients with a rapidly progressive infection or a systemic inflammatory response from their infection warrant imaging and possible surgical evaluation. Gas gangrene, necrotizing fasciitis, and soft tissue infections caused by toxin-producing strains of *S. aureus* and group A *Streptococcus* are surgical emergencies.

Soft tissue infections and osteomyelitis are common in hospitalized patients. This chapter describes common characteristics of both soft tissue infections and osteomyelitis and includes alternative diagnoses that should be considered. Approaches to evaluating and treating patients with these conditions are outlined.

Soft Tissue Infections

I. EPIDEMIOLOGY

1. Cellulitis is most commonly caused by *S. aureus* and *Streptococcus* species. Less common etiologic agents often are associated with specific clinical scenarios elucidated in the history (Table 60-1).
2. Risk factors for cellulitis include both local and host factors (Box 60-1).[1]

II. CLINICAL PRESENTATION

1. The timing and tempo of symptoms in patients presenting with soft tissue infection are important in generating a differential diagnosis. Infections that come on rapidly or spread quickly are worrisome and merit immediate attention.
2. **Cellulitis.**
a. Localized pain, warmth, and induration are the classic complaints of cellulitis. These complaints may not be as obvious if the patient has compromised sensation of the affected area, as occurs with diabetic patients or those with spinal cord injuries. Physical examination demonstrates an erythematous, confluent macular rash with ill-defined borders, most often involving the extremities. If bullae and blisters are seen, toxin-producing streptococcal species and gram-negative

TABLE 60-1

CLINICAL SITUATIONS AND ASSOCIATED PATHOGENS IN CELLULITIS

Situation	Pathogenic Organism	Comments
Hot tub exposure	*Pseudomonas aeruginosa*	Often causes folliculitis.
Venectomy or lymphedema	*Streptococcus* spp.	
Aquarium exposure	*Mycobacterium marinum*	Often causes nodular cellulitis.
Freshwater exposure	*Aeromonas* spp.	
Saltwater exposure	*Vibrio* spp.	Life-threatening in cirrhotic patients.
Fingertips	*Herpes simplex*	Health care workers at risk.
Dermatomal rash with vesicles	*Herpes zoster*	
Cellulitis surrounding diabetic foot ulcer	Polymicrobial	Management entails wound care and evaluation of vascular supply.

BOX 60-1

RISK FACTORS FOR DEVELOPMENT OF SOFT TISSUE INFECTIONS

LOCAL FACTORS

Trauma

Injection drug use

Tinea pedis

HOST FACTORS

Diabetes mellitus

Cirrhosis

Impaired lymphatic drainage (e.g., after mastectomy)

Venous stasis

Neutropenia

organisms should be considered. Fever, hemodynamic compromise, and mental status change may accompany severe infection.

b. Erysipelas is cellulitis caused by group A *Streptococcus* that has prominent lymphatic involvement. Erysipelas will typically have a more homogenous appearance with well-demarcated and raised borders. It commonly occurs in areas of lymphatic disruption, such as surgical sites and areas of trauma, and is characterized by a painful, often bright red area with a peau d'orange appearance from lymphatic obstruction.

c. Cellulitis adjacent to a diabetic foot ulcer often is polymicrobial and can be difficult to treat if arterial insufficiency is present. Deeper infections such as osteomyelitis should be ruled out. A history of antibiotic exposure should be obtained to help determine the likelihood of infection by resistant organisms.

3. **Necrotizing fasciitis** is an infection that occurs in a deeper tissue plane than cellulitis and spreads rapidly along the fascial surface (see Plate 16). This infection has a high mortality and should be considered a surgical emergency because antibiotics are considered an adjunct to rapid surgical debridement. Findings that raise suspicion of necrotizing fasciitis include tenderness out of proportion to other clinical signs of inflammation; loss of sensation in the affected area; bullae; crepitus; skin that appears shiny, indurated, brawny, or dark in color; or any unexplained vital sign abnormality. Fournier's gangrene is an equivalent deep tissue infection in the perineal region. Necrotizing fasciitis caused by group A *Streptococcus* is particularly fulminant. Toxins produced by strains of group A *Streptococcus* upregulate inflammatory cytokines, leading to a syndrome similar to staphylococcal toxic shock syndrome.

4. **Gas gangrene** (or clostridial myonecrosis) is a deep tissue infection caused by *Clostridium* species that has a fulminant presentation.

5. **Pyomyositis** is a rare entity of deep muscle abscesses typically caused by *S. aureus.* Clinical hallmarks are mild systemic symptoms, normal creatinine phosphokinase levels, and induration of muscle without fluctuance.

III. DIAGNOSIS

1. The differential diagnosis of cellulitis includes venous stasis dermatitis, necrotizing fasciitis, gas gangrene, cutaneous anthrax, deep venous thrombosis, drug reactions and hypersensitivity responses, Sweet's syndrome, and acute gout flares (see Plate 16).[1]

2. The diagnosis of cellulitis is made by history and physical examination. Imaging and cultures typically are low yield and not cost-effective in most cases. Bacteremia is a rare event in cellulitis, and blood cultures are recommended only in patients who appear to be systemically infected. A patient with soft tissue infection should undergo imaging if a deeper infection is suspected or if history and physical examination cannot differentiate between infection and deep venous thrombosis. An exception to the empiric therapy of cellulitis is blistering disease. If an intact bullous lesion is present, sterile aspiration at the bedside can yield a pathogenic organism that can guide therapy.

3. Cellulitis may show as swelling or haziness of subcutaneous fat on plain radiographs. Radiographs with radiolucent foci indicate the presence of gas. Ultrasound is most helpful when an abscess is suspected. If an abscess contains debris, however, it may not be discernible from surrounding tissue. Doppler ultrasound should be obtained to evaluate for deep venous thrombosis.

4. Computed tomography (CT) and magnetic resonance imaging (MRI) are the most helpful imaging modalities when deeper infection is suspected because of their higher resolution. CT with intravenous contrast can detect abscesses, phlegmons, or fluid accumulations.[2,3]

IV. MANAGEMENT

1. Cellulitis can be treated with intravenous or oral antibiotics; the extent of infection and the general clinical status of the patient determine which route of administration is appropriate. Drugs with antistaphylococcal and antistreptococcal spectra are preferred for cellulitis in the immunocompetent host. Antibiotic coverage should be broadened in patients who appear systemically ill, diabetics with cellulitis surrounding an ulcer, neutropenic patients, and patients with end-stage liver disease. See Table 60-2 for antibiotic recommendations.
2. Local wound care is a critical component of treatment. Clinical experience dictates that patients should always elevate the affected extremity. If the site of the break in the cutaneous barrier is an ulcer, devitalized tissue must be debrided. This can be performed surgically or with wound care preparations that have debriding qualities.
3. Risk factor reduction is also an important consideration.
a. Diabetic patients should be educated on the importance of foot care, daily inspection, and proper footwear.
b. Bed-bound patients should be repositioned frequently and put in a bed designed to prevent ulcers.
c. Intractable venous insufficiency ulcers can be helped by compression stockings.

TABLE 60-2
ANTIMICROBIAL THERAPY FOR CELLULITIS AND SOFT TISSUE INFECTIONS

Cellulitis Variant	Organisms	Recommended Antibiotics
Healthy host	Staphylococcus aureus Streptococcus spp.	Cephalexin, dicloxacillin Clindamycin (for penicillin allergy)
Recent antibiotic or hospital exposure	Consider methcillin-resistant S. aureus	Vancomycin Depending on susceptibility patterns, trimethoprim-sulfamethoxazole, minocycline, clindamycin
Ill-appearing patient	S. aureus Streptococcus spp.r	Intravenous cefazolin, oxacillin, o clindamycin
Diabetic foot ulcer	Polymicrobial, including gram-negative rods and anaerobes	Piperacillin-tazobactam, or ciprofloxacin plus metronidazole
Neutropenic patient	Fungal species Pseudomonas	Antifungals Piperacillin-tazobactam
Postoperative patient	Usually Staphylococcus, Streptococcus spp., Clostridium perfringens	Oxacillin, cefazolin, cefotetan Add clindamycin if Clostridium suspected
Cirrhotic patient	Gram-negative rods Vibrio spp.	Cefotetan or piperacillin-tazobactam Add doxycycline if Vibrio vulnificus suspected

d. All patients should be examined for the presence of tinea pedis because treating this infection reduces recurrence.

Osteomyelitis

I. EPIDEMIOLOGY

1. Osteomyelitis is an infection of bone that arises from bloodborne or local microbial infection. Risk factors include trauma to bone or surrounding soft tissue, foreign body insertion or manipulation, vascular insufficiency, and diabetes mellitus.[4]
2. Hematogenous osteomyelitis typically has an acute presentation. It is seen most often in children and adolescents and is most commonly caused by *S. aureus*. Osteomyelitis caused by *Mycobacterium tuberculosis* (Pott's disease) has a predilection for the spine and should be considered in the differential diagnosis of any patient with spinal osteomyelitis.
3. Osteomyelitis caused by local spread of soft tissue infection can be further classified as acute or chronic. Acute infections of bone occur with penetrating trauma or as a result of a complex fracture. They also are seen in the surgical setting as postoperative infections or subsequent seeding of surgically implanted prosthetics and other foreign bodies.
4. Chronic osteomyelitis adjacent to an ulcer is the form most commonly encountered by the internist. This occurs often in the feet of patients with diabetes or vascular insufficiency or at the site of a pressure ulcer in older adults or immobilized patients. Infections often are polymicrobial. Table 60-3 reviews some of the pathogens that are associated with osteomyelitis.[5-7]

II. CLINICAL PRESENTATION

1. Hematogenous osteomyelitis typically presents with localized pain and edema, malaise, fever, and chills. Patients may have a history of recent

TABLE 60-3

CLINICAL SITUATIONS AND ASSOCIATED PATHOGENS IN OSTEOMYELITIS

Osteomyelitis Variant	Pathogenic Organism	Comments
Healthy host	Staphylococcus aureus	Most common cause.
Foreign body or prosthetic	Coagulase-negative Staphylococcus	
Nosocomial infections	Enterobacteriaceae or Pseudomonas aeruginosa	Gram-negative coverage determined by hospital resistance patterns.
Diabetic or pressure ulcers	S. aureus, streptococci, gram-negative rods, anaerobes	
Sickle cell disease	Salmonella, Streptococcus pneumoniae	Hematogenous seeding.

intravenous catheters or injection drug use, although the source of infection often is unidentifiable. Blood cultures can be helpful in guiding therapy. Osteomyelitis caused by acute injury or fracture often presents with localizing complaints.

2. In contiguous osteomyelitis, the infection tends to have a subtle clinical presentation. A high clinical suspicion should be maintained with diabetic foot ulcers because early detection and treatment have been shown to reduce the need for amputation.[8]

3. The suspicion of vertebral osteomyelitis mandates a thorough neurologic examination to look for evidence of spinal cord compromise caused by vertebral destruction or epidural abscess.

III. DIAGNOSIS

1. In patients with a known ulcer, the clinician must determine whether bone infection is present beneath the soft tissue injury. Probing to bone with a blunt instrument in a diabetic foot ulcer has a sensitivity of 66% and a specificity of 85% for osteomyelitis.[9] However, the low sensitivity often necessitates additional diagnostic testing.

2. Erythrocyte sedimentation rate (ESR) and C-reactive protein (CRP) are serum markers of systemic inflammation that are often used in osteomyelitis, although both lack sensitivity and specificity. Despite these limitations, they can be used to follow a patient's response to treatment when obtained in serial fashion.

3. Microbiology.

a. In hematogenous osteomyelitis, blood cultures occasionally are positive and can help guide therapy.

b. Culture of an ulcer or drainage from a sinus tract has not been shown to be useful in determining a pathogenic organism.[10] Culturing an ulcer may be beneficial only to search for clinically significant resistant organisms such as methicillin-resistant *S. aureus* when empiric treatment is being used.

c. Culture of infected bone is the gold standard in the diagnosis of osteomyelitis. Given the often subtle clinical picture associated with chronic osteomyelitis, noninvasive imaging is diagnostically important.[11]

4. Imaging in osteomyelitis is well studied, but there is no consensus on the best modality.[12,13] Table 60-4 reviews the options for imaging in osteomyelitis. In general, all of these imaging modalities lack specificity in diagnosing osteomyelitis in patients with contiguous inflammation. Compared with nuclear bone scans, MRI has superior specificity and adds the ability to characterize the surrounding soft tissue. The choice of modality varies according to the experience of a particular institution, and consultation with radiology and nuclear medicine specialists is recommended. In vertebral osteomyelitis, MRI is the image modality of choice because it detects marrow inflammation and has superior spatial resolution in imaging the spinal cord and nerve roots.[14]

TABLE 60-4
COMPARISON OF IMAGING MODALITIES IN OSTEOMYELITIS[14]

Modality	Findings	Advantages	Disadvantages	Comments
Plain radiograph	Soft tissue edema Cortical erosion	Readily available Inexpensive	30-50% loss of bone density before becomes abnormal (~2 wk into infection)	Poor sensitivity Specificity equal to that of nuclear scans
CT	Same as plain radiograph but with better resolution	Detects bony sequestra, foreign bodies in chronic osteomyelitis	Lacks sensitivity of MRI	
MRI	Low signal on T1 High signal on T2	Good delineation of bone marrow, soft tissue	Hard to distinguish trauma, neoplasm from infection, new from old disease	Sensitivity 60-100% Specificity 50-90%
Technetium bone scan	Increased signal from osteoblastic activity, hyperemia	Scans whole skeleton Sensitive earlier in disease than radiograph and CT	Expense Timing of test (3 phases, takes 24 hr)	Sensitivity 95% Specificity 85%
Indium WBC scan	Increased signal from indium-labeled WBCs	Sensitivity high, can effectively rule out diabetic foot osteomyelitis	Hard to distinguish overlying soft tissue infection	Sensitivity 65-100% Specificity 23-100%

CT, computed tomography; MRI, magnetic resonance imaging; WBC, white blood cell.

IV. MANAGEMENT

1. Antibiotics.
   a. Osteomyelitis is traditionally treated with 4 to 6 weeks of parenteral antibiotics directed against biopsy-proven pathogens. Unless the patient is unstable, antibiotics can wait until microbiologic data are obtained.
   b. Hematogenous osteomyelitis is caused most often by a single organism and can be treated with antibiotics specific for that organism.
   c. Diabetic foot ulcers with underlying osteomyelitis often are infected with gram-negative organisms and anaerobes, in addition to gram-positive organisms, and warrant broad coverage guided by culture information.
   d. Clinicians may choose to complete a course of therapy with oral agents. This should be considered only after the patient is fully evaluated with appropriate cultures, diagnostic imaging, and debridement, which usually entails in-hospital evaluation. The choice of oral therapy should be on the basis of culture data, ability of agents to reach appropriate concentrations in bone, and consultation with infectious disease experts.
2. The treatment of osteomyelitis often warrants a multimodality strategy including antibiotics, surgical debridement, and possibly revascularization.[15] Cure can be difficult to achieve in patients with untreated vascular insufficiency. Amputation of a portion of the affected extremity deserves consideration when systemic infection is uncontrollable, when the vascular supply to the area cannot be improved with surgical or radiologic intervention, or when the ulcer does not heal despite local wound care and appropriate antibiotics.

PEARLS AND PITFALLS

- Patients often have recurrence of cellulitis or osteomyelitis with the same organism; previous culture data can help guide therapy. Duration and efficacy of prior therapy should be evaluated because osteomyelitis can recur if not fully treated.
- Community-acquired methicillin-resistant *S. aureus* has been reported in several countries, including the United States. It has been associated with skin and soft tissue infections and with necrotizing pneumonia. This pathogen's antibiotic resistance patterns and virulence factors appear to be different from those of nosocomial methicillin-resistant *S. aureus*.
- Anthrax has become an entity of increased clinical importance. The clinical hallmarks of cutaneous anthrax, a primarily toxin-mediated reaction, include a painless papulovesicular lesion with massive surrounding edema that progresses to an eschar within 2 to 5 days (see Supplemental PDA Chapter 8).

60

SOFT TISSUE AND BONE INFECTION

REFERENCES

1. Swartz MN: Clinical practice. Cellulitis, *N Engl J Med* 350(9):904-912, 2004. C
2. Levine SE, Neagle CE, Esterhai JL, et al: Magnetic resonance imaging for the diagnosis of osteomyelitis in the diabetic patient with a foot ulcer, *Foot Ankle Int* 15(3):151-156, 1994. B

3. Sella EJ, Grosser DM: Imaging modalities of the diabetic foot, *Clin Podiatr Med Surg* 20(4):729-740, 2003. C

4. Lew DP, Waldvogel FA: Osteomyelitis, *N Engl J Med* 336(14):999-1007, 1997. C

5. Bennett OM, Namnyak SS: Bone and joint manifestations of sickle cell anaemia, *J Bone Joint Surg Br* 72(3):494-499, 1990. B

6. Kak V, Chandrasekar PH: Bone and joint infections in injection drug users, *Infect Dis Clin North Am* 16(3):681-695, 2002. C

7. Givner LB, Luddy RE, Schwartz AD: Etiology of osteomyelitis in patients with major sickle hemoglobinopathies, *J Pediatr* 99(3):411-413, 1981. B

8. Newman LG, Waller J, Palestro CJ, et al: Unsuspected osteomyelitis in diabetic foot ulcers. Diagnosis and monitoring by leukocyte scanning with indium in 111 oxyquinoline, *JAMA* 266(9):1246-1251, 1991. B

9. Grayson ML, Gibbons GW, Balogh K, et al: Probing to bone in infected pedal ulcers. A clinical sign of underlying osteomyelitis in diabetic patients, *JAMA* 273(9):721-723, 1995. A

10. Mackowiak PA, Jones SR, Smith JW: Diagnostic value of sinus-tract cultures in chronic osteomyelitis, *JAMA* 239(26):2772-2775, 1978. B

11. Mader JT, Ortiz M, Calhoun JH: Update on the diagnosis and management of osteomyelitis, *Clin Podiatr Med Surg* 13(4):701-724, 1996. C

12. Gross T, Kaim AH, Regazzoni P, Widmer AF: Current concepts in posttraumatic osteomyelitis: a diagnostic challenge with new imaging options, *J Trauma* 52(6):1210-1219, 2002. C

13. Tomas MB, Patel M, Marwin SE, Palestro CJ: The diabetic foot, *Br J Radiol* 73(868):443-450, 2000. C

14. Tehranzadeh J, Wong E, Wang F, Sadighpour M: Imaging of osteomyelitis in the mature skeleton, *Radiol Clin North Am* 39(2):223-250, 2001. C

15. Haas DW, McAndrew MP: Bacterial osteomyelitis in adults: evolving considerations in diagnosis and treatment, *Am J Med* 101(5):550-561, 1996. C

FAST FACTS

- *Candida* isolated from blood is never a contaminant and must always be treated.
- Fluconazole, amphotericin B, and caspofugin have shown similar efficacy in treating candidemia, especially in nonneutropenic patients. However, most experts recommend initial therapy with amphotericin B or caspofungin in a clinically unstable patient with an unspeciated isolate, especially if he or she was given azole prophylaxis.
- All patients with candidemia need a formal ophthalmologic examination and follow-up.
- Mortality from candidemia increases if central venous catheters are left in place.
- The endemic mycoses often present with nonspecific symptoms. A high index of suspicion should be maintained in areas in which these fungi are known to be endemic.
- Itraconazole and amphotericin are the mainstays of treatment for endemic mycoses. Immunocompetent patients with acute histoplasmosis or coccidioidomycosis often are asymptomatic and do not need treatment.

61

Infection with *Candida* spp. or endemic fungi often presents in a nonspecific manner and causes significant morbidity and mortality. *Candida* spp. account for 5% to 10% of all blood stream infections and are the fourth leading organism isolated (behind coagulase-negative staphylococcal species, *Staphylococcus aureus* and enterococci). In addition to candidemia, infections with fungi such as *Histoplasma capsulatum, Coccidioides immitis,* and *Blastomyces dermatitidis* are a significant cause of illness in endemic areas, infecting anywhere from 100,000 to 500,000 people throughout the United States each year.

Candidemia

I. EPIDEMIOLOGY

A. INCIDENCE

1. Candidemia most commonly occurs in immunosuppressed patients (especially those who are neutropenic) and patients with prolonged intensive care unit stays. Invasive candidiasis accounts for 17% of hospital-acquired infections.[1]

2. *Candida albicans* is the most common candida species isolated, accounting for about 45% to 60% of isolates. The incidence of non-*albicans* species and fluconazole-resistant candidal species has been

increasing in recent years and is thought to be caused in part by increasing use of fluconazole prophylaxis. The relative frequency of other candida species is *Candida glabrata* > *Candida parapsilosis* > *Candida tropicalis* > *Candida krusei.*[2]

B. RISK FACTORS

1. Factors that affect the host's level of immunosuppression, such as neutropenia, corticosteroid use, chemotherapy (especially with agents that cause excessive gastrointestinal mucosal damage), and malignancy predispose patients to candidemia.

2. Other patients at risk for developing candidemia include those with indwelling central lines, multisite candidal colonization, acute renal failure, recent antibiotic or parenteral nutrition use, or recent surgery (especially gastrointestinal surgery).

3. Risk factors for breakthrough candidemia, defined as persistently positive cultures despite antifungal agents, include intensive care unit admission, neutropenia, and corticosteroid use.

II. CLINICAL PRESENTATION

1. *Candida* spp. are considered normal flora on the skin, gastrointestinal tract, and genitourinary tract and often colonize the upper respiratory tract.

2. *Candida* causes a wide spectrum of clinical manifestations depending on the site of the body infected (Box 61-1).

3. Candidemia often presents in a very nonspecific manner, with the only clue to diagnosis being a sepsis syndrome or fever. Several clues include a positive funduscopic examination (white infiltrative lesions on the retina or vitreous haze present in 3.7% to 25% of cases) or typical skin lesions (clusters of painless pustules on an erythematous base). Certain forms of candidiasis may manifest as neutropenia resolves (e.g., hepatosplenic candidiasis).

III. DIAGNOSIS

1. Diagnosis of candidemia is based on positive blood cultures. Speciation and susceptibility testing should be performed on all candidal isolates because of the increasing rates of fluconazole-resistant *C. albicans* and the increasing incidence of *C. glabrata* (relatively resistant to fluconazole) and *C. krusei* (resistant to fluconazole).

2. A diagnosis of candidemia remains problematic mainly because of the long incubation time needed (1 to 4 days) for candidal cultures to become positive. Clinical suspicion is important to diagnosis. An autopsy review showed that only 22% of invasive fungal infections were suspected or documented before death.[3]

IV. MANAGEMENT

1. Several randomized controlled trials have shown the equivalency of fluconazole to amphotericin B in treating candidal bloodstream

BOX 61-1

CANDIDA INFECTIONS IN HUMANS: SPECTRUM OF DISEASES

HEMATOGENOUS INFECTIONS

Candidemia

Endophthalmitis

Vascular access–related infection

Septic thrombophlebitis

Infectious endocarditis

Arthritis

Osteomyelitis

Spondylodiscitis

Meningitis

Pyelonephritis

Pulmonary candidiasis

Hepatosplenic candidiasis

NONHEMATOGENOUS INFECTIONS

Superficial Infections

Cutaneous candidiasis

Oropharyngeal candidiasis

Vaginitis

Deep-Seated Infections

Esophageal candidiasis

Cystitis

Peritonitis

Tracheitis and bronchitis

Modified from Eggimann P, Garbino J, Pittet D: *Lancet Infect Dis* 3(11):685-702, 2003.

infections in nonneutropenic patients.[4,5] Traditionally, in neutropenic patients who are unstable, have a visceral source of infection, or have received fluconazole prophylaxis, amphotericin B is used. Because of the rising prevalence of fluconazole-resistant candidal species, consideration should also be given to using amphotericin B or caspofungin in treating any non-*albicans*, germ tube–negative yeast until sensitivities are available.

2. More recently, caspofungin has been compared with amphotericin B and has been found to have similar efficacy in treating both azole-resistant and azole-sensitive candidemia (Table 61-1).[6] Caspofungin must be used with caution in patients with hepatotoxicity.

3. Antifungal treatment should continue for 14 days after the date of either the last positive blood culture and resolution of signs and symptoms of infection.[7]

4. Neutropenic patients should also receive granulocyte colony-stimulating factor or granulocyte-macrophage colony-stimulating factor in addition to antifungal therapy.

TABLE 61-1
SENSITIVITIES OF *CANDIDA* SPP. TO VARIOUS ANTIFUNGALS

Species	Fluconazole	Itraconazole	Voriconazole	Posaconazole	Ravuconazole	Caspofungin	Flucytosine	Liposomal Amphotericin B
C. albicans	S	S	S	S	S	S	S	S
C. tropicalis	S	S	S	S	S	S	S	S
C. parapsilosis	S	S	S	S	S	S	S	S
C. glabrata	S-DD to R	S-DD to R	S	S	S	S	S	S to I
C. krusei	R	S-DD to R	S	S	S	S	I to R	S to I
C. lusitaniae	S	S	S	S	S to R	S	S	S to R

S, sensitive; S-DD, sensitive-dose dependent; R, resistant; I, intermediate. Modified from Eggimann P, Garbino J, Pittet D: *Lancet Infect Dis* 3(11):685-702, 2003.

5. All central venous catheters should be removed.[7]
6. Because about 26% of patients with candidemia develop ocular candidiasis, all patients should undergo a formal ophthalmologic examination and be followed with serial eye examinations for at least 2 weeks after clearance of *Candida* from the bloodstream.[8]

V. PROGNOSIS

1. In all patients, candidemia carries an overall mortality of about 50%.
2. Mortality increases if a patient has a higher APACHE II score at the time of diagnosis or persistently positive blood cultures. Mortality also increases when central venous lines are not changed or there is a delay in treatment with appropriate antifungal agents.

Zygomycosis

See Supplemental PDA Chapter 6.

Aspergillosis

I. EPIDEMIOLOGY AND PATHOGENESIS

1. *Aspergillus fumigatus* causes about 90% of cases of invasive aspergillosis. Other species including *Aspergillus niger*, *Aspergillus terreus* (high mortality), *Aspergillus flavus* (often causes paranasal sinus disease), and *Aspergillus nidulans* (common in patients with chronic granulomatous disease) occasionally cause disease.
2. *Aspergillus* organisms are ubiquitous; however, disease caused by tissue invasion occurs mainly in patients who are neutropenic or undergoing corticosteroid treatment. Other high-risk populations include patients with the human immunodeficiency virus, bone marrow transplant patients, and lung transplant recipients.
3. Invasive aspergillosis is characterized by vascular invasion with subsequent infarction and necrosis.
4. Allergic bronchopulmonary aspergillosis (ABPA) is the result of type I and III hypersensitivity reactions to *A. fumigatus* growing in airway mucus and is discussed in detail elsewhere (see Chapter 81).[9]

II. CLINICAL PRESENTATION

1. Chronic invasive aspergillosis and aspergillomas usually present in patients with underlying lung disease (e.g., bullous emphysema) with symptoms that include cough, low-grade fever, and hemoptysis. Lesions typically are unilateral and located in the upper lobes.[9]
2. Invasive pulmonary aspergillosis typically presents as fever, cough, hemoptysis, and pleuritic chest pain. Chest radiography and computed tomography can be variable, with nodular infiltrates, cavities, or patchy infiltrates. A characteristic early finding on computed tomography is the halo sign: ground-glass attenuation surrounding a soft tissue nodule (caused by hemorrhage around the central necrotic nodule). Ten percent of chest films appear normal on initial evaluation.

61

FUNGUS

3. Disseminated aspergillosis often presents with sepsis. The most common extrapulmonary sites of infection include the central nervous system (CNS), liver, kidney, spleen, and skin.
4. *Aspergillus* can also cause sinusitis (similar to zygomycetes), tracheobronchitis, endocarditis, and endophthalmitis.

III. DIAGNOSIS

1. Diagnosis is often difficult. The isolation of *Aspergillus* from respiratory secretions or its presence on Gram stain preparation often can be misleading because the fungus may be a colonizing organism in the respiratory tract. For this reason, histopathology of tissue is necessary.
2. Narrow, septated hyphae with acute angle branching suggest aspergillosis but are also characteristic of other organisms (e.g., *Pseudoallescheria boydii*).
3. *Aspergillus* rarely grows from blood cultures but usually grows in culture from tissues within 3 days. However, if the inoculum is small, longer culture times may be necessary.

IV. TREATMENT

1. **Aspergilloma.** Optimal treatment is unknown. Surgical removal of the aspergilloma is definitive but reserved for patients at extremely high risk (i.e., life-threatening hemoptysis, severe immunosuppression).
2. **Invasive aspergillosis.** Voriconazole has become the standard of care for treating invasive aspergillosis. A recent study comparing voriconazole and amphotericin B showed successful outcomes in 53% of patients treated with voriconazole and 32% of patients treated with amphotericin B.[10]

Endemic Mycoses: *Histoplasma capsulatum*

I. EPIDEMIOLOGY

1. *Histoplasma capsulatum* is a dimorphic fungus that is highly endemic in the Ohio and Mississippi river valleys. Approximately 50% of adults in endemic areas have been infected.
2. Risk factors include exposure to bird and bat excrement. Immunosuppressed patients are at higher risk for developing symptomatic or disseminated infection.
3. Transmission of the organism is via inhaled spores in the mold phase, which subsequently germinate into yeast at body temperature.

II. CLINICAL PRESENTATION

1. Between 50% and 90% of immunocompetent people infected with histoplasmosis are asymptomatic.
2. Symptomatic disease can have various presentations.
a. Acute pulmonary syndrome usually presents with a flulike illness with general malaise, cough, fevers, chills, and fatigue. This presentation

usually is self-limited and develops about 2 weeks after exposure. Pericarditis can occur in 10% of patients with acute pulmonary histoplasmosis. Complications that occur years after initial infection include lymphadenopathy and fibrosing mediastinitis.

b. Chronic pulmonary histoplasmosis occurs almost exclusively in patients with emphysema or underlying structural lung disease. Characteristic findings include fibrotic apical infiltrates with cavitation on chest radiography.

c. Disseminated histoplasmosis occurs mainly in immunosuppressed patients (especially those with the human immunodeficiency virus) but can occur in older immunocompetent patients. It typically presents with chronic, progressive fevers, night sweats, weight loss, anorexia, fatigue, and dyspnea. Adrenal involvement occurs in 50% of patients, but less than 10% of these develop adrenal insufficiency. Oral ulcers often are seen.

d. CNS histoplasmosis causes symptoms that range from subacute or chronic meningitis to focal strokelike symptoms caused by embolic or vascular phenomena. Basilar meningeal involvement is typical, and 20% of patients with CNS involvement will develop nonobstructing hydrocephalus. Cerebrospinal fluid generally shows a lymphocytic pleocytosis, elevated protein, and low glucose.

III. DIAGNOSIS

1. Culture is the gold standard for diagnosis but is limited by a long (2- to 4-week) incubation period and low sensitivity in self-limited disease. Even in disseminated disease a false negative rate of about 20% can be expected. Fungal staining of blood or tissue is more rapid but less sensitive (50%).
2. Antigen detection (urine more sensitive than blood) is useful in detecting disseminated disease or acute pulmonary histoplasmosis.[11]
3. Common associated laboratory abnormalities include markedly elevated lactate dehydrogenase, anemia, leukopenia, thrombocytopenia, and elevated liver function tests. Chest radiography is abnormal in 70% of patients.

IV. MANAGEMENT

1. Indications for treatment are listed in Box 61-2.
2. Treatment.
a. Amphotericin B or itraconazole can be used to treat acute pulmonary (6 to 12 weeks with or without steroids), chronic pulmonary (12 to 24 months), and disseminated (6 to 18 months) histoplasmosis.
b. Meningitis is treated with amphotericin B for 3 months and then fluconazole for 1 year.[12]
c. In general, except in CNS infection, itraconazole is more effective than fluconazole.[13]

61

FUNGUS

BOX 61-2

INDICATIONS FOR ANTIFUNGAL TREATMENT IN PATIENTS WITH HISTOPLASMOSIS[12]

TREATMENT INDICATED

Acute pulmonary histoplasmosis with hypoxemia

Acute pulmonary histoplasmosis for >1 mo

Chronic pulmonary histoplasmosis

Esophageal compression or ulceration

Granulomatous mediastinitis with obstruction or invasion of tissue

Disseminated histoplasmosis

TREATMENT NOT INDICATED

Acute self-limited syndromes

Acute pulmonary histoplasmosis, mildly ill

Rheumatologic

Pericarditis

Histoplasmoma

Broncholithiasis

Fibrosing mediastinitis

Modified from Wheat J, Sarosi G, McKinsey D, et al: *Clin Infect Dis* 30:688-695, 2000.

Endemic Mycoses: *Coccidioides immitis*

I. EPIDEMIOLOGY

1. *C. immitis* is a dimorphic fungus highly endemic in the southern San Joaquin Valley of California and southern Arizona, New Mexico, Nevada, Texas, northern Mexico, and parts of Central and South America.

2. The incidence and prevalence of *C. immitis* infection range from 3% to 10% depending on the season and natural events (i.e., earthquakes or windstorms), which may increase the amount of airborne fungal spores.

3. Risk factors for extrapulmonary dissemination include male sex, immunosuppressed state, and Filipino or African American race.[14]

II. CLINICAL PRESENTATION

1. Sixty percent of people infected with *C. immitis* remain asymptomatic.

2. Approximately 40% have a flulike illness with symptoms of cough, fever, night sweats, pleuritic chest pain, and dyspnea 1 to 3 weeks after inhalation of spores. Coccidioidomycosis sometimes is called desert rheumatism because of the prominence of associated arthralgias and myalgias. Five percent of these patients develop residual pulmonary lesions such as nodules or cavities (thin walled, near the pleura).

3. Less than 1% of patients develop disseminated extrapulmonary disease; the most common form is skin changes (especially verrucous plaques, nodules, or papules, which can be located anywhere but are commonly found in the nasolabial folds or sternoclavicular area). Other

extrapulmonary sites of infection include bones, joints, CNS, and very rarely thyroid, eye, larynx, or genitourinary tract.

III. DIAGNOSIS

1. Biopsy for culture and histopathology (i.e., bronchoalveolar lavage with or without biopsy or skin or bone biopsy) should be performed for definitive diagnosis. Growth on culture generally can be seen in less than 7 days.
2. Serologic tests for tube precipitin-reacting antigen and the complement-fixing antigen are important diagnostic aids.
3. Chest radiography most often shows infiltrates with ipsilateral adenopathy. Pulmonary nodules, cavities, and pleural effusions can also be seen.

IV. MANAGEMENT

1. Uncomplicated primary pulmonary infection, asymptomatic pulmonary nodules, and asymptomatic pulmonary cavities in healthy, immunocompetent hosts can be managed without antifungal therapy as long as the patient has close follow-up.
2. Diffuse pneumonia, disseminated disease, or any presentation in an immunosuppressed patient can be treated with amphotericin B, fluconazole, or itraconazole. Randomized, controlled trials comparing fluconazole and itraconazole show equivalent efficacy.[15]
3. CNS coccidioidomycosis should be treated with fluconazole. Data are limited on the efficacy of intrathecal amphotericin. Itraconazole may have equivalent efficacy.[16] Hydrocephalus is common, and many patients need placement of an intraventricular shunt.

Endemic Mycoses: *Blastomyces dermatitidis*

I. EPIDEMIOLOGY

1. Endemic areas include the Mississippi and Ohio river basins, areas surrounding the Great Lakes, and the St. Lawrence River valley. Transmission occurs via inhalation of conidia.
2. The incidence and prevalence are unknown. Exposure to moist soil appears to be a risk factor.

II. CLINICAL PRESENTATION

1. Clinical presentation is highly variable. Many patients have nonspecific symptoms including fevers, chills, night sweats, weight loss, dyspnea, and cough, but others are asymptomatic. Pneumonia is the most common presentation, and chest radiography most often shows alveolar infiltrates, lesions, or reticulonodular infiltrates. The incubation period is 30 to 45 days.
2. Extrapulmonary involvement occurs in 25% to 40% of cases. Cutaneous blastomycosis with verrucous or ulcerative lesions is the most common extrapulmonary manifestation. Other extrapulmonary

manifestations include osteomyelitis, prostatitis, epididymo-orchitis, meningitis, or epidural or cranial abscesses.

III. DIAGNOSIS

1. Definitive diagnosis requires culture or identification of the organism in tissue or exudate. However, culture may take 2 to 5 weeks of growth to show positive results.[17]
2. Cytology often is useful in diagnosis.

IV. TREATMENT

1. Mortality approaches 60% if untreated.
2. Treatment of choice is amphotericin B (if severely ill or immunocompromised) or itraconazole for a minimum of 6 months.[18]

PEARLS AND PITFALLS

- *Candida* endocarditis often results in large valvular vegetations and embolic events (often to large vessels). Risk factors for *Candida* endocarditis include prosthetic valves, indwelling central lines with prolonged fungemia, and intravenous drug use.
- Ninety-five percent of *C. albicans* isolates are germ tube positive. Therefore, germ tube–negative status increases the probability of a fluconazole-resistant species.
- Antigen detection of circulating galactomannan may aid in the early identification of invasive aspergillosis in certain patient populations. False positive tests may occur in patients being treated with piperacillin-tazobactam.
- Amphotericin B is ineffective against *Pseudoallescheria boydii* (voriconazole is the drug of choice). *Fusarium* species are less responsive to amphotericin and may warrant the addition of 5-flucytosine or use of voriconazole.
- The presence of eosinophils in the cerebrospinal fluid may suggest *Coccidioides* infection.

REFERENCES

1. Eggimann P, Garbino J, Pittet D: Epidemiology of *Candida* species infections in critically ill non-immunosuppressed patients, *Lancet Infect Dis* 3(11):685-702, 2003. C
2. Abi-Said D, Anaissie E, Uzon O, et al: The epidemiology of hematogenous candidiasis caused by different species, *Clin Infect Dis* 24(6):1122-1128, 1997. B
3. Groll AH, Shah PM, Mentzel C, et al: Trends in the postmortem epidemiology of invasive fungal infections at a university hospital, *J Infect* 33:23-32, 1996. C
4. Rex JH, Bennett, Sugar AM, et al: A randomized trial comparing fluconazole with amphotericin B for the treatment of candidemia in patients without neutropenia, *N Engl J Med* 331:1325-1330, 1994. A
5. Phillips P, Shafran S, Garber G, et al: Multicenter randomized trial of fluconazole versus amphotericin B for treatment of candidemia in non-neutropenic patients, *Eur J Clin Microbiol Infect Dis* 16:337-345, 1997. A

6. Mora-Duarte J, Betts R, Rotsteinn C, et al: Comparison of caspofungin and amphotericin B for invasive candidiasis, *N Engl J Med* 347(25):2020-2029, 2002. A

7. Rex JH, Walsh TJ, Sobel JD, et al: Practice guidelines for the treatment of candidiasis. Infectious Diseases Society of America, *Clin Infect Dis* 30(4):662-678, 2000. D

8. Krishna R, Amuh D, Lowder CY, et al: Should all patients with candidaemia have an ophthalmic examination to rule out ocular candidiasis? *Eye* 14(Pt 1):30-34, 2000. B

9. Marr KA, Patterson T, Denning D: Aspergillosis: pathogenesis, clinical manifestations and treatment, *Infect Dis Clin North Am* 16(4):875-894, 2002. C

10. Hebrecht R, Denning DW, Patterson TF, et al: Voriconazole versus amphotericin B for primary therapy of invasive aspergillosis, *N Engl J Med* 347:408-415, 2002. B

11. Wheat J, French ML, Kohler RB, et al: The diagnostic laboratory tests for histoplasmosis: analysis of experience in a large urban outbreak, *Ann Intern Med* 97(5):680-685, 1982. B

12. Wheat J, Sarosi G, McKinsey D, et al: Practice guidelines for the management of patients with histoplasmosis. Infectious Diseases Society of America, *Clin Infect Dis* 30:688-695, 2000. B

13. LeMonte AM, Washum KE, Smedema ML, et al: Amphotericin B combined with itraconazole or fluconazole for treatment of histoplasmosis, *J Infect Dis* 182(2):545-550, 2000. B

14. Chiller TM, Galgiani JN, Stevens DA: Coccidioidomycosis, *Infect Dis Clin North Am* 17(1):41-57, 2003. C

15. Galgiani JN, Catanzaro A, Cloud GA, et al: Comparison of oral fluconazole and itraconazole for progressive, nonmeningeal coccidioidomycosis. A randomized, double-blind trial. Mycoses Study Group, *Ann Intern Med* 133(9):676-686, 2000. A

16. Tucker RM, Denning DW, Dupont B, Stevens DA: Itraconazole therapy for chronic coccidioidal meningitis, *Ann Intern Med* 112(2):108-112, 1990. B

17. Martynowicz MA, Prakash UB: Pulmonary blastomycosis: an appraisal of diagnostic techniques, *Chest* 121(3):768-773, 2002. B

18. Chapman SW, Bradsher RW Jr, Campbell GD Jr, et al: Practice guidelines for the management of patients with blastomycosis. Infectious Diseases Society of America, *Clin Infect Dis* 30(4):679-683, 2000. D

61

FUNGUS

Infection in the Solid Organ Transplant Recipient

David Lim, MD, PhD; and Aruna Subramanian, MD

FAST FACTS

- The two inexorably linked fundamental goals in the transplant recipient are immunosuppression to prevent and treat rejection and antimicrobial intervention to prevent and treat infection.
- After the patient's net state of immunosuppression is assessed, the overall risk of infection is determined by the intensity of pathogenic exposure (community vs. nosocomial), organism virulence (e.g., drug resistance), and postsurgical anatomy (e.g., fluid collection, vascular access, vascular thrombus).
- Typical signs and symptoms of infection often are masked by immunosuppression-induced attenuation of the inflammatory response.
- Transplant recipients may have multiple infections simultaneously and may have concomitant allograft rejection.
- Empiric antimicrobial therapy for the toxic-appearing transplant recipient should be broad, covering gram-positive, gram-negative, and anaerobic infections. In addition, consideration should be given to adding appropriate coverage for resistant gram-positive organisms (e.g., methicillin-resistant *Staphylococcus aureus,* vancomycin-resistant *Enterococcus*), highly resistant gram-negative rods, cytomegalovirus, and fungi.
- For the critically ill, immunosuppressive agents usually are continued until assessment for concomitant rejection is complete; however, dosage reduction or discontinuation should be considered in life-threatening infections.

Over the last two decades there has been a dramatic improvement in the success of transplantation. Despite this success, 50% to 75% of recipients contract infection within the first year after transplantation with both direct (e.g., pneumonia) and indirect sequelae.[1,2] The latter encompasses the process by which cytokines, chemokines, and growth factors induced by microbial infection decrease the net state of immunosuppression, worsen acute and chronic allograft injury, and increase the risk of malignancy. This chapter provides an approach to understanding both immunosuppression and the risk of infection in the transplant recipient.

I. GENERAL PRINCIPLES OF IMMUNOSUPPRESSION

A. ANTILYMPHOCYTE ANTIBODIES

1. Antibody therapy is used both for induction therapy immediately after transplantation (thus avoiding nephrotoxic calcineurin inhibitors for kidney transplants) and for therapy of steroid-resistant acute rejection. Antibodies are potent pan–T lymphocyte–depleting agents. Both polyclonal and monoclonal preparations are available. Polyclonal preparations include antithymocyte globulin and antilymphocyte serum, and the monoclonal preparations include OKT-3, a murine antibody to the CD3 T cell receptor.

2. Use of these agents increases risk infection from reactivation of herpes viruses (especially cytomegalovirus [CMV]), fungus, and mycobacteria.

3. Major side effects of polyclonal preparations include nonspecific antibody-mediated neutropenia, thrombocytopenia, and hemolysis, which are not observed with the monoclonal OKT-3 preparation. Both preparations can cause allergic reactions ranging from fevers to anaphylaxis. Both also initiate the release of interleukin-1 and tumor necrosis factor (TNF), which can cause fevers, chills, hypotension, and malaise. Finally, immune responses to the murine portion of OKT-3 can interfere with T cell depletion (thus reducing overall immunosuppression). OKT-3 also can cause an aseptic meningitis and encephalopathy.

4. Two monoclonal antibodies to the interleukin-2 receptor were approved recently: daclizumab and basiliximab. Both are non–lymphocyte-depleting, non–cytokine-releasing antibodies. Data are pending on the efficacy of these agents in preventing chronic rejection.

B. IMMUNOSUPPRESSANTS

1. Standard immunosuppression regimens usually consist of three drugs: corticosteroids, a purine synthesis inhibitor (mycophenolate mofetil or azathioprine), and a calcineurin inhibitor (tacrolimus or cyclosporine).

a. **Corticosteroids.** Corticosteroids inhibit cytokine production, leukocyte function, arachidonic acid metabolites, platelet-activating factor, and vascular permeability. The net immunosuppressive effect is inhibition of T cell activation and proliferation. As a result, patients on corticosteroids are at greater risk of infection from bacteria, mycobacteria, *Pneumocystis jiroveci* pneumonia (PCP), herpes, hepatitis B and C, fungi, and *Strongyloides stercoralis*. Clinical signs and symptoms (including radiographic findings) are greatly diminished until late into infection. In addition, microbial burden is much higher than in normal hosts.

b. **Purine synthesis inhibitors.**
   (1) **Azathioprine.** Azathioprine is a purine synthesis and salvage inhibitor, which results in inhibition of DNA and RNA synthesis. Its greatest effect is in actively dividing lymphocytes, thus increasing the risk of infection from herpes viruses, papillomaviruses, fungi, mycobacteria, *S. stercoralis,* and other intracellular organisms. In

addition to its immunosuppressive effects, azathioprine causes bone marrow suppression and neutropenia.

(2) **Mycophenolate mofetil (MMF).** MMF is a prodrug of mycophenolic acid that effectively inhibits both B and T lymphocyte proliferation by its selective, reversible inhibition of guanosine synthesis. MMF often is substituted for azathioprine both because it is a more potent antirejection agent and because the added immunosuppression is not associated with a major increase in infection or lymphoma. When compared with azathioprine, MMF usage is associated with the same infectious organisms but has less risk of neutropenia. Side effects include cramps and diarrhea.

c. **Calcineurin inhibitors (cyclosporine and tacrolimus).** Calcineurin inhibitors prevent T cell activation and proliferation by preventing the nuclear translocation of the transcription factor nuclear factor of activated T cells, which in turn prevents the production of T cell–activating cytokines. Tacrolimus is 10 to 100 times more potent than cyclosporine. Calcineurin inhibitors are associated with a higher risk of infection by replicating herpes group viruses: CMV and Epstein-Barr virus (EBV). Major side effects include hypertension (cyclosporine > tacrolimus), hyperlipidemia, nephrotoxicity, and diabetes (tacrolimus > cyclosporine).

d. **Rapamycin.** Rapamycin prolongs cell cycle G_1 to S phase progression by inhibiting ribosomal protein synthesis and progression to DNA synthesis. Although it is a less potent cytokine inhibitor than the calcineurin inhibitors, it inhibits B cell immunoglobulin synthesis, antibody-dependent cellular cytotoxicity, lymphocyte-activated killer cells, and natural killer cells. It can be used synergistically with cyclosporine. Rapamycin is associated with a higher incidence of aphthous ulcers and PCP. Major side effects include hyperlipidemia, hypertension, bone marrow suppression, and the potential to potentiate cyclosporine nephrotoxicity. A newly recognized syndrome of pulmonary toxicity has recently been reported.

2. Drug interactions in the transplant recipient are summarized in Table 62-1.

II. POSTTRANSPLANT TIMELINE OF INFECTION (Fig. 62-1)

A. LESS THAN 4 WEEKS AFTER TRANSPLANTATION

1. Infection can be derived from either the donor or the recipient, underscoring the importance of pretransplant evaluation.

2. In addition, transplant recipients can develop infection from surgical complications such as obstructed stents, devitalized tissues, and fluid collections. Finally, patients can develop nosocomial infections such as aspiration pneumonia, line sepsis, and urinary tract infections.

B. TWO TO SIX MONTHS AFTER TRANSPLANTATION

1. Infection can arise from residual problems from the perioperative period such as hematoma, lymphocele, and ischemic tissue.

TABLE 62-1

ANTIMICROBIAL INTERACTIONS WITH CNIS

Agents	Net Effect on CNIs	Complications
Rifampin Isoniazid Nafcillin	↓ CNI concentration	Insufficient immunosuppression Allograft rejection
Macrolides (erythromycin > clarithromycin > azithromycin)	↑ CNI concentration	Supratherapeutic immunosuppression
Azoles (ketoconazole > itraconazole and voriconazole > fluconazole)	↑ CNI concentration	Nephrotoxicity Infection
High-dose fluoroquinolones Bactrim Amphotericin B Aminoglycosides (avoid last 2 drugs when possible)	No change	Renal failure (sometimes occurring after single dose)

CNI, calcineurin inhibitor.

2. In addition, patients are at risk of developing infection both from opportunistic infections (e.g., PCP) and from the reactivation of latent viruses (e.g., CMV). PCP prophylaxis (e.g., trimethoprim-sulfamethoxazole) usually is administered for about 6 months after transplantation. The advantage of trimethoprim-sulfamethoxazole is that it also prevents infections with *Nocardia, Listeria,* toxoplasmosis, and many urinary tract pathogens. Of note, the routine use of CMV and PCP prophylaxis has resulted in the occurrence of some of these infections beyond the 2- to 6-month period.

C. MORE THAN 6 MONTHS AFTER TRANSPLANTATION

1. Category 1: 80% of patients have posttransplant infectious disease problems similar to those in the community (e.g., urinary tract infections). Opportunistic infections generally are not a problem.

2. Category 2: 10% of patients have chronic or progressive immunomodulating viral infections (hepatitis B and C viruses [HBV, HCV], CMV, EBV, papillomavirus, BK virus, or human immunodeficiency virus). Left untreated, these infections lead to destruction of the transplanted organ or malignancy.

3. Category 3: 10% of patients have chronic transplant infectious disease problems. Poor allograft function caused by rejection necessitates higher-dose immunosuppression, thus placing patients at the highest risk for opportunistic infections (e.g., *Cryptococcus,* PCP). In addition, they have high rates of recurrent *Clostridium difficile* colitis. These patients usually need prophylactic antimicrobial therapy beyond the standard 6-month period.

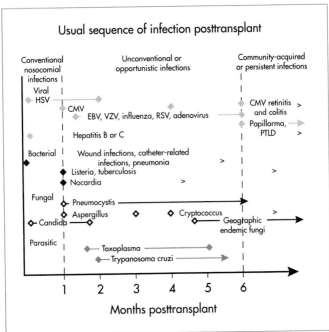

Usual sequence of infection posttransplant

| Conventional nosocomial infections | Unconventional or opportunistic infections | Community-acquired or persistent infections |

Viral
◆ HSV
CMV
EBV, VZV, influenza, RSV, adenovirus
CMV retinitis and colitis >
Papillorma, PTLD >
Hepatitis B or C

Bacterial
Wound infections, catheter-related infections, pneumonia >
Listeria, tuberculosis >
Nocardia >

Fungal
◇ Pneumocystis
◇ Aspergillus ◇ Cryptococcus >
◇ Candida ◇ Geogtaphic endemic fungi

Parasitic
Toxoplasma
Trypanosoma cruzi

Months posttransplant
1 2 3 4 5 6

FIG. 62-1

Usual sequence of infection after transplantation. Exceptions to the usual sequence of infections after transplantation suggest the presence of unusual epidemiologic exposure or excessive immunosuppression. Solid lines indicate the most common period for the onset of infection; dotted lines and arrows indicate periods of continued risk at reduced levels. *CMV,* cytomegalovirus; *EBV,* Epstein-Barr virus; *HSV,* herpes simplex virus; *PTLD,* posttransplantation lymphoproliferative disease; *RSV,* respiratory syncytial virus; *VZV,* varicella-zoster virus. *(Redrawn from Fishman JA et al: N Engl J Med 338:1741-1751, 1998.)*

III. COMMON INFECTIONS

A. CYTOMEGALOVIRUS

1. **Epidemiology.** CMV is the single most important pathogen in transplant recipients because of its prevalence; the variable route of infection from primary, reactivated, or superinfected states; and the direct and indirect effects of viral replication. Time course for infection usually is 1 to 4 months after transplantation but may occur later in patients on prophylactic antiviral therapy. The risk of developing active disease is related to donor and recipient CMV exposure status (Table 62-2).
2. **Presentation.**

TABLE 62-2

RISK OF CYTOMEGALOVIRUS CLINICAL DISEASE

Donor	Recipient	Immunosuppression	Risk (%)
+	−	Conventional	>50
+/−	+	Conventional	15-20
+/−	+	Conventional + induction ALA	25-35
+/−	+	Conventional + antirejection ALA	65
−	−	Any	Almost 0

Adapted from Rubin RH: *Transpl Infect Dis* 3(suppl 2):1-5, 2001.
ALA, antilymphocyte antibody; *conventional*, calcineurin inhibitor, azathioprine, or mycophenolate mofetil + prednisone.

a. CMV infects a wide variety of cells, causing direct injury with varied symptomatic presentation. Presenting symptoms typically include fever, leukopenia, thrombocytopenia, mild hepatitis, anorexia, and malaise. In addition, virus-induced immune modulation results in an increased state of immunosuppression. The additional immunosuppression increases the risk of superinfection from opportunistic infections such as PCP, *Nocardia*, and *Listeria*.

b. In addition to systemic infection, CMV can cause preferential infection of the allograft. See the individual organ transplantation chapters for more details.

3. **Diagnostic criteria.** CMV infection is diagnosed by the presence of CMV antigenemia, hybrid capture, positive polymerase chain reaction (PCR), histology, and culture from sterile sites (not urine or sputum). It is important to note that CMV serologies are useful only for risk factor assessment and not active viremia or infection.

4. **Management.**

a. CMV prophylaxis is used in all CMV-negative transplant recipients who receive organs from CMV-positive donors and is often used in CMV-positive recipients as well. Some centers administer prophylaxis to all recipients of cadaveric organs regardless of donor or recipient CMV status. Dosing is 50% of therapeutic intravenous ganciclovir (GCV) or oral valganciclovir (note that oral valganciclovir has not been approved by the U.S. Food and Drug Administration for liver transplant recipients). Prophylaxis is administered for 3 to 6 months and should begin within 10 days after transplant. It is also administered for patients undergoing antilymphocytic antibody therapy for acute rejection beyond the initial posttransplant period.

b. Preemptive therapy is used by some centers in lower-risk patients (e.g., for CMV seropositive recipients). Surveillance should be started within 10 days after transplantation and performed weekly for 3 months. Treatment is begun if low-level viremia is detected.

c. Treatment of active CMV disease entails a minimum of 2 weeks of induction with intravenous GCV or, if there is no evidence of tissue-invasive disease, oral valganciclovir. Induction may stop once antigenemia, hybrid capture, or PCR tests are negative and should be followed by 3 months of maintenance therapy with oral valganciclovir to reduce the risk of recurrence. Anti-CMV hyperimmune globulin can be used for severe or relapsing disease.

d. GCV-resistant CMV may develop with low-level viremia in the face of inadequate levels of drug therapy. This should be suspected if the CMV viral load is rising despite 2 weeks of adequate GCV therapy. The diagnosis is made by CMV genotyping. Certain mutations confer low-level GCV resistance and may be overcome by higher dosages of intravenous GCV. There are reports of success with the combination of GCV with foscarnet in cases of high-level GCV resistance. Given its risk of nephrotoxicity, foscarnet should be used with caution in transplant recipients.

B. OTHER HERPES VIRUSES.

1. Herpes simplex virus 1 and 2 infection occurs in the first month after transplantation in the absence of prophylaxis (acyclovir or GCV) and can present both in a localized dermatologic form and as an invasive infection. Dermatologic manifestations include orolabial, genital, and perianal lesions. Invasive infections include esophagitis, hepatitis, and pneumonitis. Diagnosis is by viral culture or direct immunofluorescence from lesion swabs. Treatment of severe disease is with intravenous acyclovir. Limited disease may be treated with oral acyclovir, famciclovir, or valacyclovir.

2. Varicella zoster virus (VZV) typically presents more than 3 months after transplantation as a dermatomal or disseminated rash. Roughly 10% of patients on immunosuppression develop clinical infection as a result of reactivation.[1] Visceral involvement includes pneumonitis, hepatitis, or encephalitis. Diagnosis arises from viral culture of skin lesion swab, bronchoalveolar lavage, or viral PCR of cerebrospinal fluid. Primary VZV infection is associated with a high mortality in transplant recipients, underscoring the importance of pretransplant evaluation and vaccination. Treatment of disseminated or visceral disease is with intravenous acyclovir. Dermatomal disease may be treated with famciclovir or valacyclovir.

3. Human herpesvirus 6 (HHV-6) and 7 infection presents 1 to 6 months after transplantation with exanthem subitum, a high, spiking febrile illness that precedes a macular rash. In addition, patients infected with these viruses may develop a mono-like illness with neutropenia or meningitis. Infection is a risk factor for CMV activation. Diagnosis is by viral culture from blood (5 to 21 days for results) or the more rapid viral antigenemia or PCR assays. Treatment options include foscarnet, GCV, or cidofovir coupled with a reduction in immunosuppression, but optimal management remains to be determined.

4. Human herpesvirus 8 (HHV-8) infection can manifest itself in a variety of ways, including Kaposi's sarcoma, primary effusive lymphoma, Castleman's syndrome, fever, and bone marrow suppression. Risk

factors for infection include recipient or donor seropositivity and intensity of immunosuppression. Incidence approaches 30% within the first 3 years after transplantation for seropositive patients.[2] Diagnosis is made on skin biopsy and PCR of peripheral blood leukocytes. Treatment options include reduced immunosuppression, radiation therapy, chemotherapy, and antiviral medications. Viral load PCR is useful in monitoring treatment response. Optimal management is still to be determined.

C. EPSTEIN-BARR VIRUS AND POSTTRANSPLANT LYMPHOPROLIFERATIVE DISEASE

1. Epidemiology and etiology.
a. The natural reservoir for EBV is the epithelial cell of the upper respiratory tract, with transmission through intimate contact and exchange of saliva. The virus also latently infects B lymphocytes, resulting in transformation and immortalization of these cells. In the immunocompetent patient, lymphoproliferation does not ensue because of active immune surveillance by major histocompatibility complex (MHC)–restricted cytotoxic T cells. With immunosuppression, however, EBV actively replicates in epithelial cells, and because immune surveillance is effectively shut off, latently infected B cells can rapidly expand into posttransplant lymphoproliferative disease (PTLD).
b. The incidence of PTLD varies between 1% and 33% in the solid organ transplant recipient. Because 90% of the population is infected, most infections represent reactivation of latent EBV.
2. Clinical presentation may include unexplained fever, mononucleosis syndrome (fever, malaise, lymphadenopathy, pharyngitis), gastrointestinal symptoms (pain, bleeding, obstruction), hepatic disease, and either focal or global central nervous system manifestations. Time course for the appearance of PTLD is as early as 6 months after transplantation (mean = 4 years). Anatomic allograft organ involvement can be observed (e.g., hilar mass in the transplanted kidney or portal mass in the transplanted liver). Importantly, absence of lymphadenopathy on computed tomography scan does not rule out PTLD. The gold standard for diagnosis is pathologic examination of affected organs (including lymph nodes, if present). Serum EBV DNA PCR is a useful adjunct, and in adults a high viral load is highly specific but may lack sensitivity.
3. Current treatment options are limited. Roughly one third of patients improve with reduction or cessation of immunosuppression (more so in children than adults). Most centers use acyclovir, GCV, or foscarnet despite the lack of current evidence to support this approach. This is done to reduce the effect of lytic EBV infection on lymphomagenesis and to prevent CMV replication, which is thought to promote EBV-mediated B cell transformation. For patients with PTLD tumors of the gastrointestinal tract, surgery may offer effective treatment. Reduction in immunosuppression and antiviral therapy usually is given for 4 to 6

62

INFECTION IN SOLID ORGAN TRANSPLANT RECIPIENT

weeks with frequent EBV DNA monitoring. Should these measures fail, chemotherapy or the more recently developed anti–B cell (rituximab) or anti–interleukin-6 antibody therapy should be initiated.

D. HEPATITIS B AND C (See Chapter 34)

1. HBV transmission from transplants is exceedingly rare given the high sensitivity and specificity of hepatitis B surface antigen testing before transplantation. Major efforts are currently focused on management of patients infected before transplantation because corticosteroids directly stimulate virus replication. Progressive liver disease can ensue in this patient population despite normal liver function tests. In previous studies, renal transplant recipients with prior HBV infection had a much higher mortality from liver failure (54%) than those not infected with HBV (12%), making HBV infection a relative contraindication to transplantation.[3] However, outcomes are now changing with the use of nucleoside analogs such as lamivudine or adefovir in this patient population. Perioperative and long-term prophylaxis with anti–hepatitis B surface antigen hyperimmune globulin is used in HBV-infected recipients of livers from uninfected donors.

2. HCV increases the risk of liver disease in the transplant recipient but has questionable effects on overall mortality as compared with uninfected recipients. Currently, a positive HCV serology (in the donor or recipient) is not a contraindication for transplantation because of the need for immediate lifesaving measures, organ shortages, and the growing numbers of patients awaiting transplants. This practice is supported by the observation that HCV-positive patients with end-stage renal disease survive longer with renal transplantation than they do on dialysis.[4] Currently, interferon-alpha is contraindicated for therapy in the transplant recipient secondary to the high risk of developing acute organ rejection. However, one study showed that pretransplant interferon-alpha therapy for HCV-infected renal transplant recipients helped prevent membranoproliferative and membranous glomerulonephritis.[5] The role of ribavirin for HCV therapy in transplant recipients is still being investigated.

E. BK VIRUS (See Chapter 75)

PEARLS AND PITFALLS

- Serologic testing is most useful in pretransplant evaluation. Because immunosuppression attenuates antibody production during active infection, direct testing (e.g., nucleic acid PCR), tissue biopsies, cultures, and direct molecular assays are the most accurate means of establishing diagnosis of infection.
- With tissue-invasive CMV disease (especially gastrointestinal disease), CMV DNA hybrid capture, antigenemia, or PCR from blood can be negative. In this case the diagnosis is made by histology of endoscopic biopsies.
- One can have low-level viremia with CMV without symptomatic disease, which is of unknown clinical significance.

- Antimicrobial therapy is futile and potentiates drug resistance as long as there is an undrained fluid collection or necrotic tissue. Rapid surgical debridement is essential for effective and timely therapy.
- With immunosuppression-mediated attenuation of the inflammatory response, more sensitive imaging modalities usually must be performed to detect infection or malignancy (i.e., computed tomography scan or magnetic resonance imaging over conventional radiographic imaging).

REFERENCES

1. Luby JP et al: A longitudinal study of varicella-zoster virus infections in renal transplant recipients, *J Infect Dis* 135:659, 1977. B
2. Frances C et al: Outcome of kidney transplant recipients with previous human herpesvirus-8 infection, *Transplantation* 69:1776, 2000. B
3. Rao KV et al: Long-term results and complications in renal transplant recipients. Observations in the second decade, *Transplantation* 45:45, 1988. B
4. Pereira BJ et al: Effects of hepatitis C infection and renal transplantation on survival in end-stage renal disease. The New England Organ Bank Hepatitis C Study Group, *Kidney Int* 53:1374, 1988. B
5. Cruzado JM et al: Pretransplant interferon prevents hepatitis C virus–associated glomerulonephritis in renal allografts by HCV-RNA clearance, *Am J Transplant* 3:357, 2003. B

62

INFECTION IN SOLID ORGAN TRANSPLANT RECIPIENT

Urinalysis

Leslie S. Gewin, MD; and Derek M. Fine, MD

FAST FACTS

- The urinalysis consists of both chemical and microscopic analyses. Whenever there is concern about renal disorders, the physician should examine the sample personally.
- A first morning urine specimen is preferable[1] (more acidic and concentrated, thus preserving cellular elements) and should be examined within 1 hour of collection to prevent bacterial overgrowth and cast disintegration.[2]
- For proper microscopic preparation, remove 10 ml of urine, centrifuge for 5 minutes at 3000 rpm, pour off the supernatant, resuspend the pellet by tapping the tube, place 1 drop on a slide, and cover with a coverslip.[2] Scan under both low (×100) and high (×400) power, with special attention to coverslip edges, where cellular elements concentrate.

I. CHEMICAL ANALYSIS (DIPSTICK)

A. APPEARANCE[3]

1. A red appearance can be caused by blood, porphyria, urates, phenolphthalein, laxatives such as Dorbane, anthocyanin in beets and blackberries, and rifampin.
2. Brown or black discoloration comes from alkaptonuria, melanin, blood,[3] porphyria, drugs causing hemolysis, tyrosinosis, cascara, and aldomet.
3. Orange urine can indicate bile, pyridium, and sulfasalazine.
4. Green-blue urine can be produced by biliverdin, *Pseudomonas* infection, Elavil, methylene blue, Phenergan, triamterene, and phenols.
5. Turbidity is most commonly the result of phosphaturia or pyuria but is rarely caused by lipiduria, hyperoxaluria, or uricosuria.[2]

B. PH

Normal pH is 4.5 to 7.8,[1] and a pH greater than 8 should strongly raise suspicion for urinary tract infection with a urease-splitting organism such as *Proteus mirabilis*.[2] It is important to note that the reagents used in the dipstick are not accurate enough to evaluate renal tubular acidosis.

C. SPECIFIC GRAVITY[3]

Specific gravity is an estimate of relative density and can reflect renal tubular function. The failure to concentrate urine, as can occur in diabetes insipidus, severe hyperthyroidism, or sickle cell anemia, results in a diluted sample. If measured by a refractometer, specific gravity may be increased by protein, glucose, and contrast dye.[3]

D. PROTEIN

1. The source of proteinuria is either glomerular, tubular, or overflow. Potential causes are listed in Box 63-1.[2]
2. Dipstick measurements of protein are semiquantitative for albumin and lack sensitivity with low levels of protein. In one study using the Albustix strip, the sensitivity and specificity were 81% and 55%, respectively, giving almost a 50% chance of false-negative results.[1,4] Most dipsticks detect only albumin and fail to measure Bence Jones protein (unless sulfosalicylic acid is added).[3] Therefore, if proteinuria is suspected, a spot protein and creatinine ratio should be obtained (see Chapter 68).

E. GLUCOSE

1. The tubular capacity for glucose reabsorption is exceeded when serum glucose levels surpass 165 to 200 mg/ml.[3]
2. False-negative results can occur with large dosages of aspirin, levodopa, beta-lactam antibiotics, 2-mercaptoethane sulfonate, ascorbic acid, and alkaptonuria.[2]
3. Positive results usually indicate hyperglycemia, but positive normoglycemic results are found in pregnancy, Fanconi's syndrome, and certain nephrotoxins (carbon monoxide, lead, mercuric chloride).[3]

F. KETONES

During diabetic or alcoholic ketoacidosis and starvation, beta-hydroxybutyric acid (78%), acetoacetic acid (20%), and acetone (2%) are produced. However, acetoacetic acid is the only one detected by the Acetest dipstick. In renal insufficiency, the kidney may be unable to filter

BOX 63-1
CAUSES OF PROTEINURIA
NONPATHOLOGIC CAUSES
Muscular exertion (e.g., in marathon runners)
Pregnancy
Orthostatic proteinuria
NONRENAL PATHOLOGIC STATES
Fever
Venous congestion (congestive heart failure)
Renal hypoxia
Hypertension
Bence Jones proteinuria
Myxedema
RENAL PATHOLOGIC STATES
Nephrotic syndromes
Glomerulonephritis
Infection of kidney or lower genitourinary tract
Parenchymal lesions

ketones into the urine despite severe ketosis. Therefore, plasma or serum ketones should also be checked.[3]

G. RED BLOOD CELLS

There is significant variation between dipsticks, but most have a sensitivity of detecting 3 red blood cells (RBC) per high-powered field of 90%.[5] A positive result indicates either RBCs, hemoglobin, or myoglobin, all of which cause a peroxidase reaction.[3]

H. LEUKOCYTE ESTERASE

Leukocyte esterase has a sensitivity of 80% to 90%[3] for detecting white blood cells (WBCs), but this number decreases as the sample sits and WBCs lyse. Other causes of false negatives include elevated specific gravity, glycosuria, medications (tetracycline), and large amounts of ascorbic acid (used as preservative in some antibiotics).[2] False positives usually result from vaginal secretions and contamination.[3]

I. NITRITE

The presence of nitrite has a sensitivity of 35% to 50% and a specificity of 90% for detecting bacteriuria.[6] The test relies on the ability of gram-negative organisms to reduce urinary nitrates to nitrites.

J. BILE AND UROBILINOGEN

Conjugated bile presents in the urine when biliary tract obstruction occurs. Unconjugated bile is not renally excreted. Urobilinogen, formed when intestinal bacteria metabolize conjugated bile, appears in the urine during hemolysis or results from an inability to metabolize normal enterohepatic reabsorption.[2]

II. MICROSCOPIC ANALYSIS

A. CELLULAR COMPONENTS

RBCs that appear dysmorphic usually originate in the kidney.[2] Other cellular elements include WBCs and bacteria. WBCs usually are present as neutrophils and indicate infection, especially if bacteria coexist. See Chapter 59 for discussion of urinary tract infections, and see Box 63-2 for the differential diagnosis of sterile pyuria.

B. CASTS

Casts are protein aggregates that outline the shape of renal tubules and capture luminal contents within the matrix.[3] With the exception of hyaline or finely granular casts that consist of the Tamm-Horsfall mucoprotein, casts reflect renal disorders.[3] See Table 63-1 for the significance of various forms of casts and Figs. 63-1 and 63-2.

C. CRYSTALS

1. Calcium oxalate crystals appear as uniform, small double pyramids and can reflect nephrolithiasis or ethylene glycol toxicity in the right clinical setting.[1] Fig. 63-3 provides illustrations of crystals found in the microscopic examination of the urine.
2. Calcium phosphate crystals are needle-like rectangular formations that clump together.
3. Uric acid crystals are reddish brown and rectangular or rhomboid.

BOX 63-2

CAUSES OF STERILE PYURIA

COMMON

Bacterial infection	Vaginitis or balanitis
Urethritis or cervicitis	Epididymitis
Prostatitis	Sexually transmitted ulcerative genitourinary diseases

LESS COMMON

Interstitial nephritis	Inflammation of adjacent organs (e.g., appendicitis)
Nephrolithiasis	
Genitourinary cancer	Glomerulonephritis
Nonbacterial cystitis	Perinephric abscess
Pregnancy	Papillary necrosis

RARE

Genitourinary tuberculosis	Corticosteroids
Atypical mycobacterial infections	Enterovesical fistula
Noncandidal fungal infection	Behçet's syndrome
Parasitic infections	

TABLE 63-1

SIGNIFICANCE OF URINARY CASTS

Type of Cast	Implications
Hyaline	Not necessarily pathologic; dehydration, pyelonephritis
Granular	Nonspecific[1]; often indicates acute tubular necrosis
Red blood cell casts	Glomerulonephritis
White blood cell casts	Interstitial nephritis, pyelonephritis, glomerulonephritis
Fatty casts or oval fat bodies	Nephrotic syndrome, tubule poisons such as mercury, hypersensitivity from insect bites, lipiduria, hypothyroidism[2]
Waxy	Further degeneration of cellular components[2]
Broad	Occurs in distal collecting tubules, reflects greater damage and more stasis

---

4. Calcium-magnesium-ammonium–pyrophosphate crystals (triple-phosphate), formed in alkaline urine often in the presence of urease-splitting organisms, are characteristically described as coffin lids.

D. MISCELLANEOUS

1. Epithelial cells generally serve as a marker for contamination. Spermatozoa can be seen in both women and men.
2. Trichomonas infection often is associated with proteinuria and pyuria. The trichomonads are easy to distinguish by the flagella.
3. Yeast often can be mistaken for RBCs, so cells should be inspected for budding and a more ovoid, homogeneous shape.

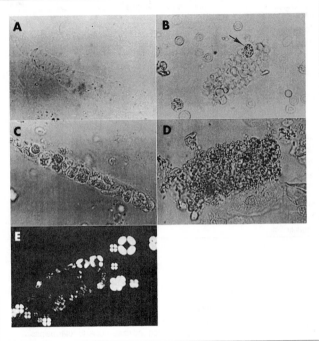

FIG. 63-1

Protein casts. **A,** Hyaline cast. Bright field microscopy (× 250). **B,** Red-cell cast with one polymorphonuclear leukocyte in the matrix *(arrow)*. Bright field microscopy (× 250). **C,** White-cell cast. Bright field microscopy (× 250). **D,** Granular cast. Only remnants of cells are present, and cell borders are not distinct. The cast is filled with coarse granules from cells that have undergone degeneration. Bright-field microscopy (× 250). **E,** Fatty cast. The fat is doubly refractile to polarized light and has a Maltese cross pattern. Polarized microscopy (× 250). *(Courtesy of the American Society of Clinical Pathologists.)*

4. Yellow-brown, coarse granules of hemosiderin can be seen in severe cases of hemochromatosis.[3]

PEARLS AND PITFALLS

- One common mistake in preparing specimens for microscopic examination is failure to adequately mix the specimen before pouring it into centrifuge tube for concentration.
- Acute tubular necrosis usually presents with muddy brown (granular) casts and, initially, a fixed specific gravity of 1.010.

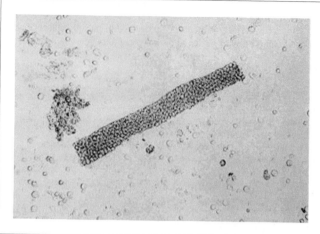

FIG. 63-2

Red cast, which strongly suggests a glomerulonephritis or vasculitis (× 160.) *(From Piccoli G, Varese D, Rotunno M: Atlas of urinary sediments: Diagnosis and clinical correlations in nephrology, New York, 1984, Raven.)*

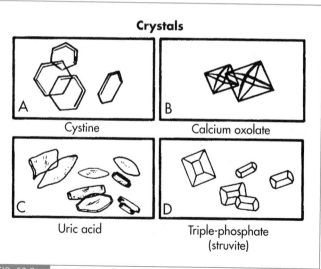

FIG. 63-3

Crystals under light microscopy. *(From Walsh P: Campbell's urology, 8th ed, St Louis, 2002, WB Saunders.)*

- If there is concern about proteinuria, a spot urine protein and creatinine ratio is much more sensitive than the dipstick. Also, microalbuminuria is an important risk factor for end-organ damage in patients with diabetes and is associated with higher cardiovascular mortality in patients with essential hypertension.

REFERENCES

1. Brenner BM: *The kidney,* 7th ed, St Louis, 2004, WB Saunders. C
2. Walsh P: *Campbell's urology,* 8th ed, St Louis, 2002, WB Saunders. C
3. Ravel R: *Clinical laboratory medicine,* 6th ed, St Louis, 1995, Mosby. C
4. Viberti GC, Jarrett RJ, Mahmud U, et al: Microalbuminuria as a predictor of clinical nephropathy in insulin-dependent diabetes mellitus, *Lancet* 1:1430-1432, 1982. B
5. Shaw ST, Pan SY, Wong ET: Routine urinalysis: Is the dipstick enough? *JAMA* 253:1956, 1985. C
6. Pels RJ, Bor DH, Woolhandler S: Dipstick urinalysis screening of asymptomatic adults for urinary tract disorders. II. Bacteriuria, *JAMA* 262:1221, 1989. C

Approach to Acute Renal Failure

Julia Scialla, MD; John J. Friedewald, MD; and Michael J. Choi, MD

FAST FACTS

- Because serum creatinine does not accurately reflect glomerular filtration rate (GFR), especially in older patients and those with preserved renal function, an estimated GFR should be calculated in all inpatients using the Modification of Diet in Renal Disease (MDRD) Study equations.[1] Note that this formula cannot be used with a serum creatinine that is rising or falling.
- Acute renal failure (ARF) may be defined as a rise in creatinine of more than 0.5 mg/dl over baseline or a decrease in GFR by 50% over a period of days to weeks.
- The differential diagnosis of ARF can be divided into prerenal, intrinsic renal, and postrenal causes. A thorough history and physical examination, urinalysis, blood work, and renal ultrasonography may help to quickly differentiate the different causes.
- The development of ARF in hospitalized patients increases mortality sixfold.[2]
- Indications for acute dialysis include severe metabolic acidosis, severe hyperkalemia, certain toxic ingestions, volume overload, and signs of uremia.
- For unstable patients needing emergent hemodialysis, the following temporizing measures can be used until renal replacement therapy is available:
  - For volume overload, intravenous nitroglycerin and high-dose intravenous diuretics can be used.
  - For hyperkalemia, calcium gluconate can be used to stabilize the cardiac cell membrane; intravenous insulin, glucose, and nebulized albuterol can be used to temporarily shift potassium into cells; and intravenous diuretics or sodium polystyrene sulfonate can be used to remove potassium.
  - For metabolic acidosis, bicarbonate infusion can be used.

I. EPIDEMIOLOGY[2]

1. ARF is a common condition, but because of varied definitions, its incidence has proved difficult to quantify in large studies.
2. Estimated to be present in 1% of patients at hospital admission, ARF develops in about 5% of hospitalized patients and up to 30% of patients in the intensive care unit.

3. Prerenal azotemia accounts for 60% to 70%, intrinsic renal disease accounts for 25% to 40%, and postrenal causes account for 5% to 10% of cases of ARF in hospitalized patients.[2]

II. CLINICAL PRESENTATION

1. Patients with ARF usually are asymptomatic if the ARF is not severe and incidentally are noted to have changes in blood urea nitrogen (BUN) and creatinine measurements. However, signs and symptoms of uremia or volume overload may be presenting complaints. Patients with uremia typically complain of anorexia; nausea; vomiting; metallic taste; altered mental status; and, occasionally, pruritus.
2. Renal failure can be classified on the basis of urine output as nonoliguric (> 400 ml/day), oliguric (100 to 400 ml/day), or anuric (< 100 ml/day).
3. Because the differential diagnosis is large, a thorough history and physical examination are the most effective tools in determining the cause of ARF.
   a. The history should focus on distinguishing the different categories of renal failure.
      (1) Postrenal causes are suggested by a history of urologic conditions such as benign prostatic hypertrophy, gynecologic malignancy, or nephrolithiasis. In addition, anuria is an important clue to a postrenal cause.
      (2) Prerenal causes would be suggested by a history of symptoms or factors predisposing to volume depletion (e.g., diarrhea) or diseases associated with poor renal perfusion such as congestive heart failure.
      (3) Intrinsic renal causes are suggested by a history of recent exposure to intravenous contrast dye, the use of nephrotoxic medications (Table 64-1), symptoms suggestive of proteinuria (anasarca and foamy urine), and symptoms of glomerulonephritis or vasculitis (palpable purpura, pulmonary hemorrhage, hematuria).
   b. Physical examination should focus on the following:
      (1) Indications for emergent hemodialysis including volume overload (hypoxia, flash pulmonary edema, and volume-related hypertensive emergency) and signs of uremia (altered cognition, depressed level of consciousness, asterixis, and pericardial friction rub).
      (2) Clues to the underlying diagnosis such as the presence of a rash, livedo reticularis, anasarca, or palpable purpura.
      (3) Stigmata of more long-standing renal disease such as Terry nails, Lindsey nails, and uremic frost.

III. PATHOPHYSIOLOGY AND DIFFERENTIAL DIAGNOSIS

1. The differential diagnosis of ARF (Table 64-2) is extensive.
2. Prerenal ARF is the result of diminished glomerular blood flow caused by actual or effective intravascular volume depletion.

TABLE 64-1

DRUGS ASSOCIATED WITH ACUTE RENAL FAILURE

Mechanism	Drug
Reduction in renal perfusion through alteration of intrarenal hemodynamics	NSAIDs, angiotensin-converting enzyme inhibitors or angiotensin receptor blockers, CNIs, radiocontrast agents, amphotericin B, interleukin-2[a]
Direct tubular toxicity	Aminoglycosides, radiocontrast agents, cisplatin, CNIs, amphotericin B, methotrexate, foscarnet, pentamidine, organic solvents, heavy metals, intravenous immune globulin[b]
Rhabdomyolysis	Cocaine, ethanol, lovastatin[c]
Intratubular obstruction by precipitation of the agent	Acyclovir, sulfonamides, ethylene glycol,[d] chemotherapeutic agents,[e] methotrexate
Allergic interstitial nephritis[f]	Penicillins, sulfonamides, ciprofloxacin, NSAIDs, phenytoin, allopurinol
Hemolytic-uremic syndrome	CNIs, mitomycin, cocaine, quinine, conjugated estrogens

Modified from Thadhani R, Pascual M, Bonventre JV: *N Engl J Med* 334:1448, 1996.
CNIs, calcineurin inhibitors; *NSAIDs,* nonsteroidal antiinflammatory drugs.
[a]Interleukin-2 produces a capillary leak syndrome with volume contraction.
[b]Mechanism unclear; may be caused by additives.
[c]Acute renal failure is most likely to occur when lovastatin is given in combination with cyclosporine.
[d]Ethylene glycol–induced toxicity can cause calcium oxalate crystals.
[e]Uric acid crystals may form as a result of tumor lysis.
[f]Many other drugs in addition to those listed here cause allergic interstitial nephritis.

a. Congestive heart failure may cause a prerenal state through ineffective forward flow.
b. Hepatorenal syndrome is a common cause of ARF in patients with moderate or severe liver disease that is effectively a prerenal state. As a result of vasodilation of the splanchnic circulation there is underfilling of the systemic circulation, leading to activation of homeostatic vasoconstrictor systems. As a result, there is renal vasoconstriction, with decreased perfusion of the kidneys, resulting in decreased GFR, extreme retention of sodium and free water, and oligoanuria (hepatorenal syndrome type I). This syndrome can be precipitated by bacterial peritonitis, large-volume paracentesis, and gastrointestinal bleeding. It is important to note that this is a diagnosis of exclusion.[3]
3. The pathophysiology of intrinsic renal disease is beyond the scope of this chapter (see Chapters 65-67).
4. Postrenal causes of ARF are listed in Table 64-2. Irreversible damage occurs unless the obstruction is removed or bypassed.

IV. DIAGNOSIS

1. Given the many causes of ARF, a complete history, physical examination, basic metabolic panel, calcium, phosphorus, albumin, uric acid, creatinine kinase, complete blood cell count with differential, liver

TABLE 64-2

DIFFERENTIAL DIAGNOSIS OF ARF

Underlying Disorder	Possible Causes
PRERENAL ARF	
Intravascular depletion	Sepsis, hemorrhage, vomiting, diarrhea
↓ Effective circulating volume	Congestive heart failure, cirrhosis or hepatorenal syndrome, nephrotic syndrome
Medications	Angiotensin-converting enzyme inhibitors, nonsteroidal antiinflammatory drugs
INTRINSIC ARF	
Acute tubular necrosis	Ischemia
	Toxins: drugs (e.g., aminoglycosides), contrast agents, pigments (myoglobin or hemoglobin)
Glomerular disease	Rapidly progressive glomerulonephritis: SLE, small vessel vasculitis (Wegener's granulomatosis or microscopic polyangiitis), Henoch-Schönlein purpura, immunoglobulin A nephropathy), Goodpasture's syndrome
	Acute proliferative glomerulonephritis: endocarditis, streptococcal infection, pneumococcal infection
Vascular disease	Microvascular disease: atheroembolic disease (cholesterol plaque microembolism), thrombotic thrombocytopenic purpura, hemolytic uremic syndrome, HELLP syndrome, or postpartum ARF
	Macrovascular disease: renal artery occlusion, severe abdominal aortic disease (aneurysm)
Interstitial disease	Allergic reaction to drugs, autoimmune disease (SLE or mixed connective tissue disease), pyelonephritis, infiltrative disease (lymphoma or leukemia)
POSTRENAL ARF	
	Benign prostatic hypertrophy, prostate cancer, cervical cancer, retroperitoneal disorders, intratubular obstruction (crystals or myeloma light chains), pelvic mass or invasive pelvic malignancy, intraluminal bladder mass, neurogenic bladder, urethral strictures

Modified from Agrawal M, Swartz R: *Am Fam Physician* 61(7):2077, 2000.
ARF, acute renal failure; *HELLP,* hemolysis, elevated liver enzymes, and low platelet count; *SLE,* systemic lupus erythematosus.

function tests, and renal ultrasound should be performed before more specific tests are ordered. A diagnostic algorithm is presented in Fig. 64-1.

2. **Laboratory studies.** See Table 66-1.
a. The fractional excretion of sodium should be calculated only in patients with oliguric renal failure. An Fe_{Na} is of limited use in the setting of conditions such as diuretic use, glucosuria, or chronic kidney disease in which sodium transport is altered.[4,5]

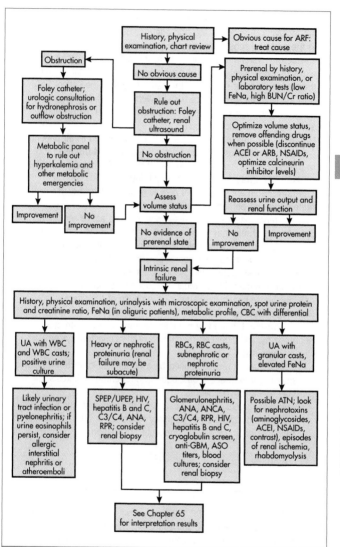

FIG. 64-1

See legend on the next page

b. Fractional excretion of urea ($[U_{un}/P_{un}]/[U_{cr}/P_{cr}]$) is useful when patients are receiving diuretics or are non-oliguric. Because urea is reabsorbed in the proximal tubule along with water, its reabsorption from urine is elevated in prerenal states, leading to a low fractional excretion. Most diuretics work distally in the loop of Henle and NaCl cotransporter and therefore do not affect Fe_{UN} in the same way that they affect Fe_{Na}. An Fe_{UN} less than 35% is consistent with prerenal azotemia.[6] Exceptions include states in which proximal tubule reabsorption is altered (e.g., osmotic diuresis).

3. **Urinalysis.** Complete urinalysis should be performed in all patients with ARF because it helps distinguish the three different disease processes. In the case of intrinsic renal disease, it directs further diagnostic workup. See Chapter 63 for additional details.

a. The urine sediment in prerenal ARF is generally bland with trace or no proteinuria and perhaps a few hyaline casts.

b. Intrinsic renal disease often presents with more active sediment. Glomerulonephritis may be suggested by the presence of dysmorphic red blood cells, red blood cell casts, or proteinuria. Granular casts can be present in acute tubular necrosis. Urine eosinophils may be seen in both acute interstitial nephritis and atheroemboli.

c. The urine sediment in postrenal ARF usually is bland. It may contain crystals whose shape may suggest the cause of the stone.

4. **Radiologic studies.**

a. Renal ultrasound is the key modality for diagnosing obstructive nephropathy, as evidenced by dilation of the collecting system (hydronephrosis).

(1) False-negative results caused by a nondilated collecting system may occur with acute obstruction, retroperitoneal fibrosis, or concomitant hypovolemia.

(2) Hydronephrosis can also been seen in conditions such as reflux nephropathy, pregnancy, papillary necrosis, or brisk diuresis and therefore does not always implicate obstruction.

Diagnosis and management of ARF. *ACEI*, angiotensin-converting enzyme inhibitor; *ANA*, antinuclear antibody; *ANCA*, antineutrophilic cytoplasmic antibody; *anti-GBM*, anti–glomerular basement membrane antibody; *ARB*, angiotensin receptor blocker; *ARF*, acute renal failure; *ASO*, antistreptolysin O; *ATN*, acute tubular necrosis; *BUN/Cr*, blood urea nitrogen/creatinine; *C3/C4*, complements 3 and 4; *CBC*, complete blood cell count; *FeNa*, fractional excretion of sodium; *HIV*, human immunodeficiency virus; *NSAIDs*, nonsteroidal antiinflammatory drugs; *RBC*, red blood cell; *RPR*, rapid plasma reagin; *SPEP*, serum protein electrophoresis; *UA*, urinalysis; *UPEP*, urine protein electrophoresis; *WBC*, white blood cell.

(3) Ultrasound also provides valuable information about renal size, echotexture, and vasculature if duplex studies are ordered.

(4) Normal renal size is 10 to 12 cm in longest diameter. Small kidneys with thin echogenic cortex imply chronic irreversible damage.[7]

b. In patients with evidence of hydronephrosis, spiral computed tomography scan without contrast media can be performed to evaluate for urolithiasis or obstructing masses (see Chapter 70).

5. **Renal biopsy.**

a. In most cases of ARF, renal biopsy is not necessary. If the aforementioned studies suggest an intrinsic cause of ARF other than acute tubular necrosis, a biopsy may be of value.

b. When performed, renal biopsy has been shown to change management in nearly 71% of cases.[8]

V. MANAGEMENT

1. Initial therapy of ARF is directed toward reversing the underlying cause and correcting fluid and electrolyte abnormalities.

a. Relief of urinary obstruction should be addressed early in the evaluation, particularly in patients with anuria. Bladder catheterization is low risk and can rule out urethral obstruction and allow accurate urine output measurement.

b. Volume-depleted states should be treated with saline infusions. However, patients with oliguria or anuria may have total volume overload at presentation. This does not necessarily imply intravascular volume overload.

c. Renal replacement therapy with hemodialysis, or continuous venovenous dialysis with or without hemofiltration, is recommended if severe metabolic derangements are encountered. The mnemonic "AEIOU" can be used to help recall the indications for acute dialysis:

(1) **Acidosis.** Life-threatening acidosis in the setting of ARF.

(2) **Electrolyte imbalances** such as severe hyperkalemia.

(3) **Ingestions.** Toxic ingestions that can be cleared by hemodialysis or charcoal hemoperfusion (e.g., ethylene glycol, lithium, paraldehyde, phenytoin, salicylates).

(4) **Overload.** Volume overload refractory to diuretic therapy.

(5) **Uremia.** Indications include a BUN level greater than 100 mg/dl, uremic pericarditis, and uremic encephalopathy.

d. For patients with intravascular hypervolemia, a trial dose of furosemide should be administered, and if an adequate response is not achieved in the first hour, the dosage should be doubled. If the volume overload is life threatening and not adequately treated with medication, ultrafiltration via dialysis may be necessary. No trials have studied the effectiveness of diuretics in modifying the course of ARF when used solely to change from an oliguric to a nonoliguric state.

e. Hyperkalemia should be monitored and treated on an urgent basis, as discussed in detail in Chapter 74.

f. Metabolic acidosis, if severe ([HCO_3^-] level less than 12 mEq/L or pH less than 7.2), can be treated with sodium bicarbonate in either oral or intravenous forms. The base deficit can be calculated as follows:

$$[HCO_3^-] \text{ deficit (mEq/L)} = 0.5 \times \text{Weight (kg)} \times (24 - \text{Measured serum } HCO_3^-).$$

This formula is conservative and may underestimate the true deficit with serum bicarbonate levels less than 10 mEq/L.[9]

2. Medications that are eliminated primarily by the kidney should be administered at appropriate dosage levels according to GFR. It is important to note that calculations of estimated GFR assume steady state.

3. Patients with a calcium phosphate product greater than 72 are at risk for metastatic calcification and should be treated aggressively with sevelamer. Note that if severe hypocalcemia is present, calcium supplementation may be necessary. Theoretically, calcium-containing phosphate binders such as calcium acetate should be avoided until the calcium phosphate product is less than 55 because these might raise total calcium levels, further precipitating calcium phosphate crystals.

4. The treatment of choice for hepatorenal syndrome is liver transplantation. The use of vasoconstrictors such as terlipressin and midodrine along with plasma expanders such as albumin has shown some promise in small studies.

VI. PREVENTION

Given the morbidity and mortality associated with ARF, preventative measures are essential.

1. Ensuring renal blood flow with appropriate volume resuscitation and maintenance of adequate blood pressure is critical in hypovolemic patients.

2. Avoiding nephrotoxic agents in patients at high risk for ARF (e.g., patients with hypovolemia, congestive heart failure, and contrast dye exposure) is also beneficial.

3. Contrast-induced nephropathy is a significant cause of morbidity and mortality for hospitalized patients and is particularly prevalent in patients with preexisting renal dysfunction, diabetic nephropathy, or hypovolemia and those taking drugs resulting in decreased renal blood flow such as nonsteroidal antiinflammatory drugs and angiotensin-converting enzyme inhibitors. A recent study suggests that hydration with sodium bicarbonate may reduce the risk of contrast nephropathy more than hydration with normal saline. The patients in this study were given 154 mEq/L of sodium bicarbonate as a 3-mL/kg/hr bolus for 1 hour before contrast, followed by infusion of 1 mL/kg/hr for 6 hours

after the procedure. Compared with saline, this resulted in an 11.9% absolute reduction in the rate of contrast nephropathy. The authors speculate that the beneficial effect of sodium bicarbonate results from the alkalosis-mediated inhibition of free radical formation in the renal tubule.[10] See Chapter 66 for additional details, including a discussion of the utility of N-acetyl cysteine.

PEARLS AND PITFALLS

- The American Society of Nephrology recommends the MDRD equation as the most accurate estimation of GFR to estimate baseline renal function. However, the value of the MDRD equation may be limited in the setting of extremes of age or body size, malnutrition, severe obesity, diseases of skeletal muscle, and pregnancy.
- Estimations of GFR assume steady state. Do not use the MDRD equation when the serum creatinine is fluctuating. As a rule, if the serum creatinine doubles in 1 day, GFR is near zero.
- An elevated serum creatinine may result from increased production (e.g., muscle breakdown) or decreased excretion (trimethoprim and cimetidine inhibit renal tubular secretion). In these conditions, BUN may not change much, reflecting stable GFR.
- An elevated BUN may be seen in patients receiving corticosteroids, those with increased catabolism, and those with gastrointestinal tract bleeding. In these states serum creatinine may not change much, reflecting stable GFR.
- In patients whose renal failure is not reversible and is expected to progress to end-stage renal disease, long-term vascular access should be a priority from the outset. Because patients receiving long-term hemodialysis often have vascular access created in an upper extremity, care should be taken to protect the nondominant arm. In particular, placement of indwelling catheters in the subclavian vein should be avoided to reduce the risk of stenosis of that vessel. Phlebotomy and intravenous access should also be avoided in the nondominant arm because venous thrombosis from venipuncture prevents graft and fistula placement.
- Uremia may result in a bleeding diathesis as a result of platelet dysfunction. Desmopressin acetate may partially reverse this dysfunction by increasing plasma levels of both von Willebrand factor and factor VIII.

64

APPROACH TO ACUTE RENAL FAILURE

REFERENCES

1. Levey, AS, Bosch JP, Lewis JB, et al: A more accurate method to estimate glomerular filtration rate from serum creatinine: a new prediction equation, *Ann Intern Med* 130:461-470, 1999. B
2. Nolan CR, Anderson RJ: Hospital-acquired acute renal failure, *J Am Soc Nephrol* 9:710, 1998. C
3. Gines P, Guevara M, Arroyo V, et al: Hepatorenal syndrome, *Lancet* 362:1819-1827, 2003. C
4. Steiner RW: Interpreting the fractional excretion of sodium, *Am J Med* 77:699, 1984. C

5. Espinel CH, Gregory AW: Differential diagnosis of acute renal failure, *Clin Nephrol* 13:73-77, 1980. B

6. Carvounis CP, Nisar S, Guro-Razuman S: Significance of the fractional excretion of urea in differential diagnosis of acute renal failure, *Kidney Int* 62:2223-2229, 2002. B

7. O'Neill CW: Sonographic evaluation of renal failure, *Am J Kidney Dis* 35(6):1021-1038, 2000. C

8. Richards NT et al: Knowledge of renal histology alters patient management in over 40% of cases, *Nephrol Dial Transplant* 9:1255, 1994. B

9. Fernandez PC, Cohen RM, Feldman GM: The concept of bicarbonate distribution space: the crucial role of body buffers, *Kidney Int* 36:747, 1989. C

10. Merten GJ, Burgess WP, Gray LV, et al: Prevention of contrast-induced nephropathy with sodium bicarbonate: a randomized controlled trial, *JAMA* 291:2328-2334, 2004. A

Glomerular Disease

Megan R. Haymart, MD; and Mohamed G. Atta, MD

FAST FACTS

- After diabetes mellitus and hypertension, glomerulonephritis is the third leading cause of end-stage renal disease (ESRD) in the United States and Europe.[1]
- Glomerulonephritis can further be divided into nephrotic syndrome and nephritic syndrome.
- Nephrotic syndrome is characterized by more than 3 g of proteinuria per day, low serum albumin, edema, and dyslipidemia.
- Nephritic syndrome is characterized by red blood cells and red blood cell casts on urine microscopy, hypertension, renal insufficiency, mild proteinuria, and edema.
- Some primary glomerular diseases fall within the continuum of nephritic and nephrotic syndrome and can present with either syndrome (e.g., membranoproliferative glomerulonephritis).
- When clinically appropriate, secondary causes of glomerular disease should be sought by checking serum protein electrophoresis and urine protein electrophoresis, human immunodeficiency virus (HIV), hepatitis B and C, complements 3 and 4 (C3 and C4), antinuclear antibody, rapid plasma reagin, antineutrophilic cytoplasmic antibody (ANCA), anti–glomerular basement membrane (anti-GBM), cryoglobulins, and antistreptolysin O titers.
- Primary glomerular disease may warrant both steroids and cytotoxic agents, which should be administered only under the supervision of a nephrologist.
- Management of glomerular disease also includes angiotensin-converting enzyme inhibitors (ACEIs) or angiotensin receptor II blockers (ARBs) to reduce proteinuria and to prevent further decline in glomerular filtration rate.[2] In addition, antihypertensive agents should be added to control blood pressure, cholesterol-lowering agents to treat dyslipidemia, and sodium restriction and diuretics to treat edema.

65

Approximately 80% of glomerular disease is classified as primary glomerulonephritis, and the remaining 20% is secondary to another illness.[1] Although multiple systemic diseases can affect the glomeruli, this chapter focuses on the major primary causes of glomerular disease.

Nephrotic Syndrome (Box 65-1)

BOX 65-1

DIFFERENTIAL DIAGNOSIS OF NEPHROTIC SYNDROMES[3]

IDIOPATHIC OR PRIMARY (INCIDENCE)

Minimal change (5-10%)	MPGN (5%)
FSGS (20-25%)	Other (15-30%)
Membranous nephropathy (25-30%)	

SECONDARY CAUSES OF NEPHROTIC SYNDROME (PATHOLOGY)

Systemic Disease

Diabetes mellitus (FSGS, MGN)

Amyloidosis (+ Congo red, polarized light apple-green birefringence)

Obesity/OSA (FSGS)

Systemic lupus erythematosus (see Table 65-2)

Vasculitic immunologic disease (MGN, MPGN)

Sickle cell anemia (FSGS, MGN)

Medication Related

Gold, mercury, heavy metals (MGN)

Captopril (MGN)

Nonsteroidal antiinflammatory drugs (MCD, MGN)

Lithium

Heroin (FSGS)

Others: probenecid, chlorpropamide, rifampin, tolbutamide, paramethadione, trimethadione (variable)

Paraneoplastic

Hodgkin's lymphoma (MCD)

Solid tumors (membranous)

Infectious

Viral

Human immunodeficiency virus (FSGS)

Hepatitis B and C (MGN, MPGN)

Parasites

Malaria (MGN, MPGN)

Schistosomiasis (FSGS, MGN, MPGN)

Filariasis (MGN)

Bacterial

Streptococcus (MPGN)

Syphilis (MGN, MPGN)

Subacute bacterial endocarditis, shunt nephritis (MPGN, MGN)

Typhoid fever (MPGN)

Leptospirosis (MPGN)

Hereditary and Metabolic Conditions

Alport's syndrome

Fabry's disease

Familial nephrotic syndrome

Nail patella

Other

Pregnancy

Transplant rejection

Serum sickness

Accelerated hypertensive nephrosclerosis

Unilateral renal artery stenosis

Reflux nephropathy

FSGS, focal segmental glomerulosclerosis; *MCD*, minimal change disease; *MGN*, membranous nephropathy; *MPGN*, membranoproliferative glomerulonephritis; *SBE*, subacute bacterial endocarditis.

Minimal Change Disease

I. EPIDEMIOLOGY AND ETIOLOGY

Minimal change disease (MCD) causes more than 90% of idiopathic nephrotic syndrome in children younger than age 6 but only 30% of nephrotic syndrome in adults.[4] Believed to be caused by an uncharacterized nephrotoxic lymphokine, MCD is equally common in women and men. Secondary causes of MCD include nonsteroidal antiinflammatory drugs, Hodgkin's disease, and other lymphoproliferative disorders.

II. CLINICAL PRESENTATION

Patients often present with acute onset nephrotic syndrome after an upper respiratory infection.[5] It is more likely to present with hypertension, impaired renal function, and acute renal failure in adults than in children.

III. DIAGNOSIS

1. Urinalysis typically is acellular, although oval fat bodies may be seen.
2. Biopsy reveals normal glomeruli on light microscopy, but foot process effacement and fusion of podocytes are seen on electron microscopy.

IV. MANAGEMENT

Treatment with prednisone induces remission in almost all patients with MCD. However, adults often have relapsing disease, and cytotoxic agents such as cyclophosphamide and chlorambucil can be added to the regimen after relapse occurs.[5]

V. PROGNOSIS

MCD has a worse prognosis in adults than in children and typically relapses.

Membranous Nephropathy

I. EPIDEMIOLOGY AND ETIOLOGY

Membranous nephropathy is the most common cause of adult-onset nephrotic syndrome in the United States.[6] Secondary causes of membranous nephropathy include infection (e.g., chronic hepatitis B infection), rheumatologic disorders (e.g., systemic lupus erythematosus [Table 65-1]), drugs (e.g., gold), and paraneoplastic manifestations of neoplasms (e.g., carcinoma of the lung, colon, and breast; leukemia; and non-Hodgkin's lymphoma).

II. CLINICAL PRESENTATION

Most patients present with nephrotic syndrome. Approximately 30% to 50% of patients have hypertension.[6]

III. DIAGNOSIS

1. The urinalysis typically is acellular, but occasionally patients have microscopic hematuria.
2. Light microscopy of kidney biopsy shows thickened capillary walls. Immunofluorescence microscopy reveals diffuse granular capillary wall staining with anti-immunoglobulin G antibody. Electron microscopy shows that the immune deposits are subepithelial.

65

GLOMERULAR DISEASE

TABLE 65-1

WORLD HEALTH ORGANIZATION PATHOLOGIC CLASSIFICATION OF LUPUS NEPHRITIS[3,10]

Class	Pathology	Clinical Features	Treatment
I	Normal glomeruli (LM, IF, EM)	No renal disease.	None.
IIa	Minimal mesangial lupus nephritis: normal glomerulus on LM but mesangial deposits by IF and EM	Mild clinical renal disease with mild or moderate proteinuria and minimally active sediment with serologic activity.	None.
IIb	Mesangial proliferative GN: mesangial hypercellularity and deposits	As in IIa.	None.
III	Focal proliferative GN: < 50% of glomeruli on LM with active or inactive segmental or global GN and mesangial involvement	More active sediment pattern with elevated proteinuria (25% nephrotic) and often active serology. Hypertension may be present. May evolve into class IV.	Mycophenolate mofetil, cyclophosphamide, steroids, azathioprine.
IV	Diffuse proliferative GN: > 50% of glomeruli on LM with segmental or global GN and mesangial involvement	Severe renal involvement with active sediment, hypertension, heavy proteinuria, reduced glomerular filtration, and active serology.	Mycophenolate mofetil, cyclophosphamide, steroids, azathioprine.
V	Membranous GN: subepithelial immune deposits that can occur with any of the first 4 classes	Significant proteinuria with less active serology.	Steroids, cyclosporine, cyclophosphamide, azathioprine. Note: In patients with both type V and a proliferate pathology, therapy is guided by the proliferate lesion.
VI	Advanced sclerosing lupus nephritis: > 90% glomerular sclerosis	Bland sediment; end-stage renal disease.	Dialysis.

EM, electron microscopy; *ESRD,* end-stage renal disease; *GN,* glomerulonephritis; *IF,* immunofluorescence; *LM,* light microscopy.

IV. MANAGEMENT

1. Patients with normal creatinine at presentation, subnephrotic proteinuria, and stable renal function for 6 months are considered to be at low risk. Spontaneous remission is common in this low-risk group, and so only symptomatic treatment is recommended (i.e., control blood pressure with ACEIs or ARBs, treat dyslipidemia and edema).[6]
2. Patients with normal creatinine at presentation, 4 to 8 grams of proteinuria per day, and stable renal function for 6 months are considered to be at medium risk. Although spontaneous remission may occur within 2 years in 30% of this group, patients with persistent nephrotic syndrome typically are treated with corticosteroids alone or in combination with immunosuppressive or cytotoxic agents such as mycophenolate, cyclophosphamide, or cyclosporine.[6–8]
3. High-risk patients with more than 8 g of proteinuria per day or impaired renal function generally are treated with corticosteroids and a cytotoxic agent.[6,9]

V. PROGNOSIS

The 10-year survival of patients with membranous nephropathy is 65% to 85%. Spontaneous remission occurs in 20% to 30% of patients.[6] Subnephrotic proteinuria and female sex correlate positively with spontaneous remission. Poor outcome is more common in older patients, men, patients with hypertension, and patients with impaired renal function.[6,8]

Focal Segmental Glomerulosclerosis

I. EPIDEMIOLOGY AND ETIOLOGY

Focal segmental glomerulosclerosis (FSGS) is the most common cause of idiopathic nephrotic syndrome in African Americans.[6] Secondary causes of FSGS include processes that cause hyperfiltration such as obesity and hypertension. Systemic illnesses such as sickle cell disease and HIV are also known to cause FSGS. HIV-associated nephropathy is a common cause of progressive renal insufficiency in patients with HIV and is characterized pathologically by microcystic tubulointerstitial disease and the collapsing variant of FSGS.

II. CLINICAL PRESENTATION

Eighty-two percent of patients with FSGS present with nephrotic syndrome, about one third with hypertension, and about one third with hematuria. Renal function can be impaired (average creatinine clearance, 90 ml/min).[6]

III. DIAGNOSIS

1. The urinalysis typically is acellular, although there may be fat oval bodies.
2. Light microscopy reveals segmental sclerosis of glomeruli in a focal distribution, and electron microscopy may show foot process effacement.

IV. MANAGEMENT

1. As with other cases of nephrotic syndrome, ACEIs, ARBs, and symptomatic control are the standard of care.
2. Corticosteroid treatment is standard. Response in adults is highly dependent on the duration of treatment, with a minimum course of 12 weeks. Approximately 40% of nephrotic patients respond to steroids with complete remission. In patients with frequent relapse or steroid resistance, cyclosporine can be added.[11] Mycophenolate is another treatment option.[7]
3. Patients with HIV-associated nephropathy should be strongly considered for initiation of HAART therapy.

V. PROGNOSIS

Poor prognostic indicators include creatinine greater than 1.5 mg/dl and kidney biopsy demonstrating interstitial fibrosis and more than 20% tubular atrophy. In addition, resistance to treatment correlates with progression to ESRD, whereas remission correlates with a good outcome.[12]

Membranoproliferative Glomerulonephritis

I. EPIDEMIOLOGY AND ETIOLOGY

1. Type I membranoproliferative glomerulonephritis (MPGN) is an immune complex–mediated glomerulonephritis associated with activation of the complement pathway. The disease incidence is equal in males and females, with the majority of cases, up to 80%, associated with chronic hepatitis C. Other diseases associated with type I MPGN include systemic lupus erythematosus, Sjögren's syndrome, mixed cryoglobulinemia, endocarditis, leukemia, lymphoma, and sarcoidosis.
2. Type II MPGN occurs through activation of the alternative complement pathway. This form is less common than type I MPGN but is thought to be more aggressive.
3. Type III MPGN is similar to type I except that immune complexes favor localization in the subepithelial space.

II. CLINICAL PRESENTATION

MPGN occurs primarily in older children and young adults and may present as nephrotic syndrome with minimally decreased renal function in 35%, a nephritic picture in 35%, as chronic progressive glomerulonephritis in 20%, or as rapidly progressive variant with renal failure.[13] Systemic hypertension is present in the majority of patients and may be severe at the time of presentation.

III. DIAGNOSIS

1. Complement levels typically are low (Box 65-2).
2. The urinalysis can have red blood cells and red blood cell casts typical of nephritic syndrome.
3. Renal biopsy results vary according to the type of MPGN.

IV. MANAGEMENT

Steroids and cytotoxic agents such as cyclophosphamide are used to treat idiopathic MPGN, although the efficacy of this therapy in adults is unknown. Secondary MPGN warrants treatment of the underlying disease in order to prevent disease progression.

V. PROGNOSIS

Response to therapy generally is poor, and most patients develop ESRD. The 10-year survival rate is 50% to 60%.[13]

Immunoglobulin A Nephropathy

I. EPIDEMIOLOGY AND ETIOLOGY

Immunoglobulin A (IgA) nephropathy is the most common primary glomerular disease worldwide, with a male to female ratio that ranges from 2:1 in Japan to 6:1 in the United States.[14] Incidence varies greatly by ethnicity and geographic location. Approximately 50% of glomerular disease in Japan is IgA nephropathy, whereas in some regions of the United States the incidence is as low as 2%.[15] Secondary causes of IgA nephropathy include celiac sprue, dermatitis herpetiformis, connective tissue disease, ulcerative colitis, and sarcoidosis.

BOX 65-2

COMPLEMENT LEVEL AS A DIAGNOSTIC MARKER IN GLOMERULONEPHRITIS

LOW SERUM COMPLEMENT

Disorders Confined to the Kidney
Postinfection GN (↓C3 in 90%)
Membranoproliferative glomerulonephritis (↓C4 in type 1, ↓C3 in type II)
Systemic Disorders
Systemic lupus erythematosus (↓C4 in 70-90%)
Cryoglobulinemia (↓C4 in 80%)
Endocarditis (↓C3 in 90%)
Shunt nephritis (↓C3 in 90%)

NORMAL SERUM COMPLEMENT

Disorders Confined to the Kidney
Immunoglobulin A nephropathy
Renal limited antiglomerular basement membrane disease
Idiopathic rapidly progressive glomerulonephritis
Systemic Disorders
Henoch-Schönlein purpura
Goodpasture's syndrome
Pauci-immune GN (microscopic polyangiitis, Wegener's granulomatosis)
Churg-Strauss syndrome

C3, C4, complements 3 and 4; *GN,* glomerulonephritis.

II. CLINICAL PRESENTATION

Approximately 40% to 50% of patients present with painless macroscopic hematuria at the time of an infectious illness such as pharyngitis. The gross hematuria may last from 24 hours to 1 week. Another 30% to 40% of patients present with microscopic hematuria and mild proteinuria. Nephrotic range proteinuria occurs in less than 5%.[14]

III. DIAGNOSIS

1. Urinalysis shows red blood cells, red blood cell casts, proteinuria, and possibly hemoglobin.
2. Light microscopy of the kidney biopsy can vary from minor mesangial changes to crescents. Immunohistology reveals IgA deposits in the mesangium. Glomerular sclerosis, interstitial fibrosis, and involvement of the glomerular capillary wall are poor prognostic signs.[14]

IV. MANAGEMENT

If a patient does not have hypertension, renal insufficiency, or more than 0.5 g of proteinuria per day, conservative therapy with an ACEI or ARB may be sufficient.[5,15] For patients with poor prognostic indicators, such as nephrotic range proteinuria and progressive renal failure, treatment with steroids is recommended. Fish oil has been shown to be beneficial in progressive IgA disease in several, but not all, studies.[6,16] The use of mycophenolate mofetil is currently under investigation.

V. PROGNOSIS

1. ESRD develops in one third of patients with IgA nephropathy.
2. Poor prognosis is associated with hypertension, more than 1.5 g of proteinuria per day, renal insufficiency, and the absence of macroscopic hematuria.[14]

Goodpasture's Syndrome and Anti-GBM Disease

I. EPIDEMIOLOGY AND ETIOLOGY

Goodpasture's syndrome and anti-GBM disease are characterized by antibodies directed against the glomerular basement membrane. One third of patients have only kidney involvement (anti-GBM disease), and two thirds of patients have both kidney and lung involvement (Goodpasture's syndrome). Incidence is bimodal, with peaks at around age 30 and 60. The syndrome occurs all year but peaks during spring and early summer, suggesting that an infection is the inciting event.[17]

II. CLINICAL PRESENTATION

1. Patients with Goodpasture's syndrome may present with pulmonary symptoms such as shortness of breath, cough, or hemoptysis. Malaise, weight loss, or fever may accompany the respiratory symptoms.

2. Pulmonary hemorrhage can precede renal involvement by years, or it can occur after the diagnosis of glomerulonephritis. Patients almost always have nephritic syndrome but not nephrotic range proteinuria. They may have mild hypertension at the time of diagnosis.
3. Rapidly progressive glomerulonephritis can occur with either anti-GBM disease or Goodpasture's syndrome. Rapid doubling of creatinine (in less than 3 months) should alert the clinician to this possibility.

III. DIAGNOSIS

1. The urinalysis usually has active sediment with red blood cells and red blood cell casts.
2. Creatinine varies between normal and rapidly rising.
3. The diagnosis is made by identification of anti-GBM antibodies in kidney glomeruli on immunofluorescence of the biopsy.

IV. MANAGEMENT

Treatment typically involves both plasma exchange and immunosuppressive agents such as steroids and cyclophosphamide.

V. PROGNOSIS

A creatinine less than 5 mg/dl and a kidney biopsy with less than 50% crescents portend a good response to treatment. Conversely, for patients with a creatinine more than 5 mg/dl and a biopsy with more than 50% crescents, the prognosis is poor.[17]

Wegener's Granulomatosis

I. EPIDEMIOLOGY AND ETIOLOGY

Wegener's granulomatosis involves necrotizing and granulomatous inflammation of the upper and lower respiratory tract, glomerulonephritis, and systemic vasculitis. Sixty percent of patients diagnosed with Wegener's granulomatosis are male. The patients are primarily of Caucasian descent, with an average age at time of diagnosis of 35 to 54 years.[18]

II. CLINICAL PRESENTATION

1. Patients may present with abrupt renal failure and pulmonary symptoms, or they may describe a long course of constitutional and upper respiratory symptoms followed by renal insufficiency. The onset of constitutional symptoms such as fever, fatigue, and weight loss may precede the official diagnosis of Wegener's granulomatosis by several months.[18]
2. Classically, up to 80% of patients with Wegener's granulomatosis have nasal involvement including sinusitis, rhinitis, or epistaxis. Forty-five to seventy-five percent have disease of the lower respiratory tract and present with symptoms of dyspnea, cough, hemoptysis, or pleuritic chest pain. Anywhere from 50% to 95% of patients have renal involvement. Approximately 85% of patients with Wegener's

granulomatosis have arthralgias; 20% to 50% have a rash; 65% have ocular involvement such as proptosis, uveitis, and conjunctivitis; and 25% to 50% have nervous system involvement such as mononeuritis multiplex.[18]

III. DIAGNOSIS

1. Urinalysis typically shows red blood cells and red blood cell casts in addition to mild proteinuria.
2. Laboratory studies are remarkable in that more than half of patients have anemia of chronic disease and up to three fourths of patients have an elevated erythrocyte sedimentation rate. C-ANCA is elevated in 90% of patients with Wegener's granulomatosis, whereas P-ANCA is more likely to be positive in microscopic polyangiitis, another form of pauci-immune glomerulonephritis.
3. Chest radiography often reveals single or multiple cavitated nodules. Less commonly it shows an infiltrate or pleural effusions.
4. Biopsy of the kidney often reveals crescents with granulomatous inflammation, focal segmental necrotizing glomerulosclerosis or global glomerulosclerosis, interstitial inflammation, and inflammation of small and medium vessels on light microscopy. Microscopic polyangiitis has a similar appearance on light microscopy, but interstitial granulomas are more common with Wegener's. Wegener's granulomatosis and microscopic polyangiitis are both classified as pauci-immune because when electron dense particles are seen on electron microscopy they are sparse and small.[18]

IV. MANAGEMENT

Cyclophosphamide combined with corticosteroids is the standard treatment regimen.

V. PROGNOSIS

The addition of cyclophosphamide to the treatment regimen has improved survival dramatically. Five-year survival is about 75%.[19]

Churg-Strauss Syndrome

I. EPIDEMIOLOGY

1. Churg-Strauss syndrome is defined by development of asthma, granulomatous vasculitis, eosinophilic infiltrate of multiple organs, and peripheral eosinophilia.
2. Churg-Strauss is a rare disorder that is equally prevalent in men and women. The average age of onset of asthma is 35 years, and the average age of onset of vasculitis is 38 years. However, it is not uncommon for the diagnosis of asthma or allergic rhinitis to occur 30 years before the onset of eosinophilia and subsequent vasculitis.[18]

II. CLINICAL PRESENTATION

Patients with Churg-Strauss syndrome often have a prodrome of weight loss, fatigue, and fever. The asthma and allergic rhinitis usually occur before the peripheral eosinophilia and vasculitis. Patients may also have skin lesions, mononeuritis multiplex, and arthralgias.

III. DIAGNOSIS

1. Microscopic hematuria and mild proteinuria are noted on urinalysis.
2. The complete blood cell count is remarkable for eosinophilia.
3. Kidney biopsy light microscopy varies from no significant change to severe glomerulosclerosis, vasculitis, and interstitial inflammation with eosinophils. Eosinophils may be visible in the artery wall and surrounding connective tissue.

IV. MANAGEMENT

Initial treatment is corticosteroids, but if the patient is resistant, immunosuppressive medications such as cyclophosphamide can be added.

V. PROGNOSIS

The advent of effective therapies has significantly altered the course of the disease, with a 5-year survival rate currently greater than 70%. Cardiac, neurologic, gastrointestinal, and renal (proteinuria or elevated creatinine) involvement portend a worse prognosis.

PEARLS AND PITFALLS

- Glomerular disease causes less than 10% of hematuria, whereas bladder, prostate, and urethral disease account for about 80%. Clues indicating glomerular origin include dysmorphic red blood cells and red blood cell casts visible on urine microscopy.
- In addition to the primary glomerular diseases and diabetes mellitus, AL-amyloidosis is another cause of nephrotic range proteinuria. AL-amyloidosis is characterized by both mild elevation of monoclonal plasma cells in the bone marrow and amyloid deposition in multiple organs. Amyloid deposition in the kidneys can lead to subnephrotic to nephrotic range proteinuria, hematuria, monoclonal light chains in urine or blood, and renal insufficiency.
- Complications of nephrotic syndrome include infection, accelerated atherosclerosis, thrombosis (including renal vein thrombosis), and malnutrition.
- All patients with nephrotic syndrome should receive the Pneumovax.
- The loss of antithrombin III in patients with nephrotic syndrome results in a hypercoagulable state. Therefore, all inpatients with nephrotic syndrome should receive venous thromboembolism prophylaxis.

65

GLOMERULAR DISEASE

REFERENCES

1. Maisonneuve P, Agoda L, Gellert R, et al: Distribution of primary renal diseases leading to end-stage renal failure in the United States, Europe, and Australia/New Zealand: results from an international comparative study, *Am J Kidney Dis* 35(1):157-165, 2000. B

2. The GISEN Group: Randomized placebo-controlled trial of effect of ramipril on decline in glomerular filtration rate and risk of terminal renal failure in proteinuric, non-diabetic nephropathy, *Lancet* 349:1857-1863, 1997. A

3. Appel G: Glomerular disorders, *Cecil textbook of medicine,* 22nd ed, Saunders, 2004, Philadelphia. D

4. Nolasco F, Cameron JS, Heywood EF, et al: Adult-onset minimal change nephrotic syndrome: a long-term follow-up, *Kidney Int* 29:1215-1233, 1986. B

5. Bargman JM: Management of minimal lesion glomerulonephritis: evidence-based recommendations, *Kidney Int* 55(s):3-16, 1999. C

6. Cattran D: Outcomes research in glomerulonephritis, *Semin Nephrol* 23(4):340-354, 2003. C

7. Choi MJ, Eustace JA, Giminez LF, et al: Mycophenolate mofetil treatment for primary glomerular diseases, *Kidney Int* 61:1098-1114, 2002. B

8. Cattran DC, Appel GB, Hebert LA, et al: Cyclosporine in patients with steroid-resistant membranous nephropathy: a randomized trial, *Kidney Int* 59(4):1484-1490, 2001. A

9. Schieppati A, Mosconi L, Perna A, et al: Prognosis of untreated patients with idiopathic membranous nephropathy, *N Engl J Med* 329:85-89, 1993. B

10. Weening JJ, D'Agat VD, et al: The classification of glomerulonephritis in systemic lupus erythematosus revisited, *Kidney Int* 65(2):521-530, 2004. C

11. Cattran DC, Appel GB, Hebert LA, et al: A randomized trial of cyclosporine in patients with steroid-resistant focal segmental glomerulosclerosis, *Kidney Int* 56(6):2220-2226, 1999. A

12. Shiiki H, Dohi K: Primary focal segmental glomerulosclerosis: clinical course, predictors of renal outcome and treatment, *Intern Med* 39:606-611, 2000. C

13. Holley KE, Donadio JV: Membranoproliferative glomerulonephritis. In Tisher CC, Brenner BM, eds: *Renal pathology with clinical and functional correlations,* 2nd ed, Philadelphia, 1994, Lippincott. C

14. Donadio JV, Grande JP: IgA nephropathy, *N Engl J Med* 347:738-748, 2002. C

15. Praga M, Gutierrez E, Gonzales E, et al: Treatment of IgA nephropathy with ACE inhibitors: a randomized controlled trial, *J Am Soc Nephrol* 14(6):1578-1583, 2003. A

16. Donadio JV, Bergstralh EJ, Offord KP, et al: A controlled trial of fish oil in IgA nephropathy, *N Engl J Med* 331:1194-1199, 1994. A

17. Bolton WK: Goodpasture's syndrome, *Kidney Int* 50:1753-1766, 1996. C

18. D'Agati VD, Appel GB: Polyarteritis nodosa, Wegener's granulomatosis, Churg-Strauss syndrome, temporal arteritis, Takayasu arteritis and lymphomatoid granulomatosis. In Tisher CC, Brenner BM, eds: *Renal pathology with clinical and functional correlations,* 2nd ed, Philadelphia, 1994 Lippincott. C

19. Booth AD, Almond MK, Burns A, et al: Outcome of ANCA-associated renal vasculitis: a 5-year retrospective study, *Am J Kidney Dis* 41(4):776-784, 2003. B

Renal Tubulointerstitial Diseases

Adam R. Berliner, MD; and Michael J. Choi, MD

FAST FACTS

- The renal tubulointerstitial diseases are a heterogeneous group of disorders with characteristic features that may include sterile pyuria and white blood cell casts, parenchymal concentrating defects resulting in polyuria and nephrogenic diabetes insipidus, and tubular defects such as renal tubular acidosis.
- Acute interstitial nephritis (AIN) can be caused by drugs, infection, and immunologic disease. Findings on urinalysis may include pyuria, eosinophils, white blood cell casts, hematuria, and proteinuria. Treatment of drug-induced AIN is supportive, with corticosteroids reserved for recalcitrant cases.
- Acute tubular necrosis (ATN) is the most common cause of in-hospital acute renal failure (ARF) and often is caused by medications, iodinated contrast dye, and hypotension. The urinary sediment typically is bland with muddy brown granular casts. Treatment is supportive.
- Patients with preexisting renal dysfunction, diabetes mellitus, multiple myeloma, and advanced age are at high risk for contrast nephropathy (CN). Pericontrast hydration, N-acetylcysteine, and sodium bicarbonate administration have been shown to reduce its incidence.
- Rhabdomyolysis leads to ARF via intratubular obstruction and ATN. Large hemoglobin on urine dipstick without concomitant hematuria on microscopic examination is a diagnostic clue and should prompt total serum creatinine phosphokinase measurement. Copious intravenous hydration to maintain vigorous urine output is the cornerstone of management, with urinary alkalinization (pH higher than 6.5) being an additional step to decrease cast formation and intratubular obstruction.

The tubulointerstitial diseases of the kidney are a heterogeneous group of diseases. Their unifying feature is involvement of the renal tubules and their supporting structures. These disorders can be classified by pace (acute vs. chronic), pathogenic mechanism (e.g., infectious, toxic), or by whether the disease process represents primary involvement of the kidney or renal manifestation of a systemic disease. Given the vast territory this topic encompasses, the aim of this chapter is to highlight a few diseases both relevant to inpatient medicine and representative of the diversity of the tubulointerstitial diseases.

Acute Interstitial Nephritis

I. EPIDEMIOLOGY AND ETIOLOGY

1. The prevalence of biopsy-proven AIN varies from 1% in a series of Finnish male military recruits with proteinuria or hematuria to 15% of patients with ARF.[1,2]
2. Drugs are the predominant cause of AIN, with the mechanism of injury believed to be immune-mediated hypersensitivity. Dozens of drugs are known to cause AIN, including penicillin derivatives, cephalosporins, sulfa-containing drugs (including furosemide), rifampin, allopurinol, mesalamine, and nonsteroidal antiinflammatory drugs (NSAIDs).
3. Other precipitants of AIN include infection, immunologic diseases (e.g., Sjögren's syndrome), sarcoidosis (rare), and secondary interstitial nephritis from primary glomerulonephritides. As in drug-induced AIN, the mechanism of injury in infection-related AIN is thought to be secondary to systemic immune response.

II. PRESENTATION

1. The temporal relationship between ARF and drug exposure can range from days or weeks (e.g., methicillin) to months or years (e.g., NSAIDs). Previous tolerance of a drug does not exclude it as a cause of AIN.
2. Symptoms include flank pain (from capsular stretch by the inflamed renal parenchyma), fever, and rash. The traditionally quoted triad of fever, maculopapular rash, and eosinophilia is uncommon (< 5% of cases of non–methicillin-induced AIN), and it is most commonly seen with beta-lactam antibiotics. NSAID-induced AIN is typified by the paucity of these findings but is often associated with significant proteinuria.
3. Urinalysis and culture often show sterile pyuria, leukocyte casts, and erythrocytes.
   a. Either Hansel's stain or Wright's stain may be used to examine urinary sediment for eosinophiluria (considered positive when > 1% of urinary leukocytes show positive staining). In one series of 200 patients with urinary eosinophils, the sensitivity, specificity, and positive predictive value for AIN were only 40%, 72%, and 38%, respectively. Other conditions associated with eosinophiluria include prostatitis, rapidly progressive GN, bladder cancer, and renal atheroembolic disease.[3]
   b. Gross or microscopic hematuria may be present in some cases.
   c. Proteinuria may be present at levels up to 1 g/24 hours, with the notable exception of NSAID-induced AIN, which usually is associated with concomitant glomerular pathology and proteinuria that can enter the nephrotic range (3-3.5 g/24 hours).
   d. It is important to note that the urinalysis may be completely unrevealing.

4. Renal ultrasound shows normal-sized kidneys, occasionally enlarged, with greater echogenicity.

III. DIAGNOSIS

1. The gold standard for diagnosis is renal biopsy, which characteristically shows inflammatory interstitial infiltrates.
2. Most patients in whom AIN is suspected do not undergo biopsy but rather are initially managed by discontinuation of the suspected offending agent. Renal biopsy is reserved for patients who do not improve as expected, patients in whom the diagnosis is uncertain, and patients for whom immunosuppressive therapy is being contemplated.

IV. MANAGEMENT

1. Suspected drugs should be discontinued immediately.
2. If a conservative approach ultimately fails, immunosuppressive therapy may be considered.
a. Corticosteroids are the most common immunosuppressants used to treat drug-induced AIN, with very little supportive data. In an often-quoted retrospective study of 14 patients with AIN (8 cases biopsy proven), the 8 patients who took an average dosage of 60 mg of prednisone daily for about 10 days were compared with the 6 patients who did not receive steroids. Patients who received steroids were found to have a lower average serum creatinine at follow-up and to achieve this new baseline faster than patients who did not receive steroids.[4] Optimal dosing and duration of corticosteroids are not well defined. One regimen is oral prednisone 1 mg/kg daily for 4 weeks, with continuation of therapy if there is some response.[2]
b. Adjunctive therapy with cyclophosphamide is supported only by small anecdotal reports.

V. PROGNOSIS

If the offending drug is discontinued within 1 week of the onset of ARF, prognosis for return to baseline renal function generally is good. The longer the patient is exposed to the offending agent, the lower the chance of complete or even partial recovery because tubular atrophy and interstitial fibrosis increase.

Acute Tubular Necrosis[5]

I. EPIDEMIOLOGY AND ETIOLOGY

1. ATN is the result of either a toxic (Box 66-1) or ischemic insult to the renal tubular epithelium and is the most common cause of ARF in patients in the hospital or intensive care unit (38% and 76%, respectively).
2. Advanced age and preexisting renal disease are strong risk factors for development of ATN after exposure to a potential insult. The dosage and duration of nephrotoxin administration also correlate directly with risk for ATN.

BOX 66-1

COMMON CAUSES OF TOXIC ACUTE TUBULAR NECROSIS

EXOGENOUS TOXINS

Antibiotics: aminoglycosides, amphotericin B, acyclovir, pentamidine, foscarnet

Other: organic solvents, intravenous immune globulin, intravenous iodinated
contrast agents, chemotherapeutic agents, nonsteroidal antiinflammatory drugs,
bacterial toxins, ethylene glycol

ENDOGENOUS TOXINS

Myoglobin: rhabdomyolysis

Hemoglobin: massive hemolysis, hemolytic anemia

Uric acid: in the setting of tumor lysis syndrome

---

3. Although it usually appears in concert with multiple comorbid illnesses,
   ATN has been shown to be an independent predictor of survival, with
   mortality in patients with ATN who need dialysis support between 50%
   and 80%.

II. PRESENTATION

1. ATN presents with either oliguric or nonoliguric ARF.
2. Urinalysis generally is devoid of red cells, white cells, or protein; major
   urine findings include renal tubular epithelial cells, hyaline casts, and
   muddy brown granular casts.

III. DIAGNOSIS

1. The presence of potential antecedent ischemic or nephrotoxic insults
   should be sought in the history and medical record. Toxins typically
   cause an increase in serum creatinine within 3 days after the insult,
   especially if there is concomitant vasoconstriction (as with contrast dye
   and amphotericin B), although drugs whose metabolites accumulate in
   the interstitium (e.g., aminoglycoside antibiotics) may not manifest ATN
   until 5 to 10 days after initiation of the drug.
2. Urinary obstruction and intrinsic renal disease should be excluded.
3. Distinguishing ATN from a prerenal state can be challenging. Urine
   studies useful in distinguishing the two are presented in Table 66-1.
4. Renal biopsy is not necessary to diagnose ATN.

IV. MANAGEMENT

1. Except for ARF from iodinated contrast dye, few preventive strategies
   exist other than avoidance of nephrotoxins and situations predisposing
   to renal ischemia. For established ATN, care is largely supportive.
2. "Renal-dose" dopamine infusion (< 5 µg/kg/min) increases the
   glomerular filtration rate (GFR) and urine output when infused into
   healthy volunteer subjects. Despite these physiologic effects, low-dose
   dopamine has not been shown to be clinically beneficial. In a recent
   randomized trial, low-dose dopamine did not show any benefit in
   mortality, need for dialysis, or length of hospitalization in patients
   with ATN.[6]

TABLE 66-1

URINE INDICES USED TO DISTINGUISH PRERENAL AZOTEMIA FROM ACUTE TUBULAR NECROSIS

Diagnostic Index	Prerenal Azotemia	Acute Tubular Necrosis
Fractional excretion of Na^+ [(Urinary sodium × Plasma creatine)/(Urinary creatine × Plasma sodium)] × 100	<1%	>2%
Fractional excretion of urea [(Urinary urea nitrogen × Plasma creatine)/ (Urinary creatine × Plasma urea nitrogen)] × 100	<35%	>50%
Urinary [Na^+]	<10	>40
Urine specific gravity	>1.018	<1.012
Urine osmolality (mOsm/kg H_2O)	>500	<250
Blood urea nitrogen/creatinine ratio	>20	<10-15
Urine sediment	Bland; hyaline casts	Bland; muddy brown granular casts, tubular epithelial cells, hyaline casts

66

RENAL TUBULOINTERSTITIAL DISEASES

3. Although loop diuretics are useful for managing hypervolemia associated with ARF, converting oliguric to nonoliguric ATN with high-dose loop diuretics does not reduce mortality or the need for dialysis.

V. PROGNOSIS

1. ATN may be categorized into an **initiation** phase lasting hours to days, during which the toxic or ischemic insult is sustained; a **maintenance** phase, typically lasting 1 to 2 weeks but in some cases for months, during which GFR remains extremely low (GFR less than 10 mL/min); and a **recovery** phase, when the renal tubular epithelium is repaired and regenerated with return of renal function.
2. The onset of the recovery phase often is associated with a return of normal urinary output or a robust post-ATN diuresis as excessive sodium and water accumulated during the illness are excreted.
3. About 50% to 60% of patients with ATN, even those needing temporary dialysis, can expect full renal recovery. Five to eleven percent need long-term dialysis.

Radiographic Contrast Nephropathy

I. EPIDEMIOLOGY

1. CN is defined as either an absolute increase of more than 0.5 mg/dl or a relative increase of more than 25% of serum creatinine within 48 hours of administration of contrast.
2. CN occurs in 10% to 15% of patients exposed to intravenous contrast and accounts for about 10% of hospital-acquired ARF. Roughly 8% of

patients need hemodialysis (usually temporary), and more than 7000 deaths ultimately are attributed to CN annually.[7]

II. ETIOLOGY AND RISK FACTORS

1. Free radical–induced apoptosis and alteration in renal hemodynamics are the two pathogenic mechanisms that underlie CN. Experimental data show a biphasic response to contrast media, with an initial increase in renal blood flow followed by a sustained decrease in GFR.
2. The strongest patient risk factors for CN are preexisting renal insufficiency, diabetes mellitus, and advanced age. Other patient risk factors include female sex, concurrent administration of other nephrotoxins, dehydration, decreased left ventricular ejection fraction, class III or IV New York Heart Association classification heart failure, myocardial infarction in the preceding 24 hours, contrast exposure in the preceding 48 hours, and multiple myeloma.
3. Contrast-related factors also contribute to risk. Lower osmolality and nonionic contrast media result in a lower incidence of CN, although this benefit has been demonstrated only in patients with preexisting renal insufficiency. The volume of contrast administered directly correlates with risk of CN. In one study of 7000 patients, each 100 ml of dye correlated with a hazard ratio for CN of 1.12.[8]

III. DIAGNOSIS[9]

The diagnosis should always be entertained when ARF ensues 1 to 2 days after exposure to intravenous contrast. No specific physical signs or symptoms exist, and the biochemical evaluation of blood and urine is consistent with ATN. Urine output often is normal. It is imperative to be vigilant for other causes of ARF, especially those associated with intravascular procedures, such as renal atheroemboli or interruption of renal perfusion from iatrogenic aortic dissection.

IV. MANAGEMENT

1. There is no specific therapy for CN other than supportive care and avoidance of further nephrotoxic or ischemic insults. Temporary dialysis may be necessary.
2. **Prevention.** In addition to discontinuing NSAIDs, angiotensin-converting enzyme inhibitors, and diuretics the day before the procedure whenever possible, the following preventive measures have been studied:
a. **Hydration with normal saline.** Precontrast and postcontrast hydration have been widely studied, with study protocols varying in terms of the properties of the fluid, duration, and rate of infusion. To summarize the data broadly, periprocedure hydration is better than not hydrating, and isotonic solutions (typically 0.9% sodium chloride) are better than hypotonic solutions. The benefit of hydration is thought to reflect enhanced renal perfusion, which counteracts renal hypoperfusion from contrast-induced vasoconstriction.

b. **Hydration with sodium bicarbonate.** A recent randomized trial of 119 patients undergoing procedures with iodinated contrast demonstrated a substantially lower incidence of CN (1.7% vs. 13.6%) when 154 mEq/L sodium bicarbonate (3 ml/kg for 1 hour before the procedure and 1 ml/kg for 6 hours after the procedure) was compared with 0.9% sodium chloride infusion. The authors postulate that the beneficial effect results from urinary alkalinization, which theoretically decreases free radical formation.[10]

c. **N-acetylcysteine.** Several studies[11,12] in patients undergoing contrast-enhanced CT or coronary angiography have shown that N-acetylcysteine can significantly reduce the incidence of CN in patients with preexisting renal disease. Although some studies have failed to show a benefit, N-acetylcysteine is safe and therefore is recommended in patients with serum creatinine greater than 1.5 mg/dl or a GFR of less than 60 ml/min. The most common dosage used is 600 mg orally twice daily, with two doses before and two doses after the procedure.

d. **Other measures.** Prevention of renal vasoconstriction with calcium channel blockers, dopamine, the dopamine agonist fenoldopam, angiotensin-converting enzyme inhibitors, and theophylline has not been proven effective. Prophylactic hemodialysis begun after contrast administration in patients with baseline serum creatinine greater than 2.3 mg/dl was shown to be of no benefit and potentially harmful.[13] Pericontrast hemofiltration has been shown to decrease both the incidence of CN and mortality, although several methodologic flaws of this study have been cited.[14] Additionally, hemofiltration is expensive, timeconsuming, and impractical on a large scale.

V. PROGNOSIS

A retrospective analysis of more than 16,000 patients showed in-hospital mortality rates of about 34.0% in patients who developed CN, compared with about 7.0% of patients who did not have ARF. Prognosis is generally worse in patients with preexisting renal disease and those needing dialysis.

Rhabdomyolysis[15-18]

I. EPIDEMIOLOGY AND ETIOLOGY (Box 66-2)

1. Approximately 26,000 cases of rhabdomyolysis are reported yearly, about 15% of which are complicated by ARF.
2. Rhabdomyolysis causes ARF via myoglobin's direct toxic effects on the tubular epithelium, intratubular obstruction, and reduction in hydrostatic glomerular filtration pressure. In addition, rhabdomyolysis causes an overwhelming state of renal hypoperfusion from third-space fluid losses into injured skeletal muscle. Preexisting volume depletion and sepsis increase the risk of ARF.
3. It is important to note that there is no absolute threshold at which creatinine phosphokinase levels predispose to ARF, although it is

---

BOX 66-2

COMMON CAUSES OF RHABDOMYOLYSIS

Muscle injury: trauma, electric shock, hypothermia, hyperthermia (e.g., malignant hyperpyrexia)

Extreme muscular exertion: seizures, delirium tremens, physical exercise

Muscle ischemia: prolonged compression (e.g., coma), compromise of major vessels (e.g., thromboembolism, dissection)

Metabolic disorders: hypokalemia, hypophosphatemia, (less likely: hyponatremia or hypernatremia, diabetic ketoacidosis, hyperosmolar states)

Infections: influenza, infectious mononucleosis, Legionnaires disease, tetanus

Toxins: ethanol, isopropyl alcohol, ethylene glycol, toluene, snake and insect bites

Drugs: cocaine, statins, amphetamines, phencyclidine, succinylcholine

Inherited diseases: deficiency of myophosphorylase, phosphofructokinase, carnitine palmitoyltransferase, or myoadenylate deaminase

---

Modified from Brenner and Rector's *The Kidney.*

generally held that higher levels correlate with higher risk, with most cases of ARF being associated with creatinine phosphokinase levels of 10,000 to 15,000 U/L.

II. DIAGNOSIS

1. Diagnosis is based on the development of ARF in the setting of severely elevated serum creatinine kinase.
2. Urinalysis reveals red-brown urine that is markedly positive for hemoglobin by dipstick. Microscopy reveals zero or few urinary erythrocytes and the characteristic urinary muddy brown casts of ATN.
3. Urine dipstick testing for myoglobin is an insensitive marker of rhabdomyolysis; negative dipstick for urinary myoglobin should never be used to rule out the diagnosis.

III. TREATMENT

1. Aggressive intravenous fluid resuscitation is critical for both preventing ARF and managing established ARF. Fluid resuscitation restores renal perfusion to correct prerenal azotemia and helps maintain tubular urinary flow to avoid stasis of myoglobin and Tamm-Horsfall protein crystals.
2. Early studies of rhabdomyolysis demonstrated that aggressive intravenous hydration reduces the risk of ARF. Normal saline should be used initially at a rate of 1 to 1.5 L/hr to induce urinary output of about 200 to 300 ml/hour. Once adequate urinary output is achieved, alkalinizing the urine (pH higher than 6.5) with intravenous sodium bicarbonate (one common formulation is 5% dextrose in water with 150 mEq of sodium bicarbonate per liter of fluid) theoretically attenuates precipitation of intratubular myoglobin and Tamm-Horsfall protein casts. However there are no clear data to support the superiority

of this technique over hydration with normal saline, and in the setting of oliguria or anuria, sodium bicarbonate infusion can create a metabolic alkalosis or worsen the hypocalcemia that usually accompanies rhabdomyolysis.

IV. PROGNOSIS

1. When needed, dialysis usually is temporary.
2. Mortality from rhabdomyolysis-induced ARF is about 20%.

PEARLS AND PITFALLS

- Aminoglycosides cause ATN in 10% to 20% of patients; preferential accumulation in the renal cortex is thought to account for this effect, which can be delayed even several days after drug discontinuation.
- Atheroembolic renal disease occurs in 1% to 2% of patients after cardiac catheterization, renal arteriography, or aortic procedures and can be mistaken for contrast nephropathy. Clues that suggest atheroemboli as cause of ARF include hypocomplementemia, eosinophilia or eosinophiluria, and other evidence of microembolization (e.g., ischemic toes, livedo reticularis).
- Rhabdomyolysis often is accompanied by hypocalcemia because extracellular calcium is shifted into damaged skeletal muscle. Avoid correcting hypocalcemia unless it is symptomatic (i.e., tetany, cardiac arrhythmias) because the later phases of rhabdomyolysis are characterized by calcium efflux from muscle back into blood, with possible resultant hypercalcemia.
- The hypercalciuria associated with sarcoidosis leads to progressive nephrocalcinosis and nephrolithiasis, although overt signs of renal failure are the exception rather than the rule. Sarcoid nephropathy rarely occurs in isolation, and concurrent pulmonary, ocular, dermatologic, or other organ system disease usually is evident. Acute and chronic granulomatous interstitial nephritis is thought to be an uncommon complication of sarcoidosis. Corticosteroids can slow the progression.
- Cystic diseases of the kidney are some of the hereditary tubulointerstitial diseases; autosomal dominant polycystic kidney disease is the most common and accounts for about 5% of cases of end-stage renal disease in the United States. Hypertension, hematuria, and chronic flank pain make up the clinical spectrum. Intracerebral aneurysms complicate a small percentage of cases; patients with autosomal dominant polycystic kidney disease and a family history of intracerebral aneurysm or subarachnoid hemorrhage, severe headaches, or high-risk occupation (e.g., airplane pilot) should be screened with brain magnetic resonance angiography.
- Analgesic nephropathy is an insidious progressive form of chronic tubulointerstitial disease that results from years of sustained antipyretic analgesic use, usually in combination. Diagnosis is difficult because the history of chronic analgesic ingestion often is concealed. Noncontrast abdominal computed tomography scanning is highly sensitive

66

RENAL TUBULOINTERSTITIAL DISEASES

and specific for diagnosis; typical findings include renal papillary calcification, small kidneys, and irregular renal contours. Uroepithelial malignancies of the renal pelvis, ureters, and bladder develop in about 10% of patients with analgesic nephropathy. Yearly screening for hematuria is warranted, with urine cytology and cystoscopic or other urologic imaging if hematuria is present.

REFERENCES

1. Peterson E: et al: Nephritis among young Finnish men, *Clin Nephrol* 22:217-222, 1984. B
2. Neilson EG: Pathogenesis and therapy of interstitial nephritis, *Kidney Int* 35:1257-1270, 1989. C
3. Ruffing K et al: Eosinophils in urine revisited, *Clin Nephrol* 41(3):163-166, 1994. C
4. Galpin JE et al: Acute interstitial nephritis due to methicillin, *Am J Med* 65(5):756-765, 1978. B
5. Esson ML, Schrier RW: Diagnosis and treatment of acute tubular necrosis, *Ann Intern Med* 137:744-752, 2002. C
6. Bellomo R et al: Low-dose dopamine in patients with early renal dysfunction: a placebo-controlled randomized trial. Australian and New Zealand Intensive Care Society (ANZICS) Clinical Trials Group, *Lancet* 356(9248):2139-2143, 2000. A
7. Gami AS, Garovic VD: Contrast nephropathy after coronary angiography, *Mayo Clin Proc* 79:211-219, 2004. C
8. Rihal CS, Textor SC, Grill DE, et al: Incidence and prognostic importance of acute renal failure after percutaneous coronary intervention, *Circulation* 105:2259-2264, 2002. B
9. McCullough PA et al: Contrast-induced nephropathy, *Crit Care Clin* 21:261-280, 2005. A
10. Merten GJ et al: Prevention of contrast-induced nephropathy with sodium bicarbonate: a randomized controlled trial, *JAMA* 291(19):2328-2334, 2004. A
11. Tepel M et al: Prevention of radiographic-contrast-agent-induced reductions in renal function by N-acetylcysteine, *N Engl J Med* 343:180-184, 2000. A
12. Kay J, Chow WH, Chan TM, et al: Acetylcysteine for prevention of acute deterioration of renal function following elective coronary angiography and intervention: a randomized controlled trial, *JAMA* 289:553-558, 2003. A
13. Vogt B, Ferrari P, Schonholzer C, et al: Prophylactic hemodialysis after radiocontrast media in patients with renal insufficiency is potentially harmful, *Am J Med* 111:692-698, 2001. B
14. Marenzi G, Marana I, Lauri G, et al: The prevention of radiocontrast-agent-induced nephropathy by hemofiltration, *N Engl J Med* 349(14):1333-1340, 2003. B
15. Sauret JM et al: Rhabdomyolysis, *Am Fam Physician* 65(5):907-912, 2002. C
16. Holt SG, Moore KP: Pathogenesis and treatment of renal dysfunction in rhabdomyolysis, *Intensive Care Med* 27:803-811, 2001. C
17. Allison RC, Bedsole DL: The other medical causes of rhabdomyolysis, *Am J Med Sci* 326(2):79-88, 2003. C
18. Grover DS, Atta MG, Eustace JA, et al: Lack of clinical utility of urine myoglobin detection by microconcentrator ultrafiltration in the diagnosis of rhabdomyolysis, *Nephrol Dial Transplant* 19(10):2634-2638, 2004. B

Renovascular Hypertension

Leslie S. Gewin, MD; and Paul Scheel, MD

> ## FAST FACTS
>
> - Stenosis greater than 75% in one or both renal arteries (or 50% residual stenosis after dilation procedure) is necessary for a diagnosis of renal artery stenosis and may suggest renovascular hypertension.[1]
> - Renovascular hypertension is defined retrospectively when blood pressure control improves after revascularization of a stenotic lesion.
> - Approximately 90% of renal artery stenosis is caused by atherosclerosis and about 10% by fibromuscular dysplasia (FMD).[2]

67

Renovascular hypertension is a secondary cause of hypertension that results from poor renal perfusion secondary to flow-limiting lesions. Among unselected patients with mild to moderate hypertension, renovascular hypertension occurs in 0.6% to 3.0%, but the frequency increases to 10% to 45% among patients with acute, severe, or refractory hypertension.[3,4] Animal models of unilateral renovascular hypertension suggest a three-phase model. During the first phase, flow-limiting lesions elevate renin levels, leading to hypertension. In the second phase, renin levels normalize but hypertension persists. The hypertension is reversible if the stenosis is fixed. In the final phase, blood pressure does not respond to removal of the stenosis, presumably because of injury caused by prolonged hypertension.[5] In contrast, in bilateral renal artery stenosis, hypertension is volume dependent rather than renin dependent. As in unilateral stenosis, the renin level initially rises, but there is no normally functioning kidney to perform natriuresis. Therefore, sodium and volume retention lead to reduced renin levels but increase blood pressure. This chapter provides an approach to the diagnosis and management of the two most common causes of renovascular hypertension: atherosclerosis and FMD.

I. RENAL ARTERY ATHEROSCLEROSIS

A. EPIDEMIOLOGY

1. The presence of atherosclerosis in the renal artery increases with age and is more likely among those with risk factors for atherosclerosis (e.g., diabetes, hypertension) or evidence of vascular disease elsewhere (e.g., coronary artery disease).[2]
2. Atherosclerotic stenosis generally involves the ostium, periaortic region, and proximal one third of the main renal artery, although distal disease can be found in more severe cases.[2]
3. Studies indicate that atherosclerotic renal artery disease is progressive in about 50% of patients over a 2- to 5-year period.[6]

B. CLINICAL PRESENTATION

1. Renal artery stenosis from atherosclerosis can present asymptomatically or cause one of two syndromes: hypertension or ischemic nephropathy.[2] Hypertension is not a prerequisite for ischemic nephropathy, which commonly presents as acute renal failure or unexplained chronic or progressive azotemia.[2] Creatinine levels usually do not rise until bilateral involvement occurs. End-stage renal disease resulting from atherosclerotic renal disease carries higher mortality rates than other causes of renal failure.

2. Given the high prevalence of essential hypertension, it may be difficult to determine which patients need further workup. See Box 67-1 for factors in the clinical presentation that should raise suspicion for renovascular hypertension.

C. DIAGNOSIS

Diagnosis is made by radiographic imaging.

D. MANAGEMENT (Fig. 67-1)

1. Medical treatment with angiotensin-converting enzyme (ACE) inhibitors, aspirin, cholesterol-lowering drugs, and smoking cessation to limit atherosclerosis is imperative.[2]

2. Percutaneous transluminal renal angioplasty (PTRA) with stent placement is the treatment of choice. Angioplasty alone is suboptimal because the extensive recoil of the plaques often leads to restenosis. A review of 14 case series demonstrates that renal artery stent placement results in the "cure" of hypertension in 17%, improvement in 47%, and absence of change in 36%.[5] The effect on renal function was more equivocal, with improvement in 30%, stabilization in 42%, and worsening in 29%.[5] Although the rates of renal improvement and decline are approximately equal with PTRA with endovascular stenting,

---

BOX 67-1

CLINICAL CLUES TO RENOVASCULAR HYPERTENSION

Severe or refractory hypertension including retinal hemorrhages or papilledema

Acute rise in blood pressure over a stable baseline (includes baseline essential hypertension)

Proven age of onset before puberty or age > 50

Acute elevation in creatinine after institution of angiotensin-converting enzyme inhibitor

Moderate to severe hypertension in patient with diffuse atherosclerosis or incidentally discovered asymmetry in renal disease

Negative family history for hypertension

Moderate to severe hypertension in patients with recurrent episodes of flash pulmonary edema or unexplained heart failure

Modified from Mann SJ, Pickering TG: *Ann Intern Med* 117:845, 1992.

there is evidence that among those with stabilization, there is a slowing in the deterioration of renal function. The largest randomized, prospective trial (DRASTIC) comparing medical therapy with percutaneous revascularization revealed only a decrease in antihypertension medications conferred by PTRA.[7] However, 44% of those assigned to medical therapy crossed over to revascularization because of medical failure.[7]

3. Surgical options include aortorenal bypass surgery and extraanatomic bypass (bypass from mesenteric or celiac artery rather than aorta). Surgical intervention has largely been replaced by PTRA.

II. RENAL ARTERY FMD

67

A. EPIDEMIOLOGY

1. FMD is a noninflammatory and nonatherosclerotic lesion that generally affects women aged 15 to 50.[8] Of patients with FMD, about 60% to 75% have renal involvement, 25% to 30% have extracranial cerebrovascular involvement, and 28% have involvement of more than one vascular bed.[8] Unlike atherosclerotic disease, FMD usually involves the middle to distal portions of the renal artery.[8] Medial fibroplasia is the most common dysplastic lesion. Other forms of FMD, named based on the anatomic involvement, together make up less than 12% of FMD and include medial hyperplasia, intimal fibroplasia, and adventitial hyperplasia.

2. Although cigarette smoking and genetic factors are associated with higher risk of FMD, the exact mechanisms have yet to be elucidated.[10]

B. PRESENTATION

1. Presentation is similar to that caused by renal artery atherosclerosis.

2. Disease progression, the development of a new lesion, worsening stenosis, or enlargement of an aneurysm occurs in 37% of patients with renal FMD.[6] There is often an associated reduction in renal size, but impaired excretory function leading to renal failure is very rare.

C. DIAGNOSIS

The diagnosis is made radiographically. Classically, it looks like a string of beads when medial fibroplasia is present.[11]

D. MANAGEMENT

1. Percutaneous transluminal angioplasty without stent placement has emerged as the modality of choice for revascularization.[8] If necessary, stents or surgery can be used, although angioplasty alone is associated with only a 10% risk of restenosis.[9] The rate of hypertension "cure," defined as no antihypertensive medications needed to maintain a blood pressure less than 140/90, is 60% after revascularization of FMD, compared with less than 30% for atherosclerotic renal artery stenosis.[10]

2. Because of the high cure rate offered by angioplasty, some advocate it for all young patients with FMD and renovascular hypertension. Good responses are particularly noted in the population younger than 50

RENOVASCULAR HYPERTENSION

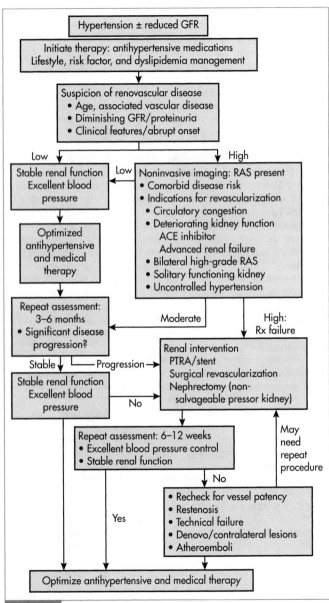

Hypertension ± reduced GFR

Initiate therapy: antihypertensive medications
Lifestyle, risk factor, and dyslipidemia management

Suspicion of renovascular disease
• Age, associated vascular disease
• Diminishing GFR/proteinuria
• Clinical features/abrupt onset

Low → Stable renal function
Excellent blood pressure

High → Noninvasive imaging: RAS present
• Comorbid disease risk
• Indications for revascularization
  • Circulatory congestion
  • Deteriorating kidney function
    ACE inhibitor
    Advanced renal failure
• Bilateral high-grade RAS
• Solitary functioning kidney
• Uncontrolled hypertension

Low →

Optimized antihypertensive and medical therapy

Repeat assessment: 3–6 months
• Significant disease progression?

Moderate →

High: Rx failure →

Stable → Stable renal function
Excellent blood pressure

Progression →

Renal intervention
PTRA/stent
Surgical revascularization
Nephrectomy (non-salvageable pressor kidney)

No →

Repeat assessment: 6–12 weeks
• Excellent blood pressure control
• Stable renal function

May need repeat procedure

No →

• Recheck for vessel patency
• Restenosis
• Technical failure
• Denovo/contralateral lesions
• Atheroemboli

Yes →

Optimize antihypertensive and medical therapy

FIG. 67-1

See legend on the opposite page

years old, without coronary or carotid stenosis, and with hypertension for less than 8 years.[9]

III. DIAGNOSTIC IMAGING

1. **Renal angiography.** The gold standard for diagnosis is renal arteriography. Advancements in technology are improving the sensitivity and specificity of many less invasive imaging modalities. In the near future, magnetic resonance angiography (MRA), duplex ultrasound, and spiral computed tomography (CT) with angiography may supplant renal arteriography.

2. **MRA.** For evaluation of the main renal arteries, studies have shown a sensitivity of 100% and a specificity ranging from 70% to 96%.[11] This diagnostic test is less useful in accessory renal arteries, although breath-hold MRA with gadopentetate dimeglumine promises to improve evaluation.[12]

3. **Spiral CT with angiography.** This diagnostic test uses intravenous contrast injection (unlike the riskier intraarterial injection of arteriography) in concert with spiral CT. The sensitivity and specificity of spiral CT and angiography are 98% and 94%, respectively, unless the creatinine exceeds 1.7 mg/dl.[13] With renal insufficiency, the sensitivity drops to 93% and specificity to 81% because of reduced blood flow.[13]

4. **Duplex ultrasound.** This modality allows both visualization of the arteries and measurement of the velocity of flow, which increases with the degree of stenosis. For patients with a high pretest probability, the positive predictive value is 99% and the negative predictive value is 97% compared with arteriography.[14] Duplex ultrasound can also be used to calculate a resistance index that predicts success after angioplasty.[15] Disadvantages include technical difficulty and interoperator variability.[14]

5. ACE-inhibitor–stimulated renography and renin measurements have also been used in the past as diagnostic modalities but have now been largely supplanted by the above imaging studies.

PEARLS AND PITFALLS

- Complications of renal artery angioplasty include contrast-induced renal failure and atheroemboli. Associated findings of atheroemboli include eosinophilia, eosinophiluria, and hypocomplementemia.
- FMD is associated with spontaneous carotid dissection.

67

RENOVASCULAR HYPERTENSION

Management algorithm. *ACE,* angiotensin-converting enzyme; *GFR,* glomerular filtration rate; *PTRA,* percutaneous transluminal renal angioplasty; *RAS,* renal artery stenosis; *Rx,* medication. (*Modified from Textor SC: Renovascular hypertension and ischemic nephropathy. In Brenner BM, ed:* The kidney, *7th ed, St Louis, 2004, WB Saunders.*)

- Angiography remains the gold standard for diagnosis of renovascular disease, but MRA and spiral CT with angiography have great utility as noninvasive screening tests.
- Realistic goals for revascularization include reduction in antihypertensive medication needs and stabilization of renal function.[5]
- Predictors of good outcomes after revascularization include young age, recent deterioration of renal function, or recent progression of hypertension.[5] Predictors of poor renal function after PTRA with endovascular stenting include resistance index greater than 80 on Doppler ultrasonography,[15] creatinine > 3 mg/dl,[16] and kidney size less than 8 cm.[17]

REFERENCES

1. Kaplan NM, Rose BR: Screening for renovascular hypertension, *UpToDate,* January 13, 2004. D
2. Safian RD, Textor SC: Renal-artery stenosis, *N Engl J Med* 344:431, 2001. C
3. Lewin A, Blaufox MD, Castle H, et al: Apparent prevalence of curable hypertension in the Hypertension Detection and Follow-up Program, *Arch Intern Med* 145:424-427, 1985. B
4. Working Group on Renovascular Hypertension: Detection, evaluation and treatment of renovascular hypertension: final report, *Arch Intern Med* 147:820-829, 1987. D
5. Textor SC: Renovascular hypertension and ischemic nephropathy. In Brenner BM, ed: *The kidney,* 7th ed, St Louis, 2004, WB Saunders. D
6. Schreiber MJ, Pohl MA, Novick AC: The natural history of atherosclerotic and fibrous renal artery disease, *Urol Clin North Am* 11:383-392, 1984. B
7. van Jaarsveld BC, Krijnen P, Pieterman H, et al: The effect of balloon angioplasty on hypertension in atherosclerotic renal-artery stenosis, *N Engl J Med* 342:1007-1014, 2000. A
8. Slovut DP, Olin JW: Fibromuscular dysplasia, *N Engl J Med* 1862-1871, 2004. C
9. Tegtmeyer CJ, Selby JB, Hartwell GD, et al: Results and complications of angioplasty in fibromuscular disease, *Circulation* 83(suppl):I155-I161, 1991. B
10. Novick AC, Ziegelbaum M, Vidt DG, et al: Trends in surgical revascularization for renal artery disease: ten years' experience, *JAMA* 257:498-501, 1987. C
11. Postma CT, Joosten FB, Rosenbusch G, Thien T: Magnetic resonance angiography has a high reliability in the detection of renal artery stenosis, *Am J Hypertens* 10:957, 1997. B
12. de Haan MW, Kouwenhoven M, Thelissen GRP, et al: Renovascular disease in patients with hypertension: detection with systolic and diastolic gating in three-dimensional, phase-contrast MR angiography, *Radiology* 198:449, 1996. B
13. Olbricht CJ, Paul K, Prokop M, et al: Minimally invasive diagnosis of renal artery stenosis by spiral computed tomography angiography, *Kidney Int* 48:1332, 1995. B
14. Olin JW, Piedmonte MR, Young JR, et al: The utility of duplex ultrasound scanning of the renal arteries for diagnosing significant renal artery stenosis, *Ann Intern Med* 122:833, 1995. B
15. Radermacher J, Chavan A, Bleck J, et al: Use of Doppler ultrasonography to predict the outcome of therapy for renal-artery stenosis, *N Engl J Med* 344:410, 2001. B

16. Hallett JW, Textor SC, Kos PB, et al: Advanced renovascular hypertension and renal insufficiency: trends in medical comorbidity and surgical approach from 1970 to 1993, *J Vasc Surg* 21:750-759, 1995. C
17. Lamawansa MD, Bell R, Kumar A, House AK: Radiological predictors of response to renovascular reconstructive surgery, *Ann R Coll Surg Engl* 77:337-341, 1995. B

Chronic Kidney Disease

Martin F. Britos, MD; and Mohamed G. Atta, MD

FAST FACTS

- Chronic kidney disease (CKD) is defined as the presence of structural or functional kidney damage for more than 3 months with or without a decrease in glomerular filtration rate (GFR) or a decreased GFR (< 60 ml/min/1.73 m^2) for 3 months or more, with or without kidney damage, irrespective of diagnosis.[1]
- Features of early CKD include hypertension, proteinuria, elevated blood urea nitrogen (BUN) and creatinine, nephrotic or nephritic syndrome, and gross hematuria.
- Evaluation of patients with suspected CKD includes estimation of GFR, risk stratification by CKD stage, assessment of structural and functional damage through imaging studies, examination of the urine sediment, and determination of the spot urine albumin/creatinine ratio.
- Management aims at identifying and treating the reversible causes of renal dysfunction, slowing the progression of renal damage, treating the complications of CKD, and preparing patients with end-stage renal disease (ESRD) for renal replacement therapy.
- All patients with GFR less than 30 ml/min/1.73 m^2 should be referred to a nephrologist.

I. EPIDEMIOLOGY AND ETIOLOGY[1]

1. The incidence and prevalence of ESRD have doubled in the past 10 years and are expected to continue to rise steadily. In the United States about 400,000 people have ESRD, of whom about 70% are treated with dialysis and about 30% with functioning kidney transplants. The annual mortality rate of patients on dialysis is greater than 20%.

2. CKD exists on a spectrum from asymptomatic renal dysfunction to ESRD. Ongoing nephron loss in CKD forces the surviving nephrons to adapt and enlarge. Solute handling and creatinine clearance markedly increase in the remaining nephrons in an attempt to maintain the whole kidney GFR and postpone uremia. Intraglomerular hypertension and glomerular hypertrophy lead to mesangial hyperproliferation and focal glomerulosclerosis (scarring) of nephrons, with consequent worsening in proteinuria and systemic hypertension. This ultimately leads to renal failure.

3. Adverse outcomes from CKD can be prevented or delayed through interventions during earlier stages of CKD, irrespective of the cause. Unfortunately, CKD is underdiagnosed and undertreated in the United States.

TABLE 68-1

PREVALENCE OF CKD IN PATIENTS WITH END-STAGE RENAL DISEASE

Underlying Disorder	Prevalence in Patients with End-Stage Renal Disease
Diabetic glomerulosclerosis	50%
Glomerular diseases	13%
Renovascular diseases	27%
Tubulointerstitial diseases	4%
Cystic diseases	6%

4. Table 68-1 classifies the etiology and prevalence of CKD in patients with ESRD.

II. CLINICAL PRESENTATION

1. Because patients are asymptomatic in the early stages of CKD, most patients do not come to medical attention until most of their kidney function has been lost.

2. Features of advanced CKD [(GFR < 15 ml/min/1.73m^2, BUN > 60 mg/dl) include fatigue, anorexia, nausea, morning vomiting, malnutrition, pruritus, bone pain, impotence, amenorrhea, epistaxis, easy bruising, myopathy, muscle twitching and cramps, nail changes, uremic frost on skin surfaces, pleurisy, pericarditis, edema, volume overload, lethargy, confusion, asterixis, peripheral neuropathy, seizures, and coma. Laboratory findings include normocytic anemia, hyperkalemia, hyperphosphatemia, and metabolic acidosis.

3. Hypertension and proteinuria are the most common features of CKD and are present at all stages of the disease. Hypertension is caused by NaCl retention and inappropriately high renin levels. Glomerular injury and dysfunction lead to proteinuria.

4. Progressive metabolic acidosis develops when renal ammoniagenesis fails and impairs tubular acid excretion. If untreated, metabolic acidosis leads to osteodystrophy (through bone buffering), skeletal muscle breakdown, and diminished albumin synthesis.

5. Hematologic abnormalities include anemia secondary to decreased erythropoietin production and shortened red cell survival; it is usually normocytic and normochromic. Uremic coagulopathy, caused by platelet abnormalities and abnormal factor VIII function, is characterized by a prolonged bleeding time with normal prothrombin and partial thromboplastin times and platelet counts.

6. Gastrointestinal bleeding may occur secondary to platelet dysfunction and diffuse mucosal erosions through the gut.

7. Uremia leads to impaired capillary permeability, fluid accumulation, and uremic serositis, a syndrome characterized by pericarditis, pleural effusions, and ascites.

8. Renal osteodystrophy results from secondary hyperparathyroidism (caused by hyperphosphatemia and hypocalcemia, marked parathyroid

68

CHRONIC KIDNEY DISEASE

hypertrophy, and bony resistance to the action of parathyroid hormone) and metabolic acidosis. The principal types of bone disease in CKD are osteitis fibrosis (resulting mainly from secondary hyperparathyroidism) and adynamic bone disease (resulting from oversuppression of parathyroid hormone).

9. Urinary tract symptoms (dysuria, frequency, polyuria) are unusual, although occasionally patients with tubulointerstitial disorders may have polyuria and nocturia caused by impaired renal concentrating ability (see Chapter 66).

10. Patients with progressive glomerular or tubulointerstitial disorders caused by systemic disease may have particular clinical presentations depending on the underlying disorders (see Chapters 65 and 66).

11. Malnutrition is common and is caused primarily by a lowered caloric intake (mainly due to anorexia), a decrease in intestinal absorption and digestion, and metabolic acidosis.

III. DIAGNOSIS

In 1999 the National Kidney Foundation introduced a set of guidelines for evaluating, classifying, stratifying, and treating patients with CKD. These guidelines, called the Kidney Disease Outcomes Quality Initiative (K/DOQI), have become the standard of care for this patient population. The salient points of the practice guidelines for evaluation and classification are summarized in this section.

A. EVALUATION[1]

1. As part of all routine health encounters, all patients should be assessed for susceptibility factors (older age, family history), initiation factors (diabetes, high blood pressure, autoimmune diseases, urinary tract infections, urinary stones, lower urinary tract obstruction, drug toxicity), and progression factors (higher degrees of proteinuria, poor blood pressure control, poor glycemic control, and smoking) for CKD.

2. Patients with the aforementioned risk factors should undergo periodic evaluation for evidence of renal injury and an estimation of GFR.

3. Evaluation should aim to determine the patient's diagnosis (type of kidney disease), comorbid conditions, severity (assessed by GFR), complications related to CKD, risk of disease progression, and risk of cardiovascular disease.

4. All patients with CKD should be assigned to a particular CKD stage on the basis of their estimated GFR. Stratification by GFR should occur irrespective of diagnosis (Table 68-2) and will dictate the goals of management and clinical plan of action for that patient.

5. All patients with CKD with a GFR less than 30 ml/min/1.73 m^2 should be referred to a nephrologist in order to prepare for renal replacement therapy.

B. ESTIMATION OF GFR[1]

1. Estimates of GFR are the best overall indexes of kidney function. The serum creatinine concentration alone should not be used to assess the level of kidney function.

TABLE 68-2

NATIONAL KIDNEY FOUNDATION STAGES OF CHRONIC KIDNEY DISEASE

Stage	Description	GFR (ml/min/1.73 m²)	Action
1	Kidney damage with normal or ↑ GFR	≥ 90	Diagnose and treat
			Treat comorbid conditions
			Slow progression
			Reduce cardiovascular disease risk
2	Kidney damage with mild ↓ GFR	60-89	Estimate progression
3	Moderate ↓ GFR	30-59	Evaluate and treat complications
4	Severe ↓ GFR	15-29	Prepare for kidney replacement therapy
5	Kidney failure	< 15 (or dialysis)	Replacement therapy

GFR, glomerular filtration rate.

2. In adults, the GFR should be estimated by using equations that estimate the GFR based on the serum creatinine, such as the Modification of Diet in Renal Disease (MDRD) Study or Cockcroft-Gault equations (available at www.kdoqi.org).

3. Equations that use the serum creatinine to estimate GFR rely on a steady state of creatinine production and clearance. Therefore, estimates will be unreliable if the GFR is changing or if the muscle mass or dietary creatine intake is unusually high or low.

4. Measuring creatinine clearance using timed (e.g., 24-hour) urine collections does not improve the estimate of GFR over that provided by the prediction equations (MDRD, Cockcroft-Gault) but may be useful in estimating the GFR in patients with exceptional dietary intake (vegetarians, creatine supplements) or decreased muscle mass (amputation, malnutrition, muscle wasting).

5. All four variants of the MDRD equation perform similarly and consistently better than the Cockcroft-Gault equation, which overestimates GFR by up to 23%.[2]

C. ASSESSMENT OF PROTEINURIA[1]

1. Albuminuria and proteinuria are early and sensitive markers of kidney damage (Table 68-3).

2. When screening adults at elevated risk of CKD, albumin rather than total protein should be measured in a spot urine sample using either an albumin-specific dipstick or the albumin/creatinine ratio. Albumin is a more sensitive marker than total protein for CKD.

3. Patients with a positive dipstick test (1+ or greater) should undergo confirmation of albuminuria by a quantitative measurement (spot urine albumin/creatinine ratio) within 3 months. Two or more positive quantitative methods spaced by 1 to 2 weeks are diagnostic of persistent albuminuria.

4. Total spot urine protein/creatinine ratio is acceptable if the spot urine albumin/creatinine ratio is high (500 to 1000 mg/g).

TABLE 68-3

ASSESSMENT OF PROTEINURIA

	Urine Collection Method	Normal	Microalbuminuria	Albuminuria or Clinical Proteinuria
Total protein	24-hour excretion	< 300 mg/day	NA	> 300 mg/day
	Spot urine protein/ creatinine ratio	< 200 mg/g	NA	> 200 mg/g
Albumin	24-hour excretion	< 30 mg/day	30-300 mg/day	> 300 mg/day
	Spot albumin-specific dipstick	< 3 mg/dl	> 3 mg/dl	NA
	Spot urine albumin/ creatinine ratio*	< 17 mg/g (men) < 25 mg/g (women)	17-250 mg/g (men) 25-355 mg/g (women)	> 250 mg/g (men) > 355 mg/g (women)

*Current recommendations from the American Diabetes Association define cutoff values for spot urine albumin/creatinine ratio for microalbuminuria and albuminuria as 30 mg/g and 300 mg/g, respectively, without regard to sex.

D. MARKERS OF CKD OTHER THAN PROTEINURIA[1]

1. Markers of kidney damage other than proteinuria include abnormalities in the urine sediment and abnormalities on imaging studies.
2. Urine sediment examination or dipstick for red blood cells and white blood cells should be performed in all patients with CKD or in patients at risk for CKD (see Chapter 63).
3. Imaging of the kidneys should be performed in all patients with CKD to evaluate for structural abnormalities, impaired renal blood flow, and urinary obstruction. Imaging should begin with renal ultrasonography but may also include computed tomography or magnetic resonance imaging. Computed tomography has largely supplanted intravenous pyelography.

IV. MANAGEMENT

A. TREATING REVERSIBLE CAUSES OF RENAL DYSFUNCTION

Patients with CKD with a recent decrease in GFR may be suffering from a reversible process in addition to their underlying primary renal disorder, such as decreased renal perfusion. See Chapter 67 for additional discussion.

B. SLOWING THE RATE OF PROGRESSION

Further renal injury may result from secondary factors that are unrelated to the initial disease.

1. There is clear evidence that in diabetic and nondiabetic renal disease, the administration of angiotensin-converting enzyme inhibitors or angiotensin

II receptor blockers slows the progression of CKD. The benefit is greatest when these medications are initiated early in the course of the disease and in patients with higher degrees of proteinuria.[3]

2. Aggressive control of proteinuria and blood pressure as recommended by both the Joint National Committee on Prevention, Detection, Evaluation, and Treatment of High Blood Pressure and K/DOQI[4,5]:

a. Angiotensin-converting enzyme inhibitors and angiotensin II receptor blockers are recommended as first-line agents for treating hypertension and proteinuria. Goal blood pressure is less than 125/75 mmHg (even lower systolic pressures in patients with spot protein/creatinine ratios greater than 1000 mg/g),[3] and the goal protein excretion is less than 1000 mg/day or at least 60% of baseline values.

b. If blood pressure goals are not met, a calcium channel blocker or a beta-blocker should be added.

c. If the proteinuria goal is not reached after the blood pressure goals are met, an angiotensin-converting enzyme inhibitor or an angiotensin II receptor blocker should be added (whichever was not used initially).

3. Hyperlipidemia and metabolic acidosis should be treated because there is evidence that they may promote progression of CKD.

C. TREATING THE COMPLICATIONS OF CKD

1. **Anemia.**[6] All patients with GFR less than 60 ml/min/1.73 m^2 should be evaluated for anemia (see Chapter 41 for evaluation). Patients on hemodialysis lose an average of 2 g of iron per year. Iron deficiency develops in all patients receiving erythropoietic agents unless supplemental iron is given.

a. An erythropoietic agent should be given to patients with hemoglobin concentrations less than 11 g/dl (target hemoglobin is 11 to 12 g/dl).

b. Adequate iron stores should be confirmed before erythropoietic agents are started. Supplemental iron therapy (oral or parenteral) should be used to keep transferrin saturation greater than 20% and serum ferritin level greater than 100 ng/ml). Most patients eventually need parenteral iron (sodium ferric gluconate) to maintain these goals. This is especially true if the transferrin saturation is less than 20%.

2. **Dyslipidemia.** CKD is considered a coronary artery disease equivalent. On the basis of data from trials, some experts suggest reducing low-density lipoprotein cholesterol to less than 80 mg/dl.[7]

3. **Hyperkalemia.** See Chapter 74 for management.

4. **Hyperphosphatemia.**

a. K/DOQI guidelines recommend that the calcium phosphate should not exceed 55 in patients with stage 3 to 5 CKD. Measurement of serum calcium and phosphate in patients with CKD stages 3, 4, and 5 should be done every year, 3 months, and 1 month, respectively.

b. In patients with stage 5 CKD who remain hyperphosphatemic (serum phosphate > 5.5 mg/dl) despite use of either calcium-based or non–calcium-based phosphate binding agents, a combination of both should be used (see Supplemental PDA Chapter 10).

5. **Hypertension.** See Chapter 67.
6. **Malnutrition.**
a. Body weight and serum albumin should be checked periodically.
b. Diets should provide 30 to 35 kcal/kg/day.
c. For patients with CKD, protein intake should be limited to 0.8 to 1.0 g/kg/day. Conversely, patients on hemodialysis should not be protein restricted.
d. Water-soluble (B complex) vitamins are lost with dialysis and should be supplemented on a daily basis.
7. **Metabolic acidosis.**
a. If untreated, CKD-associated metabolic acidosis usually results in serum bicarbonate levels of 12 to 20 mEq/L (rarely falling below 10 mEq/L).
b. Serum bicarbonate should be kept above 22 mEq/L with sodium bicarbonate (0.5 to 1 mEq/kg/day). If this is not tolerated because of bloating, sodium citrate can be used if the patient strictly avoids aluminum-containing antacids (there is increased intestinal absorption of aluminum when sodium citrate is administered, and this may lead to aluminum toxicity).
8. **Renal osteodystrophy.**[8]
a. Treatment of metabolic acidosis is crucial in order to prevent bone resorption.
b. Prevention in predialysis patients consists mainly of dietary phosphate restriction and oral phosphate binders. Later stages of CKD require the administration of calcitriol or vitamin D analogs to directly suppress the secretion of parathyroid hormone.
c. Serum 25(OH)-vitamin D should be greater than 30 ng/ml; otherwise, the patient should receive supplemental oral vitamin D.
d. For patients with CKD stage 3, the serum intact parathyroid hormone (PTH) should be checked every year; in stages 4 and 5 it should be checked every 3 months.
e. Target serum levels of intact PTH:
(1) 35 to 70 pg/ml for stage 3 CKD
(2) 70 to 110 pg/ml for stage 4 CKD
(3) 150 to 300 pg/ml for stage 5 CKD

D. PREPARING FOR RENAL REPLACEMENT THERAPY
All patients with GFR less than 30 ml/min/1.73 m^2 should be referred to a nephrologist for specialized care and for preparation and education in anticipation of dialysis (see Chapter 69).

PEARLS AND PITFALLS
- The uremic syndrome is rare with BUN less than 60 mg/dl. It occurs more commonly but not invariably when the BUN is greater than 100 mg/dl. With severe protein restriction or muscle wasting, the uremic syndrome may occur at lower BUN levels.
- Urea itself is nontoxic but is a good surrogate measure of the toxicity of the end products of protein metabolism.

- Other cardiovascular risk factors secondary to CKD include high PTH levels, increased vascular and myocardial calcification (caused by an increase in the calcium phosphate product), left ventricular hypertrophy, dyslipidemia, hyperhomocysteinemia, and insulin resistance.
- Uremic patients should be regarded as immunocompromised because their neutrophil function and cellular immunity are impaired.
- There is increasing evidence that uremia and ESRD cause an increased systemic inflammatory state (elevated C-reactive protein levels, erythrocyte sedimentation rate, tumor necrosis factor-α, and interleukin-6) that may contribute to impaired protein metabolism, negative nitrogen balance, malnutrition, and atherosclerosis.
- Pruritus is a common complication caused in part by hyperparathyroidism and a high calcium phosphate product with increased microscopic calcifications of subcutaneous tissue.
- Platelet dysfunction responds to dialysis and infusion of desmopressin.
- As CKD progresses, diabetic patients often need less exogenous insulin because of a decrease in insulin degradation by renal insulinase. Nondiabetic patients may demonstrate uremic pseudodiabetes secondary to peripheral insulin resistance.
- On average, after the age of 30, creatinine clearance decreases by approximately 1 ml/min/1.73 m^2 per year (from a baseline of approximately 120 ml/min/1.73 m^2).

68

CHRONIC KIDNEY DISEASE

REFERENCES

1. NKF-K/DOQI clinical practice guidelines for chronic kidney disease: evaluation, classification and stratification, *Am J Kidney Dis* 39(Suppl 1): S1, 2002. D
2. Levey AS et al: A more accurate method to estimate glomerular filtration rate from serum creatinine: a new prediction equation. Modification of Diet in Renal Disease Study Group, *Ann Intern Med* 130:461-470, 1999. A
3. Jafar TH et al: Progression of chronic kidney disease: the role of blood pressure control, proteinuria, and angiotensin-converting enzyme inhibition: a patient meta-analysis, *Ann Intern Med* 139:244, 2003. C
4. Chobanian AV et al: The seventh report of the Joint National Committee on Prevention, Detection, Evaluation, and Treatment of High Blood Pressure: the JNC 7 report, *JAMA* 289(19):2560-2571, 2003. D
5. NKF-K/DOQI clinical practice guidelines on hypertension and antihypertensive agents in chronic kidney disease, *Am J Kidney Dis* 43:5(Suppl 1):S1, 2004. D
6. NKF-K/DOQI clinical practice guidelines for anemia of chronic disease: update 2000, *Am J Kidney Dis* 37:1(Suppl 1):S182-S238, 2001. D
7. Grundy SM et al: Implications of recent clinical trials for the National Cholesterol Education Program Adult Treatment Panel III guidelines, *Circulation* 110(2):227-239, 2004. C
8. K/DOQI clinical practice guidelines for bone metabolism and disease in chronic kidney disease, *Am J Kidney Dis* 42(Suppl 3):S1, 2003. D

Dialysis

Michelle Estrella, MD; Jennifer S. Myers, MD; and Paul Scheel, MD

FAST FACTS

- In chronic kidney disease, renal replacement therapy should be initiated when the glomerular filtration rate decreases to 15 ml/min, a stage at which patients are considered to have end-stage renal disease.[1]
- Common conditions in which hemodialysis (HD) is used in patients with or without end-stage renal disease include drug overdose, uremia, hyperkalemia, volume overload, and metabolic acidosis refractory to conservative treatment.
- Native arteriovenous fistulas are the preferred form of vascular access for patients undergoing long-term HD.

I. MODES OF DIALYSIS

A. HEMODIALYSIS

1. HD is the most common form of renal replacement therapy in the United States and is accomplished by the countercurrent flow of blood and dialysate over a dialysis membrane. HD with ultrafiltration (UF) serves three functions: removal of toxins, restoration of electrolyte and acid-base balance, and removal of excess volume.

a. The removal of solutes is accomplished by both diffusive and convective mechanisms.

b. Concentration gradients for calcium, potassium, and bicarbonate can be individualized to the patient's metabolic derangements by choosing the appropriate dialysate.

c. Ultrafiltration (movement of cell-free fluid from the blood side to dialysate side) occurs when a hydrostatic pressure gradient is established between the blood and dialysate compartments. The rate of UF can be adjusted by changing the transmembrane pressure across the dialyzer.

d. Drugs that can be removed by HD include ethanol, methanol, isopropanol, barbiturates, theophylline, lithium, salicylates, and atenolol.

2. Complications of HD.

a. Hypotension is the most common complication of HD and usually is caused by UF-related volume depletion, osmolar shifts, excess heat retention and consequent vasodilation from dialysate temperature, reflex sympathetic inhibition, autonomic neuropathy, sepsis, tamponade, and membrane reaction. Several different interventions can be used to manage UF-related volume depletion including slowing the UF rate, administering intravenous saline, sodium profiling (in which hypertonic sodium concentration is gradually decreased to an isotonic concentration during HD), and cooling the dialysate temperature to 34° C to 36° C.

b. Occasionally, a systemic reaction consisting of hypotension, nausea, shortness of breath, and chest pain can be caused by a reaction to the dialysis membrane. This first-use syndrome results from activation of the complement system and is more common with the use of cellulose membranes.

c. Hypersensitivity reactions can occur to either the ethylene oxide used to sterilize the dialyzer or to polyacrylonitrile, a synthetic membrane used in continuous renal replacement. Patients taking angiotensin-converting enzyme inhibitors (especially catopril) are particularly susceptible to the latter, given the ability of polyacrylonitrile to promote the formation of bradykinin.

d. Disequilibrium syndrome presents with nausea, vomiting, and headache but can evolve to seizures and coma. It is thought to result from cerebral edema, as plasma becomes hypotonic relative to brain cells during HD. The risk of this syndrome is minimized by limiting reduction of plasma urea nitrogen by only 30% during each HD session, and by avoiding low-sodium dialysate.

B. PERITONEAL DIALYSIS

1. Peritoneal dialysis (PD) is the preferred method of dialysis outside the United States. A plastic catheter is surgically tunneled under the skin and inserted into the peritoneal cavity. Dialysate is then infused into the peritoneum, where it is left to dwell for several hours. Solute transport takes place by diffusion across the peritoneal membrane and depends on the properties of the peritoneal membrane (e.g., surface area and permeability), dialysate flow, concentration gradients, and dwelling time. An osmotic gradient for UF is created by the addition of glucose to the dialysate.

2. Two thirds of patients use continuous ambulatory PD, in which the dialysate is exchanged four times each day. The other one third use automated PD, in which a mechanical cycler infuses and drains dialysate at night. The latter method allows the patient more freedom during the day and can be augmented, if necessary, with one or two daytime exchanges.

3. Complications: peritonitis.

a. The most serious complication of PD is peritonitis, which accounts for two thirds of PD catheter losses and one third of conversions to HD. It should be suspected when abdominal pain, fever, or a cloudy dialysate develops in a patient receiving PD. It is diagnosed by the presence of white blood cells (more than 100 cells/mm^3 with more than 50% polymorphonuclear cells) in the dialysate.

b. Sixty to seventy percent of peritonitis cases are caused by gram-positive cocci; the remaining cases are caused by gram-negative rods and fungi. Fungal peritonitis is a more difficult infection to clear and often necessitates catheter removal.

c. Empiric therapy generally consists of a first-generation cephalosporin and ceftazidime. Once culture data are available, antibiotic therapy may be tailored accordingly. Routes of administration are oral, intraperitoneal, or intravenous, according to the severity of the infection.

d. Recurrence of peritonitis with the same organism within 4 weeks of treatment indicates relapsing peritonitis. Relapse with *Staphylococcus* suggests catheter tunnel infection, whereas relapse with gram-negative organisms suggests an intraabdominal abscess.[2]

e. Exit site infections can be treated with local wound care and antibiotics. Failure to resolve the infection after prolonged treatment should prompt catheter removal.

f. Patients on PD who are *Staphylococcus aureus* nasal carriers should receive prophylactic mupirocin intranasally or topically to reduce the incidence of peritonitis and exit site infection.[2]

4. Noninfectious complications.

a. **Metabolic abnormalities.** Patients on PD lose 4 to 7 g of albumin per day. Glucose absorption leads to hyperglycemia, hypertriglyceridemia, and weight gain.[3]

b. **Abdominal wall hernia.** These develop in up to one fourth of all patients on PD and may lead to dialysate leakage into soft tissue and fascial planes.

c. **Hydrothorax.** This occurs when the dialysate moves across the diaphragm via lymphatics or through diaphragmatic defects. It usually presents within the first month of PD initiation, and the majority of cases occur in the right pleural space. Diagnosis is established by the presence of a transudative pleural effusion containing a high glucose concentration.

d. **Sclerosing encapsulating peritonitis.** This rare complication is characterized by thick-walled membranes enclosing the bowel loops. It presents with abdominal pain, nausea, vomiting, and bowel obstruction; patients have poor solute clearance and ultrafiltration. Sclerosing encapsulating peritonitis is associated with a 50% mortality rate despite medical and surgical intervention.[3]

C. **CONTINUOUS RENAL REPLACEMENT THERAPIES**

1. Continuous renal replacement therapy (CRRT), such as continuous venovenous hemodialysis (CVVHD), can be performed as dialysis (solute removal) or filtration (convection-based solute and water removal). Continuous hemodialysis uses dialysate that circulates through the circuit, thereby removing solutes primarily by diffusion. In contrast, continuous hemofiltration uses a large volume of replacement fluid that infuses into the inflow or outflow line, clearing solutes by convection. Continuous hemofiltration removes middle molecules more effectively than continuous hemodialysis. Continuous hemodialysis and continuous hemofiltration may be combined into one process, continuous hemodiafiltration. Slow continuous ultrafiltration simply removes fluid slowly without metabolic clearance.[4]

2. Continuous venovenous hemofiltration is the CRRT modality of choice because of its lower rates of complications and morbidity as compared with continuous arteriovenous hemofiltration.[5]
3. The major advantage of CRRT over traditional HD, which is conducted in 4- to 6-hour sessions, is its slower rate of volume removal, which is essential for hemodynamically unstable patients.
4. Indications.
a. CRRT is commonly used in critically ill patients because it provides greater hemodynamic stability and more effective control of electrolytes, volume, and acid-base status.
b. In patients with elevated intracranial pressure (acute brain injury, recent neurosurgery, intracranial infection, or fulminant hepatic failure), CRRT is preferred because it is not associated with decreased cerebral perfusion or increased cerebral edema, as is conventional intermittent HD.[6]
c. Slow continuous ultrafiltration has been used in a small number of patients with congestive heart failure refractory to fluid restriction and diuretics. In these patients, subsequent increased diuresis and responsiveness to diuretics were observed.[5]
d. Although CRRTs generally are not used for acute drug intoxications, they may be considered for drugs that have slow extracellular-intracellular equilibration, such as lithium.[5]

II. VASCULAR ACCESS
A. TYPES
1. Arteriovenous (AV) fistulas are the preferred forms of long-term vascular access not only because of their lower incidence of thrombosis and stenosis but also because of the lower risk of infection. These benefits outweigh the disadvantages of long maturation times (i.e., 1 to 4 months) and potential failure for the fistula to mature.
2. An AV graft constructed of polytetrafluoroethylene is the next preferred type of vascular access if a primary AV fistula cannot be established. The main advantages of this access type are large surface area for cannulation and short maturation time.
3. A tunneled cuffed venous catheter (e.g., Devol catheters) is the method of choice for temporary access needed for more than 3 weeks. The preferred site is the right internal jugular vein. The catheter should not be placed ipsilateral to the maturing AV fistula, and placement into the subclavian vein should be avoided. It may be used immediately and does not entail venipuncture; however, it is associated with higher rates of thrombosis and infection and carries the risk of permanent central venous stenosis or occlusion.[7]
4. Noncuffed tunneled catheters (e.g., Shiley catheters) are used when immediate vascular access is necessary. They are generally inserted into the internal jugular or femoral vein.

69

DIALYSIS

B. COMPLICATIONS

1. Limb ischemia.

a. Limb ischemia distal to an AV access can occur a few hours to several months after access placement. Patients at highest risk are older adults, those with diabetes mellitus, or those with multiple attempts at access in the same limb.

b. Mild ischemia presents with cold sensation and paresthesia along the effected limb. It is treated symptomatically; however, these patients should undergo frequent examination. Severe ischemia is considered a surgical emergency.[7]

2. Stenosis, thrombosis, and pseudoaneurysms.

a. A hemodynamically significant graft stenosis (greater than 50%) manifests itself as elevated venous dialysis pressures, decreased blood flow, increased recirculation, and extremity edema. Stenosis predisposes to graft thrombosis, which shortens long-term graft patency even after repair by angioplasty.

b. In patients with thrombosed AV access, thrombectomy or thrombolysis may be performed; however, thrombosed AV accesses have low treatment success rates.

c. With time patients develop pseudoaneurysms and subsequently delayed hemostasis with needle removal. These can ultimately result in graft or fistula rupture, which is a surgical emergency.[7]

3. Central vein stenosis.

a. Central vein stenosis develops in patients with previous arm, neck, and chest surgery or trauma or multiple subclavian access placements and typically manifests itself as upper extremity edema, pain, and tortuous superficial veins.

b. Percutaneous angioplasty is the preferred treatment. Stent placement is considered in patients with restenosis within 3 months of angioplasty.[7]

4. Access-related infection.

a. AV fistula infections are rare and are treated with 6 weeks of antibiotics.

b. AV graft infections.

   (1) Typically, AV graft infections present with pain, erythema, warmth, and skin breakdown along the AV graft. They are treated with 3 to 4 weeks of antibiotics and partial or total surgical resection. Initial antibiotic treatment should cover gram-positive organisms (including *Enterococcus*) and gram-negative organisms.[7]

   (2) Old clotted AV grafts may harbor silent infections in patients with fever or bacteremia and no other obvious sources. A white blood cell scan may be helpful in making the diagnosis.

c. Catheters.

   (1) Patients with diabetes mellitus and poor hygiene are at high risk for exit site infections, which can be treated with topical antibiotics. If tunnel drainage is present, the catheter should be removed and parenteral antibiotics administered. The new catheter should be placed at a different site.[8]

(2) Because catheter-related bacteremia usually is caused by either staphylococcal species or gram-negative organisms, empiric antibiotics should cover both gram-positive and gram-negative microbes. The catheter should be removed if the patient is clinically unstable.

PEARLS AND PITFALLS

- Physical examination of AV grafts is a highly sensitive screening test for identifying grafts with low flows at risk for occlusion. The presence of a thrill at three sites (the arterial, midpoint, and venous portions of the AV graft) correlates with blood flow volumes greater than 450 ml/min.[9]
- Unlike in HD, phosphate is efficiently cleared by continuous venovenous hemofiltration and should be checked regularly in patients undergoing CRRT.
- Approximately 30% of patients with end-stage renal disease on HD have an elevated troponin level, which may be a marker for higher mortality.[10]
- Because residual renal function is critical to the successful clearance of toxins in patients on PD, great care should be taken not to prescribe nephrotoxic medications to these patients.

69

DIALYSIS

REFERENCES

1. NKF-K/DOQI: Clinical practice guidelines for chronic kidney disease, Am J Kidney Dis 39(suppl 1), 2002. D
2. Keane WF: Adult peritoneal dialysis related peritonitis treatment recommendations: update 2000, Perit Dial Int 20:396-430, 2000. D
3. Teitelbaum I, Burkart J: Peritoneal dialysis, Am J Kidney Dis 42:1082-1096, 2003. D
4. Daugirda JT, Blake PG, Ing TS: Handbook of dialysis, 3rd ed, Philadelphia, 2001, Lippincott, Williams & Wilkins. D
5. Manns M, Sigler MH, Teehan BP: Continuous renal replacement therapies: an update, Am J Kidney Dis 32:185, 1998. C
6. Davenport A: Renal replacement therapy in the patient with acute brain injury, Am J Kidney Dis 37:457-466, 2001. C
7. NKF-K/DOQI: Clinical practice guidelines for vascular access, Am J Kidney Dis 37:S137-S181, 2001. D
8. Nassar GM, Ayus JC: Infectious complications of the hemodialysis access, Kidney Int 60:1-13, 2001. C
9. Trerotola SO, Scheel PJ Jr, Powe NR, et al: Screening for dialysis access graft malfunction: comparison of physical examination with US, J Vasc Interv Radiol 7(1):15-20, 1996. B
10. Dierkes J, Domrose U, Westphal S, et al: Cardiac troponin T predicts mortality in patients with end-stage renal disease, Circulation 102(16):1964-1969, 2000. B

Acute Renal Colic

John A. Dooley, MD; and Michael J. Choi, MD

> **FAST FACTS**
>
> - *Nephrolithiasis, urolithiasis, urinary tract stones,* and *kidney stones* are synonymous terms for the crystallization of solutes from urine. Acute renal colic is the painful episode that results from movement of the stone through the urinary tract.
> - Noncontrast helical computed tomography (CT) is the gold standard for diagnosis.
> - Indications for urgent intervention are acute renal failure, high-grade obstruction of a single or transplanted kidney, concurrent urinary tract infection with obstruction, and intractable symptoms.
> - In the absence of indications for urgent intervention, initial management consists of supportive care.
> - Stones smaller than 5 mm are likely to pass spontaneously; these patients can be followed for stone passage as outpatients. Stones larger than 5 mm usually warrant elective removal.

I. EPIDEMIOLOGY AND ETIOLOGY[1,2]

1. Renal stones have a lifetime incidence of about 12%. They occur most often in 20- to 40-year-old men, and women are affected somewhat less often. Rates are higher in whites than in blacks. A family history of renal stones is present in 55% of cases.
2. Half of patients with calcium stones suffer additional episodes. White, middle-aged men with a positive family history are at elevated risk, as are patients with malabsorption, chronic diarrhea, gout, and those who needed a procedure to remove a previous stone. Patients with uric acid, cystine, and struvite stones also are at high risk for recurrence.
3. Table 70-1 lists the common types of stones and the disorders associated with each. Most stones contain calcium and are associated with hypercalciuria (urinary excretion > 300 mg/day in men, > 250 mg/day in women). Stones often are composed of mixtures of minerals and are associated with multiple underlying biochemical abnormalities.
4. Indinavir, an antiretroviral drug, can crystallize in the urine to form stones.
5. Inadequate fluid intake leads to a low volume of urine supersaturated with stone-forming compounds. Volume depletion explains why nephrolithiasis is more common in warm climates.

70

TABLE 70-1
TYPES OF RENAL STONES

Type of Stone (composition)	Frequency[3,4] (% of all stones)	Radiopaque by Plain Film Radiography?	Pathophysiology and Associated Conditions[5,6]
Calcium (calcium oxalate or calcium phosphate)	~80%	Yes	Hypercalciuria (32-59%), hyperuricosuria (16-36%), hyperoxaluria (5-25%), hypocitraturia (22-44%), primary hyperparathyroidism (2-5%), type I renal tubular acidosis (1-10%), and sarcoidosis. Low fluid intake (23%) and diet high in animal protein or sodium are commonly implicated as well.
Uric acid	~10%	No (when pure)	Crystallization is promoted by hyperuricosuria, low urine volumes, and urine pH < 5.5. Associated conditions include gout (20%), myeloproliferative diseases, and chronic diarrhea.
Struvite (magnesium-ammonium-phosphate)	~10%	No	Chronic or recurrent urinary tract infection by urease-producing bacteria (59%).*
Cystine	~1%	No	Cystinuria, an autosomal recessive disorder of excessive urinary cystine excretion (100%).

*These include *Proteus, Pseudomonas, Providencia, Klebsiella, Staphylococci,* and *Mycoplasma. Escherichia coli* does not produce urease and therefore is not responsible for struvite stones.

ACUTE RENAL COLIC

II. PRESENTATION

1. Classic symptoms include severe flank pain, developing over the course of minutes to hours, and hematuria. As the stone moves into the lower third of the ureter, referred pain may migrate to the groin and genitalia. Intermittent ureteral spasm around the stone may cause colic. Stones that lodge in the intramural segment of the ureter cause irritative bladder symptoms such as dysuria, urgency, and urinary frequency. Nausea and vomiting may occur. Renal colic does not induce peritoneal signs.

2. Stones can be asymptomatic, usually discovered incidentally on radiographs. Nephrolithiasis is also a cause of isolated hematuria.

III. DIAGNOSIS

1. The following should be performed in all patients in whom nephrolithiasis is suspected: full history and physical, with careful attention to urine output and evidence of infection; serum electrolytes, creatinine, calcium, and uric acid; and urinalysis with microscopy.

2. Although hematuria is a classic finding, in isolation it is unreliable for diagnosis. One study of patients with acute flank pain found that hematuria (> one red blood cell per high-power field) had a sensitivity of 86% and specificity of 29% for acute renal colic. Therefore, a normal urinalysis cannot exclude nephrolithiasis.[7]

3. Clinical features may suggest the diagnosis but do not obviate confirmatory imaging. In one study of adults with acute abdominal pain, a diagnostic score factoring in hematuria, normal appetite, duration of pain less than 12 hours, and renal or loin tenderness yielded a sensitivity of 89% and specificity of 99% for acute renal colic.[8]

4. Radiographic studies.

a. As a single test, noncontrast helical CT scan is the gold standard. It has a high sensitivity (98%) and specificity (98%) in patients with acute flank pain.[9] CT is also likely to suggest an alternative diagnosis when no stone is seen. Contrast may be necessary to diagnose indinavir stones, which are not readily seen on noncontrast CT.

b. Conventional intravenous pyelogram (IVP) is fairly accurate but is more timeconsuming than CT and exposes patients to the risks of intravenous contrast. IVP is the diagnostic test of choice for medullary sponge kidney, an anatomic abnormality associated with calcium stone formation. A direct comparison of CT and IVP in 106 patients who underwent both studies found that CT had a sensitivity of 96% and specificity of 100%, whereas IVP was only 87% sensitive and 94% specific.[10] Noncontrast helical CT is comparable to IVP for the diagnosis of obstruction.[11]

c. Plain radiography alone is insensitive. Compared with IVP or stone retrieval, plain films had a sensitivity of only 58% and specificity of 69%.[12] If the stone is visible, serial plain films—rather than CT—are

sufficient to follow the stone's passage. Radiolucency on plain film can help predict stone composition (see Table 70-1).
d. Ultrasonography is specific but poorly sensitive for nephrolithiasis. It is an excellent test for hydronephrosis when other studies are inconclusive. Its utility for renal colic generally is limited to pregnant women, in whom avoidance of radiation is especially desirable.
5. The differential diagnosis is broad and includes retroperitoneal bleeding, ectopic pregnancy, pyelonephritis, and many other causes of abdominal, flank, and back pain.

IV. RISK STRATIFICATION AND PROGNOSIS
1. The major complications from renal stones are loss of renal function and sepsis. Early urologic intervention to relieve obstruction can prevent or reverse these sequelae. Therefore, the critical step in risk stratification is to identify patients at risk for sepsis or renal insufficiency.
2. See Fig. 70-1 for an approach to risk stratifying and managing renal colic.

V. MANAGEMENT
A. SHORT-TERM MANAGEMENT AND TREATMENT
1. Nonsteroidal antiinflammatory drugs (NSAIDs) are first-line agents for analgesia. In addition to providing effective pain relief, these agents reduce ureteral edema and spasm. At typical dosages, NSAIDs are not likely to cause renal impairment unless there is significant obstruction or preexisting renal dysfunction. In clinical trials, NSAIDs have proven equivalent or superior to narcotics for pain relief, but the latter are necessary when NSAIDs are inadequate or contraindicated.[13]
2. Intravenous hydration is not generally warranted in patients without volume depletion. Overhydration may induce diuresis, worsening ureteral spasm and pain.
3. Treat concomitant urinary tract infections aggressively with broad-spectrum antibiotics. Struvite stones should be removed promptly.
4. Uric acid stones are unique in their tendency to dissolve readily in alkaline urine. Treat with potassium citrate, up to 80 mEq/day in two or three divided doses. The patient should monitor his or her urine pH to ensure that it is 6.5 at some point during the day. If the stone persists on imaging repeated after a month of medical therapy, refer for intervention.
5. Patients with stones judged unlikely to pass spontaneously should be referred promptly for stone extraction, usually with lithotripsy or ureteroscopy. The choice of procedure is best left to the urologist, but ureteroscopy is generally preferred for proximal ureteral stones larger than 1 cm. Smaller proximal stones are better treated with lithotripsy. The two approaches have similar success rates for distal stones (those beyond the iliac vessels).[14]

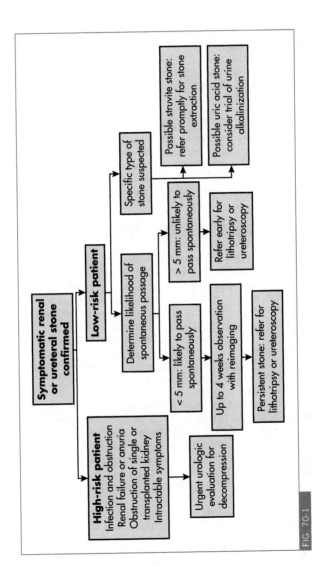

FIG. 70-1

Management of acute renal colic.

6. For stones smaller than 5 mm, expectant observation with repeated imaging in 4 weeks is appropriate. If the stone has not moved after 4 weeks, the likelihood of complications increases (particularly if the patient remains symptomatic), and the patient should be referred to a urologist for possible intervention.

B. LONG-TERM MANAGEMENT

1. The priority in long-term management is to identify the cause of the patient's stones. Patients should strain their urine until the stone has passed and submit recovered fragments for composition analysis. The composition of noncalcium stones correlates well with underlying metabolic abnormalities.[6]

2. The timing of metabolic assessment is controversial; some experts advocate evaluating all patients with a first calcium stone, whereas others reserve evaluation for patients at high risk for recurrence.

3. In addition to the studies obtained at initial diagnosis, metabolic stone evaluation includes a 24-hour urine collection for volume, pH, calcium, oxalate, uric acid, phosphate, sodium, citrate, creatinine, and sulfate or urea nitrogen (markers of animal protein intake). Experts generally recommend deferring the urine collection until at least 3 weeks after stone passage to minimize the risk that urinary tract inflammation may influence the results.[1]

4. The long-term management goal is to prevent recurrence (Table 70-2). Repeat a 24-hour urine collection 1 to 2 months after dietary or medical intervention to assess the response to therapy.

5. Note that dietary calcium restriction usually is ineffective therapy for hypercalciuria and may lead to bone demineralization. Therefore, calcium restriction should not be routinely prescribed.

6. Patients with asymptomatic stones have a 50% chance of developing symptoms over 5 years. The ideal management strategy for these patients depends on an individual risk assessment.

PEARLS AND PITFALLS

- Common names for the minerals that form stones are as follows: whewellite is calcium oxalate monohydrate, weddellite is calcium oxalate dihydrate, and apatite and brushite are two forms of calcium phosphate.
- The absence of hematuria does not exclude the diagnosis of acute renal colic.
- Hyperoxaluria results from increased intestinal absorption of oxalate in a variety of disorders. In the case of fat malabsorption, for example, fatty acids precipitate with calcium in the ileal lumen. Because less calcium is available to complex oxalate, the latter is absorbed into the bloodstream and ultimately excreted in the urine. This mechanism reveals how dietary calcium restriction exacerbates hyperoxaluria and thereby promotes stone formation.
- About 20% of uric acid stones are radiopaque because they form in combination with calcium oxalate. Only pure uric acid stones fully dissolve with urine alkalinization.

70

ACUTE RENAL COLIC

TABLE 70-2
PREVENTION OF STONE RECURRENCE

Type of Stone or Biochemical Abnormality	Intervention	Notes and Rationale
All patients	Daily fluid intake ≥ 2 L/day	Drinking ≥ 2 L/day of water reduces recurrence of idiopathic calcium stones from 27% to 12% over 5 years.[15] Apple and grapefruit juices may increase stone risk; water, coffee, lemonade, and alcoholic beverages are safe.[16]
Hypercalciuria	Low-salt (< 2 g sodium/day) and low–animal protein (< 1 g/kg ideal body weight/day) diet	For patients with recurrent calcium oxalate stones and idiopathic hypercalciuria, a low-salt, low-protein diet reduced recurrence rates from 38% to 20% over 5 years compared with a low-calcium diet.[17]
Persistent hypercalciuria despite diet modification	Chlorthalidone 25 mg qd, indapamide 2.5 mg qd, or hydrochlorothiazide 25 mg qd	Thiazides reduce the relative risk of recurrent stone formation by about 55%.[18] Watch for treatment-related hypokalemia, which in turn can cause hypocitraturia. Sodium restriction is necessary.
Hyperoxaluria	Calcium supplements, 400 mg PO before meals; low-oxalate diet	Hyperoxaluria is defined as urinary excretion > 35 mg/d. Foods rich in oxalate should be avoided; these include nuts, chocolate, tea, beans, and megadose vitamin C.
Calcium stones with hypocitraturia	Potassium citrate, 30-80 mEq/d in divided doses	Hypocitraturia is defined as urinary excretion < 320 mg/d. Citrate treatment reduces annual stone recurrence risk by 92%.[19]
Calcium oxalate stones with hyperuricosuria	Dietary purine restriction ± allopurinol	Hyperuricosuria is defined as urinary excretion > 800 mg/d in men, > 750 mg/d in women. Combined with increased fluid intake, allopurinol reduces the annual risk of stone recurrence by 81%, significantly better than placebo.[20]

- Urine normally contains a variety of factors that inhibit stone formation; these include Tamm-Horsfall mucoprotein, citrate, nephrocalcin, and glycosaminoglycans.
- Conditions associated with pure calcium phosphate stones include type 1 renal tubular acidosis, medullary sponge kidney, and primary hyperparathyroidism.

REFERENCES

1. Teichman JM: Clinical practice. Acute renal colic from ureteral calculus, *N Engl J Med* 350(7):684-693, 2004. C
2. Stoller ML, Carroll PR: Urinary stone disease. In *Current medical diagnosis and treatment,* 43rd ed, New York, 2004, McGraw-Hill. C
3. Gault MH, Chafe L: Relationship of frequency, age, sex, stone weight and composition in 15,264 stones: comparison of results for 1980 to 1983 and 1995 to 1998, *J Urol* 164:302-307, 2000. B
4. Mandel NS, Mandel GS: Urinary tract stone disease in the United States veteran population. II. Geographical analysis of variations in composition, *J Urol* 142(6):1516-1521, 1989. B
5. Brenner BM, ed: *Brenner & Rector's The Kidney,* 7th ed, Philadelphia, 2004, WB Saunders. C
6. Pak CY, Poindexter JR, Adams-Huet B, Pearle MS: Predictive value of kidney stone composition in the detection of metabolic abnormalities, *Am J Med* 115(1):26-32, 2003. B
7. Bove P, Kaplan D, Dalrymple N, et al: Reexamining the value of hematuria testing in patients with acute flank pain, *J Urol* 162(3 Pt 1):685-687, 1999. B
8. Eskelinen M, Ikonen J, Lipponen P: Usefulness of history-taking, physical examination and diagnostic scoring in acute renal colic, *Eur Urol* 34:467-473, 1998. B
9. Dalrymple NC, Verga M, Anderson KR, et al: The value of unenhanced helical computerized tomography in the management of acute flank pain, *J Urol* 159:735, 1998. B
10. Miller OF, Rineer SK, Reichard SR, et al: Prospective comparison of unenhanced spiral computed tomography and intravenous urogram in the evaluation of acute flank pain, *Urology* 52(6):982-987, 1998. B
11. Smith RC, Rosenfield AT, Choe KA, et al: Acute flank pain: comparison of non–contrast-enhanced CT and intravenous urography, *Radiology* 194(3):789-794, 1995. B
12. Mutgi A, Williams JW, Nettleman M: Renal colic. Utility of the plain abdominal roentgenogram, *Arch Intern Med* 151:1589-1592, 1991. B
13. Larkin GL, Peacock WF IV, Pearl SM, Blair GA, D'Amico F: Efficacy of ketorolac tromethamine versus meperidine in the ED treatment of acute renal colic, *Am J Emerg Med* 17(1):6-10, 1999. B
14. Executive summary: Report on the management of ureteral calculi. The American Urological Association, 1997. Retrieved May 12, 2004, at http://www.auanet.org/timssnet/products/guidelines/main_reports/UreStnMain8_16.pdf. D
15. Borghi L, Meschi T, Amato F, Briganti A, Novarini A, Giannini A: Urinary volume, water and recurrences in idiopathic calcium nephrolithiasis: a 5-year randomized prospective study, *J Urol* 155(3):839-843, 1996. B

70

ACUTE RENAL COLIC

16. Curhan GC, Willett WC, Rimm EB, Spiegelman D, Stampfer MJ: Prospective study of beverage use and the risk of kidney stones, *Am J Epidemiol* 143(3):240-247, 1996. B

17. Borghi L, Schianchi T, Meschi T, et al: Comparison of two diets for the prevention of recurrent stones in idiopathic hypercalciuria, *N Engl J Med* 346:77-84, 2002. B

18. Ettinger B, Citron JT, Livermore B, Dolman LI: Chlorthalidone reduces calcium oxalate calculous recurrence but magnesium hydroxide does not, *J Urol* 139(4):679-684, 1988. A

19. Barcelo P, Wuhl O, Servitge E, Rousaud A, Pak CY: Randomized double-blind study of potassium citrate in idiopathic hypocitraturic calcium nephrolithiasis, *J Urol* 150(6):1761-1764, 1993. A

20. Ettinger B, Tang A, Citron JT, Livermore B, Williams T: Randomized trial of allopurinol in the prevention of calcium oxalate calculi, *N Engl J Med* 315:1386-1389, 1986. A

Acid-Base Disorders

John A. Dooley, MD; and Stephen D. Sisson, MD

FAST FACTS

- Both an arterial blood gas and a basic metabolic panel are necessary to determine a patient's acid-base status.
- Analysis of a patient's acid-base disorder includes identification of the primary disorder, calculation of the anion gap (AG), evaluation for the presence of excess acid or base, comparison of the expected and actual compensation, and explanation of the cause of each identified acid-base disorder.

71

Acid-base disorders are defined by abnormalities in the serum concentrations of hydrogen ion (H^+), bicarbonate ion (HCO_3^-), or carbon dioxide (CO_2). Although acidemia or alkalemia can cause symptoms and disrupt homeostasis, the primary clinical importance of acid-base analysis is to generate a differential diagnosis and identify the underlying disorder.

I. OVERVIEW OF ACID-BASE PHYSIOLOGY

1. Normal metabolism generates endogenous acid, including CO_2 and sulfuric and phosphoric acids. Acids such as lactic acid and ketoacids accumulate in pathologic states.
2. Rapid shifts in pH are prevented by the buffering properties of HCO_3^-, proteins, and bone.
3. The lungs excrete CO_2. The kidneys excrete or retain HCO_3^- and nonvolatile acids. Together these organs maintain acid-base homeostasis.

II. DEFINITIONS OF FUNDAMENTAL ACID-BASE DISORDERS

1. Derangements in acid-base equilibrium are classified by changes in pH, PCO_2, and $[HCO_3^-]$; their relationships are summarized by the Kassirer and Henderson-Hasselbalch equations (Box 71-1). There are four primary acid-base disorders:
   a. Primary increase in PCO_2: respiratory acidosis
   b. Primary decrease in PCO_2: respiratory alkalosis
   c. Primary decrease in $[HCO_3^-]$: metabolic acidosis
   d. Primary increase in $[HCO_3^-]$: metabolic alkalosis
2. Compensatory (secondary) processes restore pH toward normal in response to one or more primary acid-base abnormalities; the kidneys compensate for primary respiratory disorders, and the lungs compensate for primary metabolic disorders.
3. A **simple** acid-base disorder is caused by a single **primary** abnormality with appropriate physiologic compensation.

BOX 71-1

FORMULAS IN ACID-BASE ANALYSIS

Kassirer: $[H^+] = 24 \times Pco_2/[HCO_3]$

Henderson-Hasselbalch: $pH = 6.1 + log([HCO_3]/0.03 \times Pco_2)$

Anion gap $= [Na] - ([Cl] + [HCO_3])$

Urine anion gap $= U_{Na} + U_K - U_{Cl}$

Delta $-$ delta $= (Anion\ gap/HCO_3) = (AG_{Measured} - AG_{Normal}/HCO_{3Measured} - HCO_{3Normal})$

Calculated osmolarity $= 2[Na] + [Glucose]/18 + [BUN]/2.8 + [Ethanol]/4.6$

Osmolar gap $= Osmolarity_{Measured} - Osmolarity_{Calculated}$

---

4. **Mixed** acid-base disorders result from multiple **primary** processes. Up to three of the four primary processes can coexist, but respiratory acidosis and respiratory alkalosis are mutually exclusive.

5. Metabolic acidosis is further classified into normal AG and elevated AG varieties.

6. Metabolic alkalosis is further classified into saline-responsive and saline-resistant varieties.

III. PRESENTATION (Box 71-2)

IV. STEP-BY-STEP ANALYSIS

Analysis of acid-base status should follow a stepwise approach. The initial analysis defines the acid-base abnormality. Subsequent investigation is necessary to determine the cause of the abnormalities.

1. Collect necessary data: arterial blood gas and basic metabolic panel.

a. The arterial blood gas is the standard means of directly measuring pH and PCO_2. Arterial and venous values correlate in most cases, but results may deviate in the setting of severe circulatory failure.[3-5] Compared with arterial values, venous pH typically is lower by 0.03 and PCO_2 higher by 5 mmHg.

b. The $[HCO_3^-]$ reported with a blood gas is calculated from the Henderson-Hasselbalch equation (see Box 70-1). The $[HCO_3^-]$ reported on an electrolyte panel is actually total CO_2 content, of which about 95% is in the form of bicarbonate and 5% dissolved carbon dioxide gas. The two reported $[HCO_3^-]$ values should not differ by more than 3 mEq/L.

2. Assess the pH and primary disorder.

a. First evaluate pH to define the presence of acidemia or alkalemia. If the pH is less than 7.4, a primary acidosis is present. A pH greater than 7.4 indicates a primary alkalosis.

b. Abnormalities in Pco_2 or $[HCO_3^-]$ that are consistent with the pH indicate a primary process (Fig. 71-1).

c. Occasionally, coexisting acidosis and alkalosis offset each other and result in a normal pH. You can still identify the component processes from the changes in PCO_2 and $[HCO_3^-]$.

BOX 71-2

SYMPTOMS AND CONSEQUENCES OF ACIDEMIA AND ALKALEMIA[1,2]

ACIDEMIA

Cardiovascular
  Decreased myocardial contractility
  Diminished catecholamine
    responsiveness
  Arrhythmia
  Venoconstriction
  Arteriolar dilation
Pulmonary
  Hyperventilation
  Dyspnea

Central nervous system
  Obtundation
  Coma
Metabolic
  Hyperkalemia
  Decreased adenosine triphosphate
    synthesis
  Insulin resistance
  Protein catabolism

ALKALEMIA

Increased mortality
Cardiovascular
  Arrhythmia
  Decreased coronary and cerebral
    blood flow
Pulmonary
  Hypoventilation
  Decreased peripheral oxygen delivery

Neurologic
  Neuromuscular irritability
  Tetany
Metabolic
  Hypokalemia
  Hypocalcemia (decreased ionized
    calcium)
  Hypomagnesemia

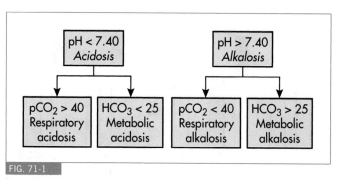

FIG. 71-1

Determining the primary acid-base abnormality.

3. Calculate the AG.
a. The AG is an accounting tool used to demonstrate the presence of
   organic acids and thus reveal metabolic acidoses. AG is defined as
   the difference between measured cations and measured anions (AG =
   [Na] − [Cl] − [HCO$_3$]).
b. The normal AG is 10 to 14 mEq/L, reflecting physiologic concentrations
   of unmeasured anions such as albumin, phosphorus, and sulfate.

Marked hypoalbuminemia may mask an elevated AG, so it is good practice to compensate for the [albumin]. A useful guideline is that the normal (reference) AG is three times the [albumin]. Alternatively, adjust the calculated AG by adding 2.5 mEq/L for every 1 g/dl decrement in [albumin] below 4 g/dl.

c. An elevated AG generally indicates the presence of a pathologic anion such as lactate. This defines an elevated AG metabolic acidosis regardless of the pH or [HCO_3^-]. Rarely, an elevated AG is the only laboratory evidence of a mixed acid-base disorder.

d. In the context of a metabolic acidosis, a normal AG defines a normal AG acidosis.

4. Calculate the excess acid or base relative to an elevated AG.

a. In a pure elevated AG metabolic acidosis, [HCO_3^-] is theoretically reduced by the exact amount by which the AG is increased because each unit of organic acid is neutralized by one unit of HCO_3^-.

b. The delta-delta equation ($\Delta/\Delta = \Delta AG/\Delta[HCO_3^-]$) assesses the relationship between the changes in AG and HCO_3 to identify the presence of other disorders (Fig. 71-2; see Box 71-1).

    (1) If the Δ/Δ is less than 1, there is acid in excess of the AG, indicating a coexisting normal AG metabolic acidosis.

    (2) If the Δ/Δ equals 1, there is a pure elevated AG metabolic acidosis.

    (3) If the Δ/Δ is greater than 2, there is excess HCO_3^- relative to the AG, indicating a concomitant metabolic alkalosis.

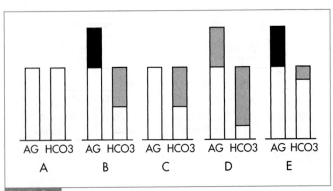

FIG. 71-2

Comparison of anion gap (AG) and serum HCO_3^- changes in different acid-base states. **A,** Normal. **B,** Elevated AG metabolic acidosis: AG increases by the same amount HCO_3^- decreases; $\Delta/\Delta = 1$. **C,** Normal AG metabolic acidosis: HCO_3^- decreases, but AG is unchanged. **D,** Combination of elevated AG metabolic acidosis and normal AG metabolic acidosis: HCO_3^- falls by more than AG increases; $\Delta/\Delta < 1$. **E,** Combination of elevated AG metabolic acidosis and metabolic alkalosis: AG increases by more than HCO_3^- decreases; $\Delta/\Delta > 1$.

c. The delta-delta equation oversimplifies the pathophysiology of metabolic acidosis. In lactic acidosis, for example, only some of the H^+ is neutralized by HCO_3^-; the remainder is buffered by bone and intracellular anions. However, all lactate remains in the extracellular space. The net result is a Δ/Δ that is typically about 1.6, not 1.[6]

5. Calculate and compare expected and actual compensation (Table 71-1).

a. For a primary respiratory acidosis, buffers provide acute compensation in the initial minutes to hours. Chronic compensation requires a gradual increase in renal acid excretion, a process that takes 3 to 5 days.

b. For a primary respiratory alkalosis, there are also acute and chronic compensatory changes. Changes in pH are difficult to predict accurately, but respiratory alkalosis is the only primary acid-base disorder for which chronic compensation may restore a normal pH.

c. In patients with a primary metabolic acidosis, respiratory compensation (hyperventilation) occurs within hours. If the PCO_2 is higher than expected, there is a concomitant respiratory acidosis; if the PCO_2 is lower than expected, there is a concomitant respiratory alkalosis.

d. In primary metabolic alkalosis, the degree of expected respiratory compensation is less predictable because hypoxemia limits the degree of hypoventilation necessary to elevate PCO_2. Changes substantially more or less than predicted suggest a concomitant primary respiratory acidosis or alkalosis.

71

ACID-BASE DISORDERS

TABLE 71-1

PREDICTED COMPENSATORY CHANGES AND LIMITS OF COMPENSATION

Primary Disorder and Compensatory Mechanism	Predicted Values	Limit of Compensation
Respiratory acidosis with metabolic compensation	Acute: For every 10–mmHg rise in PCO_2, $[HCO_3^-]$ rises by 1 mEq/L and pH falls by 0.08.	
	Chronic: For every 10–mmHg rise in PCO_2, $[HCO_3^-]$ rises by 3-4 mEq/L and pH falls by 0.03.	$[HCO_3^-] = 45\text{-}55$
Respiratory alkalosis with metabolic compensation	Acute: For every 10–mmHg fall in PCO_2, $[HCO_3^-]$ falls by 2.5 mEq/L and pH increases by 0.1.	
	Chronic: For every 10–mmHg fall in PCO_2, $[HCO_3^-]$ falls by 5 mEq/L; pH may normalize.	$[HCO_3^-] = 15$
Metabolic acidosis with respiratory compensation	$PCO_2 = [HCO_3^-] \times 1.5 + 8 \pm 2$ (Winters's formula).	$PCO_2 = 20$
Metabolic alkalosis with respiratory compensation	PCO_2 rises ~0.5-1.0 mmHg for every 1-mEq/L rise in $[HCO_3]$.	$PCO_2 = 55$

BOX 71-3

DIFFERENTIAL DIAGNOSIS OF RESPIRATORY ACIDOSIS

LUNG AND AIRWAY

Pneumonia	Mechanical obstruction
Pulmonary edema	Foreign body
Bronchospasm; laryngospasm	Mucus plugging
Chronic obstructive pulmonary disease	Tumor

CHEST CAVITY

Neurologic disorders	Pleural effusion
Muscular disorders	Severe chest wall deformity
Pneumothorax	

CENTRAL

Sedation, narcotics	Respiratory center hypofunction
Obstructive sleep apnea	Infection
	Ischemia
	Infarction

---

e. **Important limitation.** Predictions of compensation apply to simple acid-base disorders only; they are unreliable for known mixed acid-base disorders.

V. SPECIFIC ACID-BASE DISORDERS

A. RESPIRATORY ACIDOSIS

1. See Box 71-3 for differential diagnosis of respiratory acidosis (hypoventilation).
2. Treatment is directed at the underlying disorder.

B. RESPIRATORY ALKALOSIS

1. See Box 71-4 for the differential diagnosis of respiratory alkalosis (hyperventilation).
2. Treatment for pathologic causes is directed at the underlying disorder.

C. ELEVATED AG METABOLIC ACIDOSIS

1. Most causes of elevated AG metabolic acidosis are potentially life-threatening processes that warrant urgent evaluation. A careful history, physical examination, and selected laboratories (blood urea nitrogen and creatinine, lactate, ketones, and salicylate levels) will identify most clinically significant causes of elevated AG acidosis. The differential diagnosis is shown in Box 71-5.
2. Uncommon causes of elevated AG metabolic acidosis include ingested toxins that are metabolized to organic acids. Some toxins can be detected by the presence of an elevated osmolar gap. If the difference between measured and predicted (see Box 71-1) serum osmolality exceeds 10 mOsm/L, screen for volatile toxins such as methanol and ethylene glycol. Isopropyl alcohol and mannitol cause osmolar gaps but not elevated AGs.
3. Lactic acid itself has a broad differential diagnosis (Box 71-6).

BOX 71-4

DIFFERENTIAL DIAGNOSIS OF RESPIRATORY ALKALOSIS

PULMONARY

Mechanical (hyper)ventilation	Pulmonary embolism
Hypoxemia	Restrictive lung disease

SYSTEMIC

Sepsis	Liver failure
Salicylate intoxication	Pregnancy
Hyperthyroidism	High-altitude living

NEUROLOGIC

Stroke	Central nervous system infection
Central nervous system tumor	Anxiety

BOX 71-5

DIFFERENTIAL DIAGNOSIS OF ELEVATED ANION GAP METABOLIC ACIDOSIS

NORMAL OSMOLAR GAP

Lactic acidosis*

Diabetic ketoacidosis*

Renal failure: phosphates, sulfates, urate, and other anions accumulate*

Alcoholic and starvation ketoacidosis*

Rhabdomyolysis

Salicylate ingestion (metabolized to lactate and ketones)

Iron ingestion

Isoniazid ingestion

ELEVATED OSMOLAR GAP

Methanol ingestion (metabolized to formic acid)

Ethylene glycol ingestion (metabolized to oxalic and glycolic acids)

Toluene ingestion (metabolized to hippuric acid; AG disappears quickly as
  hippurate is excreted by kidney)

---

*These are by far the most common causes.

4. It is not always possible to identify the unmeasured anions responsible
   for an elevated AG. A cause can almost always be found for an AG
   greater than 30, but smaller gaps sometimes are less easily
   characterized. One study found that 29% of all AGs between 20 and
   29 could not be explained even with extensive laboratory analysis.[7]
5. Treatment of elevated AG metabolic acidosis is directed at the
   underlying cause. Whether an acute elevated AG metabolic acidosis
   itself should be treated with supplemental bicarbonate is a matter of
   debate.[8]

D. OTHER CONSIDERATIONS REGARDING METABOLIC ACIDOSIS

1. As shown in Table 71-2, ionic species other than measured cations and
   anions contribute to the AG. Significant abnormalities in unmeasured

---

BOX 71-6

DIFFERENTIAL DIAGNOSIS OF LACTIC ACIDOSIS

TYPE A: CAUSED BY TISSUE HYPOXIA

Seizures

Severe exercise

Shock: cardiogenic, neurogenic, septic, anaphylactic

Severe hypoxemia: CO poisoning, severe anemia, methemoglobinemia, acute
  respiratory failure

TYPE B: NOT CAUSED BY TISSUE HYPOXIA

Drugs and toxins: metformin, ethanol, salicylates, cyanide, methanol, isoniazid,
  nitroprusside, streptozocin, ethylene glycol, nalidixic acid, topiramate, nucleoside
  reverse transcriptase inhibitors

Inherited enzyme defects

Malignancy: leukemia, lymphoma, solid tumors

Diabetes mellitus

Liver failure

Renal failure

Systemic infection

TABLE 71-2

FACTORS AFFECTING THE ANION GAP

	Increased Unmeasured Anions	Decreased Unmeasured Cations
Elevated anion gap	Lactate, ketoacids	Hypocalcemia
	Hyperalbuminemia	Hypomagnesemia
	Sulfate, phosphate, and urate	
	Formate	
	Glycolate and oxalate	
	Decreased Unmeasured Anions	Increased Unmeasured Cations
Low anion gap	Hypoalbuminemia	Hypercalcemia
		Hyperkalemia
		Paraproteinemia

---

ions such as calcium, phosphate, and albumin can increase or
decrease the AG. For example, one study of patients with cholera and
hypovolemic shock found that electrolyte and protein concentration
abnormalities contributed more to the AG than did lactate.[9]

2. It is possible that the AG will be normal in a patient with an organic
   acidosis if renal function is well preserved. For example, if the ketoacids
   formed in diabetic ketoacidosis are promptly excreted (as sodium salts)
   in the urine, the unmeasured anions do not accumulate, and the
   patient will have a normal AG metabolic acidosis. In fact, one review
   of patients presenting with diabetic ketoacidosis found a wide spectrum
   of acid-base patterns ranging from pure elevated AG acidosis to pure

BOX 71-7

DIFFERENTIAL DIAGNOSIS OF NORMAL ANION GAP METABOLIC ACIDOSIS

NEGATIVE URINE ANION GAP (NH_4^+ PRESENT)

Acid gain
  Exogenous acid administration (e.g., NH_4Cl)
Bicarbonate loss
  Type 2 renal tubular acidosis (proximal)
  Diarrhea
  External pancreatic or small bowel drainage
  Ureteral diversion
  Loss of bicarbonate equivalent (e.g., ketonuria)
  Toluene poisoning
Dilutional acidosis

POSITIVE URINE ANION GAP (NH_4^+ ABSENT)

Acid gain or retention
  Type 1 renal tubular acidosis (distal)
  Type 4 renal tubular acidosis
  Renal failure (some cases; see text)
  Amphotericin B administration

71

ACID-BASE DISORDERS

normal AG acidosis. Patients with impaired renal function had a higher
degree of ketoacid retention and, on average, a higher AG.[10]

E. NORMAL AG METABOLIC ACIDOSIS

1. A normal AG metabolic acidosis is caused by loss of bicarbonate or
   retention of hydrochloric acid. Neither mechanism results in
   accumulation of an unmeasured anion.
2. These processes are classified by their origin as renal or nonrenal
   (Box 71-7). When the cause is nonrenal, such as diarrhea, the kidney
   responds by excreting the excess acid as ammonium chloride ($NH_4^+Cl^-$).
   In contrast, acidoses of renal origin result in a low urine $NH_4^+Cl^-$
   because the kidney itself cannot appropriately excrete acid.
3. To distinguish between renal and nonrenal causes of normal gap
   metabolic acidosis, we measure a surrogate marker of $NH_4^+Cl^-$
   excretion, the urine AG ($UAG = U_{Na} + U_K - U_{Cl}$). If the UAG is
   negative, additional unmeasured cations must be present in the urine.
   This unmeasured cation is inferred to be NH_4^+, and the acidosis must
   be of nonrenal origin. A positive gap indicates the absence of NH_4^+ and
   therefore an acidosis of renal origin.
4. See Chapter 72 for discussion of the types of renal tubular
   acidosis.
5. Treatment is directed at the underlying disease.

F. LIMITATIONS ON THE USE OF THE URINE AG

1. The urine AG generally is a reliable indicator of the cause of normal AG
   metabolic acidosis. One study found that normal people given NH_4Cl
   and patients with diarrhea all had negative urine AGs; the gap was

positive in all patients with renal tubular disorders or aldosterone deficiency.[11]

2. Occasionally the UAG is misleading. For example, diarrhea may induce a state of marked volume depletion in which sodium and chloride are reabsorbed to such an extent that no chloride remains in the tubular lumen to be excreted with NH_4^+. Although the primary problem is diarrhea, the kidney cannot excrete NH_4^+, and the UAG is positive.

3. The UAG may be spuriously positive when large amounts of unmeasured anions are excreted in the urine. For example, in ketoacidosis the filtration of nonreabsorbed ketoacid anions compels natriuresis and kaluresis. Although NH_4^+ excretion may be appropriately high for the acidosis, the elevation in urine sodium and potassium predominates and causes the UAG to be positive. For this reason, use of the UAG in the setting of a known elevated AG metabolic acidosis is not recommended. An elevation in the urine osmolar gap (see Box 71-1) is a clue that ketoacid salts or similar compounds are present in large quantities.

G. SPECIAL TYPES OF NORMAL AG ACIDOSIS

1. Dilutional acidosis. Rapid infusion of intravenous fluids (such as saline or dextrose in water) lowers $[HCO_3^-]$ through dilution without contributing unmeasured anions and therefore causes a normal gap metabolic acidosis. The effect is opposite that of contraction alkalosis. With normal renal function, dilutional acidosis is short lived.

2. In some cases, ketoacidosis and lactic acidosis manifest partially as normal AG metabolic acidosis.

H. METABOLIC ALKALOSIS: DIFFERENTIAL DIAGNOSIS, CLASSIFICATION, AND PATHOPHYSIOLOGY

1. Metabolic alkalosis is initiated by bicarbonate gain or acid loss. The kidney normally has a robust capacity for excreting excess HCO_3^-, so a metabolic alkalosis can be maintained only if this homeostatic system is impaired, usually by elevated aldosterone levels. Aldosterone promotes both excretion of H^+ and coabsorption of sodium and HCO_3^-.

2. Hyperaldosteronism may be primary, as in the case of a Conn's tumor, but is more commonly the result of volume depletion or other processes that activate the renin-angiotensin system.

3. To narrow the differential diagnosis of metabolic alkalosis, measure the urine chloride concentration. Levels less than 10 mEq/L imply that volume depletion is the sustaining force behind the alkalosis and that giving saline should resolve the problem (saline responsive). When urine chloride is greater than 10 mEq/L, volume contraction is not the primary abnormality, and giving saline will not correct the alkalosis. Exceptions to this guideline are states in which the kidneys excrete sodium and chloride despite volume contraction (e.g., ongoing diuretic use). See Fig. 71-3 for the differential diagnosis of metabolic alkalosis.

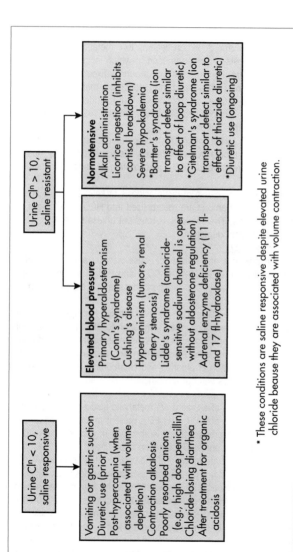

Urine Cl⁻ > 10, saline resistant

Normotensive
Alkali administration
Licorice ingestion (inhibits cortisol breakdown)
Severe hypokalemia
*Bartter's syndrome (ion transport defect similar to effect of loop diuretic)
*Gitelman's syndrome (ion transport defect similar to effect of thiazide diuretic)
*Diuretic use (ongoing)

Elevated blood pressure
Primary hyperaldosteronism (Conn's syndrome)
Cushing's disease
Hyperreninism (tumors, renal artery stenosis)
Liddle's syndrome (amioride-sensitive sodium channel is open without aldosterone regulation)
Adrenal enzyme deficiency (11 ß and 17 ß-hydroxlase)

Urine Cl⁻ < 10, saline responsive

Vomiting or gastric suction
Diuretic use (prior)
Post-hypercapnia (when associated with volume depletion)
Contraction alkalosis
Poorly resorbed anions (e.g., high dose penicillin)
Chloride-losing diarrhea
After treatment for organic acidosis

* These conditions are saline responsive despite elevated urine chloride beause they are associated with volume contraction.

FIG. 71-3

Differential diagnosis of metabolic alkalosis.

I. SPECIAL TYPES OF METABOLIC ALKALOSIS

1. In posthypercapnia alkalosis, the kidney compensates for hypercapnia by increasing acid excretion. If hypercapnia is rapidly corrected (as with mechanical ventilation), the compensatory process may persist if there is concomitant volume depletion, leading to a metabolic alkalosis.
2. Contraction alkalosis is a phenomenon in which volume depletion causes extracellular fluid to "contract" around a fixed quantity of bicarbonate, raising $[HCO_3^-]$ and thus inducing a metabolic alkalosis.
3. Easily overlooked sources of exogenous alkali include citrate, used as an anticoagulant in transfused blood, and acetate, administered in parenteral nutrition solutions.
4. Renal filtration of certain poorly reabsorbed anions, such as penicillin, renders the renal tubular lumen relatively electronegative and thus facilitates H^+ excretion and HCO_3^- reabsorption, leading to metabolic alkalosis.
5. When the underlying cause of lactic acidosis or ketoacidosis is corrected quickly, the organic anions are metabolized into HCO_3^-, yielding a metabolic alkalosis. The alkalosis is transient unless there is concomitant volume depletion.

PEARLS AND PITFALLS

- Clues to the presence of a mixed acid-base disorder are normal pH with abnormal PCO_2 or $[HCO_3^-]$; $[HCO_3^-]$ and Pco_2 move in opposite directions; pH changes in the direction opposite that expected from a known primary disorder.
- When calculating the AG in the setting of marked hyperglycemia, it is important to not correct sodium concentration for that of glucose. This adjustment is commonly done as a means of assessing hydration status, but it is inappropriate for the AG determination because hyperglycemia affects the concentration of chloride and bicarbonate, as well as sodium. Correcting one species without the others leads to an incorrect result.[12,13]
- An uncommon cause of elevated AG metabolic acidosis is phosphate intoxication. This can occur if NaH_2PO_4, present in some enemas and oral bowel cleansing preparations, is absorbed in excess of the kidney's ability to excrete phosphate. Dissociation into H^+ and HPO_4^{2-} results in markedly high phosphate levels and a proportionately elevated AG.[14]
- In diabetic ketoacidosis, a normal gap metabolic acidosis usually develops because ketoacid anion excretion by the kidney is equivalent to loss of bicarbonate. With insulin therapy, ketoacidosis resolves quickly; ketoacids are metabolized into bicarbonate. The normal gap metabolic acidosis takes longer to correct because the kidney must regenerate lost bicarbonate.
- In most cases of renal failure, accumulation of organic acids leads to an elevated AG metabolic acidosis. However, in some cases of renal failure, renal tubular dysfunction predominates, causing a normal AG metabolic acidosis.

- Sepsis and salicylate intoxication both may present with mixed respiratory alkalosis and elevated AG metabolic acidosis.

REFERENCES

1. Kokko JP: Fluids and electrolytes. In Goldman L, Bennett JC, eds: *Cecil textbook of medicine,* 21st ed, Philadelphia, 2000, WB Saunders. C
2. Effros RM, Widell JL: Acid-base balance. In Murray JF, Nadel JA, eds: *Textbook of respiratory medicine,* 3rd ed, Philadelphia, 2000, WB Saunders. C
3. Adrogue HJ, Rashad MN, Gorin AB, et al: Assessing acid-base status in circulatory failure. Differences between arterial and central venous blood, *N Engl J Med* 320(20):1312-1316, 1989. B
4. Brandenburg MA, Dire DJ: Comparison of arterial and venous blood gas values in the initial emergency department evaluation of patients with diabetic ketoacidosis, *Ann Emerg Med* 31(4):459-465, 1998. B
5. Chu YC, Chen CZ, Lee CH, et al: Prediction of arterial blood gas values from venous blood gas values in patients with acute respiratory failure receiving mechanical ventilation, *J Formos Med Assoc* 102(8):539-543, 2003. B
6. DiNubile MJ: The increment in the anion gap: overextension of a concept? *Lancet* 332(8617):951-953, 1988. C
7. Gabow PA et al: Diagnostic importance of an increased serum anion gap, *N Engl J Med* 303:854-858, 1980. B
8. Forsythe SM, Schmidt GA: Sodium bicarbonate for the treatment of lactic acidosis, *Chest* 117:260-267, 2000. C
9. Wang F, Butler T, Rabbani GH, Jones PK: The acidosis of cholera. Contributions of hyperproteinemia, lactic acidemia, and hyperphosphatemia to an increased serum anion gap, *N Engl J Med* 315:1591-1595, 1986. B
10. Adrogue HJ, Wilson H, Boyd AE, et al: Plasma acid-base patterns in diabetic ketoacidosis, *N Engl J Med* 307:1603-1610, 1982. B
11. Battle DC, Hizon M, Cohen E, et al: The use of the urinary anion gap in the diagnosis of hyperchloremic metabolic acidosis, *N Engl J Med* 318:594-599, 1988. B
12. Tomer Y: Calculating the anion gap for patients with acidosis and hyperglycemia [Letter], *Ann Intern Med* 129(9):753, 1998. D
13. Beck LH: Should the actual or the corrected serum sodium be used to calculate the anion gap in diabetic ketoacidosis? *Cleve Clin J Med* 68(8):673-674, 2001. C
14. Kirschbaum B: The acidosis of exogenous phosphate intoxication, *Arch Intern Med* 158:405-408, 1998. B

71

ACID-BASE DISORDERS

Renal Tubular Acidosis

Adam R. Berliner, MD; and Michael J. Choi, MD

FAST FACTS

- Renal tubular acidosis (RTA) is a common finding in many of the tubulointerstitial diseases and is characterized by a normal anion gap metabolic acidosis.
- RTAs are subdivided into distal RTA (types I and IV) and proximal RTA (type II).
- The urine anion gap is essential in distinguishing distal RTA from the other major cause of a normal anion gap metabolic acidosis, namely gastrointestinal bicarbonate loss.
- Treatment depends on the type of RTA and is important to prevent osteoporosis, nephrolithiasis, and hyperkalemia.

Urinary excretion of acid generated by metabolism of ingested proteins and from endogenous metabolic processes is critical to the maintenance of proper acid-base balance. Proximal tubular bicarbonate (HCO_3^-) resorption and distal tubule and collecting tubule excretion of hydrogen ions (H^+) in the form of ammonium ion (NH_4^+) are the basic processes in this homeostasis. Net H^+ excretion in urine can be expressed as the sum of titratable acid and NH_4^+ excretion, minus the urinary HCO_3^-. The type I, II, and IV renal tubular acidoses (type III is no longer thought to be a separate disorder) represent dysfunction of these different homeostatic mechanisms. These disorders are independent of glomerular filtration rate, as opposed to the metabolic acidosis associated with advanced renal failure, which usually reflects decreased renal ammoniagenesis.

I. CLASSIFICATION

1. **Proximal (type II) RTA** (Box 72-1). This uncommon form of RTA reflects impaired HCO_3^- resorption in the proximal tubule, with resultant bicarbonaturia. This defect usually coexists with generalized proximal tubule dysfunction and manifests as Fanconi's syndrome in which glucose, amino acids, and phosphate are also wasted in the urine. The disorder is self-limiting because once serum HCO_3^- falls below 15 mmol/L, compensatory mechanisms of reabsorption in the distal collecting duct limit further urinary HCO_3^- wasting.
2. **Distal (type I) RTA** (Box 72-2). Type I RTA results in decreased net H^+ excretion in the cortical collecting duct by one of four mechanisms.[1]
   a. Permeability defects induced by tubular damage prevent the establishment of a [H^+] gradient. Amphotericin B is a classic offender.
   b. Secretory defects from defective H^+/ATPase pumps prevent excretion of H^+.

BOX 72-1

CAUSES OF PROXIMAL (TYPE II) RENAL TUBULAR ACIDOSIS

SELECTIVE DEFECTS (UNASSOCIATED WITH FANCONI'S SYNDROME)

Primary: transient (infants); idiopathic or genetic; carbonic anhydrase deficiency, inhibition, or alteration

Drugs: acetazolamide

GENERALIZED DYSFUNCTION (ASSOCIATED WITH FANCONI'S SYNDROME)

Primary: genetic (e.g., Wilson's disease, methylmalonic acidemia) or sporadic

Dysproteinemic states: multiple myeloma; monoclonal gammopathy; secondary hyperparathyroidism with chronic hypocalcemia

Drugs or toxins: ifosfamide, outdated tetracycline, 3-methylchromone, streptozocin, lead, mercury

Modified from Brenner, BM: *The kidney,* 7th ed, Philadelphia, 2004, WB Saunders.

72

BOX 72-2

CAUSES OF CLASSIC DISTAL (TYPE I) RENAL TUBULAR ACIDOSIS

IDIOPATHIC

Autoimmune Diseases
Hyperglobulinemic purpura
Cryoglobulinemia
Sjögren's syndrome
Polyarteritis nodosa
Thyroiditis
Human immunodeficiency virus
Chronic active hepatitis
Primary biliary cirrhosis
Hypercalciuria and Nephrocalcinosis
Primary hyperparathyroidism
Hyperthyroidism
Medullary sponge kidney
Fabry's disease
Hereditary fructose intolerance
Wilson's disease
X-linked hypophosphatemia

Vitamin D intoxication
Idiopathic hypercalciuria
Drug and Toxin-Induced Diseases
Amphotericin B
Ifosfamide
Toluene
Foscarnet
Classic analgesic nephropathy
Lithium
Mercury
Associated with Genetic Disorders
Ehlers-Danlos syndrome
Sickle cell anemia
Marfan's syndrome
Medullary cystic disease
Hereditary sensorineural deafness

Modified from Brenner, BM: *The kidney,* 7th ed, Philadelphia, 2004, WB Saunders.

c. A decreased electrical gradient for H^+ entry into the tubular lumen. This is classically seen in severe volume depletion and with potassium-sparing diuretics such as amiloride and triamterene, where diminished sodium delivery and resorption leads to a relatively electropositive tubule lumen, resulting in decreased H^+ excretion.

d. Ammonium synthesis or transfer defects.

BOX 72-3

CAUSES OF DISTAL (TYPE IV) RENAL TUBULAR ACIDOSIS

MINERALOCORTICOID DEFICIENCY

Primary Mineralocorticoid Deficiency

Addison's disease

Congenital enzymatic defects

Isolated aldosterone deficiency

Heparin in critically ill patient

Persistent ↓ blood pressure or ↓ PaO_2 in critically ill patient

Angiotensin II-converting enzyme inhibition or angiotensin receptor blockade

Familial hypoaldosteronism

Secondary Mineralocorticoid Deficiency

Hyporeninemic hypoaldosteronism

Diabetic nephropathy

Tubulointerstitial nephropathies

Immunoglobulin M monoclonal gammopathy

Nephrosclerosis

Nonsteroidal antiinflammatory drugs

Acquired immunodeficiency syndrome

MINERALOCORTICOID RESISTANCE

Drugs Interfering with Na^+ Channel Function in Collecting Tubule

Amiloride

Triamterene

Trimethoprim

Pentamidine

Drugs That Inhibit Aldosterone

Spironolactone

Calcineurin inhibitors

Modified from Brenner, BM: *The kidney,* 7th ed, Philadelphia, 2004, WB Saunders.

3. **Distal (type IV) RTA** (Box 72-3). This other form of distal RTA results from endogenous aldosterone deficiency or resistance or from the use of aldosterone antagonists (e.g., spironolactone).

II. DIAGNOSIS

1. The differential diagnosis of normal anion gap hyperchloremic metabolic acidosis includes RTAs; gastrointestinal HCO_3^- losses; acetazolamide use, which causes a proximal RTA; and rarely acid ingestion with excretion of anions (treatment phase of diabetic ketoacidosis and toluene exposure).

2. The urinary anion gap ($UAG = U_{Na} + U_K - U_{Cl}$) estimates urinary NH_4^+ excretion and is both sensitive and specific for distinguishing distal acidification defects (types I and IV RTA) from the metabolic acidosis of gastrointestinal HCO_3^- losses. It is important to note that when urinary pH is 6.5 or higher, urine [HCO_3^-] should be considered a significant

TABLE 72-1

DIAGNOSTIC STUDIES IN RENAL TUBULAR ACIDOSIS

Finding	Type of Renal Tubular Acidosis		
	Proximal (Type II)	Distal (Type I)	Distal (Type IV)
Plasma [K$^+$]	Low	Low	High
Urine pH	< 5.5	> 5.5	Usually < 5.5
Urine anion gap	Negative	Positive	Positive
Fanconi's lesion	Present	Absent	Absent
Fractional HCO$_3$ excretion	> 10%	< 5%	< 10%
Response to alkali therapy	Least readily	Readily	Less readily

urinary anion and included in UAG calculations. Of note, the urine anion gap should be used only when the serum anion gap is not extremely elevated.

a. The UAG is positive in distal RTA and negative in gastrointestinal-related acidosis.

b. Although the UAG usually is negative in proximal RTA, this generalization is unreliable because many proximal RTAs are associated with decreased ammoniagenesis and therefore may give a positive UAG.

3. **Urinary pH.** Although the inability to acidify the urine to a pH of 5.5 or less in the face of systemic acidosis suggests distal RTA, the urine pH should be interpreted with caution. Urinary infection with urea-splitting organisms, severe hypokalemia, and severe sodium depletion can all raise urine pH. Similarly, appropriate urinary acidification does not exclude type IV RTA. In general, the urine pH does not reflect renal ability to excrete the complete daily acid load.

4. Fractional urinary excretion of HCO$_3^-$ is the most reliable test for diagnosis of proximal RTA and is measured during the intravenous infusion of HCO$_3^-$. This test is infrequently used, however. A more practical approach in suspected proximal RTA is a challenge with oral alkali followed by measurement of urine pH.

5. Table 72-1 compares common features of the RTAs.

III. MANAGEMENT

1. Patients with RTAs usually are asymptomatic. However, treatment is warranted because buffering of chronic acidosis by bone leads to osteopenia and osteoporosis.

2. Treatment is tailored to the specific RTA, but replacement of bicarbonate is necessary in all forms. Sodium citrate liquid (15 ml two or three times daily) or sodium bicarbonate tablets (650 to 1300 mg two to four times daily) is commonly used. The former may not be as effective in patients with severe liver dysfunction because it requires hepatic conversion of citrate to bicarbonate. RTA-specific treatment is as follows:

a. **Type II (proximal) RTA** often necessitates very large amounts (e.g., 10 to 15 mEq of alkali/kg/day) of oral alkali to overcome the reduced absorptive capacity of the proximal tubule. This can lead to heavy bicarbonaturia and potassium wasting. To decrease the burden of oral alkali and improve compliance, a thiazide diuretic may be used to increase HCO_3^- resorption. Associated hypophosphatemia or vitamin D deficiency should be treated appropriately.

b. **Type I (distal) RTA** often is associated with hypercalciuria and nephrolithiasis, either as a primary disorder causing the RTA or as a result of the RTA (elevated urine pH favors calcium-phosphate precipitation). Citrate-based salts are preferred in these cases because the citrate anion binds with calcium, making it more soluble in urine. **Potassium citrate** is preferred over sodium citrate because it both treats the hypokalemia often associated with type I RTA and avoids the natriuresis and calciuresis that result from a sodium load.

c. **Type IV RTA.** In addition to alkali therapy for acidosis, treatment with fludrocortisone may be useful for correcting both the acidemia and hyperkalemia associated with type IV RTA. Resultant hypertension or edema may limit its use; concurrent use of a loop diuretic may mitigate these effects.[2]

PEARLS AND PITFALLS

- Fanconi's syndrome can occur in patients infected with the human immunodeficiency virus who are being treated with tenofovir.
- Because about 15% of patients with type 2 diabetes mellitus have a type IV RTA (hyporeninemic hypoaldosteronism), mild metabolic acidosis with concomitant hyperkalemia in these patients should not be overlooked. Further evaluation includes obtaining a urine anion gap and a transtubular potassium gradient.

REFERENCES

1. Smulders Y et al: Renal tubular acidosis: pathophysiology and diagnosis, *Arch Intern Med* 156:1629-1636, 1996. C
2. Penney, MD Oleeskey DA: Renal tubular acidosis, *Ann Clin Biochem* 36:408-422, 1999. C
3. Brenner, BM: *The kidney,* 7th ed, Philadelphia, 2004, WB Saunders. D

Disorders of Sodium Balance

Emily L. Schopick, MD; Kerri L. Cavanaugh, MD;
and Derek M. Fine, MD

> ## FAST FACTS
>
> - Disorders of sodium balance typically indicate problems with water balance; hyponatremia (Na < 135 mEq/L) usually is caused by an excess of free water, and hypernatremia (> 145 mEq/L) usually is caused by a deficit of free water.[1,2]
> - Severe hyponatremia occurs at serum sodium concentration less than 120 mEq/L.
> - Treatment is based on the severity of symptoms and the rate of development of hyponatremia. Too rapid correction of the serum [Na$^+$] may result in development of the osmotic demyelination syndrome and eventually central pontine myelinolysis.[3]
> - Treatment and prognosis of hypernatremia are based on the severity of symptoms and the rate of development of hypernatremia. Too rapid a correction of serum [Na$^+$] may result in the development of cerebral edema.
> - For hypernatremia to occur, there must be a combination of water loss and lack of access to water for repletion of that loss.

Hyponatremia[1,4,5]

I. EPIDEMIOLOGY

The prevalence of hyponatremia varies from 2.5% in hospitalized patients to 30% in patients in the intensive care unit.[3,6] Populations at high risk for acute neurologic symptoms include premenopausal women,[7] postoperative patients, patients taking thiazide diuretics, elderly hospitalized patients, endurance exercise participants, and patients with psychogenic polydipsia.

II. CLINICAL PRESENTATION

1. Symptoms of hyponatremia are related to both the absolute concentration of sodium and the rate of development of the hyponatremia. Acute hyponatremia refers to onset within 48 hours (Table 73-1).
2. Symptoms and physical findings are caused by excess water entry into cells of the brain and other tissues.[3] As a result, cerebral edema develops and can result in intracranial hypertension, particularly if the rate of development of hyponatremia is too rapid for the brain to adapt.

TABLE 73-1		
SYMPTOMS OF HYPONATREMIA		
Level of Hyponatremia	Serum [Na$^+$] (mEq/L)	Symptoms
Mild	125-135	Anorexia, apathy, restlessness, nausea, lethargy, muscle cramps
Moderate	120-125	Agitation, disorientation, headache
Severe	< 120	Seizures, coma, ↓ reflexes, Cheyne-Stokes breathing, incontinence, death

III. CAUSES

A. HYPOVOLEMIC HYPONATREMIA

1. This usually results from loss of both solute and fluid, with the replacement of fluid losses with water, in the presence of nonosmotic antidiuretic hormone (ADH) secretion. It occurs in the context of gastrointestinal losses, renal losses, excessive sweating, and third spacing of fluid.

2. Diuretic therapy can also cause acute, severe, hypovolemic hyponatremia in the setting of volume repletion with free water. In addition to direct volume depletion from the diuretic, thiazide diuretics cause hyponatremia by another mechanism: impairment of urinary dilution by diminishing distal NaCl reabsorption.[8]

B. EUVOLEMIC HYPONATREMIA

1. Syndrome of inappropriate AHD secretion (SIADH). Box 73-1 lists the causes and defining features of SIADH. There are four different osmoregulatory defects believed to cause SIADH[1]:

a. ADH secretion appears to be independent of osmoreceptor control, or a nonosmotic stimulus is present (e.g., paraneoplastic ADH release).

b. The osmostat is reset so that the threshold value for the stimulus of ADH secretion is below the normal range ([Na$^+$] about 125 to 130 mEq/L).

c. Urinary dilution is impaired because of a constant and nonsuppressible "leak" of ADH.

d. The osmoregulation response is normal, but the patient cannot excrete a water load, possibly because of renal sensitivity or another antidiuretic stimulus.

2. Cortisol deficiency results in ADH release. In addition, because ADH is co-secreted with corticotropin-releasing hormone by cells in the paraventricular nucleus, in the cortisol-deficient state the lack of a negative feedback may result in excessive ADH secretion.[4]

3. Severe hypothyroidism also can cause hyponatremia by an unknown mechanism.[4]

4. Primary polydipsia is a condition most commonly found in patients with psychiatric disorders such as schizophrenia. It manifests when a patient

---

BOX 73-1

SYNDROME OF INAPPROPRIATE ADH SECRETION

CAUSES

Enhanced hypothalamic ADH production
  Infections: meningitis, encephalitis, abscess, varicella-zoster virus
  Vascular: subarachnoid hemorrhage, cerebrovascular accident, temporal arteritis
  Other: neoplasm, psychosis, human immunodeficiency virus, Guillain-Barré
    syndrome, acute intermittent porphyria, hypothalamic sarcoidosis
Waldenström's macroglobulinemia
Pulmonary disease
Postoperative state
Severe nausea
Oxytocin during labor
Ectopic ADH production (small cell carcinoma of the lung)
Prolactinoma
Drugs: chlorpropamide, intravenous cyclophosphamide
Head trauma
Shy-Drager syndrome
Delirium tremens
Idiopathic

FEATURES

Hyponatremia and hypoosmolality
Urinary osmolality >100 mOsm/kg
Urinary sodium level >20 mEq/L
Hypouricemia in some cases
Normovolemia
Normal renal, adrenal, and thyroid function
Normal acid-base and potassium balance

ADH, antidiuretic hormone.

takes in more free water (about 12 to 20 L/day) than the kidney can excrete.

5. Irrigant absorption. During a transurethral resection of the prostate or with endoscopic urologic or gynecologic procedures, large volumes of hypotonic or isotonic solution (e.g., glycine) are used and can cause hyponatremia. Although there can be large fluctuations in serum [Na^+], plasma osmolality remains constant, and therefore cerebral edema is not a major problem.

C. HYPERVOLEMIC HYPONATREMIA

As with hypovolemic hypernatremia, decreased effective circulating volume leads to excessive secretion of ADH. This is seen with congestive heart failure, cirrhosis, and nephrotic syndrome, where total body Na^+ is elevated but total body water is elevated further. In the presence of a decreased effective circulating volume, the combination of thirst stimulation and ADH release with associated water retention results in hyponatremia.[5]

D. HYPERTONIC HYPONATREMIA

1. Although most hyponatremia is reflected by a hypotonic state, there are a few exceptions. Elevated serum osmolality can be associated with hyperglycemia, mannitol administration, or intravenous immune globulin administration with concurrent renal failure. These cases often are classified as translocational hyponatremia because they are caused by fluid shifts out of cells to adjust for the increased serum osmolality.
2. The correction for hyperglycemia is a 1.6 mEq/L reduction in plasma $[Na^+]$ for every 100 mg/dl elevation in plasma glucose.

IV. DIAGNOSIS

1. Diagnosis is based on laboratory assessment, specifically serum $[Na^+]$.
2. Plasma osmolarity (P_{osm}) can be used to distinguish between hypertonic hyponatremia and the other causes of hyponatremia. In the case of a normal P_{osm}, pseudohyponatremia (e.g., from hyperlipidemia, hyperproteinemia) should be considered.
3. Once it is determined that the P_{osm} is low, it is important to assess the patient's volume status, to categorize as hypovolemic, euvolemic, or hypervolemic. Other useful laboratories to determine the cause of the hyponatremia are urine osmolality, urine $[Na^+]$, and a full chemistry panel[1] (Table 73-2).

V. MANAGEMENT

A. GENERAL PRINCIPLES

1. Caution in the treatment of hyponatremia is driven by concern for the risk of developing osmotic demyelination syndrome and central pontine

TABLE 73-2

APPROACH TO HYPOOSMOTIC HYPONATREMIA BY VOLUME STATUS

Hypovolemia		Euvolemia	Hypervolemia	
$U_{Na} > 20$ mEq/L *Renal Losses*	$U_{Na} < 20$ mEq/L *Extrarenal Losses*	$U_{Na} >$ 20 mEq/L	$U_{Na} >$ 20 mEq/L	$U_{Na} <$ 20 mEq/L
Diuretic losses	Gastrointestinal	Glucocorticoid	Renal	Cirrhosis
Mineralocorticoid	losses (vomiting,	deficiency	failure	Pregnancy
deficiency	diarrhea)	Hypothyroidism		Nephrotic
Salt-losing	Burns	Drugs		syndrome
nephropathy	Pancreatitis	Syndrome of		Heart
Cerebral salt-wasting	Trauma	inappropriate		failure
syndrome	Marathon running	antidiuretic		
Bicarbonaturia with		hormone		
renal tubular		secretion		
acidosis and		Reset osmostat		
metabolic alkalosis				
Ketonuria				
Osmotic diuresis				

U_{Na}, urinary sodium.

myelinolysis (CPM). In the hyponatremic state, the brain initially swells as fluid shifts to equalize osmolality. As a compensatory mechanism, the brain produces intracellular solutes (e.g., taurine) that restore homeostasis. When hyponatremia is corrected too rapidly, fluid shifts out of the cells without allowing the brain time to adjust its solute contents. Through poorly understood mechanisms this results in demyelination of the central pons and other extrapontine sites. CPM is characterized by spastic quadriparesis, pseudobulbar palsy, swallowing dysfunction, and mutism.[3]

2. Because of the concern for the development of CPM, hyponatremia is treated aggressively only if it is severe or the patient is symptomatic.
3. If the hyponatremia is not severe and the patient not symptomatic, treatment is aimed at the underlying cause.

B. SEVERE, SYMPTOMATIC HYPONATREMIA (ANY CAUSE)

1. With symptomatic hyponatremia, the replacement rate should be no faster than 1 mEq/L/hr. See Box 73-2 for equations used in the management of sodium imbalances and Box 73-3 for an example of how to apply them.
2. Once the patient becomes asymptomatic, the desired rate of correction decreases to 0.5 to 1 mEq/L, with a maximum correction of 12 mEq/L in 24 hours.

BOX 73-2

FORMULAS TO GUIDE THERAPY FOR HYPONATREMIA

$P_{osm} = 2 \times [Na^+] + [Glucose]/18 + [BUN]/2.8$

$TBW = 0.6$ (men) or 0.5 (women) $\times$ Body weight (kg)

Sodium deficit (estimate) $= TBW \times$ (Desired [Na] – Plasma [Na])

Osmolal gap $=$ Measured P_{osm} – Calculated P_{osm} (normal <10 mOsm/L)

BUN, blood urea nitrogen; *P_{osm},* plasma osmolality; *TBW,* total body water.

BOX 73-3

EXAMPLE CALCULATION FOR THE TREATMENT OF SEVERE HYPONATREMIA

PATIENT INFORMATION

Sex, male; weight, 70 kg; serum sodium, 110 mEq/L.

STEP 1

Estimate TBW:

TBW = Weight in kg × 0.6 if male, 0.5 if female.

Therefore, in our patient, TBW = 70 kg × 0.6 = 42 L.

STEP 2

Calculate the effect of 1 L of 3% saline ($[Na^+] = 513$ mEq/L) on serum $[Na^+]$:

Δ in serum $[Na^+]$ per liter infused $=$ ([Infusate Na] – [Serum Na])/(TBW + 1).

Therefore, Δ in serum $[Na^+] = (513 - 110)/(42 + 1) = 9.4$ mEq/L.

STEP 3

Calculate the hourly infusion rate to raise serum $[Na^+]$ 1-2 L/hr:

To raise serum $[Na^+]$ 2 mEq/L/hr: 2/9.4 = 0.213 L/hr.

TBW, total body water.

DISORDERS OF SODIUM BALANCE

73

3. Once the serum sodium reaches 125 mEq/L, simple fluid restriction can correct the remaining deficit.

C. HYPOVOLEMIC HYPONATREMIA

1. Medications causing volume depletion should be discontinued.
2. The patient's hypovolemia should be corrected with normal saline. Once the intravascular volume is partially replenished, the nonosmotic signal for ADH secretion is inhibited, allowing the patient to maximally dilute urine and reverse hyponatremia.
3. Replace all electrolytes needed in the correction process. Depending on the cause of the hypovolemia, aggressive replacement of electrolytes such as potassium may be necessary.

D. EUVOLEMIC HYPONATREMIA

1. SIADH.
a. Treatment of SIADH includes fluid or free water restriction so that the total daily intake of free water is less than urinary free water excretion.
b. Loop diuretics can help induce excretion of hypotonic urine.
c. In chronic SIADH, demeclocycline (300 mg twice daily) can help by inducing nephrogenic diabetes insipidus (DI).
d. Use of isotonic saline can worsen hyponatremia in SIADH. Because osmotic urine losses are maintained in SIADH, the solute load may be excreted at a greater rate than ongoing water losses, resulting in net water retention and exacerbation of hyponatremia.
2. If the hyponatremia is caused by cortisol deficiency or hypothyroidism, correction of the underlying disorder leads to normalization of serum sodium.
3. If the hyponatremia is caused by psychogenic polydipsia, limiting free water intake will normalize serum sodium.

E. HYPERVOLEMIC HYPONATREMIA

1. Fluid or free water restriction.
2. Treatment of the underlying disease. Loop diuretics may help by mobilizing fluid and inducing excretion of hypotonic urine.

F. HYPERTONIC HYPONATREMIA

Treating the underlying cause of hypertonicity will restore Na^+ balance.

Hypernatremia[2,4,5]

I. EPIDEMIOLOGY

1. Sixty to eighty percent of hypernatremia develops in hospitalized patients. In hospitalized patients, hypernatremia usually is iatrogenic, occurring in intubated patients or patients with mental status changes who do not have the ability to access free water. In contrast, patients presenting to the hospital with hypernatremia usually have an underlying infection and typically are older, female, and nursing home residents.

2. The mortality rate associated with hypernatremia is high. A serum [Na$^+$] greater than 160 mEq/L is associated with a 75% mortality. The risk of mortality rises as the [Na$^+$] increases.

II. CLINICAL PRESENTATION

1. Symptoms of hypernatremia vary with the severity of the Na$^+$ elevation. Because hypernatremia often is associated with dehydration, patients with mild hypernatremia may present with symptoms such as tachycardia, orthostasis, hypotension, and dry mucous membranes.
2. Symptoms of severe hypernatremia include restlessness, irritability, lethargy, muscle twitching, hyperreflexia, and spasticity.
3. Cerebral edema develops when hypernatremia is corrected too rapidly. This is characterized by deterioration of neurologic symptoms after initial improvement and can eventually lead to coma, convulsions, and death.

III. CAUSES

A. HYPOVOLEMIC HYPERNATREMIA

1. This is the most common cause of hypernatremia, often characterized by decreased water intake in combination with impaired renal urinary concentration, hypotonic gastrointestinal losses, or increased insensible losses. Homeostatic mechanisms attempt to compensate for increased osmolarity by increasing the sensation of thirst, thereby increasing water ingestion. Hypernatremia occurs with any breakdown in this feedback system.
2. **Decreased access to free water.** In hospitalized patients, there is often increased free water loss (e.g., from fevers). Many of these patients have limited access to fluids and therefore are at risk for hypernatremia.
3. **Decreased sensation of thirst.**
a. In older adults, the sensitivity of thirst sensors declines, placing these patients at high risk for hypernatremia.
b. Primary hypodipsia is a condition in which thirst centers in the hypothalamus are destroyed. This most commonly results from metastatic cancer (about 50%), vascular abnormalities (about 15%), and trauma.
4. **Impaired free water reabsorption.**
a. Central DI is a condition of deficient vasopressin secretion in the hypothalamus (Box 73-4).
b. Nephrogenic DI is a condition of decreased kidney collecting duct response to ADH and the resulting failure to absorb water and concentrate urine (see Box 73-4).

B. EUVOLEMIC HYPERNATREMIA

Many of the causes of hypotonic hypernatremia can also cause euvolemic hypernatremia. For instance, a patient with DI or primary hypodipsia may not appear hypovolemic.

BOX 73-4

CAUSES OF DIABETES INSIPIDUS

Central: idiopathic, head trauma, suprasellar and infrasellar tumors (e.g., craniopharyngioma), cerebral hemorrhage, central nervous system infections (e.g., meningitis, encephalitis), granulomatous disorders (e.g., tuberculosis, sarcoid, Wegener's, histiocytosis)

Nephrogenic: congenital renal disorders, obstructive uropathy, renal dysplasia, polycystic disease

Systemic disease with renal involvement: sickle cell disease, sarcoidosis, amyloidosis

Drugs: amphotericin B, phenytoin, lithium, aminoglycosides, methoxyflurane

---

C. HYPERVOLEMIC HYPERNATREMIA

1. This is a very rare cause of hypernatremia. It can occur in patients with severe intravascular volume depletion with underlying congestive heart failure, liver cirrhosis, or nephrotic syndrome, causing hypotonic fluid to shift into extravascular spaces.[5]
2. Hypervolemic hypernatremia can also occur with large infusions of hypertonic solutions. Some of these solutions include increased sodium in total parental nutrition, sodium bicarbonate during cardiac arrest, and intravenous hypertonic saline during abortions. All of these solutions cause hypernatremia only in the setting of decreased water intake or renal impairment of water reabsorption.

IV. DIAGNOSIS

1. See Fig. 73-1.[9]
2. The following should be noted:
a. Urine osmolality is inappropriately low (< 150 mmol/kg) in cases of renal losses such as DI and appropriately high (> 700 mmol/kg) with extrarenal hypotonic losses. Urine often is isotonic with the use of diuretics.
b. Urine [Na$^+$] is high with renal losses and low with extrarenal losses as the kidney works to reabsorb sodium. In cases of increased sodium infusion causing hypervolemic hypernatremia, urine [Na$^+$] often is high.

V. MANAGEMENT

A. GENERAL PRINCIPLES

Proper management depends on both the acuity of hypernatremia and the patient's symptoms. In the absence of severe [Na$^+$] elevations or symptoms, treatment should be directed at the underlying cause.

B. ACUTE OR SYMPTOMATIC HYPERNATREMIA

1. In acute hypernatremia that has developed over the course of hours, rapid correction improves prognosis, and there is very little risk of cerebral edema. In these patients, the goal is to lower the serum

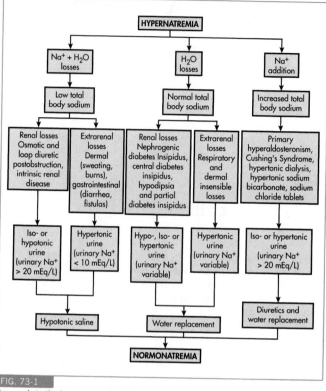

FIG. 73-1

Approach to the hypernatremic patient. (*Modified from Walsh PC et al, eds: Campbell's urology, 8th ed, Philadelphia, 2002, WB Saunders.*)

[Na$^+$] by 1 mEq/L/hour to a goal of 145 mmol/L (see Box 73-2 and Box 73-5).

2. Once the patient is no longer symptomatic, correction can be slowed to 0.5 mEq/L/hr, with a goal of no more than 10 mEq/L/day.

C. CHRONIC HYPERNATREMIA

In chronic hypernatremia, developed over the course of more than 24 hours, or in hypernatremia of unknown duration, correction should be much slower in order to reduce the risk of cerebral edema. The maximal rate of correction should be 0.5 mEq/L/hr, and the target reduction in 24 hours is 10 mEq/L/hr. The formulas in Box 73-2 can also be used.

D. DIABETES INSIPIDUS

1. In hypothalamic, or central, DI treatment includes hormone replacement with desmopressin acetate. The most common route is 5 to 20 μg

---

BOX 73-5

EXAMPLE CALCULATION FOR THE TREATMENT OF SEVERE HYPERNATREMIA

PATIENT INFORMATION

Sex, male; weight, 70 kg; serum sodium, 160 mEq/L.

STEP 1

Estimate TBW:

TBW = Weight in kg × 0.6 in males, 0.5 in females.

Therefore, in our patient, TBW = 70 kg × 0.6 = 42 L.

STEP 2

Determine the effect on serum $[Na^+]$ of 1 L of D5W:

Δ serum $[Na^+]$ per liter D5W = ([Infusate Na] − [Serum Na])/(TBW + 1).

Therefore, Δ in serum $[Na^+]$ per liter of D5W = (0 − 160)/(42 + 1) = 3.72 mEq/L.

STEP 3

Determine hourly infusion rate to decrease $[Na^+]$ 1 mEq/L/hour:

1/3.72 = 0.269 L/hr or 269 mL/hour.

D5W, 5% dextrose in water; *TBW,* total body water.

twice daily intranasally, although it is also possible to administer 1 to 2 µg intravenously or subcutaneously every 12 to 24 hours.

2. In nephrogenic DI, treatment involves a low-salt diet and a thiazide diuretic to induce a mildly negative Na^+ balance. Culprit medications should be discontinued.

PEARLS AND PITFALLS

- Beer potomania or "tea and toast syndrome" is a phenomenon seen in patients who drink excessive amounts of beer or tea (hypotonic solutions) and do not consume a protein- and solute-rich diet. Without solute, the maximal urine volume capacity is significantly reduced, and the patient cannot excrete sufficient amounts of water.[1]

- Risk factors for central pontine myelinolysis include more than 12 mEq/L elevation in plasma sodium in the first 24 hours, overcorrection of plasma sodium to more than 140 mEq/L in the first 48 hours, hypoxic or anoxic episodes, hypercatabolism (burns), and malnutrition (alcohol).

- Overcorrection of hyponatremia sometimes occurs because of failure to recognize exogenous sources of sodium (e.g., fluid administered in the emergency room before admission) or an electrolyte shift caused by concomitant administration of potassium. Overcorrection can be addressed by free water infusion.[10]

- Isotonic saline should not be used to correct hypernatremia unless the patient has hemodynamic compromise from volume loss. Although the concentration often is less than the patient's serum $[Na^+]$, it is often not sufficient to correct the hypernatremia.[2]

- Patients with DI do not develop hypernatremia unless water access is restricted or thirst sensing is not intact.

- Given their inability to retain free water, administering normal saline to patients with DI will worsen hypernatremia.

REFERENCES

1. Adrogue JH, Madias NE: Hyponatremia, *N Engl J Med* 342:1581, 2000. C
2. Adrogue JH, Madias NE: Hypernatremia, *N Engl J Med* 342:1493-1499, 2000. C
3. Laureno R, Karp BI: Myelinolysis after correction of hyponatremia, *Ann Intern Med* 126(1):57, 1997. C
4. Rose BD et al: *Clinical physiology of acid-base and electrolyte disorders,* New York, 1994, McGraw-Hill. C
5. Kumar S, Berl T: Sodium, *Lancet* 352:220, 1998. C
6. Lee CT, Guo HR, Chen JB: Hyponatremia in the emergency department, *Am J Emerg Med* 18:264, 2000. B
7. Ayus JC, Wheeler JM, Arieff AI: Postoperative hyponatremia encephalopathy in menstruant women, *Ann Intern Med* 117:891, 1992. B
8. Ashraf N, Locksley R, Arieff AI: Thiazide-induced hyponatremia associated with death or neurologic damage in outpatients, *Am J Med* 70:1163, 1981. C
9. Blumenfeld JD, Vaughan ED Jr: Renal physiology and pathophysiology. In Walsh PC et al, eds: *Campbell's urology,* 8th ed, Philadelphia, 2002, WB Saunders. B
10. Phuong-Chi TP, Chen PV, Phung-Thu TP: Overcorrection of hyponatremia: where do we go wrong? *Am J Kidney Dis* 36:1, 2000. C

73

Disorders of Potassium Homeostasis

Deidra C. Crews, MD; Patty P. Chi, MD; and Michael J. Choi, MD

> **FAST FACTS**
>
> - Hyperkalemia most commonly occurs in patients with impaired kidney function.
> - Cardiac arrhythmia is the major complication of hyperkalemia. An electrocardiogram (ECG) should be obtained to look for peaked T waves, PR prolongation, ST segment depression, widening of QRS complexes, and flattening of P waves.
> - Treatment options for hyperkalemia include intravenous calcium gluconate or chloride to stabilize the myocardium, 50% dextrose in water and insulin to cause temporary transcellular shifts, inhaled albuterol as adjunctive treatment with insulin and glucose, and diuretics and sodium polystyrene sulfonate (Kayexalate) for permanent removal of potassium. Patients with severe hyperkalemia and severe electrocardiographic abnormalities with renal failure should be treated with dialysis.
> - The most common cause of hypokalemia in hospitalized patients is the use of loop or thiazide diuretics.
> - Symptoms of severe hypokalemia include muscle fatigue and arrhythmias.
> - The quickest method of potassium repletion is with enteral formulations. Care must be exercised in replenishing potassium in patients with a low glomerular filtration rate.

The plasma potassium level is determined by potassium intake, equilibration of potassium across cell membranes, and urinary potassium excretion. Alterations in any one of these factors can result in a change in the serum concentration. Most potassium is excreted by the kidneys. Potassium secretion into the urine is regulated primarily at the cortical collecting tubule. This secretion is stimulated by elevated plasma potassium concentration, aldosterone, and sodium and water delivery to the distal nephron.[1]

I. HYPERKALEMIA

A. EPIDEMIOLOGY AND ETIOLOGY

Although hyperkalemia can be seen in a number of settings, the patients at greatest risk are those with impaired renal function. Since the publication of the Randomized Aldactone Evaluation Study in 1999, which showed a substantial reduction in morbidity and mortality in patients with severe heart failure who were treated with the aldosterone antagonist spironolactone, the rate of hospitalization for hyperkalemia has risen from 2.4 per 1000 patients in 1994 to 11 per 1000 patients in 2001.[2]

B. PRESENTATION

Hyperkalemia can affect multiple organ systems (Table 74-1).

C. DIAGNOSIS

1. Hyperkalemia is defined as a serum [K^+] greater than 5 mEq/L and can be life threatening when severe (serum [K^+] > 6.5 mEq/L).[3,4] It is important to repeat an abnormal value to ensure that no laboratory error has occurred and that hyperkalemia is not factitious.

2. Obtaining an ECG is imperative in the evaluation of hyperkalemia. It is important to note that there is wide variability between potassium levels and electrocardiographic manifestations. For example, one patient with a potassium level of 6 mEq/L may have no electrocardiographic changes, another may have peaked T waves, whereas a third patient with the same potassium level may have sine wave morphology. Generally, however, peaked T waves are seen in mild hyperkalemia, and sine wave morphology is seen in severe hyperkalemia. Patients with chronic hyperkalemia (i.e., chronic kidney disease) may have few or no electrocardiographic changes and usually can tolerate hyperkalemia better than those with acute hyperkalemia.

3. See Box 74-1 for the differential diagnosis of hyperkalemia.

D. MANAGEMENT OF HYPERKALEMIA

If serum K^+ rises above 6.5 mEq/L or if the ECG shows conduction abnormalities, urgent treatment to lower the serum K^+ should be initiated. The goals of treatment of acute hyperkalemia are to stabilize the cardiac myocyte cellular membrane with calcium and decrease the serum K^+, either temporarily through cellular shifts with insulin and glucose or permanently via diuresis or K^+-binding medications. Inhaled albuterol can be used to shift K^+ intracellularly if intravenous access is not available (however, this has failed in 40% of patients on hemodialysis).[7] Inpatients with hyperkalemia (especially if acute) should be placed on telemetry to monitor potential electrocardiographic changes. See Table 74-2 for further treatment measures, their effects on serum K^+ concentration, and their duration of action.

TABLE 74-1	
PATHOPHYSIOLOGIC EFFECTS OF HYPERKALEMIA[3]	
Cardiovascular	Electrocardiographic manifestations: peaked T waves, PR prolongation, ST segment depression, loss of P waves, QRS widening to sine-wave
	Arrhythmia (e.g., ventricular fibrillation, asystole)
Neuromuscular	Muscle weakness, paralysis, and paresthesia
Gastrointestinal	Nausea, vomiting, and ileus
Renal	Natriuresis, decreased ammonia production
Endocrine	Increased aldosterone and insulin secretion

BOX 74-1

DIFFERENTIAL DIAGNOSIS OF HYPERKALEMIA[4-6]

FACTITIOUS

Thrombocytosis (platelets $>1,000,000/mm^3$)

Leukocytosis (white blood cell count $>100,000/mm^3$)

Hemolysis

Repeated fist clenching with tourniquet in place

INCREASED POTASSIUM LOAD

Potassium supplements

Herbal remedies (e.g., noni juice, alfalfa, dandelion, horsetail, nettle)

Stored packed red blood cells (after >10 d of storage)

Penicillin G potassium (1.7 mEq/10^6 U)

IMPAIRED K^+ EXCRETION

Renal insufficiency or failure

Decreased effective circulating volume (e.g., congestive heart failure)

Tubulointerstitial disorders (e.g., lupus nephritis, amyloidosis, sickle cell anemia)

Ureterojejunostomy (absorption of urinary potassium by the jejunum)

MINERALOCORTICOID DEFICIENCY

Addison's disease

Hyporeninemic hypoaldosteronism (type IV renal tubular acidosis)

Isolated hypoaldosteronism

Hereditary enzyme deficiencies

Pseudohypoaldosteronism

MEDICATIONS THAT IMPAIR K^+ EXCRETION

K^+-sparing diuretics that block Na^+ channels (triamterene, amiloride)

Trimethoprim, pentamidine (block Na^+ channels, which impairs exchange with K^+)

Spironolactone (competitive inhibitor of aldosterone)

Angiotensin-converting enzyme inhibitors and angiotensin receptor blockers

Nonsteroidal antiinflammatory drugs (impair release of renin)

Heparin (inhibits aldosterone production)

Cyclosporine, tacrolimus (multiple mechanisms)

IMPAIRED K^+ ENTRY INTO CELLS

Metabolic acidosis (transcellular shift of K^+ out of cells, mineral $>$ organic acidosis)

Insulin deficiency

Hypertonicity (uncontrolled diabetes)

Massive tissue breakdown (rhabdomyolysis, burns, trauma)

Familial hyperkalemic periodic paralysis

DRUGS THAT IMPAIR K^+ ENTRY INTO CELLS

β-blockers (decrease activity of sodium-potassium adenosine triphosphatase)

Digoxin (at toxic levels)

Succinylcholine

Arginine

Lysine

TABLE 74-2

TREATMENT OF HYPERKALEMIA[7,8]

EMERGENT TREATMENT

Intervention	Change in [K⁺]	Response Time	Duration
Calcium gluconate or chloride (10 ml of 10% solution). Note: Intravenous calcium should not be given in the setting of digoxin toxicity.	No effect on serum K^+	Immediate	15-30 min
Glucose (50 ml of 50% solution) + regular insulin 10 U intravenously.	0.5-1.2 mmol/L	10-20 min	2-3 hr
Albuterol 10-20 mg by inhaler over 10 min.	0.9-1.4 mmol/L	20-30 min	2-3 hr
NaHCO₃⁻, only if metabolic acidosis present.		Delayed	
Kayexalate 15-30 g with sorbitol:			
By mouth.	Binds 0.5-1.2 mEq K^+ in exchange for 2-3 mEq Na^+	4-6 hr	Permanent
As retention enema.	As above	1 hr	Permanent
Loop diuretic (intravenous).	Variable	1 hr	Permanent
Hemodialysis	1.2-1.5 mmol/L during the 1st hour	15-30 min	Permanent

LONG-TERM MANAGEMENT

Dietary K^+ restriction 2-3 g/d (avoid orange juice, melons, bananas, tomatoes)
Discontinue supplemental K^+ (salt substitutes)
Discontinue drugs that interfere with K^+ homeostasis (see Box 74-1)
Augment K^+ excretion
Loop, thiazide diuretics
Fludrocortisone, if hypoaldosteronism present
Chronic sodium polystyrene sulfonate therapy (in patients without gastrointestinal disease)

II. HYPOKALEMIA

A. EPIDEMIOLOGY AND ETIOLOGY

Hypokalemia is a common problem in patients prescribed diuretics and in patients with diarrhea.

B. PRESENTATION

1. Mild hypokalemia is generally well tolerated except in patients with ischemic or scarred cardiac muscle, in whom ectopy and arrhythmias may occur, and in those treated with digoxin.[9,10]

2. Severe hypokalemia (i.e., serum $[K^+] < 2.5$ mEq/L) can result in rhabdomyolysis or even respiratory arrest secondary to diaphragmatic paralysis (seen with serum $[K^+] < 2.0$ mEq/L).

C. DIAGNOSIS

Hypokalemia is most commonly defined as a serum $[K^+]$ less than 3.6 mEq/L and is most commonly caused by either inadequate intake (rare) or increased losses, with the most common cause being the use of diuretics.[8] See Box 74-2 for a differential diagnosis of hypokalemia.

D. MANAGEMENT OF HYPOKALEMIA (Box 74-3)

1. Treatment for hypokalemia should include stopping or reducing the offending agent (i.e., diuretics) and repleting K^+ to a normal value.
2. In cases of severe hypokalemia (serum $[K^+] < 2.0$ mEq/L), wherein cardiac arrhythmias, myopathy, or paralysis may be present, intravenous potassium administration is warranted. In cases of intravenous potassium use, a cardiac monitor should be used.
3. Oral replacement therapy should be attempted in other cases. The preferred salt for repletion is KCl (except in cases of renal tubular acidosis), given in divided doses (10 to 40 mEq per dose).
4. If low, magnesium should also be replenished because hypomagnesemia impairs the ability to replenish potassium.[4]

BOX 74-2

DIFFERENTIAL DIAGNOSIS OF HYPOKALEMIA[4]

INADEQUATE INTAKE (< 40 mEq/d)

INCREASED EXCRETION

Diarrhea, laxative abuse

Renal losses

   Loop, thiazide diuretics

   Metabolic alkalosis (vomiting, nasogastric drainage)

   Osmotic diuresis (uncontrolled diabetes)

   Nonresorbable anions (penicillins)

   Mineralocorticoid excess: primary hyperaldosteronism, glucocorticoid-responsive aldosteronism, congenital adrenal hyperplasia

Apparent mineralocorticoid excess: Liddle's syndrome, 11β-hydroxysteroid dehydrogenase deficiency, licorice

Glucocorticoids (high dose)

Bartter's and Gitelman's syndromes

Magnesium depletion

Renal tubular acidosis (types 1 and 2)

SHIFT OF K^+ INTO CELLS

Medications: β-adrenergic agonists (e.g., albuterol), theophylline, insulin

Delirium tremens

Treatment of megaloblastic anemia, neutropenia

Familial hypokalemic periodic paralysis

Barium (soluble) poisoning

BOX 74-3

TREATMENT OF HYPOKALEMIA[4]

INTRAVENOUS KCl

Dosage: maximum rate of 20 mEq/hr with cardiac monitoring; reassess after 60 mEq.

Indications: cardiac arrhythmias with rapid ventricular response, cardiac arrhythmias caused by digoxin toxicity, severe diarrhea, severe myopathy with muscle necrosis, and paralysis.

ORAL KCl

Dosage: 20-80 mEq/day in divided doses.

Indications: all other settings except renal tubular acidosis.

ORAL $KHCO_3$, CITRATE

Dosage: 20-80 mEq/day in divided doses.

Indications: renal tubular acidosis.

PEARLS AND PITFALLS

- One clue to the presence of hemolysis (and thus factitious hyperkalemia) is an elevated aspartate aminotransferase (AST).
- Administration of excessive sodium bicarbonate should be avoided because alkalosis may exacerbate arrhythmia.
- The transtubular potassium gradient (TTKG) is a way to distinguish impaired renal potassium excretion from other causes of hyperkalemia: TTKG = (Urine K)/(Urine osmolality/Plasma osmolality)(Plasma K). A TTKG less than 7 suggests decreased K^+ excretion, usually resulting from aldosterone deficiency or resistance.
- Bicarbonate generally is not effective in treating hyperkalemia in patients with end-stage renal disease unless there is severe metabolic acidosis.
- Sodium polystyrene sulfonate should not be given to patients with impaired gastrointestinal motility or constipation because it has been associated with acute colonic necrosis.
- Volume overload may be a problem with sodium polystyrene sulfonate use because potassium is bound in exchange for sodium.[10]

REFERENCES

1. Rose BD, Post TW: *Clinical physiology of acid-base and electrolyte disorders,* 5th ed, New York, 2001, McGraw-Hill. C
2. Juurlink DN et al: Rates of hyperkalemia after publication of the randomized Aldactone evaluation study, *N Engl J Med* 351(6):543-551, 2004. B
3. Johnson RJ, Feehally J: *Comprehensive clinical nephrology,* St Louis, 2000, Mosby. C
4. Gennari FJ: Disorders of potassium homeostasis: hypokalemia and hyperkalemia, *Crit Care Clin* 18(2):273-288, 2002. C
5. Wiederkehr MR, Moe OW: Factitious hyperkalemia, *Am J Kidney Dis* 36(5):1049-1053, 2000. C
6. Perazella MA: Drug-induced hyperkalemia: old culprits and new offenders, *Am J Med* 109:307-314, 2000. C

7. Greenberg A: Hyperkalemia: treatment options, *Semin Nephrol* 18:46-57, 1998. C
8. Brenner B: *The kidney,* 7th ed, Philadelphia, 2004, WB Saunders. C
9. Gennari FJ: Hypokalemia, *N Engl J Med* 339:451-458, 1998. C
10. Schulman M, Narins RG: Hypokalemia and cardiovascular disease, *Am J Cardiol* 65:4E-9E, 1990. C

Allograft Dysfunction in Renal Transplantation

Timothy Scialla, MD; and Milagros Samaniego, MD

FAST FACTS

- The differential diagnosis of kidney allograft dysfunction includes acute rejection, drug-induced toxicity, infection, recurrence of disease, surgical or mechanical complications, and chronic dysfunction.
- The most common cause of acute renal allograft dysfunction after transplantation is reversible ischemic acute tubular necrosis.
- The most common feature of allograft dysfunction is an elevation in the serum creatinine of more than 20% baseline value.
- The initial evaluation of allograft dysfunction includes measuring immunosuppressant drug levels; duplex ultrasonography; biopsy and, in certain cases, renal scintigraphy.
- High-dose corticosteroids are used initially to treat new episodes of acute cellular rejection. Episodes that are steroid resistant are treated with anti–T cell antibodies such as OKT3 or antithymocyte globulin (Thymoglobulin). Occasionally, steroid-resistant rejection can be caused by antibodies.

75

In 2002, more than 14,000 people in the United States received a transplanted kidney; 6236 patients received a living donor kidney, with the remaining receiving cadaveric transplants. The most common indications for transplantation were diabetes mellitus, hypertensive nephrosclerosis, and glomerular diseases.[1] Although many issues factor into successful kidney transplantation, clear risk factors for poor outcomes include previous transplantation, human leukocyte antigen (HLA) mismatch, prior HLA sensitization with more than 50% panel reactive antibodies, the presence of delayed graft function, the number of rejection episodes, and allograft dysfunction after transplantation. This chapter provides an approach to allograft dysfunction in a kidney transplant recipients.

I. PHYSIOLOGY OF THE TRANSPLANTED KIDNEY

1. The physiologic function of the transplanted kidney correlates with both glomerular filtration rate and nephron mass. The nephron mass of the transplanted kidney is affected by donor factors (i.e., age of donor and comorbidities), cold and warm ischemia time of the allograft, recipient factors (e.g., hypertension, hepatitis C), nephrotoxic drugs, and episodes of acute rejection.[2]

2. The metabolic function of the transplanted kidneys leads to improvement in the recipient's erythropoiesis and calcium and phosphate homeostasis. Erythropoietin levels increase in the early postoperative period, leading to increased red blood cell mass. In addition, the transplanted kidney restores the levels of 1,25-dihydroxy vitamin D, thus helping to normalize parathyroid hormone levels in most cases.

3. Both proximal and distal tubular injury in the transplanted kidney can occur. Causes include preservation injury, acute rejection, and tertiary hyperparathyroidism. Manifestations include glucosuria in the absence of hyperglycemia, Fanconi's syndrome, and hyperkalemia. Hyperkalemia is believed to be multifactorial, with cyclosporin, tacrolimus, and sulfas playing a major role.

II. DIAGNOSIS (Fig. 75-1)

1. **Serum creatinine.** The most common feature of allograft dysfunction is an asymptomatic elevation in the serum creatinine to more than 20% baseline value. Such an elevation warrants prompt evaluation.

2. **Immunosuppressant levels.** Because high concentrations of calcineurin inhibitors (CNIs) and rapamycin are associated with allograft dysfunction (e.g., cyclosporine > 350 ng/ml, tacrolimus levels > 20 ng/ml, rapamycin levels > 15 ng/ml), trough levels should be determined early in the evaluation.

3. **Duplex ultrasound.** Ultrasound is a noninvasive test often used during episodes of allograft dysfunction. It provides information about the vascular supply to the allograft with a sensitivity of 100% and specificity of 86% for detecting renal artery stenosis. In addition, it is useful for detecting hydronephrosis, perigraft fluid collections, and masses.[3]

4. **Renal biopsy.** When no mechanical or drug-related cause for an increase in creatinine is found, biopsy is needed to examine the histology of the allograft and tailor appropriate therapy.

5. **Renal scintigraphy.** Renal scintigraphy is a three-phase nuclear medicine study used to assess perfusion, function, and excretion. In the first phase, perfusion to the allograft is assessed. The second phase is the parenchymal phase, during which tracer accumulates in the graft and the clearance of the transplant is evaluated. The third phase is the excretory phase, which assesses the integrity of the ureteral system.[3]

III. CAUSES OF ALLOGRAFT DYSFUNCTION

A. HYPERACUTE REJECTION

1. **Epidemiology.** Hyperacute rejection is now rare because of better crossmatching techniques. It is caused by preformed antibodies against donor antigens that arise from pretransplant blood transfusions, pregnancy, or previous transplantation.

2. **Presentation.** The ischemic damage to the kidney often is manifested on the operating table as thrombosis, cyanosis, and anuria.

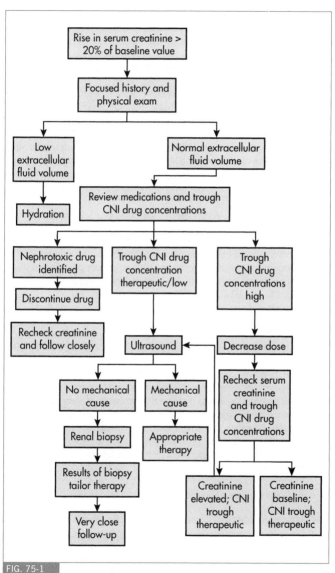

FIG. 75-1

Approach to the transplant recipient with an elevated creatinine. *CNI,* calcineurin inhibitor. *(Modified from Peddi RV, First MR: In Norman DJ, Turka LA, eds: Primer on transplantation, 2nd ed, Mt Laurel, NJ, 2001, American Society of Transplantation.)*

3. **Diagnosis.** Minimal or absent perfusion can be seen radiographically. Fibrin tissue necrosis is seen histologically.
4. **Management.** There is no effective treatment. The transplanted kidney should be removed promptly.

B. **ACCELERATED ACUTE REJECTION AND ACUTE HUMORAL REJECTION**

1. **Epidemiology.** Acute humoral rejection occurs in recipients presensitized to donor alloantigens, which are below the crossmatch detection threshold. After transplantation, the antibody levels increase dramatically and lead to allograft destruction.
2. **Presentation.** Rejection typically occurs 2 to 5 days after transplantation and can occur in both an initially functioning graft and one recovering from peritransplant acute tubular necrosis.
3. **Diagnosis.** Diagnosis is made through repeat crossmatch results and biopsy. Findings include thrombosis of glomeruli and small vessels, neutrophil infiltration of peritubular capillaries, and C4d staining in peritubular capillaries.[4]
4. **Management.** Traditional treatment with immunosuppressive antibodies and corticosteroids had a response less than 50%. Newer modalities that incorporate plasmapheresis, intravenous gamma-globulin, and enhanced immunosuppression have yielded better results.

C. **ACUTE CELLULAR REJECTION**

1. **Epidemiology.** Acute cellular rejection typically occurs in the first 3 months after transplantation and involves T cell–mediated mechanisms of injury. There has been a decline in the reported incidence of early acute rejection (0 to 6 months after transplantation) from 37% in 1991 to 18% in 1998.[4]
2. **Presentation.** The most common presentation is an elevation in the serum creatinine more than 20% baseline. With current immunosuppressive drugs, the cardinal symptoms of fever, allograft tenderness, and oliguria are rarely pronounced but can still be present.
3. **Diagnosis.** Diagnosis is made on biopsy. Histologically, the most common findings are mononuclear infiltration of an edematous interstitium and lymphocytic infiltration of the tubular epithelium.
4. **Management.** Treatment is with high-dose corticosteroids (500 to 1000 mg/day of methylprednisolone for 3 to 5 days). Immunosuppressive antibodies are used in cases of steroid resistance (e.g., OKT3).

D. **CHRONIC REJECTION**

1. **Epidemiology.** Chronic rejection is the most common cause of late allograft failure and results in a dramatic decrease in allograft half-life (5.2 vs. 17 years). Although the pathophysiology is poorly understood, there are clearly defined risk factors[4] (Box 75-1).
2. **Presentation.** The clinical presentation is that of a low and gradual decline in renal function, as evidenced by elevation in serum creatinine, persistent proteinuria, and hypertension.

BOX 75-1

RISK FACTORS FOR THE DEVELOPMENT OF CHRONIC RENAL ALLOGRAFT REJECTION

Delayed graft function
Ischemia reperfusion injury
Human leukocyte antigen mismatching
Acute rejection episodes
Inadequate renal mass
Hypertension
Hyperlipidemia
Cytomegalovirus infection

3. **Diagnosis.** The diagnosis is based on characteristic histologic changes seen on renal biopsy in conjunction with a gradual decline in renal function. Histologic changes include interstitial fibrosis with lymphocytic infiltrates, tubular atrophy, and obliterative arteriopathy with both medial intimal fibrosis, and glomerular changes.

4. **Management.** Treatment has been disappointing. Supportive measures include strict control of hyperlipidemia and blood pressure, the use of angiotensin-converting enzyme inhibitors or angiotensin-II receptor blockers for proteinuria and hypertension, aggressive treatment of all episodes of acute rejection, and reduction or discontinuation of CNIs.

E. **INFECTION: HUMAN POLYOMAVIRUS (BK, JC, AND SV40)**

1. **Epidemiology.** Polyomaviruses (e.g., BK virus) are ubiquitous DNA viruses to which 80% of the adult population has serologic evidence of exposure. Reactivation is estimated to occur in 10% to 60% of transplant recipients.

2. **Presentation.** The clinical features associated with infection include asymptomatic infection, acute graft dysfunction (secondary to interstitial nephritis), and hemorrhagic cystitis.

3. **Diagnosis.** Although the finding of decoy cells on urine cytology suggests infection, allograft biopsy is needed for definitive diagnosis of polyomavirus-associated interstitial nephritis. Light microscopy findings include the presence of intranuclear tubular cell inclusions. Immunohistochemistry confirms the diagnosis. Plasma sample polymerase chain reaction testing is an emerging diagnostic tool.[4]

4. **Management.** Treatment of BK nephropathy is challenging because decreasing immunosuppression can lead to rejection and cytokine production, which stimulates viral replication. Conversely, increasing immunosuppression decreases the host's ability to control the viremia. The best initial treatment option is to attempt to reduce immunosuppression with the hope of improving host viral clearance. Cidofovir, a nephrotoxic antiviral agent, has been used because of its antipolyomavirus effect. Its role in renal transplant recipients is not clear. Leflunomide is actively being investigated as a suitable option for

TABLE 75-1

RECURRENT DISEASES AFTER RENAL TRANSPLANTATION

Disease	Recurrence Rate in Graft	Time to Recurrence	Treatment of Recurrence	Living Donor Transplant?	Comments
Primary focal segmental glomerulosclerosis	40-50%	Hours to weeks	Plasmapheresis, steroids, ACE-Is.	No, if very high risk of recurrence	Elevated risk in recipients with rapid progression to end-stage renal disease or previous allograft loss from this condition.
MPGN	MPGN-I, 15-30% MPGN-II, 80%	Weeks to years	Plasmapheresis, high-dose MMF.	No, if very high risk of recurrence	Elevated risk in patients with low complement titers at the time of treatment.
IgA nephropathy	35%	2 mo onward	ACE-Is; fish oil; if crescentic GN, cytotoxics.	Yes	Overall graft survival is equivalent to that of other renal diseases.
Membranous nephropathy	9.6%	Weeks to years	High-dose MMF. Rituximab?	Yes	High risk for renal vein thrombosis in patients with nephrotic syndrome.
Anti-glomerular basement membrane disease	Rare	Immediately	Plasmapheresis, cyclophosphamide.	Yes	Hold transplant until clinical remission and negative serology for 6-12 mo.

Systemic lupus erythematosus	< 10%	From 1st wk onward	Increased steroids; MMF or cyclophosphamide.	Yes	Severe recurrence is rare.
Antiphospholipid antibody syndrome	30%	Immediately onward	Prevention with anticoagulation is best.	Yes	Can be associated with large vessel thrombosis and thrombotic microangiopathy.
Wegener's granulomatosis	10%	From 1st wk	Cyclophosphamide.	Yes	Avoid transplantation if disease is active.
HUS and TTP	Atypical > classic HUS	Immediately onward	Plasma exchange only in TTP cases or patients with factor H deficiency.	Yes, if not familial	Recurrence is associated with poor prognosis for graft; hold transplant until disease is quiescent > 6 mo.

Modified from Kotanko, et al: *Transplantation* 63: 1045-1050, 1997.

ACE-I, angiotensin-converting enzyme inhibitor; *GN*, glomerulonephritis; *HUS*, hemolytic uremic syndrome; *MMF*, mycophendate mofetil; *MPGN*, membranoproliferative glomerulonephritis; *TTP*, thrombotic thrombocytopenic purpura.

75

ALLOGRAFT DYSFUNCTION IN RENAL TRANSPLANTATION

both antiviral treatment and immunosuppression of patients with BK nephritis.[4]

F. CYTOMEGALOVIRUS INFECTION

Cytomegalovirus (CMV) infection usually occurs 1 to 6 months after transplantation and can occur systemically or in the allograft. Allograft infection can present with tubulointerstitial nephritis, ureteral inflammation, and thrombotic microangiopathy (hemolytic-uremic–like syndrome). Although a causal relationship between CMV infection and renal allograft dysfunction has been difficult to prove, patients who develop CMV after transplantation or receive an organ from a CMV-positive donor have worse outcomes than those who do not (see Chapter 62).

G. CNI TOXICITY

1. **Epidemiology.** CNIs, especially at high dosages, cause an acute reversible decrease in glomerular filtration rate by renal vasoconstriction.
2. **Presentation.** CNI toxicity is manifested by reversible, concentration-dependent increases in plasma creatinine.
3. **Diagnosis.** Diagnosis is based on a combination of clinical, laboratory, and histologic evidence. Clinical and laboratory findings supporting a diagnosis of CNI toxicity include signs of extrarenal toxicity such as severe tremor, a moderate increase in plasma creatinine (< 25% over baseline), and high CNI concentrations (e.g., cyclosporine > 350 ng/ml or tacrolimus levels > 20 ng/ml). Because acute CNI nephrotoxicity is mainly vasomotor and prerenal, histologic changes in this setting may be unimpressive. Nonspecific findings on biopsy include tubule vacuolization; more prolonged toxicity is associated with hyaline thickening of arterioles. Occasionally, CNI toxicity can present as thrombotic microangiopathy, which is clinically indistinguishable from hemolytic uremic syndrome and thrombotic thrombocytopenic purpura.
4. **Management.** Because it is very difficult to distinguish acute allograft rejection from acute CNI nephrotoxicity, proper management is difficult. A trial of lowering the CNI dosage and monitoring for improvement in allograft function is reasonable. If function does not improve, renal biopsy is indicated to redirect therapy.

H. SURGICAL AND MECHANICAL COMPLICATIONS

Surgical and mechanical complications of transplantation occur in the immediate peritransplant period with the exception of renal artery stenosis of the allograft. Improved surgical techniques and better diagnostic tools have decreased the incidence and severity of surgical complications after renal transplantation. However, they still account for a small percentage of graft losses. The most common surgical complications are urologic. Duplex ultrasound is very helpful in screening patients with possible surgical complications.[4]

I. RECURRENT DISEASE

Diseases that recur after transplantation are listed in Table 75-1. As overall allograft survival increases, recurrent disease is likely to be increasingly diagnosed. The recurrence of diabetic nephropathy is currently not a major issue after transplantation. This is probably because of the slow progression of diabetic nephropathy.

PEARLS AND PITFALLS

- Great care should be taken when prescribing medications that alter P-450 metabolism (e.g., macrolides, azoles, seizure medications) because this can dramatically change the clearance rate of CNIs. Increased clearance can lead to acute rejection, and decreased clearance can result in CNI toxicity.
- Grapefruit juice inhibits the activity of the intestinal P-450 system and can increase the level of CNIs.
- Because of the increased risk of acute humoral rejection, blood transfusions should be avoided, if possible, in potential transplant recipients.
- For unclear reasons, surgical correction of tertiary hyperparathyroidism can result in rapid allograft dysfunction.
- Anemia in a renal transplant recipient may be caused by tertiary hyperparathyroidism or erythropoietin resistance.

REFERENCES

1. *2003 annual report of the U.S. Organ Procurement and Transplantation Network and the Scientific Registry of Transplant Recipients: transplant data 1993-2002,* Rockville, Md, Department of Health and Human Services, Health Resources and Services Administration, Office of Special Programs, Division of Transplantation; Richmond, Va, United Network for Organ Sharing; Ann Arbor, Mich, University Renal Research and Education Association. B
2. Weir M: Physiology of the transplanted kidney. In Norman DJ, Turka LA, eds: *Primer on transplantation,* 2nd ed, Mt Laurel, NJ, 2001, American Society of Transplantation.
3. Hricak H, Meux M, Reddy G: Radiologic assessment of the kidney. In Brenner BM, ed: *Brenner and Rector's the kidney,* 7th ed, St Louis, 2004, WB Saunders. D
4. Magee CC, Milford E: Clinical aspects of renal transplantation. In Brenner BM, ed: *Brenner and Rector's the kidney,* 7th ed, St Louis, 2004, WB Saunders. D

75

ALLOGRAFT DYSFUNCTION IN RENAL TRANSPLANTATION

Delirium

*Susan Cheng, MD; Nadine Jackson, MD, MPH; Cynthia Brown, MD;
and Linda Fried, MD*

FAST FACTS

- Delirium is a neuropsychiatric syndrome that is acute in onset and fluctuating in course and involves a disturbance in consciousness and a change in cognition.
- Delirium increases a patient's risk of complications during hospitalization and the long-term risk of institutionalization and death.[1-3]
- In addition to poorer outcomes, delirium is associated with greater length of stay for patients regardless of medical illness or severity of underlying medical condition.[4] Delirium accounts for half of all hospital stays for patients older than 65 years.[5]
- Delirium is preventable in many cases and reversible in most cases. Accordingly, management should focus on identifying and treating the underlying cause, as well as environmental and pharmacologic measures to promote the patient's safety and recovery.[4-6]
- The overall approach to delirium should include focusing on prevention and early recognition, using validated assessment tools for assessing and monitoring mental status, searching for the underlying cause of delirium to facilitate prompt reversal, providing a supportive and reassuring environment for the patient, and using psychotropic agents sparingly where indicated.

I. EPIDEMIOLOGY

1. Delirium is extremely common, occurring in 15% to 20% of general hospital admissions and in up to 40% of hospitalized older adults.[7]
2. Age and underlying dementia are the strongest predictors for the development of delirium.[8]
3. The incidence of delirium is also affected by the presence of multiple individual, pharmacologic, and environmental risk factors (Box 76-1), not the least of which are medical comorbidities in a vulnerable patient. In addition, delirium is exceedingly common in the intensive care unit, with a prevalence of more than 80% in mechanically ventilated patients.[9]
4. Although delirium is common, up to two thirds of cases go unrecognized.[4,10]

II. PRESENTATION

1. By definition, delirium involves disturbance in consciousness and change in cognition.[6]

BOX 76-1

MEDICAL CAUSES OF DELIRIUM

PHARMACOLOGIC

Drugs of abuse: alcohol, cocaine, heroine, amphetamines, phencyclidine, hallucinogens

Narcotics: meperidine, opioids, codeine

Benzodiazepines: alprazolam, chlordiazepoxide, triazolam, diazepam, lorazepam

Anticholinergics: diphenhydramine, tricyclic antidepressants, scopolamine, quinidine, thioridazine, benztropine

Cardiac agents: digoxin, β-blockers

Antimicrobials: voriconazole, fluoroquinolones

Psychiatric agents: antiparkinsonian agents, lithium

Miscellaneous: corticosteroids, histamine 1 and 2 receptor blockers (e.g., ranitidine), anticonvulsants

INFECTIOUS

Urinary tract infection, pneumonia, sepsis, meningitis, encephalitis, skin infections

METABOLIC

Acid-base disorders, uremia, electrolyte disturbances, hepatic encephalopathy, vitamin deficiency (thiamine, niacin), porphyria

CARDIAC

Hypotension, hypertensive emergency, acute myocardial infarction, congestive heart failure, arrhythmia

PULMONARY

Hypoxia, hypercarbia, pulmonary embolism

ENDOCRINE

Hypoglycemia or hyperglycemia, hypothyroidism or hyperthyroidism, hyperparathyroidism, hypoadrenalism or hyperadrenalism

NEUROLOGIC

Seizures, postictal states, subdural hemorrhage, cerebrovascular accident, transient ischemic attack, migraine, tumors

ONCOLOGIC

Neoplastic and paraneoplastic syndromes (carcinoid)

MISCELLANEOUS

Dehydration, urinary retention, fecal impaction, postoperative states, sleep deprivation, undertreated pain

---

a. Disturbance in consciousness can manifest as increased or, more often, decreased alertness; easy distractibility; impaired ability to focus, shift, or maintain attention; or perseveration.[6]

b. Change in cognition can have varied presentations, from slight memory impairment to disorientation and from subtle misinterpretations of stimuli to frank hallucinations.[6]

2. The clinical presentation of delirium varies widely, which is why the definition of delirium should be interpreted with caution. Common

findings of delirium include acute onset, usually over hours to days; fluctuation of symptoms throughout the day, often increased at night; alterations in sleep-wake cycle; psychomotor agitation, retardation, or both over the course of the day, ranging from lethargy and unresponsiveness to threatening behavior with staff or climbing out of bed; emotional disturbances such as anxiety or fear; and nonthreatening delusions or hallucinations, often involving people or animals.

3. **Laboratory findings.** Delirium is a clinical diagnosis. There are no laboratory findings that are specific to the diagnosis. However, many investigational tests can be used to identify possible underlying causes of delirium.

4. Electroencephalogram often shows diffuse slowing, but this is nonspecific.

III. ETIOLOGY

1. The occurrence of delirium requires both a predisposition, or the presence of risk factors, and a trigger, or an acquired condition that allows the manifestation of delirium.

a. **Risk factors that confer vulnerability.** A number of intrinsic factors place patients at high risk for delirium while in the hospital.[4,11] These include advanced age, dementia, perioperative state, comorbid psychiatric conditions, comorbid medical conditions (e.g., malnutrition), polypharmacy, and certain environmental factors (e.g., vision and hearing deficits, social isolation).

b. **Precipitating causes** (Table 76-1; see Box 76-1). Multiple acquired conditions trigger the manifestation of delirium in patients with risk factors, and up to half of all cases of delirium have more than one cause (average of three per patient).[12] Of note, medications are implicated in 20% to 40% of cases and infections in 34% of cases.[13,14]

2. **Classification.** The fourth edition of the *Diagnostic and Statistical Manual of Mental Disorders* (DSM-IV) lists four subcategories of delirium: delirium caused by a general medical condition, delirium caused by substance abuse or withdrawal, delirium with multiple causes, or not otherwise specified.[6]

IV. DIAGNOSIS

A. APPROACH
See Box 76-2 for an approach to the patient with delirium.

B. DIAGNOSTIC TOOLS
A number of diagnostic tools have been used to aid providers in diagnosing and managing delirium, including the Confusion Assessment Method (CAM) and the Mini-Mental Status Examination (MMSE).

1. The CAM is a simple, validated, and widely used screening and diagnostic tool that identifies three main elements required for the diagnosis of delirium: acute onset and fluctuating course, inattention,

TABLE 76-1

FACTORS THAT COMMONLY PRECIPITATE DELIRIUM[11]

Factor	Relative Risk
Physical restraints	4.4
Malnutrition	4
Bladder catheter	2.4
> 3 medications	2.9
Iatrogenic event	1.9

BOX 76-2

WORKUP OF DELIRIUM

FOR ALL PATIENTS

Vital signs (blood pressure, pulse, temperature, oxygen saturation)

Review of all medications

FOR MOST PATIENTS

Electrolytes

Fingerstick or serum glucose

Complete blood cell count

Urinalysis and urine culture

Blood urea nitrogen and creatinine

FOR SELECTED PATIENTS

Arterial blood gases

Therapeutic drug levels (digoxin, anticonvulsants, theophylline)

Blood cultures

Electrocardiogram

Creatinine kinase, troponin

Thyroid function tests

Chest radiography

Urine and blood toxicology

Lumbar puncture

Electroencephalogram

Computed tomography of head

Ammonia

and either disorganized thinking or altered level of consciousness. When compared with a diagnosis made by a psychiatrist, the CAM has a sensitivity of 94% to 100% and specificity of 90% to 95%; the CAM also has high interobserver reliability, positive likelihood ratio of 8.8, and negative likelihood ratio of 0.2.[15]

2. The MMSE is a standardized tool used to help diagnose dementia. However, it can also be used in the diagnosis of delirium. Studies show that a four-point change or more between serial MMSEs indicate a significant change of cognition in stable patients.[16] Therefore, serial MMSE testing over a short period of time may help point to a diagnosis of delirium.

TABLE 76-2

DIFFERENTIAL DIAGNOSIS OF DELIRIUM[4]

	Delirium	Dementia	Depression	Psychosis
Onset	Acute	Insidious	Variable	Variable
Course	Fluctuating	Progressive	Diurnal variation	Variable
Consciousness and orientation	Clouded and disoriented	Clear until late stages	Usually unimpaired	Unimpaired except in acute stages
Attention and memory	Poor short-term memory with inattention	Poor short-term memory without inattention	Poor attention but memory intact	Poor attention but memory intact
Presence of psychosis	Common; psychotic ideas are fleeting and simple in content	Less common	Rare	Common; psychotic ideas are complex and often paranoid
Electroencephalogram	Abnormal in 80-90%; 80% show diffuse slowing	Abnormal in 80-90%; 80% show diffuse slowing	Generally normal	Generally normal

C. DIFFERENTIAL DIAGNOSIS

Although the presentation of delirium can be confused with dementia, depression, and psychotic disorders, a number of key features can be used to help distinguish between these conditions (Table 76-2).

D. IDENTIFYING THE UNDERLYING CAUSE

Once the diagnosis of delirium is made, the aim is to rapidly identify the underlying condition that triggered the episode (Boxes 76-1 and 76-3).

V. MANAGEMENT AND PREVENTION

The approach to managing delirium should include multiple strategies. In many cases, there are multiple underlying causes, the cause is not rapidly correctable, or the mental status lags behind physical recovery. In such cases, the treatment strategy should focus on providing general supportive measures and correcting precipitants.

1. Reverse any identified causes: Treat acute medical conditions as indicated, remove offending or unnecessary medications, and use patient-controlled analgesia, especially in the postoperative setting.

2. In addition to treating any identified causes, it is important to also optimize environmental factors for patients with delirium. Providing

BOX 76-3

CAUSES OF DELIRIUM: I WATCH DEATH MNEMONIC

I	Infectious (meningitis, encephalitis, urinary tract infection, pneumonia)
W	Withdrawal (ethyl alcohol, barbiturates, benzodiazepines)
A	Acute metabolic (electrolyte imbalance, hepatic or renal failure)
T	Trauma (head injury, postoperative state)
C	Central nervous system disorder (stroke, bleed, tumor, seizure, Parkinson's disease)
H	Hypoxia (anemia, congestive heart failure, pulmonary embolus)
D	Deficiencies (folate, vitamin B_{12}, thiamine)
E	Endocrinopathies (thyroid, glucose, parathyroid, adrenal)
A	Acute vascular (shot, vasculitis, hypertensive encephalopathy)
T	Toxins, substance abuse, medications
H	Heavy metals (arsenic, lead, mercury)

76

DELIRIUM

familiarity, orientation, and stimulation are the primary goals of environmental strategies.[12,17]

a. **Provide orientation.** Have a clock and a calendar in each patient room. Try to maintain staff consistency, and have staff reinforce information as to day, location, and condition during interactions with patients. Encourage the presence of family or friends, or have familiar objects in the room to help patients maintain a connection to their usual environment.[17] Facilitate participation in usual activities such as feeding and grooming; early involvement in physical and occupational therapy is important to limit debilitation and provide stimulation.[4,12]

b. **Maintain a consistent environment.** A sense of timelessness often pervades medical environments; providing clear day-night clues such as dimming hallway and room lights and minimizing ambient noise during the night helps to maintain usual sleep-wake cycles.[12] Control excess noise and stimulation, and provide a single room if possible. Speak in plain language and in the patient's native language when possible. Attempt to maintain consistent and comfortable room temperature and lighting.

c. **Maintain competence.** Correct sensory impairments with glasses and hearing aids to improve a patient's ability to interact with the environment and decrease the patient's risk of misinterpreting environmental clues.[4] Avoid mechanical restraints unless the patient's behavior risks harm to self or others. Always consider using a sitter if needed, especially as an alternative to mechanical restraints.

3. Pharmacologic intervention should be used only for patients who may harm themselves or others. Pharmacologic therapies should be limited to medications specifically indicated for the underlying cause of delirium.[4]

a. Use caution when prescribing any medication because almost all medication classes have been implicated as causes of delirium.

  b. Antipsychotic medications are the primary class of drugs used to treat delirium and have been shown to be superior to benzodiazepines, except in cases of seizures or withdrawal from alcohol or sedatives.[12] Antipsychotic medications are indicated for manifestations such as hallucinations or violent behaviors, but these should be used sparingly and in low dosages. Use of psychotropic medications may impair ongoing assessment and monitoring of delirium, limit the patient's ability to cooperate with treatment, and increase risk of falls.[4]

  c. Therapy selection (Box 76-4)

    (1) Neuroleptics are very effective in controlling delirium that is not caused by withdrawal from alcohol or sedatives. Primary side effects are extrapyramidal symptoms, neuroleptic malignant syndrome, and prolongation of the QT interval, particularly at higher dosages. Before prescribing neuroleptics, review the patient's baseline electrocardiogram.[12] Haloperidol is preferred over chlorpromazine or droperidol because of its ease of administration (intramuscular or intravenous) and fewer active metabolites, as well as fewer anticholinergic, sedative, and hypotensive effects. Dosing depends on patient factors and level of disturbance, ranging from 0.5 to 10 mg, with onset of action in 20 minutes. Dosages may be repeated every 20 to 30 minutes until behavior is adequately controlled and every 2 to 4 hours thereafter as needed. More extrapyramidal symptoms are seen with intramuscular administration; more QT prolongation and arrhythmias are seen with intravenous administration.

    (2) Benzodiazepines are effective for patients with delirium caused by withdrawal from alcohol or sedatives. Benzodiazepines are not recommended as monotherapy for treating delirium because studies have shown that they are less effective than antipsychotic medication overall. However, they may provide an important adjunctive treatment for delirium. With their use the antipsychotic

---

BOX 76-4

PHARMACOLOGIC TREATMENT OF DELIRIUM

ANTIPSYCHOTIC MEDICATIONS

Haloperidol (preferred) 0.5-10 mg IV or IM q2-4h prn agitation (maximum 100 mg q24h)

Droperidol 0.625-2.5 mg IV or IM q8h prn; cardiac monitoring needed to watch QTc

Risperidone 0.5-2.5 mg PO q12h prn; not well validated and has long dose interval

BENZODIAZEPINES

Adjunctive treatment with antipsychotics or in alcohol or sedative withdrawal

Lorazepam (preferred) 1-2 mg IV or IM q4h prn

TABLE 76-3
TARGET RISK FACTORS FOR PREVENTING DELIRIUM[5,18]

Risk Factor	Intervention
Cognitive impairment (Mini-Mental Status Examination < 20)	Environmental orientation cues, continuing reorientation via communication, cognitively stimulating activities
Sleep deprivation	Warm drink at bedtime, sleep hygiene measures, nighttime noise and light reduction
Immobility	Ambulation, range-of-motion exercises, minimal use of restraints (provide a sitter instead, if possible)
Visual impairment (< 20/70)	Visual aids, adaptive equipment
Hearing impairment (< 6/12 whispers when tested)	Portable amplifying device, disimpact earwax
Dehydration (blood urea nitrogen/creatinine > 18)	Volume repletion, encourage oral fluid intake

dosage can be reduced, limiting side effects of the neuroleptic medications.

4. Prevention is important for all patients with risk factors for delirium, particularly those with a history of delirium. Target major modifiable risk factors in vulnerable patients (Table 76-1). Compared with usual care, an intervention that involved standardized protocols for managing six risk factors for delirium (listed in Table 76-3) in hospitalized patients more than 70 years old reduced the incidence of delirium by 33%, the duration of delirium, and the number of delirium episodes.[5] When delirium developed, however, the multicomponent strategy had no effect on its severity or likelihood of recurrence, suggesting that primary prevention is the best strategy.

VI. PROGNOSIS
A. MORBIDITY
Patients who develop delirium have longer hospital stays regardless of underlying medical illness. These longer stays are likely to be associated with an increased rate of complications such as aspiration pneumonia and decubitus ulcers.[12] Patients with delirium also have a higher frequency of complications from immobility, falls, and agitation. Not surprisingly, multiple studies have shown delirium to be a risk factor for readmission or nursing home placement.[1]

B. MORTALITY
Patients with delirium have a higher risk of death caused by failure to treat the underlying medical condition, such as infection, or by outcomes associated with delirium, such as falls, fractures, decubitus ulcers, and pneumonia.[7] In a recent study, delirium was shown to increase long-term mortality from all causes at 3 years, with a risk ratio of 2:2.[3]

PEARLS AND PITFALLS

- Severity of delirium is not determined by the level of patient activity. However, hyperactive, agitated patients often have better outcomes than underactive, sedated patients, possibly because the underlying medical condition is more treatable.[4]
- Beware of using medications to treat delirium in patients with impaired liver function. These patients are at higher risk not only of delirium but also of adverse effects from the treatment of delirium. This greater susceptibility is conferred by a low albumin level and impaired medication metabolism.
- Many of the medications used to treat delirium are metabolized by the liver, but no recommendations have been made for specific dosage alterations of most drugs. This is because no test accurately measures the amount of liver impairment, and pharmacodynamics cannot be readily assessed.[19] However, haloperidol generally is thought to have similar pharmacokinetics in patients with liver dysfunction and in normal patients because glucuronidation is important in its metabolism.[12]
- Special consideration should be given to medications with anticholinergic side effects because these effects are especially prominent in the older adults. Medications commonly used for nonpsychiatric indications often are culprits, including ranitidine, diphenhydramine, and digoxin.
- Lower dosages of medication are recommended for treating older adults.[12] For instance, 0.5 mg of haloperidol or lorazepam can be used as a starting dosage rather than the usual 1-2 mg dosage.
- Benzodiazepines can cause a paradoxical reaction in older patients, resulting in agitation instead of sedation.
- Up to half of patients diagnosed with delirium have not recovered by the time of hospital discharge.[7] Symptoms of delirium that often are not completely resolved by discharge include disturbances in attention and orientation.

REFERENCES

1. Inouye SK, Rushing JT, Foreman MD, et al: Does delirium contribute to poor hospital outcomes? A three-site epidemiologic study, *J Gen Intern Med* 13(4):234-242, 1998. B
2. Lewis LM, Miller DK, Morley JE, et al: Unrecognized delirium in ED geriatric patients, *Am J Emerg Med* 13(2):142-145, 1995. B
3. Curyto KJ, Johnson J, TenHave T, et al: Survival of hospitalized elderly patients with delirium: a prospective study, *Am J Geriatr Psychiatry* 9(2):141-147, 2001. B
4. Meagher DJ: Delirium: optimising management, *BMJ* 322(7279):144-149, 2001. C
5. Inouye SK, Bogardus ST Jr, Charpentier PA, et al: A multicomponent intervention to prevent delirium in hospitalized older patients, *N Engl J Med* 340(9):669-676, 1999. B

6. American Psychiatric Association Task Force on DSM-IV: *Diagnostic and statistical manual of mental disorders: DSM-IV-TR,* 4th ed, Washington, DC, 2000, American Psychiatric Association. D
7. Brown TM, Boyle MF: Delirium, *BMJ* 325(7365):644-647, 2002. C
8. Elie M, Cole MG, Primeau FJ, Bellavance F: Delirium risk factors in elderly hospitalized patients, *J Gen Intern Med* 13(3):204-212, 1998. C
9. Ely EW, Shintani A, Truman B, et al: Delirium as a predictor of mortality in mechanically ventilated patients in the intensive care unit, *JAMA* 291(14):1753-1762, 2004. B
10. Inouye SK: The dilemma of delirium: clinical and research controversies regarding diagnosis and evaluation of delirium in hospitalized elderly medical patients, *Am J Med* 97(3):278-288, 1994. C
11. Inouye SK, Charpentier PA: Precipitating factors for delirium in hospitalized elderly persons. Predictive model and interrelationship with baseline vulnerability, *JAMA* 275(11):852-857, 1996. B
12. American Psychiatric Association: *Practice guideline for the treatment of patients with delirium,* Washington, DC, 1999, American Psychiatric Association. D
13. George J, Bleasdale S, Singleton SJ: Causes and prognosis of delirium in elderly patients admitted to a district general hospital, *Age Ageing* 26(6):423-427, 1997. B
14. Francis J: Delirium in older patients, *J Am Geriatr Soc* 40(8):829-838, 1992. C
15. Inouye SK, van Dyck CH, Alessi CA, et al: Clarifying confusion: the confusion assessment method. A new method for detection of delirium, *Ann Intern Med* 113(12):941-948, 1990. B
16. Tangalos EG, Smith GE, Ivnik RJ, et al: The Mini-Mental State Examination in general medical practice: clinical utility and acceptance, *Mayo Clin Proc* 71(9):829-837, 1996. B
17. Meagher DJ, O'Hanlon D, O'Mahony E, Casey PR: The use of environmental strategies and psychotropic medication in the management of delirium, *Br J Psychiatry* 168(4):512-515, 1996. B
18. Reuben DB, American Geriatrics Society: *Geriatrics at your fingertips,* 2002 ed. Malden, Mass, 2002, Blackwell. C
19. Rodighiero V: Effects of liver disease on pharmacokinetics. An update, *Clin Pharmacokinet* 37(5):399-431, 1999. C

76

DELIRIUM

Status Epilepticus

Andrew Mammen, MD, PhD; and Ronald Lesser, MD, PhD

FAST FACTS

- Status epilepticus (SE) is a medical emergency that often occurs in one of three contexts: in patients with an acute or chronic process affecting the brain (e.g., metabolic disturbances, head injury, central nervous system infection, hypoxia, drug intoxication or withdrawal, stroke, brain tumor); as an acute exacerbation in known epileptic patients, often as a consequence of poor compliance with antiepileptic drug regimens; and as the first seizure in a patient who will go on to develop epilepsy (12% to 30% of adult patients who develop epilepsy present with SE).
- The initial management of a patient in SE includes placing the patient in lateral decubitus position with supplemental oxygen and appropriate monitors, establishing intravenous access, and checking blood glucose. If the patient is still seizing 3 minutes after onset, lorazepam (0.1 mg/kg) can be given intravenously.
- Patients with prolonged seizures and severe physiologic disturbances have higher morbidity and mortality rates.
- Neuropsychometric testing has shown that prolonged status epilepticus leads to cognitive decline.

I. EPIDEMIOLOGY

1. The estimated incidence of SE in the United States is 102,000 to 152,000 cases per year, with about 55,000 deaths.[1,2]
2. SE occurs most often in younger age groups and in people older than 60 years.
3. The mortality rate associated with SE is 3% to 35%.[3] Young age is a favorable prognostic indicator.

II. CLINICAL PRESENTATION

A. TYPES OF SEIZURES

Seizures may be classified as being partial or generalized. Any type of seizure may evolve into a generalized seizure with impaired consciousness.

1. Partial seizures.
   a. With partial seizures, only limited areas of the brain are affected, and dysfunction may likewise be limited (e.g., clonic movements and paresthesias of a single limb, aphasia, visual changes).
   b. During **simple partial** seizures consciousness remains unimpaired.
   c. If the patient experiences an alteration of consciousness, the seizures are **complex partial**.

2. Generalized seizures.

a. In generalized seizures the entire brain is involved, and the patient experiences loss of consciousness.

b. During a **convulsive generalized seizure** the patient demonstrates tonic, clonic, or tonic-clonic movements. Generalized tonic-clonic seizures sometimes are described as progressing through five phases, but it is unusual for all these phases to occur in a given patient (Table 77-1).

c. **Absence seizures** also result from generalized seizure activity affecting both hemispheres of the brain. Absence seizures usually begin in childhood and manifest as a brief lapse in awareness with generalized brain involvement on an electroencephalogram (EEG) at seizure onset.

d. Note that complex partial seizures also manifest as decreased awareness but begin with more localized brain involvement at seizure onset.

B. DEFINITIONS

1. **Status epilepticus**[4] is defined as any seizure lasting more than 30 minutes or more than two seizures occurring within 30 minutes if the patient does not return to a normal level of consciousness between seizures. Prolonged SE may have significant long-term adverse effects on cognitive function. Therefore, SE is regarded as a medical emergency, and most clinicians choose to treat seizures before 30 minutes is allowed to elapse.

2. When generalized tonic-clonic seizures persist, the condition is called **overt generalized convulsive SE** (overt GCSE). As overt GCSE seizures evolve, the clonic activity may become less pronounced, and patients may have only twitching movements in a restricted distribution. These patients are still having generalized seizures, as reflected in the EEG, and are said to be having **subtle GCSE seizures.**

3. At the extreme end of this spectrum, some patients with impaired consciousness and seizure activity on EEG have no observable repetitious movements. This state, called **nonconvulsive SE** (NCSE),

77

STATUS EPILEPTICUS

TABLE 77-1
PHASES OF GENERALIZED TONIC-CLONIC SEIZURES

Phase	Description and Symptoms
Premonitory	Headache, irritability; may precede seizures by hours to days.
Myoclonic jerks, brief tonic-clonic seizures	Generally precede generalized tonic-clonic seizures by a few minutes.
Tonic	Contraction of axial musculature and limbs, often with epileptic cry as respiratory muscles contract.
Clonic	Jerking at a frequency of about four jerks per second; at end of clonic phase, which typically lasts < 3 min, relaxation of sphincter muscles may result in bladder or bowel incontinence.
Postictal	Patient may be asleep or confused.

should be considered in patients with altered mental status that cannot be explained otherwise.
4. It is important to recognize that although subtle GCSE and NCSE seizures may be less alarming to onlookers, they may be just as harmful to the central nervous system as overt GCSE seizures.

III. DIAGNOSIS
1. Electroencephalography. Overt GCSE tonic-clonic seizures are easily recognized, and electroencephalographic confirmation is not necessary before treatment begins. In contrast, subtle GCSE and NCSE seizures usually warrant electroencephalographic evaluation.
2. The differential diagnosis of SE includes myoclonus secondary to metabolic compromise (e.g., hypercarbia, hypoxia), medication side effect (e.g., tardive dyskinesia), and psychogenic nonepileptic seizures.

IV. MANAGEMENT
A. TREATMENT OF ONGOING SEIZURES
See Fig. 77-1, making note of the following:
1. Laboratory tests that should be ordered include electrolytes, complete blood cell count, ammonia, toxicology screen, and anticonvulsant levels (if applicable).
2. If the fingerstick reveals a low glucose level, 100 mg of intravenous thiamine should be administered before 1 ampule of 50% dextrose (D-glucose) so as to prevent precipitating Wernicke-Korsakoff syndrome.
3. If no intravenous access can be obtained, lorazepam may be given intramuscularly.
4. Lorazepam should be administered 1 to 3 mg at a time, with a delay of 1 to 2 minutes between infusions to allow the seizure to subside. The entire dose of benzodiazepine should be given only if the seizure persists. Diazepam is equally effective at terminating seizures,[5] although its antiseizure duration is only 15 to 30 minutes. In contrast, lorazepam's antiseizure duration is 12 to 24 hours.
5. Respiratory depression is a possibility with either benzodiazepine. Additional doses are associated with a higher risk of respiratory depression.
6. In patients who have been taking phenytoin and whose blood levels are thought to be low, half this dosage may be given.
7. During infusion of phenytoin the electrocardiogram should be monitored continuously and the blood pressure checked. If the electrocardiogram changes or the patient becomes hypotensive, the infusion should be slowed or stopped until these complications resolve.
B. REFRACTORY SE
1. Seizures that do not respond to phenobarbital should be considered refractory, and the patient should be treated with anesthesia induction.
2. The patient should be intubated and ventilated and in an intensive care unit with cardiovascular monitoring.

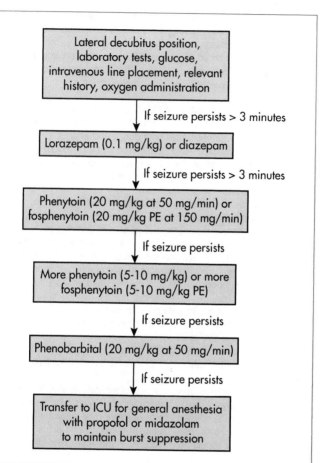

FIG. 77-1

Management approach for patients with status epilepticus. *ICU,* intensive care unit;
PE, phenytoin equivalents.

3. Arterial and central venous catheters should be placed, and continuous
   electroencephalographic monitoring should be initiated.
4. A loading dose of propofol, 1 to 2 mg/kg intravenously, should be
   administered followed by infusion at a rate of 2 to 10 mg/kg/hr.
   Alternatively, midazolam at a loading dose of 0.2 mg/kg intravenously
   should be followed by 0.75 to 10 μg/min.
5. The rate of maintenance infusion should be titrated to maintain a burst
   suppression electroencephalographic pattern.

6. Hypotension is treated with intravenous fluids, low-dose dopamine, and low-dose dobutamine. The rate of propofol or midazolam infusion can be reduced if necessary.

7. Anesthesia is maintained for at least 12 hours, then the infusion is tapered to assess for evidence of clinical or electroencephalographic seizure activity. Repeated anesthesia administration may be necessary if seizures recur.

C. DETERMINE THE CAUSE OF STATUS EPILEPTICUS

1. Seizures often are a symptom of an underlying problem. It is important to look for the cause of seizures both during and after SE.

2. Metabolic and electrolyte abnormalities should be corrected. However, keep in mind that arterial blood gases obtained during and immediately after SE probably will reveal hypoxia and acidosis; these should resolve spontaneously once the seizure is over.

3. Check drug levels in patients on antiepileptic medications. Low anticonvulsant levels are a common cause of SE.

4. Infection predisposes those with known seizure disorders to breakthrough seizures. Always obtain urinalysis and a chest radiograph in patients who have seized. Consider blood cultures in febrile patients.

5. Febrile patients with no other obvious source of infection should undergo a lumbar puncture for cerebrospinal fluid analysis if it is safe to do so.

6. Even if they are not febrile, patients with human immunodeficiency virus infection and a seizure should undergo cerebrospinal fluid examination if it is safe to do so.

7. A head computed tomogram to look for structural lesions should be considered in patients without an obvious explanation for their seizure.

8. Although some patients have focal neurologic deficits after a seizure (i.e., Todd's paralysis), their presence should always raise the suspicion of an underlying brain lesion. Because stroke may present with a seizure, magnetic resonance imaging of the brain with diffusion-weighted imaging should be considered in the appropriate clinical context.

9. Consider obtaining a nonemergent EEG in patients once SE has resolved.

PEARLS AND PITFALLS

- Parenteral valproate has a broad spectrum of activity and may be loaded rapidly. Although its use may be considered in SE patients with a known allergic reaction to phenytoin, it is not approved by the U.S. Food and Drug Administration for treating SE.

- Usually about 90% of phenytoin is bound to albumin and other serum proteins, but only unbound drug crosses the blood-brain barrier and is pharmacologically active. However, patients with hypoalbuminemia, those with renal failure, or those taking medications that compete for protein-binding sites may have a higher proportion of unbound, active phenytoin. These patients may have adequate unbound levels and good seizure control with "subtherapeutic" total phenytoin levels. For this reason, it is helpful to obtain simultaneously total and free phenytoin levels at least once in order to determine the correlation between total and free levels.

- The concept of therapeutic range is widely misunderstood. Some patients do well with levels below the ranges quoted on the laboratory slips, and others need higher levels. For example, a patient whose seizures are not controlled with a phenytoin level of 19 µg/ml may have seizures controlled with a phenytoin level of 27 µg/ml.

- Unlike phenytoin, fosphenytoin is water soluble and does not contain propylene glycol. Consequently, fosphenytoin infusion does not carry the same risk of adverse cardiovascular events that phenytoin infusion does (e.g., hypotension). The use of fosphenytoin should especially be considered in patients with known cardiovascular disease or who are critically ill. Fosphenytoin is converted to phenytoin in the body and can be monitored in the same way as phenytoin.

- As many as one third of women with epilepsy have an increase in seizure frequency during pregnancy.[6] The physiologic changes of pregnancy, stress, and sleep deprivation may all contribute to this. Furthermore, the rate of antiepileptic drug noncompliance has been found to increase during and after pregnancy, perhaps because of concerns regarding fetal antiepileptic drug exposure and breastfeeding. Because seizures in pregnancy can be harmful to both mother and fetus, SE should be treated as outlined previously. In pregnancy, the total phenytoin level may decrease, whereas the unbound level remains stable. Therefore, obtaining both an unbound and a total phenytoin level in a pregnant patient is advisable.

- NCSE should be considered in the differential diagnosis of patients with altered mental status that cannot be otherwise explained. Forced gaze deviation, episodic rhythmic movements, and acute changes in blood pressure may be signs of NCSE. When NCSE is suspected, an EEG should be obtained as soon as possible.

- After a generalized seizure, examination of the cerebrospinal fluid may reveal a pleocytosis of about 9 to 80 white blood cells per milliliter. This pleocytosis is transitory and peaks about 24 hours after the seizure. Nonetheless, cerebrospinal fluid pleocytosis should never be attributed to seizures until all cultures are negative.

- Serum prolactin levels often rise transiently (for only 15-30 minutes) after generalized tonic-clonic seizures and some complex partial seizures. Therefore, their measurement occasionally is used to help distinguish epileptic seizure activity from pseudoseizures. However, not all seizures are accompanied by a rise in serum prolactin. Furthermore, prolactin levels may rise after other "spells" that may be confused with seizures, such as vasovagal syncope.[7] For these reasons, the routine measurement of prolactin levels after seizures is unnecessary.

77

STATUS EPILEPTICUS

REFERENCES

1. Bradley WG et al: *Neurology in clinical practice,* Newton, Mass, 2000, Butterworth-Heinemann. C
2. DeLorenzo RJ et al: Epidemiology of status epilepticus, *J Clin Neurophysiol* 12:316, 1995. C
3. Dodson WE et al: Treatment of convulsive status epilepticus: recommendations of the Epilepsy Foundation of America's Working Group on Status Epilepticus, *JAMA* 270:854, 1993. D
4. Lowenstein DH, Allredge BK: Status epilepticus, *N Engl J Med* 338:970, 1998. C
5. Leppik IE et al: Double-blind study of lorazepam and diazepam in status epilepticus, *JAMA* 249:1452, 1983. A
6. Zahn CA et al: Management issues for women with epilepsy: a review of the literature, *Neurology* 51:949, 1998. C
7. Lusic I et al: Serum prolactin levels after seizure and syncopal attacks, *Seizure* 8:218, 1999. B

Stroke

Thomas E. Lloyd, MD, PhD; Benjamin Greenberg, MD;
and Eric Aldrich, MD

FAST FACTS

- Transient ischemic attacks (TIAs) are analogous to unstable angina and should be treated with similar urgency.
- Metabolic abnormalities (e.g., hypoglycemia) can mimic stroke by presenting with focal neurologic findings, especially in patients with a prior stroke.
- There are four basic questions to address in patients who present acutely with neurologic deficits: Is this an ischemic stroke? Is the patient eligible for tissue plasminogen activator (t-PA)? What can be done to protect the ischemic penumbra (i.e., minimize the area of infarction)? What can be done to prevent further strokes?
- All patients with suspected acute stroke should have an emergent noncontrast head computed tomography (CT) to evaluate for intracranial hemorrhage.
- Intravenous (IV) t-PA should be considered in patients with significant neurologic deficit presenting within 3 hours of symptom onset and no contraindications. Intraarterial thrombolysis may be considered up to 6 hours after symptom onset except in cases of basilar artery thrombosis, where the time window may be extended.
- Hyperglycemia should be treated aggressively in patients with acute ischemic stroke, whereas hypertension usually should not be treated unless the blood pressure exceeds 220/115.
- Daily aspirin is the most cost-effective antiplatelet agent for secondary prevention of ischemic stroke.
- No randomized controlled trials have demonstrated benefit with IV heparin in acute stroke; however, it may be considered in cases of crescendo TIAs from symptomatic carotid artery or basilar artery stenosis.

Ischemic Stroke

I. EPIDEMIOLOGY

1. Stroke is an acute neurologic deficit caused by either ischemia (80%) or hemorrhage (20%).
2. Stroke is the leading cause of disability and the third leading cause of death among adults in the United States. The prevalence of stroke has been increasing with the aging of the population; however, the incidence of stroke has decreased predominantly because of the

treatment of atherosclerosis and hypertension. Twenty-five percent of patients with stroke are younger than 65 years old.

II. RISK FACTORS AND PRIMARY PREVENTION[5]

The risk factors for ischemic stroke are similar to those for atherosclerosis and coronary artery disease. Older age; family history of premature cardiovascular events; and prior history of coronary artery disease, TIA, or stroke all significantly increase risk of stroke.[1]

1. **Hypertension** is the single greatest modifiable risk factor for stroke.[2] Lowering diastolic blood pressure by as little as 5 mmHg can reduce stroke risk by 42%.[3] Reduction of isolated systolic blood pressure in older adults similarly has been shown to dramatically reduce stroke rates.[4]

2. **Hyperlipidemia** has been shown in multiple clinical trials to be an independent risk factor for stroke. Meta-analyses of lipid-lowering trials have shown that statins reduce the incidence of first stroke by about 25%.[3]

3. **Diabetes** is a well-recognized risk factor for stroke. Although tight glycemic control has been shown to reduce microvascular complications, only management of hypertension and hyperlipidemia has been shown to significantly reduce stroke risk.[5]

4. **Alcohol** use in moderation (1 or 2 drinks/day) results in up to a 50% reduction in risk of stroke, whereas excessive alcohol intake (> 6 drinks per day) is associated with an increased risk.

5. **Hyperhomocysteinemia** is an independent risk factor for stroke, but it is unclear whether vitamin B_6, B_{12}, and folate supplementation reduces the incidence.

6. **Cardiac disease**.

a. **Atrial fibrillation** is the most common cause of cerebral embolism, resulting in an average annual risk of stroke of about 5%. Increased risk of stroke is present with increasing age, hypertension, heart failure, diabetes, or left atrial enlargement. Patients younger than 65 years old with atrial fibrillation and no other risk factors may be treated with aspirin monotherapy (0.5% risk of stroke/year), whereas patients older than 75 years old or with the aforementioned risk factors should be anticoagulated with warfarin (goal international normalized ratio 2 to 3) unless contraindicated.[6]

b. **Systolic dysfunction** is a common cause of intracardiac thrombus formation. Myocardial infarction increases the risk of thrombus formation and embolic stroke, particularly when causing ventricular akinesis or involving the anteroapical ventricular wall. Anticoagulation for primary stroke prevention often is considered in patients with an ejection fraction less than 20%.

c. **Patent foramen ovale (PFO)** may lead to paradoxical embolization of venous thromboembolism. However, PFOs are present in 7% to 20% of the general population, and treatment with antiplatelet agents or anticoagulation generally is not warranted for primary prevention of stroke. The relative value of closing a PFO has not been conclusively determined, but, in general, large PFOs with aneurysmal change or associated clots should be evaluated for closure.

d. **Bacterial endocarditis** may give rise to multiple septic emboli, which are at high risk for hemorrhagic conversion. Thus there is no role for t-PA, heparin, or antiplatelet agents in treating or preventing strokes in such patients. Early IV antibiotics and valve replacement, if necessary, are critical in preventing embolization.

e. **Valvular disease** may increase the risk of thrombus formation caused by turbulent blood flow.

f. **Carotid artery stenosis.** The origin of the internal carotid artery is the most common site of atherosclerosis leading to TIA or stroke.

(1) **Symptomatic.** The North American Symptomatic Carotid Endarterectomy Trial (NASCET) studied the benefit of carotid endarterectomy (CEA) in patients with symptomatic carotid stenosis greater than 70%.[7] This study demonstrated that CEA reduces the 2-year risk of stroke from 26% to 9% and suggests that CEA should be performed if the perioperative mortality risk is less than 6%. With regard to stenosis of 50% to 70%, the 5-year risk reduction of CEA was more modest, from 22% to 16%. CEA may be considered in these patients, but potential benefit must be weighed against the risks of surgery. Recently, the SAPPHIRE trial demonstrated the noninferiority of carotid artery stenting in high-risk patients.[8]

(2) **Asymptomatic.** The Asymptomatic Carotid Atherosclerosis Study demonstrated a 6% absolute reduction in stroke risk in asymptomatic patients with carotid artery stenosis greater than 60%, with a greater benefit seen in men. In these patients, the surgical complication rate should be less than 3% for the benefit of CEA to outweigh the risk.

(3) **Screening.** There has been no proven benefit to routine carotid artery auscultation or screening carotid ultrasounds in asymptomatic patients.

III. CLINICAL PRESENTATION

1. The clinical presentation of ischemic stroke depends on the mechanism of vascular insult (thrombosis, embolus, or other), the duration of ischemia, and the vascular distribution affected.

2. **Pathophysiology.**

a. Several mechanisms of arterial occlusion can cause stroke. Atherosclerosis is the most common vascular disease of large extracranial or intracranial arteries, whereas small and medium-sized arteries are more commonly affected by lipohyalinosis (or arteriosclerosis).

b. **Thrombotic strokes (25% of ischemic strokes).** Thrombotic strokes typically cause fluctuating or progressive symptoms. In contrast to coronary artery disease, total occlusion of large intracranial arteries by thrombosis is uncommon (1% to 5% of strokes). Occlusion of small to

78

STROKE

medium-sized arteries, on the other hand, is commonly caused by thrombosis due to lipohyalinosis or microatheroma. These **lacunar strokes** (15%) often affect small penetrating arteries and usually are associated with hypertension.

c. **Embolic strokes (75% of ischemic strokes).** In embolic strokes, neurologic deficits usually are greatest at onset of symptoms and may involve deficits of multiple vascular territories. **Cardioembolic** (< 30%) strokes often are caused by intracardiac thrombi. **Artery-to-artery** thromboembolism (about 20%) occurs when large artery thrombi break off and embolize to downstream vessels. The most common sites of thrombus formation leading to embolization are the carotid bifurcation and aortic arch. Approximately 40% of embolic strokes (and about 20% of all strokes) are cryptogenic, and thorough evaluation does not reveal an obvious source.

3. **TIAs** are classically defined as focal neurologic deficits lasting less than 24 hours (and usually < 1 hour) that are attributed to ischemia. With the widespread use of imaging, TIA has been redefined to exclude patients with evidence of infarction on magnetic resonance imaging (MRI) or CT.[9] A large proportion of patients with classic TIAs (i.e., rapidly reversible neurologic deficits) have evidence of infarction on MRI. Stroke and TIA share the same pathophysiology, but the ischemic injury in stroke is irreversible. The cause of TIAs should be urgently identified because there is a 5% risk of subsequent stroke within the next 48 hours.[10]

4. **Vascular distribution** (Table 78-1).

IV. DIAGNOSIS

A. DIFFERENTIAL DIAGNOSIS

1. Common vascular and nonvascular causes of focal neurologic deficits are listed in Table 78-2.

2. A thorough history and physical examination usually can distinguish stroke from nonvascular causes of focal neurologic deficits. A history of a sensory aura or migraine headaches with neurologic deficit may suggest complicated migraine, but care must be taken because migraine patients are at a marginally higher risk for stroke. A history of seizures may suggest postictal (Todd's) paralysis. Auscultation of a bruit on carotid examination or a murmur or irregular heartbeat on cardiac examination may suggest a carotid or cardiac source of thromboembolism, respectively. A fingerstick glucose should always be checked to evaluate for hyperglycemia or hypoglycemia.

3. An electrocardiogram should be performed routinely to look for evidence of an arrhythmia (especially atrial fibrillation) or old myocardial infarction to suggest a cardioembolic source.

4. Routine laboratory studies should include measurement of serum glucose, electrolytes, blood urea nitrogen, creatinine, complete blood cell count, prothrombin time, partial thromboplastin time, serologic tests

TABLE 78-1

VASCULAR DISTRIBUTION AND ACUTE STROKE

Vascular Territory	Predominant Symptoms	Comments
Anterior cerebral artery	Contralateral leg weakness	
Middle cerebral artery	Contralateral face and arm weakness and numbness Aphasia (dominant) or neglect	Most common site of embolic stroke
Internal carotid artery	Above symptoms and monocular blindness	Often asymptomatic if competent circle of Willis
Posterior cerebral artery	Contralateral hemianopsia (visual field cut)	Often unnoticed by patient
Basilar or vertebral artery	Diplopia, dysphagia, ataxia, vertigo, hearing loss with "crossed" sensory and motor deficits	"Top of the basilar" and "locked-in" syndromes
Superior cerebellar	Ipsilateral ataxia	
Posterior inferior cerebellar	Ipsilateral vertigo, nystagmus, dysphagia, diplopia	Wallenberg syndrome
Global hypoperfusion (e.g., caused by hypotension), affects watershed areas	Bilateral visual loss Weakness of shoulders and thighs ("man in a barrel")	May be unilateral if underlying atherosclerotic disease
Penetrators	Pure motor or sensory symptoms	Lacunar infarct

TABLE 78-2

DIFFERENTIAL DIAGNOSIS OF STROKE AND TRANSIENT ISCHEMIC ATTACK

Nonvascular Causes	Vascular Causes (i.e., Stroke)
Metabolic (glucose, Na^+, Ca^{2+}, blood urea nitrogen)	Thrombosis (large vessel, lacunar stroke)
Demyelinating disease (e.g., multiple sclerosis)	Embolic (artery-to-artery, cardioembolic, paradoxical embolus, endocarditis)
Seizure with postictal deficit (Todd's paralysis)	Hypercoagulable disorder: hereditary and acquired (e.g., anticardiolipin antibody and oral contraceptives)
Tumor	Venous sinus thrombosis
Migraine (complicated)	Fibromuscular dysplasia
Infections (meningitis, encephalitis, abscess)	Vasculitis (PAN, Wegner's, Takayasu's, GCA, primary central nervous system)
Trauma	Vasculitis caused by meningitis (e.g., syphilis)
Psychogenic	Sickle cell anemia or polycythemia vera
Drugs and toxins (e.g., cocaine, amphetamine)	Global hypoperfusion

PAN, polyarteritis nodosa; *GCA,* giant cell arteritis.

for syphilis, homocysteine, serum lipid profile, thyroid-stimulating hormone, erythrocyte sedimentation rate, and urinalysis.

5. Other laboratory studies may be appropriate in the correct clinical context. A hypercoagulable workup often is performed in young patients or patients with recurrent strokes or thrombi of unclear origin. A lumbar puncture may be helpful to exclude subarachnoid hemorrhage, meningeal inflammation, or demyelination. An electroencephalogram may be performed if postseizure (Todd's) paralysis is considered. In young adults, uncommon genetic or vascular malformations should be considered as causes of stroke.

B. IMAGING

The American Heart Association recommends brain imaging in all patients with suspected stroke or TIA. The ideal imaging modality (CT or MRI) depends on the clinical presentation. If embolic stroke is suggested on initial imaging (e.g., large artery distribution or multiple wedge-shaped infarcts), intracranial and extracranial arterial and cardiac imaging should be performed to determine the likely source of embolus.

1. **CT scan** usually is performed first in acute stroke or TIA to exclude hemorrhage or mass lesions that can mimic stroke. Although it is only about 50% sensitive for identifying acute ischemic infarcts, noncontrast CT scanning is fast, inexpensive, and highly sensitive for identifying intraparenchymal hemorrhage (lesions appear hyperdense). However, CT is poor at imaging posterior fossa lesions (because of bony artifact) and small lesions such as lacunar strokes. Though not routinely done, IV contrast can be used in performing a CT angiogram, which may identify occlusion of large blood vessels.

2. **MRI** is highly sensitive and specific for identifying acute ischemic stroke. Although it takes longer to perform than CT and is more expensive, it is now considered an integral part of the stroke evaluation. When combined with diffusion-weighted and perfusion-weighted imaging, MRI often can identify the age of infarction, the ischemic territory at risk for infarction, and the type of stroke: lacunar (< 2 cm^2 lesion), thrombotic, or embolic (often more than one lesion on MRI). Furthermore, magnetic resonance angiography (MRA) can be performed at the same time and may identify significant thrombosis of large intracranial or extracranial arteries as a source of artery-to-artery embolism. Although MRA is sensitive for detecting thrombosis, it is nonspecific and often exaggerates the degree of stenosis.

3. **Carotid ultrasound and transcranial Dopplers** are useful in evaluating for extracranial and intracranial atherosclerotic lesions, respectively. Compared with MRA, ultrasound is less expensive but is inferior in imaging the intracranial large arteries.

4. **Angiography** is considered the gold standard in diagnosing cerebrovascular occlusion. Conventional angiography is invasive and associated with a 1% incidence of stroke and therefore is used only when screening tests identify the need for a more detailed examination

of the cerebral vasculature. However, in institutions where it is routinely performed and associated with a low complication rate, angiography may be both diagnostic and therapeutic.

5. **Cardiac imaging and monitoring.** Intracardiac thrombus formation should be considered as a cause in all cases of embolic stroke. A 48-hour Holter monitor or inpatient cardiac monitoring is recommended to screen for paroxysmal atrial fibrillation or other arrhythmias that predispose to thrombus formation. Echocardiography is also recommended to evaluate for thrombi, left ventricular dysfunction, valvular disease, and a PFO. Transesophageal echocardiography generally is more sensitive than transthoracic echocardiography in detecting left atrial thrombi, atrial septal aneurysms, and some valvular abnormalities; it can often identify plaques or thrombi in the aortic arch. However, because transesophageal echocardiography is invasive, transthoracic echocardiography may be sufficient when the suspicion of a cardiac source is low.

V. MANAGEMENT

A. ACUTE MANAGEMENT

Acute management of ischemic stroke focuses on preventing further ischemic injury and attempting thrombolysis, if indicated. Patients with significant neurologic deficits should be managed acutely in an inpatient stroke unit if possible.

1. **Medical management** of acute stroke includes the ABCs, supplemental O_2, and emergent CT scanning to exclude cerebral hemorrhage. Surrounding most areas of infarction is an ischemic penumbra involving brain that is ischemic but potentially salvageable. The extent of hypoperfused tissue at risk for infarction can be estimated using MRI by determining mismatch between diffusion imaging (infarct) and perfusion imaging (ischemia).

2. **Intravenous thrombolysis.** The National Institute of Neurological Disorders and Stroke IV t-PA trial demonstrated that IV thrombolysis is beneficial if given within 3 hours of stroke onset.[11] The primary risk of IV t-PA is intracerebral hemorrhage (ICH), and this risk increases with the size and age of the infarct. The primary benefit observed was an increase in the number of patients without disability (26% vs. 39%, as compared with placebo). There was a trend toward reduced mortality, but this was not significant. Numerous phase IV studies have confirmed the benefit of t-PA when given less than 3 hours after symptom onset and have shown that the earlier it is given, the greater the benefit. Two trials, the Atlantis and the European Cooperative Acute Stroke Study II trials, demonstrated that when IV t-PA is given beyond the 3-hour window, the risk of ICH outweighs the potential benefit.[12,13] Additional contraindications to IV t-PA include a history of ICH, stroke or head trauma in the preceding 3 months, recent surgery or bleeding, coagulopathy, and thrombocytopenia.

78

STROKE

3. **Intraarterial t-PA.** In patients who are not candidates for IV t-PA, intraarterial thrombolysis can be considered. Emergent MRI (diffusion and perfusion only) and angiography often are performed to demonstrate diffusion-perfusion mismatch and the site of vascular occlusion. Several studies have shown benefit of intraarterial thrombolysis when given within 12 hours of stroke onset. The PROACT II trial randomized 180 patients with MCA occlusion to intraarterial urokinase (121) or placebo (59) and found that 67% of patients given intraarterial thrombolysis had clot lysis, compared with 18% of controls.[14] At Johns Hopkins Hospital, intraarterial t-PA is considered in patients with anterior circulation stroke within 6 hours, central retinal artery occlusion within 12 hours, and posterior circulation stroke within 24 hours.

4. **Hypertension** generally should not be treated because ischemic tissue is hypoperfused and has impaired cerebrovascular autoregulation. The American Stroke Association recommends treating blood pressure greater than 220/115 mmHg with short-acting agents such as intravenous labetalol or enalapril. Hypotension generally is more detrimental than hypertension and should be aggressively treated with normal saline and vasopressors.

5. **Hyperglycemia** has been shown to worsen outcome after stroke. Therefore, the patient should have frequent glucose checks and a tight sliding-scale insulin regimen.

6. **Hyperthermia** has also been shown to worsen stroke outcome and should be treated aggressively with acetaminophen. Hypothermia protocols are currently under investigation.

7. **Aspirin** has been shown to be beneficial in the acute management of stroke. The Chinese Acute Stroke Trial enrolled 20,000 patients and demonstrated that 160 mg aspirin given for 4 weeks after acute stroke resulted in a small but significant reduction (3.9% vs. 3.3%) in stroke and death when compared with placebo.[15] A similar benefit was seen in the International Stroke Trial.[16]

8. **Anticoagulation.** A large number of studies have evaluated the acute use of heparin in stroke. On the basis of the data, the American Academy of Neurology has concluded that there is no evidence that heparin lowers the risk of early recurrent stroke, including in patients with cardioembolism.[17] Despite lack of evidence, heparin sometimes is used acutely in crescendo TIAs from symptomatic carotid stenosis, progressing stroke, and posterior circulation stroke.

B. SECONDARY PREVENTION

1. Even if a patient presents several days after an ischemic stroke, an urgent workup should be performed to determine the cause of the ischemic event because the risk of a second stroke is greatest in the days or weeks after the event. The goals of secondary prevention depend on the likely mechanism of injury. If the infarcted territory is consistent with an embolic source and a cardiac source of emboli is

identified, anticoagulation should be initiated promptly. If carotid or vertebral artery thrombosis or dissection is identified, surgical or interventional radiologic intervention should be considered promptly.

2. **Statins** have been shown to be effective in secondary stroke prevention in several studies.[18,19]

3. **Hypertension** probably is the single most important modifiable risk factor for secondary prevention. Although elevated blood pressure should not be treated aggressively in the first several days after ischemic stroke, a stroke reduction rate up to 42% can be achieved with aggressive long-term blood pressure control.[20] Angiotensin-converting enzyme inhibitors appear to be especially effective at lowering stroke risk, even in patients without hypertension.[21]

4. **Antiplatelet agents.** Numerous studies have shown that aspirin has a benefit in the secondary prevention of stroke and myocardial infarction. Meta-analyses show no difference between high-, medium-, and low-dose aspirin for prevention of major vascular events.[17] The current recommendation is 50 to 325 mg per day. Ticlopidine, clopidogrel, and dipyridamole are newer antiplatelet agents that have all been shown to be more effective than aspirin in secondary prevention of stroke. In a study of 20,000 patients, clopidogrel was associated with an 8.7% relative risk reduction for the combined endpoint of myocardial infarction, ischemic stroke, or vascular death when compared with aspirin (5.83% vs. 5.32%, absolute risk reduction = 0.5%).[22] In the Clopidogrel in Unstable Angina to Prevent Recurrent Events trial, which enrolled more than 12,000 patients presenting with unstable angina, a 20% relative risk reduction in the combined endpoint of cardiovascular mortality, nonfatal myocardial infarction, or stroke was seen in the combination of clopidogrel and aspirin compared with aspirin alone.[23] However, a more recent trial of 7600 patients with prior TIA or stroke suggests that clopidogrel is equivalent to clopidogrel and aspirin in reducing cardiovascular mortality.[24] In both trials, the risk of major bleeding increased. Dipyridamole with aspirin (Aggrenox) was shown to be more effective than aspirin (50 mg per day) in reducing stroke.[25] A head-to-head trial between dipyridamole (Aggrenox) and clopidogrel (Plavix) is under way. Thus, the optimal antiplatelet agent for secondary stroke prevention is unclear. Generally, aspirin 325 mg daily is recommended initially, with consideration of changing to clopidogrel or dipyridamole if strokes continue on aspirin.

5. **Anticoagulation** has been shown to be effective only in reducing the risk of cardioembolic stroke. Warfarin should be used unless contraindicated in patients with atrial fibrillation or known intramural thrombus. The use of warfarin in patients with severely reduced left ventricular function is controversial and institution dependent. In cases of cryptogenic embolic stroke in which the patient is found to have a PFO, it is unclear whether patients benefit most from anticoagulation with warfarin, antiplatelet agents, or PFO closure.[26] In noncardioembolic

78

STROKE

stroke or in cases of intracranial stenosis where there is presumed artery-to-artery embolus, warfarin and aspirin have been shown to be equivalent in secondary prevention.[27,28]

Hemorrhagic Stroke

I. EPIDEMIOLOGY AND ETIOLOGY

Intracranial hemorrhage usually is classified on the basis of location of blood as epidural, subdural, subarachnoid, intraparenchymal (also called intracerebral hemorrhage, or ICH), or intraventricular. Epidural and subdural hemorrhages usually are secondary to trauma and are not discussed further here. Intraventricular hemorrhage in adults usually occurs as an extension of subarachnoid or ICH.

1. **ICH** accounts for two thirds of hemorrhagic stroke and usually is classified as primary or secondary, based on whether the bleeding was spontaneous or due to a specific underlying cause (e.g., tumor). Primary ICH often is called hypertensive hemorrhage because of its strong association with hypertension. The pathophysiologic mechanisms of spontaneous ICH are thought to be related to those of lacunar stroke and involve microaneurysms of small penetrating arteries that have been weakened by lipohyalinosis. Secondary ICH can have many causes, as outlined in Box 78-1.

2. **Subarachnoid hemorrhage (SAH)** accounts for one third of hemorrhagic stroke and is most commonly caused by trauma or rupture of intracranial aneurysms. Risk factors for aneurysm rupture include aneurysm diameter, smoking, hypertension, heavy alcohol use, and cocaine or amphetamine use. The incidence of SAH peaks in the sixth decade of life. Cerebral artery aneurysms are common in a number of hereditary diseases, including autosomal dominant polycystic kidney disease and Ehlers-Danlos type IV. Nonaneurysmal causes of SAH include head trauma, arteriovenous malformations, cocaine or amphetamine abuse, arterial dissection, moyamoya disease, and coagulopathy.

II. PRESENTATION

1. **ICH** can present with symptoms ranging from nonspecific changes in mental status to focal neurologic deficits. The most common locations of hypertensive (primary) ICH include the basal ganglia, pons, cerebellum, and cortex. A high index of suspicion should be maintained in patients presenting with rapid onset of neurologic symptoms or with rapid deterioration in level of consciousness.

2. **SAH** classically presents as the sudden onset of "the worst headache of my life." Symptoms of meningeal irritation often are present and include stiff neck, nausea, vomiting, and photophobia. A sentinel headache from a small aneurysmal leak is present in up to 70% of patients developing SAH. The Hunt-Hess grading scale has been used to

---

BOX 78-1

COMMON CAUSES OF INTRACRANIAL HEMORRHAGE

Trauma
Vascular malformations
  Intracranial aneurysm
  Arteriovenous malformation
  Cavernous or venous angiomas
Drug related
  Anticoagulation
  Antiplatelet agents
  Thrombolytics (recombinant tissue-type plasminogen activator)
  Drug or substance abuse (e.g., cocaine and alcohol)
Infections (e.g., mycotic aneurysms)
Systemic hypertension
Cerebral vessel occlusion
  Hemorrhagic conversion of ischemic stroke
  Cerebral venous thrombosis
Neoplastic disorders
  Primary intracranial tumor (e.g., glioblastoma multiforme)
  Metastasis
Eclampsia
Amyloid angiopathy
Autoimmune disorders
  Systemic collagen vascular disorders
  Primary cerebral vasculitis
Hematologic or platelet disorders
  Renal failure
  Liver failure
  Coagulopathy
  Hemolytic disorders

---

determine prognosis and is based on the degree of neurologic impairment from grade I (mild headache) to grade V (comatose).

III. DIAGNOSIS

1. **Noncontrast head CT** scan is the test of choice in patients with suspected intracranial hemorrhage. Ischemic and hemorrhagic strokes cannot be reliably distinguished clinically, and imaging is always indicated with acute onset or change in neurologic symptoms. CT is up to 95% sensitive for detecting acute SAH if performed hours after aneurysmal rupture, but sensitivity decreases about 10% per day after rupture. Critical findings on CT that affect management of ICH include hematoma size, supratentorial or infratentorial location, signs of midline shift or herniation, and the presence or absence of intraventricular extension with hydrocephalus.

2. **Angiography** is the gold standard for identifying cerebral aneurysms and is also helpful in diagnosing vascular malformations that may cause ICH. MRAs or CT angiograms are alternative imaging modalities. Magnetic resonance venogram often is performed in cases of hemorrhage that have suspected secondary causes including cerebral venous occlusion and underlying tumors.

3. **Lumbar puncture** should be performed in cases of suspected SAH with a negative head CT. The diagnosis is made on the basis of persistent red blood cells in the sampled cerebrospinal fluid or xanthochromia. Therefore, more than one tube of collected cerebrospinal fluid should always be sent for cell counts in order to rule out "traumatic taps" as the cause of red cells in the fluid.

4. **MRI** is particularly useful in identifying tumors, vascular malformations, and amyloid angiopathy as the cause of ICH. A gradient echo (or heme sequence) should be performed to identify old hemorrhage.

IV. MANAGEMENT

1. **Medical management** of ICH focuses on minimizing bleeding by carefully controlling both arterial blood pressure and hemostatic factors. Any coagulopathy should be corrected immediately. Most patients with SAH or ICH should be monitored acutely in a critical care environment. Frequent neurologic examinations should be performed to evaluate for signs of elevated intracranial pressure. Because blood is epileptogenic, patients should be monitored for seizure activity and given antiepileptic prophylaxis. The calcium channel blocker nimodipine is used for vasospasm prophylaxis in SAH.

2. **Surgical management.** In ICH, neurosurgical intervention is considered in large hematomas associated with mass effect or herniation and any cerebellar hematoma caused by proximity to the brainstem. Early neurosurgical intervention should be considered in any patient with SAH caused by a ruptured aneurysm. Both aneurysm clipping and endovascular aneurysm coiling are treatment options.

PEARLS AND PITFALLS

- Beware of conditions that can mimic stroke, including hypoglycemia and hyperglycemia, seizure, and migraine. Pain, headaches, and symptoms moving from one part of the body to the next are uncommon in ischemic stroke. On the other hand, the sensation of heaviness is considered to be caused by stroke until proven otherwise.

- Symptoms of basilar artery thrombosis often are nonspecific, are easily misdiagnosed, and can be life threatening. Transient symptoms of vertebrobasilar insufficiency such as hearing loss, diplopia, ataxia, or vertigo should be evaluated aggressively because these symptoms may represent brainstem TIAs. Patients with stroke risk factors and more than two symptoms or signs referable to the posterior circulation should be evaluated for vertebrobasilar stenosis.

- The brain likes blood. An early indication of brain ischemia is hypertension, often a neurogenic reflex to increase cerebral perfusion pressure. Although sudden hypertension should alert the clinician to the possibility of an intracerebral event, reactive hypertension generally should not be treated aggressively, if at all ("permissive hypertension"). On the other hand, aggressive treatment of chronic hypertension in the absence of brain ischemia is the single greatest means of stroke prevention. Once a hemorrhagic stroke has been identified, aggressive blood pressure control is indicated.

- If at all possible, personally review head CT scans and MRIs with neurologists or neuroradiologists because knowledge of the clinical presentation often allows identification of subtle abnormalities otherwise missed.

- Dedicated stroke units have been shown to decrease morbidity and mortality after stroke, primarily by preventing complications such as aspiration pneumonia and deep vein thrombosis. A bedside swallowing evaluation should be performed on all stroke patients before they are allowed to eat. Early physical and occupational therapy is critical in expediting recovery.

REFERENCES

1. Sacco RL et al: Survival and recurrence following stroke: the Framingham Study, Stroke 13:290, 1982. B
2. O'Brien AA, Rajkumar C, Bulpitt CJ: Blood pressure lowering for the primary and secondary prevention of stroke: treatment of hypertension reduces the risk of stroke, J Cardiovasc Risk 6:203, 1999. C
3. Gorelick PB et al: Prevention of a first stroke: a review of guidelines and a multidisciplinary consensus statement from the National Stroke Association, JAMA 281:1112, 1999. D
4. SHEP Cooperative Research Group: Prevention of stroke by antihypertensive drug treatment in older persons with isolated systolic hypertension, JAMA 265:3255, 1991. A
5. Davis TME et al: Risk factors for stroke in type 2 diabetes mellitus (UKPDS 29), Arch Intern Med 159:1097, 1999. B
6. Stroke Prevention in Atrial Fibrillation Investigators: Warfarin versus aspirin for prevention of thromboembolism in atrial fibrillation. Stroke Prevention in Atrial Fibrillation II Study, Lancet 343:687, 1994. A
7. North American Symptomatic Carotid Endarterectomy Trial (NASCET) Collaborators: Beneficial effect of carotid endarterectomy in symptomatic patients with high-grade stenosis, N Engl J Med 325:445, 1991. B
8. Yadav JS et al: Protected carotid-artery stenting versus endarterectomy in high-risk patients, N Engl J Med 351:1493, 2004. B
9. Albers GW et al: Transient ischemic attack: proposal for a new definition, N Engl J Med 347:1713, 2002. D
10. Johnston SC: Transient ischemic attack, N Engl J Med 347:1687, 2002. D
11. The National Institute of Neurological Disorders and Stroke rt-PA Stroke Study Group: Tissue plasminogen activator for acute ischemic stroke, N Engl J Med 333:1581, 1995. A
12. Clark WM et al: Recombinant tissue-type plasminogen activator (alteplase) for ischemic stroke 3 to 5 hours after symptom onset. The ATLANTIS study, JAMA 282:2019, 1999. A

78

STROKE

13. Hacke W et al: Randomised double-blind placebo-controlled trial of thrombolytic therapy with intravenous alteplase in acute ischaemic stroke (ECASS II), *Lancet* 352:1245, 1998. A

14. Furlan A et al: Intra-arterial prourokinase for acute ischemic stroke. The PROACT II study: a randomized controlled trial, *JAMA* 282:2003, 1999. B

15. CAST (Chinese Acute Stroke Trial) Collaborative Group: CAST: randomized placebo-controlled trial of early aspirin use in 20,0000 patients with acute ischaemic stroke, *Lancet* 349:1641, 1997. A

16. International Stroke Trial Collaborative Group: The International Stroke Trial (IST): a randomized trial of aspirin, subcutaneous heparin, both, or neither among 19,435 patients with acute ischaemic stroke, *Lancet* 349(9065):1569-1581, 1997. A

17. Coull BM et al: Anticoagulants and antiplatelet agents in acute ischemic stroke, *Neurology* 59:13, 2002. C

18. Sacks FM et al: The effect of pravastatin on coronary events after myocardial infarction in patients with average cholesterol levels. Cholesterol and Recurrent Events Trial investigators, *N Engl J Med* 335:1001, 1996. A

19. The Long-Term Intervention with Pravastatin in Ischaemic Disease (LIPID) Study Group: Prevention of cardiovascular events and death with pravastatin in patients with coronary heart disease and a broad range of initial cholesterol levels, *N Engl J Med* 339:1349, 1998. A

20. Staessen JA et al for Systolic Hypertension in Europe Trial Investigators: Randomised double-blind comparison of placebo and active treatment for older patients with isolated systolic hypertension *Lancet* 350:757, 1997. A

21. Heart Outcomes Prevention Evaluation (HOPE) Study Investigators: Effects of ramipril on cardiovascular and microvascular outcomes in people with diabetes mellitus: results of the HOPE study and MICRO-HOPE substudy, *Lancet* 355:253, 2000. A

22. CAPRIE Steering Committee: A randomized, blinded trial of clopidogrel versus aspirin in patients at risk of ischemic events (CAPRIE), *Lancet* 348:1329, 1996. A

23. The Clopidogrel in Unstable Angina to Prevent Recurrent Events Trial Investigators: Effects of clopidogrel in addition to aspirin in patients with acute coronary syndromes without ST-segment elevation, *N Engl J Med* 345:494, 2001. A

24. Diener HC et al: Aspirin and clopidogrel compared with clopidogrel alone after recent ischaemic stroke or transient ischaemic attack in high-risk patients (MATCH): randomised, double-blind, placebo-controlled trial, *Lancet* 364:331, 2004. A

25. Diener HC et al: European Stroke Prevention Study 2. Dipyridamole and acetylsalicylic acid in the secondary prevention of stroke, *J Neurol Sci* 143:1, 1996. A

26. Wu LA et al: Patent foramen ovale in cryptogenic stroke, *Arch Intern Med* 164:950, 2004. C

27. The Warfarin-Aspirin Symptomatic Intracranial Disease (WASID) Study Group: Prognosis of patients with symptomatic vertebral or basilar artery stenosis, *Stroke* 29:1389, 1998. B

28. Mohr JP et al: A comparison of warfarin and aspirin for the prevention of recurrent ischemic stroke (WARSS), *N Engl J Med* 345:1444, 2001. A

Substance Abuse

Jonathan R. Murrow, MD; Michol Rothman, MD;
and Yngvild Olsen, MD, MPH

FAST FACTS

- More than one third of patients in primary care and hospital settings have alcohol-related problems that warrant treatment.
- Complications from alcohol withdrawal include autonomic hyperactivity, agitation, seizures, and delirium; if untreated, delirium tremens carries up to a 20% mortality rate.
- Benzodiazepines are the therapy of choice for preventing alcohol withdrawal symptoms.
- However unpleasant, opiate withdrawal is not life threatening.
- Tapering dosages of a mixed opioid receptor agonist and antagonist, such as buprenorphine, can mitigate the symptoms of opiate withdrawal without producing intoxication.
- Depressed consciousness, miotic pupils, and respiratory depression in the setting of suspected opiate use establish the diagnosis of opiate overdose.
- Adequacy of airway and respiration should be established on patient presentation.
- Parenteral boluses of opiate receptor antagonists such as naloxone should be given only for signs of inadequate ventilation.

Substance abuse complicates the inpatient management of patients from all socioeconomic backgrounds. Lack of recognition of intoxication and withdrawal syndromes can lead to significant morbidity and mortality. This chapter provides an inpatient approach to dealing with substance abuse, focusing on alcohol withdrawal and opiate abuse.

Alcohol Withdrawal Syndromes

I. EPIDEMIOLOGY

1. The use of alcohol varies greatly across the U.S. population, but estimates of lifetime prevalence of abuse range from 13.7% to 23.5%. Studies suggest that up to 40% of medical and surgical patients in primary care or hospitalized settings have problems caused by alcohol that warrant treatment.[1]
2. Alcohol withdrawal occurs upon abrupt cessation or reduction in alcohol consumption after a period of prolonged, heavy use. Lack of access to alcohol coupled with lack of identification of alcohol abuse predisposes inpatients to alcohol withdrawal syndromes.
3. Alcohol withdrawal syndromes include seizures (occurring in 25% to 33% of chronic alcohol users); hallucinations (10% to 25% of

hospitalized chronic alcohol users); and delirium tremens, a potentially fatal form of alcohol withdrawal (5% of patients hospitalized with withdrawal syndromes).

II. PRESENTATION

A. SYMPTOMS

1. Major and minor symptoms are separated by degree of autonomic hyperactivity and cognitive dysfunction.
2. Minor symptoms include mild autonomic hyperactivity (sweating or pulse > 100 beats/min), tremor, insomnia, nausea, vomiting, and agitation.
3. Major symptoms include severe autonomic hyperactivity, hallucinations, delirium, and seizures. Withdrawal symptoms, including seizures, may occur while blood alcohol is still detectable.[2]

B. SIGNS AND PHYSICAL EXAMINATION

1. Autonomic hyperactivity may present with tachycardia, hypertension, or hyperthermia. Agitation, sweating, and tremor often are present on general examination.
2. Stigmata of alcohol abuse including telangiectasia, palmar erythema, gynecomastia, and testicular atrophy may be present.
3. Mental status examination can show tactile, auditory, and visual disturbances, as well as disorientation, confusion, and anxiety.[2]
4. Delirium tremens is characterized by symptoms that progress beyond the usual symptoms of alcohol withdrawal to altered mental status and seizures.

C. LABORATORY FINDINGS[1,2]

1. Anemia, high mean corpuscular volume, thrombocytopenia, elevated transaminases (aspartate aminotransferase/alanine transaminase ratio about 2:1), and elevated gamma glutamyl transpeptidase can be seen in chronic alcohol use. Low serum Mg^{2+} may suggest a lowered seizure threshold.
2. Serum volatile screen probably will be negative for ethanol. Calculation of the osmolar gap can help to diagnose other toxic ingestions.

D. OTHER STUDIES

1. Chest films may show infiltrates from aspiration, "barstool fractures" or other trauma, or cardiomegaly from alcoholic cardiomyopathy.
2. A definitely abnormal electroencephalogram suggests epilepsy or symptomatic seizures unrelated to alcohol withdrawal. The predictive value of a normal electroencephalogram in the setting of evaluation alcohol withdrawal seizures is limited.[3]

III. DIAGNOSIS

1. The diagnosis of alcohol withdrawal syndromes involves establishing a history of alcohol consumption and cessation and excluding other medical causes.

BOX 79-1

CAGE QUESTIONNAIRE

Have you ever felt as though you should **C**ut down on your drinking?

Have you felt **A**nnoyed at other people criticizing your drinking?

Have you felt **G**uilty about your drinking?

Have you ever taken a drink in the morning (an **E**ye-opener) in order to steady your nerves or to get rid of a hangover?

From Rakel R: *Conn's current therapy 2004*, 56th ed, Amsterdam, 2004, Elsevier.

a. Establishing a history of alcohol consumption and cessation is best accomplished via history obtained from the patient and the patient's family. Aspects of the history of particular interest include quantity, frequency, and duration of use. The time of the patient's last drink is also useful because it helps predict the timing of potential complications.

b. Because alcoholics are immunocompromised and prone to trauma, it is important to exclude other medical causes that may mimic withdrawal. Evaluation of seizures with brain imaging and lumbar puncture with spinal fluid analysis should be pursued in patients with a temperature higher than 38° C, known recent head trauma, focal seizures, or seizures developing after the onset of delirium.

2. Several different screening tests have been developed for identifying alcohol abuse and predicting the likelihood of developing a withdrawal syndrome. Because of its ease of use, the most prominent of these is the CAGE questionnaire (Box 79-1). For the diagnosis of alcohol abuse, CAGE is 60% to 95% sensitive and 40% to 95% specific when the cut off is more than 2 positive questions (lower specificity found in patients 60 years and older and pregnant patients).[2]

IV. RISK STRATIFICATION AND PROGNOSIS

1. Withdrawal symptoms, including seizures and delirium, are more common and severe in patients with comorbid illnesses or a prior history of withdrawal.[4]

2. Risk factors for developing delirium tremens include a prior history of delirium tremens and history of withdrawal seizures.

3. Although previous studies reported a 20% mortality rate for delirium tremens, current treatment lowers that risk to about 1%.[5] Poor outcomes are associated with intercurrent illnesses, fluid shifts, and metabolic disarray.

V. MANAGEMENT AND TREATMENT

A. SUPPORTIVE AND NUTRITIONAL THERAPY

1. Supportive care includes maintaining a quiet and safe environment. One-to-one observation or enclosed beds should be used when the patient is delirious and posing a safety risk to self or to others.[5]

2. Because of malnourishment, alcoholics often have thiamine, folate, and magnesium deficiencies.

a. Thiamine deficiency places alcoholics at high risk for developing Wernicke-Korsakoff syndrome, which is typified by ataxia, cognitive impairment, oculogyric crises, and confabulation. It is often precipitated by high-concentration glucose solutions. A replacement dosage is typically thiamine 100 mg orally, intramuscularly, or intravenously daily.[2,6]

b. Folate deficiency may present as a megaloblastic anemia. Vitamin B_{12} deficiency should be excluded to avoid masking the neurologic manifestations of B_{12} deficiency with folate repletion.

c. Alcoholics often have significant depletion of total body magnesium.[6]

B. PHARMACOLOGIC THERAPY

1. Benzodiazepines are first-line therapy for alcohol withdrawal.

a. Studies show that most benzodiazepines are effective in reducing clinical manifestations of withdrawal while preventing seizures. Less is known about comparable efficacy in treating delirium.[6]

b. Longer-acting benzodiazepines (e.g., chlordiazepoxide) may be more effective in preventing seizures but carry a risk of more marked and prolonged sedation in older adults and in patients with liver dysfunction. Short-acting benzodiazepines (e.g., alprazolam) have the advantage of rapid symptom control because of rapid onset of action, although they carry a higher potential for abuse in outpatients. In patients with hepatic dysfunction, lorazepam has the benefit of the renal contribution to drug clearance.

c. Fixed-schedule versus symptom-triggered therapy[6]:

(1) Fixed-schedule dosing (Box 79-2) is preferred for patients at high risk for seizures or delirium tremens. This is also preferred in facilities in which the staff is not trained in using formal clinical assessment tools.

(2) Symptom-triggered dosing is preferred in patients at low risk for seizures or delirium tremens and in patients with mild to moderate symptoms of withdrawal. Importantly, this is also the preferred approach in patients showing evidence of active delirium or convulsions, for whom monitoring should be intensified and continuous infusion of benzodiazepines may be necessary.

BOX 79-2

SAMPLE FIXED-SCHEDULE BENZODIAZEPINE TAPERS[6]

LONG-ACTING AGENTS

Oxazepam 45 mg PO q6h × 4 doses, then 30 mg PO q6h × 4 doses, then 15 mg PO q6h × 4 doses, then 15 mg PO q12h × 2 doses

Chlordiazepoxide 50 mg PO q6h × 4 doses, then 25 mg PO q6h × 8 doses

SHORT-ACTING AGENTS

Diazepam 10 mg q6h × 4 doses, then 5 mg q6h × 8 doses

Lorazepam 2 mg q6h × 4 doses, then 1 mg q6h × 8 doses

(3) In a retrospective study by Jaeger et al., symptom-triggered therapy was as effective as usual care (fixed dosing with as-needed doses of benzodiazepines as directed by the medical staff).[7] Outcomes measured were the duration of treatment, equivalent benzodiazepine dosage, occurrence of delirium tremens, or presence of any complication of withdrawal.

d. For active seizures or delirium, intravenous benzodiazepines can be administered every 5 to 10 minutes until sedation is achieved. Intensive care unit monitoring and continuous infusion of intravenous benzodiazepines may be necessary.

e. Benzodiazepine dosing can be tapered once symptoms are controlled and the patient is adequately sedated. Recovery from sedation may be prolonged, and the patient should be watched for recurrence of withdrawal symptoms.

2. Beta-blockers can reduce manifestations of withdrawal by blunting autonomic responses. However, beta-blockers may mask autonomic manifestations of withdrawal, thereby delaying the diagnosis.[6]

3. Carbamazepine has been shown to be equal to oxazepam in mild to moderate withdrawal. Although it has well-described anticonvulsant activity, evidence in comparing efficacy in preventing withdrawal or delirium tremens is limited.[6]

4. Phenytoin has not been shown to decrease the incidence of recurrent alcohol withdrawal seizures when compared with placebo.[8,9] In patients with a history of epilepsy or head trauma, phenytoin may have a role in treating withdrawal seizures thought to be related to alcohol.[10]

5. Clinical experience suggests that neuroleptics such at haloperidol and phenothiazines reduce signs and symptoms of withdrawal, treating agitation in particular. However, phenothiazines increase the incidence of seizures when compared with placebo.[6]

Opiate Withdrawal

I. EPIDEMIOLOGY

1. **Opiate abuse** is a maladaptive pattern of opiate use manifested by failure to fulfill major life obligations, recurrent use in hazardous settings, recurrent legal problems, and interpersonal problems related to use.[11] Patients have some control over their use and may use opiates sporadically in comparison to patients with opiate dependence.

2. **Opiate dependence** is a maladaptive pattern of use typified by tolerance, withdrawal, inability to control amount of use, desire to change use, increased time spent using, neglect of other activities due to use, and continued use despite knowledge of the adverse consequences.[11]

3. For the 900,000 people dependent on heroin in the United States, mortality is 6 to 20 times higher than in the general population.[12]

79

SUBSTANCE ABUSE

4. Formulations
a. Illicit heroin is a white or brownish powder sold in bags or pills and adulterated with various substances, including sugar or quinine, leading to an inconsistent amount of drug delivery.[13]
b. Prescription pain medications often are abused. It is estimated that about 1.5 million people older than 12 years abuse or depend on them.[14]

II. PRESENTATION

A. SYMPTOMS
1. Symptoms reflect physiologic rebound of organ systems affected by opiates. Nonspecific findings include restlessness, irritability, insomnia, nausea, vomiting, abdominal cramps, diarrhea, yawning, tearing, and rhinorrhea.[13]
2. Withdrawal symptoms begin 4 to 6 hours after last use, peak between 36 and 72 hours, and persist for up to 2 weeks.[4,13] Withdrawal from longer-acting opiates such as methadone can begin after 1 or 2 days and last for weeks.

B. SIGNS AND PHYSICAL EXAMINATION
1. Physical findings include pupillary dilation, tachycardia, hypertension, vomiting, diarrhea, and piloerection ("gooseflesh").[13]
2. Cutaneous findings such as needle tracks, cellulitis, or skin ulcers can help support a diagnosis of injection drug use if the patient does not provide such a history. Other protean manifestations include venous insufficiency and subcutaneous nodules.[15]

C. LABORATORY FINDINGS
Urine toxicology screening demonstrates the presence of opiates for several days after last use.

III. DIAGNOSIS

1. The diagnosis of opiate withdrawal syndrome is made by correlating a recent history of cessation or reduced use of an opiate in a chronic user with clinical symptoms and signs.
2. No diagnostic tests exist, although the diagnosis is supported by a response to treatment with opiate receptor agonists.

IV. RISK STRATIFICATION AND PROGNOSIS

1. Though unpleasant for the patient, opiate withdrawal syndromes are not associated with fatal outcomes except in the setting of profound dehydration or medical comorbidity associated with the underlying illicit drug abuse.[4]
2. Unless comorbid illnesses are present, patients typically do not need hospital admission for withdrawal of opiates.
3. Patients with a history of severe withdrawal are thought to be at risk for future withdrawal syndromes of increased severity.[16]

V. MANAGEMENT AND TREATMENT

A. ACUTE MANAGEMENT

1. Detoxification is based on the principle of cross-tolerance, in which the abused opiate is replaced with decreasing dosages of another opiate with a longer half-life and less abuse potential.[13]

a. Buprenorphine is a partial mu-opioid receptor agonist and a weak kappa-opioid receptor antagonist, yielding a profile with treatment of withdrawal symptoms and less potential for abuse, respiratory depression, and overdose. Although it can be administered intramuscularly and intravenously and via sublingual routes, the intravenous forms are currently preferred for treatment of pain in patients withdrawing from opiates.

b. Methadone is a synthetic long-acting mu-opioid receptor agonist given orally or parenterally for acute opiate detoxification, maintenance of heroin abstinence, and treatment of severe pain. It is a second-line therapy for opiate withdrawal in acute, inpatient settings. On an outpatient basis, methadone can be prescribed for detoxification and maintenance use by physicians with special registration from the Drug Enforcement Administration.

2. Symptom-based treatment regimens treat the myalgias and gastrointestinal complaints often experienced during opioid withdrawal. It is a less favored approach because it only partially addresses the underlying pathophysiology of withdrawal.

a. Clonidine is an alpha-2-agonist that diminishes the autonomic symptoms of opiate withdrawal by decreasing norepinephrine activity. However, studies have shown very little benefit in treating the subjective symptoms of withdrawal. Because of its antihypertensive effects, blood pressure should be carefully monitored during its use.[17]

b. Nonsteroidal antiinflammatory medications (e.g., ibuprofen) for myalgias, hypnotics (e.g., diphenhydramine) for insomnia, and antiemetics (e.g., promethazine) for vomiting are useful adjunctive therapies.[13]

3. The physician should be alert for illnesses, such as endocarditis, that often accompany intravenous drug abuse. Serologic testing should be performed to screen for hepatitis B, hepatitis C virus infection, and human immunodeficiency virus. Given the higher incidence of prostitution in this patient population, patients should be screened for syphilis, gonorrhea, and chlamydia. Finally, a purified protein derivative test should be administered to screen for tuberculosis.[15]

4. Injection drug users should be counseled to discontinue injecting drugs, to avoid needle sharing, and to practice safe sex.

B. THERAPY SELECTION

1. For acute treatment of opioid withdrawal, detoxification works well in suppressing symptoms and interrupting drug use. However, pharmacologic detoxification for opioid dependence produces inferior long-term outcomes than maintenance therapy. Rates of relapse to drug

79

SUBSTANCE ABUSE

BOX 79-3

TAPERING SCHEDULE FOR TREATING OPIOID WITHDRAWAL

SUBLINGUAL BUPRENORPHINE

Mild or moderate symptoms: 4 mg SL q4-6h

Severe symptoms: 8 mg SL q4-6h

Dosage decreases are done in 2- to 4-mg increments

INTRAMUSCULAR BUPRENORPHINE

0.9 mg IM q6h × 4 doses, then

0.6 mg IM q6h × 4 doses, then

0.6 mg IM q12h × 2 doses, then

0.6 mg IM q24h × 1 dose

Withdrawal symptoms should be reevaluated regularly at 4-hr intervals.

---

use are higher and retention in substance abuse treatment is lower for patients receiving detoxification than for those on maintenance therapy.

2. Opiate receptor agonists and antagonists such as buprenorphine can be administered intramuscularly or sublingually in tapering dosages to address withdrawal symptoms (Box 79-3).

3. Only one type of opiate should be chosen for replacement therapy. If the patient participates in a methadone maintenance program, then his or her methadone dosing should be continued. Given the long half-life of methadone, missing a single dose is unlikely to result in significant withdrawal symptoms. It is important to note that giving buprenorphine to patients on methadone or other long-acting opiates can precipitate severe withdrawal symptoms.

C. OTHER ISSUES

1. Pain management in a patient with opioid dependence can be challenging. Given adequate dosages, patients receiving prescribed opiates for treatment of acute pain should not have symptoms of opiate withdrawal. Mixed opiate receptor agonists and antagonists such as buprenorphine block the action of other opiate analgesics and should be avoided. Treatment of pain in opiate-abusing patients follows similar guidelines as for other patients, where scheduled doses and patient-controlled analgesia are preferred to as-needed dosing, long-acting oral formulations are preferred to short-acting parenteral forms, and analgesia is tapered gradually as symptoms permit.[15]

2. Consideration should be given to the fact that patients may be withdrawing from multiple substances, including alcohol.

3. Upon discharge, patients should be referred for treatment of substance abuse or receive information on where to obtain treatment.

PEARLS AND PITFALLS

- Toxidromes and their management are listed in Table 79-1.
- Patients admitting to consumption of illegally distilled grain alcohol, or "moonshine," should be screened for lead toxicity.[18]

TABLE 79-1

TOXIDROMES AND THEIR MANAGEMENT

Substance	Toxidrome	Complications	Management
Opiates[12,19-23]	Depressed mental status Miosis Hypoventilation Hypotension Bradycardia	Respiratory depression Noncardiogenic pulmonary edema	Respiratory support Naloxone
Cocaine[24]	Vital sign lability Diaphoresis Pupillary dilation Chest pain Nausea or vomiting Agitation or confusion Seizures Abnormal movement or weakness	Acute myocardial infarction Cardiac arrhythmias Aortic dissection Cerebrovascular accident Seizures Abruptio placentae Intestinal ischemia	Benzodiazepines
Depressants (i.e., gamma hydroxybutyrate, barbiturates, benzodiazepines)[25]	Acute confusional state Slurred speech Apnea	Respiratory depression	Respiratory support Urinary alkalization for phenobarbital Flumazenil for benzodiazepines
Hallucinogens (i.e., lysergic acid diethylamide, phencyclidine, tetrahydrocannabinol)	Hallucinations or psychosis Fever Mydriasis	Psychosis	Benzodiazepines
Stimulants (i.e., amphetamines, MDMA, ketamine)[26]	Agitation Hyperthermia Hypertension Rhabdomyolysis Serotonin syndrome (MDMA)	End-organ damage (renal failure, hepatic failure, rhabdomyolysis)	Benzodiazepines for agitation Cooling for hyperthermia Hydration for rhabdomyolysis Cyproheptadine or chlorpromazine for serotonin syndrome

MDMA, 3,4-methylenedioxymethamphetamine.

- Alcohol withdrawal seizures can occur in the absence of autonomic instability; they may be focal or generalized.
- Fever generally is not a feature of delirium tremens.
- Opiate analgesics should not be withheld in opiate-abusing patients complaining of pain.

- Complications of opiate overdose such as noncardiogenic pulmonary edema typically manifest within 2 hours after initial presentation.
- Some patients without an opiate overdose syndrome may show clinical response to naloxone. Conversely, lack of response to naloxone does not exclude opiate withdrawal.
- Patients with a history of ingesting long-acting opiate analgesics such as methadone warrant a longer period of observation.

REFERENCES

1. O'Connor PG, Schottenfeld RS: Patients with alcohol problems, *N Engl J Med* 338:592-602, 1998. C
2. Lohr RH: Treatment of alcohol withdrawal in hospitalized patients, *Mayo Clin Proc* 70:777-782, 1995. C
3. Sand T et al: Clinical utility of EEG in alcohol related seizures, *Acta Neurol Scand* 105:18-24, 2002. B
4. Kosten TR, O'Connor PG: Management of drug and alcohol withdrawal, *N Engl J Med* 348:1786-1795, 2003. C
5. Chang PH, Steinberg MB: Alcohol withdrawal, *Med Clin North Am* 85: 1191-1212, 2001. C
6. Mayo-Smith MF et al: Pharmacological management of alcohol withdrawal: a meta-analysis and evidence-based practice guideline, *JAMA* 278: 144-151, 1997. C
7. Jaeger TM et al: Symptom-triggered therapy for alcohol withdrawal syndrome in medical inpatients, *Mayo Clin Proc* 76:695-701, 2001. B
8. Rathlev NK et al: The lack of efficacy of phenytoin in the prevention of recurrent alcohol-related seizures, *Ann Emerg Med* 23:513-518, 1994. A
9. Chance JF: Emergency department treatment of alcohol withdrawal seizure with phenytoin, *Ann Emerg Med* 21:520-522, 1991. A
10. Holbrook AM et al: Diagnosis and management of acute alcohol withdrawal, *CMAJ* 160:675-680, 1999. C
11. American Psychiatric Association: *Diagnostic and statistical manual: text revision* (DSM-IV-TR), Washington, DC, 2000, American Psychiatric Association. C
12. Warner-Smith M et al: Heroin overdose: causes and consequences, *Addiction* 96:1113-1125, 2001. C
13. O'Connor PG, Fiellin DA: Pharmacologic treatment of heroin-dependent patients, *Ann Intern Med* 133:40-54, 2000. C
14. National Survey on Drug Use and Health: *Nonmedical use of prescription pain relievers, 2004*, Rockville, Md, 2004, U.S. Department of Health and Human Services, Substance Abuse and Mental Health Services Administration. B
15. Hopper JA, Shafi T: Management of the hospitalized injection drug user, *ID Clin NA* 16:571-587, 2002. C
16. Cami J, Farré M: Drug addiction, *N Engl J Med* 349:975-986, 2003. C
17. Gowing LR et al: α_2-Adrenergic agonists in opiate withdrawal, *Addiction* 97:49-58, 2002. C
18. Montgomery R et al: A brief review of moonshine use, *Psychiatr Serv* 50:1088, 1999. C
19. Sporer KA: Acute heroin overdose, *Ann Intern Med* 130:584-590, 1999. C
20. Ghuran A, Nolan J: Recreational drug misuse: issues for the cardiologist, *Heart* 83:627-633, 2000. C

21. Kaplan JL, Marx JA: Effectiveness and safety of intravenous nalmefene for emergency department patients with suspected narcotic overdose, *Ann Emerg Med* 22(2):187-190, 1993. A
22. Clarke S, Dargan P: Intravenous or intramuscular/subcutaneous naloxone in opioid overdose, *Emerg Med J* 19:249-250, 2002. A
23. Clarke S, Dargan P: Intravenous bolus or infusion of naloxone in opioid overdose, *Emerg Med J* 19:249-250, 2002. A
24. Cregler L, Mark H: Medical complications of cocaine abuse, *N Engl J Med* 315:1495-1500, 1986. C
25. Mokhlesi B et al: Adult toxicology in critical care, *Chest* 123:577-592, 2003. C
26. Gahlinger PM: Club drugs: MDMA, gamma-hydroxybutyrate (GHB), Rohypnol, and ketamine, *Am Fam Physician* 69:2619-2626, 2004. C

Pulmonary Function Tests

Jenna D. Goldberg, MD; Anna Hemnes, MD;
and Charles M. Wiener, MD

FAST FACTS

- Obstructive ventilatory defect is defined by a decrease in the expiratory flow rate.
- Restrictive ventilatory defect is defined by a decrease in total lung capacity (TLC).
- Diffusion capacities of lung carbon monoxide (DLCO) of < 50% and < 40% are predictive of oxygen desaturation with exercise and pulmonary hypertension, respectively.
- Postbronchodilator forced expiratory volume at 1 second (FEV_1) and age are the most important mortality predictors in chronic obstructive pulmonary disease.

Many pulmonary function tests (PFTs) are available, but this chapter focuses on those most commonly used. A full set of PFTs generally consists of spirometry, helium lung volume measurements, and measurement of the DLCO. These tests are useful for characterizing and quantifying pulmonary dysfunction. Other tests include a bronchodilator challenge test to detect reversible airway obstruction or a methacholine challenge test to detect airway hyperreactivity. The addition of flow-volume loops to spirometry can further characterize pulmonary physiology. Individual values are compared with those predicted by patient height, age, sex, and race. Fig. 80-1 and Table 80-1 illustrate and define the various lung volumes and capacities important in PFTs. Indications include diagnosing pulmonary disease, assessing severity or progression of known disease, and risk stratifying patients for surgery. PFTs may have a role in screening certain populations such as current or former cigarette smokers and patients with a history of exposure to lung irritants.[1] This chapter will provide a framework for interpreting PFTs and identifying obstructive ventilatory defects, restrictive ventilatory defects, and gas exchange defects.

I. OBSTRUCTION

1. The hallmark of an obstructive defect is a decrease in the expiratory flow rate; therefore, spirometry is the best test for its evaluation.[2] First, the ratio of FEV_1 to forced vital capacity (FVC) ratio should be considered. A consensus statement on spirometry put forth in 1994 by the American Thoracic Society dictates that establishing normal values and standardizing interpretation are the job of the director of a PFT laboratory.[3] At Johns Hopkins, if the measured ratio is less than 5% of the predicted ratio, obstruction is present. Once obstruction is detected,

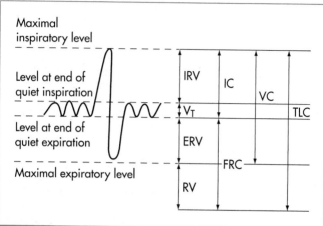

FIG. 80-1

Inspired and expired volumes during normal quiet breathing. Most lung volumes and capacities can be measured by spirometry. (TLC, FRC, and RV are not determined by spirometry.) *ERV,* expiratory reserve volume; *FRC,* functional residual capacity; *IC,* inspiratory capacity; *IRV,* inspiratory reserve capacity; *RV,* residual volume; *TLC,* total lung capacity; *VC,* vital capacity; V_T, tidal volume. (*Adapted from Honig EG, Ingram RH Jr: Sci Am WebMD, retrieved January 29, 2003, from www.samed.com.*)

TABLE 80-1

MOST COMMON PULMONARY FUNCTION TESTS

Test	Technique	Data Obtained
Spirometry	Maximal inhalation followed by maximal exhalation, measuring volume of air and time	FVC, FEV_1, FEV_1/FVC, VC
Diffusing capacity of the lung for CO	Inhalation of fixed concentration of CO and helium, breath holding for 10 s, then expiration with measurement of end-tidal CO and helium	Uptake and diffusing capacity of CO
Helium lung volumes	Maximal expiration, then inhalation of a known concentration of helium until steady state is reached	RV, ERV, IRV, TV with calculation of TLC, VC, FRC, IC

CO, carbon monoxide; *ERV,* expiratory reserve volume; FEV_1, forced expiratory volume in 1 second; *FRC,* functional reserve capacity; *FVC,* forced vital capacity; *IC,* inspiratory capacity; *IRV,* inspiratory reserve volume; *RV,* residual volume; *TLC,* total lung capacity; *TV,* tidal volume; *VC,* ventilatory capacity.

it must be quantified by a determination of the absolute value of FEV_1 in liters. If the FEV_1 is greater than 2 L, the obstruction is mild; between 1 and 2 L, it is moderate; and less than 1 L, it is severe. If obstruction is present, TLC may be greater than normal because of hyperinflation. Vital capacity sometimes is diminished as residual volume (RV) is significantly enlarged because of air trapping. It is possible to detect early air trapping with PFTs if RV is elevated. On flow-volume loops patients with obstruction appear to have a concave expiratory flow pattern with nearly normal inspiration as compared with normal subjects (Fig. 80-2). Common causes of obstruction are chronic obstructive pulmonary disease, asthma, cystic fibrosis, and bronchiolitis obliterans.

2. Bronchodilators can be used to differentiate fixed obstruction (e.g., emphysema) from reversible obstruction (e.g., asthma). If FEV_1 or FVC increases by more than 12% and an absolute improvement of 200 ml occurs in response to bronchodilation, the obstruction has a reversible component.[4] Most patients who respond to bronchodilators during this test also respond clinically, but many people who have no response to bronchodilators in the PFT laboratory demonstrate some clinical improvement; therefore, the decision to treat a patient with bronchodilators remains a clinical one.[5] The patient should not use any bronchodilator for more than 48 hours before this test.

3. Intermittent obstruction from bronchospasm may not be manifested as a decrease in FEV_1/FVC if the test is performed at a time when no bronchospasm is present. In this situation methacholine challenge testing is used to assess airway hyperreactivity. If FEV_1 decreases by 20% or more in response to methacholine at a concentration of 16 mg/ml or more dilute, bronchial hyperreactivity is present. Not all people with bronchial hyperreactivity have asthma: False positive results may be seen with allergic rhinitis, cystic fibrosis, congestive heart failure, chronic obstructive pulmonary disease, and bronchitis.[6,7] In an asymptomatic person, a positive methacholine challenge test may predict future development of asthma.[8] However, a normal methacholine test result has a negative predictive value of 95% if no bronchodilators were used before the test.

4. Flow-volume loops (which incorporate both forced inspiratory and expiratory maneuvers) can be helpful in localizing and characterizing an obstruction. Extrathoracic obstructions can be differentiated from intrathoracic obstructions by the presence of truncated inspiratory curves. Comparisons of various curves can help to differentiate fixed from variable obstructions. Fig. 80-2 illustrates examples of variable and fixed intrathoracic and extrathoracic obstructive flow-volume loops.

II. RESTRICTION

1. The hallmark of a restrictive defect is decreased lung volumes. To evaluate a patient for restriction, the physician should first measure

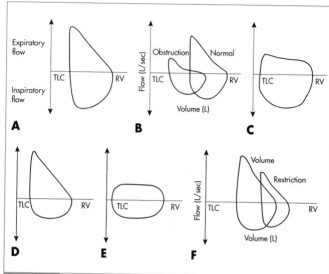

FIG. 80-2

Flow-volume curves. Flow is shown on the ordinate, with expiration above and inspiration below the intercept. Volume is shown on the abscissa, from total lung capacity (TLC) to residual volume (RV). **A,** Normal expiratory flow-volume curve. **B,** In variable intrathoracic obstruction the expiratory flow-volume curve has a scooped-out appearance resulting from progressive decreases in flow as lung volume becomes smaller. Obstruction is volume dependent. Flow rates at any given lung volume (isovolumic flow) are reduced. Because of air trapping, the entire curve may be shifted to a higher lung volume (leftward). This pattern is typical of chronic obstructive pulmonary disease of asthma. **C,** Expiratory flow-volume curve showing a decreased flow that is the same at all lung volumes. Obstruction, which is not dependent on lung volume, is caused by upper airway obstruction, not disease of the lung parenchyma. **D,** Disproportionate reduction of inspiration airflow is indicative of variable extrathoracic upper airway obstruction. **E,** Fixed airway obstruction, the site of which is undetermined, shows volume-independent reduction of flow in both inspiration and expiration. **F,** Expiratory flow-volume curve in a patient with a restrictive disorder. Isovolumic flow rates are increased, whereas the volume axis is compressed and shifted toward lower volume (rightward). *(From Honig EG, Ingram RH Jr: Functional assessment of the lung and diagnostic techniques,* Sci Am WebMD, *retrieved January 29, 2003, from www.samed.com.)*

TLC. If the TLC is less than 80% of the predicted value, restriction is present. Between 65% and 80% the restrictive ventilatory defect is mild, between 50% and 65% it is moderate, and less than 50% it is severe.

2. There are three basic categories of restrictive lung disease: intrinsic disease, chest wall deformities, and neuromuscular disorders. The other lung volume measurements (RV, functional residual capacity [FRC]) may help delineate between these conditions. Decreased FRC and RV characterize intrinsic defects such as parenchymal lung disease. FRC is also decreased in chest wall deformities such as morbid obesity and kyphoscoliosis. However, RV, which measures mainly airway closure in adults, is normal in association with chest wall disease. A restrictive ventilatory defect with a normal FRC should raise suspicion of neuromuscular diseases such as amyotrophic lateral sclerosis. In this situation, RV may be increased.

III. GAS TRANSFER

1. The diffusion of gas across the alveolar-capillary membrane is measured by assessment of carbon monoxide diffusion. CO has a high affinity for hemoglobin, so it has a virtually unlimited reservoir in the pulmonary vascular bed, and the pressure gradient for CO diffusion depends solely on the partial pressure of CO in the alveolus. Thus resistance to diffusion depends on the resistance across the alveolar-capillary membrane. Therefore, the measurement of DLCO reflects the surface area between alveolus and capillary and the thickness of the membrane.

2. Other factors affecting DLCO include the pulmonary capillary blood volume, ventilation-perfusion mismatching, and hemoglobin levels. Often the measured DLCO is corrected to adjust for the patient's hemoglobin level before it is compared with standard predicted values for age, height, and sex or for alveolar volume. The measurement of DLCO helps narrow the differential diagnosis when used in conjunction with other PFT parameters (Box 80-1).

PEARLS AND PITFALLS

- Abnormal PFT results in obese patients have been shown to indicate intrinsic respiratory dysfunction and not merely dysfunction secondary to obesity, except in the morbidly obese.
- On the basis of the test descriptions, it is clear that patient effort greatly affects the results of PFTs and is an important determinant of accuracy and reproducibility. A statement about the quality of the test (e.g., good, fair, or poor) should accompany each test result.[11] Fair- and poor-quality tests should be interpreted with caution.
- Forced expiratory volumes may be underestimated in older patients and in patients with airway obstruction. A more accurate determination of ventilatory capacity in this case may be obtained by determining the relaxed vital capacity.[3]

BOX 80-1

DIFFERENTIAL DIAGNOSIS FOR GAS EXCHANGE DEFICITS

↓ DLCO WITH NORMAL PULMONARY FUNCTION TESTS

Anemia

Pulmonary hypertension

Chronic pulmonary thromboembolism

Pulmonary vasculitis

↓ DLCO WITH OBSTRUCTION

Emphysema

Cystic fibrosis

Allergic bronchopulmonary aspergillosis

Bronchiolitis (virus, drugs)

Graft versus host disease

↓ DLCO WITH RESTRICTION

Interstitial lung disease

Hypersensitivity pneumonitis

Neoplastic lymphangitic spread

Drug toxicity (e.g., amiodarone)

↑ DLCO

Asthma

Alveolar hemorrhage

Congestive heart failure (usually mild)

Polycythemia

Left → right shunting

Exercise

DLCO, diffusing capacity of the lung for carbon monoxide.

- A DLCO measurement of < 50% of the predicted value is predictive for desaturation with exercise.[10]
- A difference between supine and erect FVC of > 10% suggests diaphragmatic weakness.
- Because age, sex, race, and especially height affect normal values, selection of the appropriate reference values is imperative. The American Thoracic Society has published guidelines for selecting such values, and in general the lower limit of normal ranges should be used.[4,12]

REFERENCES

1. Petty TL, Weinmann GG: Building a national strategy for the prevention and management of and research in chronic obstructive pulmonary disease, *JAMA* 277:246, 1997. D
2. Fergusson GT et al: Office spirometry for lung health assessment in adults: a consensus statement from the National Lung Health Education Program, *Chest* 117:1146, 2000. D
3. American Thoracic Society: Standardization of spirometry, 1994 update, *Am J Respir Crit Care Med* 152:1107, 1995. D

4. American Thoracic Society: Lung function testing: selection of reference values and interpretative strategies, *Am Rev Respir Dis* 144:1202, 1991. D
5. Crapo RO: Pulmonary-function testing, *N Engl J Med* 331:25, 1994. C
6. American Thoracic Society: Guidelines for methacholine and exercise challenge testing: 1999, *Am J Respir Crit Care Med* 161:309, 2000. D
7. Laprise C et al: Asymptomatic airway hyperresponsiveness: relationships with airway inflammation and remodeling, *Eur Respir J* 14:63, 1999. C
8. Morrison NJ et al: Comparison of single breath carbon monoxide diffusing capacity and pressure-volume curves in detective emphysema, *Am Rev Respir Dis* 139:1179, 1989. B
9. Ray CS et al: Effects of obesity on respiratory function, *Am Rev Respir Dis* 128:501, 1983. B
10. Owens GR: The diffusing capacity as a predictor of arterial oxygen desaturation during exercise in patients with COPD, *N Engl J Med* 310:1218, 1984. B
11. American Thoracic Society: Standardization of spirometry—1987 update: statement of the American Thoracic Society, *Am Rev Respir Dis* 136:1285, 1987. D
12. Screening for adult respiratory disease: official American Thoracic Society statement, March 1983, *Am Rev Respir Dis* 128:768, 1983. D

Asthma

*Anandi N. Sheth, MD; Tatiana M. Prowell, MD;
and Jerry A. Krishnan, MD*

FAST FACTS

- Essential features of asthma are chronic airway inflammation, airway hyperresponsiveness, and airflow obstruction with episodic respiratory symptoms (dyspnea, wheeze, cough, chest tightness). Airflow obstruction in asthma is reversible, either partially or completely, with bronchodilator therapy.
- Asthma exacerbations are associated most often with respiratory viral infections (> 50%). Other causes include environmental exposures to allergens (e.g., cockroaches) or irritants (e.g., tobacco smoke). Nonadherence to controller therapy is common in patients with severe asthma exacerbations.
- Spirometry is the gold standard test for diagnosing airflow obstruction.
- Signs of a severe acute asthma attack include inability to speak in full sentences, accessory muscle retraction, paradoxical movement of the abdomen, carbon dioxide retention, and pulsus paradoxus.

81

I. EPIDEMIOLOGY

1. Asthma occurs in 7% of the U.S. population; half of these cases develop in childhood. Overall mortality from asthma is 2 per 100,000 people.[1]
2. Morbidity and hospitalization rates from asthma are rising, especially among women and in urban populations.[2] African-Americans 15 to 24 years of age have the highest asthma-related mortality rate.[3]
3. Access to appropriate primary care can obviate hospitalization in asthmatic patients. Of asthmatic adults hospitalized for an asthma flare, 50% are not receiving chronic antiinflammatory therapy. Approximately 75% of patients have no plan for treating exacerbations.[4]

II. CLINICAL PRESENTATION

A. SYMPTOMS

1. Symptoms include intermittent wheezing, cough, chest tightness, and dyspnea.
2. Symptoms are episodic and often worse overnight because of increased bronchomotor tone and circadian variations of catecholamines, cortisol, and other inflammatory mediators.
3. Common triggers, usually identifiable by the patient, include respiratory infections (mostly viral), allergens (e.g., animal dander), environmental exposures (e.g., tobacco), exercise, cold air, and emotional stress.

4. Most patients with allergic asthma have a personal or family history of allergic rhinitis, sinusitis, atopy, or asthma.
5. In an acute exacerbation, it is important to assess how symptoms compare with previous exacerbations, prior hospitalizations, and exacerbations necessitating mechanical ventilation.

B. PHYSICAL FINDINGS

1. Physical examination findings are most helpful in the setting of an acute flare, when patients present with polyphonic expiratory wheezes, cough, prolonged expiratory phase, hyperinflation of the thorax, and decreased breath sounds.
2. Other important physical findings include nasal polyps, rhinorrhea, sinus tenderness, nasal mucosal edema, pallor, erythema, and dry skin with lichenification or excoriation suggestive of eczema.
3. It is important to exclude stridor or monophonic wheeze over the glottis because it suggests upper airway obstruction; crackles suggest an alternative pulmonary process.
4. Red flags for severe obstruction include upright posture, use of accessory muscles, and pulsus paradoxus.
5. Chest radiograph often shows hyperinflation. It is also important to assess for concomitant pneumonia.

III. DIFFERENTIAL DIAGNOSIS (Table 81-1)

IV. DIAGNOSIS
A. PEAK EXPIRATORY FLOW

1. The most cost-effective test to support the diagnosis of asthma is peak expiratory flow (PEF) monitoring using a peak flow meter.
2. With normal diurnal variation, PEF reaches its nadir in the early morning and peaks in early afternoon, a pattern that is exaggerated in asthmatic patients.
3. Patients should be asked to keep a diary of PEF measurements on waking, after use of a beta-agonist, and in the afternoon after use of a beta-agonist. Variability of more than 20% between any two measurements strongly suggests asthma.[5]

B. SPIROMETRY

1. Spirometry is the gold standard test for establishing obstructive lung disease in asthma (Fig. 81-1). It is superior to PEF because low PEFs can result from poor patient effort, muscle weakness, restrictive lung disease, or other obstructive lung diseases.
2. Reduced forced expiratory volume in 1 second (FEV_1) and the FEV_1/forced vital capacity ratio (fractional lung emptying in 1 second) suggests an obstructive ventilatory defect.
3. Decreased forced vital capacity in a patient without restrictive lung disease reflects an elevated residual volume, suggesting air trapping.
4. Spirometry with flow volume loops should be obtained in patients who do not improve despite inpatient therapy to confirm the presence of

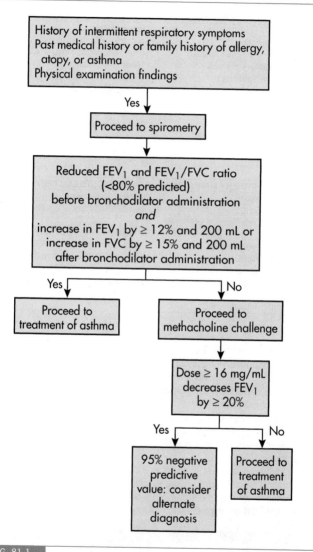

FIG. 81-1

Management approach to the patient with a possible diagnosis of asthma. *FEV₁*, forced expiratory volume in 1 second; *FVC*, forced vital capacity.

TABLE 81-1

DIFFERENTIAL DIAGNOSIS OF ASTHMA

Condition	Diagnostic Test
Vocal cord dysfunction	Spirometry with flow volume loops
Eosinophilic lung disorders (allergic bronchopulmonary aspergillosis, Churg-Strauss syndrome)	Serum immunoglobulin E, ANCA, serum eosinophil count
Gastroesophageal reflux disease	24-hour pH probe or empiric therapy
Pulmonary embolism	Ventilation-perfusion imaging or helical computed tomography
Sinusitis	Sinus computed tomography

ANCA, antineutrophilic cytoplasmic antibody.

TABLE 81-2

EXAMPLE OF INPATIENT MANAGEMENT PLAN FOR ACUTE EXACERBATION

Inpatient Medications	Discharge Medications
Albuterol nebulizer 2.5 mg q4h (or albuterol MDI w/spacer 2-4 puffs q4h)	Albuterol MDI w/spacer 2 puffs q4h PRN
Albuterol nebulizer 2.5 mg q1h PRN (or albuterol MDI w/spacer 2-4 puffs q1h)	Prednisone 50 mg PO qd for 7 d
Prednisone 60 mg PO qd (or methylprednisolone 48 mg IV qd)	Advair 250/50 Diskus 1 inhalation BID
Supplemental oxygen for SaO$_2$ >93%	Instructions about appropriate use of MDI, spacer, and Advair Diskus
Advair 250/50 Diskus (fluticasone and salmeterol) 1 inhalation BID	

BID, twice a day; *MDI,* metered-dose inhaler; *PRN,* as needed.

obstructive ventilatory defect. The lack of airflow obstruction during an exacerbation rules out asthma as the underlying cause.

C. BRONCHIAL PROVOCATION TEST

1. Bronchial provocation tests provide objective evidence of airway hyperresponsiveness.
2. FEV_1 is measured serially as the patient inhales increasing concentrations of a provocative agent (e.g., methacholine). Patients with airway hyperresponsiveness experience airway constriction and a decreased FEV_1.
3. Although a positive test (defined as a decrease in FEV_1 of > 20% with methacholine < 8 mg/ml) is not specific for asthma, a negative test has a predictive value of more than 95% and can exclude the diagnosis in a patient with an atypical history or normal FEV_1.

V. MANAGEMENT

A. INPATIENT MANAGEMENT OF ACUTE EXACERBATION (Table 81-2)

1. **Oxygen.** Hypoxemia occurs secondary to ventilation-perfusion mismatch, and so bronchodilators may transiently worsen hypoxemia. Oxygen should be administered to asthmatic patients, with a goal oxygen saturation of 92% or higher. Even patients with severe

exacerbations generally can be oxygenated with 28% to 32% supplemental oxygen.

2. **Bronchodilator therapy.**
a. The short-acting inhaled beta-2-agonists (e.g., albuterol) are the mainstay of therapy for breakthrough symptoms and acute asthma exacerbations.
b. Onset of action occurs within 5 minutes, with duration of action of 6 hours. The recommended dosage of albuterol in an acute flare is four puffs by metered-dose inhaler (MDI) and spacer every 10 minutes or 2.5 mg nebulized every 20 minutes. For equivalent dosage, an MDI with spacer (used correctly) is as effective as nebulized albuterol.[6]
c. A recent meta-analysis showed equivalent outcomes with intermittent and continuous nebulizer treatments,[7] except in the subpopulation of patients with the most severe flares (PEF of < 200 L/min or < 50% of predicted).[8]
d. No good data exist on the use of subcutaneous terbutaline or epinephrine. Because of their cardiovascular side effects, use is discouraged unless the patient is not responding to inhaled medications.
e. No evidence is available to guide the tapering of bronchodilator treatments. Patients should be evaluated frequently for signs of improvement or fatigue. Generally, treatments should not be tapered until the PEF is more than 50% of predicted or baseline values. Then, treatments may be decreased to every 4 hours, with additional treatments every 2 hours on an as-needed basis. Patients may be discharged when lung function is at least 60% baseline or predicted.

3. **Corticosteroid therapy.**
a. Multiple studies have shown that systemic corticosteroids (e.g., methylprednisolone, prednisone) decrease the rate of relapse after an acute exacerbation.[9] However, there is no benefit to steroid dosages exceeding 50 mg/day (prednisone equivalent).[10]
b. Evidence supports discharging the patient with a 5- to 10-day course of 40 to 60 mg oral prednisone,[11] with no need to involve tapering dosages.[12]
c. The addition of inhaled corticosteroids to oral prednisone can further decrease beta-2-agonist use, likelihood of relapse, and symptoms after an acute exacerbation.

4. **Anticholinergic therapy (ipratropium).** Ipratropium is preferred therapy for beta-blocker–induced bronchospasm and may have a role in treating severe asthma exacerbations. Data on the addition of ipratropium to standard therapy are contradictory and limited by small patient populations and short follow-up times. Subgroup analysis of the most severe asthma flares has shown statistically significant but clinically modest effects on PEF and hospitalization rate.[13] The dosage is four puffs by MDI and spacer every 10 minutes or 500 µg nebulized every 20 minutes.

5. **Magnesium sulfate.** There is no clinically significant benefit to the routine use of magnesium in terms of PEF or hospitalization rate. However, it has possible benefit in the subgroup with the most severe exacerbations. In this subgroup, magnesium sulfate (2 g intravenously over 20 minutes) has been shown to increase PEF by about 50 L/min and to modestly decrease hospitalization rates.[14]

6. **Other acute therapy.**
   a. Theophylline is a bronchodilator with a narrow therapeutic window and minimal efficacy in acute exacerbations. It does not add a significant benefit when given in addition to beta-2-agonists, but it does increase side effects.
   b. Antibiotics do not play a role in managing an acute asthma flare unless the patient has evidence of a concomitant bacterial infection (pneumonia or sinusitis).

7. **Noninvasive positive-pressure ventilation.** Small studies have shown a reduction in $PaCO_2$ and symptomatic improvement in asthmatic patients admitted to intensive care units with noninvasive positive-pressure ventilation.[15] On the basis of experience in other forms of respiratory failure, considering its early use in high-risk, cooperative patients as an alternative to mechanical ventilation is reasonable, with initial settings at about 8 cm H_2O inspiratory pressure and 5 cm H_2O expiratory pressure (see Chapter 19).

8. **Mechanical ventilation.** Mechanical ventilation should be considered in patients with worsening fatigue despite the aforementioned treatment or impending cardiopulmonary compromise. The goal is to minimize lung hyperinflation with low minute ventilation, decreased inspiratory time, and goal plateau airway pressures less than 35 cm H_2O until response to pharmacologic therapy decreases airway obstruction.

B. OUTPATIENT MANAGEMENT OF CHRONIC ASTHMA (Table 81-3)

1. **Inhaled corticosteroids.**
   a. Inhaled corticosteroids are the cornerstone of asthma management. Beneficial effects include improvement in FEV_1 or PEF, frequency and severity of exacerbations, and rate of relapse. Inhaled corticosteroids are the most effective single therapy for adults with asthma.[16]
   b. It is important to advise patients to rinse the mouth and to use a spacer with these medications in order to minimize local side effects (e.g., thrush, hoarseness) and systemic absorption across the gastrointestinal tract.
   c. Serious systemic side effects are uncommon in adults receiving moderate dosages but include adrenal suppression, cataracts, glaucoma, and decreased bone mineral density.

2. **Long-acting bronchodilators.** Long-acting bronchodilators include beta-2-adrenergic agonists (salmeterol) and phosphodiesterase inhibitors (theophylline and aminophylline).
   a. Salmeterol is well tolerated and has demonstrated superiority over albuterol in terms of symptom reduction and improvement in FEV_1 or

TABLE 81-3
CLASSIFICATION AND MANAGEMENT OF CHRONIC ASTHMA BY SEVERITY

Category	Symptoms	Nocturnal Symptoms	Pulmonary Function	Preferred Controller Agents	Rescue Agents
Mild intermittent	Symptoms < 2×/wk Activity unlimited Flares brief and rare	< 2×/mo	FEV_1 or PEF ≥ 80% predicted PEF varies by ≤ 20%	None	Inhaled β_2-agonist PRN*
Mild persistent	Symptoms > 2×/wk Activity mildly limited Flares once a week	< 2×/mo	FEV_1 or PEF > 80% predicted PEF varies by 20-30%	Low-dose inhaled steroid	Inhaled β_2-agonist PRN*
Moderate persistent	Symptoms daily Activity mildly limited Flares > 2×/wk	> 1×/wk	FEV_1 or PEF 60-80% predicted	Low- or medium-dose inhaled steroid with long-acting β_2-agonist†	Inhaled β_2-agonist PRN*
Severe persistent	Symptoms constant Activity severely limited Flares frequent and prolonged	Often	FEV_1 or PEF 60% predicted PEF varies by > 30%	High-dose inhaled steroid and long-acting β_2-agonist, with systemic steroids if needed	Inhaled β_2-agonist PRN*

Modified from National Heart, Blood and Lung Institute: *Guidelines for the diagnosis and management of asthma.* Expert Panel Report 2. National Asthma Education and Prevention Program, NIH Pub No 97-4051, Bethesda, Md, 1997, National Institutes of Health; and Sin DD et al: Pharmacological management to reduce exacerbations in adults with asthma: a systematic review and meta-analysis. *JAMA* 292:367-376, 2004.

FEV_1, forced expiratory volume in 1 s; *PEF*, peak expiratory flow; *PRN*, as needed.

*Daily or increasing use of short-acting inhaled β_2-agonist indicates suboptimal asthma control and the need to reevaluate environmental triggers (e.g., pets) and to advance to the next phase of controller agents.

†Alternative: increased inhaled steroid or inhaled steroid with leukotriene modifier or theophylline.

81

ASTHMA

PEF.[17] The use of long-acting beta-agonists without concomitant inhaled corticosteroids has been associated with a higher risk of death, so they should be used only with inhaled corticosteroid maintenance therapy.[18] However, when beta-agonists are added to inhaled corticosteroids, the combination is more effective than either inhaled corticosteroids alone or higher-dose inhaled corticosteroids.[16]

b. Theophylline is rarely used in adults except in cases of refractory asthma because of its narrow therapeutic window. Adverse reactions include gastrointestinal intolerance, dose-related arrhythmias, seizures, and drug interactions.

3. **Leukotriene modifiers.** Leukotriene modifiers include agents that decrease leukotriene production (zileuton) or block leukotriene receptors (zafirlukast, montelukast).

a. Beneficial effects include prevention of airway smooth muscle contraction, decrease in vascular permeability, and prevention of inflammatory cell migration. Although leukotriene modifiers have a clear benefit in terms of symptoms and PEF compared with placebo,[19] inhaled corticosteroids produce greater improvement in symptoms and PEF and decrease in frequency of exacerbations.[16]

b. Leukotriene modifiers are recommended in mild persistent asthma as an alternative to inhaled corticosteroids or in moderate persistent asthma in addition to inhaled corticosteroids. They are beneficial in patients with aspirin-sensitive asthma.

c. Reported side effects include hepatotoxicity, gastrointestinal intolerance, angioedema or anaphylaxis, and rarely Churg-Strauss syndrome (controversial).

4. **Systemic corticosteroids.** Systemic corticosteroids should be used as long-term controller medications only in patients with severe, persistent asthma after other therapies have been exhausted. Patients who appear to be glucocorticoid resistant often have alternative diagnoses (see Table 81-1). These agents have significant long-term toxicities (see Chapter 26).

5. **Antiimmunoglobulin E (IgE) therapy (omalizumab).** Omalizumab is a recombinant monoclonal humanized antibody that binds free IgE, preventing IgE from binding cells. Studies show that parenteral administration decreases serum IgE levels. Omalizumab decreases symptoms, use of oral corticosteroids and rescue medications, and frequency of exacerbations in patients with moderate persistent to severe persistent allergic asthma.[20] Drawbacks include its expense and the need for in-office biweekly to monthly subcutaneous injections.

6. **Steroid-sparing agents.** Steroid-sparing agents include methotrexate, cyclosporine, and gold. However, reduction in steroid dosage often is minimal.[21] At present, there is insufficient evidence to recommend these agents for asthma control.

7. **Short-acting bronchodilators.** Short-acting bronchodilators have less of a role in the long-term management of asthma and should be used only as rescue medications, not as scheduled treatment. Albuterol on an as-needed basis is equivalent to scheduled dosage in terms of PEF, symptoms, and exacerbations in mild disease.[22] Albuterol use has been associated with an increase in fatal and near-fatal outcomes, even after adjustment for disease severity.[23]

C. NONPHARMACOLOGIC MANAGEMENT OF ASTHMA

1. **Allergy history.**
a. All asthmatic patients should be screened for a history of allergies. Common household allergens include dust mites (often found in carpets and bedding materials), pollen, cockroaches, molds, and pets.
b. Surprisingly, studies have failed to demonstrate a significant benefit of decreasing allergen exposure.[24] Immunotherapy using identified patient-specific allergens has been shown to significantly reduce symptoms and bronchial hyperreactivity, although data are controversial.[25] Adverse reactions such as atopic dermatitis and rhinitis are common, and anaphylactic reactions can occur.
2. **Asthma triggers.** Common triggers, usually identifiable by the patient, include respiratory infections (mostly viral), allergens (dust mites, animal dander, mold, pollen), environmental exposures (tobacco, exhaust, ozone), exercise, cold air, emotional stress, gastroesophageal reflux disease, and postnasal drip. Avoiding or modifying triggers appears to reduce symptoms but may not produce a significant improvement in measures of pulmonary function.[26]
3. **Patient education and self-monitoring.**
a. Every patient should have a peak flow meter and should be educated about the differences between controller and rescue medications.
b. Staff should confirm correct technique with MDIs, spacer devices, and peak flow meters.
c. A written plan for the diagnosis of an exacerbation and actions to take based on the patient's personal best or predicted PEF should be developed, including specific PEF values for each zone of severity and specific directions on how to alter medications (Table 81-4).

PEARLS AND PITFALLS

- Worsening tachypnea, tachycardia, diaphoresis, accessory muscle use, and inability to complete full sentences despite maximal therapy (short-acting bronchodilators, systemic corticosteroids, supplemental oxygen) suggest a severe asthma flare and warrant immediate treatment in the intensive care unit.
- Other clinically established markers of a life-threatening flare include pulsus paradoxus of more than 25 mmHg (inspiratory fall in systolic blood pressure, compared with normal decrease of < 10 mmHg), bradycardia, hypotension, mental status changes, pneumothorax, diminishing respiratory effort, and cyanosis.

TABLE 81-4

EXAMPLE OF ASTHMA FLARE ACTION PLAN

Zone	Interpretation	Action
Green zone: 80-100% predicted PEF	Good control	No change needed
Yellow zone: 50-79% predicted PEF	Inadequate control	Add rescue medications Increase dosage of controllers
Red zone: < 50% predicted PEF	Medical emergency	Add or increase rescue medications Call physician immediately

Modified from National Heart, Lung and Blood Institute: *Guidelines for the diagnosis and management of asthma*, Expert Panel Report 2, National Asthma Education and Prevention Program, NIH Pub No 97-4051, Bethesda, Md, 1997, National Institutes of Health.
PEF, peak expiratory flow.

- Pulsus paradoxus depends on inspiratory and expiratory effort, so it may fall with respiratory fatigue.
- Arterial blood gases should be assessed when the PEF is less than 50% of the predicted value or if there is any suspicion of respiratory failure.
- Early in an asthma flare, patients have a respiratory alkalosis caused by dyspnea and hyperventilation. As respiratory muscles become fatigued, pseudonormalization of CO_2 tension and pH occurs as CO_2 retention and respiratory acidosis develop. Although oxygenation may still be normal, this is worrisome for impending respiratory failure.
- Persistent hypoxemia despite oxygen therapy should prompt consideration of an alternative diagnosis with shunt physiology (e.g., pneumonia).
- Because mechanical ventilation is always preferable on an elective rather than an emergency basis, any patient with evidence of respiratory muscle fatigue deserves early evaluation by the intensive care unit staff and frequent reevaluation by a physician.
- Exercise-induced bronchospasm may be an isolated problem or one of many asthma triggers in a given patient. Patients generally report cough, shortness of breath, wheezing, or chest tightness during exercise, with symptoms peaking about 10 minutes after cessation of activity and resolving spontaneously within 30 minutes of activity.
- Exercise-induced asthma is most commonly a clinical diagnosis but may be confirmed by a decrease of more than 15% in PEF or FEV_1 after exercise.
- Therapeutic options for exercise-induced asthma include albuterol or salmeterol taken 30 minutes before exercise; salmeterol has a more prolonged effect. Nedocromil can be taken shortly before exercise for a 1- to 2-hour effect. An inhaled steroid should be used on a regular basis in an attempt to reduce use of short-acting agents.[16]

- When appropriately managed, exercise-induced asthma should not prevent an athlete from participating in recreational or competitive sports.
- Allergic bronchopulmonary aspergillosis is a complex hypersensitivity disorder often seen in patients with severe asthma and cystic fibrosis when their airways become colonized with *Aspergillus*. It should be considered when patients with asthma have recurrent fever, malaise, eosinophilia, and pulmonary infiltrates.
- Diagnostic criteria for allergic bronchopulmonary aspergillosis include the presence of asthma, positive skin test for *Aspergillus,* elevated total serum IgE level (> 1000 ng/ml), *Aspergillus*-specific IgE or IgG antibodies, and pulmonary infiltrates or central bronchiectasis seen on computed tomography.
- With increasing recognition of the prevalence of allergic bronchopulmonary aspergillosis among asthmatic patients, a skin test for *Aspergillus fumigatus* is indicated in patients with worsening asthma control with no other explanation.
- Treatment includes systemic corticosteroids, although some studies suggest a benefit from the antifungal itraconazole.[27]

81

ASTHMA

REFERENCES

1. Sly RM, O'Donnell R: Stabilization of asthma mortality, *Ann Allergy Asthma Immunol* 78(4):347-354, 1997. B
2. American Lung Association: *Trends in asthma morbidity and mortality,* http://www.lungusa.org/data/asthma, 2003. C
3. McFadden ER Jr, Warren EL: Observations on asthma mortality, *Ann Intern Med* 127(2):142, 1997. B
4. National Heart, Lung and Blood Institute: *Guidelines for the diagnosis and management of asthma,* Expert Panel Report 2, National Asthma Education and Prevention Program, NIH Pub No 97-4051, Bethesda, Md, 1997, National Institutes of Health. D
5. Tierney LM Jr et al: *Current medical diagnosis and treatment 2000,* New York, 2000, Appleton & Lange. C
6. Cates CJ et al: *Holding chambers versus nebulizers for β-agonist treatment of acute asthma (Cochrane Review),* Cochrane Library, Issue 4, Oxford, UK, 2002, Update Software. C
7. Rodrigo GJ et al: Continuous vs. intermittent β-agonists in the treatment of acute adult asthma: a systematic review with meta-analysis, *Chest* 122:160-165, 2002. C
8. Lin RY et al: Continuous versus intermittent albuterol nebulization in the treatment of acute asthma, *Ann Emerg Med* 22:1847, 1993. A
9. Rowe BH et al: The effectiveness of corticosteroids in the treatment of acute exacerbations of asthma: a meta-analysis of their effect on relapse following acute assessment. In Cates C et al, eds: *Airway Review Group module: Cochrane Library,* May 1997, Cochrane Collaboration. C
10. Bowler SD et al: Corticosteroids in acute severe asthma: effectiveness of low doses, *Thorax* 47(8):584-587, 1992. B

11. Hasegawa T et al: Duration of systemic corticosteroids in the treatment of asthma exacerbation; a randomized study, *Intern Med* 39 (10):794-797, 2000. A

12. O'Driscoll B et al: Double blind trial of steroid tapering in acute asthma, *Lancet* 341:324, 1993. A

13. Rodrigo G et al: A meta-analysis of the effects of ipratropium bromide in adults with acute asthma, *Am J Med* 107:363, 1999. C

14. Rowe BH et al: Intravenous magnesium sulfate treatment for acute asthma in the emergency department: a systematic review of the literature, *Ann Emerg Med* 36(3):181, 2000. C

15. Silverman RA et al: IV magnesium sulfate in the treatment of acute severe asthma: a multi-center randomized controlled trial, *Chest* 122:489-497, 2002. A

16. Soroksky A et al: A pilot prospective, randomized, placebo-controlled trial of bilevel positive airway pressure in acute asthmatic attack, *Chest* 123:1018-1025, 2003. A

17. D'Alonzo GE et al: Salmeterol xinafoate as maintenance therapy compared with albuterol in patients with asthma, *JAMA* 271:1412, 1994. A

18. Rickard K: http://www.fda.gov/medwatch/SAFETY/2003/serevent.htm. A

19. Reiss TF et al: Montelukast, a once-daily leukotriene receptor antagonist, in the treatment of chronic asthma: a multicenter, randomized, double-blind trial, *Arch Intern Med* 158(11):1213-1220, 1998. A

20. Soler M et al: The anti-IgE antibody omalizumab reduces exacerbations and steroid requirement in allergic asthmatics, *Eur Respir J* 18(2):254-261, 2000. A

21. Marin MG: Low-dose methotrexate spares steroid usage in steroid-dependent asthmatic patients: a meta-analysis, *Chest* 112:29, 1997. C

22. Drazen JM et al: Comparison of regularly scheduled with as-needed use of albuterol in mild asthma, *N Engl J Med* 335:841, 1996. A

23. Spitzer WO et al: The use of β-agonists and the risk of death and near death from asthma, *N Engl J Med* 326:501, 1992. B

24. Gotzsche PC et al: House dust mite control measures in the management of asthma: meta-analysis, *BMJ* 317:1105, 1998. C

25. Abramson MJ et al: Is allergen immunotherapy effective in asthma? A meta-analysis of randomized controlled trials, *Am J Respir Crit Care Med* 151(4):969-974, 1995. C

26. Field SK, Sutherland LR: Does medical antireflux therapy improve asthma in asthmatics with gastroesophageal reflux? A critical review of the literature, *Chest* 114:275, 1998. C

27. Stevens DA et al: A randomized trial of itraconazole in allergic bronchopulmonary aspergillosis, *N Engl J Med* 342:756, 2000. A

Chronic Obstructive Pulmonary Disease

David Cosgrove, MD; Majd Mouded, MD; and Robert Wise, MD

FAST FACTS

- Chronic obstructive pulmonary disease (COPD) is underdiagnosed. The Longcope Spirometry Investigation Team recently demonstrated that only one third of inpatients with evidence of severe obstruction on spirometry carry the diagnosis of COPD.[1]
- Oxygen is the only therapy that has been shown to reduce mortality in advanced COPD, and smoking cessation is the only intervention that has been shown to slow the progression of COPD.
- Initial management of acute COPD exacerbations includes supplemental O_2 (goal SaO_2 88% to 92%), aggressive use of inhaled bronchodilators, steroids (methylprednisolone 125 mg intravenously or equivalent), and antibiotics if there is evidence of infection or increased sputum production.
- Noninvasive positive-pressure ventilation can be used to temporarily stabilize an alert, cooperative patient at risk for impending respiratory failure, thus allowing time for response to pharmacologic intervention.
- Indications for intubation include respiratory muscle fatigue, worsening acidosis or hypoxemia, worsening mental status, and cardiovascular instability.

I. EPIDEMIOLOGY AND ETIOLOGY

1. COPD is characterized by progressive airflow obstruction resulting from chronic bronchitis (productive cough for > 3 months for 2 consecutive years) or emphysema (abnormal, permanent enlargement of airspaces distal to the terminal bronchioles with destruction of the airway walls). Most patients exhibit a combination of chronic bronchitis and emphysema.
2. COPD is the fourth leading cause of death in the United States and affects an estimated 16 million people.[2] The mortality rate is higher in whites than nonwhites and inversely related to socioeconomic factors. In the year 2000, COPD mortality in women exceeded male mortality for the first time.[3]
3. Risk factors.
a. Age. Normal individuals exhibit a progressive decline in lung capacity with age, reflected in a decreasing 1-second forced expiratory volume (FEV_1) of about 20 ml per year.

b. Environmental exposures. Cigarette smoking is by far the most important risk factor for the development of COPD in the United States and is associated with a 2.5-fold faster rate of decline in FEV_1.

c. Genetic predisposition. Alpha-1-antitrypsin deficiency is the most common genetic cause of COPD but accounts for less than 1% of cases in the United States. The PiZZ genotype accounts for 95% of cases and is found most often in whites of northern European descent but is present throughout Europe and in all populations of European descent.[4] Alpha-1-antitrypsin screening is indicated in patients with COPD who are younger than 45 years, do not have a smoking history, or have a strong family history.

4. Pathophysiology.

a. Three major mechanisms have been implicated in the accelerated decline in FEV_1 and increased severity of disease.[5]

(1) Loss of elasticity and destruction of alveolar attachments of airways within the lung, caused by emphysema, resulting in a loss of support and closure of small airways during expiration.

(2) Narrowing of small airways as a result of inflammation and scarring within airway walls.

(3) Blockage of small airway lumens with mucus secretions.

b. These alterations in the lung architecture are induced by inflammation of the terminal airspaces consequent to cigarette smoking and inhalation of noxious agents. Together, they combine to produce hyperinflation of the lungs, producing the characteristic dyspnea of COPD.

II. CLINICAL PRESENTATION

A. SYMPTOMS

1. Mild COPD manifests most often as an intermittent cough, especially in the morning. In addition, patients experience recurrent respiratory infections and dyspnea with vigorous exertion. Symptoms often vary from day to day.

2. In severe COPD, dyspnea progresses; weight loss, morning headache, drowsiness (caused by hypercapnia), and lower extremity edema may develop as a result of cor pulmonale.

3. Symptoms of an acute exacerbation include dyspnea, wheezing, agitation, confusion, and drowsiness.

B. PHYSICAL EXAMINATION

1. **Pulmonary.** On inspection, patients may demonstrate hyperinflation ("barrel chest"), accessory muscle use, and pursed lip breathing. Percussion of the lung fields often demonstrates hyperresonance and decreased diaphragmatic excursion. Auscultatory findings include decreased breath sounds, prolonged expiratory phase, and expiratory wheezing.

2. **Other.** Cardiovascular examination findings may reflect underlying pulmonary hypertension (e.g., right ventricular heave, loud P_2,

tricuspid regurgitation). Other findings include clubbing and cyanosis.

3. Physical examination findings of an acute exacerbation include tachypnea, increased work of breathing (e.g., accessory muscle use), polyphonic expiratory wheezing with a decreased inspiratory to expiratory ratio, and pulsus paradoxus.

III. DIAGNOSIS

A. RADIOGRAPHY AND COMPUTED TOMOGRAPHY

1. The chest radiograph is neither sensitive nor specific for COPD, except in very advanced disease. It should not be used to exclude the diagnosis. It is most useful to assess other causes of dyspnea and complications of COPD such as pneumonia and pneumothorax. Chest radiograph findings in advanced disease can demonstrate hyperinflation with flattened hemidiaphragms, increased retrosternal airspace, and narrow cardiac silhouette.

2. Emphysematous changes may cause the lung parenchyma to be hyperlucent, with rapid tapering of the pulmonary vasculature.

3. High-resolution chest computed tomography is the most sensitive and specific study for identifying the bullous changes associated with emphysema.

B. PULMONARY FUNCTION TESTS AND ARTERIAL BLOOD GAS

1. Pulmonary function tests are essential in the diagnosis, prognosis, and staging of COPD.

a. **Spirometry.** Evidence of airway obstruction is reflected in a ratio of FEV_1 to forced vital capacity < 70%. FEV_1 is the single most important variable in quantifying COPD severity and predicts long-term mortality.[6]

b. **Lung volumes.** Air trapping from COPD may cause an increase in total lung capacity, residual volume, and the ratio of residual volume to total lung capacity.

c. **Carbon monoxide diffusion.** Alveolar destruction associated with emphysema decreases the area for gas exchange, resulting in a lower diffusing capacity.

2. Arterial blood gas analysis often demonstrates hypercapnia and hypoxemia.

IV. CLASSIFICATION OF DISEASE SEVERITY

1. The Global Initiative for Chronic Obstructive Lung Disease summary is a consensus statement from the World Health Organization[7] that classifies disease severity and supersedes previous classification systems from other organizations (Table 82-1).

2. The Global Initiative for Chronic Obstructive Lung Disease summary recommends that initial pulmonary function tests be performed both before and after bronchodilator therapy to exclude the diagnosis of asthma and to evaluate the degree of bronchodilator responsiveness.

TABLE 82-1

GLOBAL INITIATIVE FOR CHRONIC OBSTRUCTIVE LUNG DISEASE STAGING
CRITERIA FOR CHRONIC OBSTRUCTIVE PULMONARY DISEASE

Stage	FEV_1 (percentage of predicted value)	Symptoms
0	> 80%	None
I	> 80%	Variable symptoms
II	50-79%	Mild to moderate symptoms
III	30-49%	Symptoms that limit exertion
IV	< 30%	Symptoms that limit daily activities

Modified from Sutherland ER, Cherniack RM et al: *N Engl J Med* 350:2689-2697, 2004.

3. All further pulmonary function tests for the purpose of severity
   stratification should then be done only after bronchodilator therapy to
   minimize the reversible component of the FEV_1.

V. MANAGEMENT

A. ACUTE EXACERBATIONS

Treatment of an acute exacerbation involves reducing bronchospasm,
treating reversible precipitants, and ensuring tissue oxygenation.

1. Pharmacologic methods of reducing bronchospasm.
a. Beta-2-adrenergic agonists.
   (1) Short acting beta-2-adrenergic agonists (e.g., albuterol) are first-line
       treatment during an acute COPD exacerbation and can be delivered
       via metered-dose inhaler (MDI) with a spacer or in nebulized form
       every 30 to 60 minutes. The initial use of a nebulizer may improve
       pulmonary function earlier than with an MDI and is preferred in
       patients unable to use an MDI. The safety and value of continuous
       nebulization have not been demonstrated, but it may be used in
       the setting of impending respiratory failure in an attempt to avoid
       mechanical ventilation.
   (2) Once the patient's condition has stabilized, the frequency of
       treatments may be decreased gradually.
   (3) There are no data to support the use of long acting beta-agonists
       during acute exacerbations.
b. Anticholinergic agents.
   (1) Anticholinergic agents reduce the parasympathetic tone of the
       airways and should be used early in the management of an acute
       COPD exacerbation in conjunction with beta-2-agonists.
   (2) Similar to beta-agonists, inhaled anticholinergics such as
       ipratropium bromide may be used in an MDI (1 puff = 18 µg) or a
       nebulized solution (500 µg in each 2.5-ml treatment every 6
       hours). Underdosage with the MDI is common, and up to 12 MDI
       inhalations can be given every 4 hours.
c. Corticosteroids

(1) Several randomized clinical trials have shown that systemic corticosteroids improve FEV_1 and reduce the duration of acute flares. Although the most effective dosage and duration of therapy have not been established, both high-dose methylprednisolone (125 mg intravenously every 6 hours for 72 hours followed by a 2-week steroid taper) and prednisone (30 mg orally daily for 14 days) have been shown to be effective. A prolonged 6-week taper appears to offer no benefit.[8] However, management must be tailored to the patient's clinical situation.

(2) High-dose, prolonged steroid treatment should be avoided whenever possible.

(3) Inhaled corticosteroids have no role in an acute COPD exacerbation.

d. Theophylline is a second-line agent used to treat COPD whose role is limited by its narrow therapeutic window and significant toxicities. The use of theophylline to treat acute exacerbations is controversial and generally not recommended.[9]

2. Correction of precipitants.

a. Environmental irritants, gastroesophageal reflux, heart failure, and viral infection may exacerbate COPD. The cause of the exacerbation should be treated when possible.

b. Bacterial colonization is difficult to distinguish from active infection in patients with COPD. However, recent data using molecular typing of bacterial strains have demonstrated that acquisition of a new bacterial strain increases the risk of a COPD exacerbation approximately twofold.[10] *Haemophilus influenzae*, *Moraxella catarrhalis*, and *Streptococcus pneumoniae* account for more than 70% of the bacteria isolated from the sputum of patients with COPD exacerbations. Antibiotics are recommended for patients who have an exacerbation characterized by an increase in the volume or purulence of sputum.[11] Doxycycline, amoxicillin, and trimethoprim-sulfamethoxazole have all been shown to be effective. Depending on local resistance patterns and the severity of the exacerbation, macrolide or fluoroquinolone antibiotics may be used.

3. Oxygenation and respiratory support.

a. Oxygen therapy.

(1) Adequate tissue oxygenation ($PaO_2 > 60$ mmHg; SaO_2 about 90% to 93%) is the primary goal in COPD management. Because the primary respiratory defects are ventilation-perfusion mismatch and decreased diffusing capacity of the lung for carbon monoxide (DLCO), most COPD exacerbations do not necessitate supplementation with high concentrations of oxygen. If hypoxemia is not corrected by low concentrations of O_2, other causes of hypoxia should be considered, including pneumonia, pulmonary edema, pulmonary embolism, and intracardiac shunt.

(2) Close monitoring of oxygenation in patients with COPD and CO_2 retention is important in preventing hypercapnia, respiratory

82

CHRONIC OBSTRUCTIVE PULMONARY DISEASE

acidosis, and respiratory failure.[11] When CO_2 retention occurs in response to oxygen, it is the consequence of altered breathing patterns with smaller tidal volumes rather than reduction in total minute ventilation.

(3) Patients with a history of CO_2 retention should be treated only with a known concentration of O_2 by Venturi mask to prevent worsening retention and respiratory depression. Because O_2 concentration delivered by nasal cannula *increases* as the minute ventilation falls, use of a nasal cannula can precipitate a cycle of worsening ventilatory failure.

(4) Arterial blood gas monitoring is indicated after changes in FIO_2 until a stable PaO_2 greater than 60 mmHg with a pH greater than 7.30 is achieved.

b. Noninvasive positive-pressure ventilation (Chapter 19). In alert patients with severe COPD exacerbations, use of noninvasive positive-pressure ventilation to improve hypercapnia is associated with lower rates of intubation and shorter hospitalizations. However, the patient must be alert and cooperative. Once noninvasive positive-pressure ventilation is started, the patient must be monitored closely for signs of clinical deterioration.

c. Mechanical ventilation (Chapter 19). Patients with severe respiratory compromise may need intubation for ventilatory support. Indications include respiratory muscle fatigue, worsening acidosis, hypoxemia, cardiovascular instability, and worsening mental status.

B. STABLE SYMPTOMATIC COPD

1. Once an acute exacerbation of COPD has resolved, a regimen for managing stable COPD should be instituted (Table 82-2).[11]

2. Smoking cessation is the most effective preventive treatment for COPD and is the only treatment shown to alter the rate of progression.[15] Once a patient stops smoking, the rate of decline of FEV_1 returns to the original rate. However, damage is not reversed. The most effective strategy to date involves bupropion paired with the use of nicotine replacement and dedicated smoking cessation counseling.[16]

3. Pulmonary rehabilitation involves education and exercise programs to aid performance of activities of daily living in patients with COPD. Quality of life, well-being, and health status improvements have been reported, including better exercise tolerance, reduced respiratory symptoms, increased independence, and less anxiety.[11]

4. Long-term O_2 therapy (Box 82-1) improves survival in patients with severe COPD and hypoxemia.[17] Beneficial effects include reversal of secondary polycythemia, improved neurocognitive performance, increased body weight, and improvement in right-sided heart function caused by decreased pulmonary vasoconstriction.

5. Both pneumococcal and yearly influenza vaccinations are recommended by the American Thoracic Society.[11]

6. Lung volume reduction surgery.

TABLE 82-2

STEP-UP PHARMACOLOGIC THERAPY FOR PATIENTS WITH COPD

Symptoms	Intervention
Mild, variable	β_2-agonist MDI aerosol, 1-2 puffs q2-6h PRN; not to exceed 12 puffs/24 hr
Mild or moderate, persistent	Ipratropium MDI aerosol, 2-6 puffs q6-8h *Plus* β_2-agonist MDI aerosol, 1-4 puffs qid PRN or as regular supplement *Consider* Sustained-release β_2-agonist (e.g., salmeterol 50 µg inhaled bid) Sustained-release anticholinergic (e.g., tiotropium 18 µg inhaled qd)* Inhaled corticosteroid (e.g., fluticasone 100-500 µg inhaled bid)[†]
Exacerbation	Add prednisone (up to 40 mg/d for 10-14 d)[‡]
Severe exacerbation	Refer to the emergency department

COPD, chronic obstructive pulmonary disease; MDI, metered-dose inhaler; PRN, as needed.

*Recent studies suggest that tiotropium is superior to ipratropium in preventing exacerbations.[12]
[†]Use of inhaled corticosteroids in stable COPD continues to be controversial but may improve forced expiratory volume in 1 second and also may improve airway reactivity and prevent exacerbations in some patients.[13,14]
[‡]There is no role for long-term oral steroids in COPD.

BOX 82-1

INDICATIONS FOR LONG TERM O_2 THERAPY* IN CHRONIC OBSTRUCTIVE PULMONARY DISEASE

Absolute indications: $PaO_2 \leq 55$ mmHg or $SaO_2 \leq 88\%$
Indications in cor pulmonale:
  PaO_2 55-59 mmHg or $SaO_2 \leq 89\%$
  Electrocardiographic evidence of P pulmonale
  Hematocrit > 55%
  Congestive heart failure

Modified from American Thoracic Society: *Am J Respir Crit Care Med* 152:S77, 1995.
*If patient meets criteria at rest, O_2 should also be prescribed during sleep and exercise.

a. Lung volume reduction surgery can improve lung mechanics by removing diseased, poorly ventilated areas of lung. The National Emphysema Treatment Trial demonstrated that this approach yields a survival advantage over medical therapy for patients with predominantly upper-lobe emphysema and low baseline exercise capacity (risk ratio for death 0.47, p = 0.005) but is associated with increased mortality in patients with non–upper lobe emphysema, low diffusing capacity, and high exercise tolerance (risk ratio for death 2.1, p = 0.02).[18,19]

b. It is important to note that although some patients benefit greatly, lung function appears to deteriorate more quickly in the 5 years after volume reduction despite initial improvement.

c. Data regarding long-term morbidity and mortality and duration of benefit are not yet complete.

7. Lung transplantation.

a. COPD is the leading reason for lung transplantation referrals.[20] Current indications for transplantation are $FEV_1 < 25\%$ of predicted value (without reversibility), $PaCO_2 > 55$ mmHg, and elevated pulmonary artery pressure with progressive deterioration (e.g., cor pulmonale).

b. The most recent statistics show that 1-, 3-, and 5-year survival rates after transplantation are 83.1%, 65.3%, and 44.7%, respectively.

PEARLS AND PITFALLS

- Data suggest that patients with mild COPD who do not need frequent bronchodilators benefit from beta-blockade after myocardial infarction.
- The same mortality benefit is not conferred by the use of beta-blockers in patients with moderate to severe COPD, presumably because of bronchospasm.[21]
- Only selective beta-blockers should be used in patients with COPD.
- There are no large clinical trials analyzing cardiac function and arrhythmia potential in patients taking beta-agonists.
- Reports exist of arrhythmias induced by beta-agonist bronchodilators. However, these data are not controlled and do not take into account patient comorbidities. One study of patients with severe COPD ($FEV_1 < 1$ L) showed no difference in either supraventricular tachycardia or ventricular ectopy in patients using placebo or salbutamol four times a day.[22]
- Cardiac monitoring should be used in any patient with an arrhythmia or at risk of developing an arrhythmia if beta-agonist bronchodilators are needed.
- Anticholinergic dosage should be maximized because these agents have less arrhythmogenic potential.
- Hypoxia can contribute to the development of arrhythmias.
- About 50% of patients with a DLCO of 50% of predicted or less will meet criteria for continuous oxygen.
- A DLCO of less than 40% predicted correlates with the presence of pulmonary hypertension.

REFERENCES

1. Zaas D, Wise R, Wiener C: Longcope Spirometry Investigation Team. Airway obstruction is common but unsuspected in patients admitted to a general medical service, *Chest* 125(1):106-111, 2004. B
2. Halbert RJ: Interpreting COPD prevalence estimates: what is the true burden of disease? *Chest* 123(5):1684-1692, 2003. C
3. Mannino DM, Homa DM, Akinbami LJ, Ford ES, Redd SC: COPD disease surveillance: United States, 1971-2000, *MMWR Surveill Summ* 51:1-16, 2002. C

4. Luisetti M, Seersholm N: Alpha$_1$-antitrypsin deficiency 1: epidemiology of alpha$_1$-antitrypsin deficiency, *Thorax* 59(2):164-169, 2004. C

5. Hogg JC et al: The nature of small airways obstruction in COPD, *N Engl J Med* 350:2645-2653, 2004. C

6. Schunemann HJ et al: Pulmonary function is a long-term predictor of mortality in the general population: 29 year follow-up of the Buffalo Health Study, *Chest* 118(3):656, 2000. A

7. Pauwels RA et al: Global strategy for the diagnosis, management and prevention of chronic obstructive pulmonary disease. NHLB/WHO Global Initiative for Chronic Obstructive Lung Disease (GOLD) Workshop Summary, *Am J Respir Crit Care Med* 163:1256, 2001. C

8. Davies L, Angus RM, Calverley PMA: Oral corticosteroids in patients admitted to hospital with exacerbations of chronic obstructive pulmonary disease: a prospective randomized controlled trial, *Lancet* 354:456, 1999. A

9. Rice KL et al: Aminophylline for acute exacerbations of COPD. A controlled trial, *Ann Intern Med* 107(3):305-309, 1987. A

10. Sethi S et al: New strains of Bacteria and exacerbations of chronic obstructive pulmonary disease, *N Engl J Med* 347:465-471, 2002. C

11. American Thoracic Society: Standards for the diagnosis and care of patients with chronic obstructive pulmonary disease, *Am J Respir Crit Care Med* 152:S77, 1995. D

12. Tashkin D, Cooper C: The role of long-acting bronchodilators in the management of stable COPD, *Chest* 125(1):249-259, 2004. C

13. Burge PS, Calverley PM, et al: Randomized, double blind, placebo-controlled study of fluticasone propionate in patients with moderate to severe chronic obstructive pulmonary disease: the ISOLDE trial, *BMJ* 320:1297-1303, 2000. A

14. Lung Health Study Research Group: Effect of inhaled triamcinolone on the decline in pulmonary function in chronic obstructive pulmonary disease, *N Engl J Med* 343:1902, 2000. B

15. Anthonisen NR et al: Effect of smoking intervention and the use of an inhaled anticholinergic bronchodilator on the rate of decline of FEV_1. The Lung Health Study, *JAMA* 272:1497, 1994. B

16. Jorenby DE et al: A controlled trial of sustained-release bupropion, a nicotine patch, or both for smoking cessation, *N Engl J Med* 340:685, 1999. A

17. Medical Research Council Working Party: Long-term domiciliary oxygen therapy in chronic hypoxic cor pulmonale complicating chronic bronchitis and emphysema, *Lancet* 1:681, 1981. D

18. National Emphysema Treatment Trial Research Group: A randomized trial comparing lung-volume-reduction surgery with medical therapy for severe emphysema, *N Engl J Med* 348:2059-2073, 2003. A

19. Fessler HE, Wise RA: Lung volume reduction surgery: is less really more? *Am J Respir Crit Care Med* 159:1031, 1999. C

20. United Network for Organ Sharing (UNOS): *SR & OPTN annual reports 1993-2002,* retrieved July 2004 from www.unos.org. D

21. Chen J et al: Effectiveness of beta-blocker therapy after acute myocardial infarction in elderly patients with chronic obstructive pulmonary disease or asthma, *J Am Coll Cardiol* 37(7):1950, 2001. C

22. Hall IP, Woodhead MA, Johnston IDA: Effect of high-dose salbutamol on cardiac rhythm in severe chronic airflow obstruction: a controlled study, *Respiration* 61:214, 1994. A

82

Pleural Effusions

M. Bradley Drummond, MD; and Peter B. Terry, MD

FAST FACTS

- Indications for urgent diagnostic and therapeutic thoracentesis include unexplained unilateral pleural effusion with fever, respiratory compromise, or hemodynamic instability.
- Pleural fluid should always be analyzed for lactate dehydrogenase (LDH), protein, pH, Gram stain, culture, and differential cell count.
- Light's original criteria for exudative effusions include fluid to serum protein ratio greater than 0.5, fluid to serum LDH ratio greater than 0.6, or fluid LDH level more than two thirds of the upper limit of the normal serum value.
- Indications for tube thoracostomy include pH less than 7.2, purulent aspirate, positive Gram stain, hemothorax, large pneumothorax, and evidence of tension pneumothorax.
- Routine chest radiograph after uncomplicated diagnostic thoracentesis is not needed.

Pleural effusions are a common finding on chest radiography that arise as a result of disrupted homeostatic mechanisms in the pleural space. The need for diagnostic thoracentesis depends on the patient's clinical presentation and hospital course.

I. EPIDEMIOLOGY AND ETIOLOGY

1. Approximately 1.3 million people in the United States present with pleural effusions each year, which in most cases are attributable to congestive heart failure (CHF), pneumonia, and cancer.[1]
2. Less common causes of pleural effusions include pulmonary embolism, viral and mycobacterial infection, rheumatologic disease, esophageal rupture, pancreatitis, and vascular trauma.
3. Pleural fluid analysis helps distinguish transudative from exudative fluid.
a. Transudative pleural effusions arise from an imbalance between oncotic and hydrostatic pressures and are most commonly caused by CHF (90%), cirrhosis, and nephrotic syndrome.
b. Exudative pleural effusions result from the accumulation of proteinaceous material in the pleural space and often are caused by pneumonia, malignancy, and pulmonary embolism.

II. PRESENTATION

A. SYMPTOMS

Dyspnea, cough, and pleuritic chest pain are the most common presenting complaints. Weight loss, night sweats, and malaise may suggest systemic illness (malignancy, tuberculosis).

B. SIGNS

Physical examination findings associated with an effusion depend on size because effusions less than 250 ml generally are difficult to appreciate on physical examination.

1. Percussion and palpation often reveal dullness and decreased tactile fremitus.
2. Auscultation may reveal diminished breath sounds and egophony, which suggests underlying atelectasis.
3. Physical examination may also provide clues to the cause of the effusion:
   a. Distended neck veins, S_3 gallop, and edema suggest that the effusion is a result of CHF.
   b. A right-sided effusion in the setting of ascites suggests hepatic hydrothorax.
   c. Evidence of right heart strain (electrocardiographic $S_1Q_3T_3$, elevated neck veins, lower extremity edema) in the setting of a new pleural effusion suggests pulmonary embolism.

C. RADIOGRAPHIC IMAGING

1. **Chest radiograph.** The chest radiograph remains the main imaging modality for identifying a pleural effusion, determining whether it is loculated, and generating a preliminary differential diagnosis. A posterior-anterior upright radiograph will have costophrenic angle blunting if there is more than 500 ml of pleural fluid. In contrast, a lateral upright radiograph can detect as little as 200 ml fluid. Further imaging with lateral decubitus films can help distinguish between loculated and free-flowing fluid. Any effusion larger than 10 mm layering on a lateral decubitus film is a clinically significant effusion for which thoracentesis should be considered.
2. **Computed tomography.** Though not generally needed in the initial evaluation of a pleural effusion, a thoracic computed tomogram offers better characterization of the lung parenchyma, mediastinum, and effusion. The addition of intravenous contrast can help distinguish pleural fluid from atelectasis. In addition, computed tomography can lend insight into the cause of the effusion (e.g., pleural calcification and thickening suggest asbestos exposure, increasing the likelihood of a malignant effusion or benign asbestosis effusion).
3. **Ultrasound.** Though not often used to diagnose an effusion, bedside ultrasound can assist in reducing complications associated with the thoracentesis of loculated or small (< 10 mm thickness on lateral decubitus film) effusions.

III. DIAGNOSIS

Thoracentesis remains the central diagnostic modality for differentiating a transudative from an exudative effusion; see Chapter 2 for a description of the technique. The only absolute contraindication to diagnostic thoracentesis is an uncooperative patient. Relative contraindications include abnormal bleeding time, positive-pressure ventilation, or effusion less than 10 mm thick on radiograph.

A. GROSS APPEARANCE OF FLUID

1. Transudates generally are clear to yellowish.
2. Bloody fluid suggests cancer, pulmonary embolism, and trauma.
3. A milky white appearance suggests chylous effusions. Causes include trauma to the thoracic duct, malignancy, and lymphangioleiomyomatosis.

B. CHEMICAL ANALYSIS

All pleural fluid should be sent to the laboratory for total protein, LDH, glucose, and pH. Additional tests are guided by clinical suspicion. Several different criteria have been proposed to distinguish transudative from exudative effusions; see Table 83-1 for the relative sensitivity and specificity of each criterion. In addition, the following clues are useful in determining the cause of the effusion:

1. A glucose concentration that is less in the effusion than in the serum typically is seen in infection, malignancy, and rheumatoid disease.
2. A pH < 7.2 suggests empyema, esophageal rupture, or hemothorax. This is an indication for tube thoracostomy drainage.
3. High levels of adenosine deaminase and lysozyme are seen in tuberculous effusions and can distinguish them from malignancy-associated effusions.[2]
4. The ratio of pleural fluid complement levels to serum complement levels is less than 0.4 in lupus and rheumatoid-associated effusions.[3]
5. A pleural fluid triglyceride concentration > 110 mg/dl supports the diagnosis of chylothorax; a level < 50 mg/dl excludes it. Detection of chylomicrons confirms the diagnosis.

TABLE 83-1

SENSITIVITY AND SPECIFICITY OF TESTS TO DISTINGUISH EXUDATIVE FROM TRANSUDATIVE EFFUSIONS

Biochemical Test	Sensitivity for Exudate (%)	Specificity for Exudate (%)
Pleural fluid protein/serum protein ratio > 0.5	98	83
Pleural fluid LDH/serum LDH ratio > 0.6	86	84
Pleural fluid LDH > 2/3 upper limit of normal serum LDH level	82	89
Pleural fluid cholesterol > 60 mg/dl	54	92
Pleural fluid cholesterol > 43 mg/dl	75	80
Pleural fluid cholesterol to serum cholesterol level > 0.3	89	81
Serum albumin − pleural albumin level ≤ 1.2 g/dl	87	92

From Light R: *N Engl J Med* 346:1971-1977, 2002.
LDH, lactate dehydrogenase.

C. BACTERIOLOGY SMEARS AND CULTURE

1. All pleural fluid should be sent to the laboratory for Gram stain and culture for both aerobic and anaerobic organisms.
2. In addition, samples should be sent to the laboratory for fungal and acid-fast bacilli. However, acid-fast bacilli cultures have a low sensitivity for diagnosing tuberculosis unless the patient has a tuberculous empyema or is immunocompromised.
a. Pleural fluid culture has a sensitivity of less than 40% for tuberculosis, whereas the sensitivity of a pleural biopsy demonstrating pleural granulomas is 70%. Multiple pleural biopsies increase the sensitivity to almost 80%. Combining pleural fluid culture and histologic examination of the pleura yields a diagnosis in 90% of cases and is considered the most sensitive testing modality.
b. Additional tests such as adenosine deaminase, lysozyme, and interferon-gamma levels are useful in the minority of patients with a high clinical suspicion but negative pleural fluid culture and histology; however, they are not indicated as part of the initial evaluation of a suspected tuberculous effusion.

D. CELLS

1. Pleural effusions caused by a chronic disease process contain predominantly mononuclear cells.
2. Eosinophils in the pleural fluid usually are a result of air or blood in the pleural space. Other causes include pulmonary infarction, benign pulmonary asbestosis, drug-induced effusions, and parasitic infections.
3. The presence of mesothelial cells (> 5%) in the pleural fluid virtually excludes tuberculosis as the cause of the effusion.
4. Pleural fluid should be sent to the laboratory for cytology from any patient with an undiagnosed exudative pleural effusion. Depending on the tumor type, three separate specimens have a combined sensitivity of up to 90% if a tumor is the cause of effusion.[4]

IV. PROGNOSIS

The natural course and prognosis of an effusion generally depend on its origin.

1. Malignant pleural effusions portend poor prognosis.
2. Parapneumonic effusions can be risk stratified by size, bacteriology, and pH.[5]
a. Small to moderate (< half of the hemithorax) pleural effusions with a pH 7.2 or higher and negative culture and Gram stain have a low risk of poor outcome and should not be drained unless clinical status worsens, at which time the fluid should be resampled.
b. Large effusions (half or more of the hemithorax) or loculated effusions with positive culture and Gram stain or pH < 7.2 have a moderate to high risk of poor outcome and should be drained.
3. Hepatic hydrothorax is refractory to large-volume drainage and typically recurs.

83

PLEURAL EFFUSIONS

V. MANAGEMENT

The management of an effusion depends on both the patient's presentation and the presumed cause of the effusion.

1. Therapeutic thoracentesis is indicated for any patient with evidence of respiratory compromise, hemodynamic instability, or evidence of massive effusion with contralateral mediastinal shift. Removal of more than 1000 ml pleural fluid in a single sitting should be avoided because this increases risk of pulmonary reexpansion syndrome, which can cause further pulmonary decompensation.
2. Tube thoracostomy is indicated if pleural fluid analysis demonstrates pH < 7.2, presence of pus or hemothorax (fluid hematocrit > 50% peripheral hematocrit), or positive Gram stain.
3. The presence of bilateral pleural effusions and evidence of CHF in the absence of fever warrants a trial of diuresis before sampling of pleural fluid. However, if the effusion is not getting smaller 3 days after diuresis, diagnostic thoracentesis is indicated. Analyzing fluid-serum gradients for albumin and protein is useful in this setting for distinguishing transudative from exudative effusions.[6]
4. Liver transplantation is the definitive treatment for refractory hepatic hydrothorax, although transjugular portosystemic shunt can be used as a bridge while the patient awaits transplantation.
5. Chemical pleurodesis often is used to treat patients with recurrent, symptomatic pleural effusions caused by malignancy.
6. Routine chest radiograph is not indicated after uncomplicated diagnostic thoracentesis.[7] Risk factors for pneumothorax from thoracentesis include aspiration of air, use of vacuum bottle to withdraw fluid, operator inexperience, increased number of needle passes to obtain fluid, and persistent symptoms after the procedure.[8]

PEARLS AND PITFALLS

- Pulmonary embolism can present with either a transudative or an exudative effusion.
- Pleural fluid pH should be collected in an arterial blood gas syringe and analyzed immediately.
- Any change in clinical status after thoracentesis should be considered a pneumothorax until proven otherwise and be rapidly evaluated with a chest radiograph.
- Bilateral pleural effusions with a normal-size heart on chest radiograph usually are caused by malignancy, collagen vascular disease, or viral infection and are less likely to be caused by heart failure.
- A pleural effusion occupying more than half of a thorax usually is caused by tumor, tuberculosis, trauma, or hepatic hydrothorax.

REFERENCES

1. Light R: Pleural effusions, *N Engl J Med* 346:1971-1977, 2002. D

2. Villegas MV et al: Evaluation of polymerase chain reaction adenosine deaminase and interferon-gamma in pleural fluid for the differential of PTB, *Chest* 118:1355-1364, 2000. B
3. Pettersson T et al: Chemical and immunological features of pleural effusions: comparison between rheumatoid arthritis and other diseases, *Thorax* 37:354-361, 1982. B
4. Ong K et al: The diagnostic yield of pleural fluid cytology in malignant pleural effusions, *Singapore Med J* 41:19-23, 2000. B
5. Colise G et al: Medical and surgical treatment of parapneumonic effusions: an evidence-based guideline, *Chest* 118:1158-1171, 2000. D
6. Romero-Candeira S et al: Influence of diuretics on the concentration of proteins and other components of pleural transudates in patients with heart failure, *Am J Med* 110:681-686, 2001. B
7. Doyle J et al: Necessity of routine chest roentgenography after thoracentesis, *Ann Intern Med* 124:816-820, 1996. B
8. Petersen WG et al: Limited utility of chest radiograph after thoracentesis, *Chest* 117:1038-1042, 2000. B

83

PLEURAL EFFUSIONS

Hemoptysis

Adlah Sukkar, MD; Sarah Noonberg, MD, PhD;
and Edward Haponik, MD

> ### FAST FACTS
>
> - In immunocompetent patients, hemoptysis is most commonly caused by bronchitis, bronchiectasis, and lung cancer.
> - The volume of blood expectorated does not correlate with the gravity of the underlying cause of hemoptysis, but it is the strongest predictor of short-term mortality.
> - The cause of death in massive hemoptysis is almost always asphyxiation.
> - Initial management of life-threatening hemoptysis should focus on ensuring adequate airway protection, ventilation, and oxygenation, protecting the nonbleeding lung, and monitoring hemodynamic status.

Hemoptysis is the expectoration of blood or blood-tinged sputum and is common, although its precise frequency is undefined. This chapter provides an approach to the evaluation and management of hemoptysis and concludes with a discussion of the management of both life-threatening hemoptysis and diffuse alveolar hemorrhage.

I. EPIDEMIOLOGY

A. OCCURRENCE AND MORTALITY

1. Most cases are caused by minor mucosal erosions arising from respiratory infections, are self-limited, and have favorable outcomes.
2. In less than 5% of cases, hemoptysis is massive or life-threatening (variably defined as 100 to 1000 ml blood/24 hours) and carries a mortality rate of up to 80%.[1,2]

B. ETIOLOGY

1. The epidemiology and etiology of hemoptysis have changed greatly over the past 50 years.[3,4] Until the 1960s, hemoptysis usually was caused by tuberculosis (TB), lung abscesses, or bronchiectasis.[3] In the present era, the most common causes of hemoptysis are bronchitis, bronchogenic carcinoma, and bronchiectasis.[3-5] TB remains an important cause in developing countries, where the prevalence of TB remains high.
2. Community-acquired pneumonia is a less common cause of hemoptysis, accounting for 10% of cases; hemoptysis occurs in 16% to 20% of patients with pneumococcal pneumonia.[6]
3. Up to 30% of cases of hemoptysis have no identifiable cause despite careful evaluation.[7] Bleeding usually is self-limited in such cases.

4. Limited data suggest that among patients with the human immunodeficiency virus, 80% of cases of hemoptysis have infectious causes. Roughly half of these cases are caused by bacterial pneumonias; other infectious causes include TB, *Pneumocystis carinii* pneumonia, *Mycobacterium avium,* and fungal infections.[8] Kaposi's sarcoma is a rare cause of hemoptysis but can cause severe hemorrhage.

II. CLINICAL PRESENTATION AND PATHOPHYSIOLOGY

1. The clinical presentation and outcome of patients with hemoptysis depend on the rate, degree, and source of blood loss and the patient's physiologic reserve.
2. The bronchial circulation generally arises from the aorta or intercostal arteries and operates under systemic pressures. It is usually (in > 80% of cases) the source of bleeding in hemoptysis. Less often, hemoptysis originates from the lower-pressure pulmonary arterial bed.
3. There are numerous causes of hemoptysis (Box 84-1).[1,2]

III. DIAGNOSIS

A. SOURCE OF BLEEDING

1. The first step in evaluating a stable patient with hemoptysis is to rule out an upper airway or gastrointestinal source (pseudohemoptysis).
2. Once a pulmonary source of bleeding is confirmed, a detailed history often can reveal clues to the possible cause and contributing factors.

B. PHYSICAL EXAMINATION

Although the physical examination may assist in diagnosis, it is notoriously unreliable for identifying the site of bleeding. Special attention should be directed to the vital signs, including the patient's pulmonary reserve, effectiveness of cough, respiratory rate, and presence of accessory respiratory muscle recruitment. Sinus tachycardia or orthostasis may indicate hemodynamically significant hemorrhage. A thorough examination of the head and neck should be conducted, including nasopharyngeal and oropharyngeal inspection.

C. LABORATORY STUDIES

1. Initial laboratory studies should include a complete blood cell count with differential, coagulation studies, and electrolyte panel. Urinalysis should be performed in patients with suspected pulmonary-renal syndrome.
2. Arterial blood gas analysis should be considered for patients with tachypnea, altered mental status, or lower extremity swelling and those in whom hypoxemia or hypoventilation is suspected.
3. When obtainable, sputum samples should be sent for bacterial, fungal, and mycobacterial culture as well as cytologic tests. Sputum induction or chest percussion may exacerbate bleeding.

84

HEMOPTYSIS

BOX 84-1

CAUSES OF HEMOPTYSIS

PULMONARY

Bronchiectasis*

Bronchitis (acute or chronic)*

Cystic fibrosis*

Sarcoidosis

Cryptogenic organizing pneumonia

Hypersensitivity pneumonitis

INFECTIOUS

Necrotizing bacterial pneumonia*

Fungal infections*

Tuberculosis*

Lung abscess

Septic embolism

Pneumocystis carinii pneumonia

COLLAGEN-VASCULAR DISORDERS

Systemic lupus erythematosus*

Wegener's granulomatosis*

Goodpasture's syndrome*

Microscopic polyarteritis

Churg-Strauss syndrome

Idiopathic pulmonary hemosiderosis

CARDIAC

Mitral stenosis*

Congestive heart failure*

Severe pulmonary hypertension

Eisenmenger's syndrome

HEMATOLOGIC

Coagulopathy*

Thrombocytopenia*

Platelet dysfunction

Disseminated intravascular coagulation

IATROGENIC

Bronchoscopy*

Transbronchial or percutaneous biopsy*

Pulmonary artery rupture (Swan-Ganz catheter trauma)

NEOPLASTIC

Bronchogenic carcinoma*

Bronchial adenoma*

Kaposi's sarcoma

Metastatic carcinoma or sarcoma

Angiosarcoma

VASCULAR

Pulmonary arteriovenous malformation*

Pulmonary embolism with infarction*

Aortic aneurysm

Bronchovascular fistula

TRAUMA

Blunt or penetrating chest injury*

Foreign body aspiration

Fat embolism

DRUGS AND TOXINS

Anticoagulants

Antiplatelet agents

Thrombolytics

Cocaine

OTHER

Catamenial (pulmonary endometriosis)

Cryptogenic*

Amyloidosis

Munchausen syndrome

Broncholithiasis

*More common cause of hemoptysis.

4. Although chest radiography is normal in up to 30% of patients with hemoptysis, it may demonstrate infiltrates, lymphadenopathy, or cavitary or mass lesions.

5. Purified protein derivative tests and respiratory isolation are mandatory in patients with risk factors for TB exposure.

D. FURTHER EVALUATION

1. No standard algorithms have been established for the workup of patients whose source of bleeding remains unknown after initial assessment.

2. The clinician's task is to use the initial history, physical examination, laboratory data, and chest radiograph to risk stratify patients and guide further evaluation (Fig. 84-1).

E. COMPUTED TOMOGRAPHY

1. Computed tomography (CT) imaging should be obtained before invasive procedures. If the CT shows widespread metastatic disease, bronchiectasis, or a benign process, an invasive procedure may be avoided.

a. If a peripherally located lesion is found, percutaneous biopsy is the most appropriate initial invasive study.

b. If CT does not provide a diagnosis and risk factors are present, bronchoscopy is generally indicated.

2. The type of CT scan (high-resolution CT, spiral CT, or conventional CT) should be chosen on the basis of clinical suspicion of underlying disease (e.g., bronchiectasis, pulmonary embolism, or lung abscess).

F. BRONCHOSCOPY

1. Bronchoscopy complements CT in the evaluation of patients with hemoptysis.[9,10] The combination of bronchoscopy and CT leads to a diagnosis in 93% of patients, whereas each study alone is diagnostic in only 42% and 67% of patients, respectively.[5]

2. In most cases of cryptogenic or idiopathic hemoptysis, both patient and clinician often are concerned about underlying malignancy; however, the risk of occult malignancy generally is less than 5%.[4,11]

a. Age older than 40 years, male sex, smoking history of more than 40 pack-years, and hemoptysis of more than 1 week's duration predict a neoplasm with bronchoscopy.[4,11,12]

b. In the absence of these risk factors, the likelihood of malignancy is low, and a more conservative, watchful approach is warranted.

3. The optimum timing of diagnostic bronchoscopy has not been defined. Early bronchoscopy does not ensure a better outcome.

G. OTHER STUDIES

1. Echocardiography, radionuclide ventilation-perfusion imaging, and urine and serum toxicology may be useful but are cost-effective only when pretest probability is sufficiently high.

2. Serologic tests (e.g., antinuclear antibodies, antineutrophil cytoplasmic antibodies, anti–glomerular basement antibodies) are obtained if the

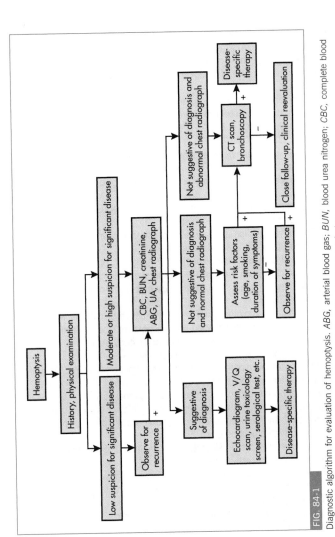

FIG. 84-1

Diagnostic algorithm for evaluation of hemoptysis. *ABG*, arterial blood gas; *BUN*, blood urea nitrogen; *CBC*, complete blood cell count; *CT*, computed tomography; *UA*, urinalysis; *V/Q*, ventilation-perfusion.

diagnosis of diffuse alveolar hemorrhage or a pulmonary renal syndrome is strongly suspected.

3. Radionuclide imaging with technetium-99m and sulfur colloid or labeled red blood cells is rarely of benefit.[13]

IV. MANAGEMENT OF LIFE-THREATENING HEMOPTYSIS

The expectoration of large quantities of frank blood (> 200 ml/day) can be alarming for both patient and physician. Such an event is life-threatening and should be treated as a medical emergency in an intensive care setting. Because the clinical course can be unpredictable, pulmonologists, anesthesiologists, interventional radiologists, and thoracic surgeons should be consulted early. Overall mortality in massive hemoptysis ranges from 7% to 80%. The mortality rate is 58% when the rate of bleeding exceeds 1000 ml/24 hours, compared with 9% if bleeding is less than 1000 ml/24 hours.[1,2,14]

A. INITIAL EVALUATION

1. Initial assessment should focus on airway patency, oxygenation, ventilation, and hemodynamic status.
2. Early elective intubation is needed for all patients in whom an adequate airway cannot be ensured, with use of an **8-mm or larger endotracheal tube to allow subsequent bronchoscopy.**
3. When possible, the bleeding lung should be placed in a dependent position to avoid compromise of the nonbleeding lung.
4. Selective lung intubation and double-lumen intubation may be considered at the discretion of an experienced intensivist.[1,2,14]
5. Large-bore intravenous access is imperative (two 18-gauge or larger peripheral intravenous lines or a 7-Fr or larger central catheter).
6. Blood should be sent immediately for complete blood cell count, type and screen, and coagulation studies.
7. Any significant thrombocytopenia (goal platelet count > 50,000) or coagulopathy (goal international normalized ratio < 1.4) should be corrected.

B. OTHER MEASURES

1. Bronchoscopy is performed early in most patients with massive hemoptysis because it can be both diagnostic and therapeutic.
2. Adequate bleeding control may be achieved with topical thrombin or fibrinogen, iced saline, epinephrine injections, laser photocoagulation, balloon tamponade, cryotherapy, or electrocautery, as indicated by endobronchial findings.[15-17]
3. Once the patient is stable, bronchial arteriography with embolization usually (in > 80% of cases) achieves hemostasis, although rebleeding may recur.[18,19]
4. If bleeding continues despite these measures, surgical resection of the localized bleeding site may be warranted. Every effort should be made to stabilize the patient before surgery because perioperative mortality is much higher with active bleeding.[20]

84

HEMOPTYSIS

V. DIFFUSE ALVEOLAR HEMORRHAGE

1. Patients with hemorrhage from pulmonary capillaritis syndromes may have rapid clinical deterioration despite only modest blood loss, necessitating rapid diagnosis and initiation of treatment.[21]

2. Most patients receive pulsed methylprednisolone (30 mg/kg intravenously over 20 minutes every other day for three doses followed by daily oral prednisone [1 mg/kg/day]).

3. Second-line immunosuppressants include cyclophosphamide and azathioprine; it is important to note that data on these agents' effectiveness are limited.[21]

4. Plasmapheresis has been used with success in Goodpasture's syndrome but has not proven effective in other diffuse hemorrhagic syndromes.

5. Prompt treatment is important in reducing the probability of progression to pulmonary fibrosis and in preventing irreversible renal damage. Despite treatment, morbidity and mortality are still high, from both the disease and the complications of immunosuppressive therapy.

PEARLS AND PITFALLS

- No established guidelines define which patients with hemoptysis warrant admission. It is reasonable to admit all patients with documented hemoptysis of frank blood of at least 50 ml for observation when the cause is unknown. Patients with coagulopathy, serious cardiopulmonary conditions, hypoxia, or hypoventilation should also be hospitalized.

- Public health concerns mandate that when TB is strongly suspected, patients should be placed in isolation until the sputum is analyzed.

- For patients who smoke, hemoptysis may represent a unique opportunity to intervene with cessation efforts.

REFERENCES

1. Cahill BC, Ingbar DH: Massive hemoptysis: assessment and management, *Clin Chest Med* 15:147, 1994. C

2. Thompson AB, Teschler H, Rennard SI: Pathogenesis, evaluation, and therapy for massive hemoptysis, *Clin Chest Med* 13:69, 1992. C

3. Santiago S, Tobias J, Williams AJ: A reappraisal of the causes of hemoptysis, *Arch Intern Med* 151:2449, 1991. C

4. Johnston H, Reisz G: Changing spectrum of hemoptysis: underlying causes in 148 patients undergoing diagnostic flexible fiberoptic bronchoscopy, *Arch Intern Med* 149:1666, 1989. B

5. Hirshberg B, Biran I, Glazer M, Kramer MR: Hemoptysis: etiology, evaluation, and outcome in a tertiary referral hospital, *Chest* 112:440, 1997. B

6. Brandenburg JA et al: Clinical presentation, processes and outcomes of care for patients with pneumococcal pneumonia, *J Gen Intern Med* 15:638, 2000. B

7. Adelman M et al: Cryptogenic hemoptysis: clinical features, bronchoscopic findings, and natural history in 67 patients, *Ann Intern Med* 102:829, 1985. B

8. Nelson JE, Forman M: Hemoptysis in HIV-infected patients, *Chest* 110:737, 1996. C

9. Haponik EF et al: Computed chest tomography in the evaluation of hemoptysis: impact on diagnosis and treatment, *Chest* 91:80, 1987. B

10. McGuinness G et al: Hemoptysis: prospective high resolution CT/bronchoscopic correlation, *Chest* 105:1155, 1994. B
11. O'Neil KM, Lazarus AA: Hemoptysis: indications for bronchoscopy, *Arch Intern Med* 151:171, 1991. D
12. Jackson CV, Savage PJ, Quinn DL: Role of fiberoptic bronchoscopy in patients with hemoptysis and a normal chest roentgenogram, *Chest* 87:142, 1985. D
13. Haponik EF et al: Radionuclide localization of massive pulmonary hemorrhage, *Chest* 86:208, 1984. B
14. Dweik RA, Stoller JK: Flexible bronchoscopy in the 21st century: role of bronchoscopy in massive hemoptysis, *Clin Chest Med* 20:89, 1999. C
15. Edmonstone WM et al: Life-threatening hemoptysis controlled by laser photocoagulation: short report, *Thorax* 38:788, 1983. B
16. Saw EC et al: Flexible fiberoptic bronchoscopy and endobronchial tamponade in the management of massive hemoptysis, *Chest* 70:589, 1976. B
17. Tsukamoto T, Sasaki H, Nakamura H: Treatment of hemoptysis patients by thrombin and fibrinogen-thrombin infusion therapy using a fiberoptic bronchoscope, *Chest* 96:473, 1989. B
18. Haponik EF et al: Managing life-threatening hemoptysis: has anything really changed? *Chest* 118:1431, 2000. C
19. Mal H et al: Immediate and long-term results of bronchial artery embolization for life threatening hemoptysis, *Chest* 115:996, 1999. B
20. Endo S et al: Management of massive hemoptysis in a thoracic surgical unit, *Eur J Cardiothorac Surg* 23:467, 2003. B
21. Green RJ et al: Pulmonary capillaritis and alveolar hemorrhage, *Chest* 110:1305, 1996. B

84

HEMOPTYSIS

Pulmonary Hypertension

Amar Krishnaswamy, MD; Reda Girgis, MD;
and Hunter C. Champion, MD, PhD

> **FAST FACTS**
>
> - Pulmonary hypertension is defined by pulmonary artery pressures greater than 25 mmHg at rest or greater than 30 mmHg during exercise. It can be divided into five disease categories: pulmonary artery hypertension (PAH), disorders of the respiratory system or hypoxemia, left-sided heart disease, chronic thromboembolic disease, and miscellaneous causes.
> - Symptoms that bring patients to attention can include fatigue, dyspnea, syncope, and other signs of right-sided heart failure.
> - Right heart catheterization is essential to confirm diagnosis, determine prognosis, and assign therapy.
> - Maintaining euvolemia and hemodynamic stability can be difficult because of the interplay between preload dependence and interventricular interdependence. Care should be taken to avoid overdiuresis and agents that can lower systemic arterial pressure.
> - Hypotension in the setting of pulmonary hypertension and right ventricular failure may warrant diuresis, not intravenous fluids, in order to relieve impingement of the right ventricle on the left ventricle.
> - Maintenance therapy with calcium channel blockers or prostacyclin infusion must not be interrupted.
> - Because of abrupt changes in hemodynamics, medical arrest is almost uniformly fatal.

Pulmonary hypertension comprises a rare group of diseases that result in elevated pulmonary arterial pressure and right-sided heart failure. However, with the recent awareness of the disease entity, the widespread use of less invasive diagnostic techniques, and improvements in treatment modalities, the diagnosis of pulmonary hypertension is being made more often at the primary care level. This chapter provides an approach to the diagnosis and treatment of pulmonary hypertension, with the majority of the discussion focusing on PAH.

I. EPIDEMIOLOGY AND ETIOLOGY

1. There are five distinct disease categories, recently revised at the third World Conference on Pulmonary Hypertension in Venice in 2003 (Box 85-1). Although pulmonary hypertension as a whole is rare, its incidence is increasing as recognition of the disease entity increases

---

BOX 85-1

2003 VENICE CLASSIFICATION OF PULMONARY HYPERTENSION

PAH

Idiopathic PAH

Familial PAH

Associated with PAH

  Collagen vascular disease

  Congenital systemic-pulmonary shunts

  Portal hypertension

  Human immunodeficiency virus infection

  Drugs and toxins (e.g., anorexigens)

  Other (e.g., hemoglobinopathies, myeloproliferative disorders, thyroid disease)

Significant venous or capillary involvement

  Pulmonary venoocclusive disease

  Pulmonary capillary hemangiomatosis

MISCELLANEOUS

Sarcoidosis

Histiocytosis X

Lymphangiomatosis

Compression of the pulmonary vessels

PULMONARY HYPERTENSION CAUSED BY HYPOXIA OR LUNG DISEASE

Chronic obstructive pulmonary disease

Interstitial lung disease

Sleep-disordered breathing

Alveolar hypoventilation disorders

Chronic exposure to high altitude

Developmental abnormalities

PULMONARY HYPERTENSION CAUSED BY CHRONIC THROMBOTIC OR EMBOLIC DISEASE

Thromboembolic obstruction of proximal pulmonary arteries

Thromboembolic obstruction of distal pulmonary arteries

Nonthrombotic pulmonary embolism (e.g., tumor, parasites or ova)

PULMONARY HYPERTENSION WITH LEFT-SIDED HEART DISEASE

Left-sided atrial or ventricular disease

Left-sided valvular heart disease

Classification modified from Simonneau et al: *J Am Coll Cardiol* (43)12:5S-12S, 2004.
PAH, pulmonary artery hypertension.

and secondary causes are further elucidated. For instance, recent evidence suggests that the incidence of disease secondary to venous thromboembolism is underappreciated. In their prospective study of 314 patients with acute pulmonary embolism, Pengo and colleagues found that the incidence of symptomatic pulmonary hypertension increased from 1% at 6 months to 3.8% at 2 years.[2]

2. In contrast to the other forms of pulmonary hypertension, PAH produces characteristic abnormalities in the wall of small distal pulmonary

arteries. These abnormalities involve narrowing of the vessel lumen, smooth muscle hypertrophy, and intimal proliferation.[3-7] PAH can be a primary disorder associated with genetic or environmental factors (e.g., bone morphogenic protein II gene mutations, human immunodeficiency virus, and the vasculotropic human herpesvirus 8) or secondary to other diseases (e.g., scleroderma).[8]

II. CLINICAL PRESENTATION

1. Symptoms include shortness of breath, dyspnea on exertion, fatigue, chest pain, syncope, and lethargy. Less common symptoms include Raynaud's phenomenon, cough, hemoptysis, and hoarseness caused by impingement on the left recurrent laryngeal nerve by a dilated main pulmonary artery.
2. The physical examination is characterized by features of right ventricular hypertrophy including a right ventricular heave, a pronounced (and sometimes palpable) pulmonic component to S_2 (P_2), a right ventricular S_4 gallop with early disease, an S_3 gallop with advanced disease, and tricuspid regurgitation. Inspection of the jugular venous pulse may reveal a prominent A wave secondary to impaired emptying of the right atrium against a hypertrophied right ventricle and a prominent V wave secondary to tricuspid regurgitation. Other signs of right ventricular failure include peripheral edema, hepatomegaly, and bowel congestion.[3,6]

III. DIAGNOSIS

The diagnostic evaluation of a patient with suspected pulmonary hypertension seeks to place patients in one of the five distinct categories in order to guide therapy (Fig. 85-1).

A. ELECTROCARDIOGRAPHY

1. Findings in patients with chronic right ventricular overload may include right axis deviation, an R/S ratio greater than 1 in lead V_1, P pulmonale, and incomplete or complete right bundle branch block.
2. These findings tend to have high specificity but low sensitivity.

B. CHEST RADIOGRAPHY

1. Chest radiographs typically show enlargement of the central pulmonary arteries and attenuation of the peripheral vessels, resulting in oligemic lung fields. Right ventricular and right atrial dilation are observed on chest radiographs in later stages of disease and result in a decrease in the retrosternal space on the lateral view.
2. The chest radiograph may demonstrate evidence of the underlying disease process, such as interstitial fibrosis.

C. TWO-DIMENSIONAL ECHOCARDIOGRAPHY

1. An echocardiogram provides a noninvasive way to estimate pulmonary artery pressure, evaluate the function of the right ventricle, and exclude certain causes of pulmonary hypertension, such as mitral valve stenosis. Stress on the right side of the heart initially results in

85

PULMONARY HYPERTENSION

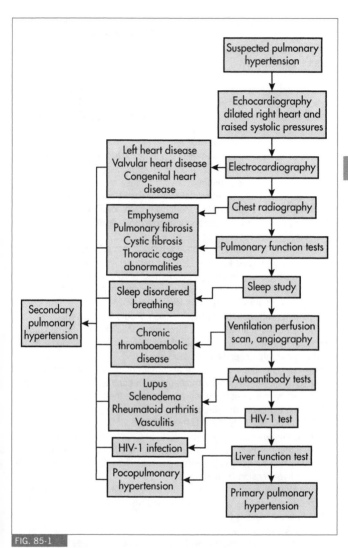

FIG. 85-1

Algorithm for diagnostic evaluation of suspected pulmonary hypertension. *HIV,* human immunodeficiency virus. *(Reproduced from Gaine S, Rubin L:* Lancet *352:719-725, 1998.)*

hypertrophy and hyperkinesis. As the disease progresses, however, right ventricular dilation and hypokinesis ensue. Additionally, the septum may be seen to bow to the left as the right ventricle dominates the pericardial space.

2. Right ventricular systolic pressure is estimated by Doppler examination of tricuspid regurgitation and can serve as a proxy for pulmonary artery pressure. This method usually underestimates right ventricular systolic pressure (by as much as 20%) when correlated with pressures obtained during catheterization of the right side of the heart.

D. PULMONARY FUNCTION TESTS

A full set of pulmonary function tests (spirometry, helium lung volumes, and diffusing capacity) may reveal obstructive disease, parenchymal disease, or thoracic cage abnormalities as a cause of pulmonary hypertension. Only severe interstitial lung disease (lung volume < 50% of predicted) results in pulmonary hypertension. Moreover, a mildly restrictive pattern can be caused by pulmonary hypertension itself.

E. SLEEP STUDY

In patients who are overweight, have a history of loud snoring (usually a historical fact gleaned from the sleeping partner), and exhibit hypersomnolence, a sleep study is performed to rule out obstructive sleep apnea, a potentially reversible cause of pulmonary hypertension.

F. PULMONARY VENTILATION-PERFUSION SCAN

1. All patients with pulmonary hypertension should have a ventilation-perfusion (V/Q) scan to rule out thromboembolic disease. Spiral chest computed tomography with contrast media alone is not adequate to rule out chronic thromboembolic disease.

2. If the results of the V/Q scan are abnormal, pulmonary angiography and spiral chest computed tomography with contrast dye are obtained to define the extent of the disease and explore the feasibility of thromboendarterectomy surgery.

G. SEROLOGIC TESTING AND LUNG BIOPSY

1. Human immunodeficiency virus infection is associated with the development of PAH, with a frequency estimated at 0.5%, which is clinically and pathologically indistinguishable from idiopathic pulmonary arterial hypertension (IPAH).

2. Lung biopsy is rarely necessary, generally poorly tolerated by patients with severe pulmonary hypertension, and reserved for cases in which the clinical diagnosis is unclear.

H. MISCELLANEOUS

1. The 6-minute walk test is used to obtain an objective measure of exercise tolerance, to assess response to therapy, and to forecast prognosis.

2. Portal hypertension is associated with the development of pulmonary hypertension, a condition called portopulmonary hypertension. The presence of portal hypertension may be demonstrated on abdominal imaging using Doppler ultrasonography or by obtaining the hepatic wedge pressure at the time of catheterization.[3,6]

IV. PROGNOSIS

The prognosis of PAH generally is regarded to be poor, although there is a wide range of outcomes. A National Institutes of Health registry conducted in the early 1980s showed that the 1-, 3-, and 5-year survival rates were 68%, 48%, and 34%, respectively.[9] The investigators also provided an equation to gauge prognosis on the basis of catheterization parameters they found most significant: mean pulmonary artery pressure, mean right atrial pressure, and cardiac index. Later work has shown that mean right atrial pressure may be of greatest prognostic significance. Furthermore, clinical markers of disease severity such as New York Heart Association (NYHA) functional class and the 6-minute walk test are regarded as good prognostic indicators and correlate with mortality data. It should be noted that patients with PAH associated with the scleroderma spectrum of disease have poorer outcomes than those with IPAH (both with and without prostacyclin therapy).[9]

V. MANAGEMENT (FIG. 85-2)

Early in the course of PAH, the pathologic features of the predominant lesion are smooth muscle hypertrophy and vasoconstriction. During this stage of the disease, treatment with oral vasodilator therapy relaxes the vascular smooth muscle and reduces pulmonary vascular resistance. Later in the disease course, proliferative features predominate, leaving no room for conventional vasodilator therapy. Unfortunately, more than 75% of people with PAH are in the proliferative stage at the time of presentation. Therefore, right-heart catheterization with an acute vasodilator trial is necessary to determine the appropriate treatment strategy.[3] Inhaled nitric oxide is an ideal vasodilatory agent because it is short acting, is specific to the pulmonary vasculature, and is inactivated by hemoglobin once it enters the bloodstream. Adenosine or intravenously administered epoprostenol can also be used.

1. Vasodilators.
a. Patients who are said to respond to the vasodilator challenge demonstrate a reduction in pulmonary vascular resistance of > 20% and a drop in pulmonary artery pressure of > 10 mmHg. These patients may be initiated on calcium channel blocker therapy. Verapamil is generally is avoided because of its negative inotropic properties).[3] Unfortunately, calcium channel blockers are useful in only 10% to 15% of patients who respond to the vasodilator challenge.[10,11]
b. Vasodilator-unresponsive patients with IPAH who have NYHA class III or IV symptoms (marked limitation in activity or symptoms at rest, respectively) experience improved exercise tolerance, decreased pulmonary vascular resistance (PVR), and improved survival from continuous infusion of epoprostenol (prostacyclin/prostaglandin I_2, a short-acting vasodilator and platelet inhibitor).[12,13] Other types of PAH also appear to benefit from epoprostenol (although less favorably). A recent randomized trial in patients with PAH related to the scleroderma

85

PULMONARY HYPERTENSION

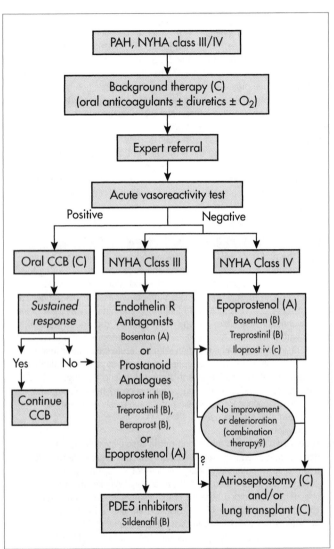

FIG. 85-2

See legend on the opposite page

spectrum of disease demonstrated that epoprostenol increased exercise tolerance and improved hemodynamics, although an effect on mortality was not demonstrated.[14]

c. It is important to note that epoprostenol therapy is not suitable for causes of pulmonary hypertension other than PAH because it can worsen the underlying disease. For instance, patients with significant parenchymal lung disease may experience worsening V/Q mismatch in response to epoprostenol. Additionally, prostacyclin can precipitate acute pulmonary edema in patients with left atrial pressures greater than 15 mmHg.

d. An inhaled prostacyclin, iloprost, has been studied in two trials (one lasting 3 months and the other 12 months) for the treatment of IPAH with good effect on exercise tolerance, NYHA class, and hemodynamics.[15,16] Benefits also include ease of administration and the certainty that intravenous treatment (as needed for epoprostenol) will not be interrupted, which can cause rebound pulmonary hypertension and death.

e. More recently, treprostinil, a prostacyclin analog administered in a continuous subcutaneous fashion, was approved for treatment of patients with PAH with NYHA class II-IV symptoms. In a 12-week randomized, placebo-controlled study of patients with IPAH and PAH associated with connective tissue disease, treprostinil was shown to improve exercise capacity, symptoms of pulmonary hypertension, and cardiopulmonary hemodynamics.[16] Patients have also been successfully transitioned from epoprostenol to treprostinil if necessary because of intolerable side effects or complications of epoprostenol therapy.

f. Sildenafil, an agent that indirectly increases nitric oxide–mediated vasodilation, is an emerging treatment for pulmonary hypertension. Recent studies of sildenafil administration have shown promising results by decreasing pulmonary vascular resistance and improving exercise tolerance.[17,18] Though sometimes used, sildenafil is not yet approved by the Food and Drug Administration for this indication.

g. Bosentan, an endothelin-1 antagonist, was recently approved as a therapy for pulmonary hypertension in patients with NYHA class III or IV heart failure symptoms. Two placebo-controlled trials have demonstrated the effectiveness of this oral medication in pulmonary

85

PULMONARY HYPERTENSION

Management algorithm for pulmonary arterial hypertension. The level of evidence is given in parentheses (A, multiple randomized trials or meta-analysis; B, single randomized trial or multiple randomized trials with heterogeneous results; C, small nonrandomized studies or expert consensus opinion). *CCB,* calcium channel blocker; *inh,* inhaler; *IV,* intravenous; *NYHA,* New York Heart Association; *PAH,* pulmonary artery hypertension; *PDE5,* phosphodiesterase 5. *(Modified from Galiè N et al: J Am Coll Cardiol 43(12):81S-88S, 2004.)*

hypertension (primary or associated with connective tissue disease), with resultant improvement in 6-minute walk test, hemodynamics, and decrease in clinical events.[19,20]

2. Adjunctive therapy.

a. Several nonrandomized studies suggest that anticoagulation increases survival in patients with IPAH and PAH caused by anorexigen use.[21,22] Unless a contraindication exists, patients should undergo anticoagulation with warfarin (goal international normalized ratio about 2).

b. Diuretics are important in the treatment of right ventricular dilation and failure, although care must be given during diuresis to maintain the balance between preload dependence and right ventricular volume overload.

c. Cardiac glycosides may produce a modest increase in cardiac output in patients with PAH and right ventricular failure and a significant reduction in circulating norepinephrine levels.

d. In patients with borderline systemic blood pressure, low-dose dopamine can maintain systemic blood pressure while enhancing natriuresis. It may also be administered on a long-term basis as a bridge to lung transplantation.[3,6,7]

e. Balloon atrial septostomy may be a bridge to transplantation or in patients who are refractory to all medical therapies. The rationale for the procedure is to allow right-to-left shunting, thereby increasing left ventricular preload and systemic output. Several small series have shown decreased symptoms, improved hemodynamics, and improved survival.[23]

f. Single or bilateral lung transplantation is performed for patients who have not responded to medical therapy for pulmonary hypertension. Patients with NYHA class III or IV should be evaluated for transplantation if they do not show improvement after 3 to 6 months of intravenous prostacyclin therapy and have a right atrial pressure greater than 15 mmHg and a pulmonary artery pressure greater than 55 mmHg.[24] Right ventricular dysfunction improves significantly on restoration of normal pulmonary vascular resistance. Heart-lung transplantation is reserved for patients with significant heart disease on the left side or complicated structural abnormalities associated with congenital heart disease. The 5-year survival rate after lung transplantation is between 45% and 50%.[3]

PEARLS AND PITFALLS

- Vasoactive medications must be added to a pulmonary hypertension regimen with great care. Whereas conventional heart failure therapy seeks to minimize stress and strain on the left ventricle, these treatments often have a deleterious effect on the patient with pulmonary hypertension, whose right ventricle is dominant. Because approximately 75% of patients with PAH do not respond to an acute vasodilator trial, it is important to prescribe these medications carefully—they will only decrease systemic blood pressure without improving pulmonary hemodynamics. Decreases in systemic blood pressure decrease left ventricular afterload and can worsen right ventricular impingement on the left ventricle, thus worsening hypotension. Additionally, right ventricular coronary perfusion will be compromised as systemic blood pressure drops while pulmonary pressure remains elevated, resulting in right ventricular ischemia.[3]

- Use of vasoconstricting agents, such as nasal decongestants, should be avoided.
- Because the right ventricle is preload dependent, great care must be taken not to overly diurese the patient with pulmonary hypertension.
- Hypotension in patients with severe pulmonary hypertension may be caused by impingement of the massively dilated right ventricle on a small and underfilled left ventricle. In this situation, hypotension should be treated with diuretics, not intravenous fluids, if the right atrial pressure is clearly elevated.
- Sedation, when needed, should be administered with caution, avoiding any agents known to decrease systemic blood pressure.
- Once calcium channel blockers have been successfully initiated in a patient with pulmonary hypertension, abrupt discontinuation can result in syncope and death because of rebound pulmonary hypertension. This is also true with patients receiving intravenous prostacyclin therapy. Abrupt discontinuation of the drug, even if only for a few seconds, can lead to syncope and death. Should central access be lost while the patient is in the hospital, intravenous prostacyclin can be administered via a peripheral vein until central access is again achieved.[3]
- Transfusion with platelets or fresh frozen plasma often is poorly tolerated because of the combination of a significant volume load and the presence of vasoactive compounds, such as thromboxane and serotonin, in these products.

85 PULMONARY HYPERTENSION

REFERENCES

1. Simonneau G et al: Clinical classification of pulmonary hypertension, *J Am Coll Cardiol* 43(12):5S-12S, 2004. D
2. Pengo V et al: Incidence of chronic thromboembolic pulmonary hypertension of pulmonary embolism, *N Engl J Med* 350(22):2257-2264, 2004. A
3. Gaine S: Pulmonary hypertension, *JAMA* 284:3160-3168, 2000. A
4. Gailie N et al: Primary pulmonary hypertension: insights into pathogenesis from epidemiology, *Chest* 114:184S-194S, 1998. B
5. Gaine S, Rubin L: Primary pulmonary hypertension, *Lancet* 352:719-725, 1998. A
6. Brij S, Peacock AJ: Pulmonary hypertension: its assessment and treatment, *Thorax* 54:S28-S32, 1999. B
7. Rubin LJ: Primary pulmonary hypertension, *N Engl J Med* 336:111-117, 1997. A
8. Lane KB et al: Heterozygous germline mutations in BMPR2, encoding a TGF-beta receptor, cause familial primary pulmonary hypertension, *Nature Genet* 26:81-84, 2000. A

9. McLaughlin VV et al: Prognosis of pulmonary arterial hypertension: ACCP evidence-based clinical practice guidelines, *Chest* 126:78S-92S, 2004. D
10. Galiè N et al: Comparative analysis of clinical trials and evidence-based treatment algorithm in pulmonary hypertension, *J Am Coll Cardiol* 43(12):81S-88S, 2004. D
11. Rich S et al: The effect of high doses of calcium channel blockers on survival in primary pulmonary hypertension, *N Engl J Med* 327:76-81, 1992. A
12. McLaughlin VV et al: Reduction in pulmonary vascular resistance with long-term epoprostenol (prostacyclin) therapy in primary pulmonary hypertension, *N Engl J Med* 338:273-277, 1998. B
13. Barst RJ et al: A comparison of continuous intravenous epoprostenol (prostacyclin) with conventional therapy for primary pulmonary hypertension, *N Engl J Med* 334:296, 1996. A
14. Badesch DB et al: Continuous intravenous epoprostenol for pulmonary hypertension due to the scleroderma spectrum of disease: a randomized, controlled trial, *Ann Intern Med* 132(6):425-434, 2000. A
15. Hoeper MM et al: Long-term treatment of primary pulmonary hypertension with aerosolized iloprost, a prostacyclin analogue, *N Engl J Med* 342:1866-1870, 2000. A
16. Simonneau G et al: Continuous subcutaneous infusion of treprostinil, a prostacyclin analogue, in patients with pulmonary arterial hypertension: a double-blind, randomized, placebo-controlled trial, *Am J Respir Crit Care Med* 165(6):800-804, 2002. A
17. Ghofrani HA et al: Sildenafil for treatment of lung fibrosis and pulmonary hypertension: a randomized controlled trial, *Lancet* 360(9337):895-900, 2002. A
18. Sastry BKS et al: Clinical efficacy of sildenafil in primary pulmonary hypertension, *J Am Coll Cardiol* 43:1149-1153, 2004. A
19. Rubin LJ, Badesch DB, Barst RJ: Bosentan therapy for pulmonary arterial hypertension, *N Engl J Med* 346:896-903, 2002. A
20. Channick RN, Simonneau G, Sitbon O, et al: Effects of the dual endothelin-receptor antagonist bosentan in patients with pulmonary hypertension: a randomised placebo-controlled study, *Lancet* 358:1119-1123, 2001. A
21. Fuster V et al: Primary pulmonary hypertension: natural history and the importance of thrombosis, *Circulation* 70:580-587, 1984. C
22. Frank H et al: The effect of anticoagulant therapy in primary and anorectic drug-induced pulmonary hypertension, *Chest* 112:714-721, 1997. C
23. Sandoval J et al: Graded balloon dilation atrial septostomy in severe primary pulmonary hypertension, *J Am Coll Cardiol* 32(2):297-304, 1998. C
24. International guidelines for the selection of lung transplant candidates, *Am J Respir Crit Care Med* 158:335, 1998. D

Venous Thromboembolism

Eric Schmidt, MD; David Zaas, MD; and David Pearse, MD

FAST FACTS

- Of patients with proximal lower extremity deep venous thrombosis (DVT), more than half have pulmonary embolism (PE).
- Lower extremity compression ultrasound is highly (> 95%) sensitive and specific for symptomatic proximal DVT but is only 30% to 60% sensitive for asymptomatic proximal DVT.
- A negative D-dimer test has an excellent negative predictive value for venous thromboembolism (VTE) if there is low clinical suspicion for PE.
- A normal PaO_2 (> 80 mmHg) on arterial blood gas analysis does not rule out PE.
- Spiral computed tomography (CT) angiography, although highly sensitive for proximal PE, has limited specificity and sensitivity for subsegmental emboli.
- Because delays in anticoagulation are associated with increases in mortality from PE, treatment should be initiated before diagnostic testing in patients with a high clinical suspicion of PE.
- In an inpatient population, the first manifestation of PE often is sudden death, so DVT prophylaxis is essential in high-risk patients.

In 1889 Rudolph Virchow identified DVT as the source of PE, thus establishing that they are both manifestations of a singular disease process: VTE. Despite improvements in diagnosis and treatment, VTE remains a source of morbidity and mortality.

I. EPIDEMIOLOGY

1. Venous thrombosis usually originates in the lower extremities. Other, less common sources of thrombus include the pelvic, renal, and axillary veins and the inferior vena cava. Although calf thromboses rarely embolize, 12% to 20% extend into the deep veins of the thigh. From these proximal positions, the risk of PE is about 50%.[1] Contrary to common belief, it is estimated that one third of upper extremity DVTs lead to PE.
2. It is estimated that more than 500,000 cases of VTE occur annually in the United States. Incidence has decreased over the past 20 years, presumably because of advances in prophylaxis.
3. Risk factors for the development of VTE often act synergistically.
a. Virchow's classic triad of VTE risk is venous stasis, vascular endothelial damage, and hypercoagulability. The presence of one or more of these states accounts for the increased VTE risk attributed to classic clinical risk factors (Box 86-1).[2]

BOX 86-1

RISK FACTORS FOR VENOUS THROMBOEMBOLISM

STRONG RISK FACTORS (ODDS RATIO >10)

Fracture (hip or leg)

Hip or knee replacement

Major trauma

Spinal cord injury

Major general surgery

MODERATE RISK FACTORS (ODDS RATIO 2:9)

Malignancy

Oral contraceptives, hormone replacement therapy

Pregnancy, postpartum

Chemotherapy

Paralytic stroke

Arthroscopic knee surgery

Central venous lines

Congestive heart failure or respiratory failure

Previous venous thromboembolism

Thrombophilia

WEAK RISK FACTORS (ODDS RATIO < 2)

Bed rest > 3 d

Age > 40

Varicose veins

Obesity

Pregnancy, antepartum

Laparoscopic surgery

Prolonged sitting (e.g., "economy class syndrome")

Modified from Anderson FA, Spencer FA: *Circulation* 107:I9-I16, 2003.

---

b. Advancing age is a powerful predictor for the development of DVT and PE. The incidence of VTE in people older than 80 years approaches 1% per year.

c. Hypercoagulability is believed to exist in a majority of patients with VTE. Increased tendency for thrombosis can arise from malignancy, pregnancy, a coagulation pathway abnormality, or smoking.

II. CLINICAL PRESENTATION

PE can have a variety of presentations because its manifestations are nonspecific. As a result, the differential diagnosis is broad, and the diagnosis often is missed (see Chapter 7).

A. SYMPTOMS

1. Dyspnea and pleuritic chest pain are the most common symptoms, present in 73% and 66% of patients, respectively. Other symptoms, such as cough, hemoptysis, leg pain and swelling, palpitations, and wheezing, are present in a minority of patients.

2. Massive PE can present as syncope or hemodynamic instability.
3. The absence of pleuritic chest pain, dyspnea, and tachypnea is 97% specific for the absence of PE.[3]

B. PHYSICAL SIGNS

The most common physical signs of PE are tachypnea, crackles, and tachycardia, present in 70%, 51%, and 30% of patients, respectively. Signs present in less than 25% of patients with PE include fever, diaphoresis, cyanosis, pleural friction rub, rales, wheezes, Homans' sign, an S_4, a loud P_2, and an S_3.

C. BASIC TESTING

1. **Arterial blood gas analysis.**
a. The increased dead space ventilation arising from pulmonary arterial obstruction is compensated (and often overcompensated) by an increase in minute ventilation. Consequently, patients with PE are rarely hypercapnic at presentation unless they are unable to increase their minute ventilation (e.g., as in hemodynamic collapse, mechanical ventilation).
b. Hypoxemia, found in only 80% of patients with PE, results from a combination of a right-to-left shunt from atelectasis and a patent foramen ovale, ventilation-perfusion (V/Q) mismatch, or a low mixed-venous O_2 partial pressure (PvO_2).
c. An abnormal alveolar-arterial O_2 (PAO_2-PaO_2) gradient is more sensitive than hypoxemia alone in PE evaluation because most patients with normal arterial oxygenation are hypocapnic. However, a normal PAO_2-PaO_2 gradient does not rule out a diagnosis of PE, particularly in younger patients with normal cardiopulmonary reserve.

2. **Chest radiograph.** Findings on chest radiography are most helpful in excluding other causes of hypoxemia. The most common radiographic abnormalities are atelectasis, small pleural effusions, and peripherally based infiltrates. Classic but rare (< 7%) findings include Westermark's sign (prominent central pulmonary artery with decreased pulmonary vascularity), Hampton's hump (wedge-shaped peripheral-based infiltrates just above the diaphragm), and Palla's sign (enlargement of the right descending pulmonary artery).

3. **Electrocardiogram.**
a. The electrocardiogram often is abnormal, but the changes are nonspecific. The most common abnormalities are nonspecific ST segment and T wave changes and sinus tachycardia.
b. Electrocardiographic findings indicative of elevated right-sided heart pressures, such as P pulmonale, right ventricular (RV) hypertrophy, right axis deviation, right bundle branch block, and $S_1Q_3T_3$, are found in less than 6% of patients with PE. Therefore, their absence is not helpful in the diagnostic evaluation of PE.
c. Electrocardiographic evidence of RV ischemia may be found consequent to severe RV strain with massive PE. Furthermore, strain may lead to

compression of the right coronary artery, prompting electrocardiographic findings such as (rarely) T wave inversions in V_1 to V_4.

4. **Echocardiogram.** With the exception of right heart thrombus, echocardiographic abnormalities rarely are of sufficient specificity to diagnose PE. Recently described findings, such as the McConnell sign (RV free wall hypokinesia with concurrent apical normokinesia), may indicate the presence of acute RV strain. The absence of RV overload in a patient with hypotension suggests an alternative diagnosis.

III. DIAGNOSIS

1. Because of the absence of pathognomonic signs and symptoms, PE cannot be diagnosed reliably by clinical observation alone. Likewise, imaging modalities by themselves (with the possible exception of the invasive and often inconvenient pulmonary angiogram) are insufficiently sensitive or specific to allow a diagnosis to be made. If incorporated together into rational algorithm, however, clinical suspicion and diagnostic testing can be used to diagnose PE. Multiple diagnostic algorithms have been validated prospectively; most begin with the clinical determination of a pretest probability of PE. This probability is then used to guide the choice of further diagnostic interventions. One typical algorithm is detailed in Fig. 86-1.[4]

2. Initially defined by the PIOPED investigators as a qualitative clinical sense (inferred from the patient's history, physical examination, chest radiograph, and electrocardiogram), the pretest probability has since been quantified by a number of predictive clinical criteria, such as the Wells scoring system.[5] Despite prospective validation, these scoring systems have not yet demonstrated diagnostic superiority to the qualitative clinical judgment first proposed in the PIOPED study.

3. Once clinical risk is defined, the choice of further testing can be made rationally in accordance with a diagnostic algorithm. Such tests include the following:

a. **V/Q scan.** The value of the V/Q scan was investigated in the multicenter prospective PIOPED study.[6] This study demonstrated that the combination of V/Q scan findings and pretest probability assessment improved overall diagnostic accuracy.

   (1) A high-probability scan was useful in diagnosing PE (positive predictive value of 88%) if pretest probability was intermediate or higher. The combination of a low pretest probability and a high-probability scan pattern was associated with a positive predictive value of only 50% and therefore should not be considered diagnostic of PE.

   (2) A normal- or very low–probability scan, though rare (accounting for only 14% of scan results), had a 91% negative predictive value (NPV). In the setting of a high pretest clinical suspicion, however, this finding is not sufficient to rule out PE. However, a completely

normal perfusion scan excludes the diagnosis of PE regardless of the pretest probability.

(3) A low-probability scan had an overall NPV of 86% and therefore was capable of ruling out PE only if the pretest probability was low.

(4) Intermediate-probability scans, though common (particularly in those with preexisting parenchymal or vascular lung disease), were not useful in diagnosing PE.

(5) Unfortunately, in a majority of patients, clinical assessment and V/Q scanning alone are not adequate to diagnose PE. Further testing often is necessary.

b. **Spiral CT.**

(1) Use of contrast-enhanced spiral CT in the diagnosis of PE has dramatically increased in the past decade. Despite this popularity, few prospective data exist to support the use of helical CT alone in evaluating PE.

(2) Studies report a wide variety of sensitivities (53% to 100%). This lack of consensus reflects not only interobserver variability but also intertrial heterogeneity in the detection of emboli affecting small, subsegmental pulmonary arteries. Although a new generation of multidetector helical CT scanners has promised improved sensitivity for these subsegmental emboli, no randomized prospective data exist to support these claims.

(3) A proximal pulmonary arterial filling defect identified on spiral CT is highly specific for the presence of thrombus. The specificity of a filling defect in smaller, subsegmental vessels is much lower for the diagnosis of PE.

(4) Spiral CT is useful for the simultaneous evaluation of the lung parenchyma. It is important to recognize that many pulmonary parenchymal abnormalities (infiltrate, mass, effusion) can be associated with a concurrent embolism.

(5) Disadvantages of spiral CT include the contrast dye load, with its associated risks of allergy and nephrotoxicity.

c. **Magnetic resonance imaging.**

(1) Noncontrast magnetic resonance venography is thought to be highly sensitive and specific for the diagnosis of both symptomatic and asymptomatic lower extremity DVT. Magnetic resonance venography can also be used to diagnose thrombosis in areas not easily accessed by ultrasonography (e.g., pelvic vessels).

(2) Gadolinium-enhanced magnetic resonance arteriography (MRA) is thought to be highly sensitive and specific for the diagnosis of PE. Nonenhanced MRA is limited by cardiac and pulmonary motion artifact.

(3) MRA can be performed rapidly, without the risks associated with contrast material used for spiral CT and pulmonary angiography. Therefore, MRA may be useful in patients with iodinated contrast allergy or renal failure. Despite its promise, the utility of MRA in

86

VENOUS THROMBOEMBOLISM

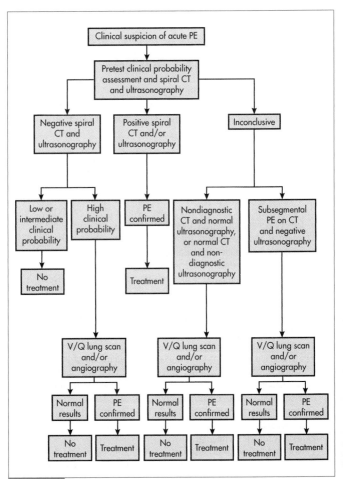

FIG. 86-1
Diagnostic algorithm for pulmonary embolism. Note that D-dimer detection is not included in the diagnostic algorithm. This exclusion is appropriate because of the low prevalence of useful (e.g., negative) D-dimer results in a medical inpatient population. *CT,* computed tomography; *PE,* pulmonary embolism; *V/Q,* ventilation-perfusion. *(Modified from Musset D et al:* Lancet *360(9349):1914-1920, 2002.)*

diagnosing PE has not yet been validated by randomized, prospective trial data.

d. **Pulmonary angiography.**
   (1) Pulmonary angiography is the gold standard for the diagnosis of PE. Morbidity and mortality of pulmonary angiography often are overstated; in the PIOPED study, morbidity was less than 2% and mortality less than 0.5%. Pulmonary angiography should be performed when the diagnosis remains in doubt after a workup with noninvasive modalities.
   (2) Limitations include the need for a skilled and experienced interventional radiologist, significant interobserver variability, and exposure to nephrotoxic contrast dye.

e. **D-dimer.**
   (1) D-dimers are specific degradation products of cross-linked fibrin. They may be detected in a patient's blood up to 12 days after a VTE event.
   (2) Though highly sensitive for VTE, D-dimer tests are nonspecific. In the appropriate setting, a negative D-dimer test may help exclude a diagnosis of VTE, but a positive D-dimer test is of no diagnostic utility. In most inpatient populations, the prevalence of negative D-dimers is low, particularly after surgery and in patients being treated for liver failure or cancer. Therefore, the utility of the test in these populations is limited.
   (3) Several assay systems are available to detect D-dimers.
      (a) Studies report a high sensitivity (> 95%) of D-dimer enzyme-linked immunosorbent assays (ELISAs) and a useful NPV (> 95%). A negative ELISA thus excludes PE in patients with low or intermediate pretest probability. Unfortunately, D-dimer ELISA assays are time consuming and therefore are not used clinically at many institutions.
      (b) Agglutination assays are widely available because of their relative ease and rapidity of testing. They are less sensitive than ELISA. As a result, the NPV of the test is acceptable only if it is used in populations with a low prevalence of PE. A negative agglutination assay therefore can rule out PE only in the setting of low pretest probability, a risk category typically found only in outpatients.

f. **Lower extremity compression ultrasonography.**
   (1) Venography, though remaining the gold standard for the diagnosis of DVT, has been largely replaced by compression ultrasonography in clinical practice.
   (2) Ultrasonography is 95% sensitive and 96% specific for detecting symptomatic DVT in the popliteal or more proximal lower extremity veins. Sensitivity for asymptomatic proximal DVT is only 30% to 60%; however, specificity remains high. Similar results are noted in the detection of upper extremity DVT.[7]

86

VENOUS THROMBOEMBOLISM

(3) Serial lower extremity ultrasonography (at days 1, 4, and 7) without therapeutic anticoagulation has been used to rule out VTE after an indeterminate V/Q scan or negative contrast-enhanced spiral CT. However, patient compliance with this regimen often is suboptimal and a delay in the diagnosis of VTE may be risky in patients with poor cardiopulmonary reserve.

IV. MANAGEMENT

A. ANTICOAGULATION

1. Anticoagulation is used to prevent new clot formation while the body degrades existing clots. The classic regimen of anticoagulation for DVT or PE is the intravenous administration of unfractionated heparin followed by orally administered warfarin.

2. When the diagnosis of VTE is suspected and no contraindications to anticoagulation are present, heparin should be started using a weight-based algorithm. Initially, the activated partial thromboplastin time must be measured every 6 hours to confirm adequate heparin dosing. The goal activated partial thromboplastin time, although typically 45 to 70 seconds, can vary depending on the method used by individual laboratories.

3. Low molecular weight heparin, an attractive alternative to unfractionated heparin, allows greater ease of administration, less strict monitoring, and a lower incidence of heparin-induced thrombocytopenia in comparison to unfractionated heparin. The use of low molecular weight heparin to treat DVT allows highly cost-effective management of a clinically stable outpatient.

4. Warfarin should be initiated with concurrent heparin administration to avoid the transient hypercoagulability associated with warfarin's rapid reduction of protein C and protein S levels. Warfarin should be started at 5 mg/day and adjusted to reach an international normalized ratio of 2 to 3. Once the goal international normalized ratio has been reached, heparin should be continued for an additional 48 hours to ensure continued therapeutic oral anticoagulation. The major risk of long-term oral anticoagulation is bleeding, with a 3% yearly risk of major hemorrhage.

5. VTE in the absence of major risk factors (Box 86-1) indicates an insidious predisposition for thrombosis and hence the need for a longer duration of therapy[8] (Table 86-1). However, the optimal length of treatment remains unclear because patients with idiopathic VTE remain at elevated risk for recurrent thrombosis. Patients at particular risk for recurrence may be identified by persistently abnormal D-dimer levels or compression ultrasonography after cessation of standard anticoagulation. The continuation of low-dose (goal international normalized ratio 1.5 to 2) anticoagulation after the completion of a standard course of therapy for idiopathic VTE has been shown to

TABLE 86-1

DURATION OF ANTICOAGULATION IN VTE

	Duration
TRANSIENT STRONG RISK FACTOR PRESENT	
Isolated distal DVT	6 wk
Proximal DVT or pulmonary embolism	3 mo
Concurrent thrombophilia, cancer, IVC filter	6 mo
NO TRIGGERING STRONG TRANSIENT RISK FACTOR IDENTIFIED	
Isolated distal DVT or DVT at any site in a patient at high risk of bleeding	3 mo
Weak reversible risk factor (any site) or DVT at any site in patient with a moderate risk of bleeding	6 mo
Recurrent VTE, active cancer, concurrent thrombophilia, poor cardiopulmonary reserve	Indefinite

Modified from Kearon C: *Clin Chest Med* 24:63-72, 2003.
DVT, deep vein thrombosis; *VTE,* venous thromboembolism.

decrease the risk of recurrent thrombosis with little increase in the
risk of bleeding complications.[9]

B. THROMBOLYTIC AGENTS

Urokinase, streptokinase, and tissue plasminogen activator have
been shown to cause more rapid clot lysis and quicker resolution
of hemodynamic changes than does heparin. However, there is no
convincing evidence of morbidity or mortality benefits to justify the greater
bleeding risk of thrombolysis. The only widely accepted indication is shock
in a patient with a large, hemodynamically significant PE. However, data
supporting this use are mostly anecdotal. Thrombolytic agents have been
investigated in the treatment of submassive PE, a state defined by the
presence of acute RV overload in the absence of hypotension. The
mortality and morbidity benefits of thrombolysis in this population are
unclear and controversial.[10,11]

C. VENA CAVAL FILTERS

1. Vena cava filters are used to prevent the progression of a DVT into a
   PE. Traditional indications include an inability to tolerate anticoagulation
   and the failure of anticoagulation.
2. No head-to-head trials have compared filter placement with
   anticoagulation, and only one randomized controlled trial evaluated
   vena cava filters as an adjunct to anticoagulation. In 400 patients
   randomly assigned to filters plus at least 3 months of anticoagulation or
   to anticoagulation alone, vena cava filters decreased the incidence of PE
   within the first year. However, these benefits were offset by an increase
   in recurrent DVT.[12] Furthermore, no significant benefit in PE incidence
   or mortality was seen after 1 year.
3. On the basis of the lack of data supporting caval filter placement,
   anticoagulation is the first choice in treatment of VTE. The use of filters
   should be considered only for patients in whom anticoagulation is either
   contraindicated or ineffective.

86

VENOUS THROMBOEMBOLISM

D. EMBOLECTOMY

The surgical removal of a PE may be considered in hemodynamically unstable patients with contraindications to thrombolysis. In some centers, embolectomy can be pursued via a percutaneous approach. This typically relies on a catheter-directed mechanical clot disruption.

V. PREVENTION

1. Approximately two thirds of patients with PE are diagnosed only at autopsy. The bulk of VTE mortality arises from such missed antemortem diagnosis and the consequent failure to initiate treatment. Given these shortcomings, VTE prophylaxis is vital, particularly in patients at elevated thrombotic risk.
2. Medical patients admitted for the treatment of congestive heart failure, chronic obstructive pulmonary disease, or infections are considered to be at a moderate risk of developing VTE. In these patients, the combination of subcutaneous low-dose unfractionated heparin and mechanical lower extremity compression devices usually provides sufficient VTE prophylaxis.[13,14]
3. Surgical patients are at much higher risk of developing VTE and may need more aggressive prophylaxis.

VI. PROGNOSIS

1. Ten percent of PEs are fatal within the first hour of symptom onset.
2. In patients who survive long enough to reach medical attention, the presence of hemodynamic instability (massive PE) carries a poor prognosis (25% to 50% in-hospital mortality).
3. If hemodynamically stable PE is diagnosed and treated properly, the long-term prognosis is good, with survival rates determined primarily by the underlying state that triggered venous thrombosis. If PE is misdiagnosed and proper treatment is not initiated, 26% of PE survivors will have a fatal second PE, and another 26% will have a nonfatal recurrence.[15]
4. In hemodynamically stable patients with PE, signs of right heart failure (submassive PE) may suggest an elevated risk of recurrent PE or death. Consequently, intact RV systolic function on echocardiography, low brain natriuretic peptide levels, or normal cardiac troponin levels may indicate a good short-term prognosis.[16,17]

PEARLS AND PITFALLS

- A hypercoagulable workup cannot be conducted accurately in the setting of acute thrombosis or during anticoagulation (see Chapter 46).
- Postphlebitic syndrome is a common sequela of DVT. To prevent venous stasis and its attendant complications, all patients with DVT should be prescribed stockings with 30 mmHg of compression on discharge (thromboembolic disease hose provide insufficient compression).
- Approximately 4% of patients will develop pulmonary hypertension after a pulmonary embolism (see Chapter 85).

REFERENCES

1. Dalen JE: Pulmonary embolism: what have we learned since Virchow? Natural history, pathophysiology, and diagnosis, *Chest* 122:1440-1456, 2002. C
2. Anderson FA, Spencer FA: Risk factors for venous thromboembolism, *Circulation* 107:I9-I16, 2003. C
3. Stein PD et al: Clinical, laboratory, roentgenographic, and electrocardiographic findings in patients with acute pulmonary embolism and no pre-existing cardiac or pulmonary disease, *Chest* 100(3):598, 1991. B
4. Musset D, Parent F, Meyer G, et al: Diagnostic strategy for patients with suspected pulmonary embolism: a prospective multicentre outcome study, *Lancet* 360(9349):1914-1920, 2002. B
5. Wells PS, Anderson DR, Ginsberg RM, et al: Derivation of a simple clinical model to categorize patients probability of pulmonary embolism: increasing the models utility with the SimpliRED D-dimer, *Thromb Haemost* 83(3):416-420, 2000. B
6. PIOPED Investigators: Value of the ventilation/perfusion scan in acute pulmonary embolism, *JAMA* 263(20):2753, 1990. A
7. Kearon C, Ginsberg J, Hirsch J: The role of venous ultrasound in diagnosis of suspected deep venous thrombosis and pulmonary embolism, *Ann Intern Med* 128(12):1044, 1998. B
8. Kearon C: Duration of therapy for acute venous thromboembolism, *Clin Chest Med* 24:63-72, 2003. C
9. Ridker PM, Goldhaber SZ, Danielson E, et al: Long-term, low-intensity warfarin therapy for the prevention of recurrent venous thromboembolism, *N Engl J Med* 348:1425-1434, 2003. B
10. Konstantinides S, Geibel A, Heusel G, et al: Heparin plus alteplase compared with heparin alone in patients with submassive pulmonary embolism, *N Engl J Med* 347:1143-1150, 2002. A
11. Hamel E, Pacouret G, Vincentelli D, et al: Thrombolysis or heparin therapy in massive pulmonary embolism with right ventricular dilation, *Chest* 120:120-125, 2001. B
12. Descous H et al: A clinical trial of vena caval filters in the prevention of pulmonary embolism in patients with proximal deep vein thrombosis, *N Engl J Med* 338(7):409, 1998. A
13. Geerts WH, Pineo GF, Heit JA, et al: Prevention of venous thromboembolism: the Seventh ACCP Conference on Antithrombotic and Thrombolytic Therapy, *Chest* 126:338S-400S, 2004. D
14. Mismetti P, Laporte-Simitsidis S, Tardy B, et al: Prevention of VTE in internal medicine with unfractionated or low molecular-weight heparins: a meta-analysis of randomized clinical trials, *Thromb Haemost* 83:14-19, 2000. C
15. Kearon C: Natural history of venous thromboembolism, *Circulation* 107:I22-I30, 2003. C
16. Grifoni S, Olivotto I, Cecchini P, et al: Short-term clinical outcome of patients with pulmonary embolism, normal blood pressure, and echocardiographic right ventricular dysfunction, *Circulation* 101:2817-2822, 2000. B
17. Kucher N, Goldhaber SZ: Cardiac biomarkers for risk stratification of patients with acute pulmonary embolism, *Circulation* 108:2191-2194, 2003. B

86

VENOUS THROMBOEMBOLISM

Interstitial Lung Disease

Neil Aggarwal, MD; Kerry Dunbar, MD; and Albert J. Polito, MD

87

FAST FACTS

- The interstitial lung diseases (ILDs) are a diverse group (Box 87-1) of lung disorders characterized pathologically by varying degrees of chronic inflammation and progressive fibrosis of the pulmonary interstitium and physiologically by a restrictive pattern and gas transfer defect on pulmonary function tests (PFTs).
- The most common interstitial disorder, idiopathic pulmonary fibrosis (IPF), represents 44% to 46% of all ILDs and requires the presence of usual interstitial pneumonia (UIP) on biopsy.[1] IPF belongs to a subcategory of ILD known as idiopathic interstitial pneumonias (IIPs), which are the focus of this chapter.
- Surgical lung biopsy is the diagnostic gold standard in determining the pathologic subtype of IIP. However, high-resolution chest computed tomography scan (HRCT) demonstrates about 61% to 80% accuracy in diagnosing ILD and may obviate invasive procedures in certain cases.
- Prognosis and response to treatment are related to the pathologic characteristics seen on biopsy and appear to be inversely related to the degree of fibrosis and number of fibroblast foci seen.

Idiopathic ILDs are only one subset of the more than 200 causes of ILD. The history is crucial in delineating potential environmental or occupational exposures, and the physical examination may identify extrapulmonary manifestations such as arthritis and rashes that support a secondary cause of ILD (Fig. 87-1).

I. EPIDEMIOLOGY

1. The incidence of ILD is estimated to be 31.5 cases per 100,000 people per year for men and 26.1 cases per 100,000 people per year for women.[1]
2. Familial forms of IPF are transmitted in an autosomal dominant pattern.[2]
3. The incidence of the different ILDs varies by age, sex, and risk factors (Table 87-1).

II. CLINICAL PRESENTATION

Most patients present with the variable onset of progressive dyspnea and cough and generally have inspiratory crackles on examination. See Table 87-1 for a comparison of the different presentations, physical examination findings, radiographic features, and biopsy findings of the idiopathic interstitial pneumonias.

BOX 87-1

DIFFERENTIAL DIAGNOSIS OF INTERSTITIAL LUNG DISEASE

ENVIRONMENTAL AND OCCUPATIONAL

Organic dusts (farmer's lung, etc.)

Asbestosis

Silicosis

Pneumoconiosis

Berylliosis

Talcosis

COLLAGEN-VASCULAR DISEASE AND VASCULITIS

Rheumatoid arthritis

Systemic lupus erythematous

Scleroderma

Polymyositis and dermatomyositis

Sjögren's syndrome

Goodpasture's syndrome

Mixed connective tissue disease

Wegener's granulomatosis

Churg-Strauss syndrome

SYSTEMIC DISEASES (OTHER THAN COLLAGEN-VASCULAR)

Langerhans cell granulomatosis

Gaucher's disease

Lymphangioleiomyomatosis

Amyloidosis

Tuberous sclerosis

Sarcoidosis

DRUGS AND THERAPIES

Radiation

Nitrofurantoin

Methotrexate

Phenytoin

Gold

Penicillamine

Amiodarone

Heroin

Bleomycin

Melphalan

Chlorambucil

IDIOPATHIC PULMONARY DISORDERS

Usual interstitial pneumonia and idiopathic pulmonary fibrosis

Respiratory bronchiolitis–associated interstitial lung disease and desquamative interstitial pneumonia

Acute interstitial pneumonia

Cryptogenic organizing pneumonia

Chronic eosinophilic pneumonia

87

INTERSTITIAL LUNG DISEASE

TABLE 87-1
FEATURES OF IDIOPATHIC INTERSTITIAL PNEUMONIA

	UIP	RB-ILD	DIP	AIP	NSIP	COP
Male/female	2:1	2:1	2:1	1:1	2:3	1:1
Average age at onset (yr)	59	36	45	49	49	58
Symptoms	Symptoms over 1-4 yr, mistaken for prolonged viral illness	Mild complaints of dyspnea, new or changed cough	Milder presentation with insidious onset of dyspnea and cough	In 50%, a viral illness precedes rapid onset of respiratory failure	Subacute onset of dyspnea and cough	4-8 wk of new, nonproductive cough and flulike illness
Physical examination	Crackles, clubbing in 25-50%, cor pulmonale with late stages	Rales or crackles, occasional inspiratory squeaks	Crackles and clubbing are common, rarely right-sided heart failure	Crackles on examination, but cor pulmonale or clubbing extremely rare	Inspiratory squeaks, crackles, fever in a third	Inspiratory squeaks and crackles
High-resolution computed tomography scan	Patchy bilateral reticular infiltrates; subpleural and basal predilection; traction bronchiectasis; honeycombing	Diffuse involvement of bronchial wall thickening, centrilobular nodules, and patchy ground-glass opacity	Bilateral patchy ground-glass infiltrates in a mosaic pattern; basal predominance	Diffuse bilateral ground-glass infiltrates with or without consolidation	Bilateral patchy ground-glass infiltrates with interlobular interstitial thickening; rare honeycombing	Patchy, unilateral or bilateral areas of airspace or ground-glass consolidation, half with subpleural or peribronchial distribution, rare honeycombing

87

INTERSTITIAL LUNG DISEASE

Biopsy findings	Temporal heterogeneity with fibroblast foci, patchy inflammation, honeycomb changes, normal lung; subpleural distribution	Patchy, pigmented and Prussian blue staining macrophages in lumen of respiratory bronchioles, bronchiolocentric distribution; preserved distal airspaces	Macrophages with yellow-brown pigment in alveolar spaces representing smokers' histiocytes; no fibroblast foci; no honeycombing	Interstitial fibrosis; active, diffuse, homogenous fibroblast proliferation; septa lined with atypical type II pneumocytes; resembles diffuse alveolar damage seen with acute respiratory distress syndrome	Chronic inflammatory mononuclear cell infiltrate in alveolar septa; rare areas of homogenous fibrosis or fibroblast foci; normal lung may be seen	Proliferating fibroblasts and myofibroblasts within alveolar ducts, with airway occlusion but preservation of architecture; rare fibrosis and honeycombing
Temporal heterogeneity?	Yes	No	No	No	No	No
Mortality (%)	59-70	Rare	27.5	62	16	Rare
Mean survival	2.8-5.6 yr	Normal	12 yr	1-2 mo	13 yr	Normal
Response to treatment	Poor	Good	Good	Poor	Good	Good

AIP, acute interstitial pneumonia; *COP*, cryptogenic organizing pneumonia; *DIP*, desquamative interstitial pneumonia; *NSIP*, nonspecific interstitial pneumonia; *RB-ILD*, respiratory bronchiolitis–associated interstitial lung disease; *UIP*, usual interstitial pneumonia.

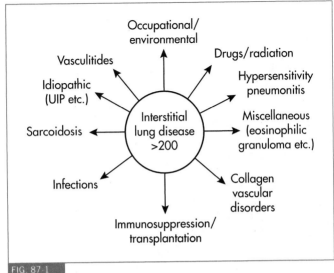

FIG. 87-1

Causes of interstitial lung disease. *UIP*, usual interstitial pneumonia. *(Modified from Green FHY: Chest 122:334S-339S, 2002.)*

1. **UIP or IPF.** Also called cryptogenic fibrosing alveolitis, IPF is the most common cause of idiopathic ILD and serves as the prototype for all interstitial disorders. UIP is the pathologic equivalent of the clinical diagnosis of IPF. Although some patients may respond to immunosuppressive therapy, life expectancy is about 28 months from the time of diagnosis. On pathology, UIP is defined by temporal heterogeneity, with normal lung, interstitial inflammation, fibroblast foci, and honeycombing all appearing in the same biopsy. In patients with biopsy-proven UIP, increased fibroblast foci have been associated with shorter survival, indicating the possibility that IPF is a disease of disordered fibroblast regulation rather than active inflammation.

2. **Respiratory bronchiolitis-associated interstitial lung disease (RB-ILD).** There is a direct link between cigarette smoking and RB-ILD, with at least a 30 pack-year history in affected patients. On pathology, it can mimic UIP, but the fibrotic changes are mild, and there is no honeycombing. Respiratory bronchiolitis to RB-ILD to desquamative interstitial pneumonia (DIP) represents a spectrum of disease from mild to severe.

3. **DIP.** About 90% of patients with DIP have a history of smoking. DIP does not progress to UIP if left untreated, and it tends to produce less severe restrictive disease on PFTs than does UIP.

4. **Acute interstitial pneumonia (AIP).** Hamman and Rich provided the first pathologic description of idiopathic ILD in four patients, all of whom had AIP based on pathology and the acute onset of their symptoms.[3] Patients with AIP display a temporally homogenous appearance of extensive interstitial fibroblast proliferation. Analogous to acute respiratory distress syndrome in presentation and pathology, AIP is characterized by the rapid onset of severe dyspnea, cough, and fever with quick progression to respiratory failure; many patients need intensive care and mechanical ventilation. A virus-like prodrome precedes the development of AIP in about 50% of patients.

5. **Cryptogenic organizing pneumonia (COP).** Also known as bronchiolitis obliterans organizing pneumonia (BOOP). COP can be idiopathic or can occur in association with other disorders, including infections, drug reactions, eosinophilic lung disease, inflammatory bowel disease, collagen-vascular disease, and aspiration pneumonia. It also can develop as a reparative reaction around other processes. Inspiratory crackles and squeaks on examination are characteristic of bronchiolitis. Pathology is significant for polypoid plugs of fibroblasts in the distal airspaces with preservation of the lung architecture.

6. **Nonspecific interstitial pneumonia (NSIP).** Although NSIP occasionally may represent a precursor to UIP, it is clearly distinguished from UIP by temporal uniformity on pathology and a better prognosis. The presence of honeycombing on pathology may indicate less responsiveness to treatment and an overall course similar to that of UIP. Most cases of NSIP are idiopathic, but 20% to 40% occur in association with other conditions, including collagen-vascular disease, drug-induced pneumonitis, infection, and hypersensitivity pneumonitis.

III. DIAGNOSIS

A specific diagnosis of ILD is made through composite assessment of the history, physical examination, PFTs, high-resolution computed tomography (HRCT), and lung biopsy.

A. LABORATORY STUDIES

1. Few laboratory studies are useful for the diagnosis of ILD, but laboratory tests may help rule out secondary causes of ILD. Routine testing should include a complete blood cell count with differential, hepatic and renal function panels, urinalysis, arterial blood gas, antinuclear antibody, rheumatoid factor, antineutrophil cytoplasmic antibody, anti-Scl70, anti-Jo-1, creatine kinase, aldolase, and erythrocyte sedimentation rate.

2. Up to 20% of patients with IPF have a positive rheumatoid factor or a low positive antinuclear antibody titer (< 1:160).[4] Higher titers suggest an autoimmune cause.

3. A number of serum markers suggestive of ILD have been identified, including surfactant proteins A and B, monocyte chemoattractant

protein-1, and KL-6.[5] KL-6 is a glycoprotein expressed by type II pneumocytes; it had the highest sensitivity and specificity for the presence of ILD in a study evaluating both collagen-vascular disease–associated ILD and idiopathic ILD.[6]

B. PULMONARY FUNCTION TESTS

1. In most patients with ILD, PFTs show a restrictive pattern, with reduction in vital capacity, total lung capacity, and residual volume.
2. The diffusing capacity of the lung for carbon monoxide (DLCO) is reduced, often out of proportion to the degree of restriction.
3. In early disease, arterial O_2 levels may be normal at rest and may decline during exercise, but patients with end-stage disease generally show resting hypoxemia.[7] In a study designed to assess the prognostic value of desaturation during a 6-minute walk test, mortality was greater in patients with UIP and NSIP who desaturated.[8]
4. Low DLCO and declines in forced vital capacity at 6 and 12 months are associated with increased mortality.[9]

C. RADIOGRAPHIC FINDINGS

1. HRCT is the standard of care in the evaluation of ILD and can establish the disorder in 61% to 80% of patients. Ten percent of patients with ILD have a normal appearance on chest radiograph.
2. When trained observers made a confident diagnosis of IPF on HRCT, 80% to 90% of the time a subsequent biopsy confirmed UIP.[10] However, of all biopsies that showed UIP, in only two thirds was a confident diagnosis made from HRCT and clinical presentation. In the other third, the diagnosis could have been missed without biopsy.[11]
3. Data on the accuracy of HRCT in diagnosing ILD vary, partly because many patients do not undergo open lung biopsy, the gold standard.

D. LUNG BIOPSY

1. Lung biopsy is the most definitive way to diagnose different pathologic subtypes of ILD, differentiating the treatable secondary causes and steroid-responsive primary causes from the more life-threatening IPF. In certain circumstances, however, the clinical picture and radiographic findings are enough to make a specific diagnosis and establish a treatment plan.
2. Indications for biopsy include atypical clinical features (age < 50, fever, weight loss, hemoptysis, signs of vasculitis); progressive course; a normal, atypical, or rapidly changing HRCT; pulmonary vascular disease of unclear origin; and unexplained extrapulmonary manifestations. Other situations favoring a biopsy include a physician- or patient-directed need to determine prognosis and a concern about ruling out an infectious or neoplastic process, especially when the patient's symptoms include hemoptysis.
3. Transbronchial lung biopsy often is the initial procedure of choice, especially when secondary causes of ILD such as sarcoidosis, Goodpasture's syndrome, or eosinophilic pneumonias are suspected, because the yield is fairly high and the procedure less invasive.

Unfortunately, transbronchial biopsies obtained by fiberoptic bronchoscopy are too small to permit identification of the idiopathic ILDs and are further hindered by sampling variation.[12]

4. Video-assisted thoracoscopic surgery and open lung biopsy provide larger pieces of tissue; between the two techniques, video-assisted thoracoscopic surgery is preferred because it is believed to have less associated morbidity. In cases of severe pleural disease or when hemostasis might be difficult to achieve, open thoracotomy is preferred.

5. Relative contraindications to biopsy include radiologic evidence of honeycombing without areas of milder disease activity, severe cardiovascular or pulmonary dysfunction, advanced age, and other risks of major surgery or general anesthesia.

IV. MANAGEMENT

Optimal therapy for IPF has been difficult to determine for several reasons. Historically, biopsies were not routinely performed, and studies on patients with "IPF" probably included diseases other than UIP. Because the various diseases demonstrate different responses to therapy, with NSIP and DIP responding better than UIP and AIP, the quoted response rates for patients with "IPF" from older studies must be questioned. There are very few randomized, placebo-controlled trials of treatment, even in the newer literature.

A. CORTICOSTEROIDS AND IMMUNOSUPPRESSANTS

The American Thoracic Society and European Respiratory Society (ATS/ERS) issued an international consensus statement on IPF in 2000 and recommended a combination of corticosteroids and other immunosuppressants as first-line therapy for IPF.[7] However, the ATS/ERS recommendations are based more on theoretical benefits of individual drugs than on evidence.

1. Corticosteroids traditionally have been used in the treatment of IPF to reduce inflammation and prevent fibrosis.

2. When used as part of a combination regimen, the recommended prednisone dosage is 0.5 mg/kg/day (based on lean body weight) for 4 weeks, 0.25 mg/kg/day for 8 weeks, and then a taper down to 0.125 mg/kg/day. The response rate has been reported to be 10% to 30%; however, the data were collected when biopsies were not performed on all patients, some of whom certainly had subtypes of IIP other than UIP.[7]

3. Few controlled trials of corticosteroid therapy in IPF are available, and several studies showed little or no improvement in patients treated with steroids.[13]

4. In terms of immunosuppressive agents, azathioprine used in conjunction with corticosteroids may be steroid-sparing and may improve survival, but data are limited.[14] Cyclophosphamide has been used with corticosteroids as a steroid-sparing agent and may improve survival, although results are mixed.[15,16] Current ATS/ERS

recommendations for initial IPF treatment are for combination therapy with prednisone and either azathioprine 2 to 3 mg/kg/day (maximum of 150 mg) or cyclophosphamide 2 mg/kg/day (maximum of 150 mg).

5. Therapy is continued for 3 to 6 months and is then adjusted or discontinued if the patient has not responded. In general, therapy should continue if the patient's symptoms and objective tests are stable or improved.

6. The side effects of these therapies should not be discounted. In one study of 41 patients with biopsy-proven, previously untreated IPF, all patients experienced at least one steroid-related side effect.[17] See Chapter 25 for a discussion of the long-term management of patients on high-dose steroids (e.g., *Pneumocystis carinii* pneumonia prophylaxis).

B. OTHER MEDICATIONS

1. The antifibrotic agents colchicine and D-penicillamine show no benefit over steroids alone.[18]

2. A large, multicenter, randomized, placebo-controlled trial of interferon-gamma-1b in patients with IPF concluded that interferon-gamma-1b did not affect progression-free survival, pulmonary function, or quality of life.[19] However, there was a trend toward greater survival in those receiving interferon-gamma-1b compared with placebo, but the study was not powered to detect a statistically significant difference.

3. Other cytotoxic agents, including cyclosporine and methotrexate, have shown no benefit.

C. LUNG TRANSPLANTATION

1. Single-lung transplantation for UIP or IPF is another treatment option, but definitive criteria for the timing of transplantation referral are still lacking.

2. Oxygen dependence, clinical deterioration, and functional limitation should prompt transplantation evaluation. Because patients with IPF have the highest mortality of all patients on the waiting list for lung transplantation, evaluation should begin early.

V. PROGNOSIS

See Table 87-1 for prognosis and response to treatment.

PEARLS AND PITFALLS

- If all clinical data support a diagnosis of UIP or IPF, a surgical lung biopsy may not be necessary. However, if there are atypical findings (e.g., lack of subpleural distribution of infiltrates on HRCT, lack of honeycombing, development of symptoms over < 6 months, young age), early surgical lung biopsy is crucial to distinguish between UIP and the other interstitial lung diseases.[20]

- The most useful objective way to track response to treatment in patients with IPF is with PFTs. In particular, DLCO and forced vital capacity are sensitive indicators of a change in pulmonary status.

- Patients with IPF have an elevated risk of lung cancer (10%). What appears to be dense fibrosis on chest radiograph may actually be a mass.

- It is difficult to distinguish between infection and progression of disease in patients with interstitial lung disease who present with respiratory failure. Bronchoalveolar lavage and transbronchial biopsy are often necessary.
- If PFTs demonstrate mixed restrictive-obstructive disease, diagnoses such as RB-ILD or secondary causes of ILD (sarcoidosis, hypersensitivity pneumonitis, lymphangioleiomyomatosis) should be considered.

REFERENCES

1. Green F: Overview of pulmonary fibrosis, *Chest* 122:334S, 2002. C
2. Bitterman PB et al: Familial idiopathic pulmonary fibrosis: evidence of lung inflammation in unaffected family members, *N Engl J Med* 314:1343, 1986. B
3. Hamman L, Rich A: Acute diffuse interstitial fibrosis of the lungs, *Bull Johns Hopkins Hosp* 74:177, 1944. C
4. Chapman JR et al: Definition and clinical relevance of antibodies to nuclear ribonucleoprotein and other nuclear antigens in patients with cryptogenic fibrosing alveolitis, *Am Rev Respir Dis* 130:439, 1984. B
5. Shimizu S, Yoshinouchi T, Ohtsuki Y, et al: The appearance of S-100 protein-positive dendritic cells and the distribution of lymphocyte subsets in idiopathic nonspecific interstitial pneumonia, *Respir Med* 96:770, 2002. B
6. Kobayashi J, Kitamura S: KL-6: A serum marker for interstitial pneumonia, *Chest* 108:311, 1995. B
7. American Thoracic Society, European Respiratory Society: Idiopathic pulmonary fibrosis: diagnosis and treatment: international consensus statement, *Am J Respir Crit Care Med* 161:646, 2000. D
8. Lama VN, Flaherty KR, Toews GB, et al: Prognostic value of desaturation during a 6-minute walk test in idiopathic interstitial pneumonia, *Am J Respir Crit Care Med* 168:1084, 2003. B
9. Nicholson AG, Fulford LG, Colby TV, et al: The relationship between individual histologic features and disease progression in idiopathic pulmonary fibrosis, *Am J Respir Crit Care Med* 166:173-177, 2002. B
10. Wells AU et al: The predictive value of appearances on thin-section computed tomography in fibrosing alveolitis, *Am Rev Respir Dis* 148:1076, 1993. B
11. Raghu G: Interstitial lung disease: a diagnostic approach. Are CT scan and lung biopsy indicated in every patient? *Am J Respir Crit Care Med* 151:909, 1995. C
12. Ravini M, Ferrara G, Barbieri B, et al: Changing strategies of lung biopsies in diffuse lung diseases: the impact of video-assisted thoracoscopy, *Eur Respir J* 11:99, 1998. D
13. Raghu G et al: Azathioprine combined with prednisone in the treatment of idiopathic pulmonary fibrosis: a prospective double-blind, randomized, placebo-controlled clinical trial, *Am Rev Respir Dis* 144:291, 1991. A
14. Johnson MA et al: Randomized controlled trial comparing prednisolone alone with cyclophosphamide and low dose prednisolone in combination in cryptogenic fibrosing alveolitis, *Thorax* 44:280, 1989. A
15. Zisman DA et al: Cyclophosphamide in the treatment of idiopathic pulmonary fibrosis: a prospective study in patients who failed to respond to corticosteroids, *Chest* 117:1619, 2000. B
16. Flaherty KR, Toews GB, Lynch JP III, et al: Steroids in idiopathic pulmonary fibrosis: a prospective assessment of adverse reactions, response to therapy, and survival, *Am J Med* 110:278, 2001. B

87

INTERSTITIAL LUNG DISEASE

17. Latsi PI, Du Bois RM, Nicholson AG, et al: Fibrotic idiopathic interstitial pneumonia: the prognostic value of longitudinal functional trends, *Am J Respir Crit Care Med* 168:531-537, 2003. B
18. Selman M et al: Colchicine, D-penicillamine, and prednisone in the treatment of idiopathic pulmonary fibrosis: a controlled clinical trial, *Chest* 114:507, 1998. A
19. Raghu G, Brown K, Williamson BZ, et al: A placebo-controlled trial of interferon gamma-1b in patients with idiopathic pulmonary fibrosis, *N Engl J Med* 350:125, 2004. A
20. Katzenstein A-LA, Myers JL: Idiopathic pulmonary fibrosis: clinical relevance of pathologic classification, *Am J Respir Crit Care Med* 157:1301, 1998. B

Sarcoidosis

Homaa Ahmad, MD; and David Moller, MD

FAST FACTS

- Sarcoidosis is a multisystem disease of unknown origin. Its presentation ranges from asymptomatic to a chronic, progressive form with multiorgan involvement.
- The diagnosis of sarcoidosis is based on consistent clinicoradiologic findings, histologic evidence of noncaseating granulomas, and exclusion of other granulomatous diseases.
- Sarcoidosis can be a self-limited or chronic disease.
- African Americans may have more severe disease than Caucasians. The overall mortality from sarcoidosis is 1% to 5%.[1]
- Guidelines for starting treatment depend on disease presentation because clinical involvement is quite variable, and up to 40% of cases resolve on their own.
- Corticosteroids are the mainstay of treatment for sarcoidosis. Indications for beginning immediate treatment include ocular, neurologic, and cardiac involvement.

I. EPIDEMIOLOGY AND ETIOLOGY

1. Sarcoidosis predominantly affects people 20 to 50 years of age, although all ages can be affected. Up to two thirds of patients can be asymptomatic.
2. The prevalence of sarcoidosis is influenced by both race and sex. It is more common in women than in men, and in the United States the lifetime risk is about three times higher in African Americans than in Caucasians (2.4% vs. 0.85%).[1]
3. In addition to influencing incidence, ethnicity influences clinical presentation. For instance, hypercalcemia and erythema nodosum are found more commonly in Caucasians, whereas hematologic abnormalities, extrathoracic lymphadenopathy, and lupus pernio are more common in blacks. Notably, cardiac and ocular sarcoidosis are more common in Japan.
4. The cause of sarcoidosis is unknown, but there is increasing evidence that it is triggered by the exposure of a genetically predisposed host to certain microbial agents. So far, infectious agents that are implicated as potential causes include *Propionibacterium acnes* and mycobacterial organisms.[2] Genetic factors also play a role, as evidenced by the high incidence among first- and second-degree relatives.[3] The mode of inheritance appears to be polygenic, and recent evidence suggests that allelic variation at the HLA-DRB1 locus contributes to this genetic predisposition.

5. The activation of macrophages coupled with a CD4 T-helper-1 polarized response to tissue antigens leads to the formation of granulomatous inflammation. Untreated inflammation causes tissue injury, resulting in fibrosis and irreversible end organ damage.

II. CLINICAL PRESENTATION

1. By definition, sarcoidosis is a systemic granulomatous disease. Clinical presentation varies, with the potential for involvement of any organ system as part of a limited or more fulminant course. Manifestations can be protean, with up to one third of patients presenting with nonspecific complaints that include fever, weight loss, fatigue, anorexia, and malaise.
2. Sarcoidosis often is an interstitial lung disorder, but the bronchi, larynx, and trachea can also be involved. Pulmonary hypertension and cor pulmonale usually present in patients with severe fibrocystic sarcoidosis (about 1% to 4% of patients). Common symptoms of pulmonary sarcoidosis include a dry cough, dyspnea, and chest pain. Physical examination findings are uncommon, with rales present in less than 20% of patients.
3. For other organ system involvement, see Table 88-1.

III. DIAGNOSIS

1. The diagnosis of sarcoidosis is based on a compatible clinical picture, histologic evidence of noncaseating epithelioid granulomas, and the exclusion of other diseases capable of producing a similar histologic picture (e.g., mycobacteria). See Box 88-1 for a differential diagnosis.
2. Diagnostic modalities.
a. Chest radiographs demonstrate pulmonary involvement in more than 90% of patients (Table 88-2).
b. Pulmonary function tests may show a restrictive pattern, an obstructive pattern (30% to 50%), or both. Carbon monoxide diffusion capacity may also be impaired.
c. A biopsy demonstrating noncaseating granulomas is a prerequisite for confirming a diagnosis of sarcoidosis, with the possible exception of Lofgren's syndrome. Skin, superficial lymph nodes, nasal mucosa, and bronchi are the preferred biopsy sites because of their high yield and low morbidity. A transbronchial lung biopsy, transbronchial needle biopsy, or endobronchial biopsy has a diagnostic yield that ranges from 40% to 90%, depending on operator experience.[1] When transbronchial lung biopsy, transbronchial needle biopsy, or endobronchial biopsy is nondiagnostic, a surgical lung biopsy may be indicated.
d. Patients suspected of having cardiac involvement should be evaluated for evidence of arrhythmias, conduction disease, and myocardial involvement.
   (1) Electrocardiogram and Holter monitor are useful for identifying arrhythmias and conduction system disease.

TABLE 88-1

NONPULMONARY ORGAN SYSTEM INVOLVEMENT IN SARCOIDOSIS

Organ System (% of patients)	Symptoms and Associated Conditions
Neurologic (5%)	Cranial nerve palsy (e.g., Bell's palsy), space-occupying masses, aseptic meningitis, seizure, polyneuropathy, myelopathy, headache, ataxia, hearing loss, dementia, encephalopathy, hypothalamic hypopituitarism, hyperprolactinemia, and papilledema
Cardiac (5-10%)	Complete heart block, sudden cardiac death, arrhythmias, conduction disturbances, valvular dysfunction, cardiomyopathy, and congestive heart failure
Gastrointestinal (50-80%)	Granulomatous involvement of the liver, stomach, and pancreas; cholestasis, dysphagia, and pruritus
Rheumatologic (4-38%)	Acute or chronic arthritis that may be monoarticular or polyarticular, arthralgias, and myopathy
Dermatologic (20-35%)	Lupus pernio, erythema nodosum, papules, plaques, and alopecia
Ocular (25%)	Anterior and posterior uveitis, optic neuritis, chorioretinitis, lacrimal gland enlargement, keratoconjunctivitis sicca, and conjunctivitis
Hematologic and lymphatic (up to 90%)	Lymphadenopathy, hypersplenism (thrombocytopenia, leukopenia, anemia), and nonclonal hypergammaglobulinemia
Renal (< 5%)	Nephrocalcinosis, renal failure, and nephrolithiasis
Genitourinary	Testicular mass, epididymitis
Endocrine-metabolic (< 10%)	Hypercalciuria, hypercalcemia, central diabetes insipidus, syndrome of inappropriate antidiuretic hormone, and hypopituitarism
Psychiatric (4-30%)	Depression

88

SARCOIDOSIS

BOX 88-1

DIFFERENTIAL DIAGNOSIS OF GRANULOMATOUS DISEASES

Mycobacterial infection: tuberculosis, atypical mycobacterial infection
Fungal infection: histoplasmosis, coccidioidomycosis
Foreign body reaction: talc, beryllium, zirconium, paraffin, titanium
Other infections: brucellosis, toxoplasmosis, schistosomiasis, treponemal infections
Hypersensitivity pneumonitis
Autoimmune syndromes: Wegner's granulomatosis, primary biliary cirrhosis, Churg-Strauss syndrome
Neoplasm: lymphoma

TABLE 88-2

RADIOGRAPHIC STAGING OF PULMONARY SARCOIDOSIS

Stage	Hilar Adenopathy	Parenchymal Disease	Percentage at Onset	Percentage with Resolution
0	No	No	< 10	Not applicable
I	Yes; may be associated with paratracheal adenopathy	No	50	65
II	Yes	Parenchymal infiltration	30	20-50
III	No	Parenchymal infiltration	10-15	< 20
IV	No	Advanced fibrosis with evidence of honeycombing, hilar retraction, bullae, cysts, and emphysema	5	< 5

- (2) Nuclear imaging (i.e., gated thallium-201 myocardial scan or sestamibi myocardial scan) is more sensitive than echocardiography in showing areas of granulomatous infiltration and fibrosis.[4]
- (3) Because endomyocardial biopsy is positive in less than 20% of cases, the diagnostic utility of a biopsy is limited.
- e. Serum angiotensin converting enzyme levels can be elevated in granulomatous disorders. The test lacks both sensitivity and specificity, so it is of limited utility in the diagnosis and management of sarcoidosis.

IV. MANAGEMENT

Unfortunately, a lack of randomized, controlled trials has made it difficult to determine optimal therapy for patients with sarcoidosis. The different management strategies are described here.

A. NO INTERVENTION

Because the clinical course of sarcoidosis is uncertain, patients often are observed without therapy. This course of therapy is not recommended if there is a high risk of permanent disability (e.g., cardiac sarcoidosis, neurosarcoidosis).

B. CORTICOSTEROIDS

1. At present, there are no long-term studies that clearly show that a short course of corticosteroid therapy affects long-term patient outcome. However, patients with progressive, chronic pulmonary sarcoidosis often improve or stabilize with corticosteroid treatment.[5]
2. Oral corticosteroids are first-line treatment of severe ocular, neurologic, cardiac, or cutaneous sarcoidosis; malignant hypercalcemia; or progressive stage II or III pulmonary disease. Typical starting dosages are 20 to 40 mg/day of prednisone but may be higher in patients with neurologic, ocular, or cardiac involvement. Response typically is

assessed at 3 to 6 months, at which time an attempt can be made to taper the steroids. To prevent or reduce steroid-induced osteoporosis, patients are given bisphosphonates and calcium.

C. IMMUNOSUPPRESSIVE AGENTS

1. Methotrexate is used as a steroid-sparing agent in patients with chronic sarcoidosis. Unfortunately, it usually takes more than 6 months to see a beneficial response.
2. Azathioprine is used in chronic disease with efficacy similar to that of methotrexate.[1] The use of azathioprine is reserved for patients with progressive end organ damage that is not responsive to low-dose corticosteroid therapy.[6]

D. OTHER AGENTS

1. Hydroxychloroquine and chloroquine often are effective in treating involvement of the skin, sinuses, and larynx. In addition, they are useful in treating hypercalcemia and bone, joint, and muscle involvement. Because of the attendant ocular toxicities, patients should be monitored with serial ophthalmologic evaluations.[6]
2. Anecdotal experience suggests that anti–tumor necrosis factor drugs including infliximab and pentoxifylline may be effective in selected patients, but they have not yet been shown effective by large-scale clinical trials.

E. ORGAN TRANSPLANTATION

Organ transplantation may be considered in the management of end-stage disease that is refractory to treatment.

V. PROGNOSIS

1. Disease progression varies. About 30% to 50% of cases spontaneously remit by 3 years, about 30% show progression over 5 to 10 years, and 20% to 30% remain stable with slow progression of disease.
2. Factors that portend poor prognosis include African-American race, presentation age older than 40 years, absence of erythema nodosum, splenomegaly, involvement of more than three organ systems, and stage III and IV pulmonary disease.[4]

PEARLS AND PITFALLS

- A skin biopsy demonstrating noncaseating epithelioid cell granulomas, in the appropriate clinical context, obviates a more invasive bronchoscopic biopsy.
- Patients with cardiac sarcoidosis are at risk of sudden cardiac death. A history of palpitations or syncope in conjunction with premature ventricular contractions on electrocardiogram and evidence of cardiac sarcoidosis should lead to consideration for automatic implantable cardioverter-defibrillator placement.
- Lupus pernio is a dermatologic manifestation of sarcoidosis that appears as disfiguring nodular lesions over the cheeks, nose, lips, eyes, and ears. It has a predilection for blacks, especially West Indians and African Americans.

88

SARCOIDOSIS

- A number of different syndrome complexes have been described with sarcoidosis:
- Lofgren's syndrome is characterized by arthritis, anterior uveitis, erythema nodosum, and bilateral hilar adenopathy. It generally has a self-limited course, with more than 80% of patients having spontaneous remission. Treatment is with bed rest and nonsteroidal antiinflammatory drugs and occasionally glucocorticosteroids for severe arthritis.
- Heerfordt's syndrome, or uveoparotiditis, is characterized by fever, anterior uveitis, parotid gland swelling, and Bell's palsy.
- Granulomatous lesions of unknown significance, characterized by granulomas with B cells, are thought to be a separate disease entity.
- Given the upregulated hydroxylation of vitamin D by sarcoid granulomas, patients with sarcoidosis are at risk for developing nephrolithiasis or nephrocalcinosis.

REFERENCES

1. Statement on Sarcoidosis. Joint Statement of the American Thoracic Society (ATS), the European Respiratory Society (ERS) and the World Association of Sarcoidosis and Other Granulomatous Disorders (WASOG) adopted by the ATS Board of Directors and by the ERS Executive Committee, February 1999, *Am J Respir Crit Care Med* 160(2):736-755, 1999. C
2. Du Bois RM, Goh N, et al: Is there a role for microorganisms in the pathogenesis of sarcoidosis? *J Intern Med* 253:4-17, 2003. C
3. Rybicki BA, Iannuzzi MC, Frederick MM, et al, ACCESS Research Group: Familial aggregation of sarcoidosis. A case-control etiologic study of sarcoidosis (ACCESS), *Am J Respir Crit Care Med* 164(11):2085-2091, 2001. B
4. Sharma OP: Cardiac and neurologic dysfunction in sarcoidosis, *Clin Chest Med* 18(4):813-825, 1997. C
5. Reich JM: Adverse long-term effect of corticosteroid therapy in recent-onset sarcoidosis, *Sarcoidosis Vasc Diffuse Lung Dis* 20(3):227-234, 2003. B
6. Moller DR: Treatment of sarcoidosis: from a basic science point of view, *J Intern Med* 253:31-40, 2003. C

Approach to the Rheumatic Disorders

Ann Reed, MD; and Philip Seo, MD

FAST FACTS

- The history and physical examination are more important than laboratory studies in diagnosing rheumatic disease.
- Many patients who complain of joint pain may actually have a problem with the structures surrounding the joint.
- A useful approach to the diagnosis of arthritis is to consider the number of joints involved and the pattern of involvement, which can be used to narrow the differential diagnosis.

89

I. EPIDEMIOLOGY

1. One fourth of all Americans have arthritis.[1] Arthritis and other rheumatic diseases are the leading cause of disability in the United States.
2. Rheumatology encompasses a wide spectrum of disorders, from osteoarthritis to vasculitis, all of which have in common the presence of pain and inflammation. From a practical standpoint, these diseases may be divided into two groups: those that are predominantly articular, with some systemic manifestations (e.g., the crystalline arthropathies), and those that are predominantly systemic syndromes, with some articular manifestations (e.g., systemic lupus erythematosus [SLE]).

II. CLINICAL PRESENTATION

1. **The history and physical examination are the cornerstone of the evaluation of a patient with rheumatic complaints.** Laboratory abnormalities in the absence of appropriate clinical suspicion are notoriously unhelpful and misleading for this group of diseases.
2. The first step in the evaluation is to determine whether the patient truly has joint pain. Many patients who experience musculoskeletal discomfort localize their complaints to their joints, even when the primary process is not articular. For example, lateral epicondylitis and trochanteric bursitis commonly present as "joint pain," although neither involves the true joint. Neuropathies, myopathies, periostitis, tendonitis, hypothyroidism, and fibromyalgia may all be interpreted by a patient as "arthritis;" careful history and physical examination can do much to exclude these mimics.
3. The physical examination provides multiple clues for determining whether a patient has true joint pain. Patients with a true synovitis complain of pain on both active and passive range-of-motion exercises.

Pain that is reproduced only on active range-of-motion exercises (i.e., only when the patient moves the joint) implies that the periarticular structures, such as the tendons or the surrounding soft tissue (as in cellulitis), are the cause of pain, not the joint itself. In addition, complaints that localize to a specific joint are less likely to be caused by diffuse musculoskeletal pain syndromes, such as fibromyalgia.

III. DIAGNOSIS

A. HISTORY AND PHYSICAL EXAMINATION

1. **Once it has been determined that a patient has true joint pain, the next step is to determine whether the complaints are noninflammatory or inflammatory** (Fig. 89-1). A key question is whether there is morning stiffness. Typically, patients with noninflammatory joint conditions note morning stiffness that lasts < 30 minutes and pain that is worst at the end of the day. Conversely, patients with inflammatory joint complaints report morning stiffness that lasts > 1 hour and improves with activity during the day. Patients in this latter category often have systemic symptoms as well.

2. The most common cause of noninflammatory joint pain is osteoarthritis (which typically affects the distal interphalangeal joints and the carpometacarpal joint at the base of the thumb), but other common causes include avascular necrosis (in patients with sickle cell disease or chronic glucocorticoid use) and joint trauma. Patients who describe joint "locking" may have a torn meniscus or articular cartilage.

3. The presence of inflammatory joint pain often is frequently evidenced by an active synovitis: on examination the involved joints are swollen, warm, and tender to palpation and feel like foam rubber, a sensation often described as "boggy." Examination of the small joints of the hands is best performed with the use of one hand to isolate the joint and the other to palpate for tenderness and evaluate range of motion. The inability of the patient to make a tight fist is a good clue to the presence of arthritis in a hand that looks normal at first glance. Visual inspection and comparison to the contralateral joint often are helpful.

4. **Patients who have an inflammatory, active synovitis may be categorized in terms of the number of joints involved: a monoarthritis involves one joint, an oligoarthritis involves two to four joints, and a polyarthritis affects multiple joints.**

5. The cause of monoarthritis is limited to two major categories: infection (as in septic arthritis or Lyme disease) and crystalline arthritis (as in gout or pseudogout). Infection accounts for approximately 20% of acute monoarthritis, and crystalline disorders account for the remaining 80%.[2] Examination of synovial fluid is crucial in determining the cause of monoarthritis. The clinical picture and laboratory values associated with crystalline and septic arthritis overlap and may be difficult to separate in any particular patient.

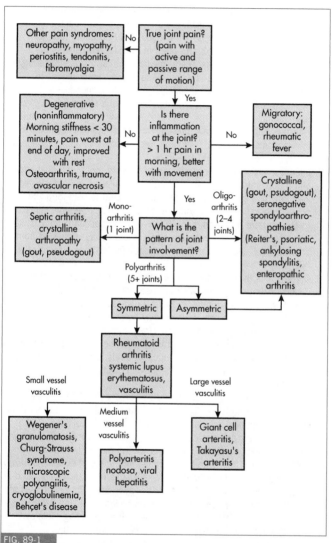

FIG. 89-1

Diagnosis of rheumatic disorders.

6. An acute gout attack presents with severe pain and swelling of one joint, classically the great toe (i.e., podagra), although any of the peripheral joints may be affected. Gout occurs in men (or postmenopausal women), and often in hospitalized patients (as a result of dehydration, changes in medications, and stress). Pseudogout occurs equally in men and women and may be associated with hyperparathyroidism, hypothyroidism, hemochromatosis, hypercalcemia, illness, and trauma. The knee is affected in 50% of cases, although other large joints also are commonly affected. Patients with pseudogout classically present with fewer systemic symptoms than patients with gout.[3,4] Notably, prosthetic joints are rarely affected by crystalline disease.

7. Infectious arthritis presents with acute swelling, pain, and erythema and merits immediate medical attention (cartilage can be destroyed in 24 to 48 hours if left untreated). Eighty percent to 90% of acute nongonococcal bacterial arthritis is monoarticular. The large joints (hip, knee) are most commonly affected, and infection usually is via hematogenous spread, although artificial joints may be seeded from infected skin.[5] Disseminated gonococcal infection may present as a migratory polyarthritis.

8. Oligoarthritis may be caused by a crystalline arthritis or a seronegative spondyloarthropathy. The latter are associated with HLA-B27 and include ankylosing spondylitis, Reiter's disease, psoriatic arthritis, and enteropathic arthritis, all of which may be associated with lower back pain, enthesopathy, and dactylitis. When gout presents as an oligoarthritis, it typically affects the joints in the lower extremities in an asymmetric pattern. Chronic pseudogout tends to involve the wrists, knees, and shoulders and may be initially misdiagnosed as rheumatoid arthritis.

9. Polyarthritis with asymmetric joint involvement has the same differential diagnosis as oligoarthritis. Causes of symmetric polyarthritis include rheumatoid arthritis (RA), SLE, and the vasculitides. RA generally affects the metacarpophalangeal and proximal interphalangeal joints and the wrists. SLE is more often associated with arthralgias than with true arthritis, and the joint examination may be benign. Jaccoud's arthropathy, a reversible ulnar deviation found in SLE, is distinct from the fixed ulnar deviation and joint deformities of RA. When considering vasculitis, the physician must simultaneously consider the mimickers of vasculitis (e.g., the hypercoagulable states and infective endocarditis) that are treated very differently.

10. The vasculitides may be classified in terms of the vessels involved: small, medium, and large vessel vasculitis. See Chapter 90 for further discussion of the vasculitides.

B. LABORATORY ANALYSIS

1. Routine laboratory tests can provide clues to the origin of a patient's rheumatic symptoms. An active sediment in a urine specimen may be

consistent with lupus nephritis or a small vessel vasculitides. Renal insufficiency may be seen with SLE, polyarteritis nodosa, or the hyperuricemia found with long-standing gout.

2. Laboratory studies often help confirm the clinical assessment but rarely are sufficient by themselves. For example, 20% of patients with RA do not have detectable rheumatoid factor (RF); in contrast, RF may be seen in association with mixed essential cryoglobulinemia, chronic infections, and malignancy, as well as RA.

3. Elevated serum uric acid levels are associated with gouty flares, but they are neither sensitive nor specific; 40% of patients have normal levels during a flare. Iron, thyroid-stimulating hormone, and parathyroid hormone levels should be checked in patients with pseudogout in the appropriate clinical setting.[2,4,6]

4. The detection of antinuclear antibody (ANA) at low titer is unhelpful by itself. Up to 30% of normal individuals have ANA that is detectable at a titer of 1:40. The assays used by different institutions demonstrate different sensitivities, but **titers less than 1:320 in the absence of appropriate signs and symptoms generally do not indicate rheumatic disease.** Very high titers are more specific for the presence of rheumatic disease but can be found not only with SLE, but also with Sjögren's syndrome, systemic sclerosis (or scleroderma), limited scleroderma (including CREST syndrome [calcinosis, Raynaud's phenomenon, esophageal dysmotility, sclerodactyly, and telangiectasia]), polymyositis, and even in some patients with RA.

5. The ANA is very helpful in ruling out SLE, which is generally not seen in the absence of ANA. If ANA is not detected, testing for antibodies to the extractable nuclear antigens (e.g., anti-Smith, anti-Ro, and anti-La) is unnecessary because these are rarely found in the absence of ANA (Table 89-1).

C. SYNOVIAL FLUID ANALYSIS

1. **A diagnostic arthrocentesis may provide a great deal of information as to the origin of joint pain and has few contraindications. Synovial fluid should be evaluated for cell count with differential, presence of crystals, and culture.**

2. Gout can be diagnosed by the presence of needle-shaped, highly birefringent urate crystals that are yellow when parallel to polarized light. Pseudogout crystals are rhomboid, blue when parallel to polarized light, and weakly birefringent. Pseudogout crystals are more difficult to visualize; their absence does not rule out this diagnosis.

3. The number of white blood cells (WBCs) in the synovial fluid can be helpful. Fewer than 200 WBCs/ml is generally considered to be noninflammatory and may be associated with degenerative joint disease, trauma, and nonarticular diseases. More than 2000 WBCs/ml is consistent with an inflammatory effusion and may be seen with the crystalline arthropathies, the seronegative spondyloarthropathies, RA, and other diseases, including sepsis. Septic arthritis generally is

associated with > 50,000 WBCs/ml, with > 100,000 WBCs/ml considered diagnostic. However, lower numbers of cells may be seen in patients with human immunodeficiency virus infection or tuberculous arthritis. Sixty percent of septic joints are infected with *Staphylococcus aureus,* 20% with aerobic *Streptococcus* species, and 18% with aerobic gram-negative rods. Other pathogens include tuberculosis, Lyme disease, and fungus, all of which may present as chronic infections that may rarely require synovial biopsy to obtain a diagnosis.[5,7]

D. RADIOGRAPHIC ANALYSIS

1. Radiographs can be helpful in assessment of the patient with joint complaints. Osteoarthritis is accompanied radiographically by the presence of osteophytes, subchondral cysts, joint sclerosis, and asymmetric joint space narrowing. Pseudogout often is accompanied by chondrocalcinosis, which is caused by deposition of calcium pyrophosphate crystals in bone cartilage and leaves a telltale linear radiodensity at the articular surfaces. Tophi and bony erosions with an overhanging edge are classic for chronic gout. Patients with long-standing RA may have erosions and destruction in the bones of the hands and feet. Ulnar deviation in the hands in the absence of erosions should alert the examiner to the possibility of a Jaccoud-like arthropathy (associated with SLE).

2. Magnetic resonance imaging may be useful to confirm the presence of a lesion not apparent on plain films, such as a torn meniscus or a small fracture. It is also useful for detecting synovitis when the physical examination is equivocal.

IV. MANAGEMENT

1. Specific elements of the management of rheumatic disease depend on the underlying diagnosis.

2. **Septic arthritis generally should be considered a medical emergency** and deserves aggressive treatment with intravenous antibiotics to prevent long-term sequelae. Patients with septic arthritis often must undergo arthrocentesis multiple times because antibiotics cannot penetrate a pus-filled joint. Emergent surgical drainage often is needed to prevent progressive joint destruction.

3. A patient with monoarthritis not caused by infection (e.g., osteoarthritis or the crystalline arthropathies) often experiences relief from aspiration of the joint (which removes pressure on the joint capsule) and injection of the joint with corticosteroids. Many practitioners use a solution of triamcinolone acetate (40 mg for a large joint, such as a knee; 20 mg for a smaller joint, such as a wrist or ankle) mixed with an equivalent volume of 1% lidocaine just before use. The latter provides rapid but transient relief of the patient's symptoms, allowing the corticosteroids time to work. At the concentrations commonly used, the addition of lidocaine to a syringe filled with triamcinolone causes the latter to precipitate if allowed to sit too long.

TABLE 89-1

AUTOANTIBODIES IN RHEUMATIC DISEASE

Disease	Antibody	Sensitivity (%)
Systemic lupus erythematosus	Antinuclear	95-100
Sjögren's disease	SSA/Ro	75
Systemic sclerosis	Scl 70	26-76
CREST syndrome	Centromere	80
Polymyositis	JO-1	20-30
Wegener's granulomatosis	c-ANCA	> 90 (for active disease)
Microscopic polyangiitis	p-ANCA	> 75
Mixed connective tissue disease	Ribonucleoprotein	100 (by definition)
Drug-induced systemic lupus erythematosus	Antihistone	90
Rheumatoid arthritis	Rheumatoid factor	80

ANCA, antineutrophilic cytoplasmic antibodies; *CREST,* calcinosis, Raynaud's phenomenon, esophageal dysmotility, sclerodactyly, and telangiectasia.

4. For any patient with arthritis, pain control is important and may be as simple as prescribing nonsteroidal antiinflammatory drugs (NSAIDs) which are excellent at relieving the pain associated with inflammation when taken on a fixed schedule and generally are well tolerated as long as the physician monitors for gastrointestinal and renal toxicity.

5. Despite their long-term toxicity, corticosteroids are excellent antiinflammatory and immunosuppressant agents. Patients who have severe symptoms of a rheumatic illness are commonly treated with corticosteroids, which are used in dosages proportional to the severity of the illness. For example, a patient with acute monoarthritis caused by crystalline arthropathy or with polyarthritis from newly diagnosed RA might be treated initially with oral prednisone 40 mg daily to achieve immediate relief and to give other, less toxic medications time to work.

6. For acute crystalline arthritis, NSAIDs are the treatment of choice. Oral and intraarticular steroids also offer rapid relief. When intraarticular injection of glucocorticoids is not practical, gout may be treated with oral prednisone 20 to 40 mg per day, tapered gradually over 2 weeks. Oral colchicine may also be used acutely, but associated diarrhea and abdominal pain make it less well tolerated. Intravenous colchicine can be lethal and is not recommended. Chronically, allopurinol is the most common prophylactic agent used in gout. Allopurinol lowers serum uric acid levels over the long term but may worsen an acute flare, so therapy should not be initiated until patients have recovered fully from their acute attack. In patients with normal renal function, oral allopurinol can be started at a dosage of 100 mg per day and titrated to effective uric acid control. **Allopurinol hypersensitivity syndrome (fever, rash, eosinophilia, and hepatic and renal dysfunction) is a rare but serious condition that may be lethal in up to 20% of patients. Immediate cessation of the drug is essential if the syndrome is**

suspected. Both allopurinol and colchicine must be dose-adjusted in renal insufficiency.[2]

PEARLS AND PITFALLS

- When the diagnosis is not completely clear, the prudent approach is to treat the patient's symptoms and follow up clinically until the disease process manifests itself more clearly.
- A positive ANA alone does not establish the diagnosis of SLE.
- Most of the rheumatic diseases are difficult to diagnose or exclude on the basis of serologic tests alone. The history is the most valuable tool for diagnosis of a rheumatic illness.
- Arthritis at the distal interphalangeal joints is commonly noted in only a handful of diseases: the seronegative spondyloarthropathies (especially psoriatic arthritis), osteoarthritis, and gout.
- Migratory arthritis (i.e., involvement of new joints as other joints improve) is seen in association with disseminated gonococcal infection and rheumatic fever.
- Osteoarthritis generally spares the wrists and the metacarpophalangeal joints; involvement of these joints should raise the suspicion of rheumatoid arthritis.

REFERENCES

1. Prevalence of doctor-diagnosed arthritis and possible arthritis: 30 states, 2002, *MMWR Morb Mortal Wkly Rep* 53(18):383, 2004. C
2. Terkeltaub RA: Gout, *N Engl J Med* 349(17):1647, 2003. C
3. Roubenoff R et al: Incidence and risk factors for gout in white men, *JAMA* 266:3004, 1991. B
4. Campion EW, Glynn RJ, DeLabry LO: Asymptomatic hyperuricemia: risks and consequences in the Normative Aging Study, *Am J Med* 82:421, 1987. B
5. Baker DG, Schumacher HR: Acute monoarthritis, *N Engl J Med* 329:1013, 1993. C
6. Chaisson CE et al: Lack of association between thyroid status and chondrocalcinosis or osteoarthritis: the Framingham Osteoarthritis Study, *J Rheumatol* 23:711, 1996. B
7. Schalapbach P et al: Bacterial arthritis: are fever, rigors, leucocytosis and blood cultures of diagnostic value? *Clin Rheumatol* 9:69, 1990. B

Vasculitis

John S. Nguyen, MD; and John A. Flynn, MD, MBA

90

The vasculitides are inflammatory disorders that affect primarily blood vessels of varying sizes. The size of the vessels affected and the vascular bed involved determine the presentation of the individual vasculitides. Although multiple organ systems may be involved in disorders such as Wegener's granulomatosis (WG) and PAN, other vasculitides such as TAO (Buerger's disease) and GCA tend to be much more limited in their systemic involvement. A brief outline of the vasculitides is listed in Table 90-1.

Takayasu's Arteritis (Pulseless Disease or Martorell's Syndrome)

I. EPIDEMIOLOGY
In the United States, the estimated incidence of TA is 2.6 per million, with a higher prevalence in Asians. TA affects primarily women (80% to 90% of all cases) and has a median age of onset of 20 to 30 years.[1]

II. PRESENTATION
1. Classically, there are three phases of TA. The first phase presents with prominent constitutional symptoms. The second phase presents with symptoms of vascular stenosis, occlusion, or aneurysm formation. The final phase is characterized by remission of disease.
2. Vascular stenosis and involvement of the carotid arteries are common and can result in carotid bruits (up to 70%), pain over the carotid area

TABLE 90-1

OVERVIEW OF THE VARIOUS SYSTEMIC VASCULITIDES

Name	Vessels Involved	Organ System Affected	Diagnostic Testing
Takayasu's arteritis	Large vessels (aorta and its main branches)	Carotid artery, brachial artery, renal artery, aortic root.	Angiography shows tapering and stenosis or aneurysmal dilation.
Giant cell arteritis	Large and medium vessels (arteries, including aorta)	Cranial artery, aorta, subclavian artery, axillary artery.	Temporal artery biopsy shows panarteritis.
Wegener's granulomatosis	Medium and small vessels (arteries and veins)	Upper airways, lower airways, kidneys, nervous system.	c-ANCA, biopsy shows vasculitis, granulomas, and necrosis.
Polyarteritis nodosa	Medium and small vessels (arteries)	Renal, skin, nervous system, gastrointestinal, heart, and lungs are spared.	Associated with hepatitis B virus, biopsy shows polymorphonuclear infiltration into vessel walls.
Thromboangiitis obliterans	Medium and small vessels (arteries and veins)	Extremities.	Positive Allen's test, arteriography will show segmental occlusive lesions.
Cryoglobulinemia syndromes	Medium and small vessels (arteries and veins)	Skin, kidney, nervous system.	Presence of cryoglobulins, associated with hepatitis C virus infection.
Churg-Strauss syndrome	Small vessels (arteries, capillaries, veins, venules)	Lungs, skin, nervous system, cardiac, gastrointestinal.	p-ANCA, eosinophilia.
Microscopic polyangiitis	Small vessels (arterioles, capillaries, and venules)	Similar to polyarteritis nodosa except there is usually lung involvement.	p-ANCA, renal biopsy shows rapidly progressive glomerulonephritis, not associated with hepatitis B virus.

ANCA, antineutrophilic cytoplasmic antibodies.

(carotodynia in 32%), vertigo or lightheadedness, blurry vision, transient ischemic attacks, and syncope.[1] Stenosis of aortic branches can result in upper or lower extremity claudication, upper extremity pulse deficit, and unequal upper extremity blood pressure measurements. Aortic involvement may result in aortic regurgitation or angina because of coronary ostial involvement. Renal artery narrowing may result in hypertension (found in 50% of cases) and audible renal bruits.

III. DIAGNOSIS

1. Laboratory findings are nonspecific in TA but often include an elevated erythrocyte sedimentation rate (ESR) and C-reactive protein (CRP), reflecting the inflammatory nature of this disease.
2. Angiography is necessary to confirm the diagnosis of TA and typically shows involvement of the aorta and its main branches, with areas of tapering, stenoses, and aneurysmal dilation. CTA or MRA imaging of the aorta are less invasive diagnostic alternatives, which may also be used to follow a patient's clinical course.
3. Other conditions that can also involve the aorta and large vessels include fibromuscular dysplasia, Ehlers-Danlos syndrome, excessive ergotamine use, and GCA.
4. The American College of Rheumatology has developed guidelines to help distinguish TA from other vasculitides (three or more criteria has sensitivity of 91% and specificity of 98% in patients with vasculitis): age ≤ 40 years, claudication of extremities, decreased pulses in one or both brachial arteries, difference of ≥ 10 mmHg in systolic blood pressure between arms, bruit over the subclavian artery or abdominal aorta, and angiographic narrowing of the aorta, its major branches, or large proximal arteries of the upper or lower extremity not caused by atherosclerosis, fibromuscular dysplasia, or other causes.[2]

IV. TREATMENT AND PROGNOSIS

Corticosteroids are the first-line drugs for the treatment of TA. If patients relapse despite corticosteroid use (which occurs in 50% of patients), cytotoxic agents such as azathioprine or methotrexate can be added. Vascular involvement tends to be progressive, but overall prognosis is good, with a 5-year survival of 80% to 90%.[3] Patients who have both a major complication (hypertension, aneurysms, aortic regurgitation, or retinopathy) and a progressive course have only a 43% survival at 15 years, compared with 100% survival in patients with neither.

Giant Cell Arteritis (Temporal Arteritis)

I. EPIDEMIOLOGY

GCA is the most common primary vasculitis, with an incidence of 15 to 25 per 100,000. There is a higher incidence among women and people older than 50 years.

90

VASCULITIS

II. PRESENTATION

1. GCA is an inflammatory vasculopathy that affects mainly medium and large arteries. Classically, the cranial arteries are affected, but other large vessels may be involved. Patients can present with fevers of unknown origin, cachexia, night sweats, and anorexia.

2. Patients with carotid artery involvement present with severe headaches, scalp tenderness, jaw claudication (which is disease specific), facial swelling, and odynophagia. Sudden and painless loss of vision heralds ophthalmic artery involvement.

3. GCA can also affect other large arteries such as the subclavian and axillary arteries. In these cases, symptoms include arm claudication, absent or asymmetric pulses or blood pressure readings, and peripheral paresthesia (similar to that found in TA). The aorta is involved in up to 15% of patients and may result in aortic dissection, aortic rupture, or aortic regurgitation.

4. Approximately 40% of patients with GCA also have polymyalgia rheumatica. Conversely, only 10% of patients with isolated polymyalgia rheumatica will develop GCA.

III. DIAGNOSIS

1. Physical examination may reveal tender or thickened temporal arteries. Bruits may be heard over the carotid, brachial, or axillary arteries.

2. Highly elevated ESR in patients older than 50 years should prompt consideration of GCA, although 3% to 6% of patients with GCA may have a low ESR (< 40), even before treatment with corticosteroids.[4]

3. Definitive diagnosis of GCA requires biopsy of an affected artery, typically the temporal artery. Temporal artery biopsy has a reasonable sensitivity (up to 79%) and high specificity (95%).[5] A negative biopsy does not rule out GCA, and a contralateral temporal artery biopsy should be performed if the clinical suspicion remains high. **The initiation of treatment should not be delayed** because temporal artery biopsies may still show evidence of arteritis in 86% of patients with GCA, even after 6 weeks of corticosteroid therapy.[6]

4. In patients in whom the temporal artery biopsy is negative but GCA is still strongly suspected, additional vascular imaging is necessary. CTA or MRA is used to evaluate subclavian, axillary, carotid, and vertebral artery involvement.

5. Criteria for the diagnosis of GCA are listed in Box 90-1.

IV. TREATMENT AND PROGNOSIS

Almost all patients with GCA respond to initial corticosteroid therapy (typically prednisone at 1 mg/kg body weight). The response to corticosteroids often occurs within 48 hours. Once symptoms remit, the steroid dosage can be tapered. Patients typically can be weaned off corticosteroids after several years. The effectiveness of corticosteroids alone

> **BOX 90-1**
>
> **1990 AMERICAN COLLEGE OF RHEUMATOLOGY CRITERIA FOR THE CLASSIFICATION OF GIANT CELL ARTERITIS[7]**
>
> Criteria (≥ 3 criteria has sensitivity 94% and specificity 91% in patients with vasculitis):
> - Age ≥ 50 at time of onset
> - Localized headache of new onset
> - Tenderness or decreased pulsation of the temporal artery
> - Erythrocyte sedimentation rate > 50 mm/hr
> - Biopsy that includes an artery and reveals a necrotizing arteritis with a predominance of mononuclear cells or a granulomatous process with multinucleated giant cells

is a feature that helps to distinguish GCA from other vasculitides. Patients with GCA have the same life expectancy as the general population.

Wegener's Granulomatosis

I. EPIDEMIOLOGY

The prevalence is approximately 3 per 100,000, with equal occurrence among men and women. The majority of patients are Caucasian (80% to 97%), and the mean age of onset is 40 to 55 years.[8]

II. PRESENTATION

1. WG is a vasculitis that involves granulomatous, inflammatory necrosis of small and medium vessels. **Classic WG involves the upper airways, lower airways and kidneys.** Limited WG usually spares the kidney and accounts for 25% of cases. Upper airway involvement, one of the main reasons patients seek medical attention, includes nasal congestion, epistaxis, sinus pain, persistent rhinorrhea, perforation of the nasal septum, serous otitis media, oral ulcers, and saddle nose deformity.

2. Lower airway involvement in WG typically affects the pulmonary parenchyma and bronchi. Patients present with cough, dyspnea, hemoptysis, or wheezing. The radiographic presentation of WG is heterogenous and may include bilateral nodular infiltrates, a solitary pulmonary nodule, cavitary disease, and diffuse alveolar hemorrhage.

3. Small vessel involvement in the kidney leads to glomerulonephritis, which can rapidly progress to complete renal failure. Although renal involvement is found in only 20% of patients on initial presentation, 80% of patients with WG ultimately develop this complication.[9]

4. WG can also present with constitutional symptoms. In addition to the classic triad of organ involvement, WG can affect the eyes and nervous system and present with conjunctivitis, optic neuritis, uveitis, scleritis, or mononeuritis multiplex.

III. DIAGNOSIS

1. The diagnosis of WG is established by the presence of appropriate organ involvement, laboratory data, and characteristic histopathology. In patients with vasculitis, the presence of ≥ 2 of the following has a sensitivity of 88% and specificity of 92%: abnormal urinary sediment (red cell casts, > 5 red blood cells per high-power field), abnormal chest radiographs (nodules, cavities, fixed infiltrates), oral ulcers or nasal discharge, and granulomatous inflammation on biopsy.[10]
2. Antineutrophil cytoplasmic antibodies (ANCA) with a predominant cytoplasmic pattern (c-ANCA) are common in patients with active WG.
3. Tissue biopsy (upper airways, kidney, or lung) is used to confirm the diagnosis in suspected cases. Histologically, the characteristic features are small and medium vessel vasculitis, granulomatous inflammation, and necrosis.

IV. TREATMENT AND PROGNOSIS

1. Combination therapy with cyclophosphamide and corticosteroids should be initiated once the diagnosis of WG has been confirmed. Ninety percent of those treated will have a significant clinical response, and up to 75% will achieve complete remission.[9]
2. Plasmapheresis should be considered in patients with WG and anti–glomerular basement membrane antibodies, dialysis-dependent renal failure on presentation, pulmonary hemorrhage, and patients who are refractory to conventional immunosuppressants.[11]
3. Untreated, WG is almost universally fatal. Historically, untreated patients usually succumb to progressive renal failure and pulmonary complications. With treatment, mortality decreases dramatically to 12% at 12 years.[12] Patients who undergo treatment and have prolonged survival may succumb to the long-term complications of therapy.

Polyarteritis Nodosa

I. EPIDEMIOLOGY

The annual incidence of PAN ranges from 4.6 to 77 per million, with a prevalence of 6.3 per 100,000.[13] Men and women are affected equally, usually in the fourth and fifth decades of life. Although it is usually idiopathic, there is a subset of patients whose PAN is secondary to hepatitis B virus (HBV) infection.

II. PRESENTATION

1. PAN is caused by inflammation of medium and small arteries and complicated by arterial aneurysms and thrombosis. Characteristically, necrotizing vasculitis, healing vasculitic lesions, and unaffected artery can be found in the same tissue specimen.[14]
2. As with other vasculitides, patients present with protean symptoms of malaise, fever, arthralgias, myalgias, and weight loss. Mononeuritis multiplex is also common.

3. **PAN typically affects multiple vascular beds in a stepwise fashion as sequential arteries become inflamed.** The cutaneous manifestations of PAN include papulopetechial purpura, subcutaneous nodules, livedo reticularis, and occasionally distal gangrene. Renal involvement is also common and may lead to hypertension. Abdominal pain can be severe and may represent gastrointestinal vasculitis with resulting ischemia. Gastrointestinal bleeding and bowel perforation can also occur. Pulmonary involvement is very rare in PAN, and if it is present, microscopic polyangiitis (MPA) should be considered instead. Orchitis is a classic symptom found more commonly in PAN secondary to HBV.

III. DIAGNOSIS

1. No single laboratory or radiologic test can establish the diagnosis of PAN. Laboratory testing should include hepatitis B surface antigen because 7% to 36% of patients with PAN are HBV positive.[15]
2. Diagnosis is confirmed by biopsy of an involved organ (skin, peripheral nerve, testis, or kidney). When biopsies are unrevealing, the diagnosis may be suggested by abdominal angiography, which can show the presence of microaneurysms (particularly in the kidneys, mesentery, and liver) and stenoses in medium-sized vessels.

IV. TREATMENT AND PROGNOSIS

High-dose corticosteroids are the mainstay of treatment for mild disease. For patients who are refractory to corticosteroids alone or who have more severe disease (renal involvement, mesenteric involvement, mononeuritis multiplex), a combination of corticosteroids and cyclophosphamide should be initiated. Relapse is uncommon. In untreated patients, 5-year survival is only 13%.[16] Treatment with corticosteroids and cytotoxic agents can improve 5-year survival to 80%.[17]

Thromboangiitis Obliterans (Buerger's Disease)

I. EPIDEMIOLOGY

The incidence of TAO is 12.6 per 100,000 in the United States.[18] The median age of onset is 30 years, with a strong male predominance. Although the cause remains unclear, tobacco use is strongly linked to the onset of disease.[19]

II. PRESENTATION

1. TAO is characterized by segmental thrombotic occlusions of small and medium arteries and veins, with sparing of the vessel walls. This disease, in comparison to the other vasculitides, is a noninflammatory vasculopathy.
2. The most common clinical presentation is ischemic pain at rest and ulceration of the forefoot. Other common signs include upper and lower extremity ulcerations, thrombophlebitis, and Raynaud's phenomenon.

90

VASCULITIS

3. **TAO should be considered when patients have severe digital ischemia without evidence of systemic vasculitis.**

III. DIAGNOSIS

1. Multiple diagnostic criteria have been proposed for the diagnosis of TAO. The most commonly used criteria are age younger than 45 years; current or recent history of tobacco use; presence of distal extremity ischemia documented by noninvasive vascular testing; exclusion of autoimmune disease, hypercoagulable state, and diabetes mellitus; and exclusion of proximal source of emboli.[20]
2. Arteriography typically demonstrates small and medium vessel involvement of the extremities with segmental occlusive lesions (i.e., diseased arteries interspersed with normal appearing arteries). More severe disease is seen distally, with proximal sparing without evidence of atherosclerosis; collateralization is seen around the areas of occlusion (corkscrew collaterals). Vascular biopsy usually is not necessary.

IV. TREATMENT

The only proven treatment to halt disease progression is cessation of all forms of tobacco use.[21] Other treatment options for TAO are unproven.

Cryoglobulinemia Syndromes

1. Cryoglobulinemia syndrome is a systemic vasculitis that damages mainly the small and medium arteries and veins through immune complex deposition.
2. The classic clinical triad (sometimes called Meltzer's triad) includes palpable purpura, arthralgias, and weakness or asthenia.[22] Characteristically, symptoms of cryoglobulinemia wax and wane over periods of years, with cutaneous manifestations, arthritis, arthralgias, and myalgias often worsening with cold exposure.
3. The diagnosis of cryoglobulinemia syndrome is based on the detection of cryoglobulin precipitate from serum in the clinical setting of vasculitis or thrombosis. Approximately 40% of normal individuals have low levels of cryoglobulins, in contrast to patients with cryoglobulinemia syndromes, who have higher concentrations (> 1 mg/dl). Other laboratory abnormalities include hypocomplementemia, elevated ESR, and elevated CRP. The incidence of hepatitis C virus infection associated with mixed cryoglobulinemia ranges from 40% to 100%.[23,24] Table 90-2 summarizes the main clinical characteristics of the various cryoglobulinemia syndromes.

Churg-Strauss Syndrome (Allergic Granulomatous Angiitis)

I. EPIDEMIOLOGY

CSS is a rare systemic vasculitis that involves small vessels, characterized by hypereosinophilia and extravascular granulomas with an annual

TABLE 90-2

CLINICAL CHARACTERISTICS OF CRYOGLOBULINEMIA SYNDROMES

Class*	Immunoglobulin Composition	Associated Conditions	Clinical Manifestations	Prognosis	Treatment
Type I	Monoclonal IgG or IgM	Waldenström's macroglobulinemia, multiple myeloma, or chronic lymphocytic leukemia	Signs and symptoms of hyperviscosity or thrombosis: digital ischemia, Raynaud's phenomenon, livedo, and palpable purpura	Dependent on underlying malignancy and treatment.	Chemotherapy and radiation therapy directed at underlying malignancy.
Type II	Mixture of polyclonal immunoglobulins and a monoclonal IgG or IgM	Chronic inflammatory conditions such as connective tissue diseases, autoimmune disorders, or chronic infections	Constitutional symptoms, hepatosplenomegaly, peripheral neuropathy, and palpable purpura; renal failure presenting as membranoproliferative glomerulonephritis.	Mean survival is 50% at 10 yr after diagnosis. 5-10% subsequently develop B cell non-Hodgkin's lymphoma.[25]	Mild symptoms: analgesics, cold avoidance, and corticosteroids. Severe symptoms: plasmapheresis, high-dose corticosteroids, cyclophosphamide. If present, associated hepatitis C virus should also be treated.
Type III	Mixture of only polyclonal immunoglobulins				

*Based on Brouet JC et al: *Am J Med* 57:775, 1974.

90

VASCULITIS

incidence of 4 per million and a mean age of onset in the 50s.[26] Patients typically have a history of asthma and allergic rhinitis.

II. PRESENTATION

1. There are three overlapping phases of CSS. The first phase, characterized by allergic rhinitis, nasal polyposis, and asthma, may last for years. The second phase is marked by peripheral hypereosinophilia with or without tissue eosinophilia (chronic pneumonitis, Loeffler's syndrome, or eosinophilic gastroenteritis). The third phase includes constitutional symptoms and manifestations of systemic vasculitis.
2. Neurologic involvement, particularly peripheral neuropathy and mononeuritis multiplex, is common and can occur in up to 75% of patients with CSS.
3. The most common skin manifestations include palpable purpura, petechiae, and subcutaneous nodules. Pulmonary infiltrates are commonly found on chest radiograph. These infiltrates usually are transient alveolar opacities in a patchy distribution. Cardiac involvement in the form of myocarditis and heart failure is common and accounts for half of the mortality seen in CSS. Gastrointestinal involvement is also common (diarrhea, gastrointestinal bleeding, cholecystitis, and bowel perforation) and is associated with a poor prognosis.

III. DIAGNOSIS

1. CSS is a clinical diagnosis established by the presence of asthma and peripheral eosinophilia in a patient with systemic vasculitis. The presence of ≥ 4 of the following in a patient with vasculitis has a sensitivity of 85% and specificity of 99% for the diagnosis of CSS: asthma, eosinophilia (> 10% of total white blood cells), mononeuropathy or polyneuropathy, migratory pulmonary infiltrates on chest radiographs, paranasal sinus abnormalities (acute or chronic pain or tenderness), and extravascular eosinophils on biopsy.[27]
2. Eosinophilia (often $> 10^9$ cells/L) is found in most cases except when patients have had recent steroid treatment for an asthma exacerbation. CSS is strongly associated (70% to 75%) with perinuclear ANCA.

IV. TREATMENT AND PROGNOSIS

Initial treatment includes high-dose corticosteroids and should be continued until all evidence of active vasculitis has resolved and tapered thereafter. If vasculitic symptoms are uncontrolled by corticosteroids alone, cyclophosphamide should be added. Untreated, only 50% of patients with CSS survive 3 months after diagnosis. With corticosteroid treatment, the survival rate is 90% at 1 year and 75% at 5 years.[28]

Microscopic Polyangiitis (Microscopic Polyarteritis)

I. EPIDEMIOLOGY

MPA is a systemic necrotizing vasculitis involving arterioles, capillaries, and venules without evidence of necrotizing granulomatous inflammation.

The annual incidence is estimated to be 3.6 per million, and the mean age of onset is 50 to 56 years.[29]

II. PRESENTATION

1. As in PAN, multiple organ systems can be affected in MPA. Renal involvement is almost universal and is characterized by rapidly progressive glomerulonephritis. Up to 46% of patients progress to oliguric renal failure necessitating hemodialysis.[30]
2. Unlike classic PAN, MPA commonly has pulmonary involvement, often presenting with hemoptysis and diffuse alveolar hemorrhage. Diffuse alveolar hemorrhage can present as bilateral alveolar infiltrates in the absence of pulmonary edema or active pneumonia and an elevated carbon monoxide diffusing capacity on pulmonary function tests.

III. DIAGNOSIS

1. MPA can be confused with other systemic vasculitides, particularly PAN and WG. MPA shares many features with WG. Both affect small vessels, cause glomerulonephropathies, and have pulmonary involvement; however, MPA does not have predominant upper airway lesions, and granulomatous lesions are not found in MPA.
2. In 25% to 50% of patients, rheumatoid factor may be positive. In contrast to the common association between PAN and HBV, patients with MPA usually are HBV negative.
3. Biopsy of affected tissue should be done to demonstrate the presence of small vessel vasculitis and establish the diagnosis of MPA. The most accessible sites include the kidneys, skin, and peripheral nerves (e.g., sural nerve).

IV. TREATMENT AND PROGNOSIS

1. Because of the rapidly progressive nature of the renal involvement, high-dose corticosteroid and cyclophosphamide should be initiated once the diagnosis is established. The rate of relapse in MPA is high (up to 38%), and patients typically need prolonged treatment courses.
2. Patients with fulminant MPA typically present with pulmonary and renal failure necessitating supportive therapy with mechanical ventilation and hemodialysis. Fulminant MPA is associated with a 35% mortality at 5 years. As in WG, plasmapheresis may be useful in patients with hemodialysis dependence and diffuse alveolar hemorrhage refractory to conventional immunosuppressive therapy.

PEARLS AND PITFALLS

- *Pneumocystis jiroveci* pneumonia prophylaxis should be prescribed to all patients on combination cyclophosphamide and corticosteroid therapy.
- The diagnosis of TA should be considered in a young woman with unclear upper thoracic chest pain, back pain, or cardiomyopathy.
- The most specific symptom of GCA is jaw claudication.

90

VASCULITIS

- A "normal" ESR does not exclude GCA because 11% of patients with GCA present with an ESR < 50 mm/hr and 5% present with an ESR < 40 mm/hr.[31]
- Patients undergoing treatment for WG who have seemingly refractory disease should also be evaluated for the presence of opportunistic infections (pneumocystic, bacterial, fungal, viral, or mycobacterial pneumonia) or drug-induced toxicity (pneumonitis secondary to methotrexate or cyclophosphamide).
- MPA is the most common cause of pulmonary-renal syndrome.
- Visceral abdominal angiography revealing multiple saccular aneurysms in more than one organ is specific but not diagnostic for vasculitis, particularly PAN.
- In patients with established chronic hepatitis C virus infection, cryoglobulins should be measured in patients with a purpuric rash, arthralgias, Raynaud's phenomenon, peripheral neuropathy, or progressive renal failure to rule out cryoglobulinemia.
- In contrast to the common association between PAN and HBV, almost all patients with MPA are HBV negative.

REFERENCES

1. Kerr GS et al: Takayasu arteritis, *Ann Intern Med* 120:919, 1994. B
2. Arend WP et al: The American College of Rheumatology 1990 criteria for the classification of Takayasu arteritis, *Arthritis Rheum* 33:1129, 1990. D
3. Ishikawa K: Natural history and classification of occlusive thromboaortopathy (Takayasu's disease), *Circulation* 57:27, 1978. B
4. Salvarani C et al: Giant cell arteritis with low erythrocyte sedimentation rate: frequency of occurrence in a population-based study, *Arthritis Rheum* 45:140, 2001. B
5. Dominguez-Castellano A et al: Usefulness of temporal artery biopsy: analysis of 100 cases, *Med Clin (Barc)* 28(92):81, 1989. B
6. Ray-Chaudhuri N et al: Effect of prior steroid treatment on temporal artery biopsy findings in giant cell arteritis, *Br J Ophthalmol* 86:530, 2002. B
7. Hunder GG et al: The American College of Rheumatology 1990 criteria for the classification of giant cell arteritis, *Arthritis Rheum* 33:1122, 1990. D
8. Cotch MF et al: The epidemiology of Wegener's granulomatosis, *Arthritis Rheum* 39:87-92, 1996. B
9. Hoffman GS et al: Wegener granulomatosis: an analysis of 158 patients, *Ann Intern Med* 116:488, 1992. B
10. Leavitt RY et al: The American College of Rheumatology 1990 criteria for the classification of Wegener's granulomatosis, *Arthritis Rheum* 33:1101, 1990. D
11. Klemmer PJ et al: Plasmapheresis therapy for diffuse alveolar hemorrhage in patients with small-vessel vasculitis, *Am J Kidney Dis* 42:1149, 2003. C
12. Reinhold-Keller E et al: An interdisciplinary approach to the care of patients with Wegener's granulomatosis: long-term outcome in 155 patients, *Arthritis Rheum* 43:1021, 2000. B
13. Hochberg MC et al: *Rheumatology*. Philadelphia, 2003, Mosby. D
14. Lie JT: Histopathologic specificity of systemic vasculitis, *Rheum Dis Clin North Am* 21:883, 1995. C

15. Guillevin L et al: Polyarteritis nodosa related to hepatitis B virus. A prospective study with long-term observation of 41 patients, *Medicine (Baltimore)* 74:238, 1995. B

16. Frohnert PP et al: Long-term follow-up study of peri-arteritis nodosa, *Am J Med* 43:8, 1967. B

17. Gayraud M et al: Long-term followup of polyarteritis nodosa, microscopic polyangiitis, and Churg-Strauss syndrome: analysis of four prospective trials including 278 patients. French Vasculitis Study Group, *Arthritis Rheum* 44(3):666, 2001. C

18. Lie JT: The rise and fall and resurgence of thromboangiitis obliterans (Buerger's disease), *Acta Pathol Jpn* 39:153, 1989. C

19. Papa M et al: Autoimmune mechanisms in thromboangiitis obliterans (Buerger's disease): the role of tobacco antigen and the major histocompatibility complex, *Surgery* 111:527, 1992. B

20. Olin JW: Thromboangiitis obliterans (Buerger's disease), *N Engl J Med* 343:864, 2000. C

21. Corelli F: Buerger's disease: cigarette smoker disease may always be cured by medical therapy alone. Uselessness of operative treatment, *J Cardiovasc Surg (Torino)* 14:28, 1973. B

22. Meltzer M, Franklin EC: Cryoglobulinemia: a study of 29 patients. I. IgG and IgM cryoglobulins and factors effecting cryoprecipitability, *Am J Med* 40:828, 1966. B

23. Misiani R et al: Hepatitis C virus infection in patients with essential mixed cryoglobulinemia, *Ann Intern Med* 117:573, 1992. B

24. Agnello V et al: A role for hepatitis C virus infection in type II cryoglobulinemia, *N Engl J Med* 327:1490, 1992. B

25. La Civita L et al: Mixed cryoglobulinemia as a possible preneoplastic disorder, *Arthritis Rheum* 38:1859, 1995. C

26. Kurland LT et al: The epidemiology of systemic arteritis. In Lawrence RC, Shulman LE, eds: *The epidemiology of the rheumatic diseases*, New York, 1984, Gower. C

27. Masi AT et al: The American College of Rheumatology 1990 criteria for the classification of Churg-Strauss syndrome (allergic granulomatosis and angiitis), *Arthritis Rheum* 33:1094, 1990. D

28. Chumbley LC et al: Allergic granulomatosis and angiitis (Churg-Strauss syndrome): report and analysis of 30 cases, *Mayo Clin Proc* 52:477, 1977. B

29. Watts RA et al: Effect of classification on the incidence of polyarteritis nodosa and microscopic polyangiitis, *Arthritis Rheum* 39(7):1208, 1996. B

30. Savage CO et al: Microscopic polyarteritis: presentation, pathology, and prognosis, *Q J Med* 56:467, 1985. B

31. Hall S et al: Takayasu arteritis. A study of 32 North American patients, *Medicine* 64:89, 1985. B

90

VASCULITIS

Systemic Lupus Erythematosus

Ann Reed, MD; Traci Thompson Ferguson, MD; and Peter Holt, MD

FAST FACTS

- The incidence of systemic lupus erythematosus (SLE) has tripled in the past four decades.
- Women are nine times more likely than men to have SLE.[1]
- Antinuclear antibody (ANA) quantification is a very sensitive test for SLE, but it has poor specificity. ANA titers may be elevated with viral infection and other rheumatologic disorders. An elevated ANA titer is neither necessary nor sufficient to diagnose SLE.
- The arthritis of SLE usually presents as an additive symmetric polyarthritis.
- In the Hopkins Lupus Cohort the most common causes of hospitalization were active SLE (35%), infection (14%), and other medical complications of SLE (including coronary artery disease). Sepsis is the most common cause of death in patients with end-stage renal disease caused by lupus nephritis.[2-4]
- Antiphospholipid antibody syndrome (APS) is common in patients with SLE.

I. EPIDEMIOLOGY

1. SLE is a chronic, systemic autoimmune disease with broad phenotypic diversity. SLE syndromes include drug-induced lupus (associated with hydralazine, procainamide, isoniazid, chlorpromazine, methyldopa, quinidine, sulfasalazine, and others, characterized by resolution of symptoms after the offending agent is withdrawn),[5] chronic cutaneous (discoid) lupus (skin lesions present without any systemic manifestations), subacute cutaneous lupus, and neonatal lupus (congenital heart block or skin lesions).
2. SLE is predominantly a disease of women of childbearing age. Disease onset generally occurs in the second to fourth decades of life.
3. Ethnicity plays an important role in the natural history of SLE. African Americans have a higher incidence and prevalence of SLE,[2] with more neurologic disease, renal disease, and higher Systemic Lupus Activity Measure scores. Native Americans also have a higher prevalence of SLE, with higher SLE Disease Activity Index scores at the time of diagnosis and a higher rate of vasculitis, renal involvement, and mortality.[6]

II. CLINICAL PRESENTATION

1. Most of the common signs and symptoms associated with SLE are nonspecific. For example, patients with SLE may have constitutional

symptoms, polyarthralgias or, less commonly, polyarthritis. More specific for the diagnosis of SLE is the presence of Jaccoud's arthropathy (a hand deformity caused by ligamentous laxity, producing a reducible deformity on physical examination. Other musculoskeletal manifestations include tenosynovitis, myositis, and corticosteroid-induced myopathy or osteonecrosis.

2. Renal involvement (lupus nephritis) may present with proteinuria or an active urinary sediment and is associated with an overall poor prognosis. The World Health Organization classifies lupus nephritis in five categories based on renal biopsy: type I (normal), type II (mesangial abnormalities), type III (focal proliferative), type IV (diffuse proliferative glomerulonephritis), and type V (membranous). Type II is the most common biopsy finding.[7] Lupus nephritis correlates with the presence of antibodies to double-stranded DNA and is significantly more common in African Americans.[4,8]

3. Cutaneous manifestations of SLE are common and include a malar rash, discoid lesions, alopecia, and oral and nasal ulcerations. Less commonly, vasculitic lesions (especially around the nail beds), urticarial lesions (painful rather than pruritic) that last > 24 hours, panniculitis that heals with a scar, and livedo reticularis may be seen.

4. SLE has multiple pulmonary manifestations, including pneumonitis, pleurisy, pleural effusions, pulmonary alveolar hemorrhage, and acute and chronic interstitial lung disease. Pulmonary embolism may be seen in association with APS.

5. Gastrointestinal signs and symptoms are less common and may include abdominal pain, anorexia, nausea, vomiting, pancreatitis, mesenteric vasculitis, serositis, ascites, and a protein-losing enteropathy. Elevated liver function tests are a recognized manifestation of lupoid hepatitis.

6. The most common neuropsychiatric manifestations of SLE are seizure and psychosis. SLE has numerous neurologic sequelae, including brainstem dysfunction, stroke, major depression, encephalopathy, cognitive impairment, chorea, transverse myelitis, aseptic meningitis, peripheral neuropathy, cranial neuropathy, mononeuritis multiplex, pseudotumor cerebri, optic neuritis, uveitis, episcleritis, and scleritis.

7. Pericarditis and pericardial effusion are common cardiac manifestations of SLE. In addition, systolic or diastolic dysfunction, myocarditis, and Libman-Sacks endocarditis (sterile verrucous vegetations on the mitral valve, highly associated with antiphospholipid antibodies [APAs]) all occur disproportionately in patients with SLE. The cardiovascular manifestation of SLE that is of most concern is coronary arteritis. Patients with SLE have premature atherosclerosis with a higher prevalence of coronary atherosclerosis,[9] carotid atherosclerosis, left ventricular hypertrophy,[10] and peripheral vascular disease.

8. Hematologic abnormalities are common and include anemia, leukopenia, lymphopenia, and thrombocytopenia.

9. The arthritis of SLE usually presents as an additive symmetric polyarthritis. The differential diagnosis of additive symmetric polyarthritis includes SLE, rheumatoid arthritis, arthritis associated with a connective tissue disease, and arthritis associated with a vasculitis such as Wegener's granulomatosis.

III. DIAGNOSIS

1. The diagnosis of SLE is based on the history and physical examination and supported by the results of standard blood analyses (e.g., complete blood cell count, electrolytes, and urinalysis), the presence of autoantibodies (including antinuclear antibodies, anti-dsDNA, anti-Sm, anti-RNP, anti SS-A [Ro], anti SS-A [La]), and other data (e.g., results of a renal biopsy or low serum complement levels). **The autoantibodies anti-dsDNA and anti-Sm are most specific for SLE. The presence of antinuclear antibodies is neither necessary nor sufficient to diagnose SLE.**

2. The most recent criteria for the diagnosis of SLE were published in 1997 (Table 91-1). A patient is classified as having SLE if ≥ 4 of the 11 criteria are present, either serially or simultaneously.[11]

IV. MORTALITY

Survival in patients with SLE has improved over time,[1] yet the overall 10-year survival rate is still only about 80%.[12] Predictors of mortality include the presence of nephritis, seizures, thrombocytopenia, and poverty.[3]

TABLE 91-1
CRITERIA FOR THE CLASSIFICATION OF SYSTEMIC LUPUS ERYTHEMATOSUS[11]

Criterion	Definition
Malar rash	Fixed erythema over the malar eminences, sparing the nasolabial folds.
Discoid rash	Erythematous raised patches with adherent keratotic scaling and follicular plugging; atrophic scarring may occur in older lesions.
Photosensitivity	Skin rash as a result of unusual reaction to sunlight.
Oral ulcers	Oral or nasopharyngeal ulceration, usually painless.
Arthritis	Nonerosive arthritis involving two or more peripheral joints.
Serositis	Pleuritis or pericarditis.
Renal disorder	Persistent proteinuria greater than 3+ or presence of cellular casts.
Neurologic disorder	Seizures or psychosis in the absence of other explanation.
Hematologic disorder	Hemolytic anemia, leukopenia ($< 4000/mm^3$), lymphopenia ($< 1500/mm^3$), or thrombocytopenia ($< 100,000/mm^3$).
Immunologic disorder	Presence of antiphospholipid antibodies or antibodies to native DNA or to Sm nuclear antigen.
Antinuclear antibody	An abnormal titer of antinuclear antibody in the absence of drugs known to be associated with "drug-induced lupus" syndrome.

V. MANAGEMENT

1. When a patient with SLE is admitted to the hospital, the clinician must determine whether the patient's symptoms are a manifestation of a lupus flare, complications of SLE, or an unrelated disease process. For example, chest pain in a patient with SLE may be caused by musculoskeletal injury, serositis from a lupus flare, or ischemia from coronary arteritis.

2. When a patient has a lupus flare, all of the patient's particular lupus manifestations usually flare at the same time.

3. When infected, patients with lupus may not develop a fever, especially if they are on corticosteroids. Invasive studies (e.g., lumbar puncture, arthrocentesis, bronchoalveolar lavage, or biopsy) may be necessary, depending on the presentation, to reliably exclude the possibility of infection. If hypocomplementemia is a manifestation of the patient's lupus, the complement levels will tend to fall when the lupus flares and rise when the patient is infected. Likewise, leukopenia is a manifestation of active lupus, whereas leukocytosis is a manifestation of active infection or corticosteroid use.

4. Serologic test results (such as anti-dsDNA, C3, or C4) are not predictive of later flares.[14] The most common finding on the day of a flare is a reduction in anti-dsDNA levels.[15]

5. Most manifestations of SLE flares respond readily to corticosteroids. Intravenous corticosteroids are commonly used to treat the more serious manifestations of SLE, such as nephritis, cerebritis, hematologic abnormalities, and vasculitis. Although there is some debate as to whether lower dosages of steroids might be equally effective in treating severe SLE flares, **intravenous methylprednisolone, administered in boluses up to 1000 mg/day for 3 days, is very effective in quickly controlling life-threatening SLE flares.**[10]

6. When a patient is admitted with acute renal failure, an active urinary sediment, and hypocomplementemia, renal biopsy should be performed to establish an accurate diagnosis and direct therapy.

   a. Intravenous cyclophosphamide usually is the treatment of choice for diffuse proliferative glomerulonephritis.[16,17]

   b. Patients with lupus nephritis treated with either intravenous or oral cyclophosphamide can achieve long-term preservation of renal function; however, complications of cyclophosphamide therapy include ovarian failure, hemorrhagic cystitis, and malignancy. A combination of corticosteroids and mycophenolate mofetil may be less toxic and as effective in some cases.[18]

7. Chronic oral corticosteroids are the mainstay of maintenance therapy for many patients with SLE. Combination therapy (steroids plus antimalarials or other immunosuppressants) often is used to limit the cumulative toxicity of long-term corticosteroid use.

8. Hydroxychloroquine is an antimalarial agent that is generally used to treat cutaneous lesions, arthritis, and serositis. In patients without

91

SYSTEMIC LUPUS ERYTHEMATOSUS

active lupus, hydroxychloroquine should be continued to maintain remission and prevent flares. Patients should be alerted to the low risk of retinopathy associated with hydroxychloroquine use.[19]

9. Multiple immunosuppressive drugs can be used for the long-term management of SLE. Azathioprine is commonly used as a steroid-sparing drug in patients with SLE. Cyclosporine is effective in limiting disease activity but is rarely used as a corticosteroid-sparing agent because of its nephrotoxicity. Weekly doses of methotrexate (15 to 20 mg) can significantly control mild cutaneous and articular symptoms and may permit gradual decreases in daily corticosteroid dosing.[20]

VI. SPECIAL CONSIDERATION: ANTIPHOSPHOLIPID SYNDROME

1. APS is called primary in the absence of autoimmune disease and secondary when diagnosed in a patient with lupus or other connective tissue disease. APS is a diagnosis with both clinical and laboratory criteria (see Chapter 46). The presence of APAs alone does not make a diagnosis of APS.

2. APAs are present at a higher rate in patients with SLE (anticardiolipin antibodies or lupus anticoagulant antibodies are present in one third of patients).[21] Patients with APAs and SLE have a 34% to 70% chance of developing APS within 20 years.[22,23]

3. The management of APAs in asymptomatic patients is debated. Hydroxychloroquine may be useful in patients with SLE and isolated APAs.[32,38] Patients with APS should be treated with warfarin (see Chapter 46).[21,24,25] Patients with catastrophic APS in conjunction with a lupus flare may be given cyclophosphamide in addition to usual therapy for catastrophic APS.[26]

PEARLS AND PITFALLS

- Diagnosis of both SLE and APS is based on the findings of a thorough history and physical examination and supported by appropriate laboratory studies.
- Renal involvement with SLE confers a poor prognosis.
- SLE flares respond quickly to high-dose intravenous steroids. However, it is important to consider other common causes of morbidity in patients with SLE presenting to the hospital, including infection and cardiac disease.
- Patients who need cyclophosphamide or chronic high-dose steroids should be considered for *Pneumocystis jirovecii* pneumonia prophylaxis.
- Offer annual influenza vaccinations and ensure that pneumococcal vaccinations are up to date in all patients with SLE.
- Patients with APS may have a false-positive Venereal Disease Research Laboratory test and a prolonged activated partial thromboplastin time.

REFERENCES

1. Uramoto KM et al: Trends in the incidence and mortality of systemic lupus erythematosus, 1950-1992, *Arthritis Rheum* 42:46, 1999. B

2. Petri M: The effect of race on incidence and clinical course in systemic lupus erythematosus: the Hopkins Lupus Cohort, *J Am Med Womens Assoc* 53:9, 1998. B

3. Petri M: Detection of coronary artery disease and the role of traditional risk factors in the Hopkins Lupus Cohort, *Lupus* 9:170, 2000. C

4. Petri M et al: Morbidity of systemic lupus erythematosus: role of race and socioeconomic status, *Am J Med* 91:345, 1991. B

5. Solinger AM: Drug-related lupus: clinical and etiologic considerations, *Rheum Dis Clin North Am* 14(1):187, 1988. C

6. Peschken CA, Esdaile JM: Systemic lupus erythematosus in north American Indians: a population based study, *J Rheumatol* 27:1884, 2000. B

7. Gladman DD et al: Kidney biopsy in SLE. I. A clinical-morphologic evaluation, *Q J Med* 73:1125, 1989. B

8. Austin HA, Balow JE: Natural history and treatment of lupus nephritis, *Semin Nephrol* 19:2, 1999. C

9. Ward MM: Changes in the incidence of end-stage renal disease due to lupus nephritis, 1982-1995, *Arch Intern Med* 160:3136, 2000. C

10. Mackworth-Young CG et al: A double blind, placebo controlled trial of intravenous methylprednisolone in systemic lupus erythematosus, *Ann Rheum Dis* 47:496, 1988. A

11. Hochberg MC: Updating the American College of Rheumatology revised criteria for the classification of systemic lupus erythematosus, *Arthritis Rheum* 40:1725, 1997. D

12. Abu-Shakra M et al: Mortality studies in systemic lupus erythematosus: results from a single center, *J Rheumatol* 22:1259, 1995. B

13. Alarcon GS et al: Systemic lupus erythematosus in three ethnic groups. VII [correction of VIII]. Predictors of early mortality in the LUMINA cohort. LUMINA Study Group, *Arthritis Rheum* 45:191, 2001. B

14. Ho A et al: A decrease in complement is associated with increased renal and hematologic activity in patients with systemic lupus erythematosus, *Arthritis Rheum* 44:2350, 2001. B

15. Ho A et al: Decreases in anti-double-stranded DNA levels are associated with concurrent flares in patients with systemic lupus erythematosus, *Arthritis Rheum* 44:2342, 2001. A

16. Austin HA III: Therapy of lupus nephritis: controlled trial of prednisone and cytotoxic drugs, *N Engl J Med* 314:614, 1986. A

17. Steinberg AD, Steinberg SC: Long-term preservation of renal function in patients with lupus nephritis receiving treatment that includes cyclophosphamide versus those treated with prednisone only, *Arthritis Rheum* 34:945, 1991. A

18. Chan TM et al: Efficacy of mycophenolate mofetil in patients with diffuse proliferative lupus nephritis. Hong Kong-Guangzhou Nephrology Study Group, *N Engl J Med* 343:1156, 2000. A

19. Petri M: Thrombosis and systemic lupus erythematosus: the Hopkins Lupus Cohort perspective, *Scand J Rheumatol* 25:191, 1996. C

20. Carneiro JR, Sato EI: Double blind, randomized, placebo controlled clinical trial of methotrexate in systemic lupus erythematosus, *J Rheumatol* 26:1275, 1999. A

21. Levine JS, Branch DW, Rauch J: The antiphospholipid syndrome, *N Engl J Med* 346:752, 2002. C

22. Somers E, Magder LS, Petri M: Antiphospholipid antibodies and incidence of venous thrombosis in a cohort of patients with systemic lupus erythematosus, *J Rheumatol* 29:2531, 2002. B

SYSTEMIC LUPUS ERYTHEMATOSUS

23. Petri M: Evidence-based management of thrombosis in the antiphospholipid syndrome, *Curr Rheumatol Rep* 5:370, 2003. B
24. Khamashta MA et al: The management of thrombosis in the antiphospholipid antibody syndrome, *N Engl J Med* 332:993, 1995. B
25. Lockshin MD, Erkan D: Treatment of the antiphospholipid syndrome, *N Engl J Med* 349:1177, 2003. D
26. Asherson RA et al: Catastrophic antiphospholipid syndrome: international consensus statement on classification criteria and treatment guidelines, *Lupus* 12:530, 2003. D

Connective Tissue Diseases

Christopher Tehlirian, MD; and Allan C. Gelber, MD, MPH, PhD

FAST FACTS

- Rheumatoid arthritis (RA) is a severe inflammatory autoimmune disorder, multifactorial in origin, that affects women and men.
- Systemic sclerosis (SSc) is a connective tissue disorder characterized by extracellular matrix deposition in skin and viscera and fibrotic vasculopathy of both the peripheral and visceral vasculature.
- Sjögren's syndrome (SS) is a slowly progressive autoimmune disease with lymphocytic infiltration of exocrine glands and is characterized by the presence of anti-Ro and anti-La autoantibodies.
- Inflammatory myopathies are a heterogenous group of disorders in adults characterized by proximal muscle weakness and nonsuppurative inflammation of skeletal muscle.
- Mixed connective tissue disorder (MCTD) is an overlap syndrome that includes features of systemic lupus erythematosus (SLE), SSc, and polymyositis in the presence of anti-U1 ribonucleoprotein (RNP) autoantibody.
- Diagnosis of specific connective tissue diseases is based on clinical signs and symptoms in combination with laboratory evidence of autoimmunity.

Connective tissue diseases (CTDs) include SLE, RA, SSc, SS, inflammatory myopathies, and MCTD. This chapter focuses on the epidemiology, clinical presentation, diagnosis, and treatment of these CTDs.

Rheumatoid Arthritis

I. EPIDEMIOLOGY

RA affects all ethnic groups worldwide, and its prevalence increases with age. Women are affected twice as often as men, and the peak incidence is between the fourth and sixth decades.

II. ETIOLOGY AND PRESENTATION

1. RA is a pleomorphic disease with varied presentations. The pathophysiology is complex and is characterized by an imbalance of B cell and T cell proinflammatory and antiinflammatory cytokines that stimulates synovial cells to proliferate. Patients who are HLA-DR4 positive are predisposed to a more severe course.
2. **The onset of the disease is marked by the insidious development of morning stiffness that lasts > 1 hour.** The duration of morning stiffness correlates with the amount of synovitis. Symmetric synovitis is a prominent early manifestation.

3. The pattern of progression may be brief (e.g., palindromic rheumatism), episodic, or prolonged and progressive. The pattern of onset does not correlate with the pattern of progression and vice versa.

III. DIAGNOSIS

1. The diagnosis of RA is a clinical one but is based on the American College of Rheumatology (ACR) revised criteria (Table 92-1). Symptoms include morning stiffness, symmetric polyarthritis, inflammatory synovitis, and the presence of rheumatoid factor (RF).
2. RF is an autoantibody (usually immunoglobulin M) that is specific for the Fc fragment of immunoglobulin G. RF is the major serologic marker of RA and is present in up to 80% of patients. Anti–cyclic citrullinated peptide (CCP) antibody is more specific, with a specificity of 90%, but is only 56% sensitive for the diagnosis of RA.[2]
3. Several pulmonary complications are frequent reasons for admission in patients with RA. These include pleural effusions, pleuritis, interstitial fibrosis, inflammation of the cricoarytenoid joint, bronchiolitis obliterans, and pulmonary nodules. Rheumatoid pleural effusions usually have a low glucose and white blood cell count $< 5000/mm^3$.
4. Fifty percent of patients with RA have cardiac involvement but may be asymptomatic.
5. Gastritis and peptic ulcer disease are common complications of RA treatment.
6. The extraarticular manifestations of RA are shown in Table 92-2.

IV. PROGNOSIS

1. Twenty percent of patients have a monocyclic pattern followed by remission in 1 year, 70% have a polycyclic pattern with intermittent

TABLE 92-1[1]
ACR CRITERIA FOR THE DIAGNOSIS OF RA

Criterion	Definition
Morning stiffness	Morning stiffness in and around the joints, lasting at least 1 hr before maximal improvement
Arthritis of 3 or more joints	Simultaneous soft tissue swelling or effusions in at least 3 joints (PIP, MCP, wrist, elbow, knee, ankle, or metatarsophalangeal)
Arthritis of hand joints	Arthritis in at least one wrist, MCP, or PIP joint
Symmetric arthritis	Simultaneous involvement of the same joint area on both sides of the body (i.e., bilateral)
Rheumatoid nodules	Subcutaneous nodules over bony prominences or extensor surfaces or in juxta-articular regions
Serum rheumatoid factor	Abnormal amounts of rheumatoid factor demonstrated by laboratory testing
Radiographic changes	Radiographic changes on the posterior hand and wrist, which include erosions and bony decalcification

MCP, metacarpal; *PIP*, proximal interphalangeal, *RA*, rheumatoid arthritis.

TABLE 92-2[3]

EXTRAARTICULAR MANIFESTATIONS OF RA

Organ System	Description
Skin	Rheumatoid nodules are present in 50% of patients with RA, but almost all patients with rheumatoid nodules are RF positive.
Ocular	Keratoconjunctivitis sicca syndrome is very common in RA. Scleritis (associated with a poor prognosis) and episcleritis (good prognosis) are less common.
Respiratory	Inflammation of the cricoarytenoid joint, pleural effusions (usually low glucose, white blood cell count < 5000/mm³), interstitial fibrosis, pleuritis, bronchiolitis obliterans, and pulmonary nodules can all affect the lung.
Cardiac	Pericardial effusion, pericarditis, aortic insufficiency secondary to aortic root dilatation, or valvular rheumatoid nodules. Fifty percent of patients have cardiac involvement but may be asymptomatic.
Gastrointestinal	Not common. Possibly xerostomia secondary to sicca syndrome or ischemic bowel secondary to vasculitis.
Renal	Glomerular disease is exceedingly rare. More commonly, interstitial renal disease secondary to Sjögren's or nonsteroidal antiinflammatory drug abuse.
Neurologic	Cervical spine instability, peripheral nerve entrapment, and vasculitis or mononeuritis multiplex.
Hematologic	Hypochromic-microcytic anemia with low serum ferritin and low to normal iron binding capacity. Felty's syndrome characterized by RA with leucopenia or neutropenia and splenomegaly.

RA, rheumatoid arthritis; *RF,* rheumatoid factor.

and smoldering activity, and 10% have a progressive pattern involving new joints. The monocyclic pattern has the best prognosis, and the progressive pattern has the worst.
2. The presence of RF and an elevated C-reactive protein (CRP) are prognostic signs of progressive joint destruction.

V. TREATMENT

1. The goals of treatment are twofold: controlling symptoms, including pain and swelling (e.g., corticosteroids and nonsteroidal antiinflammatory drugs [NSAIDs]), and slowing the progression of the disease and improving long-term outcomes with disease-modifying antirheumatic drugs (DMARDs).
2. NSAIDs, including cyclooxygenase 1 and 2 inhibitors, are the mainstay of antiinflammatory and analgesic therapy; the patient's age, sex, and medical history must be taken into account before this therapy is initiated. In one study, 15% of RA patients had an NSAID-induced gastrointestinal side effect during a 2.5-year study period,[4] so protecting the gastric mucosa is important.

3. Corticosteroids are very effective in reducing inflammation and pain; however, **RA should not be managed with corticosteroid monotherapy.** Osteoporosis prevention and *Pneumocystis jiroveci* pneumonia prophylaxis must be considered if dosages of > 20 mg of prednisone are used for > 12 weeks.[5]

4. There are two basic approaches with the use of DMARDs. The step-up approach begins with monotherapy and adds other DMARDs as needed to control the disease, and the step-down approach begins with combination therapy (two or more DMARDs) before tapering down. Either approach is acceptable.

Systemic Sclerosis

I. EPIDEMIOLOGY

SSc has a 3:1 female/male ratio. SSc affects a variety of racial and ethnic groups, but the severity and prevalence of the disease vary between them. The average age of onset is between 45 and 55 years. Notably, there is no familial aggregation or family concordance of SSc.

II. ETIOLOGY AND PRESENTATION

1. The pathogenic mechanism of SSc remains unclear. The best available experimental evidence suggests that susceptible patients are exposed to an exogenous trigger that activates the immune system and vascular endothelium. Ultimately, this process stimulates fibroblasts, leading to fibrosis and obliterative vasculopathy.

2. Patients often present with Raynaud's phenomenon and vague symptoms of fatigue and malaise. Subsequently, patients develop swelling or puffiness of the fingers and hands.

III. DIAGNOSIS

1. SSc is a multisystem disease characterized by functional and structural abnormalities of small blood vessels and fibrosis of the skin and internal organs.

2. The disease is classified into subsets by the degree of clinically involved skin: localized scleroderma (morphea), diffuse cutaneous SSc (rapid onset with prominent visceral disease), and limited cutaneous SSc (CREST syndrome [calcinosis, Raynaud's phenomenon, esophageal dysmotility, sclerodactyly, telangiectasia]).

3. A diagnosis of SSc requires 1 major and ≥ 2 minor criteria to be present.[6]

a. Major criteria: symmetric thickening, tightening, and induration of the skin of the fingers and skin proximal to the metacarpophalangeal and metatarsophalangeal joints.

b. Minor criteria: sclerodactyly, digital pitting scars or loss of substance from finger pad, bibasilar pulmonary fibrosis.

4. The clinical manifestations of scleroderma can affect every organ system.

5. Scleroderma renal crisis, a syndrome characterized by elevated blood pressure, elevated creatinine, proteinuria, and microscopic hematuria, occurs in 80% of patients within the first 5 years of diagnosis.
6. Restrictive ventilatory defects and decreased carbon monoxide diffusing capacity secondary to fibrosing alveolitis are common and often lead to end organ damage, including interstitial fibrosis and pulmonary hypertension.

IV. PROGNOSIS

Diffuse SSc has visceral involvement early on in the disease process, but the overall course is highly variable. Overall, the prognosis is poor, with a 10-year survival between 40% and 60%.[7]

V. TREATMENT

1. As with other rheumatologic diseases, treatment is directed toward ameliorating symptoms (organ specific) and improving long-term outcome. Improving long-term outcomes is more difficult in SSc because evidence-based treatment options are limited. Aggressive treatment with immunomodulating therapy may be useful early in the disease.
2. Raynaud's phenomenon should be treated with calcium channel blockers, hand warming, and smoking cessation.
3. Azathioprine, cyclophosphamide, and low-dose corticosteroids may improve lung function in early fibrosing alveolitis, and interferon-gamma may slow the progression of pulmonary fibrosis.[8-10] Pneumococcal and influenza vaccinations are recommended for all patients.
4. Pulmonary hypertension in SSc is treated in the same manner as pulmonary hypertension from other causes (i.e., with oxygen, intravenous epoprostenol, vasodilators, and bosentan; see Chapter 85).
5. Large pericardial effusions may occur, which are harbingers of scleroderma renal crisis.[11]
6. **Scleroderma renal crisis is a medical emergency and is treated with angiotensin-converting enzyme inhibitors that reverse the hyperreninemic state.** Timely recognition of malignant hypertension accompanied by acute renal failure is essential so treatment can begin immediately. Nearly 60% of patients with renal crisis need dialysis; however, half of those on dialysis will regain independent renal function if angiotensin-converting enzyme inhibitors therapy is instituted promptly.[12]
7. Musculoskeletal symptoms should be treated with NSAIDs and physical therapy.

Sjögren's Syndrome

I. EPIDEMIOLOGY

1. SS, also known as Mikulicz's disease, Gougerot's syndrome, sicca syndrome, and autoimmune exocrinopathy, is a chronic inflammatory

CONNECTIVE TISSUE DISEASES

92

autoimmune exocrinopathy that affects primarily the salivary and lacrimal glands. Primary SS occurs in the absence of another autoimmune disorder, whereas secondary SS occurs in the presence of other autoimmune disease (e.g., RA, SLE, SSc, MCTD, primary biliary cirrhosis, vasculitis, thyroiditis, mixed cryoglobulinemia).

2. SS affects patients of all ages, but it is most common among women (in a 9:1 ratio) in the fourth and fifth decades of life. The frequency of SS increases with age.

II. ETIOLOGY AND PRESENTATION

1. The pathogenesis of SS remains poorly defined.
2. The most common presentation is that of dry eyes and dry mouth. Patients may describe a sandpaper sensation in their eyes. Clinical manifestations may affect most organ systems.
a. Fifty percent of patients with SS experience joint swelling and stiffness.
b. Uncommonly, patients may develop interstitial lung disease (i.e., interstitial pneumonitis).
c. Renal manifestations include nephrocalcinosis, distal hypokalemic hyperchloremic acidosis (in 35% of SS patients), interstitial nephritis, and interstitial cystitis.
d. Patients with SS have a significantly elevated risk of lymphoma (B cell lymphomas are most common).

III. DIAGNOSIS

1. Several diagnostic studies assist in the diagnosis of SS. The Schirmer tear test, Rose Bengal staining of the corneal epithelium, and sialometry are used to evaluate tear and saliva production. Biopsy of a minor salivary gland of the lip can be performed by a dermatologist or oral surgeon.
2. Anti-Ro (SS-A) and anti-La (SS-B) autoantibodies are strongly associated with SS. The sensitivity and specificity of anti-Ro/SS-A are 53% and 100%, respectively, and for anti-La/SS-B they are 40% and 98%, respectively.[13] Almost 80% of patients have antinuclear antibodies (ANA), and 90% have a positive RF.

IV. PROGNOSIS

The prognosis is widely variable depending on the extent of disease. Overall, the mortality for patients with SS is similar to that of sex- and age-matched controls. However, 1 in 5 deaths of patients with primary SS disease is caused by lymphoma.[14,15]

V. TREATMENT

1. Keratoconjunctivitis is treated symptomatically with topical ocular lubricants, artificial tears, and hydroxypropylcellulose pellets. Topical corticosteroids are of questionable benefit.

2. Xerostomia is treated with artificial saliva and lubricants. Frequent dental care and daily fluoride are important to prevent dental caries. In addition, secretogogues such as pilocarpine often are used. Oral thrush is a common problem and can be managed with oral antifungal troches.

3. The milder systemic manifestations such as fever, rash, and arthritis can be treated with hydroxychloroquine. As with SLE, other immunomodulating therapies may be used to treat more severe systemic manifestations of SS.

Inflammatory Myositis

I. EPIDEMIOLOGY

The incidence of inflammatory myositis in the United States is estimated at 0.5 to 8 cases per million.[16] The age of onset has a bimodal pattern, with a peak between ages 10 and 15 in children and another peak between ages 45 and 60 in adults.

II. ETIOLOGY AND PRESENTATION

1. Inflammatory myopathies are immune-mediated processes triggered by environmental factors, such as viruses, in genetically susceptible people. Polymyositis (PM) and dermatomyositis (DM) differ pathogenetically. PM is a CD8 T cell–mediated attack on myofibers, whereas DM is mediated by immune complex deposition in blood vessels.

2. The idiopathic inflammatory myopathies are characterized by chronic, painless, proximal muscle weakness with an insidious onset.[17] They can be distinguished from polymyalgia rheumatica, which is usually painful, by the finding of true muscle weakness, which is absent in polymyalgia rheumatica.

3. The adult inflammatory myopathies are classified clinically into PM, DM, inclusion body myositis, paraneoplastic myositis, and myositis associated with other connective tissue disorders.

III. DIAGNOSIS

1. Diagnostic criteria for DM and PM include symmetric proximal muscle weakness, the typical rash of dermatomyositis (heliotrope rash, Gottron's papules, and "shawl sign"), elevated serum muscle (skeletal) enzymes (creatine kinase, lactate dehydrogenase, aspartate aminotransferase (AST), and aldolase), myopathic changes on electromyography, and characteristic muscle biopsy abnormalities.[18]

2. Myositis-specific autoantibodies include anti-histidyl-tRNA synthetase (anti-Jo-1 antibody), which can be detected in up to 20% of patients with PM or DM; however, ANA can be detected in up to 80% of patients with inflammatory myositis.[22]

92

CONNECTIVE TISSUE DISEASES

3. Magnetic resonance imaging can demonstrate inflammation in the soft tissues and skeletal muscle and therefore can be helpful in determining the best muscle site for electromyography and biopsy.

IV. PROGNOSIS

1. Prognosis is variable. Older age and myositis associated with cancer have worse outcomes.[20] Other clinical predictors of poor outcome include dysphagia, respiratory muscle weakness, and cardiac involvement.
2. The presence of anti-Jo-1 autoantibody tends to coexist with interstitial lung disease; these patients have a worse prognosis. Conversely, the presence of anti-Mi-2 antibody is associated with remission rates up to 40%.[21]

V. TREATMENT

Before beginning treatment, it is useful to objectively evaluate the patient's clinical status (creatine kinase, swallowing study, chest imaging, pulmonary function tests) so the patient can be monitored for improvement during therapy. Empiric corticosteroid therapy should be started with prednisone 1 mg/kg/day. More severe disease or disease that does not respond to steroids alone (after 3 months) should also be treated with methotrexate or azathioprine. Almost all patients respond at least partially to steroids alone, and nearly half achieve complete remission.

Mixed Connective Tissue Disorder

I. EPIDEMIOLOGY AND ETIOLOGY

The prevalence of MCTD is unknown; the female/male ratio is about 9:1. The cause of MCTD is also unknown, but there may be an association with exposure to vinyl chloride.

II. PRESENTATION AND DIAGNOSIS

1. MCTD is an overlap syndrome, lacking distinctive clinical features of its own; rather, it exhibits signs and symptoms characteristic of other CTDs such as SLE, SSc, and PM. There is some debate as to whether MCTD is a distinct disease with a specific autoantibody or an early manifestation of other CTDs.
2. Many of the following clinical features are common in MCTD: arthritis (95%), Raynaud's phenomenon (85%), esophageal dysmotility (67%), impaired pulmonary diffusing capacity (67%), swollen hands (66%), myositis (63%), lymphadenopathy (39%), skin rash (38%), sclerodactyly (33%), and renal involvement (20%).[22]
3. The suggested criteria for diagnosis of MCTD include positive serology (anti-U1 RNP) and ≥ 3 of the following: edema of the hands, myositis, synovitis, Raynaud's phenomenon, and acrosclerosis.[23]

III. PROGNOSIS AND TREATMENT

1. The overall prognosis of MCTD is variable; however, MCTD with progressive pulmonary hypertension carries a poor prognosis.[24]
2. There is no specific treatment for MCTD. Mild arthralgias should be managed symptomatically with NSAIDs. Severe disease, including myositis and fibrosing alveolitis, should be treated aggressively with high-dose systemic steroids and immunosuppressive therapy. Pulmonary hypertension should be treated aggressively.

PEARLS AND PITFALLS

- Many, if not all, patients with CTDs take NSAIDs or steroids. Therefore these patients should receive gastric ulcer prophylaxis with histamine 2 blockers or proton pump inhibitors.
- Patients being treated for > 4 weeks with steroid dosages of > 20 mg of oral prednisone daily should be given *Pneumocystis* pneumonia prophylaxis.
- Hydroxychloroquine is a good agent to use for the cutaneous manifestations of connective tissue diseases.
- Any patient diagnosed with an inflammatory myopathy should undergo age-appropriate cancer screening (including an evaluation for ovarian cancer in women).
- Consider steroid myopathy in all patients on chronic steroids with new or recurrent muscle weakness, regardless of previous diagnosis.

REFERENCES

1. Arnett FC et al: The American Rheumatism Association 1987 revised criteria for the classification of rheumatoid arthritis, *Arthritis Rheum* 31:315, 1988. D
2. Schellekens GA et al: Citrulline is an essential constituent of antigenic determinants recognized by rheumatoid arthritis–specific autoantibodies, *J Clin Invest* 101:273, 1998. B
3. Anderson RJ: Rheumatoid arthritis: clinical and laboratory features. In Klippel JH et al, eds: *Primer on the rheumatic diseases,* Atlanta, 2001, Arthritis Foundation. C
4. Singh G et al: Gastrointestinal tract complications of nonsteroidal anti-inflammatory drug treatment in rheumatoid arthritis. A prospective observational cohort study, *Arch Intern Med* 156:1530, 1996. B
5. Yale SH, Limper AH: Pneumocystis carinii pneumonia in patients without acquired immunodeficiency syndrome: associated illness and prior corticosteroid therapy, *Mayo Clin Proc* 71:5, 1996. D
6. Subcommittee for Scleroderma Criteria of the American Rheumatism Association Diagnostic and Therapeutic Criteria Committee: Preliminary criteria for the classification of systemic sclerosis, *Arthritis Rheum* 23:581, 1980. D
7. Scussel-Lonzetti L et al: Predicting mortality in systemic sclerosis: analysis of a cohort of 309 French Canadian patients with emphasis on features at diagnosis as predictive factors for survival, *Medicine* 81:154, 2002. B
8. Silver RM et al: Evaluation and management of scleroderma lung disease using bronchoalveolar lavage, *Am J Med* 88:470, 1990. B

9. Ziesche R et al: A preliminary study of long-term treatment with interferon gamma-1b and low dose prednisolone in patients with idiopathic pulmonary fibrosis, *N Engl J Med* 341:1264, 1999. B

10. White B et al: Cyclophosphamide is associated with pulmonary function and survival benefit in patients with scleroderma and alveolitis, *Ann Intern Med* 132:947, 2000. B

11. Steen VD et al: Factors predicting development of renal involvement in progressive systemic sclerosis, *Am J Med* 76:779, 1984. B

12. Steen VD, Medsger TA Jr: Long-term outcomes of scleroderma renal crisis, *Ann Intern Med* 133:600, 2000. B

13. Markusse HM et al: The clinical significance of the detection of anti-Ro/SS-A and anti-La/SS-B autoantibodies using purified recombinant proteins in primary Sjögren's syndrome, *Rheumatol Int* 13:147, 1993. B

14. Ioannidis JP, Vassiliou VA, Moutsopoulos HM: Long-term risk of mortality and lymphoproliferative disease and predictive classification of primary Sjögren's syndrome, *Arthritis Rheum* 46:741, 2002. B

15. Theander E, Manthorpe R, Jacobsson LT: Mortality and causes of death in primary Sjögren's syndrome: a prospective cohort study, *Arthritis Rheum* 50:1262, 2004. B

16. Hochberg MC: Epidemiology of polymyositis/dermatomyositis, *Mt Sinai J Med* 55:447, 1988. B

17. Dalakas MC, Hohlfeld R: Polymyositis and dermatomyositis, *Lancet* 362:971, 2003. B

18. Bohan A, Peter JB: Polymyositis and dermatomyositis, *N Engl J Med* 292:403, 1975. B

19. Reichlin M, Arnett FC Jr: Multiplicity of antibodies in myositis sera, *Arthritis Rheum* 27:1150, 1984. B

20. Maugars YM et al: Long-term prognosis of 69 patients with dermatomyositis or polymyositis, *Clin Exp Rheumatol* 14:263, 1996. B

21. Love LA et al: A new approach to the classification of idiopathic inflammatory myopathy: myositis-specific autoantibodies define useful homogeneous patient groups, *Medicine* 70:360, 1991. B

22. Lemmer JP et al: Clinical characteristics and course in patients with high titer anti-RNP antibodies, *J Rheumatol* 9:536, 1982. B

23. Alarcon-Segovia D, Cardiel MH: Comparison between 3 diagnostic criteria for mixed connective tissue disease. Study of 593 patients, *J Rheumatol* 16:328, 1989. B

24. Burdt MA et al: Long-term outcome in mixed connective tissue disease: longitudinal clinical and serologic findings, *Arthritis Rheum* 42:899, 1999. B

PART III

Comparative Pharmacology and Dosing Tables

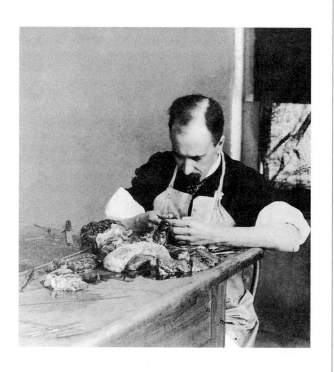

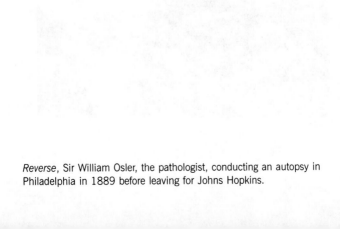

Reverse, Sir William Osler, the pathologist, conducting an autopsy in Philadelphia in 1889 before leaving for Johns Hopkins.

TABLE 1

EQUIANALGESIC DOSAGE CONVERSION FOR SELECTED OPIATES*

	Parenteral (IM/SC/IV)	Oral (PO)	Onset Route	Onset Time (min)	Duration Route	Duration Time (hr)	Comments‡
Morphine	10 mg	30 mg	PO, IR	30-60	PO	3-6	Active metabolite; adjust dosage in renal failure.
			SC, IM	10-20	R	4-5	
			IV	5-10	IM, IV	3-4	
Hydromorphone	1.5 mg	7.5 mg	PO, IR	15-30	PO, R, SC, IM, IV	3-4	
			SC, IM	10-20			
			IV	5			
Fentanyl	0.1 mg	—	OT	15	OT	2-5	25 μg/hr TD, ~45 mg PO morphine.
			IV	3-5	IV	0.5-4	
			TD	12-24 hr	TD	48-72	
Meperidine†	75 mg	300 mg	IV	5-10	PO	2-4	Active metabolite causes central nervous system excitation; adjust dosage in renal failure.
			SC, IM	10-20			
			PO	30-60			
Hydrocodone	—	30 mg	PO	30-60	PO	4-6	Used in combination with other analgesics because of adverse reactions at high dosages.
Codeine	130 mg	200 mg	PO	30-60	PO, IM	3-4	
			SC, IM	10-20			
Oxycodone	—	20 mg	PO, IR	30-60	PO	3-4	
					R	4-6	
Methadone	5 mg	10 mg	PO	30-60	PO, IV, SC, IM	4-8	Prior opiate exposure allows much lower methadone dosing. Higher dosages in chronic use tend to accumulate.
			IV	4-8	SL, IV	Unknown	
			SL	Unknown			
Propoxyphene	—	240 mg	PO	30-60	PO	4-6	Active metabolite; adjust dosage in renal failure.

cont'd

IM, intramuscular; *IR*, immediate release; *IV*, intravenous; *OT*, oral transmucosal; *PO*, oral; *R*, rectal; *SL*, sublingual; *SC*, subcutaneous; *TD*, transdermal.
*Note: This is not a chart of dosage recommendations.
*The American Pain Society does not recommend meperidine for acute or chronic pain management.
†Allergic and anaphylactic reactions are rare and poorly documented. The majority of urticaria, pruritus, and sneezing is caused by histamine release. This is a pharmacologic effect most noted with the natural (morphine, codeine) and semisynthetic (hydromorphone, hydrocodone, oxycodone) compounds.

COMPARATIVE PHARMACOLOGY AND DOSING TABLES

TABLE 2
EQUIVALENT DOSING STEROID TABLE

Drug	Relative Antiinflammatory Potency	Dosage Equivalency (mg)	Sodium Retention Capacity	Biologic Half-Life	IM, PO* (mg/d)	IV* (mg/d)
Hydrocortisone	1	20	1	8-12	PO 20-240 IM 15-240	15-240
Prednisone	4	5	0.8	18-36	5-60	—
Prednisolone	4	5	0.8	18-36	5-60	—
Methylprednisolone	5	4	0.5	12-36	PO 4-48	10-250
Triamcinolone	5	4	0	12-36	PO 4-48 IM 40-80	—
Betamethasone	25	0.6	0	36-72	0.6-9	0.6-9
Dexamethasone	30	0.75	0	36-72	0.75-9	0.5-9
Fludrocortisone	12	N/A	125	18-36	0.1-0.3	—

IM, PO, intramuscular or oral usual dosage range; *IV,* intravenous usual dosage range; *HPA,* hypothalmic-adrenal axis.
*Steroid-responsive conditions and drug dosing show wide interpatient variation. Duration of steroid tapering needed depends on three variables: disease flare (level of concern depends on which disease is being treated), duration and dosage of steroid treatment, and HPA suppression concerns.

TABLE 3

PROTON PUMP INHIBITORS

Mechanism of action	Proton pump inhibitors bind the hydrogen-potassium adenosine triphosphatase in gastric parietal cells, blocking the final step in the secretion of acid.
Drug interactions	Theoretical class effect on other substrates of 2C19 generally not clinically supported. In agents with a narrow therapeutic range, consider increased monitoring. Esomeprazole is an inducer of P-450 2C19.
Adverse reactions	Potential for proton pump inhibitors to alter absorption of pH-dependent drugs (e.g., ketoconazole, digoxin). 1-10%: diarrhea, abdominal pain, nausea, constipation, flatulence, and dry mouth. 5%: headache. Rare: pancreatitis, severe rash.

Characteristics	Esomeprazole	Lansoprazole	Omeprazole	Pantoprazole	Rabeprazole
Dosing (daily)*	PO 20-40 mg	PO 15-30 mg	PO 20-40 mg	PO 40 mg IV 40 mg ZES: maximum 80 mg q8h Upper gastrointestinal bleeding: 80-mg load, 8 mg/hr up to 72 hr PO = IV, median pH 3.8 on day 7[†]	PO 20 mg
Intragastric pH >4 (hr/d)	13 hr (20 mg) 17 hr (40 mg)	12 hr (15 mg) 16 hr (30 mg)	80-97% decrease in intragastric acidity[†]		14 hr
Bioavailability	89-90%	81-91%	30-76% depending on formulation	77%	52%
Elimination	80% urine 20% feces	20% urine 67% bile	77% urine 23% bile	81% urine 19% feces	90% urine 10% feces
Administration	1 hr before meals	30 min before meals	1 hr before meals	Before or after meals	Before or after meals
Safety in pregnancy	B	B	C	B	B

IV, intravenous; *PO*, oral.

*There are few exceptions in the literature when twice-daily dosing may be reasonable (e.g., Zollinger Ellison syndrome [ZES]).

[†]pH >4 not reported in available literature.

COMPARATIVE PHARMACOLOGY AND DOSING TABLES

WEIGHT-BASED UNFRACTIONATED HEPARIN DOSING ALGORITHM

INITIAL DOSING

Initial bolus	Depends on bleeding risk*	50-80 u/kg (maximum 7500 U)[†]
Initial infusion rate		13-18 U/kg/hr (maximum 1600 U/hr)[†]

aPTT Ratio (× control)	Rebolus	Hold Infusion	Change Infusion	Repeat aPTT
< 1.2	Repeat original weight-based bolus.[‡]	—	Add 4 U/kg/hr.	6 hr
1.2-1.4	Repeat ½ original weight-based bolus dose.[‡]	—	Add 2 U/kg/hr.	6 hr
1.5-2.5	—	—	—	6 hr[§]
2.6-3	—	—	Subtract 1 U/kg/hr.	6 hr
3.1-4	—	60 min	Subtract 3 U/kg/hr.	7 hr
4.1-5	—	120 min	Subtract 5 U/kg/hr.	8 hr
> 5	—	180 min	Subtract 7 U/kg/hr.	9 hr

Note: It is critical for each hospital to determine its specific therapeutic targets; this will in turn affect your bolus and starting infusion rates.

aPTT, activated partial thromboplastin time.

*Risk factors for bleeding include age >70 yr, postoperative, renal failure, concomitant antiplatelet or thrombolytics, liver disease, platelet count <100,000.

[†]Always round dosage to the nearest 50 U.

[‡]If bolus given when initiating heparin infusion (i.e., may not be given to neurology patients, postoperative patients, and trauma patients with venous thromboembolism; clinicians must make this judgment).

[§]Check aPTT q6h until aPTT in therapeutic range on 2 consecutive laboratory values, then check aPTT q12h × 2, then q.a.m. as long as aPTT remains in the normal range and no dosage adjustments are made.

TABLE 5A

DIRECT THROMBIN INHIBITORS

Characteristics	Argatroban	Bivalirudin	Lepirudin
Dosing (primary usage)	HIT: 2 μg/kg/min continuous (maximum 10 μg/kg/min). Initial dosage in hepatic impairment 0.5 μg/kg/min. No titration information available for HIT. Some have extrapolated lepirudin titration with mixed success. Package insert has extensive recommendations for PCI dosage titration.	PCI: 1 mg/kg IV bolus, followed by 2.5 mg/kg/hr for 4 hr, then 0.2 mg/kg/hr. Manufacturer recommends aspirin 325 mg/d given concomitantly. Reduction in infusion dosage with severe renal impairment 1 mg/kg/hr or 0.25 mg/kg/hr with hemodialysis. Titrated by provider familiar with its usage in PCI.	0.4 mg/kg bolus, followed by 0.15 mg/kg/hr continuous. Weight based up to 110 kg (maximum 0.21 mg/kg/hr suggested). Dosage adjustment in renal impairment. Cirrhosis may warrant dosage adjustment. Manufacturer-recommended titration: high aPTT, hold 2 hr, ↓ infusion 50%; low aPTT, ↑ infusion 20%.
aPTT ratio range	Affects ACT, aPTT, and PT/INR. aPTT goal: 1.5-3 × baseline. Do not exceed aPTT of 100 s.	Affects ACT, aPTT, and PT/INR.	aPTT goal: 1.5-2.5 × baseline. Do not start in patients with baseline aPTT ratio > 2.5.
Monitoring frequency	aPTT at baseline, 2 hr after initiation and dosage changes. ACT for PCI titration.	ACT at baseline, 1-2 hr after infusion.	Baseline, 4 hr after initiation and dosage changes.
Plasma half-life	IV, 45 min.	IV, 25 min.	IV, 78 min; SC, 120 min.
Route of elimination	Hepatic.	Partial renal.	Renal.
Effect on INR	Substantial.	Minimal because of short half-life.	Minimal.
Safety in pregnancy	B.	B.	B.

cont'd

COMPARATIVE PHARMACOLOGY AND DOSING TABLES

TABLE 5A

DIRECT THROMBIN INHIBITORS—cont'd

Characteristics	Argatroban	Bivalirudin	Lepirudin
Adverse reactions	2-10% hemorrhagic effects, hypotension, fever, diarrhea, nausea, cardiac arrest, pain.	5-15% hemorrhagic effects, hypotension, nausea, vomiting, pain, headache.	1-5% hemorrhagic effects, abnormal liver function, allergic skin reaction, multiorgan failure.
Safety	Bleeding consistent with historical control.[†]	Lower bleeding than with heparin.[‡]	Higher bleeding than with historical control.[§]
Conversion to oral anticoagulants	Estimate expected daily warfarin dosage; then titrate argatroban down to lowest effective dosage (i.e., aPTT 1.5 × normal); then when INR ≥ 4, hold argatroban and check INR 4-6 hr on warfarin alone; then when INR in target range, discontinue argatroban.	Not applicable.	Reduce lepirudin dosage until aPTT ratio is around 1.5. When INR in target range, discontinue lepirudin.
Drug interactions	Concomitant use of drugs that inhibit coagulation are associated with an increased risk of hemorrhage.		

ACT, activated clotting time; *aPTT*, activated partial thromboplastin time; *HIT*, heparin-induced thrombocytopenia; *INR*, international normalized ratio; *IV*, intravenous; *PCI*, percutaneous coronary intervention; *PT*, prothrombin time; *SC*, subcutaneous.

*Alteplase, amiodarone, amphotericin B, chlorpromazine, diazepam, prochlorperazine, reteplase, streptokinase, vancomycin.
[†]Argatroban PI.
[‡]*Chest* 126:265S-286S, 2004.
[§]Greinacher: *Circulation* 100:587-593, 1999.

TABLE 5B
LEPIRUDIN DOSING IN RENAL INSUFFICIENCY: BOLUS 0.2 mg/kg

Creatinine Clearance (ml/min)	Percentage of Original Infusion	Maintenance (mg/kg/hr)
45-60	50%	0.075
30-44	30%	0.045
15-29	15%	0.0225
< 15 or hemodialysis	No infusion or stop*	

*Additional bolus injections of 0.1 mg/kg every other day may be administered if the activated partial thromboplastin time ratio falls below therapeutic limits (1.5-2.5).

TABLE 5C
BIVALIRUDIN DOSING IN RENAL INSUFFICIENCY: NO CHANGE IN BOLUS

Renal Function	Glomerular Filtration Rate (ml/min)	Half-Life (min)	Reduction in Infusion Dosage (%)
Normal	>90	25	—
Mild	60-90	22	—
Moderate	30-59	34	20
Severe	10-29	57	60
Dialysis dependent*	—	3.5 hr	90

*25% of drug removed by hemodialysis.

TABLE 6
WARFARIN INITIATION IN THE HOSPITAL

	INR	Warfarin Dosage
Day 1	Baseline	5 mg is the average maintenance dosage needed in most patients. Use 2.5 mg if patient has liver disease or heart failure or is elderly, chronically malnourished, or on medications that may significantly increase INR. Use 7.5 mg if the patient weighs > 85 kg. If patient at goal INR in past, start with known dosage.
Day 2	Check INR (partially reflects 1st dose)	If INR < 1.5, give same dosage. If INR ≥ 1.5, give lower dosage (in increments of 2.5 mg).
Day 3	Check INR (partially reflects 1st 2 doses)	INR <1.5 suggests a higher than average maintenance dosage needed. INR 1.5-2 suggests an average maintenance dosage needed. INR > 2 suggests a lower than average maintenance dosage needed.

Any increase in the INR > 0.3-0.4 per day should prompt a warfarin dosage reduction.

The frequency of INR testing is determined by the patient's response and the provider's judgment of the patient's reliability and other risk factors for hemorrhage or thrombosis.

Depending on indication for warfarin, initiation of heparin product may also be needed.

INR, international normalized ratio.

TABLE 7	

WARFARIN MAINTENANCE DOSING

INR	Action
INR > 0.3 BELOW TARGET RANGE	
With removable causative factor (e.g., missed dose, more vitamin K consumption)	Remove causative risk factor, then make no change in dosage, *or* increase weekly dosage by 10-20%.
Without causative factor	Increase weekly dosage by 10-20%.
INR 0.1-0.3 BELOW TARGET RANGE	
With removable causative factor	No change in dosage.
Without causative factor	Take extra 5-10% of weekly dosage × 1 day and continue weekly dosage.
2 or 3 consecutive subtherapeutic INRs, with or without causative factor	Increase weekly dosage by 5-10%.
INR within target range	**No change in dosage**
INR 0.1-0.5 ABOVE TARGET RANGE	
With removable causative factor	No change in dosage.
Without causative factor	No change or decrease weekly dosage by 5-10%.
2 or 3 consecutive supratherapeutic INRs, with or without causative factor	Decrease weekly dosage by 5-10%.
INR 0.6 ABOVE TARGET RANGE (INR < 5)	
With removable causative factor	Consider repeat INR. If elevation confirmed, remove causative factor. Hold 0 or 1 dose and continue weekly dosage. Repeat INR in 1 wk.
Without causative factor	Consider repeat INR. If elevation confirmed, hold 0 or 1 dose and decrease weekly dosage by 10-20%. Repeat INR in 1 wk.

From Ansell J et al: *Chest* 126(Suppl):204S-233S, 2004.
INR, international normalized ratio.

TABLE 8

MANAGEMENT OF EXCESSIVE ANTICOAGULATION WITH WARFARIN

INR < 5 without significant bleeding	Review medication list for interacting medication.
	If interacting medication identified,
	  Eliminate if possible, hold warfarin, and check INR in 24 hr.
	  When INR approaches therapeutic range (INR < 4), restart warfarin at previous dosage and check INR in 2-3 d and 7 d later.
	If no interacting medication or if interacting medication cannot be eliminated,
	  Hold warfarin, recheck INR in 24 hr.
	  When INR approaches therapeutic range (INR < 4), resume warfarin at 15-20% lower weekly dosage and check INR in 2-3 d and 7 d later.

INR ≥ 5 but < 9 without significant bleeding	Review medication list for interacting medication.
	If interacting medication identified,
	  Eliminate if possible, hold warfarin and check INR in 24-48 hr.
	  When INR approaches therapeutic range (INR < 4), restart warfarin at previous dosage and check INR in 2-3 d and 7 d later.
	If no interacting medication or if interacting medication cannot be eliminated,
	  Hold warfarin, recheck INR in 24-48 hr.
	  When INR approaches therapeutic range (INR < 4), restart warfarin at 20% lower weekly dosage and check INR in 2-3 d and 7 d later.
	If at high risk for bleeding,* give vitamin K_1 1-2.5 mg PO × 1 dose.
	If patient requires reversal for an urgent invasive procedure (within 24 hr), give vitamin K_1 up to 5 mg PO × 1 dose.

INR ≥ 9 without significant bleeding	Review medication list for interacting medications and discontinue interacting medications. Hold warfarin, give higher-dose vitamin K_1 (5 mg PO), and monitor INR daily. Use additional vitamin K_1 (1-2 mg PO) if needed. If no identifiable reason for ↑ INR, reduce weekly warfarin dosage by at least 20%. Hold warfarin until INR approaches the therapeutic range (INR < 4) and check INR 2-3 d and 7 d after warfarin restarted.
Serious bleeding at any INR elevation	Hold warfarin and give vitamin K_1 (10 mg IV over 1 hr in monitored setting with an anaphylaxis kit at bedside). Consider use of fresh frozen plasma, NovoSeven (20 µg/kg IV), or FEIBA (50 U/kg IV). Monitor INR at least every 12 hr.
Life-threatening bleeding	Hold warfarin. Give NovoSeven (20-40 µg/kg IV) or FEIBA (50 U/kg IV). Give vitamin K_1 IV (10 mg IV over 1 hr) in a monitored setting with an anaphylaxis kit at bedside. Monitor INR at least every 6 hr. Vitamin K_1 can be repeated in 12 hr, depending on INR.

From Ansell J et al: *Chest* 126(Suppl):204S-233S, 2004.

INR, international normalized ratio; *IV,* intravenously; *PO,* orally.

*Bleeding risk factors include recent surgery (within 1 mo), active cancer, history of gastrointestinal bleeding or cerebrovascular accident, age >65 yr, serum creatinine >1.5 mg/dl.

COMPARATIVE PHARMACOLOGY AND DOSING TABLES

TABLE 9

COMPARISON OF ANGIOTENSIN-CONVERTING ENZYME INHIBITORS

Mechanism of action	Inhibits the conversion of angiotensin I to angiotensin II, thus interrupting the renin-angiotensin-aldosterone system. In contrast to angiotensin receptor blockers, bradykinin levels are increased.
Special populations	Most effective in high-normal renin hypertension. Additional renoprotective effects in diabetic and nondiabetic renal disease. Lower incidence of cerebrovascular disease and stroke in patients with diabetes. Less effective in African Americans and older adults.
Dosage adjustments	Adjust dosage at 1- to 2-wk intervals. A limited increase in serum creatinine of 35% is acceptable and not a reason to withhold treatment unless hyperkalemia develops.
Common side effects	Central nervous system: headache and dizziness.
	Respiratory: cough (10-44%).
	Gastrointestinal: taste disturbances and nausea.
	Renal: hyperkalemia, deterioration of renal function.
	Dermatologic: rash.
	Hematologic: neutropenia (< 0.005%).
	Obstetric: fetal abnormalities.
	Cardiovascular: hypotension.
	Rare: angioedema (0.1-0.2%; typically occurs in 1st wk of therapy but may be delayed up to 1 yr.)
Drug interactions	Antacids (more likely with captopril; separate administration by 1-2 hr), digoxin, lithium, combination use with angiotensin receptor blockers and potassium supplements, potassium-sparing diuretics, and nonsteroidal antiinflammatory drugs.
Contraindications	Pregnancy, bilateral renal artery stenosis, severe renal failure (caution if serum creatinine > 3 mg/dl).

Agent	Strength	Usual Adult Dosage Maintenance Range (hypertension)	Half-Life	Lipid Solubility	Tissue Angiotensin-Converting Enzyme Inhibition	Active Metabolite	Elimination
Benazepril	5-, 10-, 20-, 40-mg tablets	10-80 mg/d	10-11 hr	No data	Greater	Yes	Primarily renal, some biliary*
Captopril	12.5-, 25-, 50-, 100-mg tablets	75-450 mg given bid or tid	1.7 hr	Not very lipophilic	Less	No	Metabolism to disulfide, then renal*
Enalapril	2.5-, 5-, 10-, 20-mg tablets	10-40 mg/d	2 hr	Lipophilic	Less	Yes	Renal*
Fosinopril	10-, 20-, 40-mg tablets	10-80 mg/d	11-14 hr	Very lipophilic	Less	Yes	Renal (50%), hepatic (50%)
Lisinopril	5-, 10-, 20-mg tablets	10-40 mg/d, maximum 80 mg/d	12 hr	Very hydrophilic	Less	No	Renal*
Moexipril	7.5-, 15-mg tablets	7.5-30 mg/d	2-9 hr	No data	Less	Yes	Renal, fecal*
Perindopril	2-, 4-, 8-mg tablets	4-16 mg qd or bid	3-10 hr	—	Greater	Yes	Renal*
Quinapril	5-, 10-, 20-, 40-mg tablets	10-80 mg daily given qd or bid	3 hr	No data	Greatest-greater	Yes	Renal (60%), hepatic (37%)*
Ramipril	1.25-, 2.5-, 5-, 10-mg capsules	2.5-20 mg/d	13-17 hr	Somewhat lipophilic	Greater	Yes	Renal, fecal
Trandolapril	1-, 2-, 4-mg tablets	2-4 mg qd or bid	6-10 hr	Very lipophilic	Greatest	Yes	Renal (33%)

*Warrants dosage adjustment.

COMPARATIVE PHARMACOLOGY AND DOSING TABLES

TABLE 10

COMPARISON OF ANGIOTENSIN II RECEPTOR ANTAGONISTS

Mechanism of action	Selective blockade of the binding of angiotensin II to type 1 angiotensin II receptors located in brain, renal, myocardial, vascular, and adrenal tissue. Minimal agonist activity because of receptor affinity, $AT_1 >>> AT_2$.
Special populations*	Reduces progression of diabetic nephropathy; reduces both albuminuria and progression to macroalbuminuria. Also beneficial in reducing cerebrovascular disease and stroke incidence in patients with diabetes.
Common side effects	Central nervous system: dizziness, insomnia, headache, fatigue.
	Gastrointestinal: diarrhea, dyspepsia, heartburn, nausea, vomiting.
	Musculoskeletal: arthralgias, muscle cramp.
	Respiratory: upper respiratory infection, cough, nasal congestion.
	Hematologic: small decrease in hemoglobin and hematocrit.
	Lower incidence of cough, angioedema, and possibly hyperkalemia compared with angiotensin-converting enzyme inhibitors.
Dosage adjustments	Adjust dosage at 1- to 2-wk intervals. A limited increase in serum creatinine of 35% above baseline is acceptable and not a reason to withhold treatment unless hyperkalemia develops.
Drug interactions	No significant drug interactions.
Contraindications	Pregnancy, bilateral renal artery stenosis.

Agent	Strength	Usual Adult Maintenance Dosage	Half-Life	Active Metabolite	AT_1 Receptor Antagonism	Elimination	Hepatic or Renal Adjustment	CYP-450 Affinity
Candesartan	4-, 8-, 16-, 32-mg tablets	8-32 mg qd or bid	9-12 hr	Yes	Insurmountable	Renal (60%)	None.	Modest
Eprosartan	400-, 600-mg tablets	400-800 mg qd or bid	5-7 hr	No	Competitive	Renal (90%)	None.	Modest

Irbesartan	75-, 150-, 300-mg tablets	75-300 mg/d	11-15 hr	No	Insurmountable	Biliary (75%)	None.	High but no significant drug interactions
Losartan*	25-, 50-, 100-mg tablets	25-100 mg qd or bid	2 hr (metabolite, 6-9 hr)	Yes	Competitive Metabolite, insurmountable	Biliary (70%)	↓ Dosage by 50% in hepatically impaired patients.	High
Olmesartan	5-, 20-, 40-mg tablets	20-40 mg/d	12-18 hr	Yes	—	Biliary (60%)	None.	—
Telmisartan	40-, 80-mg tablets	40-80 mg/d	24 hr	No	Insurmountable	Biliary (100%)	None. Supervise patients with hepatic impairment closely.	None
Valsartan	80-, 160-, 320-mg capsules	80-320 mg/d	6 hr	No	Competitive	Biliary (80%)	None (only if creatinine clearance < 10 ml/min), mild-moderate hepatic impairment: ≤ 80 mg/d.	Modest

AT_1, angiotensin II type 1; AT_2, angiotensin II type 2.
*Losartan is unique in that it has uricosuric properties (use in patients with gout).

COMPARATIVE PHARMACOLOGY AND DOSING TABLES

TABLE 11

COMPARISON OF β-BLOCKERS

Mechanism of action		
	Cardioselective: competitive, selective inhibition of the β_1-adrenergic receptors with little or no effect on β_2 receptors except at high dosages.	
	Noncardioselective: nonselective β-adrenergic blocker, competitively blocks both β_1- and β_2-adrenergic receptors.	
	ISA: β-blockers with ISA ↓ heart rate and cardiac output to a lesser extent than those without ISA.	
Special populations	Not as effective in older adults because of reduced β receptors or in African Americans because of low renin and volume dependency. May have unfavorable effects on the blood lipid profiles (↑ triglyceride, ↓ high-density lipoprotein); nonselective > > selective agents. May mask hypoglycemic symptoms in diabetics.	
Dosage adjustments	Discontinue by tapering over 2 wk to avoid rebound hypertension. Monitor blood pressure and heart rate.	
Common side effects	Cardiovascular: bradycardia, atrioventricular block, hypotension, postural hypotension, possible deterioration of heart failure.	
	Respiratory: bronchospasm, exacerbation of asthma and chronic obstructive pulmonary disease.	
	Central nervous system: depression, sleep disturbances, insomnia (agents with high lipid solubility), fatigue, dizziness.	
	Gastrointestinal: nausea.	
	Other: hair thinning, peripheral vascular constriction (Raynaud's phenomenon), claudication, cold extremities).	
Drug interactions	Few. Medications that depress the sinoatrial or atrioventricular nodes, or with other negative inotropic agents (verapamil, diltiazem), cimetidine.	
Contraindications	Pregnancy (C/D), severe sinus bradycardia, high-degree heart block, overt left ventricular failure, cardiogenic shock, severe asthma or bronchospasm, severe depression (avoid propranolol), severe or worsening claudication, diabetes.	

Agent	Strength	Cardioselectivity	Usual Adult Maintenance Dosage (hypertension)	Lipid Solubility	ISA	Elimination (secondary)	Renal Dosage Adjustment	Active Metabolite
NONCARDIOSELECTIVE								
Propranolol	10-, 20-, 40-, 60-, 80-mg tablets 60-, 80-, 120-, 160-mg long-acting tablets	β_1 β_2	20-40 mg bid or 60-80 mg/d, mean 160-320 mg/d	High	—	Hepatic	No	Yes

Drug							
Nadolol	20-, 40-, 80-, 120-, 160-mg tablets	β_1 β_2	20-40 mg/d, maximum 320 mg/d	Low	Renal	Yes	No
Timolol	5-, 10-, 20-mg tablets	β_1 β_2	10-20 mg bid, maximum 60 mg/d	Low-moderate	Hepatic (renal)	None	No
CARDIOSELECTIVE							
Atenolol	25-, 50-, 100-mg tablets	β_1	50-200 mg/d (maximum 100 mg for blood pressure effect)	Low	Renal	Yes	No
Bisoprolol	5-, 10-mg tablets	β_1	2.5-5 mg/d	Low-moderate	Renal (hepatic)	Yes	—
Metoprolol	25-, 50-, 100-, 200-mg tablets, extended release (can be split)	β_1	100-200 mg daily, maximum 450 mg/d	Moderate	Hepatic and renal	No	No
VASODILATORY, NONSELECTIVE							
Labetalol	100-, 200-, 300-mg tablets	α_1 β_1 β_2	200-400 mg bid, maximum 2400 mg/d	Moderate-high	Renal (hepatic)	None to +	No
Carvedilol	3.125-, 6.25-, 12.5-, 25-mg tablets	α_1 β_1 β_2	Start 6.25 mg bid, maximum 25 mg bid (50 mg bid if >85 kg)	Low	Hepatic, bile into feces	None	No

ISA, intrinsic sympathomimetic activity.

COMPARATIVE PHARMACOLOGY AND DOSING TABLES

TABLE 12

COMBINATION ANTIHYPERTENSIVES

ACE inhibitor and diuretic	Accuretic (quinapril and HCTZ) 10/12.5, 20/12.5, 20/25 mg
	Capozide (captopril and HCTZ) 25/15, 25/25, 50/15, 50/25 mg
	Lotensin HCT (benazepril hydrochloride and HCTZ) 5/6.25, 10/12.5, 20/12.5, 20/25 mg
	Monopril HCT (fosinopril and HCTZ) 10/12.5, 20/12.5 mg
	Uniretic (moexipril and HCTZ) 7.5/12.5, 15/12.5, 15/25 mg
	Vaseretic (enalapril and HCTZ) 5/12.5, 10/25, 10/25 mg
	Prinzide (lisinopril and HCTZ) 10/12.5, 20/12.5, 20/25 mg
	Zestoretic (lisinopril and HCTZ) 10/12.5, 20/12.5, 20/25 mg
ACE inhibitor and calcium channel blocker	Lexxel (enalapril and felodipine) 5/2.5, 5/5 mg
	Lotrel (amlodipine and benazepril) 2.5/10, 5/10, 5/20, 10/20 mg
	Tarka (trandolapril and verapamil) 2/180, 1/240, 2/240, 4/240 mg
Angiotensin receptor blocker and diuretic	Atacand HCT (candesartan and HCTZ) 16/12.5, 32/12.5 mg
	Avalide (irbesartan and HCTZ) 150/12.5, 300/12.5 mg
	Diovan HCT (valsartan and HCTZ) 80/12.5, 160/12.5, 160/25 mg
	Hyzaar (losartan and HCTZ) 50/12.5, 100/25 mg
	Micardis HCT (telmisartan and HCTZ) 40/12.5, 80/12.5 mg
β-blocker and diuretic	Inderide (propranolol and HCTZ) 40/25, 80/25 mg tablets
	Inderide LA (propranolol LA and HCTZ) 80/50, 120/50, 160/50 mg capsules
	Lopressor HCT (metoprolol and HCTZ) 50/25, 100/25, 100/50 mg tablets
	Tenoretic (atenolol and chlorthalidone) 50/25, 100/25 mg tablets
	Timolide (timolol and HCTZ) 10/25 mg tablets
	Ziac (bisoprolol and HCTZ) 2.5/6.25, 5/6.25, 10/6.25 mg tablets

ACE, angiotensin-converting enzyme; HCT, hydrochlorothiazide; HCTZ, hydrochlorothiazide; LA, long-acting.

TABLE 13

COMPARISON OF CHOLESTEROL AGENTS

HMG CoA reductase inhibitors, mechanism of action	Inhibition of HMG CoA reductase interrupts cholesterol synthesis, increases both LDL receptor synthesis and LDL clearance. Useful for severe hypercholesterolemia and maximal lowering of LDL.
Side effects	Abdominal pain, constipation, diarrhea, dyspepsia, and nausea.
Drug interactions	Azole antifungals, diltiazem, verapamil, grapefruit juice, macrolide antibiotics, nefazodone, warfarin, fibric acids, niacin.
Monitoring	Monitor LFTs and creatine phosphokinase per manufacturer. Monitor international normalized ratio with Crestor and warfarin.

Lipid-Lowering Drug	Dosage Forms	Triglycerides	LDL	HDL	Usual Adult Maintenance Dosage Range	Dosing Instructions	Metabolism	Time to Maximum Effect
Atorvastatin	10-, 20-, 40-mg tablets	↓ 17-51%	↓ 26-60%	↑ 5-13%	10-80 mg/d	Any time of day	CYP3A4	2 wk
Rosuvastatin	5-, 10-, 20-, 40-mg tablets	↓ 28-35%	↓ 45-63%	↑ 10-13%	10-40 mg/d	Any time of day	CYP2C9	4 wk
Fluvastatin	20-, 40-mg capsules	↓ 1-15%	↓ 15-34%	↑ 2-8%	20-80 mg qd or bid	Evening	CYP2C9	3-4 wk
Fluvastatin XL	80-mg tablet	↓ 19-25%	↓ 22-36%	↑ 2-8%	80 mg/d	Evening	CYP2C9	2-4 wk
Lovastatin	10-, 20-, 40-mg tablets	↓ 10-20%	↓ 20-48%	↑ 3-11%	10-80 mg qd or bid	Evening	CYP3A4	4 wk
Pravastatin	10-, 20-, 40-mg tablets	↓ 14-26%	↓ 5-25%	↑ 5-13%	10-40 mg/d	Bedtime	Sulfation	4 wk
Simvastatin	5-, 10-, 20-, 40-, 80-mg tablets	↓ 10-36%	↓ 20-49%	↑ 5-13%	5-80 mg/d	Evening	CYP3A4	4 wk

cont'd

COMPARATIVE PHARMACOLOGY AND DOSING TABLES

TABLE 13
COMPARISON OF CHOLESTEROL AGENTS—cont'd

Bile acid sequestrants, mechanism of action	Binds bile acids in intestine, stimulating their synthesis from cholesterol in the liver. Increase LDL receptors, promoting removal of LDL from plasma. Especially useful in patients with moderately elevated LDL cholesterol.
Side effects	GI: nausea, constipation, bloating, and flatulence. Giving the drugs just before meals may improve tolerance, and increasing dietary fiber may relieve constipation and bloating. May impair absorption of fat-soluble vitamins.
Drug interactions	Acetaminophen, corticosteroids, digitalis glycosides, thiazide diuretics, thyroid hormones, warfarin. Cholestyramine can reduce the absorption of numerous medications when used concurrently. Give other medications 1 hr before or 4 hr after giving cholestyramine. May impair absorption of fat-soluble vitamins.

Lipid-Lowering Drug	Dosage Forms	Triglycerides	LDL	HDL	Usual Adult Maintenance Dosage Range	Dosing Instructions	Metabolism	Time to Maximum Effect
Cholestyramine	4-g packets	↔/↑ 3-5%	↓ 15-30%	↔/↑ 3-10%	4-24 g/d in 2 or more divided doses	None	Nonabsorbable, excreted in feces	3 wk
Colesevelam	625-mg tablets	↔/↑ 9-10%	↓ 9-20%	↑ 3-11%	3750-4375 mg qd or bid	With meals	Nonabsorbable, excreted in feces	2 wk
Colestipol	5-g packets	↔/↑ 3-5%	↓ 15-30%	↔/↑ 3-10%	5-30 g qd or bid	None	Nonabsorbable, excreted in feces	4 wk

Fibric acids, mechanism of action	Decrease synthesis of VLDL, increase lipoprotein lipase activity, increase rate of removal of triglyceride-rich lipoproteins from plasma, and decrease release of free fatty acids from peripheral adipose tissue. Most useful for patients with high triglyceride levels.
Side effects	Most common side effects of fenofibrate are rash and GI symptoms. Most common side effects of gemfibrozil are nausea, diarrhea, and abdominal pain. Risk of rhabdomyolysis when fibric acids are given with HMG CoA reductase inhibitors. Fibric acids are associated with gallstones, myositis, and hepatitis.
Drug interactions	Warfarin, HMG CoA reductase inhibitors.

Lipid-Lowering Drug	Dosage Forms	Triglycerides	LDL	HDL	Usual Adult Maintenance Dosage Range	Dosing Instructions	Metabolism	Time to Maximum Effect
Fenofibrate	54-, 160-mg tablets	↓ 15-60%	↓ 0-29%	↑ 1-34%	67-200 mg/d in up to 3 divided doses	Daily with food	Glucuronidation	2 wk
Gemfibrozil	600-mg tablets	↓ 20-60%	↓ 15-30%	↑ 10-35%	1200 mg/d in 2 doses	Twice daily 30 min before meal	Oxidation	3-4 wk

Niacin-based drugs, mechanism of action	Inhibits lipolysis, decreasing free fatty acids in plasma. Decreases synthesis of VLDL and LDL and catabolism of HDL.
Side effects	Blurred vision, flushing, gastric distress, headache, hepatotoxicity, hyperglycemia, hyperuricemia, and itching. Flushing is reduced by giving aspirin, increasing dosage gradually, and taking with meals. Should be taken with food to reduce GI upset.
Drug interactions	Increased toxicity with statins (myopathy).
Contraindications	Liver disease, active peptic ulcer disease. Used with caution in diabetes or gout.
Monitoring	Monitor LFTs, glucose, serum cholesterol.

cont'd

COMPARATIVE PHARMACOLOGY AND DOSING TABLES

TABLE 13
COMPARISON OF CHOLESTEROL AGENTS—cont'd

Lipid-Lowering Drug	Dosage Forms	Triglycerides	LDL	HDL	Usual Adult Maintenance Dosage Range	Dosing Instructions	Metabolism	Time to Maximum Effect
Niacin	375-, 500-, 750-, 1000-mg ER tablets	↓ 5-35%	↓ 3-17%	↑ 10-26%	1000-2000 mg/d	Bedtime (with food)	Conjugation	3-5 wk
Niacin	250- to 750-mg tablets or capsules, regular or SR	↓ 30-60%	↓ 10-40%	↑ 5-35%	3-8 g/d in 3 or more divided doses	Any time	Conjugation	3-5 wk

Cholesterol absorption inhibitors, mechanism of action	Selectively inhibits intestinal cholesterol and related phytosterol absorption, leading to a decrease in the delivery of intestinal cholesterol to the liver, decreased hepatic cholesterol stores, and an increase in clearance of cholesterol from the blood.
Dosing	When ezetimibe is combined with a statin, LDL is reduced by an additional 6-18%. Combining with a statin can allow use of a lower dosage of the statin, potentially reducing incidence of myopathies.
Side effects	Comparable to placebo. Gastrointestinal: diarrhea. Infection: sinusitis.

Lipid-Lowering Drug	Dosage Forms	Triglycerides	LDL	HDL	Usual Adult Maintenance Dosage Range	Dosing Instructions	Metabolism	Time to Maximum Effect
Ezetimibe	10-mg tablets	↓ 5%	↓ 19%	↑ 3%	10 mg/d.	With or without food		4-6 wk
COMBINATIONS								
Niacin ER and lovastatin	500/20, 750/20, 1000/20 mg tablets	↓ 32-44%	↓ 30-42%	↑ 20-40%	500-2000 mg/d of Niacin ER. Maximum concurrent dosage of lovastatin is 40 mg/d.	Bedtime	Conjugation, CYP3A4	4 wk
Ezetimibe and simvastatin	10/10, 10/20, 10/40, 10/80 mg tablets	↓ 23-31%	↓ 45-60%	↑ 6-10%	10/10 mg/d to 10/80 mg/d. Do not exceed 10/10 mg with concurrent cyclosporine or danazol use. Do not exceed 10/20 mg with concurrent amiodarone or verapamil use.	Bedtime		4-6 wk

ER, extended release; *GI*, gastrointestinal; *HDL*, high-density lipoprotein; *HMG CoA*, β-hydroxy-β-methylglutaryl-coenzyme A; *LDL*, low-density lipoprotein; *LFTs*, liver function tests; *SR*, slow release; *VLDL*, very low density lipoprotein.

COMPARATIVE PHARMACOLOGY AND DOSING TABLES

TABLE 14
COMPARISON OF ANTIDIABETIC MEDICATIONS

	Tablet Strengths	Usual Daily Dosage	Maximum Dosage	Duration of Action	Equivalent Dosage	Comment
Sulfonylureas						Mechanism of action: Stimulate insulin secretion through binding to membrane receptors on β cells (no effect on insulin synthesis).
						Dosage increase schedule: Every 1-2 wk.
						Typical decrease in HbA1c, monotherapy: ↓ 1.5-2% (from placebo), ↓ 1.0-2.0% (from baseline).
						Comments: Do not use in pregnancy.
						Side effects: ↓ glycemia, ↑ weight.
Acetohexamide	250, 500 mg tablets	500-750 mg/d*	1500 mg/d	10-14 hr	500 mg	
Chlorpropamide	100, 250 mg tablets	250-375 mg/d	500 mg/d	72 hr	250 mg	SIADH, disulfiram reaction. Very long t(1/2), caution in older adults.
Tolazamide	100, 250, 500 mg tablets	250-500 mg/d*	1000 mg/d	10-14 hr	250 mg	SIADH, ↓ rate of disulfiram reaction than chlorpropamide.
Tolbutamide	250, 500 mg tablets	1000-2000 mg/d*	3000 mg/d	6-12 hr	1000 mg	SIADH, ↓ rate of disulfiram reaction than chlorpropamide. No dosage adjustment in renal impairment.
Second-generation sulfonylureas						Comments: Do not use in pregnancy.
Glipizide	5, 10 mg tablets	5-20 mg/d*	40 mg	10-24 hr	5 mg	No dosage adjustment in renal impairment; dosage adjustment in hepatic impairment. Take before meals.

Drug	Preparations	Dosage	Max Dose	Duration		Side Effects/Comments
Glyburide	1.25, 2.5, 5 mg tablets	5-20 mg/d*	20 mg	18-24 hr	2.5 mg	Dosage adjustment in renal impairment. C/I in severe renal impairment. Dosage adjustment in hepatic impairment.
Third-generation sulfonylureas						
Glimepiride	1, 2, 4 mg tablets	2-8 mg/d	8 mg	24 hr	1-2 mg	Hypoglycemia, headache.
Nonsulfonylureas (secretagogues), meglitinides	Mechanism of action: stimulates insulin release from pancreatic β cells; requires presence of glucose for its action. Typical decrease in HbA1c, monotherapy: ↓ 1.7% repaglinide (from placebo); ↓ 0.7-1% nateglinide (from placebo); ↓ 1.0-2.0% (from baseline). Comments: Side effect profile similar to that of sulfonylureas; given 15 min before each meal.					
Repaglinide	0.5, 1, 2 mg tablets	0.5-4 mg with each meal	16 mg	< 4 hr		Hypoglycemia, gastrointestinal (nausea, vomiting) low. Well tolerated.
Nateglinide	60, 120 mg tablets	60-120 mg tid	360 mg/d	< 4 hr	4 hr	
Biguanides	Mechanism of action: ↓ hepatic glucose production, ↑ peripheral insulin sensitivity; does not increase insulin secretion. Dosage increase schedule: every 2 wk. Typical decrease in HbA1c, monotherapy: ↓ 1.5-2% (from placebo); ↓ 1.0-2.0% (from baseline). Comments: does not cause hypoglycemia alone; do not use in pregnancy. C/I: serum creatinine > 1.5 men, 1.4 women; CHF, 48 hr after contrast dye.					
Metformin (Glucophage) Glucophage XR	500, 850, 1000 mg tablets	500-2000 mg/d, 500-2000 mg/d, may be divided	2550 mg/d	12 hr	N/A	Development of lactic acidosis rare. Watery diarrhea, abdominal pain, nausea; minimize by taking with large meal.

cont'd

COMPARATIVE PHARMACOLOGY AND DOSING TABLES

TABLE 14
COMPARISON OF ANTIDIABETIC MEDICATIONS—cont'd

	Tablet Strengths	Usual Daily Dosage	Maximum Dosage	Duration of Action	Equivalent Dosage	Comment
Glucovance (glyburide and metformin)	500-mg tablets 1.25/250, 2.5/500, 5/500 tablets					May decrease weight.
α-Glucosidase inhibitors	Mechanism of action: reversibly inhibit the α-glucosidase enzymes in the rush border of the small intestine and delay the cleavage of oligosaccharides and disaccharides to monosaccharides. Dosage increase schedule solidus every 2-4 wk. Typical decrease in HbA1c, monotherapy: ↓ 0.5-1% (from placebo); ↓ 0.5-1% (from baseline). Comments: Alone does not cause hypoglycemia; must use glucose for management of hypoglycemia when used as dual therapy. C/I: intestinal diseases, obstructive bowel diseases, IBD.					
Acarbose	50, 100 mg tablets	25 mg tid (with meals)	< 60 kg, 50 mg tid > 60 kg, 100 mg tid	2 hr	NA	Low initial dosages and slow titration. Flatulence, cramping, diarrhea.
Miglitol	25, 50, 75 mg tablets	25 mg tid	100 mg tid	2 hr	NA	Dosage adjustment in renal impairment; not recommended serum creatinine > 2 mg/dl.
Thiazolidinediones	Mechanism of action: enhances insulin action, promoting glucose utilization in peripheral tissues; no effect on insulin secretion. Dosage increase schedule: every 3-4 wk, maximum effect 6-8 wk. Typical decrease in HbA1c, monotherapy: ↓ 1-1.5% (from placebo); ↓ 0.5-1.0% (from baseline). Comments: Instruct patients on signs and symptoms of hepatic dysfunction (nausea and vomiting, abdominal pain, jaundice, dark urine); liver function abnormalities and acute hepatic failure seen in post-marketing surveillance; resumption of ovulation in premenopausal anovulatory patients; dose-related weight gain seen.					

Rosiglitazone†	2, 4 mg tablets	4-8 mg/d; ↑ after 8-12 wk	16 mg/d	N/A	N/A	Better efficacy with divided dosing. C/I in New York Heart Association III, IV. No significant D/I to date. ↑ HDL (8-13%), ↑ LDL (18-23%), ↑ TG (≈15%).
Pioglitazone†	15, 30, 45 mg tablets; ↓ 1.9% with pioglitazone 45 mg seen in 1 dose ranging study	15-30 mg/d	45 mg/d	N/A	N/A	Metabolized by CYP4503A4 (17%). ↑ HDL (≈15-19%), ↑ LDL (7-15%), ↓ TG (9.3-12%).
Combination products: Avandamet (rosiglitazone maleate and metformin)	1/500, 2/500, 4/500, 2/1000, 4/1000 mg tablets					

C/I, contraindicated; CHF, congestive heart failure; D/I, drug interaction; HDL, high-density lipoprotein; IBD, irritable bowel disease; LDL, low-density lipoprotein; SIADH, syndrome of inappropriate antidiuretic hormone secretion; TG, triglyceride.

*May also be given in divided doses.

†May lower risk of liver function abnormalities: monitor liver function at baseline and periodically at discretion; stop when liver function tests are 1.5-2× normal, anemia, or edema.

COMPARATIVE PHARMACOLOGY AND DOSING TABLES

TABLE 15

COMPARISON OF INSULIN PRODUCTS

Product	Pharmacokinetics*	Comments
RAPID-ACTING INSULINS		
Lispro (Humalog)	Onset: 5-15 min Peak: 30-90 min Duration: 4-5 hr Absorption rate: less variable	More closely mimics the endogenous insulin response to a meal than regular insulin. Inject immediately before meal. Cost for 10 ml (100 U/ml): $55.
Aspart (NovoLog)	Onset: 5-15 min Peak: 1-3 hr Duration: 3-5 hr Absorption rate: less variable	More closely mimics the endogenous insulin response to a meal than regular insulin. Inject immediately before meal. Cost for 10 ml (100 U/ml): $65.
Glulisine (Apidra)	Onset: 20 min Peak: 30-90 min Duration: 5-6 hr Absorption rate: not available	No cost to date. Available via Early Access Program until early 2006 launch.
SHORT-ACTING INSULINS		
Regular U100, (Humulin R, Novolin R)	Onset: 30-60 min Peak: 2-3 hr Duration: 3-8 hr Absorption rate: somewhat variable	Inject 30-45 min before meal. Cost for 10 ml (100 U/ml): $25.
INTERMEDIATE-ACTING INSULINS		
NPH (Humulin N, Novolin N)	Onset: 2-4 hr Peak: 4-10 hr Duration: 10-16 hr Absorption rate: somewhat variable	NPH is a suspension and must be resuspended before each injection (gently roll bottle). Cost for 10 ml (100 U/ml): $28.
Insulin zinc (Lente, Humulin L, Novolin L)	Onset: 2-4 hr Peak: 4-12 hr Duration: 12-18 hr Absorption rate: somewhat variable	Cost for 10 ml (100 U/ml): $25.
LONG-ACTING INSULINS		
Ultralente (Humulin U)	Onset: 6-10 hr Peak: 10-16 hr Duration: 18-20 Absorption rate: more variable	Cost for 10 ml (100 U/ml): $28.
Insulin glargine (Lantus)	Onset: 2-4 hr Peak: No peak Duration: 24 hr Absorption rate: constant	Cannot be mixed with other insulins. Cannot be predrawn into syringes at this time. Can be given in AM or PM. Less nocturnal hypoglycemia than NPH and ultralente. Does not need to be resuspended. Switching: ↓ total NPH dosage by 20% for daily glargine dosage. Cost for 10 ml (100 U/ml): $46.

NPH, neutral protamine Hagedorn.

*Rate of absorption: route, IV > IM > SC; site, abdomen > arm > thigh.

PART IV

Rapid References

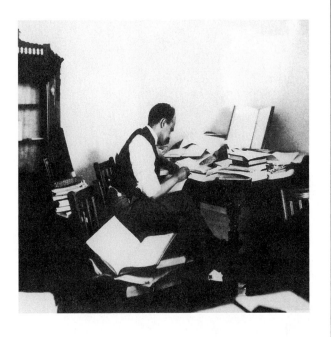

Reverse, Sir William Osler writing *The Principles and Practice of Medicine* during his tenure at the Johns Hopkins Hospital in 1891.

Rapid References

Tracy J. Warner, MD; and Matthew R. Baldwin, MD

I. CARDIOLOGY

NORMAL VALUES

Hemodynamic Parameter	Normal Value
Heart rate (HR)	60-100 beats/min
Stroke volume (SV = EDV − ESV)	60-100 ml/beat, 40-70 ml/m^2
Cardiac output (CO = HR × SV)	4-8 L/min
Body surface area (BSA)	1.73 m^2 (average 70-kg man)
Cardiac index (CI = CO/BSA)	2.6-4.2 L/min/m^2
Stroke volume index (SVI = CI/HR)	40-50 ml/beat/m^2
Systolic blood pressure (SBP)	120 mmHg
Diastolic blood pressure (DBP)	80 mmHg
Pulse pressure (PP = SBP − DBP)	40 mmHg
Mean arterial pressure (MAP = DBP + 1/3 PP)	70-105 mmHg
End diastolic volume (EDV)	70 ml/m^2
End systolic volume (ESV)	0-30 ml/m^2
Ejection fraction (EF = SV/EDV)	55-65%
Central venous pressure (CVP = RAP = RVEDP)	0-6 mmHg
Right atrial pressure (RAP)	0-6 mmHg
Right ventricular end-diastolic pressure (RVEDP)	0-6 mmHg
Right ventricular systolic pressure	15-30 mmHg
Left atrial pressure (LAP = Left ventricular end-diastolic pressure = PCWP)	5-12 mmHg
Pulmonary artery systolic pressure (PAS)	15-30 mmHg
Pulmonary artery diastolic pressure (PAD)	5-12 mmHg
Mean pulmonary artery pressure (PAP)	10-15 mmHg
Pulmonary capillary wedge pressure (PCWP)	5-12 mmHg
Coronary perfusion pressure (CPP)	60-70 mmHg
Systemic vascular resistance (SVR)	800-1200 ([dyne × s]/cm^5)
Arteriovenous O_2 difference (AVDO_2)	30-45 ml/L
Pulmonary vascular resistance (PVR)	120-250 ([dyne × s]/cm^5)

EQUATIONS

Fick principle:

$$\text{Cardiac output (L/min)} = O_2 \text{ consumption (ml/min)/AVD}O_2 \text{ (ml/L)}$$

$$\text{AVD}O_2 \text{ (ml/L)} = \text{Hg (g/dl)} \times 1.36 \times (\text{Sa}O_2 - \text{Sv}O_2)$$

SaO_2 is measured in any arterial sample, and SvO_2 is measured in right atrium, right ventricle, or pulmonary artery.

$$\text{SVR [(dyne × s)/cm}^5] = 80[\text{MAP (mmHg)} - \text{RAP (mmHg)}]/\text{CO (L/min)}$$

$$\text{PVR [(dyne × sec)/cm}^5] = 80[\text{PAP (mmHg)} - \text{PCWP}$$
$$\text{or LAP (mmHg)}]/\text{CO (L/min)}$$

Friedewald formula: Total cholesterol = LDL + HDL + Triglycerides/5

All values are in plasma or serum (mg/dl). This formula is invalid if the triglyceride level is >400 mg/dl.

(Data from Friedewald WT et al: *Clin Chem* 18:499, 1972.)

CATHETERIZATION

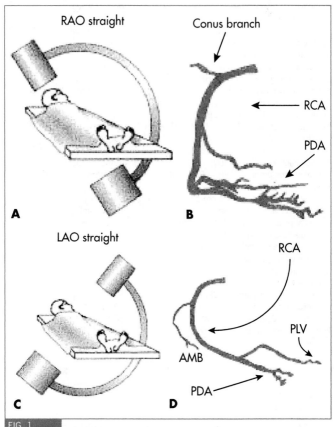

FIG. 1

Catheterization. *(From Braunwald E: Heart disease: a textbook of cardiovascular medicine, 6th ed, Philadelphia, 2001, WB Saunders.)*

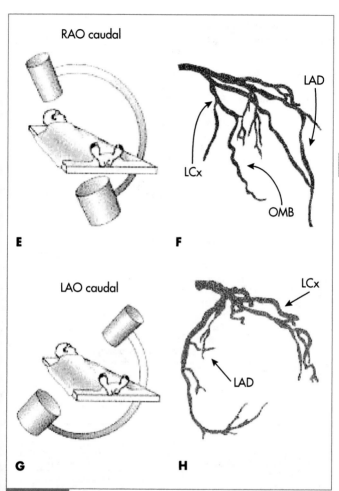

RAO caudal

LAD
LCx
OMB

E

F

LAO caudal

LCx
LAD

G

H

FIG. 1—cont'd

II. PULMONARY

Pulmonary Parameter	Equation	Normal Value
Tidal volume (V_T)	V_T = Volume of dead space (V_D) + $V_{alveolar\ space}$	~500 ml
Minute ventilation (V_E)	$V_E = V_T \times$ Respiratory rate (RR)	4-6 L/min
V_D (Bohr equation)	$V_D = V_T \times (Paco_2 - P_{expired}CO_2)/Paco_2$	~150 ml
Compliance = ΔVolume/ ΔPressure	Respiratory system compliance (CRS) = $V_T/(P_{plateau} - PEEP)$ $P_{plateau}$ = Inspiratory plateau pressure, PEEP = Positive end-expiratory pressure	> 60 ml/cm H_2O
Alveolar gas equation	$PAO_2 = FiO_2 [P_{ATM} (760\ mmHg) - P_{H2O} (47\ mmHg)] - Pco_2/$ [Respiratory quotient (0.8)] $\approx 150 - (Paco_2/0.8)$	100 mmHg
Alveolar-arterial oxygen gradient	A-a gradient (sea level, 37°C) = $PAO_2 - PaO_2$	≤ (Age/4) + 4
$Paco_2$	$Paco_2 = 0.863 \times CO_2$ production/ Alveolar ventilation	40 mmHg
Arterial O_2 content (CaO_2) (ml O_2/ml blood)	$CaO_2 = 1.36 \times Hgb \times SaO_2 + 0.003 \times PaO_2$	20 ml/100 ml
Mixed venous O_2 content (CvO_2) (ml O_2/ml blood)	$CvO_2 = 1.36 \times Hgb \times SvO_2 + 0.003 \times PvO_2$	15 ml/100 ml
Shunt fraction (QS/QT)	QS/QT (%) = $(CcO_2 - CaO_2)/(CcO_2 - CvO_2)$ CcO_2 = end-capillary O_2 content, derived from PAO_2 and O_2 dissociation curves, CaO_2 = arterial oxygen content, CvO_2 = mixed venous oxygen content	< 10%

STATIC LUNG VOLUMES

Total lung capacity (TLC)	Vital capacity (VC)	Inspiratory capacity (IC)	Inspiratory reserve volume (IRV)
			Tidal volume (TV)
		Functional residual capacity (FRC)	Expiratory reserve volume (ERV)
	Residual volume (RV)		Residual volume (RV)

OXYHEMOGLOBIN DISSOCIATION CURVE

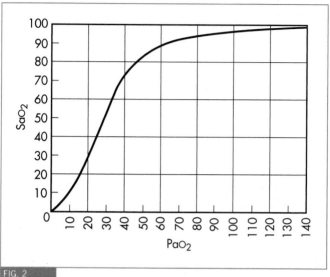

FIG. 2

Oxyhemoglobin dissociation curve. *(Data from Guinan M: Interpretation of ABGs: A four-step method, from www.rnceus.com/abgs/abgcurve.html.)*

SHIFT OF OXYHEMOGLOBIN DISSOCIATION CURVE

Left Shift (higher affinity of Hgb for O_2)	Right Shift (lower affinity of Hgb for O_2)
Alkalosis	Acidosis
Hypothermia	Hyperthermia
Decreased 2,3-diphosphoglycerate (DPG)	Increased 2,3-DPG
Fetal hemoglobin	

OXYGEN SUPPORT

Oxygen Source	Flow Rate (L/min)	FIO_2	PaO_2 at Sea Level (mmHg)
Room air	0	0.21	100
Nasal cannula	1-6	↑ by 0.04/L/min	≥ 227
Venturi mask	1-4	≥ 0.5	≥ 300
Face mask	6-15	≥ 0.6	≥ 370
Partial rebreather	5-7	≥ 0.8	≥ 512
Nonrebreather	≥ 15	≥ 1 (actual ~0.9)	≥ 655

III. RENAL

OSMOLALITY FORMULAS

Calculated osmolality = 2[Na$^+$] + Glucose/18 + BUN/2.8 + Ethanol/4.6
(Normal = 275-290 mOsm/kg)

Concentrations in mg/dl. Note: BUN is considered an ineffective osmolyte.

Osmolal gap = Measured osmolality − Calculated osmolality
(Normal < 10)

Concentrations in mg/dl.

CREATININE CLEARANCE (CrCl)

Measured CrCl = U$_{creat}$ (mg/dl)/P$_{creat}$ (mg/dl) ×
U$_{volume}$ (ml/day)/(1440 min/1 day)
= U$_{creat}$ (mg/day)/P$_{creat}$ (mg/dl) × 0.07

Modification of Diet in Renal Disease (MDRD) Study Group equation:

GFR (ml/min/1.732) = 170 × Cr$^{-0.999}$ × Age$^{-0.176}$ × BUN$^{-0.17}$
× Albumin$^{+0.318}$ × 0.762
if female × 1.18 if African American

Cockcroft-Gault equation:

CrCl = {[(140 − Age) × Weight (kg)]/(72 × P$_{creat}$)} × 0.85 if female

Online calculator: nephron.com/mdrd/default.html.

FRACTIONAL EXCRETION OF SODIUM (FE$_{NA}$)

FE$_{Na}$ = % Filtered sodium load excreted
= Urine Na/U$_{creat}$ × P$_{creat}$/Plasma Na × 100

Most helpful in oliguric patients, defined as urine volume <500 ml/day or <20 ml/hr who have not been on diuretics.

FRACTIONAL EXCRETION OF UREA (FE$_{urea}$)

FE$_{urea}$ = U$_{urea}$/BUN × P$_{creat}$/U$_{creat}$ × 100

COMPENSATION FOR ACID-BASE DISORDERS

	Expected Compensation	
	Acidosis	Alkalosis
Acute respiratory	ΔpH = −0.08 × ΔPaco$_2$	ΔpH = 0.1 × ΔPaco$_2$
	↑ HCO$_3$ = 0.1 × ΔPaco$_2$	↓ HCO$_3$ = 0.2 × ΔPaco$_2$
Chronic respiratory	ΔpH = −0.03 × ΔPaco$_2$	ΔpH—may normalize
	↑ HCO$_3$ = 0.3 × ΔPaco$_2$	↓ HCO$_3$ = 0.4 × ΔPaco$_2$
Metabolic	Paco$_2$ = 1.5 × [HCO$_3^-$] + 8 ± 2	Paco$_2$ = 0.9 × [HCO$_3^-$]
	(Winters' formula) or	+ 9 ± 2
	Paco$_2$ = last 2 digits of pH	↑ Paco$_2$ = 0.75 × HCO$_3$

IV. GASTROENTEROLOGY
MODEL FOR END-STAGE LIVER DISEASE (MELD)

$$\text{MELD} = 3.8[e^{\text{serum bilirubin (mg/dl)}}] + 11.2[e^{\text{INR}}] + 9.6[e^{\text{serum creatinine (mg/dl)}}] + 6.4$$

Any lab values < 1 are rounded to 1; serum creatinine > 4 or hemodialysis is rounded to 4.

Concurrent hepatocellular carcinoma:

- If no biopsy diagnosis, an increasing alpha-fetoprotein in a patient with chronic liver disease is an automatic MELD of 20 if the calculated MELD is less.
- American Liver Tumor Study Group (ALTSG) stage II (single tumor 2-5 cm or two to three lesions < 3 cm): automatic MELD of 24, which is then increased 4 points every 3 months thereafter even if calculated MELD is less.
- ALTSG stage I and III do not merit higher MELD priority scores.

Online calculator:
www.unos.org/resources/MeldPeldCalculator.asp?index=98.

CHILD-PUGH CLASSIFICATION

	Points Assigned		
	1	2	3
Bilirubin (mg/dl)	< 2	2-3	> 3
Albumin (g/dl)	> 3.5	2.8-3.5	< 2.8
Prothrombin time (s)	1-3	4-6	> 6
Ascites	None	Mild	Moderate
Encephalopathy*	None	Grade I-II	Grade III-IV
	Classification		
	A	B	C
Total points	5-6	7-9	> 9

Data from Pugh RN et al: *Br J Surg* 60:646, 1973.
*Encephalopathy: I = mild confusion or slowing, no asterixis; II = drowsy, asterixis present; III = marked confusion, somnolence, asterixis present; IV = unresponsive or responsive only to painful stimuli, asterixis present.

HEPATITIS DISCRIMINANT FUNCTION: MADDREY SCORE
Data from Carithers RL Jr et al: *Ann Intern Med* 110:685, 1989.

Maddrey score = 4.6 × (Prothrombin time − Control prothrombin time) + Serum bilirubin (mg/dl)

Stool osmolal gap = Plasma osmolality − 2 × (Stool [Na] + Stool [K])

V. ENDOCRINOLOGY
GLYCOSYLATED HEMOGLOBIN (HbA1c)

Mean plasma glucose (mg/dl) = (35.6 × HbA1c) − 77.3

FREE THYROXINE INDEX (FTI)

$$FTI = T_4 \times T_3RU/100 \text{ (Normal = 1-4)}$$

T_4 = thyroxine, T_3RU = triiodothyronine resin uptake.

VI. HEMATOLOGY AND ONCOLOGY

Data from Hillman et al: *Br J Haematol* 17:313, 1969.

Corrected reticulocyte count (CRC) = % Reticulocytes
$\times$ Patient hematocrit (HCT)/Normal HCT

Indicator of erythropoietic activity, corrected for differences in HCT. CRC >1.5 suggests ↑ RBC production.

Maturation factor (MF) = 1 if patient's HCT is 45 and
then ↑ 0.5 for each 10-point ↓ in HCT.

Reticulocyte distribution index = (Measured HCT/Normal HCT
$\times$ Reticulocyte count)/Maturation factor

Allows assessment of reticulocyte response for degree of anemia. In anemia, an index <2 is inadequate, 2-3 is borderline, and >3 is normal.

VII. FLUID, ELECTROLYTES, AND NUTRITION
CONTENT OF COMMON INTRAVENOUS FLUIDS

IVF Solution	Na^+ (mEq/L)	K^+ (mEq/L)	Cl^- (mEq/L)	HCO_3^- (mEq/L)	Osmolality (mOsm/L)	Dextrose (g/L)	Dextrose (kcal/L)
D_5W					278	50	170
$D_{10}W$					556	100	340
½ NS	77		77		143		
NS	154		154		286		
3% saline	513		513		1026		
LR	130	4	109	28	272	50	170

D, dextrose; *IVF*, intravenous fluid; *LR*, lactated Ringer's; *NS*, normal saline; *W*, water.

MAINTENANCE FLUIDS

	For 24-Hour Period	For an Hourly Rate
For first 10 kg	100 ml/d/kg	4 ml/hr/kg
For second 10 kg	50 ml/d/kg	2 ml/hr/kg
For each additional kg	20 ml/d/kg	1 ml/hr/kg

FREE WATER DEFICIT

$$\text{Free water deficit (L)} = \{\text{Correction factor} \times \text{Weight (kg)} \times (\text{Patient's } [Na^+] - 140)\}/140$$

Correction factor for men = 0.6, Correction factor for women = 0.5. Body weight used should be ideal body weight.

BODY FLUID DISTRIBUTION IN HEALTHY ADULTS

Parameter	Derivation	Male	Female
Total body water (TBW)	$0.6 \times$ Lean body weight (kg)	600 ml/kg	500 ml/kg
Male	$0.5 \times$ Lean body weight (kg)		
Female			
Intracellular body water	$0.4 \times$ Lean body weight (kg)	400 ml/kg	333 ml/kg
Extracellular body water	$0.2 \times$ Lean body weight (kg)	200 ml/kg	167 ml/kg
Interstitial fluid volume	$0.16 \times$ Lean body weight (kg)	160 ml/kg	160 ml/kg
Blood volume (BV)	$0.065 \times$ Lean body weight (kg)	70 ml/kg	65 ml/kg
Plasma volume (PV)	PV = BV− (BV × Hematocrit)	37 ml/kg	38 ml/kg

Data from *Documenta Geigy scientific tables*, 7th ed, Basel, Switzerland, 1970, JR Geigy SA.

$$\text{Corrected total calcium} = (4 \times \text{Albumin}) \times 0.8$$
$$+ \text{ Measured serum calcium}$$

SERUM SODIUM FORMULAS

Serum Na correction factors:

- Na increases by 1.6 mmol/L per 100 mg/dl of serum glucose above 100 mg/dl.
- Na increases by 1.0 mmol/L for each 500 mg/dl of plasma lipid (triglyceride and cholesterol).
- Na increases by 1.0 mmol/L for each 4.0 g/dl of plasma protein above 8.0 g/dl.

Estimated Na excess in hypernatremia:

$$\text{Na excess (mEq/L)} = 0.6 \times \text{Body weight (kg)}$$
$$\times (\text{Current plasma } [Na^+] - 140)$$

Estimated Na deficit in hyponatremia:

$$\text{Na deficit (mEq)} = 0.6 \times \text{Body weight} \times (\text{Desired plasma } [Na^+]$$
$$- \text{Current plasma } [Na^+])$$

BODY SURFACE AREA

$$\text{Body surface area (BSA)} = \sqrt{[\text{Height (cm)} \times \text{Weight (kg)}]/60}$$

BODY MASS INDEX

$$\text{Body mass index (BMI)} = \text{Weight (kg)}/[\text{Height (m)}]^2$$

IDEAL BODY WEIGHT (IBW)

$$\text{IBW (male)} = 50 \text{ kg} + 2.3 \text{ kg for each inch over 5 ft}$$

$$\text{IBW (female)} = 45.5 \text{ kg} + 2.3 \text{ kg for each inch over 5 ft}$$

VIII. EPIDEMIOLOGY

		Disease	
		+	−
Test	+	A	B
	−	C	D

Sensitivity = A/(A + C)   Positive predictive value = A/(A + B)

Specificity = D/(B + D)   Negative predictive value = D/(C + D)

Prevalence = (A + C)/(A + B + C + D)   Odds ratio = (A × D)/(B × C)

Index

Sn indicates supplemental content available in bonus PDA download.

A
α_1 antagonists, 117
AAI pacing mode, 185
Abdominal pain
  colicky, 445
  diagnostic testing, 351
  history of, 349-351
  initial management of, 352
  by location, 350t
  physical examination, 351
  unusual cause of, 359-360
Abdominal radiography, 49
  labeled, 50f
Acanthocytes, spur cells, 476
Accelerated acute rejection and acute
     humoral rejection
  diagnosis of, 810
  epidemiology of, 810
  management of, 810
  presentation of, 810
ACE. See Angiotensin-converting enzyme
     inhibitors
Acetaminophen
  as an antipyretic, 330
  diagnosis of, 382
  presentation of, 382
  Rumack-Matthew nomogram for
     acetaminophen poisoning,
     383f
  treatment of, 382
Acetylcysteine in preventing nephrotoxicity,
     52
Acid-base disorders, 771-782
  compensation for, 1012
  definition of fundamental, 771-772
  overview of, 771
  presentation of, 773
  step-by-step analysis, 772-776
Acquired immunodeficiency syndrome
     (AIDS), 275, S6. See also Human
     immunodeficiency virus
ACS. See Acute coronary syndrome
ACTH stimulation tests, 310
Activated partial thromboplastin time
     (aPTT), 520
Acute acalculous cholecystitis
  diagnosis of, 374
  epidemiology and pathophysiology of,
     374
  presentation of, 374
  treatment of, 374
Acute aortic dissection, 76
Acute calculous cholecystitis
  diagnosis of, 373
  pathophysiology of, 372

Acute calculous cholecystitis (*Continued*)
  presentation of, 372
  treatment of, 373
Acute cellular rejection, S2-S3
  diagnosis of, 810
  epidemiology of, 810
  in heart transplant, S2
  in liver transplant, S3
  management of, 810
  presentation of, 810
Acute chest syndrome
  definition of, 488
  management of, 488
  transfusion, 488
Acute coronary syndrome (ACS), 74, 86-
     102
  clinical presentation of, 86-88
  diagnosis of, 88
    cardiac biomarkers, 89
    electrocardiogram, 88
  ECG in, 74
    non-ST segment elevation, 88
    ST segment elevation, 88
  management of, 86
    with ST segment, 86
    without ST segment, 86
  signs and symptoms of, 87t
Acute diarrhea, 593
  approach to, 462f
  clinical presentation and diagnosis of,
     456-460
  evaluation of, 457
  history of, 457
  infectious diarrhea
    diagnosis of, 458t
    differential diagnosis of, 458t-459t
    management of, 460
Acute interstitial nephritis (AIN), 732-733
  diagnosis of, 733
  epidemiology and etiology of, 732
  management of, 733
  presentation of, 732
  prognosis of, 733
Acute liver failure (ALF), 377
  complication of, 384t-385t
Acute lymphocytic leukemias (ALLs), S5
Acute meningitis, differential diagnosis of,
     621t
Acute myeloid leukemia, S5
Acute pancreatitis, 362-368
  diagnosis of, 363-364
    imaging, 364
    laboratory evaluation, 363
  epidemiology of, 362-363
  management of, 365-367

Acute pericarditis, 165-170
    clinical presentation of, 165-166
    diagnosis of, 165-166
    epidemiology of, 165
    etiology and management of, 167-170
        infectious pericarditis, 167
        metabolic dearrangement, 168-169
        neoplastic disease, 169
        radiographic imaging, 172
        rheumatic disease, 169
Acute Physiological and Chronic Health
        Evaluation (APACHE II) tool, 212
Acute pulmonary edema and heart failure,
        nitrates role in, 137
Acute renal colic
    diagnosis of, 764
    epidemiology and etiology of, 762
    management of, 765-767
        long term, 765
        short term, 765
    presentation of, 764
    risk stratification and prognosis of, 765
Acute renal failure
    clinical presentation of, 710
    diagnosis of, 711-715
    epidemiology of, 709-710
    management of, 715-716
    oliguria and, 260
    pathophysiology and differential
        diagnosis of, 710-711
    preventive measure of, 716-717
Acute respiratory alkalosis, on arterial
        blood gas analysis, 254
Acute respiratory distress syndrome
        (ARDS), 236
Acute respiratory failure, 218-226
    cause of, 219-222
        hypercapnic, 219
        hypoxemic, 219
    clinical presentation of, 218-219
    diagnosis of, 219
    management of, 222
Acute retroviral syndrome
    diagnosis of, 562-563
    epidemiology of, 562
    management of, 563
    presentation of, 562
    symptoms and signs of, 564t
Acute tubular necrosis (ATN)
    diagnosis of, 734
    epidemiology and etiology of, 733-734
    management of, 734-735
    presentation of, 734
    prognosis of, 735
Addison's disease, 302, 304
Adefovir, a nucleotide analog, 395
Adenosine, as diagnostic tool, 189
Adrenal imaging with
        metaiodobenzylguanidine, 53
Adrenal insufficiency, 302-310
    clinical presentation of, 304
    diagnosis of, 304-308, 307f

Adrenal insufficiency (Continued)
    epidemiology of, 302
    etiology of, 304
    management of, 309
    pathophysiology of, 304
Adrenocorticotropic hormone stimulating
        testing, 260
Adult respiratory distress syndrome
    definition of, 224
    diagnosis of, 224
    epidemiology and etiology of, 223
    management of, 225
Advanced cardiopulmonary life support,
        6f
Adverse drug reactions, classification of,
        37, 38t
AF. See Atrial fibrillation
Afterload, 150
Alanine aminotransferase (ALT), 378
Alanine aminotransferase level of gallstone
        pancreatitis, 364
Alcohol withdrawal syndromes, 847-851
    diagnosis of, 848-849
    epidemiology of, 847
    management and treatment of, 849-
        851
    presentation of, 848
    risk stratification and prognosis of, 849
Alcoholic liver disease, 405
    epidemiology of, 405
    evaluation of, 405
    management of, 405
Aldosterone antagonism, 142
Alkaline phosphatase (AP), 378
Allen test, 24-25
Allergic reactions, Gell and Coombs
        classification of, 40t
Allergic rhinitis, S4
Allograft dysfunction, causes of, S3, S13
Allopurinol, 272
Alpha-1 antitrypsin deficiency, 410
Alveolar-arterial oxygen gradient equation,
        219
American Diabetes Association calorie-
        restricted diet, 293
Amiodarone
    antiarrhythmic agent, 200, 208
    thyroid dysfunction and, 322t
Amylase and lipase levels in pancreatitis,
        364
Amylase levels, 313
Anaphylaxis. See also Allergic reactions;
        Allergic rhinitis
    cause of, 37
    diagnosis of, 41
    differential diagnosis of, 41t
    epidemiology of, 37
    hypotension in, 38
    management of, 42
    manifestations of, 39f
    therapy for, 42
Androgen replacement in women, 309

Anemia
  clinical presentation of, 475-476
  diagnosis of, 476-479, 478f
  epidemiology of, 475
  management of, 479-482
Angioedema, 37
  hereditary, 43
  and urticaria, 43
  without urticaria, 37
Angioneurotic edema, 359
Angiotensin-converting enzyme inhibitors,
    42
  comparison of, 988t-989t
  in diabetic patients, 116
  in heart failure, 141
  with systolic dysfunction, 140
Angiotensin II receptor antagonists
  comparison of, 990t-991t
Anion gap
  calculation of, 314
  and serum osmolality, 314
Anisocytosis, 476
Anterior myocardial infarction, 67f
Anteroseptal leads, 63
Anthrax, S8
Antiarrhythmic drugs
  class IA agents, 207
  class IC agents, 207
  class III agents, 208
Antibiotics, broad-spectrum, 261
Anticoagulation
  in non-ST segment elevation, 92
  with warfarin, 142, 152
Antidiabetic medications, comparison of,
    1000t-1003t
Antidiuretic hormone, 250
Antimotility agents, 461
Antiphospholipid syndrome (APS), 529,
    531-534, 964
  diagnosis of, 532
  epidemiology of, 531
  etiology of, 532
  management of, 534
  presentation of, 531
  prognosis of, 534
  treatment of, 534
Antiretrovirals and common side effects,
    566t
Anti-*Sacchromyces cerevisiae* antibody
    (ASCA), 446
Anti-TSH receptor antibody, 329
Aortic dissection
  acute, 76
  background of, 76
  as chronic, 76
  classification system for, 77
  clinical presentation of, 76
    physical examination, 77
    symptoms, 76
  diagnosis of, 78
  management of, 78
  outcome of, 78

Aortic dissection (*Continued*)
  predisposing factor for, 76
  risk factor for, 76
Aortic knob, 47
Aortic regurgitation (AR), 151-153
  clinical presentation of, 152
    history and natural progression, 152
    physical examination, 152-153
  diagnosis of, 153
  epidemiology of, 152
  management of, 153
Aortic stenosis
  clinical presentation of, 150
    history and natural progression, 150
    physical examination, 150-151
  diagnosis of, 151
  epidemiology of, 150
  management of, 151-152
  pathophysiology of, 150
  symptoms of, 147
Aortic valve surgery, 151, 153
APACHE scoring, 212
APACHE-II scoring for computed
    tomography, 364
Aphthous ulcer, 279
  clinical presentation of, 279
  diagnosis of, 279
  epidemiology and etiology of, 279
  treatment of, 279
Apical murmur, in acute mitral
    regurgitation, 241
Aplastic anemia, 510
Aplastic crisis
  cause of, 490
  treatment of, 490
Apnea-hypopnea index (AHI), S12
Appendicitis
  clinical presentation of, 355
  diagnosis of, 355
  management of, 355
ARDS-net trial group, 225
Arrhythmias, reperfusion, 102
Arrhythmogenic right ventricular dysplasia, 69
Arterial blood gas (ABG), 313
  analysis, S12
  sampling, 484
Arterial stenosis, S3
Arterial thrombosis, S3
Arteriosclerotic calcifications, 49
Arteriovenous malformations (AVMs), 435
Arthrocentesis, medial approach, 15f
Ascites, 418-425
  cause of, 419t
  clinical presentation of, 418
    history, 418-420
    physical examination, 420
  diagnosis of, 421-422
    paracentesis, 421
    ultrasound, 421
  epidemiology of, 418
  low SAAG, 424
  management of, 422-425

INDEX

Aspartate aminotransferase (AST), 380
Aspergillosis, 685-686
    clinical presentation of, 685-686
    diagnosis of, 686
    epidemiology and pathophysiology of, 685
    treatment of, 686
Aspiration of nerve roots, 16
Aspiration pneumonia in lung, 48
Aspirin, 203
    in non-ST segment elevation, 92
ASSENT-2 study, 98t
Assist-control ventilation (ACV)
    advantages of, 229
    disadvantage of, 230
Asthma, 865-873, S4
    clinical presentation of, 865-866
    diagnosis of, 866
    differential diagnosis of, 868t
    epidemiology of, 865
        flare action plan, 874
    management of, 868-873
Asymptomatic patients, serial echocardiograms for, 151
Asystolic arrest
    epidemiology of, 5
    etiology of, 5t
    presentation of, 5
    treatment of, 9f
    vasopressin in, 11
Atenolol and metoprolol, β-blockers, 330
Atherosclerosis. See Renal artery atherosclerosis
Atrial abnormalities, 58
Atrial fibrillation, 188, 197-209
    acute management of, 202f-203f
    atrial rate in, 198
    cause of, 198
        cardiac, 198
        noncardiac, 198
    clinical presentation of, 198
    diagnosis of, 198
    epidemiology of, 197-198
        classification, 197
        definition, 197
        pathophysiology, 197
        prevalence, 197
    lone, 197
    management of, 200-208
    paroxysma, 197
    permanent, 197
    persistent, 197
    rate control in, 200
    secondary causes of, 199
    tachyarrhythmias and, 189
Atrioventricular nodal reentrant tachycardia (AVNRT), 188
Austin Flint murmur, 153
Autoantibodies in rheumatic disease, 945t

Autoimmune hepatitis
    clinical presentation of, 407
    epidemiology of, 406
    evaluation of, 407
    management of, 407
Autoimmune thyroiditis, 324
AV block, second-degree, 177
AV conduction disease, 178, 179t
Azathioprine, a steroidsparing drug, 964

B
β-blockers, 42. See also specific β–blockers
    and ACE inhibitors in myocardial infarction, 117
    adverse effects of, 200
    comparison of, 992t-993t
    in non-ST segment elevation, 92
    for rate control, 200
Bacillary angiomatosis
    clinical presentation of, 275
    diagnosis of, 276
    epidemiology and etiology of, 275
    treatment of, 276
Bacterial pneumonia, 577-578
    clinical presentation of, 578
    diagnosis of, 578
    epidemiology of, 577-578
    etiology of, 578
    treatment of, 578
Balloon valvotomy and valvuloplasty, 151, 155
Barium, a contrast agent, 49
Barotrauma, 236
Barrett's esophagitis, 82
Basal energy expenditure (BEE), 32
Basal metabolic rate (BMR), 32
Basic chest anatomy, 45t-46t
Behçet's syndrome, 279, 528
Bell's palsy, S6
Bernoulli's equation, modified version of, 158
Bezold-Jarisch reflex, 102, 122
Bifascicular block, 180t
Bile acid-binding resins, 464
Bile leaks, S3
Bile salt malabsorption, 453
"Biliary colic," a misnomer, 376
Biliary colic and acute cholecystitis, clinical features of, 373t
Biliary tract disease, 371-376
Biochemical liver tests, interpretation of, 377-380
Bioprosthetic valves, advantage of, 159
Bioterrorism, S8
Biphasic anaphylaxis, 38
Biventricular hypertrophy, 62t
Black wound base, 283
Bladder calculi, 49

Blastomyces dermatitidis, 689-690
  clinical presentation of, 689-690
  diagnosis of, 690
  epidemiology of, 689
  treatment of, 690
Bleeding disorders, 516-524
  clinical presentation of, 516-518
  diagnosis of, 519-521
  epidemiology of, 516
  etiology of, 518-519
  management of, 521-522
  prognosis of, 521
Blood pressure
  during chest discomfort, 83
  classification for, 108t
  control of, 143
  reduction by oral therapy, 115t
Blood sugar
  goals, 290
  monitoring, 294
Blurry vision, 108
Body mass index, formula, 1015
Body surface area, formula, 1015
Boerhaave's syndrome, 82
Bone biopsy, 290
Bone marrow aspiration, 501
Bone marrow failure, 510-514
  clinical presentation of, 510-511
  diagnosis of, 511-513
  epidemiology of, 510
  etiology of, 511
  risk stratification and prognosis of, 513
  treatment of, 513-514
Bone marrow fibrosis, S5
Botulinum toxin, S8
Bowel obstruction
  cause of, 354
  clinical presentation of, 353-354
  diagnosis of, 354
  management of, 354
Bowel perforation
  clinical presentation of, 352
  diagnosis of, 352
  management of, 353
Bradycardia
  approach to, 10f
  cause of, 177
  evaluation of, 176-177
  and pacemakers, 176-185
    epidemiology, presentation, and
      diagnosis of, 176-177
Brain and epidural abscess, 626-628
  clinical presentation of, 627
  diagnosis of, 627
  epidemiology of, 626
  management of, 627
Bronchiolitis obliterative syndrome (BOS), S13
Bronchodilator therapy for asthma, 869
Brugada syndrome, 4t, 68, 195
Budd-Chiari syndrome, 360, 386, 415,
  529

Burkitt's lymphoma, 553
Bypass of severe coronary lesions, 151

C
C-reactive protein, 446, 677
  an acute phase reactant, 366f
CABG (Coronary Artery Bypass Graft)
    Patch trial, 195
Calcineurin inhibitors toxicity
  diagnosis of, 814
  epidemiology of, 814
  management of, 814
  presentation of, 814
Calciphylaxis
  clinical presentation of, 270
  diagnosis of, 270
  epidemiology and etiology of, 270
  management of, 271
Calcium and phosphate homeostasis, 335
Calcium channel blockers, 110
  for rate control, 200
Calmette-Guérin vaccination, 645
Cancer and back pain, 543f
Candidemia, 681-685
  clinical presentation of, 682
  diagnosis of, 682
  epidemiology of, 681-682
    incidence, 681-682
    risk factors, 682
  management of, 682-685
  prognosis of, 685
Candidiasis, oropharyngeal, 587-588
  treatment, 588t
Carbohydrate, as dextrose monohydrate,
    35
Carbomedics models, 159
Cardiac arrest, 3-11
  caused by VF, 195
  diagnosis of , 3
Cardiac catheterization
  for myocardial infarction, 86
  in elderly patients, 151
Cardiac filling pressure, loss in hemorrhage
    and hypovolemia, 243
Cardiac syncope, 120
Cardiac tamponade, 170-171
  clinical presentation of, 170
  diagnosis of, 170
  management of, 171
Cardiac transplant coronary arteriopathy,
    S2
Cardiogenic shock, 240, 247
  cause of, 247
  management of, 246f
  myocardial infarction, cause of, 247
  primary defect in, 247
  represents pump failure, 248
Cardiomyopathy, 131
  causes of, 132
  ischemic, 193
  major forms of, 132

Cardiopulmonary arrest, hyperventilation during, 11
Cardiovascular disease, exercise to prevent, 142
Cardioversion, antiarrhythmic therapy for, 200
Carotid sinus massage, 127
Carvallo's sign, 158
Catheter ablation
  to cure atrial fibrillation, 208
  for patients with AF, 200
Catheterization, 1008f-1009f
CD4 count and HIV-associated complications, 601t
Central line placement
  complications for, 26
  contraindications for, 25
  indications for, 25
  in internal jugular vein, 27f
  procedure-specific equipment for, 14t
  in subclavian vein, 28f
  techniques in, 26
Central nervous system (CNS) mass lesions, 572-573
  diagnosis of, 573, 574t
  epidemiology and etiology of, 572
  management of, 572, 575t
  presentation of, 572-573
Central nervous system infection, 619-628
Central venous catheter infection, 658-661
  clinical presentation of, 659
  diagnosis of, 659-660
  epidemiology of, 658
  treatment of, 660-661
Ceralyte or Pedialyte solution, 460
Cerebral edema, 316, 319
Ceruloplasmin in acute hepatitis, 387
Charcot's triad, 375
Chest film, 88
Chest pain
  in constrictive pericarditis, 171
  differential diagnosis of, 73
  duration of, 88
  early postinfarction pericarditis, cause of, 169
  in emergency department, 72-83
  evaluation of, 72
  morbid cause of, 73
  relief of, 83
Chest radiography, 44, 134
  for heart failure or lung disease, 199
  for proper tube position, 229
Child-Pugh classification, 412t, 1013
Chlamydia, S7
Chlorhexidine, antiseptic solution, 13
Cholangiography, S3
Cholangitis
  diagnosis of, 376
  epidemiology and pathophysiology of, 374-375
  presentation of, 375
  treatment of, 376

Cholelithiasis
  diagnosis of, 372
  epidemiology and pathophysiology of, 371-372
  presentation of, 372
  treatment of, 372
Cholestasis
  and hepatocellular necrosis, 380
  markers of, 377
Cholesterol agents, comparison of, 995t-999t
Cholesterol emboli
  clinical presentation of, 271
  diagnosis of, 271
  epidemiology and etiology of, 271
  management of, 271
Chronic diarrhea
  additional studies in evaluating, 465t
  cause of, 463
  diagnosis of, 461, 593
  management of, 464, 593
  presentation of, 593
Chronic hypocalcemia
  with hypoparathyroidism, 345
  with renal insufficiency, 347
  with vitamin D deficiency, 345
Chronic kidney disease (CKD), 748-755
  clinical presentation of, 749-750
  diagnosis of, 750
  epidemiology and etiology of, 748-749
  management of, 752-755
Chronic liver disease, 506
  genetic and metabolic form of, 409-411
  manifestations of, 264t
  risk stratification and prognosis of, 411-412
Chronic myeloid leukemia, S5
Chronic obstructive pulmonary disease (COPD), 228, 877-884
  classification of, 879
  clinical presentation of, 878-879
  diagnosis of, 879
  epidemiology and etiology of, 877-878
  management of, 880-884
Chronic rejection, S3
  diagnosis of, 811
  epidemiology of, 810
  management of, 811
  presentation of, 810
Chronic wounds
  epidemiology of, 282
  management of, 282-290
  treatment of, 285
Chronotropic incompetence, a class I indication, 178
Churg-Strauss syndrome, 728-729, 954-956, S4
  clinical presentation of, 729
  diagnosis of, 729, 956
  epidemiology of, 728, 954
  management of, 729

Churg-Strauss syndrome (*Continued*)
  presentation of, 956
  prognosis of, 729
  treatment and prognosis of, 956
Chvostek's signs, 343, 347
Cine-esophagram, 51
Cinefluoroscopy, 160
Cirrhosis
  clinical presentation of, 403
  complications of, 412
  diagnostic imaging in, 404
  epidemiology of, 402
  laboratory evaluation, 404
  liver biopsy in, 404
  physical examination, 403
Clopidogrel, 93
  in percutaneous coronary intervention, 94
  in unstable angina, 93
Clostridium difficile toxin, 460
Cluster headache, S11
Coagulation factors, characteristics of, 518t
Coagulopathy, 19, 25
Coccidioides immitis, 688-689
  clinical presentation of, 688
  diagnosis of, 689
  epidemiology of, 688
  management of, 689
Cockcroft-Gault equation, 1012
Colloid and crystalloid solutions, for rapid volume resuscitation, 242
Colonoscopy, for acute lower GI bleeding, 438f
Colony-forming units (CFUs), 623
Community-acquired pneumonia (CAP), 630-636
  clinical presentation of, 631-632
  diagnosis of, 632-633
  epidemiology of, 630
  management of, 633
  prognosis of, 633-636
Comorbid risk factors, modification of, 296
COMPANION (Comparison of Medical Therapy, Pacing, and Defibrillation in Heart Failure) trial, 182
Computed tomography (CT), 19, 48, 51-52
Congenital polycythemias, 484
Congestive heart failure
  minimal, 48
  moderate, 48
  severe, 48
Conjugated bilirubin, 377
Conjugated hyperbilirubinemia, 378
Conn's grading system, 380
Constrictive pericarditis, 171-174
  clinical presentation of, 171
  diagnosis of, 172
  management of, 174
  vs restrictive cardiomyopathy, 173
Continuous positive airway pressure (CPAP), S12

Contrast media, 51
Corrigan pulse, 152
Corticosteroids, 226
  as asthma therapy, 869
  long-term management with, 300
  side effects of, 298t, 300
Corticotropin-releasing hormone (CRH), 305f
Costophrenic angles, 47
Cough and angioedema, with ACE inhibitors, 140
Creatine kinase
  with isozymes, 134
  in three isoforms, 89
Critically ill patient
  care of, 211-217
  system-based approach to, 214t-215t
Crohn's disease, 408
  clinical presentation of, 444
  diagnosis of, 444
  management of, 449
  treatment of, 451t
  vs ulcerative colitis, 443t
Cryoglobulinemia syndromes, 954
Cryptococcal meningitis
  diagnosis of, 570-571
  epidemiology and etiology of, 570
  management and treatment of, 571
  presentation of, 570
  prognosis of, 571
Cryrveilhier-Baum murmur, 404
Cullen's sign, 351, 362
Cushing's syndrome, 117
Cutaneous drug eruptions, in HIV patients, 280
Cyanosis, 226
Cytomegalovirus (CMV)
  diagnostic criteria of, 697
  epidemiology of, 696
  management of, 697-698
  presentation of, 697
Cytomegalovirus (CMV) retinitis, 598-602
  cause of, 601
  diagnosis of, 601
  epidemiology of, 598
  presentation of, 598
  prognosis and mortality of, 602
  treatment of, 602
Cytomegalovirus encephalitis
  diagnosis of, 571
  epidemiology and etiology of, 571
  presentation of, 571
  treatment of, 572

D
DANAMI-2 (Danish Trial in Acute Myocardial Infarction) study, 100
DDD(R) pacing mode, 183, 185
  timing cycle of, 185f
Decubitus film, 48

Deep vein thrombosis (DVT), 526
Defibrillation, 4
  biphasic, 4
Delirium, 816-823
  diagnosis of, 818-820
  epidemiology of, 816
  etiology of, 818
  management and prevention of, 820-
    823
  presentation of, 816-818
  prognosis of, 823
Diabetes, manifestations of, 264t
Diabetes mellitus, 292
Diabetic ketoacidosis (DKA)
  clinical presentation of
    physical examination, 313
    symptoms, 312
  common precipitant of, 314
  diagnosis of, 313
  management of
    electrolyte monitoring and
      replacement, 317
    fluid, 315
    insulin administration, 316
  risk stratification and prognosis of, 315,
    316t
Diagnostic thoracentesis, 22
Dialysis, 756-761
  mode of, 756-759
    continuous renal replacement
      therapies, 756
    hemodialysis, 756
    peritoneal dialysis, 756
  vascular access, 759-760
Diarrhea, 456-464
  acute, 593
    approach to, 462f
    clinical presentation and diagnosis of,
      456-460
    evaluation of, 457
    history of, 457
    infectious diarrhea
      diagnosis of, 458t
      differential diagnosis of, 458t-459t
      management of, 460
  chronic, 593
    diagnosis of, 593
    management of, 593
    presentation of, 593
  epidemiology of, 456
Diastolic dysfunction, evidence of systolic
  or, 134
Diffusion capacities of lung carbon
  monoxide (DLCO), 858
Digoxin, 69
  for heart failure, 142
  for rate control of atrial fibrillation,
    201
Dilated cardiomyopathy, 181t
Dilated gas-filled bowel loops, 49
Direct thrombin inhibitors, 983t-984t

Disseminated intravascular coagulation
    (DIC)
  clinical condition associated with, 507
  diagnosis of, 523
  epidemiology of, 506, 523
  etiology of, 523
  management of, 524
  presentation of, 523
  prognosis of, 524
  thrombotic microangiopathy and, 507t
Distributive shock, 240, 248, 250
  cause of, 248
  treatment of, 248
Diuretic therapy of ascites, 423
Diuretics, pharmacologic agents, 136
Diverticulitis
  clinical presentation of, 356
  diagnosis of, 356
  management of, 356
Dobutamine
  agent to improve cardiac output, 248
  a β-adrenergic agonist, 138
Dopamine
  agent to improve cardiac output, 250
  effects of, 250
  an endogenous catecholamine, 138
Doppler ultrasonography, 387
Dressler syndrome, 169
Drug rash with eosinophilia and systemic
    symptoms (DRESS), 269
Drug reaction, pruritus and fever, 267
Duke criteria, 650
Dupuytren's contractures, 403
Duration of anticoagulation in VTE, 919t
Duroziez sign, 152
Dyslipidemia, 293

E
EBV. See Epstein-Barr virus
Echocardiography, for systolic and diastolic
    function, 134
ECOG performance scale, S5t
Ectopic pregnancy, 353
Electrocardiogram analysis
  with anterior-lateral Q wave infarction,
    63f
  with inferior-lateral Q wave infarction,
    63f
Electrocardiogram (ECG), 57-70
  in acute coronary syndrome, 74
  and cardiac biomarkers, 90
  examination of axis, 58
  examination of intervals, 58
    diagnosis of, 59t-60t
  examination of rate, 57
  examination of rhythms, 57
  for myocardial ischemia, 134
  role of, 57
Electrocardiographic criteria
  for acute myocardial infarction, 65t
  for left and right atrial abnormality, 61t

Electrocardiographic criteria (*Continued*)
  for left ventricular hypertrophy, 61t
  in progressive hyperkalemia, 68f
  for right ventricular hypertrophy, 62t
Electrolyte abnormalities, 66
Encephalitis, 623-626
  clinical presentation of, 624
  diagnosis of, 624-625
  epidemiology of, 623
  management of, 625-626
Endocarditis, 162
  antibiotic prophylaxis against, 162
  suggested treatment for, 655t
  symptoms of, 162
Endomyocardial biopsy, 135
Endoscopic retrograde
      cholangiopancreatography (ERCP), 374
Endotracheal tube (ETT), 229
Enoxaparin, 93
Entecavir, a cyclopentyl guanine analog,
      395
Enteral feeding
  contraindications to, 33
  formula, 34t
Enteral nutrition, 33
Enteroclysis, 49
Eosinophilia, S4
Eosinophilic gastroenteritis, 359
Epidermoid tumors, implantation of, 16
Epidural spinal cord compression, 541-542
  clinical presentation of, 541
  diagnosis of, 541-542
  epidemiology of, 541
  management of, 541-542
Epinephrine
  intramuscular administration of, 43
  and vasopressin, 4
Eplerenone, 142
Epstein-Barr virus (EBV), 511
  clinical presentation of, 699
  epidemiology and etiology of, 699
  infections, S5
Eptifibatide, a cyclic peptide inhibitor, 94
  and tirofiban, 94
Erythema multiforme major. *See*
      Stevens-Johnson syndrome
Erythema multiforme
  clinical presentation of, 268
  diagnosis of, 269
  epidemiology and etiology of, 267-268
Erythrocyte sedimentation rate (ESR), 446
Erythrocytosis, 482-485
  clinical presentation of, 482
  diagnosis of, 482-484, 483t
  epidemiology of, 482
  management of, 484
Erythroderma
  clinical presentation of, 272
  diagnosis of, 272
  epidemiology and etiology of, 271-272
  management of, 272

Eschar, stable, 290
Esophageal disease in patients with the
      human immunodeficiency virus,
      589t-590t
Esophageal rupture
  clinical presentation of, 82
    physical examination, 82
    symptoms, 82
  diagnosis of, 82-83
  epidemiology of, 82
  management of, 83
  outcome of, 83
Estimation of
  caloric needs, 32
  protein needs, 33
Extraluminal gas, 49

F
Familial mediterranean fever of abdominal
      pain, 359
Famotidine, 36
Fanconi's anemia, 512
Febrile nonhemolytic transfusion reaction,
      471
Ferritin, major iron storage protein, 477
Fever of unknown origin (FUO), 603, 608-
      617
  classification of, 610t
  clinical presentation of, 608-614
  diagnosis of, 605f
    histologic techniques, 616
    imaging techniques, 614-616
    noninvasive laboratory testing, 614
  epidemiology of, 608
  HIV-associated, 603-606
  management of, 617
  outcome of, 617
  trends in the causes of, 609f
Fick principle, 1007
First-degree block, type of AV block, 177
Fluconazole, 310
Fluoroscopy, 51
Focal segmental glomerulosclerosis, 723-
      724
  clinical presentation of, 723
  diagnosis of, 723-724
  epidemiology and etiology of, 723
  management of, 724
  prognosis of, 724
Folate and iron regimen, pregnant women
      on, 480
Folate deficiency, causes of, 481
Foley catheter, 352
Folliculitis
  clinical presentation of, 277
  diagnosis of, 277
  epidemiology and etiology of, 277
  treatment of, 277
Foot ulcers, 282
  assessment of, 286t
Forced vital capacity, 858

Framingham Heart Study, 120
Free thyroxine index (FTI), 1014
Fresh frozen plasma (FFP), 469
Friedewald formula, 1007
Fulminant hepatic failure (FHF), 377,
    380-382, 392
  causes and survival rates of, 381t
  epidemiology of, 380
  physical examination, 381
  presentation of, 380-381
Fungal infection
  clinical presentation of, 277
  diagnosis of, 277
  epidemiology and etiology of, 276
  pulmonary, 583t-584t
  treatment of, 277
Fungus, 681-690
Furosemide, 136

G

Gallavardin's phenomenon, 151
Gallstones, 362
  as asymptomatic, 372
  classification of, 371
Gamma glutamyl transpeptidase (GGT),
    378, 405
Gastric emptying studies, requirement for, 53
Gastrografin esophagogram, 83
Gastrointestinal bleeding
  acute lower, management of, 437f
    colonoscopy and, 438f
  acute upper, causes of, 429t
Gell and Coombs classification of allergic
    reactions, 40t
Genital ulcers, characteristics of, S7t
Giant cell arteritis, 949-951
  diagnosis of, 950
  epidemiology of, 949
  presentation of, 950
  treatment and prognosis of, 950-951
Gilbert's syndrome, 371
Glargine insulin, 300
Glisson's capsule, 403
Glomerular disease, 719-729
Glossitis and cheilosis, vitamin deficiency,
    403
Glycoprotein IIb/IIIa receptor inhibitors, 94
  abciximab, tirofiban, and eptifbatide, 94
Gohn focus, 641
Gonorrhea, S7
Goodpasture's syndrome and anti-GBM
    disease, 726-727
  clinical presentation of, 726-727
  diagnosis of, 727
  epidemiology and etiology of, 726
  management of, 727
  prognosis of, 727
Graft-versus-host disease, 360, 472
Gram-negative bacteria in sepsis, 254
Gram-positive bacteria in sepsis, 254
Graves disease, 327

Graves ophthalmopathy, 328
Grey Turner's sign, 351, 362
Groin pain, hernias, 351
GUSTO-1 study, 98t
GUSTO-3 study, 98t

H

H2-receptor antagonists, for acid
    suppression, 215
HAART. *See* Highly active antiretroviral
    therapy
Haemophilus, 631
Hamwii method, 32
Harris-Benedict equation, 32
Hashimoto's thyroiditis, 323
Headache, S11
  and post-lumbar puncture, 16
Heart failure, 131-143
  acute, 135
    β-blockers, 137
    pharmacologic agents in, 136
    Swan-Ganz catheters in, 138
    vasodilators in, 137
  β-blocker therapy with, 143
  chronic, 138-143
    atenolol in, 141
    β-blockers in, 141
    pharmacologic agents in, 138-143
  classification of, 131
  clinical presentation of, 132
  device therapy for, 143
  diagnosis of, 134-135
  epidemiology of, 131-132
  hemodynamic profiles in, 133t, 135
  nonsystolic, 131
  signs of, 132
  stages in the evolution of, 139f
  treatment of, 135-143
Heart transplantation, allograft dysfunction
    in, S2
Hematuria, S9
Hemolytic anemias, 481
Hemolytic-uremic syndrome (HUS), 460, 503
Hemoptysis, 892-898
  clinical presentation of, 893
  diagnosis of, 893-897
  epidemiology of, 892-893
  management of, 897-898
Hemorrhage, and hypovolemia, 243
Hemorrhagic cystitis, 555-556
  diagnosis of, 555
  epidemiology of, 555
  grading and treatment of, 556t
  management of, 555-556
Hemorrhagic fever viruses, S8
Hemorrhagic shock, 243
Hemorrhagic stroke, 842-844
  diagnosis of, 843-844
  epidemiology and etiology of, 842
  management of, 844
  presentation of, 842

Hemorrhoids, 436
Hemosiderin-laden macrophages, 278
Heparin, low-molecular weight, 92
Heparin dosing, weight-based
    unfractionated, 982t
Heparin-induced thrombocytopenia
    diagnosis of, 506
    epidemiology and pathophysiology of, 505
    management of, 506
    presentation of, 505-506
Hepatic encephalopathy, 412
    early stages of, 413, 413t
    treatment of, 413
Hepatitis A serology, 391f
Hepatitis B, 391-396
    clinical presentation of, 392
    diagnosis of, 392
    epidemiology and virology of, 391-392
    management of, 394-395
    manifestations of, 264t
    prophylaxis of, 395
Hepatitis C
    clinical presentation of, 396
    diagnosis of, 397
    epidemiology and virology of, 396
    management of, 398
    manifestations of, 264t
    prophylaxis of, 399
Hepatitis, viral, 389-399. See also specific
        types
    clinical presentation of, 389
    diagnosis of, 389
    epidemiology and virology of, 389
    management of, 389
    prophylaxis of, 389
Hepatobiliary, requirement for, 53
Hepatocellular carcinoma (HCC), 414-415
    diagnosis of, 414
    epidemiology of, 414
    treatment of, 414
Hepatocellular injury, markers of, 378-380
Hepatorenal syndrome (HRS), 418
    diagnostic criteria for, 425
    management of, 425
Hereditary hemochromatosis
    genetic and metabolic form of, 409-410
    liver transplantation in, 410
    treatment of, 410
Herpes zoster, 265-266
    clinical presentation of, 265
    diagnosis of, 265
    epidemiology and etiology of, 265
    in HIV patients, 280
    management of, 265
Heyde's syndrome, 524
High-frequency oscillatory ventilation
        (HFOV), 225, 232
    advantage of, 232
    disadvantage of, 232
High positive end-expiratory pressure
        strategy, a ventilation strategy, 225

Highly active antiretroviral therapy
        (HAART) era, 275
Hilar opacities, 47
Hill sign, 153
Histoplasma capsulatum, 686-687
    clinical presentation of, 686-687
    diagnosis of, 687
    epidemiology of, 686
    management of, 687
Hodgkin's lymphoma, 171, S4
Holter monitoring, 127, 199
Homograft valves, 159
HOT (Hypertension Optimal Treatment)
        trial, 108
Howell-Jolly bodies, 476
HSV and varicella-zoster virus, S3
Human immunodeficiency virus (HIV)
    with anemia, 564
    associated FUO, 603-606
        cause of, 603
        diagnosis of, 604
        epidemiology of, 603
        presentation of, 603
        prognosis and mortality of, 606
    central nervous system in, 569-575
        mass lesions, 574t
    cholangiopathy
        diagnosis of, 588, 591
        epidemiology of, 588
        management of, 591
        presentation of, 588
    dementia (HIVD), 573-575
        diagnosis of, 575
        epidemiology of, 573
        management of, 575
        presentation of, 573
        prognosis of, 575
    dermatologic disorders in, 275-280
        management of, 563-565
            endocrine abnormalities, 564
            hematologic abnormalities, 563
        natural history of, 563f
        with thrombocytopenia, 565
Human polyomavirus infection
    diagnosis of, 811
    epidemiology of, 811
    management of, 811
    presentation of, 811
Hydralazine, 137
Hydroxyurea therapy, 490t
Hyperacute rejection
    diagnosis of, 810
    epidemiology of, 808
    management of, 810
    presentation of, 808
Hyperacute T waves, 62
Hyperaldosteronism, 117
Hyperbilirubinemia, cause of, 378f-379f
Hypercalcemia, 68, 549-550
    clinical presentation of, 336
    diagnosis of, 340f-341f

Hypercalcemia (*Continued*)
  epidemiology of, 335, 549
  etiology and diagnosis of, 336-337, 549
  laboratory findings, causes of, 338t-339t
  management of, 337, 549
    pharmacologic, 342t
  risk and prognosis of, 337
Hypercapnia and hypoxemia, 80
Hypercapnic respiratory failure
  diagnosis of, 223
Hypercoagulable states, 526-534
  clinical presentation of, 526-528
  diagnosis of, 529
  epidemiology of, 526
  etiology of, 528-529
  management and prevention of, 530-531
  prognosis of, 529-530
Hyperglycemia and ketoacidosis, 319
Hyperkalemia, 66
  diagnosis of, 801
  epidemiology and etiology of, 800-801
  management of, 801
  presentation of, 802
Hypermagnesemia, S10
Hypernatremia, 794-798
  cause of, 795-796
  clinical presentation of, 795
  diagnosis of, 796
  epidemiology of, 794-795
  management of, 796-798
Hyperosmolar hyperglycemic state (HHS),
    312
  clinical presentation of, 318
  diagnosis of, 318-319
  epidemiology of, 318
  management of, 319
Hyperosmolar nonketotic coma, 318
Hyperparathyroidism, 335
Hypersensitive carotid and
    neurocardiogenic syncope, 180t
Hypersensitive carotid sinus syndrome,
    182
Hypersensitivity syndrome
  clinical presentation of, 269
  diagnosis and management of, 270
  epidemiology and etiology of, 269
Hypertension
  in acute dissection, 77
  cause of, 109
  laboratory assessment of, 109
  organs involved in, 109
  risk factors for, 107
  secondary, 110
  treatment of, 111f
Hypertensive emergency, 107
Hypertensive urgency, 107
Hypertensive urgency and emergency
  clinical presentation of, 108-110
  epidemiology of, 107-108
  treatment of, 110-116
    hypertensive emergency, 112
    hypertensive urgency, 112

Hyperviscosity syndrome (HVS), 549-551
  clinical presentation of, 550
  diagnosis of, 550-551
  epidemiology of, 550
  management of, 551
Hypocalcemia
  causes of, 344t
  clinical presentation of, 343
  diagnosis of, 346f
  epidemiology of, 343
  etiology and diagnosis of, 343-345
  management of, 345
  risk and prognosis of, 345
Hypochromia, 476
Hypoglycemia
  monitoring, 296
  risk factors for, 296
  treatment of, 296
Hypokalemia, 67, 803-804
  diagnosis of, 804
  epidemiology and etiology of, 803-804
  management of, 804
Hypomagnesemia, S10
Hyponatremia, 789-794
  cause of, 789-792
    euvolemic, 790
    hypertonic, 792
    hypervolemic, 791
    hypovolemic, 790
  clinical presentation of, 789
  diagnosis of, 792
  epidemiology of, 789
  management of, 792-794
Hypophosphatemia, S10
Hypotension
  management of, 244f
  refractory, causes, 251
  symptoms of, 241
Hypothalamic-pituitary-adrenal (HPA) axis,
    302, 305f
Hypothermia, 68
  paralytic agents for, 5
Hypothyroidism
  cause of, 323t
  clinical presentation of, 323-324
  diagnosis of, 324-326
  epidemiology of, 321
  and hypoadrenalism, 309
  management of, 326
  primary, 321
Hypovolemic shock, 240, 243
Hypoxemia
  diagnosis of, 221t
  and hypercapnia, 80
  and hypoxia, 219
    diagnosis of, 220f
  troubleshooting, 234, 235f

I
Ideal body weight (IBW), formula, 1015
Idiopathic interstitial pneumonia, features
    of, 924t-925t

Idiopathic myelofibrosis, S5
Idiopathic thrombocytopenic purpura
    diagnosis of, 498
    epidemiology of, 498
    management of, 502
        acute, 502
        long-term, 502
    presentation of, 498
IgE antibodies, 41
Iliopsoas sign, 355
Immune reconstitution syndrome, 565, 567t
Immunoglobulin A nephropathy, 725-726
    clinical presentation of, 726
    diagnosis of, 726
    epidemiology and etiology of, 725
    management of, 726
    prognosis of, 726
Implantable cardioverter-defibrillators
        (ICDs), 191f
    complications of, 193
    indications for, 193
    primary and secondary prevention, 194
    VF detection in, 192
    VT detection in, 192
Infarction and ischemia, 65
Infectious colitis, 436
Infective endocarditis (IE), 650-656
    clinical presentation of, 652
        physical examination, 652
        symptoms, 652
    diagnosis of, 652-653
    epidemiology and etiology of, 650-652
    management of, 653-656
        medical therapy, 653
        prognosis, 656
        surgical theraphy, 656
Inferior myocardial infarction, 66f
Inferior vena cava filter, 25
Inflammatory bowel disease (IBD), 442-
        453
    clinical presentation of, 442
    diagnosis of, 445-447
        endoscopy, 446
        imaging, 446-447
        laboratory test, 445-446
    epidemiology of, 442
    management of, 447-453
    and pregnancy, 453
Inflammatory colitis, 436
Inflammatory myositis, 973-974
    diagnosis of, 973-974
    epidemiology of, 973
    etiology and presentation of, 973
    prognosis of, 974
    treatment of, 974
Infraumbilical approach, 20
Inhaled vasodilators, 225
Initial evaluation for thrombocytopenia,
        500f
Inotropes
    for acute HF, 138
    and vasopressors, 248, 249t

Inpatient dermatology, 263-272
Inpatient diabetes management, 292
Insulin, 35
    dosage of
        in parenteral nutrition, 35
    intravenous drip, 293-294
    preparations, 295t
    short-acting, 1004t
    therapy, intensive, 260
Insulin products, comparison of, 1004t
Intensive care unit
    admission criteria and prognostic scoring
        systems, 211
    basic principles and safety in, 213
    ethical issues in, 216
    mortality in, 211
Interleukin-6, 256
Intermediate-acting insulins, 1004t
International normalized ratio (INR), 201
International Registry of Acute Aortic
        Dissection, 76
Interstitial lung diseases, 922-930
    clinical presentation of, 922-927
    diagnosis of, 927-929
    epidemiology of, 922
    management of, 929-930
    prognosis of, 924t-925t
Intoxication with vitamin A, 337
Intraaortic balloon pump (IABP), S1
Intracranial metastases, 537-538
    clinical presentation and diagnosis of,
        537-538
    management of, 538
Intravascular catheters, examination of,
        216
Intubation, indications for, 222
Invasive and noninvasive ventilation
    clinical presentation of, 228-229
    epidemiology of, 228
    intubation in, 229
    mode of, 229, 230t
    parameter of, 231
Invasive testing, 127
Inverse ratio ventilation, 232
Iron deficiency, cause of anemia, 475
Irradiated red blood cells, 469
Irritable bowel syndrome (IBS), 355
Ischemia
    assessment and control of, 143
    and infarction, 65
Ischemia-guided management strategy, 93
Ischemic cardiomyopathy, 193
Ischemic colitis, 435
Ischemic stroke
    clinical presentation of, 835-836
    diagnosis of, 836-839
    epidemiology of, 833-834
    management of, 839-842
        acute, 839-840
        secondary prevention, 840-841
    preventive measure of, 834-835
ISIS-2 study, 98t

J

Jaundice, 404
  and coagulopathy, 402
Jugular venous pressure (JVP), 5

K

Kaposi's sarcoma
  clinical presentation of, 278
  diagnosis of, 278
  epidemiology and etiology of, 277
  treatment of, 278
Kayser-Fleischer ring, 387, 411
Kerley B lines, 134
Ketonemia, detection, 313
Killip class IV myocardial infarctions, 251
Klebsiella pneumonia, 631
Knee arthrocentesis
  complications for, 13
  contraindications for, 13
  indications for, 13
Korotkoff's sounds, 170
Kussmaul respirations, 313
Kussmaul sign, 172

L

L-thyroxine, 300
Lactate dehydrogenase (LDH) level, 553
Lactose-free diet, 463
Lamivudine, an oral nucleoside analog, 394
Laser-assisted uvulopalatoplasty, S12
Latent tuberculosis infection (LTBI), 640
Lateral chest radiograph, 45f
Lead aVR, 64
Lead poisioning of abdominal pain, 359
Left anterior descending artery (LAD), 64
Left bundle branch block (LBBB), 65
Left lower quadrant (LLQ), 355
Left ventricle and aorta, 150
Left ventricular hypertrophy, 58
Leg ulcers, assessment of, 286t-287t
Legionella pneumonia, 631
Leukoreduced red blood cells, 468
Levothyroxine, 326
Libman-Sacks endocarditis, 961
Lipid emulsions, 35
Lipid infusions, 35
Lipodystrophy
  clinical presentation of, 280
  diagnosis of, 280
  epidemiology and etiology of, 280
  treatment of, 280
Livedo reticularis, 271
  common causes of, 273
Liver biopsy, 404-405
Liver transplantation, allograft dysfunction
    in, S3
Long-acting insulins, 1004t
Loop diuretics, 136, 142, 549
  side effects of, 137
Low- and high-dose cosyntropin
    stimulation tests, 308f

Low-molecular-weight heparin, 93
Low-SAAG ascites, 424
Low tidal volume strategy, a ventilation
    strategy, 225
Lower GI bleeding (LGIB), 433-438
  clinical presentation of, 433
  diagnosis of, 434-436
  epidemiology of, 433
  evaluation and management of, 434
  independent risk factors for severe, 434t
  mortality and causes of, 434t
  outcome of, 436
  therapeutic evaluation of, 436
Ludwig's angina, S6
Lugol's solution, 330
Lumbar puncture
  complications for, 16
  contraindications for, 16
  indications for, 15
  positioning, 17f
  procedure-specific equipment for, 14t
  techniques in needle for, 16, 18f
Lung transplantation, allograft dysfunction
    in, S13
Lyme disease, 940

M

Mackler's triad, 84
Maddrey discriminant function, 382
Maddrey score, 1013
MADIT II (Multicenter Automatic
    Defibrillator Implantation Trial II)
    trial, 143
Magnesium, disorders of, S10
Magnetic resonance
    cholangiopancreatography, 352
Magnetic resonance imaging (MRI), 48,
    52, 537
  contrast agents, 53t
Malignant otitis externa, S6
Mallory Weiss tear, 429t
Management of acute pancreatitis, 366f
Marfan's syndrome, 152
Maxillofacial surgery, S12
McBurney's point, 355
Mean airway pressure (mPAW), 232
Mean corpuscular volume (MCV), 405, 476
Mechanical valves, 159f
  advantage of, 159
  lifespan of, 158
Meckel's diverticulum studies, requirement
    for, 53
Megaloblastic anemia, 480
MELD formula, 412
Membranoproliferative glomerulonephritis
    (MPGN), 724-725
  clinical presentation of, 724
  diagnosis of, 724
  epidemiology and etiology of, 724
  management of, 725
  prognosis of, 725

Membranous nephropathy, 721-723
  clinical presentation of, 721
  diagnosis of, 721
  epidemiology and etiology of, 721
  management of, 723
  prognosis of, 723
Meningitis, 619-623
  clinical presentation of, 620-621
  diagnosis of, 621-623
  epidemiology of, 619-620
  management of, 623
Mesenteric adenitis, 359
Mesenteric ischemia
  clinical presentation of, 356-357
  diagnosis of, 357
  management of, 357
Metabolic acidosis, 314
Metformin, 296
Methenamine silver stain, 277
Metoclopramide, a prokinetic agents, 36
Microbiology of infective endocarditis,
    651t
Microcytosis, 476
MICROMEDEX Healthcare Series, 118
Microscopic polyangiitis, 956-957
  diagnosis of, 957
  epidemiology of, 956
  presentation of, 957
  treatment and prognosis of, 957
Migraine, S11
Milk-alkali syndrome, 337
Milrinone
  agent to improve cardiac output, 250
  a phosphodiesterase inhibitor, 138, 250
Mineralocorticoid replacement, 309
Minimal change disease (MCD), 720-721
  clinical presentation of, 721
  diagnosis of, 721
  epidemiology and etiology of, 720-721
  prognosis of, 721
Minnesota tube, 433
Mitral regurgitation, 156-157
  acute, 157
  chronic, 157
  clinical presentation of, 156-157
    history and natural progression, 156
    physical examination, 157
  diagnosis of, 157
  epidemiology of, 156
  pathophysiology of, 156
Mitral stenosis, 154-155
  clinical presentation of, 154
    history and natural progression, 154
    physical examination, 154
  diagnosis of, 155
  epidemiology of, 154
  management of, 155
  pathophysiology of, 154
Mixed connective tissue disorder, 974-975
Model for End-Stage Liver Disease (MELD)
    score, 402

Modified Child-Pugh classification and the
    Meld Survival Model, 412t
Molluscum contagiosum
  clinical presentation of, 278
  diagnosis of, 278
  epidemiology and etiology of, 278
  treatment of, 279
Morbid chest pain, cause of, 82
Morbilliform drug eruption
  background and clinical presentation of,
    267
  diagnosis and management of, 267
Morphine, pharmacologic agents, 136
MRI. See Magnetic resonance imaging
Multiple-organ dysfunction score, 212,
    213t
Murphy's sign, 351, 373
Mushroom ingestion, 383
Musset sign, 153
Mycobacterium avium-intracellulare
    complex (MAC), 602-603
  cause of, 602-603
  epidemiology of, 602
  presentation of, 602
  prognosis and mortality of, 603
  treatment of, 603
Mycobacterium avium-intracellulare
    infection, 308
Mycobacterium tuberculosis pneumonia,
    632
Myelodysplastic syndromes, S5
  Myocardial infarction
  conduction disturbance in, 181
  and posterior wall injury, 64
Myocardial ischemia
  complications of, 102t
  and infarction, 62
Myxedema coma, 323

N
Nonalcoholic steatohepatitis
  epidemiology of, 405
  evaluation of, 406
  management of, 406
Nasogastric (NG) tube, 352
Neoplastic disease, 435
Neoplastic infiltration of the liver, 387
Neoplastic meningitis, 538-541
  diagnosis of, 539-541
  epidemiology and clinical presentation
    of, 538-539
  evaluation and treatment of, 539f-540f
  management of, 541
Nephrogenic fibrosing dermopathy, 272
Nephrotic syndrome, 529
Nesiritide, 137
  adverse effect of, 137
Neurocardiogenic syncope, 122, 182
Neurogenic syncope, 122
Neuromuscular blocking agent, 217
Neurosyphilis, S7

Neutropenic fever, 542-549
  clinical presentation of, 542-544
  diagnosis of, 544
  epidemiology of, 542
  management of, 544, 544-549
New York Heart Association (NYHA)
    classification scheme 133
NHANES III (National Health and Nutrition
    Examination Survey) data, 107
Nifedipine, 110
Nikolsky's sign, 268
"Nitrate-free" interval, 141
Nitrates
  and hydralazine in chronic heart failure,
    141
  in non-ST segment elevation, 92
Nitrogen balance in nutrition assessment,
    33
"Nonabsorbable" antibiotic, 414
Nonalcoholic fatty liver disease (NAFLD),
    402, 405, 406
Noncardiac causes of atrial fibrillation, 198
Nongap metabolic acidosis, 314
Nonglomerular hematuria CT, evaluation of,
    S9f
Non-Hodgkin's lymphoma, 399, 552, S4
Noninvasive positive-pressure ventilation
    (NPPV), 222, 232
Nonmegaloblastic anemias, 481
Non-ST segment elevation ACS
  management of, 89-90
    pharmacologic and nonpharmacologic
      intervention, 90-95
    risk stratification, 89-90, 91t
Nonsteroidal antiinflammatory drugs
    (NSAIDs), 431
Nonsystolic heart failure, 134
Nonthyroidal illness syndrome, 297
Norwegian or crusted scabies, 266
  features of, 266t
Nosocomial pneumonia (NP), 636-638
  clinical presentation of, 636
  diagnosis of, 637
  epidemiology of, 636
  management of, 637
Nuclear medicine studies, 53-54
Nutritional status, evaluation of, 32

O
Obstructive sleep apnea (OSA), S12
Ogilvie's syndrome, 354
Oliguria and acute renal failure, 260
Opiate withdrawal, 851-854
  diagnosis of, 852
  epidemiology of, 851-852
  management and treatment of, 853-854
  presentation of, 852
  risk stratification and prognosis of, 852
Opiates, equianalgesic dosage conversion
    for, 979t
Oral antihistamines, 279

Oral contrast agents, 51
Oral nutrition, 33
Orbital cellulitis, S6
Oropharyngeal candidiasis, 587-588
  epidemiology of, 587
  management of, 587-588
  presentation of, 587
  treatment options for, 588t
Orthodromic artrioventricular reciprocating
    tachycardia
  acute treatment for, 189
  medical treatment for, 189
Osborn waves, 68
Osmolality formulas, 1012
Osteomyelitis, 676-679
  clinical presentation of, 676-677
  diagnosis of, 677
  epidemiology of, 676
  management of, 679
Osteonecrosis, plain film radiography for,
    54
Otitis externa, malignant, S6
Otitis media and mastoiditis, S6
Ovarian torsion
  clinical presentation of, 356
  diagnosis of, 356
  management of, 356
Oxygen toxicity, 234
Oxyhemoglobin dissociation curve, 1011f

P
Pacemaker syndrome, 186
Pacemakers
  catheters and, S1
  and defibrillators, 128
  indication for permanent, 177
  programmable feature of, 184t
Pacing modes, common, 183
Paget-von Schrötter syndrome, 534
Palmar erythema, 403
Palpable thyroid nodules, 331
Pancreatitis, 597-598
  diagnosis of, 597-598
  epidemiology of, 597
  hematocrit for pancreatic necrosis, 367
  management of, 598
    acute, 366f
  presentation of, 597
Pancytopenia, causes of, 512
Paracentesis
  anterior abdominal anatomy, 20f
  complications for, 20
  contraindications for, 19
  indications for, 19
  procedure-specific equipment for, 14t
  techniques in, 20
Paralytic agents for shivering limits
    hypothermia, 5
Parathyroid hormone (PTH), 335
Parenteral nutrition, 35
Partial- vs full-thickness ulcers, 283

Pegylated interferon, 399
Pelvic inflammatory disease, S7
Pemberton's sign, 331
Peptic ulcer disease and gastritis, 357
    clinical presentation of, 357
    diagnosis of, 357
    management of, 357
Peptic ulcers, 432
Percutaneous coronary intervention (PCI),
        88
    vs thrombolytic therapy, 100
Pericarditis. See Acute pericarditis
Perinuclear antineutrophilic cytoplasmic
        antibody (P-ANCA), 446
Periodic acid stain diatase (PASD), 277
Peripheral parenteral nutrition, 35
Peritoneal tuberculosis
    clinical characteristics of, 420t
    diagnostic tests of, 421t
Phosphate, disorders of, S10
Phototherapy, for prurigo nodularis, 279
PiZZ variant, 410
Plague, S8
Plain film radiography, 351
Platelet transfusions, threshold for, 470f
Pleural effusions, 47, 886-890
    diagnosis of, 887-889
    epidemiology and etiology of, 886
    management of, 890
    presentation of, 886-887
    prognosis of, 889
Pneumocystis carinii pneumonia. See
        Pneumocystis jiroveci pneumonia
Pneumocystis jiroveci pneumonia, 578-
        582
    clinical presentation of, 580
    diagnosis of, 580-581
    drug therapy, 581t
    epidemiology of, 578
    treatment of, 581-582
Pneumonia, 48, 630-638. See also
        Bacterial pneumonia; Community-
        acquired pneumonia; Idiopathic
        interstitial pneumonia; Nosocomial
        pneumonia; Pneumocystis jiroveci
        pneumonia; Staphylococcal
        pneumonia
    antimicrobial therapy, 634t, 635t
    pattern of, 48
Pneumothorax, spontaneous, 48
    background of, 79
    clinical presentation of, 80
        physical examination, 80
        symptoms, 80
    diagnosis of, 80
    management of, 81
    outcome of, 81
    primary, 79
        tachycardia and tachypnea, 80
    secondary, 80
        hypoxemia and hypercapnia, 80

Poikilocytosis, 476
Polyarteritis nodosa, 952-953
    diagnosis of, 953
    epidemiology of, 952
    presentation of, 952-953
    treatment and prognosis of, 953
Polyglandular autoimmune syndrome type
        II. See Schmidt's syndrome
Polyglandular failure syndromes, types of,
        304
Polymerase chain reaction (PCR), 18
Porphyria of abdominal pain, 359
Portal vein thrombosis, S3
Positive end-expiratory pressure (PEEP),
        228
    high, as ventilation strategy, 225
Positron emission tomography, requirement
        for, 53
Post-ACS treatment
    complication of, 102
    secondary prevention of, 102
Posterior wall injury, 64
Posteroanterior radiograph, 48
    chest, 45f
Postherpetic neuralgia (PHN), 265
Post-lumbar puncture headache, 16
Postpartum thyroiditis, silent thyroiditis,
        328
Posttransfusion purpura, 473
Post-ventricular activity refractory period
        (PVARP), 183
Potassium homeostasis, disorders of, 800-
        804
Pott's disease, 676
Povidone-iodine, in lumbar punctures, 13
Pressure support ventilation (PSV), 231
    advantage of, 231
    disadvantage of, 232
Pressure ulcers, 282
    cause of, 283
    partial- vs full-thickness, 283
    staging of, 284f
Primary adrenal insufficiency, 302-303
Primary biliary cirrhosis
    diagnosis of, 408
    epidemiology and presentation of, 407-
        408
    laboratory evaluation, 408
    management of, 408
Primary central nervous system lymphoma
        (PCNSL), 570
Primary hypothyroidism, 321
Primary sclerosing cholangitis
    diagnosis of, 409
    epidemiology and presentation of, 408-
        409
    liver transplantation in, 409
    management of, 409
Prone positioning, 225
Prophylactic regimens for Pneumocystis
        jiroveci pneumonia, 581t

Prophylaxis against endocarditis, 151
Propylthiouracil and methimazole, 330
Prosthetic heart valves, 158-162
  evaluation of patient with, 159
  management of patient with, 160-162
Proton pump inhibitors, 431, 981t
  for acid suppression, 215
Prurigo nodularis
  clinical presentation of, 279
  diagnosis of, 279
  epidemiology and etiology of, 279
  treatment of, 279
Pruritus and fever, during drug reaction, 267
Pseudo-R wave, 188
Pseudo-S wave, 188
Pseudothrombocytopenia, 498
Pulmonary artery catheter (PAC), S1
Pulmonary artery catheters, pitfalls in, S1t
Pulmonary capillary wedge pressure (PCWP), S1
Pulmonary congestion and edema, control of, 143
Pulmonary embolism, cause of life-threatening chest pain, 75
Pulmonary function tests, 858-862
  gas exchange defects of, 862
  obstruction ventilatory defect of, 858-860
  restrictive ventilatory defect of, 860-862
Pulmonary fungal infections in HIV, 583t
Pulmonary hypertension, 900-908
  clinical presentation of, 902
  diagnosis of, 902-905
  epidemiology and etiology of, 900-903
  management of, 905-908
Pulmonary vascular resistance (PVR), S1
Pulse oximetry, 226
Pulseless electrical activity (PEA), 3
  epidemiology of, 5
  etiology of, 5t
  management of, 8f
  presentation of, 5
Pulses, absence of, 3
Purified protein derivative (PPD) testing, 452

Q
QRS axis, 58
Quincke pulse, 152

R
Radial arterial line
  complications for, 24
  contraindications for, 24
  indications for, 24
  procedure-specific equipment for, 14t
  techniques in, 24-25
Radiation colitis, 436

Radiographic contrast nephropathy, 735-737
  diagnosis of, 736
  epidemiology of, 735-736
  etiology and risk factor of, 736
  management of, 736
  prognosis of, 737
Radiographic imaging, 44-51
Radioiodine ablation therapy, 329
Radioiodine, measurement of, 329
Radiology, 44-54
Ranitidine, 36
Ranke complex, 644
Ranson's criteria, 365t
Ranson's score for computed tomography, 364
Rasburicase, urate oxidase, 554
Rectal examination for blood assessment, 351
Red wound base, 283
Refeeding syndrome, 36
Refractory hypotension, five main causes of, 251
Reiter's disease, 942
Renal artery atherosclerosis
  clinical presentation of, 742
  diagnosis of, 742
  epidemiology of, 741
  management of, 742-743
Renal artery fibromuscular dysplasia, 743
  diagnosis of, 743
  epidemiology of, 743
  management of, 743
  presentation of, 743
Renal artery stenosis, 116
Renal calculi, 49
Renal colic. See Acute renal colic
Renal failure, manifestations of, 264t. See also Acute renal failure
Renal insufficiency, 709-718, 748-755
  bivalirudin dosing in, 985t
  lepirudin dosing in, 985t
Renal transplantation, allograft dysfunction in, 807-814
Renal tubular acidosis, 784-788
  classification of, 784-786
  diagnosis of, 786-787
  management of, 787-788
Renal tubulointerstitial diseases, 731-740
Renovascular hypertension, 741-745
Reticulocyte count, 477
Reticulocyte indices, 477t
Revised coagulation cascade, 518f
Reye's syndrome, 387
Reynolds' pentad, 375
Rhabdomyolysis, 737-740
  diagnosis of, 737-738
  epidemiology and etiology of, 737-738
  prognosis of, 739-740
  treatment of, 738, 738-739

Rheumatic disorders, 939-945
    clinical presentation of, 939-940
    diagnosis of, 940-944
    epidemiology of, 939
    management of, 944-945
Rheumatoid arthritis, 967-970
    diagnosis of, 968
    epidemiology of, 967
    etiology and presentation of, 967-968
    treatment of, 969-970
Ribavirin side effects, 399
Right and left heart catheterization, 134
Right bundle branch block (RBBB), 68
Right heart catheterization, 172
Right lower quadrant (RLQ), 355
Right upper quadrant (RUQ), S3
Right ventricular hypertrophy, 61t
Ross procedure, 152
Roth spots, 652
Rovsing's sign, 355
Rumack-Matthew nomogram for
        acetaminophen poisoning, 383f
Ruptured ectopic pregnancy
    clinical presentation of, 353
    diagnosis of, 353
    management of, 353
Right ventricular (RV) injury, 64

S

Sarcoidosis, 933-937
    clinical presentation of, 934
    diagnosis of, 934-935
    epidemiology and etiology of, 933-934
    management of, 936-937
    prognosis of, 937
Scabies, 266-267
    clinical presentation of, 266t
    diagnosis of, 266
    epidemiology and etiology of, 266
    management of, 267
Schmidt's syndrome, 324
Schwachman-Diamond syndrome, 512
Seborrheic dermatitis, in HIV patients, 280
Secondary adrenal insufficiency, 303
Sengstaken-Blakemore techniques, 433
Sepsis, 253-260
    cause of, 254-255
    definition, 254t
    diagnosis of, 255
    epidemiology of, 253
    hemodynamic monitoring, 258
    management of, 257
    on organ systems, 259t
    presentation of, 253-254
    prognosis and mortality, 257t
    risk stratification, 256
Serum
    amylase level, 363
    biomarkers, 89
    erythropoietin level, 484
    lipase level, 364

Serum (Continued)
    myoglobin, 89
    osmolarity, 315
    sodium formulas, 1015
    sodium levels, 313
    tryptase, 41
    and urine ketones, cause of acidosis, 313
Sexually transmitted diseases, S7
Sgarbossa criteria for acute myocardial
        infarction, 67
Sheehan's syndrome, 303
Shock
    categories of, 240
    cause of, 240t
    diagnosis of, 241, 245
    management of, 244f, 246f
    organ system dysfunction, 243t
    physical examination of, 242t
    physiology of, 239
    various states of, S1
Sicca syndrome, 399
Sickle cell anemia, 487-494
Sickle cell disease (SCD)
    central nervous system, 490
    chronic sickling, 484
    epidemiology of, 487
    eyes role in, 490
    lungs role in, 490
    pain control, 489t
    vaso-occlusive crisis, 487-488
Sideroblastic anemia, S5
Sinus infections, in patients with
        nasogastric tubes, 261
Sinus node dysfunction, 178, 179t
Sinus rhythm
    control of, 143
    maintenance of, 143
Sjögren's syndrome, 967, 971-973
    diagnosis of, 972
    epidemiology of, 971-972
    etiology and presentation of, 972
    prognosis of, 972
    treatment of, 972-973
Skeletal survey, 51
Skin biopsy
    in fungal infection, 277
    to identify calcium deposition, 270
Skin prick tests, S4
Skin tests
    for drug-mediated hypersensitivity, 41
    for IgE antibodies, 41
    for penicillin allergy, 42
Sleep-disordered breathing (SDB), S12
Sliding scale insulin, 295t
Small bowel obstruction (SBO), 452
Small bowel series, 49
Smallpox, S8
Sodium balance, disorders of, 789-798
Sodium bicarbonate
    in preventing contrast-induced
        nephropathy, 52

Sodium-restricted diet, 423
Soft tissue infections, 672-675
  clinical presentation of, 672-674
  diagnosis of, 674
  epidemiology of, 672
  management of, 674
Spatial heterogeneity, 197
Sphincter of Oddi dysfunction, 359
Spider angiomata, 403
Spindle cells, 278
Spine sign, 48
Spironolactone, a potassium-sparing
        diuretic, 142
Spontaneous bacterial peritonitis (SBP), 418
ST segment elevation acute coronary
        syndromes
  management of, 95-102
    bedside stratification tool, 96t
    pharmacologic and nonpharmacologic
        intervention, 97-102
    risk stratification, 95-96
ST segment elevation, causes of, 74
ST segment elevation MI (STEMI), 62
Staphylococcal pneumonia, 631
Staphylococcus aureus infections, 254
Starr-Edwards, caged-ball models, 158
Status epilepticus (SE), 826-830
  clinical presentation of, 826-827
  diagnosis of, 828
  epidemiology of, 826
  management of, 828-830
Stem cell transplantation, S5
Sterile technique, 13
Steroid table, equivalent dosing, 979t
Steroid therapy, benefit of, 261
Steroids in the critically ill patient, 297
Stevens-Johnson syndrome, 37, 43, 557
  clinical presentation of, 268
  diagnosis of, 269
  epidemiology and etiology of, 267-268
Stewart-Hamilton equation, S1
Streptococcal toxic shock syndrome, 263
"Stress dose" steroids, 251
Stroke, 833-844
  hemorrhagic, 842-844
    diagnosis of, 843-844
    epidemiology and etiology of, 842
    management of, 844
    presentation of, 842
  ischemic, 833-842
    clinical presentation of, 835-836
    diagnosis of, 836-839
    epidemiology of, 833-834
    management of, 839-842
      acute, 839-840
      secondary prevention, 840-841
    preventive measures, 834-835
Structural thyroid disorders
  clinical presentation of, 331
  diagnosis of, 332
  epidemiology of, 331
  management of, 332

Subarachnoid hemorrhage (SAH), S11
Subclavian vein site, 26
Substance abuse, 847-854
Sucralfate for acid suppression, 215
Superficial venous thrombosis (SVT), 526
Superior vena cava (SCV) syndrome
  clinical presentation of, 552
  diagnosis of, 552
  epidemiology of, 551
  management of, 552
Supraventricular tachycardia (SVT), 188-189
  and structural heart disease, 188
  symptoms of, 188
  types of, 188
Surgical ablation with cardiac surgery, 208
Sustained virologic response (SVR), 398
Swan-Ganz catheter, 135, 256, S1f
Synchronized intermittent mandatory
        ventilation (SIMV), 229
  advantage of, 229
  disadvantage of, 229
Syncope, 120-129
  blood test in, 125
  cardiogenic, 122
  causes of, 121t
  clinical presentation and diagnosis of,
        122-128
  diagnostic tools, 123t, 124t
  echocardiography in, 125
  electrocardiogram for, 125
  epidemiology of, 120
  etiology of, 120-122
  exercise stress testing, 125
  historical point for, 126
  management of, 128-129
  manifestation of AF, 198
  pregnancy testing in, 125
  tilt table testing, 127
Systemic lupus erythematosus, 960-964
  clinical presentation of, 960-962
  diagnosis of, 962
  epidemiology of, 960
  management of, 963
  mortality of, 962
Systemic sclerosis, 970-971
  diagnosis of, 970-971
  epidemiology of, 970
  etiology and presentation of, 970
  prognosis of, 971
  treatment of, 971
Systolic and diastolic hypertension, S2
Systolic dysfunction, 150
Systolic heart failure, 134

T
T wave inversions, 62
Tachyarrhythmias and atrial fibrillation, 189
Tachy-brady syndrome, 177
Tachycardia
  diagnosis for narrow QRS, 190f
  diagnosis for wide QRS, 191f
  and tachypnea, 80

Takayasu's arteritis, 152, 947, 947-949
  diagnosis of, 949
  epidemiology of, 947
  presentation of, 947-949
  treatment and prognosis of, 949
Tamponade, diagnosis of, 5
Tamponade vs constrictive pericarditis, 172
Tenofovir, an adenine nucleoside analog, 395
Tension-type headache, S11
Therapeutic hypothermia, 4
Therapeutic thoracentesis, 22
  position of needle in, 24f
  proper positioning, 23f
Thiazolidinediones, 300
Third-degree heart block, 177
Third heart sound, 172
Thoracentesis
  complications for, 22
  contraindications for, 22
  indications for, 22
  procedure-specific equipment for, 14t
  techniques in, 22
Thromboangiitis obliterans, 953-954
  diagnosis of, 954
  epidemiology of, 953
  presentation of, 953-954
  treatment of, 954
Thrombocytopenia, 497-507
  approach to, 498
    isolated, 499f
  cause of, 507-508
  definition of, 497
  drug-induced, 503
  hereditary, 503
  with pregnancy, 503
  secondary evaluation for, 501f
Thrombolysis in Myocardial Infarction
  (TIMI) risk score assessment, 90
Thrombolytic therapy
  ACC and AHA regarding, 99
  efficacy of, 98
Thrombolytics, fibrinolytic agent, 97
Thrombotic microangiopathies, 504-505
  epidemiology of, 504
  management of, 505
  pathophysiology of, 504
  presentation of, 504
Thyroid acropachy, 328
Thyroid disorders, 321-332
Thyroid hormone levels and severity of
  nonthyroidal illness, 325f
Thyroid imaging studies, 53
Thyroid storm, management of, 330
Thyroiditis
  postpartum, 328
  silent, 328
Thyroid nodules, management of, 333f
Thyroid-stimulating hormone (TSH) level, 321
Thyroid-stimulating immunoglobulin, 329
Thyroid storm, 328

Thyrotoxicosis
  cause of, 327t
  clinical presentation of, 328
  definition of, 326
  diagnosis of, 328-329
  epidemiology of, 327
  management of, 329-330
TIMI angiographic grading system, 97t
Tirofiban, 94
  and eptifibatide, 94
Tophi and bony erosions, 944
Topical therapy for chronic wounds
  goals of, 285, 290
  guidelines for, 288t, 290
Total iron-binding capacity (TIBC), 477
Total nutrient admixture, 35
Total parenteral nutrition (TPN), 35
  complications of, 36
Toxic adenoma, 327
Toxic epidermal necrolysis (TEN)
  clinical presentation of, 268
  diagnosis of, 269
  epidemiology and etiology of, 267-268
Toxic megacolon, 444
  clinical presentation of, 354-355
  criteria for, 444
  diagnosis of, 355
  management of, 355
Toxic multinodular goiter, 327
Toxic shock syndrome
  clinical presentation of, 264
  diagnosis of, 263-264
  epidemiology and etiology of, 263
  management of, 264-265
Tracheal deviation or distended neck veins
  in goitre, 331
Tracheostomy, S12
Traditional biomarkers, 89
Transesophageal echocardiography (TEE), 199
Transfusion, an approach to, 468f
Transfusion medicine, 467-474
  components and indications, 467-471
  massive, 473
    coagulopathy, 473
    hypothermia, 473
    metabolic disturbance, 473
  risk of, 471-473
Transfusion-related acute lung injury
  (TRALI), 472
Transmural ischemia, 62
Transplanted heart, physiology of, S2
Tricuspid regurgitation, 157-158
  clinical presentation of, 158
  diagnosis of, 158
  epidemiology of, 157
  surgical valve replacement in, 158
Trifascicular block, 180t
Troponin elevation, 74
Troponin I, 89
Troponin T, 89
Trousseau's or Chvostek's signs, S10

Trousseau's sign, 343, 347
Tuberculin skin test, values for positive result, 645t
Tuberculosis, 640-647
  diagnosis of, 644-645
    active, 644
    latent, 645
  epidemiology of, 640-641
  management of, 645-647
    active, 645-647
    latent, 647
  peritoneal
    clinical characteristics, 420t
    diagnostic tests, 421t
  presentation of, 641-644
    active, 641
    latent, 644
  pathogenesis, 641
  prognosis of, 647
Tularemia, S8
Tumor lysis syndrome, 537, 553-555
  clinical presentation and diagnosis of, 553
  epidemiology of, 553
  management of, 554-555
Tumor necrosis factor, 256
Tylenol, and Rumack-Matthew nomogram for acetaminophen poisoning, 383f
Typhlitis, necrotizing enterocolitis, 360
Tzanck preparation, 272
  for diagnosing herpes zoster, 272
Tzanck smear, 265

U
Ulcerative colitis (UC)
  diagnosis of, 444
  evaluation of, 443t
  management of, 447
  presentation of, 442
  treatment of, 448f
  vs Crohn's disease, 443t
Ulcerative proctitis, 443
Ulcers
  healing of, 283
  leg, 286t-287t
  pressure
    cause of, 283
    partial- vs full-thickness, 283
    staging of, 284f
  venous stasis, 282
Ultrasonography, 332
  consideration for, 52
Unconjugated bilirubin, 377
Unconjugated hyperbilirubinemia, 377
Unfractionated heparin, 92
Upper GI bleeding (UGIB)
  acute, causes, 429t
  clinical presentation of, 428-429
  diagnosis of, 429
  epidemiology of, 428-433
  management of, 430-433

Upper GI series
  for esophageal perforation, 51
  for motility disorders, 51
Urinalysis, 313, 702-708
  chemical analysis, 702-704
  microscopic analysis, 704-706
Urinary tract infections (UTIs), 261, 663-668
  cause of, 665
  clinical presentation of, 664
  diagnosis of, 665-667
  epidemiology of, 663-664
  management of, 667-668
Urinary urea nitrogen (UUN), 33
Urticaria and angioedema, 43

V
Valvular heart disease, 147-163
  summary of severe, 148t-149t
Varicella-zoster virus, 265
Varices, esophageal, 432
Vascular or humoral rejection, S2
Vasculitis, 947-957
Vasodilators, inhaled, 225
Vasomotor autoregulation, 241
Vasopressin, 250
  in asystole, 11
  and epinephrine, 4
Vasopressors
  during cardiac arrest, 4
  for hypotensive, 259
Venoocclusive disease (VOD), 387
Venous blood gas (VBG), 313
Venous stasis ulcers, 282
Venous thromboembolism, 911-920
Venous thrombosis
  clinical presentation of, 912-914
  diagnosis of, 914-918
  epidemiology of, 911-912
  management of, 918-920
    anticoagulation, 918
    embolectomy, 920
    thrombolytic agents, 919
    vena caval filters, 919
  prevention of, 920
  prognosis of, 920
Ventilated patient, management of
  sedation and paralysis, 233
  weaning, 233
Ventilation, invasive and noninvasive
  clinical presentation of, 228-229
  epidemiology of, 228
  intubation in, 229
  mode of, 229, 230t
  parameter of, 231
Ventilator-associated lung injury, 236
Ventricular arrhythmias and ICD, 192
Ventricular fibrillation (VF), 3
  cardiopulmonary resuscitation for, 4
  defibrillation in, 4
  epidemiology of, 3
  etiology of, 4t

Ventricular fibrillation (VF) (*Continued*)
management and treatment of, 4-5, 7f
shock-refractory, 5
Ventricular pacing, 65
Ventricular rate control
pharmacologic agents available for, 204t-205t
Ventricular rate in atrial fibrillation, 198
Ventricular tachycardia (VT), 3
cardiopulmonary resuscitation for, 4
defibrillation in, 4
epidemiology of, 3
etiology of, 4t
management and treatment of, 4-5, 7f
shock-refractory, 5
Venturi masks, 222
Virchow's classic triad of VTE risk, 911
Vitamin A intoxication, 337
Vitamin D deficiency, cause of hypocalcemia, 335
Vitamin K deficiency, 519
Vitum sign, 158
Volume status, assessment, 241
Volutrauma, 236
Von Willebrand factor, 94, 471
V/Q scan, 914
VVI(R) pacing mode, 185

W

Waldenström's macroglobulinemia, 550, S5

Warfarin initiation in the hospital, 985t
Warfarin maintenance dosing, 986t
Washed red blood cells, 469
WATCH (Warfarin and Antiplatelet Therapy in Heart Failure) trial, 142
Waterhouse-Friderichsen syndrome, 303
Wegener's granulomatosis, 727-728, 951-952
clinical presentation of, 728
diagnosis of, 728, 952
epidemiology and etiology of, 727
epidemiology of, 951
management of, 728
presentation of, 951
prognosis of, 728
treatment and prognosis of, 952
Wellens T waves, 62, 65
Wells scoring system, 914
Wharton's duct, S6
Widened mediastinum, 48
Wilson's disease, 387, 411
Wolff-Parkinson-White syndrome (WPW), 68, 189, 195, 200
Wound assessment
diagnosis of, 286t-289t
history of, 282
physical examination, 283
Wright-Giemsa stain, 476

Z

Zygomycosis, 685, S6

Notes

Notes

Notes